Tabbner's Nursing Care

THEORY AND PRACTICE 9E

Tabbner's Nursing Care

THEORY AND PRACTICE 9E

VOLUME 2

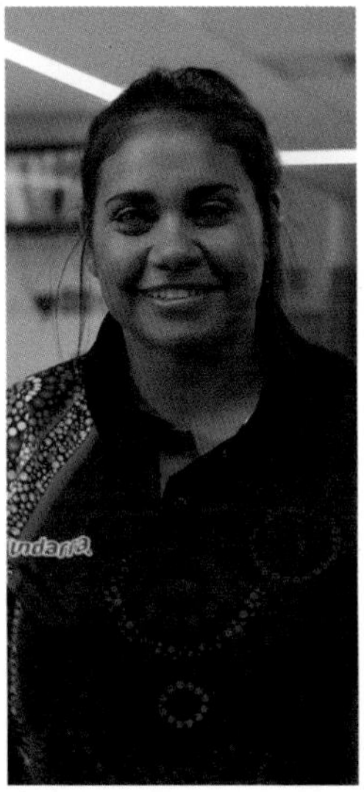
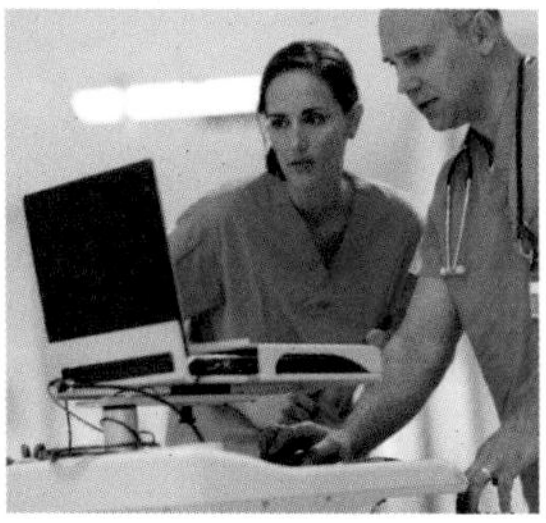
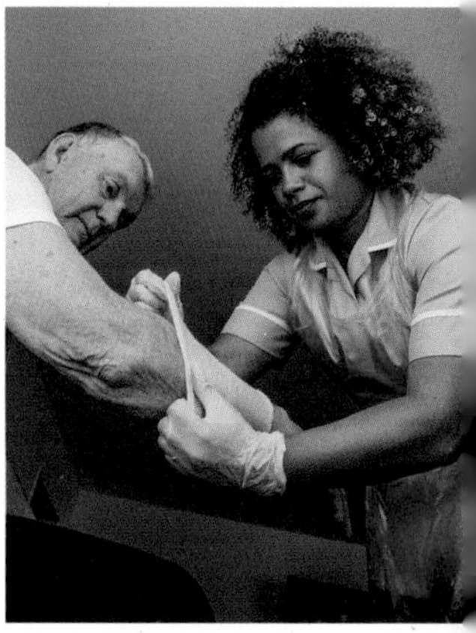
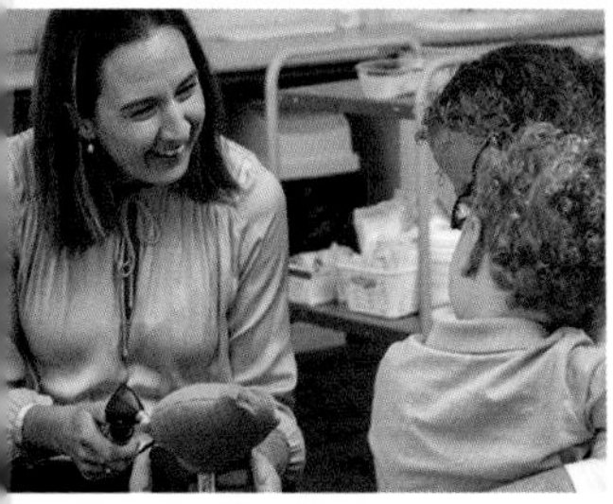
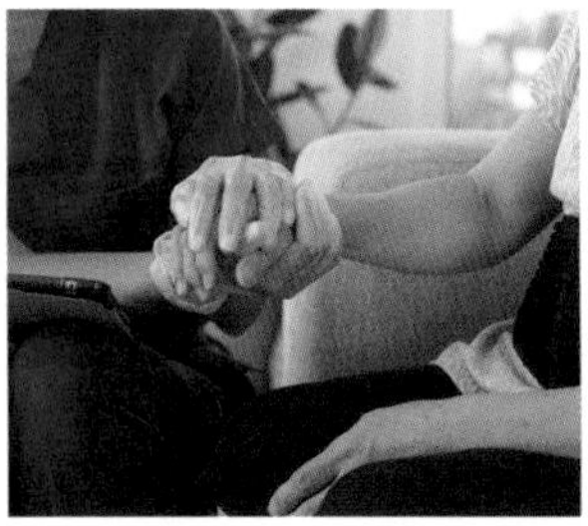
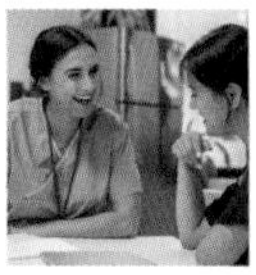
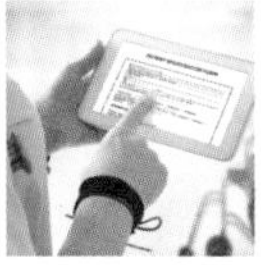

Gabrielle Koutoukidis

EdD(Research), MPH, BN(Mid), DipAppSci(Nurs), AdvDipN(Ed),
DipBus, VocGradCertBus(Transformational Management),
International Specialised Skills Institute Fellow
Dean, Faculty Health Science, Community & Social Studies, Holmesglen,
Vic, Australia

Kate Stainton

MHS(Nurs), GDipNurs(Ed), BN(Mid), DipAppSci(Nurs),
CertIV TAE, MACN
Strategy & Innovation Consultant, BaptistCare, NSW, Australia
Sessional Academic, School of Nursing & Midwifery,
University of Newcastle, NSW, Australia

ELSEVIER

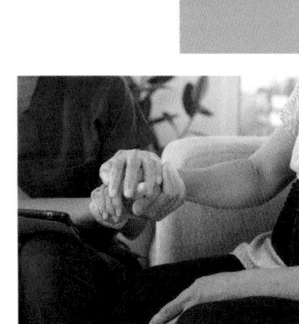

ELSEVIER

Elsevier Australia. ACN 001 002 357
(a division of Reed International Books Australia Pty Ltd)
475 Victoria Avenue, Chatswood, NSW 2067

1st edition © 1981; 2nd edition © 1991; 3rd edition © 1997; 4th edition © 2005; 5th edition © 2009; 6th edition © 2013; 7th edition © 2017; 8th edition © 2021 Elsevier Australia.

ISBN (Two-volume set): 978-0-7295-4475-7
ISBN (Volume 2): 978-0-7295-4474-0

National Library of Australia Cataloguing-in-Publication Data

NATIONAL LIBRARY OF AUSTRALIA
A catalogue record for this book is available from the National Library of Australia

Content Strategist: Elizabeth Coady
Content Project Manager: Fariha Nadeem
Edited by Scott Vanderwalk
Proofread by Annabel Adair
Copyrights Coordinator: Regina Remigius
Cover Designer: Georgette Hall
Index by Innodata
Typeset by GW Tech
Printed and bound in Singapore by Markono Print Media Pte Ltd

Last digit is the print number: 9 8 7 6 5 4 3 2 1

Short Contents

Unit 8 Specialised nursing practice

Contents

UNIT 7

Promoting health and wellbeing

CHAPTER

25

Cardiovascular and respiratory health

Kylie Porritt

Key Terms

agranular
airway
basophils
bradypnoea
cardiovascular
diffusion
eosinophils
erythrocytes
exhalation
expiration
gas exchange
granulocytes
hypercapnia
hypocapnia
hypoventilation
hypoxaemia
hypoxia
inhalation
leucocytes
lymph
lymphocytes
monocytes
neutrophils
respiration
tachypnoea
thrombocytes

Learning Outcomes

At the completion of this chapter and with further reading, learners should be able to:

- Define the key terms.
- Describe the structure of the cardiovascular and respiratory system.
- Explain the functions of the cardiovascular and respiratory system.
- Describe the position of the heart and the function of the circulatory system.
- State the factors that affect respiratory function.
- Describe the major manifestations of respiratory system disorders.
- Describe the major manifestations of circulatory system disorders.
- Briefly describe the specific disorders of the cardiac and respiratory systems outlined in this chapter.
- Assist in planning and implementing nursing care for the person with a cardiac and respiratory system disorder.
- Apply relevant principles in the planning and implementation of nursing actions to assist a person receiving oxygen therapy.

CHAPTER FOCUS

The human body relies on oxygen to survive and it is the role of the cardiac and respiratory systems to supply the body's oxygen demands. The two systems work together to achieve and maintain homeostasis. Cardiopulmonary physiology involves the delivery of oxygenated blood from the lungs to the left side of the heart, out to the tissues, and deoxygenated blood from the tissues to the right side of the heart, out to the pulmonary circulation for re-oxygenation. Blood is oxygenated through the processes of ventilation, perfusion and transport of respiratory gases.

The overall function of the cardiovascular system, which includes the lymphatic system, is to move blood around the body. The heart pumps the blood for circulation around the body through blood vessels. These blood vessels transport oxygen, nutrients and other substances to the cells and transport waste away from the cells. Blood also assists in protecting the body against infection and distributing heat evenly throughout the body, and prevents its own loss by means of a built-in clotting mechanism.

The respiratory system provides the body with the ability to absorb oxygen and excrete carbon dioxide and other waste products from the body. Oxygen from the atmosphere is delivered to the bloodstream and carbon dioxide diffused out from the bloodstream. This is achieved through the capillary alveoli membrane in the lungs.

Ventilation is the method of delivering air into and out of the lungs and is achieved through inhalation and exhalation. Respiration involves both the respiratory and the circulatory system and is the exchange of gases.

An adequate supply of blood is necessary for the normal function of every cell. Homeostasis depends on the ability of the heart to adequately circulate the required volume of blood and oxygen to the tissues. Cells temporarily deprived of blood or oxygen will not function normally, and continued disruption of blood supply causes irreversible damage or cell death. Any disorder that interferes with the distribution or delivery of blood to tissues or the uptake or excretion of gases in respiration is a potential harm to body cells and may have permanent effects on a part, or all, of the body.

The most common complication of a respiratory disorder is carbon dioxide retention. This can be a result of alveolar hypoventilation, or a cardiovascular disorder altering the ventilation or the perfusion of the lungs and other tissues.

Nursing care related to oxygenation requires an understanding of how the three systems work together to achieve oxygenation within the body. Knowledge of how to maintain and restore a clear airway is an essential component to nursing care. This includes measures directed at removing secretions by the use of suction via the nasal, oropharyngeal or endotracheal routes or by tracheostomy. The patency of airways can be assisted by the use of humidification, nebulisation and physiotherapy using isotonic or hypotonic solutions or certain medications. Education is essential to promote exercise, which maintains optimal circulation of blood, and deep breathing and coughing exercises are encouraged to minimise the retention of secretions and secondary infections. Circulation can be assisted by changes in diet, fluid, exercise, medications and positioning.

Disorders of the cardiovascular and the respiratory system are common in most communities. Population-based strategies for the prevention of cardiovascular disease are aimed at modifying the individual's lifestyle and behaviours; dietary, exercise and smoking cessation interventions are commonly recommended as a primary prevention of cardiovascular disease (Le Goff et al 2023).

LIVED EXPERIENCE

Eleanor, a 74-year-old woman, was admitted to the medical ward through the emergency department due to an acute exacerbation of congestive heart failure (CHF). Upon admission, her vital signs were relatively stable, but she was experiencing significant dyspnoea and needed assistance with her daily activities. As her nurse, I closely monitored her condition throughout my shift.

During the early hours of my shift, I noticed that Eleanor's oxygen saturation levels fell into the cautionary range on the adult observation chart. Additionally, she became increasingly lethargic and confused. Recognising the urgency, I promptly reported these changes to the charge nurse who, in turn, requested the medical team's intervention.

The resident physician ordered arterial blood gases, which revealed elevated carbon dioxide (CO_2) levels. In response, the medical team initiated an adjusted treatment plan. Eleanor was administered an additional dose of IV diuretics to manage her CHF, and her oxygen therapy was modified. To minimise the risk of CO_2 retention, I was instructed to administer low-flow oxygen at a rate of less than 3 litres per minute. Furthermore, her oxygen saturation target range was adjusted to maintain levels between 88% and 92%.

As the nursing team and medical staff closely monitored Eleanor's oxygen saturation levels, respiratory rate, and level of consciousness on an hourly basis, her condition gradually improved throughout the day. By the time my shift ended, Eleanor was showing signs of stabilisation, and the risk of CO_2 retention had been effectively managed.

Amber, Enrolled Nurse

INTRODUCTION

The respiratory system (Figure 25.1) is a complex network of organs and tissues responsible for the process of respiration, which involves the exchange of oxygen and carbon dioxide between the body and the environment. Its primary function is to provide oxygen to the body's cells and remove carbon dioxide, a waste product of cellular metabolism.

The respiratory system is composed of two main parts: the upper respiratory system and the lower respiratory system. These components work together to facilitate the process of respiration, which involves the exchange of gases between the body and the environment.

The respiratory system consists of cavities and conducting airways that begin at the nasal and oral cavity and end at the alveoli, the functional unit of the respiratory system (Berman et al 2020). The larger airways are composed of cartilage and smooth muscle that maintain their patency, and are gradually replaced with smooth muscle in the terminal airways, which allows alterations in airway diameter and ventilation. The two lungs are located in the thoracic cavity, encased by a double membrane known as the pleura, and are separated by the mediastinal cavity that contains the heart and great vessels. The thoracic cavity has ribs that aid in ventilation and protect the lungs from damage. The diaphragm and the internal and external intercostal regions are composed of skeletal muscle and constitute the main muscles of ventilation; other muscles are used when required for more forceful inhalation or expiration (Hartley 2018). The upper and lower respiratory systems work together to facilitate breathing, supply oxygen to the body's cells and remove carbon dioxide.

Upper airways

Nasal cavities

The respiratory system begins with the nose, which is the primary entry point for air. The nasal cavity filters, warms and humidifies the inhaled air, removing dust, bacteria and other impurities. The mucus lining helps trap these particles before the air continues into the rest of the system.

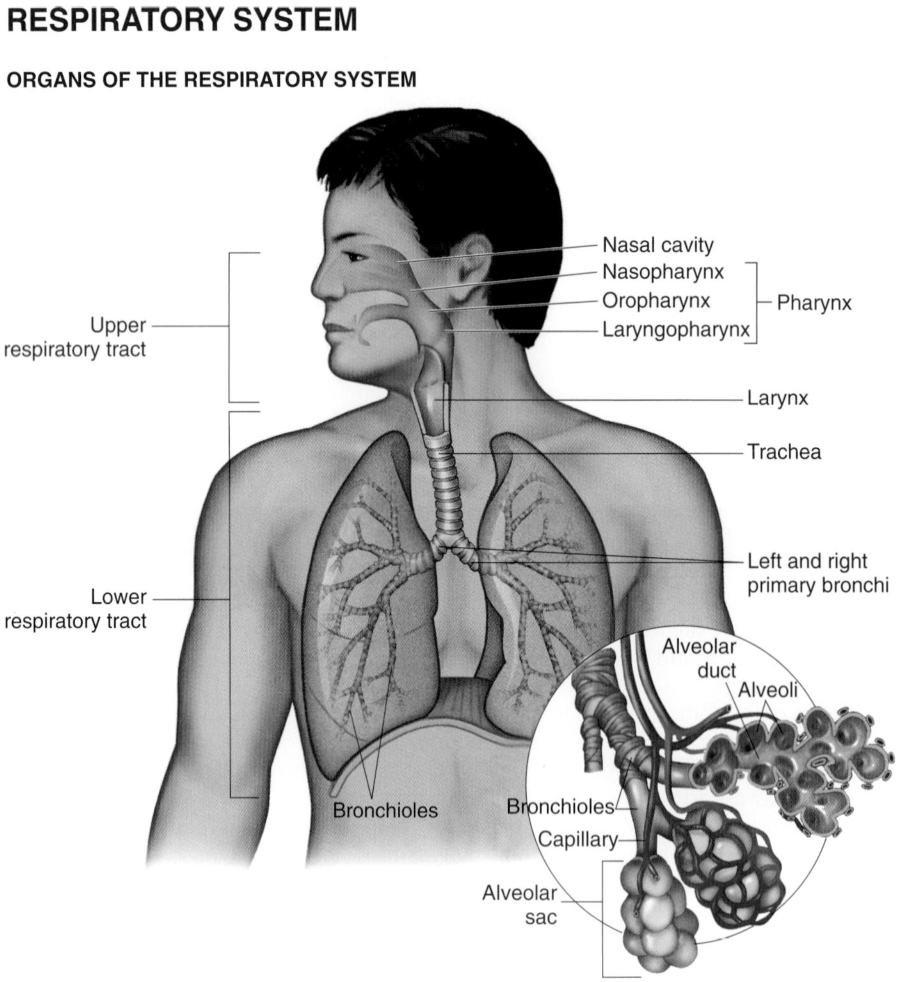

Figure 25.1 The respiratory tract

(Patton & Thibodeau 2019)

The nose is a bony cartilaginous structure divided into a right and left nasal cavity by the nasal septum. The anterior portion of the septum is cartilage and the posterior portion is bone, formed by the small thin bone separating the left and right nasal cavity and part of the ethmoid bone. Inside each nostril (nares) is a vestibule lined by skin containing sebaceous and sweat glands and coarse hairs that act as filters. Apart from the vestibules, all other areas of the nasal cavity are lined by mucous membrane. In most of the cavity, the membrane is covered by ciliated epithelium with many 'goblet' cells. Mucous cells are also present in the underlying connective tissue. The nose consists of these specific structures and cells that have the following functions:

- Hairs and cilia line the nasal cavities and filter foreign particles and pathogens from the inhaled air.
- Mucus secreted by the mucosa traps substances in inhaled air, and the cilia move particles of mucus towards the pharynx to be swallowed or expectorated.
- Inhaled air is warmed and moistened as it passes over the mucosa. The three nasal turbinate bones in each cavity cause airflow to become turbulent, which enhances contact of air with the mucosa.
- Sensory organ for the sense of smell (olfaction).

(Treuting et al 2018)

Paranasal sinus

The paranasal sinuses are a group of air-filled cavities located within the bones of the surrounding nasal cavity. There are four pairs of air-filled paranasal sinuses (Figure 25.2): frontal, maxillary, sphenoid and ethmoid sinuses.

The paranasal sinuses play a role in reducing the weight of the skull, making it easier for us to hold our heads upright. The sinuses also act as resonating chambers that affect the quality of our voice. They contribute to the resonance, pitch and tone of the sound produced during speech and singing. The mucous membranes lining the sinuses produce mucus, which helps moisten and warm the air as it passes through the nasal cavity. The mucus also serves to trap and remove dust, pollutants and other particles from the inhaled air, providing a protective function for the respiratory system. Lastly, the mucus produced by the sinuses contains antibodies and immune cells that help defend against infections, preventing pathogens from entering the respiratory system (Koeppen et al 2023).

The pharynx

The pharynx (commonly known as the throat) is a muscular tube about 13 cm long, lying in front of the cervical vertebrae and behind the nose, mouth and larynx. It is lined with mucous membrane and has three sections:

1. Nasopharynx

The nasopharynx is 2–3 cm wide and 3–4 cm long and lies behind the nose. Its functions include:

- warming and moistening inhaled air
- protecting from infection, by patches of lymphoid tissue such as the adenoids

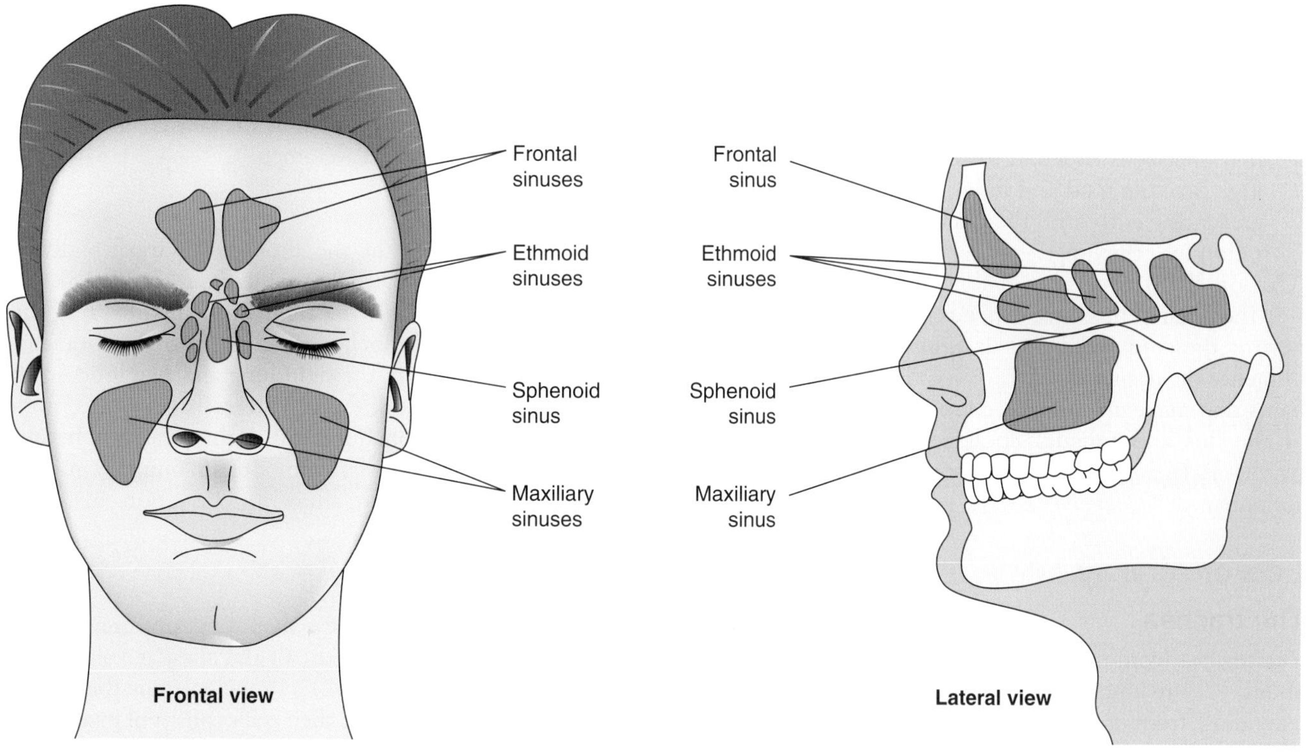

Figure 25.2 Paranasal sinus

- equalising pressure in the middle ear with the atmospheric pressure by allowing air to travel along the eustachian tubes to the middle ear.

(Koeppen et al 2023)

2. Oropharynx

This section lies behind the mouth and is separated from the cavity of the mouth by two folds of mucous membrane (the fauces). Between these folds lie the oral tonsils, which are patches of lymphoid tissue involved in the immune system. The oropharynx provides a common passage for air, food and fluids. The uvula is positioned in the middle of the soft palate and is composed of mainly glandular and connective tissue and prevents food from entering the nasal cavity (Elsherbiny et al 2018).

3. Laryngopharynx

The laryngopharynx is the section that opens into both the larynx and the oesophagus. It contains the epiglottis (see next section).

The larynx

The larynx is situated in the upper region of the neck and extends from the pharynx above to the trachea below. It is composed of pieces of cartilage connected by membranes and provides a passageway for air between the pharynx and trachea. Although an integral part of the respiratory tract, the larynx makes use of moving air for a different purpose than for respiration; it is a complex structure adapted for producing sound as well as functioning to prevent food from entering the trachea (Carlson 2018). The main cartilages that form the larynx are:

- The thyroid cartilage, which is the largest and forms a prominence known as the 'Adam's apple'.
- The epiglottis, a leaf-shaped cartilage attached to the upper part of the thyroid cartilage. During swallowing, the larynx rises and the epiglottis covers its opening, directing food and fluid into the oesophagus and preventing entry into the trachea and subsequent aspiration into the lungs.

(Carlson 2018)

The pitch of the voice depends on the length and tightness of the cords, and the air sinuses in the skull bones influence the resonance of the voice. The vowels and consonants that make up speech are formed by various positions of the lips and tongue. Speaking requires coordination of the larynx, mouth, lips, tongue, throat, lungs and abdomen.

Lower airway

The trachea

The trachea (commonly known as the windpipe) is a tube about 12 cm long that lies in front of the oesophagus, extending from the larynx to the mid-thorax, where it divides into a right and a left bronchus. The trachea consists of 15–20 C-shaped rings of cartilage joined by involuntary muscle and fibrous tissue. Posteriorly, the trachea lacks cartilage and is replaced with smooth muscle to enable the oesophagus to expand, while the cartilages maintain the patency of the airway. It thus provides a permanently open passageway for air travelling to and from the lungs. The trachea is lined with ciliated epithelium containing mucus-secreting goblet cells. The cilia sweep the mucus, cell debris and any foreign particles that enter the trachea up into the pharynx to be swallowed or expectorated. During swallowing, the larynx rises and the epiglottis covers its opening, directing food and fluid into the oesophagus and preventing its entry into the trachea and subsequent aspiration into the lungs (Carlson 2018).

The cricoid cartilage lies below the thyroid cartilage and is shaped like a wide, banded ring to provide attachments for the various muscles, cartilages and ligaments involved in opening and closing the airway and in speech production. The larynx is lined with mucous membrane, which becomes ciliated in the lower part. In the upper part, two folds of membrane containing embedded fibrous and elastic tissue form the vocal folds (cords). The vocal cords extend from the anterior wall to the posterior wall of the larynx to form the glottis, or voice box, which produces sounds (Carlson 2018).

Voice production

Sound production by the vocal cords is called phonation (Carlson 2018). During normal respiration, the vocal cords are apart. Contraction of muscles attached to the cords brings them closer together, and expired air is used to cause vibration of the cords. The brain, tongue, lips, nasal cavity and facial muscles all help to convert the resultant sounds into speech (Carlson 2018). The pitch of the voice depends on the length and tightness of the cords, and the air sinuses in the skull bones influence the resonance of the voice. Speaking requires coordination of the larynx, mouth, lips, tongue, throat, lungs and abdomen (Carlson 2018).

Bronchi

At about the middle of the thorax, the trachea divides to form the right and left bronchus (Carlson 2018). The bronchi enter the lungs: the right bronchus dividing into three, and the left bronchus dividing into two branches. There are three lobes in the right lung and two lobes in the left lung; therefore, one branch of each bronchus enters each lobe. The left bronchus is longer than the right because of the position of the heart. Smooth involuntary muscles surround the airways to allow for alteration in airway diameter (Carlson 2018).

Bronchioles

Respiratory bronchioles have a dual function: they serve as part of the airways and as part of the alveolar volume (gas exchange) (Broaddus et al 2021). Bronchioles are the smallest branches of the bronchi, and their walls consist of involuntary muscle with elastic fibrous tissue, allowing for expansion and constriction. They divide to form terminal bronchioles that give rise to microscopic alveolar ducts, which terminate in clusters of air sacs called alveoli (Carlson 2018).

Lungs

The two lungs lie in the thoracic cavity on either side of the mediastinum. The mediastinal cavity contains the heart, major blood vessels and the oesophagus. The lungs are light and spongy and consist of the bronchioles, alveoli and blood vessels and are supported by areolar tissue. There is also a great deal of elastic tissue to enable the lungs to expand and recoil freely during respiration. The base of each lung rests on the diaphragm and the apex of each extends to just above each clavicle. The right lung has three lobes and is shorter and wider than the left lung, which has two lobes (Knapp 2019). Each lobe is made up of lobules, each with its own blood, nerve and lymph supply. On the medial side of each lung is a depression called the hilus, through which the bronchi, lymphatic vessels and blood vessels enter and exit (Smith et al 2024).

Alveoli

Alveoli are microscopic air sacs in the lungs. Their walls are composed of one layer of type I, simple squamous epithelial cells, and type II cells that produce surfactant, which maintains alveolar expansion by reducing surface tension. Macrophages are present and their role is to phagocytose cell debris and pathogens. The alveoli form a surface area of about 70 m^2 for semi-permeable membrane diffusion of gases. The alveoli are surrounded by networks of capillaries, arising from the pulmonary arteries and their tributaries. The function of alveoli is the interchange of oxygen and carbon dioxide between the air in the alveoli and the blood in the capillaries (Carlson 2018) (See Figure 25.3.)

Pleura

The pleura (Figure 25.4) comprise a double layer of serous membrane, consisting of the visceral pleura, which adheres

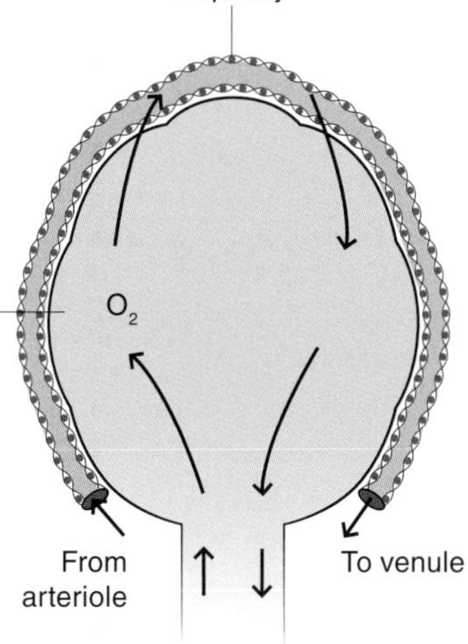

Figure 25.3 Exchange of gases in the alveoli

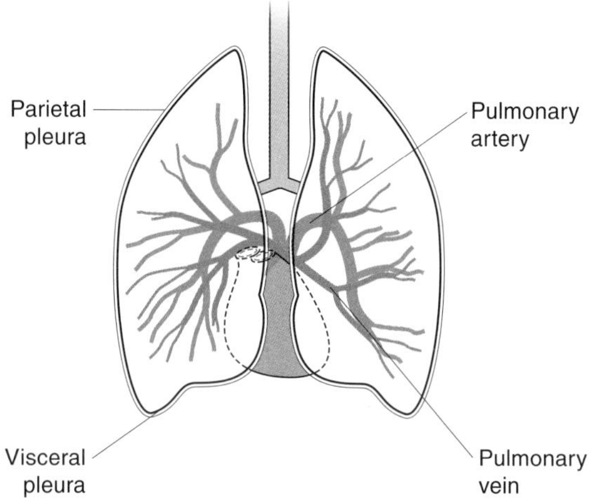

Figure 25.4 The lungs and the pleura

to the surface of the lungs, and the parietal pleura, which lines the thoracic cavity and covers the superior surface of the diaphragm (Carlson 2018). The pleura secrete a thin film of serous fluid, maintained at about 50 mL, which lies between the two layers and prevents friction between the surfaces. The pressure within the pleura is 2 mmHg below atmospheric pressure so as to prevent lung collapse.

Muscles of ventilation

The main muscles responsible for ventilation are the diaphragm and internal and external intercostal muscles. During difficult or forced breathing, accessory muscles are used, such as the muscles of the neck, thorax (e.g. sternocleidomastoid, anterior serrate, scalene) and abdominal muscles, including the rectus abdominus and transverse abdominus (Carlson 2018).

SCIENTIFIC PRINCIPLES OF VENTILATION AND RESPIRATION

The major purpose of respiration is to supply oxygen to the body and remove carbon dioxide from the cells. This is accomplished by the process of *ventilation* (movement of air in and out of the lungs), *external respiration* (exchange of gases between the atmosphere and the pulmonary capillaries) and *internal respiration* (exchange of gases between the systematic capillaries and the cell). An understanding of pressure relationships and key principles of respiration will assist in understanding the process of ventilation and respiration (Broaddus et al 2021).

Pressure

Pressure may be defined as force (or stress) per unit area applied to a surface. The concept of pressure, or force, applies equally to solids, liquids and gases. Described below are some of the principles and concepts relating to pressure that are relevant to nursing.

Atmospheric pressure

Atmospheric pressure arises by virtue of the weight of the air above the earth; it is the force per unit area exerted by the weight of the Earth's atmosphere on any object or surface in contact with it. Atmospheric pressure decreases as altitude increases because of the reduced amount of air above. Atmospheric pressure is not constant, but varies according to atmospheric conditions.

The total pressure exerted by the atmosphere is about 6.8 kg per 25 mm^2 of surface area at sea level. The atmosphere consists principally of nitrogen (N_2) 79.03%, oxygen (O_2) 20.93% and carbon dioxide (CO_2) 0.0004%, which totals 99.9604%. Other gases such as carbon monoxide (CO) are present in minute quantities. Oxygen, a colourless and odourless gas, is essential in sustaining most forms of life.

Water vapour and gases in the atmosphere have weight and, at sea level, exert a pressure defined as 1 atmosphere of pressure ('atmospheric pressure') equivalent to 760 mmHg. The terms 'negative pressure' and 'positive pressure' are used to compare a pressure to normal atmospheric pressure at sea level. Any pressure above normal atmospheric pressure is regarded as a positive pressure, and any pressure below normal atmospheric pressure is regarded as a negative pressure.

The following three laws of physics define the characteristics of gases:

1. Pascal's principle, which states that a confined liquid transmits pressure, applied to it from an external force, equally in all directions.
2. Boyle's law, which states that the volume of a given mass of gas is inversely proportional to the pressure to which it is subjected, provided that the temperature remains constant.
3. Charles' law, which states that the volume of a given mass of gas is directly proportional to its absolute temperature, provided that the pressure remains constant (e.g., as the temperature of a gas is increased (at constant pressure) the gas expands).

The combined effects of atmospheric pressure and the application of the gas laws above provide the basis for the operation of many common devices, and also of the lungs.

Boyle's law refers to pressure differentials and is able to be applied to the process of breathing. By changing the volume of the thoracic cavity, the air pressure in the lungs can be made lower or higher than atmospheric pressure, leading to inhalation or exhalation, respectively (Marieb & Hoehn 2019).

The human respiratory system relies on pressure differences between the lungs and the surrounding environment to facilitate inhalation and exhalation. When the diaphragm and chest muscles contract during inhalation, the lung volume increases, creating a lower pressure within the lungs compared to atmospheric pressure, which causes air to flow into the lungs. During exhalation, the opposite occurs.

Sensory mechanisms of the respiratory system

Every cell in the human body requires oxygen for normal metabolism and must excrete the metabolic waste product, carbon dioxide. To maintain homeostasis, cells in different locations of the body react to changes in oxygen and CO_2 levels. Sensory cells include chemoreceptors, pressoreceptors and baroreceptors.

Chemoreceptors

Chemoreceptors are specialised cells located centrally in the upper medulla of the brainstem and peripherally in bodies located in the carotid and aortic arteries. They respond to slight increases in arterial or cerebrospinal fluid CO_2 pressure (P_{CO2}) and acidity (an increased concentration of hydrogen [H^+] ions). Regulation of ventilation depends mainly on the level of CO_2 in the blood. A slight increase in CO_2 concentration stimulates chemoreceptors to increase the respiratory rate and depth until the excess CO_2 is eliminated. Conversely, a decreased CO_2 level slows the ventilatory rate (AACN & Hartjes 2022). Oxygen levels are normally sensed by the carotid bodies, which are sensitive to a fall in oxygen concentration of less than 50%. Stimulation of the carotid receptors increases the respiratory rate, the exception being individuals with chronic hypercapnia such as in emphysema.

Pressoreceptors

Pressoreceptors, or mechanoreceptors, are stretch receptors present in lung tissue and within the thoracic wall. The bronchioles and alveoli also have stretch receptors that respond to extreme over-inflation as well as extreme deflation. When over-inflation occurs, impulses are transmitted from the stretch receptors to the medulla by the vagus nerve, the expiratory centre is activated and exhalation occurs. When extreme deflation occurs impulses from the lungs activate the inspiratory centre and inhalation occurs.

Baroreceptors

Baroreceptors are cells sensitive to blood pressure, which normally monitor changes in blood pressure. When blood pressure increases, impulses are sent to the respiratory centres to cause a decrease in respiratory rate. Rate, depth and rhythm of respirations are further affected by reflex responses, chemical signals and voluntary control. For example, during actions such as swallowing, impulses from gustatory centres are conveyed to the respiratory centre, and breathing stops temporarily.

Any abnormal mechanical disturbance (e.g. the presence of chemical substances such as cigarette smoke) causes excitement of the lung irritant receptors, which induces hyperventilation and a reflex bronchoconstriction. Information from other parts of the body may also be received by the respiratory centres. For example, a rise in body temperature initiates an increase in the rate of ventilation, while a sudden cooling of the body induces a sudden inhalation followed by hyperventilation.

The respiratory centres

Respiration is controlled both voluntarily and involuntarily. The automatic control of breathing is regulated by three respiratory centres, known as the medullary centre, located in the medulla oblongata, the apneustic centre in the pons and the pneumotaxic centre in the upper pons of the brainstem. These centres receive stimuli from sensory cells described above, and from each other. Their function is to control the rate, rhythm and depth of ventilation (Carlson 2018). Impulses travel from the respiratory centres along separate nerves that exit the spinal cord at different levels to separately innervate and control the diaphragm and internal and external intercostal muscles. Impulses are also transmitted to the other centres and cause stimulation of the respiratory muscles via the phrenic nerves, to stimulate the diaphragm to contract, and the intercostal nerves, which stimulate the intercostal muscles.

VENTILATION AND RESPIRATION

Respiration is the term used to describe an interchange of gases. The main purpose of respiration is to supply the body with oxygen and dispose of carbon dioxide. The four processes involved are:

1. ventilation: movement of air containing different gases into the respiratory tract
2. external respiration: exchange of oxygen and CO_2 between the blood and the alveoli (Figure 25.3)
3. internal respiration: exchange of oxygen and CO_2 between the bloodstream and the tissues
4. cellular respiration: exchange of gases by cells.

(AACN & Hartjes 2022)

Ventilation

Ventilation has two phases (Figure 25.5): inhalation and exhalation.

Inhalation

For air to flow into the lungs, the lungs expand, creating a lower pressure in the alveoli compared to atmospheric pressure. This difference in pressure causes air to move into the lungs (Tortora et al 2021). During **inhalation**, the diaphragm contracts and flattens, enlarging the thoracic cavity lengthwise, particularly in males. In females, normal inhalations occur primarily by contraction of the external intercostal muscles, which raise the ribs and sternum, thus increasing the size of the thoracic cavity from side to side and front to back. As the chest wall moves up and outwards, the parietal pleura moves with it and, because of the 2 mmHg negative pressure within the pleura, the visceral pleura follows the parietal pleura. This causes stretching of the lungs, which expand to fill the enlarged thorax, and air is pushed into the respiratory passages (Tortora et al 2021).

Exhalation

Exhalation is normally a more passive process than inhalation except in exercise and respiratory conditions in which active expiration occurs via internal intercostal and accessory muscles. During exhalation, the diaphragm relaxes, thus decreasing the size of the thoracic cavity. The external intercostal muscles also relax, allowing the ribs and sternum to return to their former position, further decreasing the size of the thoracic cavity. The elastic tissue of the lungs allows for recoil, further forcing air out of the respiratory passages (Tortora et al 2021).

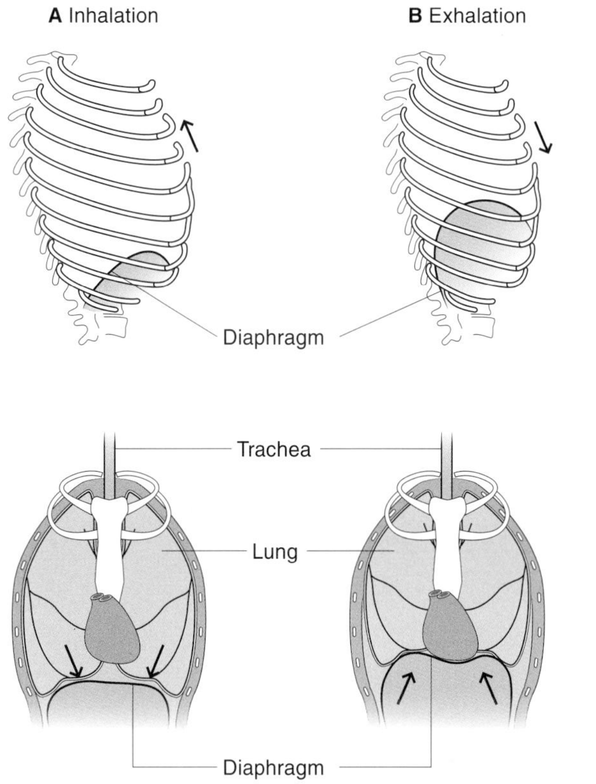

Figure 25.5 Rib cage and diaphragm positions during breathing

A: At the end of normal inhalation: chest expanded (top left) and diaphragm depressed (bottom left), **B:** At the end of a normal exhalation: chest depressed (top right) and diaphragm elevated (bottom right).

Respiration

External respiration

External respiration is the exchange of gases between air in the alveoli and the blood travelling through the capillaries surrounding the alveoli (AACN & Hartjes 2022). Branches of the pulmonary artery bring deoxygenated blood to the capillaries surrounding each alveolus. During **gas exchange**, gases normally diffuse through the semi-permeable walls of the alveoli and capillaries to the area of lowest concentration of each gas, as each gas diffuses independently of other gases, until the pressure is equal on both sides. Thus, oxygen moves from an area of higher concentration in the alveoli to an area of lower concentration in the blood capillaries, while CO_2 moves from an area of higher concentration in blood

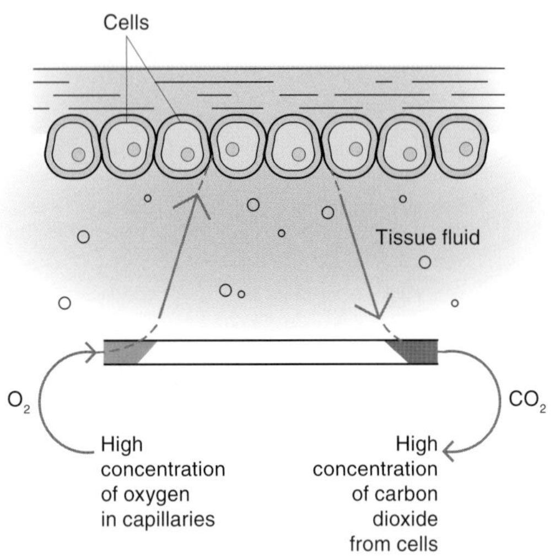

Figure 25.6 Internal respiration

capillaries to an area of lower concentration in the alveolar air. Pulmonary venules then collect the blood rich in oxygen from the capillaries and unite to form the two pulmonary veins that leave each lung to enter the left atrium of the heart (AACN & Hartjes 2022).

Internal respiration

Internal respiration (Figure 25.6) is the exchange of gases between the bloodstream and the tissues. During this exchange, the gases diffuse through the semi-permeable walls of the capillaries to equalise the concentration of gases on both sides. Oxygen moves from the blood into the tissues, down a concentration gradient, to replenish oxygen used in cellular metabolism. Carbon dioxide moves from the tissues into the blood, down a concentration gradient, to rid the tissues of waste produced by cellular metabolism (AACN & Hartjes 2022).

Cellular respiration

The gases that diffuse from the interstitial tissue into cells are used by the cells for metabolism. The metabolism of nutrients uses oxygen and produces CO_2, which diffuses from cells into the interstitial tissue. This level of respiration is termed 'cellular respiration'; while cellular respiration cannot be measured directly, it is estimated by the amount of CO_2 produced and the amount of O_2 consumed (AACN & Hartjes 2022).

Factors necessary for ventilation and respiration

The passage of oxygen from the atmosphere to the alveoli in the lungs, and the passage of carbon dioxide from the alveoli to the atmosphere, requires an unobstructed airway. In addition, the process of respiration requires:

- adequate oxygen in the atmosphere
- a patent functioning respiratory tract
- functioning thoracic muscles and nerves to control the thoracic cage and diaphragm
- capillaries in close proximity to the cells to allow the exchange of gases
- a functioning cardiovascular system that contains adequate amounts of plasma and normal erythrocytes and haemoglobin to transport the gases.

(AACN & Hartjes 2022)

Transport of oxygen

Oxygen is carried in the blood in two ways:

1. Dissolved in the plasma: Only 2–3% of oxygen is carried in this way since oxygen is not very soluble. Oxygen dissolved in plasma is measured as PaO_2.
2. Bound to haemoglobin in the red blood cells: 95–98% of oxygen is carried in this way and is measured by the percentage of oxygen saturated (SaO_2).

(Koeppen et al 2023)

Haemoglobin is composed of haem (iron) and globulin (protein). Oxygen and haemoglobin combined together form oxyhaemoglobin (Figure 25.7).

Hb that is not combined with oxygen is referred to as reduced haemoglobin. Oxyhaemoglobin refers to haemoglobin saturated with oxygen (each haemoglobin molecule is bound to four oxygen molecules) (Thomas 2018). Hb that has a mixture of Hb and HbO_2 is referred to as partially saturated haemoglobin. The percentage saturation of haemoglobin is the percentage of HbO_2 in the total haemoglobin. The percentage saturation of haemoglobin with oxygen is illustrated in the oxygen–haemoglobin dissociation curve (Figure 25.8).

The bond between haemoglobin and oxygen is affected by various physiological factors that shift the oxygen dissociation curve to the left or to the right. When the PaO_2 of blood is high, haemoglobin binds with large amounts of oxygen and is almost fully saturated. When the PaO_2 is low, the haemoglobin binds with smaller amounts of oxygen and is partially saturated (Thomas 2018).

The assessment of arterial oxygen saturation is commonly performed by using pulse oximetry. Pulse oximetry is a non-invasive medical technique that measures a person's oxygen saturation level and pulse rate. This method relies on the interaction of light with blood to provide essential health information. A pulse oximeter emits both red and infrared light through a thin, well-perfused body part like a finger or earlobe. As this light travels through the tissue, it encounters blood vessels

$$Hb + O_2 = HbO_2$$

(Uncombined or reduced haemoglobin) + oxygen = (oxyhaemoglobin or combined haemoglobin)

Figure 25.7 Haemoglobin equation

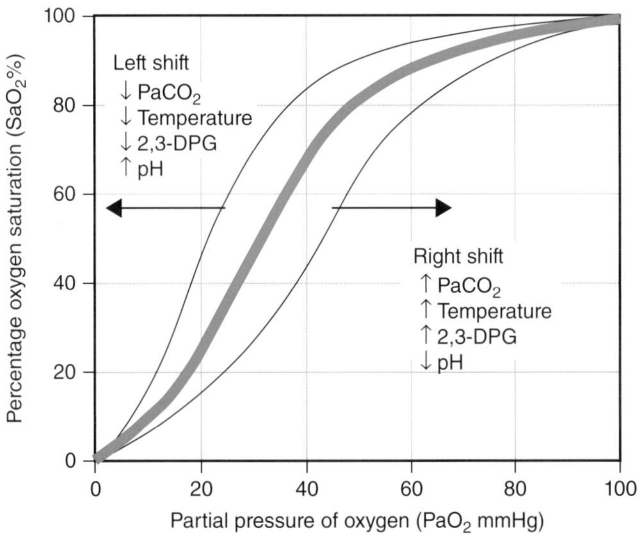

Figure 25.8 Oxygen–haemoglobin dissociation curve

(Craft et al 2023)

containing oxygenated and deoxygenated haemoglobin. These two types of haemoglobin absorb different amounts of red and infrared light. Oxygenated haemoglobin prefers infrared light and allows more red light to pass through, while deoxygenated haemoglobin has the opposite preference. On the other side of the tissue, a photodetector measures the intensity of the light that passes through. By calculating the ratio of absorbed red to infrared light, the pulse oximeter estimates the percentage of oxygenated haemoglobin, known as oxygen saturation (SpO_2) (Abraham 2023).

Factors affecting the release of oxygen from haemoglobin

Several factors affect the amount of oxygen being released from haemoglobin so that the oxygen dissociation curve is said to shift to the left or to the right (Patel & Mohiuddin 2019). When a shift occurs to the right, there is reduced binding of oxygen to haemoglobin and oxygen is released more easily into the tissues. When a shift occurs to the left, there is an increase in the binding of oxygen to haemoglobin, resulting in oxygen being less easily released into the tissues (Patel & Mohiuddin 2019). Cellular hypoxia can occur.

pH

Oxygen is released more readily from haemoglobin in an acid environment. This condition occurs often during an acute illness. During an acute illness, an increase in PaO_2 is usually present, resulting in a lower pH. This acidic environment allows the oxygen to separate more readily from the haemoglobin, allowing the tissues to have more oxygen (AACN & Hartjes 2022).

Temperature

Within limits, the amount of oxygen released from haemoglobin increases as temperature increases; therefore, hyperthermia causes a rightward shift while hypothermia causes a leftward shift (Pinsky et al 2019).

Organic phosphates

2,3-diphosphoglycerate (DPG) is a primary organic phosphate. It is an intermediate compound formed in red blood cells during the conversion of glycogen to glucose. The production of 2,3-DPG is likely an important adaptive mechanism because the production increases in several conditions where there is diminished peripheral tissue O_2 availability, such as hypoxaemia, chronic lung disease, anaemia and congestive heart failure. High levels of 2,3-DPG shift the curve to the right, while low levels of 2,3-DPG cause a leftward shift, seen in states such as septic shock and hypophosphataemia (Pinsky et al 2019).

Carbon dioxide excretion

Carbon dioxide is carried through the venous system and breathed out through the lungs. The normal level of carbon dioxide in the blood is 3.5–5.3 kPa. Carbon dioxide has a direct effect on the respiratory centre in the brain. As carbon dioxide levels rise and diffuse from the blood into the cerebrospinal fluid, the CO_2 is hydrated and carbonic acid is formed. The role of the respiratory system is to excrete carbonic acid from the lungs during expiration. Carbon dioxide stimulates respiratory rate and so high carbon dioxide levels result in a higher respiration rate (AACN & Hartjes 2022).

STRUCTURE OF THE CARDIOVASCULAR SYSTEM

The structures that make up the **cardiovascular** system are the:

- heart, which acts as a pump to circulate the blood through the body
- blood, which carries essential substances to cells and carries wastes away from cells
- blood vessels, which contain and transport the blood throughout the body
- lymphatic system, which transports tissue fluid containing electrolytes, proteins and some waste products, recognises and destroys pathogens before they reach the bloodstream and delivers nutrients from the digestive tract into the cardiovascular system.

(Carlson 2018)

The heart

The heart is a hollow, conical muscular organ situated obliquely in the thoracic cavity between the lungs and behind the sternum. One-third of the heart lies to the right and two-thirds lie to the left of the median plane. Its base is uppermost and points towards the right shoulder, and its apex is below, pointing to the left. The adult heart weighs about 0.3 kg (0.5% of body weight) (Carlson 2018).

Structure of the heart

The heart is divided into a right and a left side by a muscular partition called the septum. Each side is further divided into an upper receiving chamber, the atrium, and a lower distributing chamber, the ventricle (Figure 25.9). The walls of the heart consist of the pericardium, myocardium and endocardium:

- The pericardium is the outer coat, consisting of two layers of serous membrane. The pericardium secretes a small amount of serous fluid to moisten the surfaces in contact with each other, so that the heart can beat with minimal friction.
- The myocardium is the middle muscular layer consisting of cardiac muscle, which is a highly specialised type of muscle tissue present only in the heart. It is of varying thickness, being thicker in both ventricles than in the atria, and thicker in the left ventricle than in the right.
- The endocardium is the innermost lining of the heart, and provides a smooth surface for the flow of blood. Folds of endocardium help to form the valves of the heart.

(Carlson 2018)

Valves of the heart

Heart valves consist of flaps of fibrous tissue covered by endocardium, which allow blood to flow in one direction only, thus preventing a backward flow. The valves are the:

- bicuspid (or mitral) valve, between the left atrium and left ventricle
- tricuspid valve, between the right atrium and right ventricle
- aortic valve, between the left ventricle and the aorta
- pulmonary valve, between the right ventricle and the pulmonary artery.

Fine cords of tendons (chordae tendineae) are attached from the mitral and tricuspid valves to small projections from the muscle walls of the ventricles called papillary muscles. Contraction of the papillary muscles closes the valves, preventing blood from escaping back into the atria (Carlson 2018).

Cardiac blood vessels

Several blood vessels either enter or leave the heart. The blood vessels that enter the heart are the:

- inferior vena cava, which carries deoxygenated blood collected from the lower part of the body to the right atrium

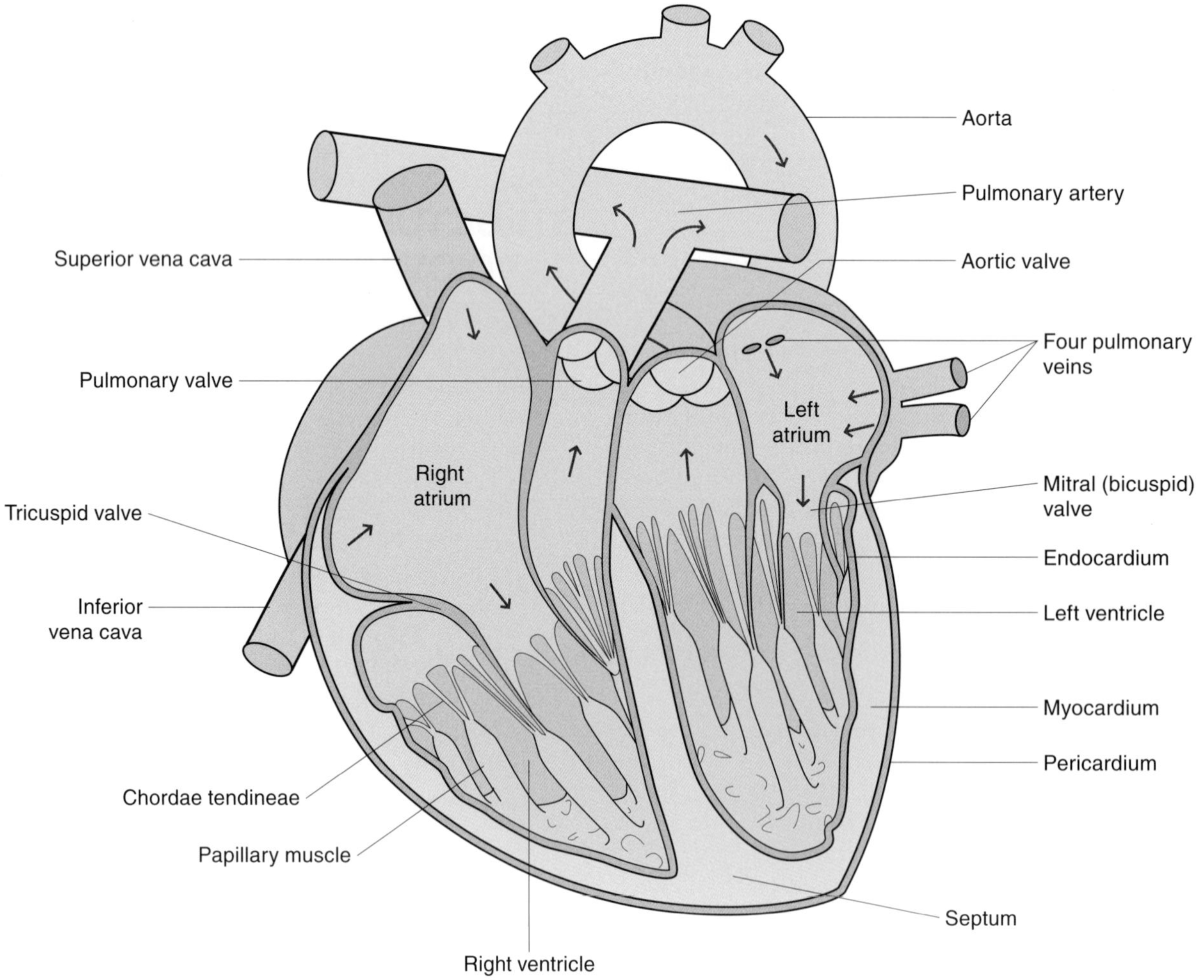

Figure 25.9 Structure of the heart

- superior vena cava, which carries deoxygenated blood collected from the upper part of the body to the right atrium
- four pulmonary veins, two from each lung, which carry oxygenated blood into the left atrium.

(Carlson 2018)

The blood vessels that leave the heart are the aorta, which carries oxygenated blood from the left ventricle for distribution to all the systems and tissues of the body, and the pulmonary artery, which leaves the right ventricle then divides into two branches that carry deoxygenated blood from the heart to each lung. Thus, the right side of the heart deals only with deoxygenated blood, and the left side deals only with oxygenated blood (Carlson 2018).

Blood supply to the heart

The heart receives its own supply of blood. As the aorta leaves the heart, it gives off two branches called the coronary arteries (right coronary). The coronary arteries divide into smaller and smaller branches, until networks of capillaries are formed in the heart wall. These arteries and their branches supply all parts of the myocardium with blood. Venules collect the deoxygenated blood from the tissues in the heart wall and unite to form a vein (coronary sinus), which opens directly into the right atrium (Carlson 2018).

The conducting system of the heart

The heart's conducting system (Figure 25.10) ensures that it contracts in a coordinated and synchronised series of events. The sinoatrial (SA) node is located in the upper part of the right atrium and acts as the pacemaker of the heart, continuously initiating impulses that innervate the rest of the heart. The atrioventricular (AV) node lies in the lower part of the interatrial septum of the heart. The AV node is connected to the bundle of His and is the only natural pathway for the impulse to travel from the atria to the ventricles. The bundle of His divides into the right and left bundle branches, which in turn divide off into tiny fibres termed Purkinje fibres. These fibres rapidly conduct the impulse throughout the myocardium from the apex to the base (Carlson 2018).

Functions of the heart

The function of the heart is to act as a pump: it pumps deoxygenated blood to the lungs to excrete carbon dioxide

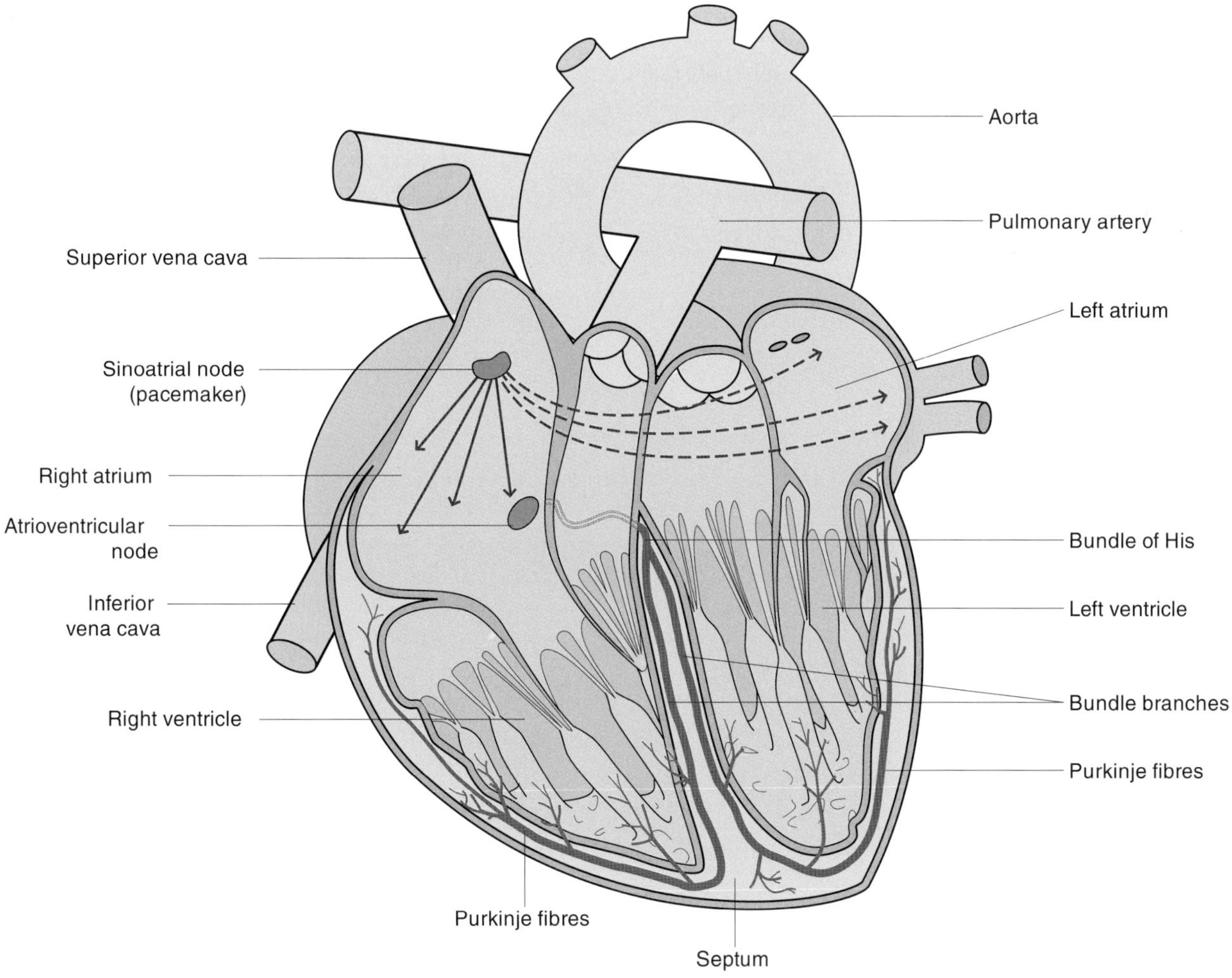

Figure 25.10 Conduction system of the heart

and pick up oxygen, and pumps oxygenated blood to all other parts of the body.

The cardiac cycle is the series of pressure changes, valve actions and electrical potentials that bring about the movement of blood through the heart during one complete heartbeat. The cardiac cycle takes about 0.8 of a second and consists of two phases: systole (the contraction phase) and diastole (the relaxation phase). During atrial systole, both atria contract at the same time, while the ventricles are relaxing after their last contraction. The combination of atria contraction and ventricular relaxation allows the flow of blood from the right atrium through the open atrioventricular (tricuspid) valve and into the right ventricle (Carlson 2018). The two ventricles then contract simultaneously, forcing their contents into the aorta and pulmonary artery. Diastole follows after each contraction occurs in the cardiac chambers (Carlson 2018).

Cardiac output is the volume of blood pumped out by each ventricle during 1 minute. It is the product of the volume of blood pumped at each beat (stroke volume) and the number of beats during 1 minute (heart rate) (Carlson 2018).

The heartbeat is controlled by the cardioregulatory centre in the central nervous system. The vagus nerve slows it and reduces the force of the beat, while sympathetic nerves quicken the beat and increase its force.

Each cardiac muscle cell is capable of spontaneous, rhythmic self-excitation known as autorhythmia. To be effective as a pump, the action of the whole heart must be coordinated. Coordination of the rhythmic movements is brought about by the specialised cells of the sinoatrial (SA) node (pacemaker) (Carlson 2018).

Blood

Blood is composed of plasma and formed elements. It is a viscous substance, heavier, thicker and more viscous than water.

Blood is classed as a connective tissue and constitutes about one-twelfth of the weight of the body. The difference between blood and other connective tissues is that its cells are not fixed but free to move in the liquid portion of the blood, known as plasma (Carlson 2018).

Depending on the weight of the individual, the average total volume of blood is about 5–6 L (Carlson 2018). Blood varies in colour, from bright red when it has a high oxygen content, to dark red when the oxygen content is low. Arterial blood normally has a pH range of 7.35 to 7.45 (AACN & Hartjes 2022).

Functions of blood

Blood has the following functions:

- transporting oxygen, nutrients, water and ions to all tissue cells
- removing waste materials to excretory organs
- transporting hormones to cells
- supplying materials from which cells and glands make their secretions
- protecting the body against infection by means of the leucocytes and antibodies
- regulating pH, body temperature and cellular content by distributing heat evenly throughout the body
- preventing loss of body fluid and blood cells by means of its clotting mechanism

(AACN & Hartjes 2022)

Plasma

Plasma, the fluid part of blood, is a straw-coloured watery fluid in which blood cells are suspended. Plasma forms about 55% of the blood volume and is composed of 90% water and 7% proteins. The remaining 3% is made up of nutrients, crystalloids, electrolytes, hormones and vitamins (Tortora et al 2021). Plasma is important in the maintenance of all body fluids and in the production of secretions.

Plasma contains:

- Water: Serves as the solvent in which the various solutes are dissolved.
- Proteins: Albumin, globulin, fibrinogen, prothrombin and heparin are some of the proteins found in plasma. The liver normally produces proteins, with the exception of serum globulin, which is derived from lymphocytes. Plasma proteins have several important functions: they assist in retaining water in the plasma and interstitial tissue; factors such as prothrombin and fibrinogen are essential for blood clotting; proteins such as heparin help to prevent abnormal clotting of blood in the blood vessels.
- Electrolytes (mineral salts): The main mineral salts found in blood plasma are sodium chloride, iodine, potassium, phosphorus, calcium, iron, magnesium and copper. Electrolytes play essential roles in maintaining fluid balance, nerve function, muscle contraction and pH regulation.
- Nutrients: Those found in blood plasma are numerous and include amino acids, glucose, fatty acids, glycerol and vitamins. They have been reduced to their simplest form by the digestive processes and absorbed from the alimentary tract into the blood and lymph for circulation to the cells.
- Waste products: Resulting from fat and protein metabolism, including urea, uric acid and creatinine are transported by plasma to be eliminated from the body.
- Gases: Includes oxygen, nitrogen and carbon dioxide. Oxygen and nitrogen enter the bloodstream after inhalation of air and carbon dioxide is an end product of oxidation in the cells.
- Hormones: Chemical substances secreted directly into the bloodstream by endocrine glands and carried to the areas of the body where they are required to stimulate activity.
- Enzymes: Produced by the body, which initiate or accelerate chemical reactions.

(Carlson 2018; Tortora et al 2021)

Formed elements

The remaining 45% of blood volume consists of blood cells and fragments suspended in the plasma and is known as formed elements (Carlson 2018). The three types of formed elements are erythrocytes, leucocytes and thrombocytes.

Erythrocytes

Erythrocytes (red cells) are biconcave non-nucleated discs measuring about 7 microns in diameter. In adults, erythrocytes are produced in the red bone marrow of cancellous bone tissue, where they pass through several stages of development (Carlson 2018). They begin as large nucleated cells but, when mature (after they have produced haemoglobin), they lose the nucleus and are liberated into the circulation. Haemoglobin is a complex protein composed of four different 'haem' chains, each containing a central atom of iron and a globulin protein. It has a strong affinity for both oxygen and carbon monoxide and gives the blood its colour. The normal haemoglobin level is about 14–16 g/100 mL of blood.

The number of erythrocytes is about 5,000,000/mm^3 of blood, and their average lifespan is 100–120 days. Since their nucleus is absent, they are unable to repair damage and become worn out in circulation, and are destroyed in the spleen and liver. The haemoglobin from the cells is split; the liver stores the iron for future use and uses the pigment in the production of bile. The primary function of erythrocytes is to carry oxygen. In the lungs, oxygen combines with haemoglobin to form oxyhaemoglobin, making the blood bright red in colour. As blood circulates through the tissues, the oxygen is released, forming deoxyhaemoglobin, and the blood becomes dark red in colour (Carlson 2018).

Leucocytes

Leucocytes (white cells) measure about 10 microns in diameter. They differ from erythrocytes in that they are larger, possess a nucleus and are less numerous. While erythrocytes remain in the bloodstream, leucocytes function outside the bloodstream and the circulatory system is merely the means by which they are carried to the extravascular locations to fulfil their duties (Carlson 2018). There are two main types of leucocytes: granulocytes and agranular leucocytes.

Granulocytes contain granules of enzymes and are classified as neutrophils, basophils or eosinophils, described as follows:

- **Neutrophils** are the most numerous of the leucocytes and are important to the body in defence against bacteria since they have the ability to engulf microorganisms or other foreign particles (phagocytosis) and digest them. Neutrophils also play an important part in the inflammatory response. Injured tissues, and other leucocytes, secrete substances that stimulate the bone marrow to release increased numbers of neutrophils.
- **Basophils** play a role in the defence against parasites. They also play a part in the allergic response and act to limit the inflammatory response.
- **Eosinophils** constitute approximately 1–3% of circulating white cells. Their main function is in the defence of the body; their cytoplasmic granules contain proteins which kill invaders.

(Carlson 2018)

Agranular leucocytes lack granules of enzymes and are classified as monocytes or lymphocytes, described as follows:

- **Monocytes** have the ability to move into the tissues, where they become macrophages and are capable of phagocytosis. They also secrete a variety of substances involved in the body's defence, and play a role in the immune response.
- **Lymphocytes** are either T-lymphocytes or B-lymphocytes, both of which divide when stimulated by antigens. T-lymphocytes are responsible for cellular immunity and adhere to cells identified as foreign to the body. They secrete cytotoxic substances that kill the foreign cells. B-lymphocytes are involved in humoral immunity since they produce antibodies and are also responsible for immunoglobulin production. While the lifespan for granular leucocytes is only about 21 days, lymphocytes may survive for up to 100 days.

The total number of leucocytes is about 8000–10,000/mm^3 of blood, but this number increases considerably (leucocytosis) when there is any infection in the body. The lifespan of a leucocyte is variable and depends to some extent on the degree of activity (Carlson 2018).

Thrombocytes

Thrombocytes (platelets) are the smallest of the formed elements. They are colourless microscopic fragments of the megakaryocyte cell. They measure about 3 microns in diameter and do not possess a nucleus. Thrombocytes are produced in the bone marrow, which is present in cancellous bone tissue. The number of thrombocytes is about 250,000–300,000/mm^3 of blood, and the average lifespan of a thrombocyte is 5–9 days. The function of thrombocytes is to play a major role in the clotting of blood to reduce blood loss when a vessel wall is injured (Carlson 2018). The process involves many substances (clotting factors) that are produced by the liver and circulate in the plasma, as well as some substances released by the platelets and injured tissues. Normally a blood clot will form within 2–6 minutes after a blood vessel wall has been damaged.

The mechanism of clotting (haemostasis) involves three phases: vasoconstriction, formation of a temporary platelet plug and formation of a clot. When a small vessel becomes damaged:

- Local vasoconstriction occurs, which reduces blood flow and therefore blood loss.
- The vessel wall becomes 'sticky' and platelets adhere to the damaged area.
- The platelets release serotonin and adenosine diphosphate (ADP), which attract other thrombocytes, leading to the formation of a temporary platelet plug.
- The temporary platelet plug is converted into a clot by the deposition of fibrin, which is formed from fibrinogen.

The conversion of fibrinogen to fibrin involves a 'cascade' of reactions that requires a number of plasma factors (numbered I to XIII). A series of reactions culminate in the conversion of prothrombin to thrombin, which converts fibrinogen to fibrin. This conversion requires the presence of platelets, factor V, factor X and calcium ions. Vitamin K is also necessary for the conversion of factors VII, IX and X.

- The fibrin forms a meshwork of fibres that traps the erythrocytes and forms the basis of a clot.
- The clot plugs the injured blood vessel, drawing the edges together.

The clotting mechanism is a complex one that will not occur if any of the necessary elements are reduced, defective or missing (Marieb & Hoehn 2019).

Blood group types

Human blood is grouped into four classifications based on immune reactivity. The groups are O, A, B, AB (Carlson 2018). The Rhesus factor (either negative or positive) is also determined. Eighty-five per cent of the population has Rh antibodies on the surface of the red blood cell (i.e. Rh positive). The blood of any one group is essentially incompatible with the blood group of another. Therefore, blood transfusions should be an exact match to the individual's blood group and Rh factor. When blood transfusions occur with mismatched blood, a haemolytic reaction can occur (Carlson 2018). To prevent a mismatch or to recognise a reaction to a transfusion it is important to follow organisational policies and procedures for the preparation, administration and monitoring of individuals undergoing a blood transfusion. See Clinical Skill 20.9 for preparing and monitoring an individual undergoing a blood transfusion.

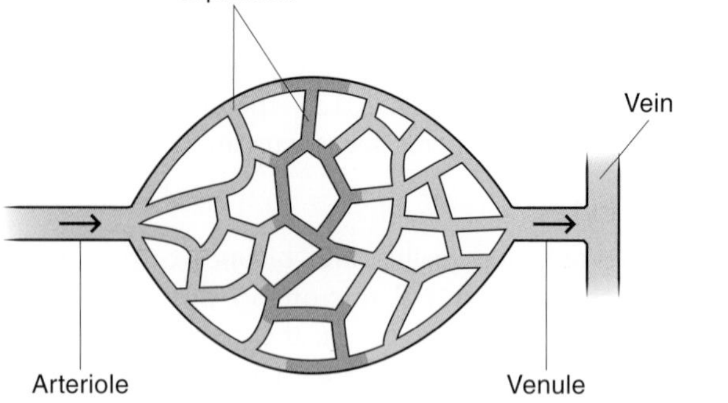

Figure 25.11 Circulation of blood through the tissues

Blood vessels

Blood is circulated throughout the body (Figure 25.11) within vessels that form a closed continuous system.

The walls of blood vessels have three layers: an outer coat of fibrous tissue, a thick middle layer of involuntary muscle with elastic fibrous tissue and an inner lining of endothelium to form a smooth surface for contact with blood (Figure 25.12). Blood vessels include the arteries, veins and capillaries (Carlson 2018).

Arteries

Arteries carry blood away from the heart (efferent). All arteries carry oxygenated (bright red) blood, with the exception of the two pulmonary arteries, which carry deoxygenated (dark red) blood from the heart to the lungs. Arteries vary in size, and large arteries divide to form smaller arteries (Figure 25.13). Further division, or branching, occurs to form the smallest arteries, called arterioles, which

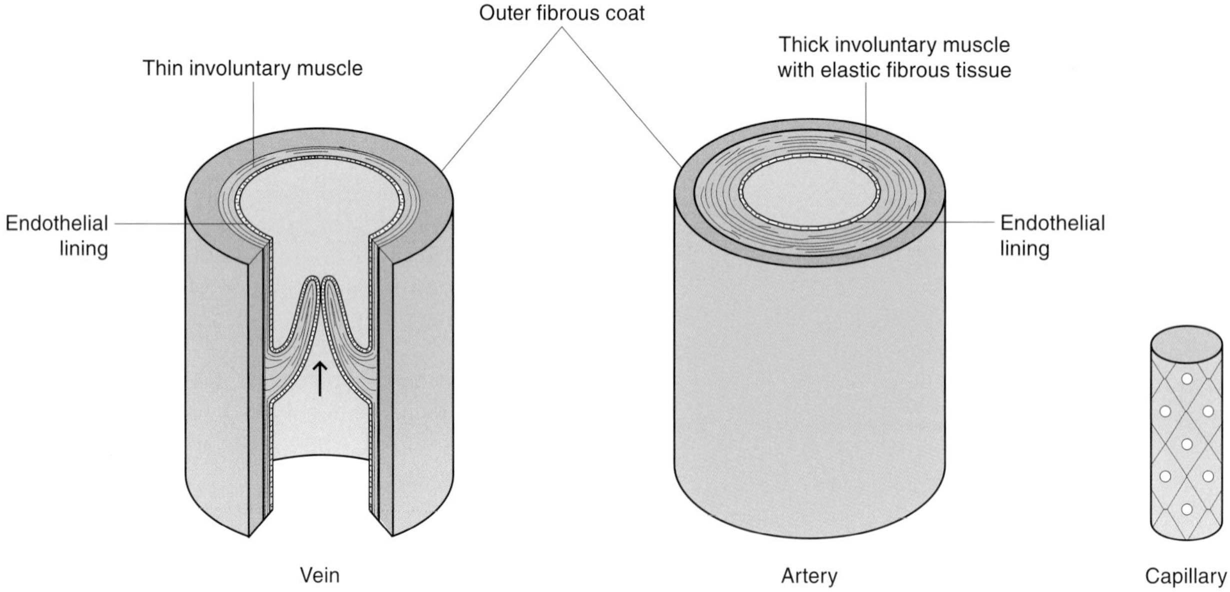

Figure 25.12 Structure of blood vessels

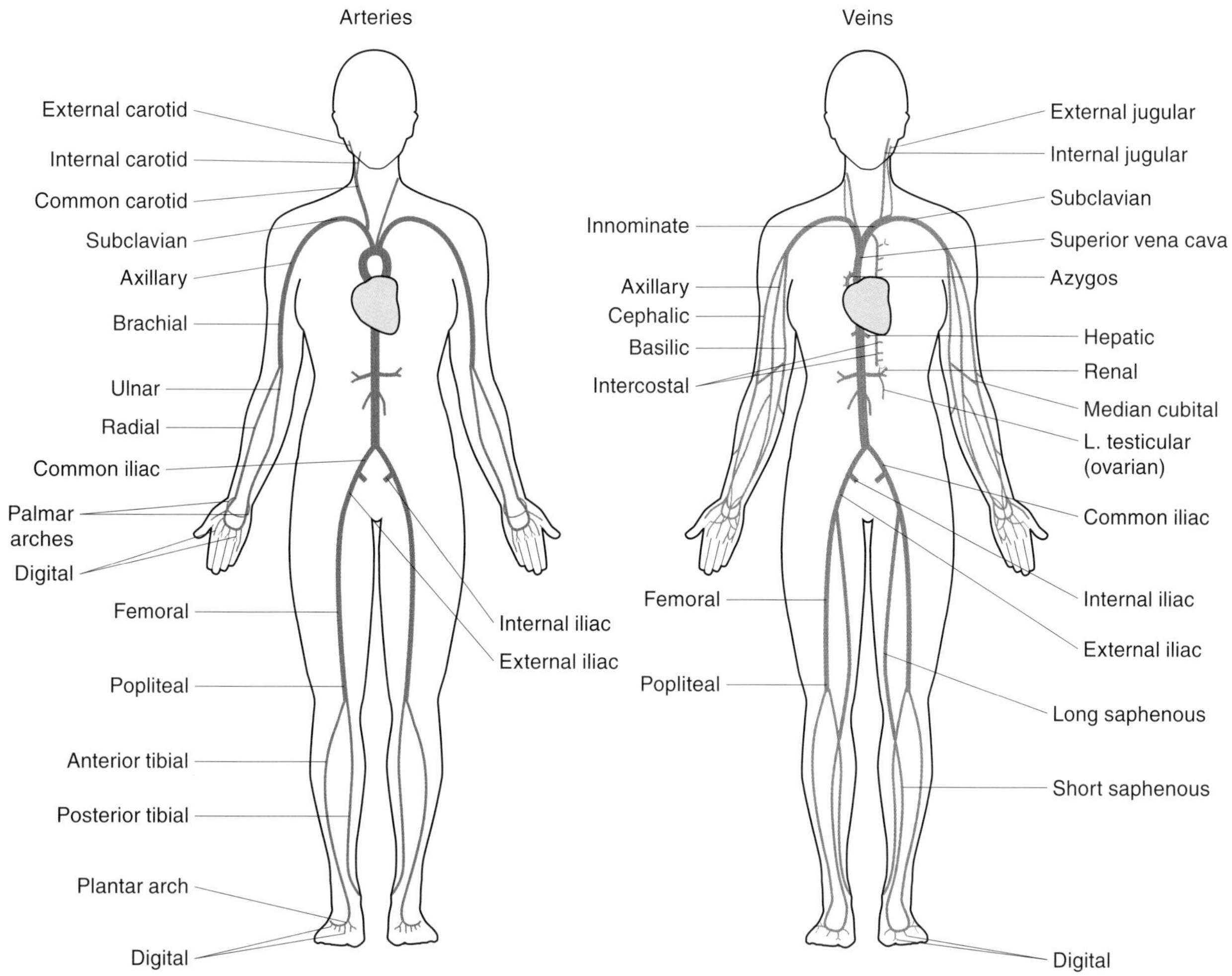

Figure 25.13 Major arteries and veins

divide into capillaries. Arteries and arterioles have the same tissue structure that allows them to stretch and recoil as the heart pumps the blood into them (Carlson 2018).

Veins

Veins carry blood towards the heart (afferent). All veins carry deoxygenated (dark red) blood, with the exception of the four pulmonary veins, which carry oxygenated blood from the lungs to the heart. Veins vary in size, and large veins divide to form smaller veins. The smallest veins are called venules, which divide into capillaries (Figure 25.13). Venules carry deoxygenated blood away from the capillary beds and unite to form veins. The walls of veins are composed of the same three layers as those of arteries, but the walls are thinner and have less elastic and muscular tissue. Veins join up until the two largest veins are formed—the superior and inferior vena cavae. These two veins empty their contents into the right atrium of the heart (Carlson 2018).

The larger veins possess pocket-like valves on their inner surfaces. These valves aid the unidirectional flow of blood towards the heart and prevent a backward flow of blood. Skeletal muscle activity also helps venous return.

Capillaries

Capillaries are microscopic vessels about 3–8 microns in diameter and are composed of a single layer of endothelium, with little surrounding connective tissue (Carlson 2018). They form closed networks through all tissues and are structurally adapted for their role in the rapid diffusion of substances between the plasma and interstitial fluid. This allows water, oxygen, nutrients and other essential substances to pass rapidly from the blood to the tissue cells, and waste products from the tissue cells pass through the capillary walls to the blood (Carlson 2018).

Blood pressure

The term 'blood pressure' refers to the pressure, or force, exerted by blood on the walls of the blood vessels. Pressure is highest in the arteries, which receive blood from the ventricles of the heart at about 120 mmHg (Carlson 2018). As the vessels divide, their cross-sectional area increases, causing the pressure to progressively reduce so that there is only very slight pressure in the capillaries (about 35 mmHg and 15 mmHg in the venules) (Carlson 2018). Systolic blood pressure is the pressure registered in a large artery as blood is forced out of the ventricle during the contracting period of the cardiac cycle (Carlson 2018). Diastolic blood pressure is the pressure registered during the relaxing period of the cardiac cycle, when there is no ejection of blood into the arteries (Carlson 2018). It is therefore lower than the systolic pressure.

CIRCULATION OF BLOOD

Blood flows continuously around the entire body. The blood vessels (of which there are two circuits—pulmonary and systemic) along with the four chambers of the heart (right and left atrium, right and left ventricle) form the closed circulatory system in which blood flows (Carlson 2018). Deoxygenated blood from all body regions is transported via the veins to the superior and inferior vena cavae, which enter the right atrium. The coronary sinus drains venous blood from the myocardium into the right atrium. At first, blood flows passively into the right ventricle as the tricuspid valve is open, then contraction of the right atrium (atrial systole) occurs to empty its entire contents. After the tricuspid valve closes, the right ventricle contracts (ventricular systole), and blood is ejected through the pulmonary valve into the pulmonary artery (Carlson 2018).

The pulmonary artery divides into the right pulmonary artery, which carries deoxygenated blood to the right lung and the left pulmonary artery, which carries deoxygenated blood to the left lung. In the lungs, oxygen is exchanged for carbon dioxide from the blood, and the oxygenated blood returns to the left atrium via four pulmonary veins. The left atrium contracts and blood passes through the mitral (bicuspid) valve into the left ventricle. After the mitral valve closes, the left ventricle contracts and blood is ejected into the aorta via the aortic valve. The aorta branches off to supply all areas of the body with oxygenated blood (Carlson 2018).

The systemic circulation

The systemic circulation is the distribution of oxygenated blood to all tissues and the return of deoxygenated blood from all tissues to the heart. When the left ventricle contracts it forces blood into the aorta under pressure (Carlson 2018). The elastic walls of the aorta distend to receive the blood. When the left ventricle relaxes, the walls of the aorta recoil and, with the aortic valve closed, the blood is driven onwards through the aorta. Branches from the aorta also distend and recoil as the blood travels through them, and this wave of distension and recoil is felt as the pulse wherever a superficial artery crosses a hard structure such as a bone (Carlson 2018).

Arterioles supply networks of capillaries with oxygenated blood, and the hydrostatic pressure behind the blood causes water and other essential substances to be pushed through the capillary walls and wash over the tissue cells to become part of the tissue fluid. Tissue cells allow certain substances they require to enter, and excrete their waste products into the tissue fluid (Carlson 2018). The pressure within the capillaries will allow only a small amount of the fluid to return through the capillary and venule wall back into the blood (Carlson 2018). The remainder of the fluid reaches the blood via the lymphatic system, which is discussed later in this chapter.

Arteries

The aorta (Figure 25.14) has four sections, each of which has a number of branches. Two coronary arteries to the heart wall branch from the ascending aorta. From the aortic arch branch the left common carotid artery to the head and neck; the left subclavian artery to the left upper limb; and the right innominate artery, which divides into the right common carotid and right subclavian arteries. From the descending thoracic aorta branch the bronchial arteries to the lungs; the oesophageal artery to the oesophagus; and 10 pairs of intercostal arteries to the intercostal muscles. From the abdominal aorta, branch the:

- phrenic arteries to the diaphragm
- coeliac trunk, which divides into the gastric artery to the stomach, the hepatic artery to the liver and the splenic artery to the pancreas and spleen
- superior mesenteric artery to the small intestine
- renal arteries to the kidneys
- ovarian or testicular arteries to the ovaries or testes
- inferior mesenteric artery to the large intestine
- two common iliac arteries to the pelvic organs and the lower limbs.

(Carlson 2018)

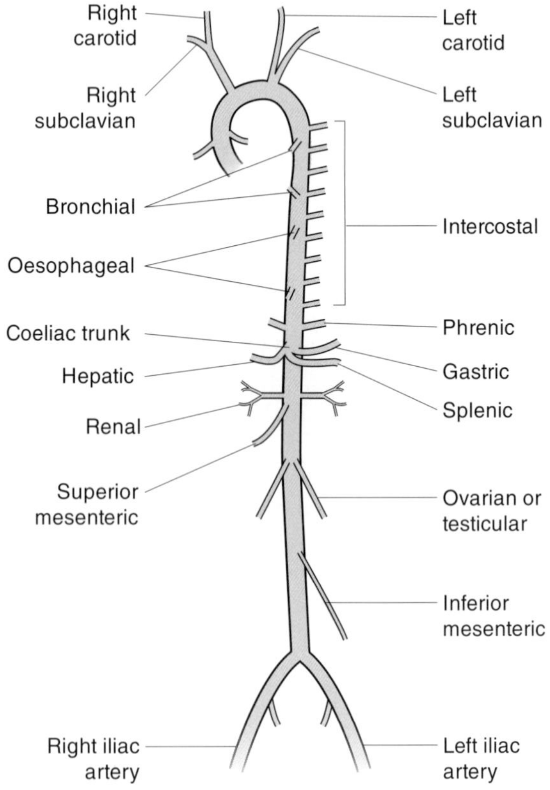

Figure 25.14 The aorta and its branches

Veins

There are two groups of veins: superficial veins (some of which can be seen as bluish lines under the skin) and deep veins (which run beside arteries and often have the same name as the arteries). Veins rely on the squeezing action of skeletal muscles to assist in pushing blood towards the heart, and on respiratory movements, which have a milking effect on the inferior vena cava as it passes through the diaphragm (Carlson 2018).

Pulmonary circulation

The pulmonary circulation (Figure 25.15) involves the transport of deoxygenated blood from the heart to the lungs and the return of oxygenated blood from the lungs to the heart (Carlson 2018). The pulmonary artery leaves the right ventricle and divides into the right and left pulmonary arteries, which carry deoxygenated blood to the lungs. In the lungs, the arteries divide until capillaries are formed (Carlson 2018). Venules collect the oxygenated blood from the capillaries and unite to form the two pulmonary veins, which leave each lung and enter the left atrium of the heart.

Hepatic–portal circulation

The hepatic–portal circulation (Figure 25.16) is a subdivision of the systematic circulation. It is responsible for carrying blood that is deoxygenated, but rich in digested nutrients, from some of the abdominal organs to the liver (Carlson 2018).

The splenic, gastric, inferior and superior mesenteric veins unite to form a large vein called the portal vein, which enters the liver. The liver converts the nutrients brought by the blood into a form to be either used by tissues throughout the body or stored for future use. The liver thus receives blood from two sources: the hepatic artery (which supplies it with oxygenated blood) and the portal vein (carrying deoxygenated blood rich in nutrients). When the oxygen has been extracted from the former and the nutrients from the latter have been processed, the blood leaves via the three hepatic veins (Carlson 2018).

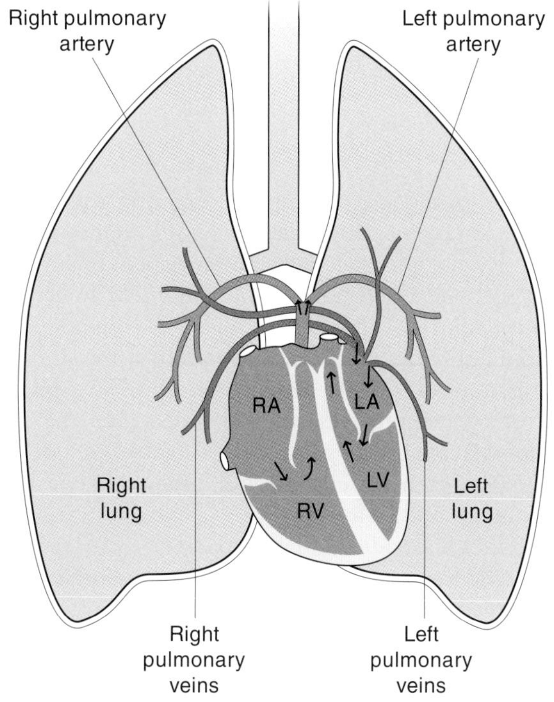

Figure 25.15 Pulmonary circulation

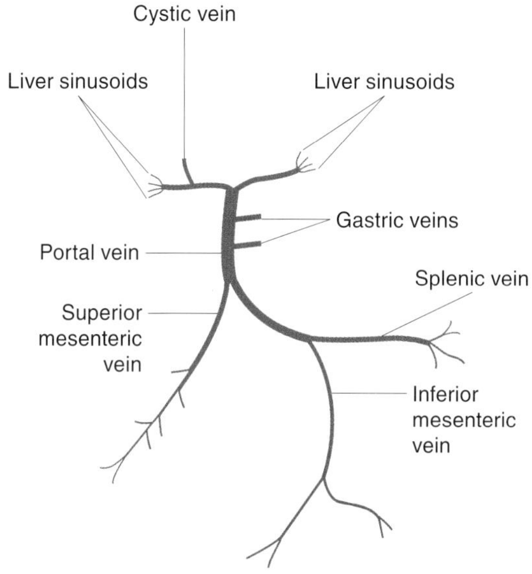

Figure 25.16 Hepatic–portal circulation

STRUCTURE OF THE LYMPHATIC SYSTEM

The lymphatic system (Figure 25.17) is closely connected with the circulation of blood and consists of an additional set of vessels through which some of the tissue fluid passes before reaching the large veins and entering the blood. Circulation within the lymphatic system is dependent upon the movement of skeletal muscles. Muscular contraction and pressure changes within the thoracic cavity during respiration assist with lymph (Carlson 2018). This system consists of lymphatic capillaries, lymphatic vessels, lymphatic nodes and lymphatic ducts. The fluid in the system is called lymph.

The lymphatics serve an important function in preventing oedema since the tiny vessels collect fluid and proteins from the interstitial spaces and promote their return to the blood circulation. They also collect the larger digested fat particles from the digestive system and empty them into the circulation. In addition, the lymphatics play a key role in the body's defence against microorganisms. They collect microorganisms in the interstitial spaces and carry them to the lymph nodes, where the lymphocytes (and macrophages) remove them from the lymph (Carlson 2018).

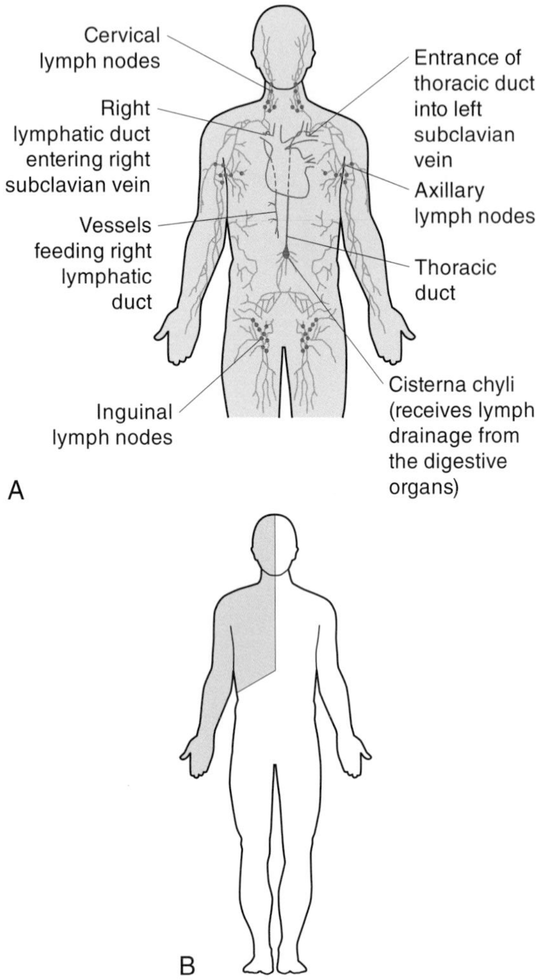

Figure 25.17 The lymphatic system

A: The distribution of lymphatic vessels and nodes, **B:** Areas drained by the right lymphatic duct (shaded) and the thoracic duct (unshaded).

Lymph

When fluid leaks out of the capillaries from the cardiovascular system, it accumulates in the tissue spaces. When this fluid is drained from the tissues and collected by the lymphatic system, it is called **lymph** and has a composition similar to the blood plasma. Lymph is normally a colourless fluid, although lymph absorbed from the intestines is saturated with fats and is milky in colour. Lymph travels slowly through the lymphatic system—approximately 2–3 litres of fluid is picked up by the lymphatic channels each day (Carlson 2018).

Lymphatic capillaries

Lymphatic capillaries are similar in size and structure to blood capillaries. They unite to form larger lymphatic vessels similar in structure to veins and, like veins, they have valves to prevent a backward flow of lymph. All lymphatic vessels pass through one or more lymph nodes. Afferent lymphatic vessels carry lymph to a node. Efferent lymphatic vessels carry lymph away from the node and empty it into the lymphatic ducts (Carlson 2018).

Lymph nodes

Lymph nodes are found mainly in groups in many parts of the body, such as the neck, thorax, abdomen, groin and the limbs. Lymphatic nodes vary in size and consist of lymphatic tissue. The functions of lymphatic nodes are to filter and destroy bacteria from the lymph passing through the node; to produce lymphocytes, which are added to the lymph; and to produce antibodies and antitoxins (Carlson 2018).

Other areas containing lymphatic tissue

In addition to the nodes already described, lymphatic tissue is found in several other anatomical structures, including the tonsils in the oropharynx, adenoids in the nasopharynx, the appendix attached to the intestines, the thymus gland in the thorax, Peyer's patches in the small intestine and the spleen in the abdomen.

Tonsils

The tonsils form part of a protective ring of tissue at the entrance to the respiratory and digestive tracts. Lymphatic vessels leave the tonsils and enter the cervical nodes (Carlson 2018).

Thymus gland

The thymus gland is a soft grey-pink gland present in the thorax behind the sternum and in front of the heart. It is large in infants and children, reaching its maximum size at puberty. After puberty this gland gradually shrinks, until in adulthood there is only a small piece of tissue left. The thymus gland functions in the production of lymphocytes (Carlson 2018).

Spleen

The spleen is the largest lymphoid organ in the body and plays a complementary role to lymph nodes (Carlson 2018). It is a purplish half-moon-shaped organ in the left hypochondriac region of the abdomen. It lies below the diaphragm and behind the lower ribs and is mainly composed of lymphoid tissue enclosed in a fibrous capsule. The functions of the spleen are to:

- Produce lymphocytes, some of which enter the bloodstream to carry out their phagocytic action.
- Destroy worn-out erythrocytes, producing bile pigments and iron.
- Produce antibodies and antitoxins.
- Provide a storage area for erythrocytes needed in emergency situations (if haemorrhage occurs, the spleen vessels contract and empty blood into the circulation in an attempt to restore normal blood volume).

(Carlson 2018)

Lymphatic ducts

The two lymphatic ducts receive the lymph from lymphatic vessels and empty it into the bloodstream via the subclavian vein (Figure 25.17). They are the thoracic duct and the right lymphatic duct.

Thoracic duct

The thoracic duct, the larger of the two lymphatic ducts, begins in the abdominal cavity at lumbar level as a dilated sac called the cisterna chyli. The duct passes upwards through the aortic opening behind the diaphragm into the thorax, where it empties its contents into the left subclavian vein so that the lymph rejoins the bloodstream. Lymphatic vessels from all parts of the body below the diaphragm, and the left side of the body above the diaphragm, empty their contents into the thoracic duct.

Right lymphatic duct

The right lymphatic duct is very small (about 1 cm long) and lies in the root of the neck. It receives lymph from the right side of the head and neck, the right side of the thorax and the right upper limb. The right lymphatic duct empties its contents into the right subclavian vein.

FACTORS AFFECTING THE RESPIRATORY SYSTEM

Oxygen concentration

Oxygen makes up approximately 21% of the air, which is normally sufficient to meet the needs of the body. A decrease in this amount of oxygen can cause problems. Two instances in which the available oxygen may be deficient are:

- High altitude: The total pressure of all gases in the air decreases as altitude increases. As the total pressure decreases, the oxygen pressure decreases proportionately, and the individual will experience difficulty in maintaining adequate tissue oxygenation (hypoxia). Acclimatising is a homeostatic response where initially the ventilatory rate is increased in an attempt to supply the body with sufficient oxygen, then later the bone marrow is stimulated to increase erythrocyte production (polycythaemia) to carry more oxygen.
- Presence of noxious gases: Some noxious gases, such as carbon monoxide, have a higher affinity for haemoglobin than does oxygen, which is displaced by them, causing a reduction in oxygen availability to tissues.

(AACN & Hartjes 2022)

Regulating mechanisms

Any factor that interferes with the respiratory centres in the brainstem or the nerves that transmit messages to and from them may cause ventilatory difficulties. Respiratory depression can be caused by increased intracranial pressure such as cerebral oedema, due to conditions such as hypercapnia, cerebral bleeds, meningitis, encephalitis, hydrocephalus, tumours, hypoalbuminaemia and ketoacidosis (AACN & Hartjes 2022). Clinical Interest Box 25.1 discusses the effect pyrexia (fever) has on oxygen regulation mechanisms. Other factors include certain medications such as analgesics (e.g. morphine), and various anticonvulsant drugs (e.g. clonazepam). Ventilation increases when the pH of the blood is lowered (a respiratory response to rid the body of the excess acid), whereas ventilation decreases when the pH increases (to retain acid) (AACN & Hartjes 2022). (Respiratory alkalosis and respiratory acidosis are described in Table 25.3.)

Exchange of gases during ventilation and respiration

The efficiency of ventilation and respiration can be affected by any factor that interferes with the patency of the respiratory tract or the actions of the ventilatory muscles. For example, an accumulation of secretions may result from respiratory conditions such as asthma, bronchitis or a reduced cough reflex (AACN & Hartjes 2022). Ventilations may also be reduced by factors that affect the actions of the ventilatory muscles, such as brainstem or spinal cord injury or motor neuron diseases such as multiple sclerosis or Guillain–Barré syndrome (AACN & Hartjes 2022). These conditions can restrict the movements of the diaphragm and/or intercostal muscles. Chest expansion and ventilation can also be affected by deformities of the chest wall or skeleton, such as scoliosis,

CLINICAL INTEREST BOX 25.1 Oxygen requirements and pyrexia

Pyrexia, or fever, can significantly influence oxygen requirements in individuals with respiratory conditions. When respiratory conditions are already present, such as chronic obstructive pulmonary disease (COPD), asthma or pneumonia, the body's ability to efficiently exchange oxygen and carbon dioxide may be compromised. During pyrexia, the increased metabolic demands for oxygen due to fever can exacerbate the challenges faced by these individuals. Respiratory conditions often involve reduced lung function, impaired gas exchange, and limited lung capacity. As a result, the combination of fever-induced higher oxygen demands and compromised lung function can lead to inadequate oxygenation of the blood and tissues. This scenario might necessitate careful monitoring and, in some cases, supplemental oxygen therapy to ensure that the body receives sufficient oxygen to support both the fever's immune response and the ongoing respiratory challenges. Healthcare professionals need to assess each individual's specific condition and oxygen saturation levels to determine the appropriate intervention in managing pyrexia in the context of respiratory conditions.

flail chest (multiple rib fractures causing instability in part of the chest wall and paradoxical breathing movements, the part of the lung underlying the injured area contracts on inspiration and bulges on expiration) and pectus excavatum (a skeletal abnormality of the chest that is characterised by a depressed sternum) (AACN & Hartjes 2022).

Diffusion of oxygen and CO_2

Any dysfunction of the lungs that affects the alveolar capillary membrane thickness or causes a reduction in their surface area will affect respiratory function. Conditions such as pulmonary oedema, alveolitis, pneumonia or chronic obstructive airways disease may reduce the diffusion of oxygen and CO_2. Information on these and other respiratory disorders is provided later in this chapter.

Transport of oxygen and CO_2 to and from the cells

Any condition affecting the efficiency of the heart, blood vessels or blood can interfere with the transportation of oxygen to the cells or CO_2 away from the cells. Such conditions include congestive cardiac failure, atherosclerosis, carbon monoxide poisoning and anaemia. Information on these and other cardiovascular disorders is provided later in this chapter.

Influences on the rate, depth and rhythm of breathing

Several factors influence the characteristics of breathing, such as pyrexia and physical activity. Oxygen requirements are greatest during exertion and least during sleep. The rate and depth of ventilations vary in response to the body's production of CO_2. For example, during strenuous exercise the volume of air drawn into the lungs with each breath may be increased from a normal tidal volume of 500 mL to as much as 2300 mL. Changes in mood, emotion and pain may also affect the rate, depth and rhythm of ventilation. For example, the ventilation rate is commonly increased during fear, anxiety or apprehension. Chronic irritation by inhaled irritants such as smoke or dust can also affect breathing and cause short-term effects such as coughing and shortness of breath, or long-term effects such as severe dyspnoea resulting from emphysema (AACN & Hartjes 2022).

Inadequate ventilation (hypoventilation)

Hypoventilation and alveolar hypoventilation is a reduction in the ventilation of the alveoli (AACN & Hartjes 2022). The causes are many and varied and include airway obstruction by oedema, inhaled foreign bodies, retained secretions (mucus, casts), polyps, tumours, bronchospasm, emphysema, neuromuscular or skeletal abnormalities and central nervous system disorders (AACN & Hartjes 2022). Hypoventilation occurs when the volume of air entering the alveoli is not adequate for the metabolic needs of the body. The reduction in ventilation causes an increase in the partial pressure of CO_2 in arterial blood ($PaCO_2$), termed **hypercapnia**, and may also cause **hypoxaemia**, a decrease in the partial pressure of oxygen in arterial blood (PaO_2).

Impaired diffusion

Diffusion is the process by which oxygen and CO_2 molecules are transported between the alveoli and the capillary network. Diffusion abnormalities can interfere with the passage of oxygen into the blood (AACN & Hartjes 2022). Such diffusion abnormalities can result from a thickening of the alveoli capillary walls (e.g. in pulmonary oedema), a reduced amount of functioning lung tissue (such as in emphysema) or fibrosis of the alveolar walls (as seen in alveolitis and pneumonitis) (AACN & Hartjes 2022).

Impaired perfusion

Not only is an adequate intake of oxygen by ventilation essential, but for oxygenation of the body tissues to occur, adequate perfusion of lung tissue with blood is essential. Any condition that decreases the circulation of blood to lung tissue may lead to ventilation–perfusion mismatches (V/Q principle) and hypoxaemia (AACN & Hartjes 2022). Such conditions include decreased blood volume, pulmonary embolism, cardiac disorders and chronic obstructive pulmonary disease (AACN & Hartjes 2022).

In addition to abnormalities of the lungs or respiratory structures, dysfunction of other body systems can adversely affect respiratory function. For example, a disease process that affects the nervous system may adversely affect respirations. When the spinal cord is damaged, the nervous system may greatly impair respiratory function. Cardiovascular dysfunction can affect respiratory function (e.g. right-sided heart failure may affect the volume of pulmonary blood circulation). A deformity of the skeletal system, such as scoliosis, may restrict movement of the thoracic cage and thus alter respiratory function. Inadequate lung expansion can also occur after abdominal surgery, as pain in the operation site may inhibit deep breathing and coughing. Not only can abnormalities of other body systems adversely affect the respiratory system, but respiratory abnormalities generally affect all other body systems.

Additional factors

Numerous other factors can modify the rate and depth of ventilation. For example, involuntary and reflex mechanisms such as exercise, pain, hiccupping, sneezing, sighing and emotions, and conscious voluntary actions such as voluntary breath holding, inhalation and exhalation. Clinical Interest Box 25.2 discusses the alteration to respirations in the older adult. Other factors that affect functioning include:

- digestive system disorders and diminished appetite, potentiating an alteration in nutritional status
- changes in renal function, which can affect erythropoietin production

CLINICAL INTEREST BOX 25.2
Respirations and the older individual

In the older population, respiratory changes become more pronounced as a result of the natural ageing process. These changes encompass a reduced lung elasticity due to the gradual loss of tissue flexibility, coupled with calcification of costal cartilage and the development of kyphosis, affecting the chest wall's ability to expand fully. Skeletal muscle fibres also experience weakening and depletion, compromising the efficiency of respiratory muscle function. Furthermore, alterations in cilia density and beating velocity, along with the thickening of alveolar membranes, collectively contribute to a decline in the respiratory system's overall ventilatory capacity. Consequently, the exchange of oxygen and carbon dioxide becomes less efficient, necessitating a higher resting respiratory rate in older individuals, as the body strives to maintain optimal oxygen levels and eliminate waste gases.

(Boltz 2021)

- osteoporosis
- circulatory disorders.

These may all combine to affect blood cell production, with subsequent anaemias. In individuals who are more sedentary, such combinations of factors and subsequent alveolar hypoventilation increase the risk of primary or secondary infections. To avoid the complications of ageing, all individuals can be educated to:

- Improve their nutritional status, including nutrients and supplementation of additional sources of vitamins as required.
- Increase their fluid intake, as permitted.
- Perform routine breathing exercises.
- Maintain their weight-bearing ability.
- Increase their exercise and mobilisation.

(AACN & Hartjes 2022)

PATHOPHYSIOLOGY RELATED TO THE RESPIRATORY SYSTEM

The signs and symptoms manifested by an individual with a respiratory disorder vary with the location and severity of the disorder. Detailed below are some common clinical features of respiratory disease.

Chest pain

Disorders of the respiratory system such as pleurisy can result in chest pain. During ventilation, friction occurs between the inflamed pleura. Chest pain may be localised or may be experienced only when the individual breathes deeply, and can vary from a continuous aching pain to a stabbing knife-like pain (Valchanov et al 2019). Pain associated with respiratory disorders may be retrosternal, lateral or posterior and is exacerbated by deep inhalation.

Cough

A cough is a common symptom of many respiratory disorders and may result from irritation or from retained secretions that obstruct some part of the airway (Valchanov et al 2019). If sputum is swallowed, expectorated or the cough sounds moist, it is described as productive. A non-productive, or dry, cough is one that sounds dry or irritating and no sputum is expectorated or swallowed. Sputum is the result of excessive mucus production and may result from inflammation, infection or congestion.

Haemoptysis (the coughing or expectoration of blood) may occur in some lung diseases. Blood-streaked sputum frequently occurs in some respiratory tract conditions, such as infections (e.g. bronchitis, tuberculosis), pulmonary oedema or bronchogenic carcinoma. The expectoration of bright red or frothy blood indicates a more serious disorder, such as pulmonary embolism or lung abscess.

Voice changes, ranging from hoarseness to aphonia (no speech), may result from numerous causes, including viral upper respiratory tract infections (e.g. laryngitis), vocal cord polyps and laryngeal tumour. Unilateral or bilateral vocal cord paralysis may also result from congenital defects, intubation or other damage to the recurrent nerve (e.g. after thyroid or cardiac surgery).

Dyspnoea (difficult or laboured breathing) may result from disorders affecting either the upper or the lower respiratory tract or surrounding structures. Disorders of the upper respiratory tract that may cause dyspnoea include obstruction of the airway by inflammation, a tumour or foreign body. Disorders of the lower respiratory tract that cause dyspnoea include airway inflammations or infections, asthma, pneumonia, pneumonitis, carcinoma of the lung and chronic obstructive pulmonary disease. Any disorder affecting the thorax, such as trauma to the chest wall, commonly causes dyspnoea. Laboured breathing may be accompanied by nasal flaring, the use of the neck and accessory chest muscles and increased ventilation rate (Valchanov et al 2019).

Changes in breathing patterns and sounds

Any disorder that affects the respiratory system may produce changes in the pattern of breathing. Examples include **tachypnoea** (increased respiratory rate), **bradypnoea** (decreased respiratory rate) and airway obstruction. For example, due to emphysema, which can result in prolonged forceful **expiration** and pursed-lip breathing (Valchanov et al 2019). Certain disorders also result in abnormal breathing sounds, such as wheezing or 'grunting' ventilations. Information on abnormal breathing sounds is provided later in this chapter.

Hypoxia

Hypoxia is a deficiency of oxygen in the tissues and may be due to lung disorders that prevent adequate supplies of

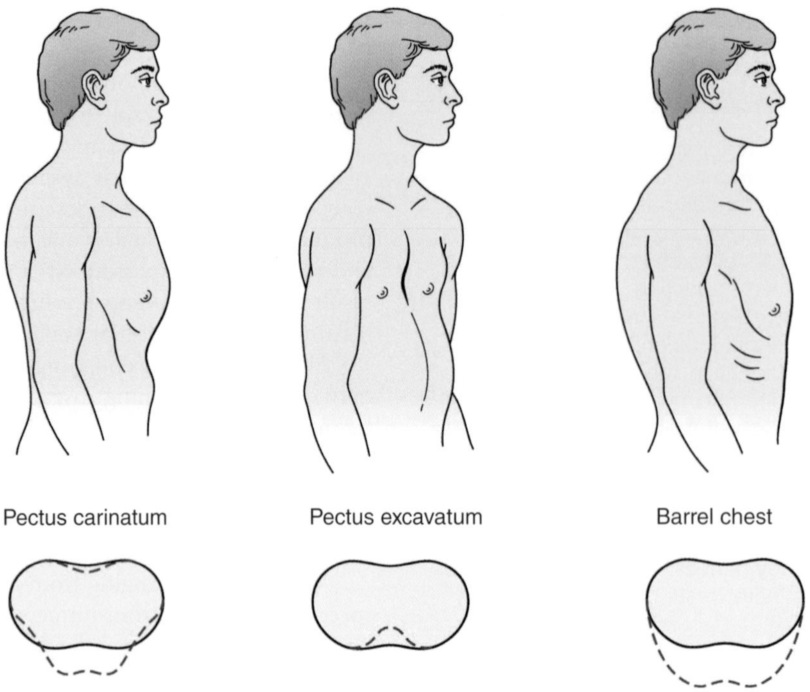

Figure 25.18 Chest deformities

(Magee 2014)

oxygen from reaching the blood (hypoxaemia). Hypoxia may also be due to hypoventilation, anaemia or impaired tissue utilisation of oxygen. The initial manifestations of hypoxia include tachycardia, tachypnoea, breathlessness, pallor, lethargy or agitation, followed by increasing confusion and deepening cyanosis (AACN & Hartjes 2022).

Thoracic abnormalities

Chest deformities refer to irregular or unusual shapes or configurations of the chest area (Figure 25.18) (Dover 2023). These deviations from the normal chest structure can be caused by various factors, including genetic conditions, developmental issues, trauma or medical procedures.

For example, a common chest deformity is pectus excavatum, where the breastbone (sternum) and rib cage are sunken into the chest, creating a concave or 'caved-in' appearance. On the other hand, pectus carinatum is a chest deformity characterised by the protrusion of the breastbone and ribs, leading to a 'pigeon chest' appearance (Dover 2023).

Chest deformities can sometimes be purely cosmetic, while in other cases, they might impact breathing, cardiovascular function, or overall physical health. Depending on the severity of the deformity and any associated complications, medical intervention may be considered.

Other manifestations

Depending on the type and severity of the disorder, other manifestations may be evident. For example, infections of the respiratory tract generally result in pyrexia, headaches, aching muscles and lethargy. Difficulty in swallowing (dysphagia) may be present in disorders such as pharyngitis and tonsillitis. In certain chronic disorders of the respiratory system, clubbing of the fingers (Figure 25.19) may be evident (AACN & Hartjes 2022). The distal portions of the fingers are abnormally enlarged by anastomosis of blood vessels in response to peripheral hypoxaemia. The nails have an increased curvature and the angle of the nail bed increases to over 85 degrees.

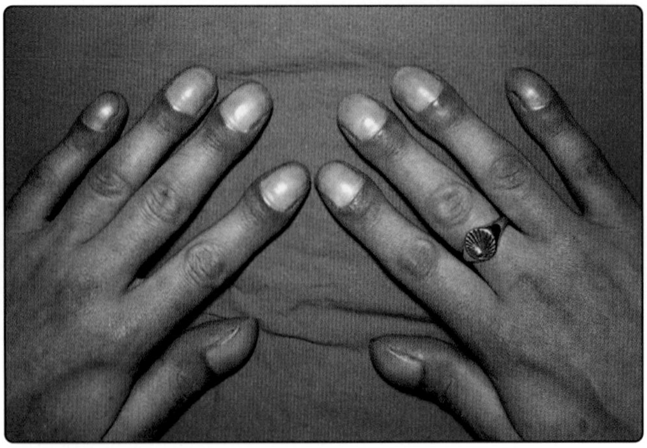

Figure 25.19 Clubbing in a patient with cyanotic congenital heart disease and secondary polycythaemia

(Haematology: An Illustrated Colour Text Fourth Edition © 2013 Elsevier Ltd)

SPECIFIC DISORDERS OF THE RESPIRATORY SYSTEM

Disorders of multiple cause

Certain disorders of the respiratory system have more than one cause and may be related to structural or functional changes, environmental conditions or a combination of factors. It is beyond the scope of this text to provide in-depth information on the various conditions related to the respiratory system. Listed below are some examples of respiratory conditions:

- rhinitis
- pleurisy
- epistaxis
- sarcoidosis
- pneumoconioses
- laryngeal oedema
- adult respiratory distress syndrome.

(AACN & Hartjes 2022)

Infectious disorders

Infectious disorders can be classed as upper or lower respiratory tract infections. Bacteria or viruses cause infections of the upper respiratory tract while a variety of microorganisms can cause lower respiratory tract infections. For more information, review the references and further reading list at the end of this chapter.

Clinical Interest Box 25.3 looks at the highly contagious viral infection COVID-19. Listed below are some examples of respiratory conditions:

- sinusitis
- influenza
- pharyngitis
- tonsillitis
- quinsy
- laryngitis
- epiglottitis
- acute bronchitis
- pneumonia
- pertussis
- croup
- tuberculosis
- empyema.

(AACN & Hartjes 2022)

CLINICAL INTEREST BOX 25.3 Severe acute respiratory syndrome (SARS)

COVID-19, caused by the novel coronavirus SARS-CoV-2, emerged as a global pandemic in late 2019, profoundly impacting every facet of human life. Characterised by its highly contagious nature, the virus spread swiftly across the world, prompting unprecedented health and socioeconomic challenges. COVID-19 primarily affects the respiratory system, often leading to symptoms ranging from mild respiratory discomfort to severe pneumonia and acute respiratory distress syndrome. The pandemic prompted widespread adoption of preventative measures, such as mask-wearing, social distancing, and lockdowns, to mitigate the virus's transmission. Governments and healthcare systems worldwide have worked tirelessly to manage healthcare resources, conduct mass testing and facilitate vaccination campaigns to curb the pandemic's impact. The COVID-19 crisis underscored the importance of global collaboration, scientific innovation, and resilience in the face of adversity, prompting a re-evaluation of public health preparedness and international cooperation for future challenges. The World Health Organization has played a central role in providing global leadership, coordination, and evidence-based guidance to navigate the challenges posed by the pandemic.

(WHO 2020)

Obstructive disorders

Obstructive disorders are lung diseases that cause a persistent obstruction of bronchial airflow (AACN & Hartjes 2022). Airway obstruction can also be due to the inhalation of a foreign body, or one or both bronchi may become obstructed by a benign or malignant tumour. Some of the more common types of airway obstruction are grouped under the term chronic obstructive pulmonary disease (COPD) or chronic obstructive airways disease (COAD) (see Nursing Care Plan 25.1). Common forms of COAD include asthma, emphysema, bronchiectasis and chronic bronchitis (AACN & Hartjes 2022). Asthma and emphysema are discussed briefly here.

Asthma

Asthma is a chronic, inflammatory disorder of the airways affecting between 1% and 29% of the population (GINA 2023). The physiology of asthma involves a complex interplay of factors. In response to triggers such as allergens, irritants, infections or exercise, the airway walls become inflamed, causing them to swell and produce excess mucus. This inflammation leads to increased sensitivity and responsiveness of the airways, making them prone to constrict and narrow in response to various stimuli. Smooth muscles surrounding the airways can contract excessively, further contributing to airway narrowing. This combination of inflammation, mucus production and muscle constriction restricts airflow, making it difficult for individuals with asthma to breathe properly (GINA 2023). (See Case Study 25.1.)

Exacerbations of asthma (commonly referred to as asthma attacks) are manifested by difficulty in breathing caused by generalised narrowing of the airways, which is characterised by wheeze, shortness of breath, chest tightness and/or cough and variable limitations in expiratory flow (GINA 2023). Exacerbations of asthma can occur as a

NURSING CARE PLAN 25.1

Assessment: Chronic obstructive pulmonary disease (COPD).
Issue/s to be addressed: Deficient knowledge on condition, treatment plan and self-management.
Goal/s: Provide information about disease process/prognosis and treatment regimen.

Care/actions	Rationale
Explain the disease process to the individual.	Decreases anxiety and can lead to improved uptake of treatment plan.
Instruct and demonstrate rationale for deep-breathing and coughing exercises.	Pursed-lip and abdominal or diaphragmatic breathing exercises strengthen muscles of respiration, help minimise collapse of small airways, and provide the individual with means to control dyspnoea.
Discuss importance of avoiding people with active respiratory infection.	Decreases exposure to and incidence of acquired acute URIs.
Discuss individual factors that may trigger or aggravate condition (excessively dry air, wind, environmental temperature extremes, pollen, tobacco smoke, aerosol sprays, air pollution).	Environmental factors can induce or aggravate bronchial irritation, leading to increased secretion production and airway blockage.
Review the harmful effects of smoking, and advise cessation of smoking.	Cessation of smoking may slow or halt progression of disease.

Evaluation:
Increased knowledge and understanding of condition.
Adherence to treatment plan.
Ability to self-manage condition.

CASE STUDY 25.1

Daniel, aged 16, is admitted to the hospital via the emergency department with an acute exacerbation of asthma. He has called for assistance and is complaining of a persistent cough, wheezing and chest tightness. He appears breathless, and his lips have a bluish tint. His last nebuliser treatment was 30 minutes ago.

1. What are the symptoms of asthma?
2. What assessments will you need to undertake?
3. What nursing measures will you implement?

first-time presentation or occur in individuals with a pre-existing diagnosis.

The long-term goal of asthma management is to achieve good control of symptoms, allowing the individual to maintain their normal level of activity, and to minimise the risk of asthma-related death, exacerbations of asthma and side effects (GINA 2023).

It is important to be aware that severe exacerbations of asthma are potentially life-threatening and the treatment requires close monitoring and careful assessment. An example of an entry in progress notes for an individual with breathing difficulties is shown in Progress Note 25.1.

Emphysema

Emphysema (pulmonary) is a chronically progressive disease characterised by over-distension and destruction of alveolar walls, resulting in a loss of lung elasticity and surface area for diffusion. The predisposing causes are the same as those for chronic bronchitis, with cigarette smoking being the major factor (Pahal et al 2023). Initially, the peripheral bronchioles become inflamed and the subsequent narrowing of the airways traps air in the alveoli. As the disease progresses, the alveolar walls become over-inflated and rupture. Because of loss of lung elasticity, the terminal bronchioles tend to collapse prematurely during exhalation, making expulsion of air from the lungs more difficult (AACN & Hartjes 2022).

Symptoms of chronic emphysema include shortness of breath, dyspnoea, cyanosis, cough, fatigue and barrel-shaped chest, from expansion of the rib cage to accommodate enlarged lungs and cyanosis due to lack of oxygen (AACN & Hartjes 2022). The individual will commonly exhale through pursed lips to prolong expiration and reduce the tendency of the airways to collapse. As the disease becomes more severe, the individual may use their accessory muscles to breathe (AACN & Hartjes 2022). The anteroposterior width of the chest usually increases because of expansion of the chest wall and loss of lung elasticity, giving the chest a barrel-shaped appearance. Distension of the neck veins may be present, as may clubbing of the fingers (AACN & Hartjes 2022). In advanced emphysema, the person fights for every breath of air.

Neoplastic disorders

Benign or *malignant* neoplasms may affect the upper or lower respiratory tract. Tumours can affect the normal functioning of the respiratory tract and, if malignant, can cause extensive tissue damage by infiltration (AACN & Hartjes 2022). The signs and symptoms of neoplastic disease vary depending on the location and extent of the lesion.

Nasal polyps are masses of hypertrophied mucosa that commonly form in response to recurrent swelling of the nasal mucosa. Obstruction of the nasal passages develops gradually as the benign polyps multiply and enlarge. The individual experiences difficulty in breathing through the nose, and the voice may have a nasal quality.

Laryngeal polyps are growths that arise from the mucous membrane of the vocal cords. The major symptom is hoarseness. Laryngeal polyps are usually benign but they may become malignant.

Laryngeal carcinoma is a malignant neoplasm arising from or around the vocal cords. Persistent hoarseness is the major symptom, and heavy cigarette smoking is believed to be a major causative factor. If the lesion is large, dysphagia may be present.

Lung cancer commonly affects a bronchus. It arises from the bronchial epithelium and rapidly invades lung tissue, causing parts of the lung to collapse. It may spread through the lymphatic network and bloodstream to form metastases in other parts of the body, such as the liver, bones or brain. The incidence of lung cancer is related to several factors, the most important being the inhalation of cigarette smoke. Other factors include exposure to atmospheric pollution and occupational pollutants.

Unfortunately, the physical manifestations of lung cancer do not generally appear until the disease is well advanced. Symptoms include persistent cough, dyspnoea, purulent or blood-streaked sputum, chest pain and repeated attacks of bronchitis or pneumonia (AACN & Hartjes 2022). Sometimes the initial symptoms are associated with organs that are the sites of metastasis, such as the liver, bones or brain. Cancer of the lung may also occur secondary to a primary malignant tumour elsewhere in the body, as a result of metastasis (AACN & Hartjes 2022).

Traumatic disorders

Injury to part of the respiratory tract can result from a variety of causes.

Laryngotracheal trauma

Laryngotracheal trauma can be minor and cause hoarseness and some dysphagia, or it may be severe, as a result of laryngeal or cricoid fracture. In a severe injury, oedema of the larynx may occur and be accompanied by signs of respiratory distress (AACN & Hartjes 2022).

Flail chest

Flail chest occurs when multiple rib fractures result in 'floating' of a segment of the rib cage. As a consequence, there may be instability in part of the chest wall and paradoxical breathing. Paradoxical breathing is characterised by the injured chest wall collapsing in during inhalation, and moving out during exhalation. The lung underlying the injury contracts on inhalation and bulges on exhalation. If uncorrected, ventilation is impaired, which may lead to hypoxia and respiratory failure. Manifestations of a flail chest are paradoxical motion of the chest wall during breathing, severe pain, dyspnoea, tachycardia and cyanosis (AACN & Hartjes 2022).

Pneumothorax

Pneumothorax is an accumulation of air in the pleural space (between the visceral and parietal pleura of the chest cavity) causing the lung on the side of the injury to collapse (Sajadi-Ernazarova et al 2022). A pneumothorax may be open or closed. In an open pneumothorax, an injury creates an opening in the chest wall, allowing air to flow into the pleural cavity. In a closed, or spontaneous, pneumothorax, the chest wall is intact and air enters the pleural space from an opening on the surface of the lung.

Depending on the severity, a pneumothorax may cause severe dyspnoea, hypoxaemia, tachypnoea and associated pain, along with ipsilateral diminished chest expansion and breath sounds. There may be subcutaneous emphysema in the neck and upper chest, and a 'sucking' sound may be heard in the region of an open pneumothorax. Tracheal deviation to the contralateral side may be observed in severe cases in some individuals (Sajadi-Ernazarova et al 2022).

Tension pneumothorax is a particularly severe form that occurs when air escapes into the pleural cavity. As a result, continuously increasing air pressure in the pleural cavity causes progressive collapse of the lung tissue. Emergency aspiration of air from the pleural cavity is necessary. In addition to chest pain and severe shortness of breath, the presence of hypoxia and hypotension suggests the presence of a tension pneumothorax (Sajadi-Ernazarova et al 2022).

CRITICAL THINKING EXERCISE 25.1

A 25-year-old male is brought into the emergency department by ambulance following a motor vehicle accident. The paramedic reports that the male's oxygen saturation levels are currently within normal limits, but they have been decreasing, and he is experiencing increasing difficulty in breathing. Upon assessment, you observe that he has an elevated respiratory rate, unusual breathing patterns, shortness of breath and reports chest tightness. What nursing procedures would you implement to alleviate his respiratory distress?

Haemothorax

Haemothorax is the accumulation of blood in the pleural space and frequently occurs as a result of trauma or acute surgery. A haemopneumothorax is a collection of air and blood in the pleural cavity. Manifestations include dyspnoea and chest tightness, and may include signs of hypovolaemia if bleeding continues. Complications can lead to shock from haemorrhage and severe pain, or respiratory failure. Management consists of observation to surgical intervention (Smith et al 2020).

FACTORS AFFECTING THE CARDIOVASCULAR SYSTEM

Changes in cardiac function

Cardiac failure occurs when the heart is unable to maintain an output of blood sufficient to meet the body's requirements and, as a result, the body tissues may become ischaemic.

Cardiac failure may result from mechanical failure due to disease of valves, obstruction to the blood flow, congenital heart disease, arteriosclerosis or hypertension. Cardiac failure can also occur as a consequence of a disease process, such as cardiomyopathy or myocardial infarction, or as the result of normal ageing. Consequently, the heart's ability to pump blood may be diminished.

When the heart fails to meet the requirements of the body, compensatory mechanisms occur in an attempt to improve cardiac output and to maintain the blood pressure. Compensatory responses include the sympathetic response, the renal response and myocardial hypertrophy. The sympathetic response is stimulated by reduced cardiac output and results in increased heart rate, dilation of the coronary and cerebral arterioles and constriction of the renal and skin arterioles. As a result, essential life functions are maintained. The renal response results in the secretion of substances that stimulate the production of aldosterone, causing vasoconstriction and retention of sodium and water. This response causes an increase in blood volume and peripheral resistance, which increases the workload of the heart.

Myocardial hypertrophy results from prolonged increase in myocardial wall tension and, while this initially maintains cardiac output, eventually cardiac output and tissue perfusion are decreased (NHFA CSANZ Heart Failure Guidelines Working Group 2018).

Changes in the blood vessels

Disturbances in the ability of the arteries to stretch and recoil as blood is pumped from the heart, or changes in the ability of the veins to return the blood to the heart, result in ischaemia of the tissues. The ability of arteries to stretch and recoil may be affected by conditions such as arteriosclerosis, obstruction from inflammation or arterial spasms or from excessive external pressure on an artery (Parrillo & Dellinger 2019). When an artery is narrowed or constricted, it is unable to transport sufficient blood to the area it supplies, resulting in ischaemia and possible tissue death (necrosis).

The ability of veins to return blood to the heart may be affected by impaired valves, a sedentary lifestyle, reduced skeletal muscle usage that normally assists venous flow or from excessive external pressure on a vein. When blood flow through a vein is impeded, pooling of blood in the vein occurs. The hydrostatic pressure inside the vein increases and causes oedema in the surrounding tissues (Parrillo & Dellinger 2019). Chronic venous insufficiency can result in thrombophlebitis, stasis cellulitis and stasis ulcers.

The formation of an embolus can cause obstruction of an artery or a vein (Parrillo & Dellinger 2019). The most common embolus is a blood clot (thrombus), although an embolus can also consist of air or fat or foreign bodies. When the thrombus, or part of it, becomes dislodged from the vessel wall it travels in the bloodstream until it reaches a blood vessel that is too narrow for its passage. As a result, blood flow beyond that area is obstructed, and the ultimate consequence may be death of the tissues deprived of adequate oxygen and nutrition (Parrillo & Dellinger 2019).

Changes in the blood

Haemoglobin in the erythrocytes is responsible for transporting oxygen in the bloodstream. Any condition that affects the normal production or function of erythrocytes may decrease the supply of oxygen to the tissues. Conditions that may impede erythrocyte formation or their ability to carry oxygen include smoking, bone marrow aplasia, metabolic abnormalities, nutritional deficiencies, chronic or acute blood loss, drugs, living at high altitudes, flying, toxins, ionising radiation and genetic abnormalities. Tissue hypoxia results in a compensatory increased production of erythrocytes (polycythaemia), which causes the blood to become viscous and increases the risk of thrombi formation.

Leucocytes protect the body from infection through phagocytosis and the production of antibodies. Any disorder that decreases the production or maturation of leucocytes renders the individual susceptible to overwhelming infection. Conditions that may impede leucocyte production or function include inadequate blood cell production, proliferation of immature leucocytes, viruses, drug reactions, radiation, nutritional deficiencies and bone marrow hypoplasia.

Thrombocytes are necessary for the clotting of blood. Any disorder that impairs thrombocyte production or function renders the individual susceptible to bleeding (Parrillo & Dellinger 2019). A decrease or increase in the formation of thrombocytes generally occurs in association with other disorders. Thrombocytopenia (decrease in thrombocyte number) is commonly due to viral infections but may be idiopathic or may result from bone marrow disease. It may also result from a condition that causes thrombocyte destruction, such as cirrhosis of the liver, or drug toxicity or continued bleeding. Thrombocythaemia (increase in thrombocyte number) is frequently idiopathic, but it may also accompany some disorders such as polycythaemia or chronic myeloid leukaemia.

Changes in the lymphatic system

The lymphatic system removes fluid and particles from the interstitial spaces, filters the lymph and returns it to the circulation (Carlson 2018). Impaired lymphatic function may result from obstruction or inflammation of the lymphatic vessels or nodes, or from neoplastic disease. When lymphatic function is impaired, fluid accumulates in the interstitial spaces, and oedema results (Carlson 2018). Because the function of lymphocytes is the key factor in immune responses, diseases of the lymphatic system, such as Hodgkin's disease, may seriously impair the immune processes. The individual with immunodeficiency is vulnerable to infection and other pathological processes that would normally be inhibited by a healthy immune system.

PATHOPHYSIOLOGY RELATED TO THE CIRCULATORY SYSTEM

The manifestations of disorders of the circulatory system vary depending on whether the disorder is one that affects the heart, the blood vessels, or the blood or blood-forming organs.

Manifestations of cardiac disorders

Cardiac disorders can present with a wide range of manifestations, often depending on the specific condition and its severity. Some common manifestations of cardiac disorders are presented below.

Dyspnoea

Dyspnoea (difficult or laboured breathing) is the most common (and often the earliest) symptom of cardiac disease (AACN & Hartjes 2022). Typically, the dyspnoea occurs with exertion although, as cardiac disease progresses, the individual may experience dyspnoea at rest. Paroxysmal nocturnal dyspnoea, which is associated with congestive cardiac failure, occurs during sleep; the individual wakes suddenly with difficulty in breathing and a sensation of suffocation (AACN & Hartjes 2022).

Chest pain

Chest pain is one of the most common causes for attending an emergency department and a frequent cause for attending a general practice (Thomsett & Cullen 2018). Chest pain (Table 25.1) may result from myocardial ischaemia or from pericarditis. Chest pain can also be caused by conditions not associated with cardiac disease, such as oesophagitis, reflux, pleurisy, musculoskeletal disorders or stress and anxiety. Missed diagnosis can have adverse outcomes when chest pain assessment is based on clinical features alone (AACN & Hartjes 2022).

Ischaemic pain is the result of a deficiency of blood to the myocardium, caused by a blocked or constricted coronary blood vessel. Angina (pectoris) is pain that results from diminished supply of oxygen to the heart, and is basically a reversible ischaemic process. Acute myocardial infarction represents the point when ischaemia becomes irreversible; blood flow to part of the heart is inadequate and unrelieved by rest, causing cardiac muscle necrosis (Valchanov et al 2019).

Palpitations

Palpitations are a sensation of fluttering in the chest or an awareness of the heart's action. The person may describe the heart's action as racing, pounding, stopping or skipping beats. Palpitations may be due to rhythm disturbances such as premature contractions (extra heartbeat), but they can also result from anxiety, stress, caffeine or nicotine, cough and cold medications and fatigue (Valchanov et al 2019).

Cough

Cough may be associated with certain cardiovascular diseases and most respiratory diseases. If cardiovascular disease is suspected, it may be caused by an accumulation of fluid in the lungs (pulmonary oedema), often made worse at night or when lying in bed (AACN & Hartjes 2022).

TABLE 25.1 | Typical patterns of cardiac pain

Angina	Myocardial infarction
Gradual or sudden onset.	Sudden onset.
Episodic and temporary, usually lasting 3–15 minutes.	Lasts longer than 15 minutes.
Substernal or anterior, not sharply localised. Radiates to back, neck, arms and jaw.	Substernal, midline or anterior. Radiates to jaw, neck, back, shoulders or one or both arms.
Sensation of mild to moderate pressure. Described as tightness, squeezing or crushing.	Persistent sensation of severe pressure. Described as crushing, heavy, vice-like, squeezing.
Precipitated by exertion, stress, ingestion of food, exposure to cold.	Not necessarily related to exertion or emotion, and may occur at rest.
Accompanied by dyspnoea, diaphoresis, nausea, apprehension.	Accompanied by nausea, vomiting, dyspnoea, apprehension, diaphoresis, a sensation of 'impending doom', pallor, cold clammy skin.
Individual keeps still to relieve the pain.	Individual moves about in search of a comfortable position.
Relieved by rest and/or glyceryl trinitrate.	Not relieved by rest or glyceryl trinitrate.

Fatigue

Fatigue frequently accompanies cardiac dysfunction and is related to inadequate cardiac output resulting in insufficient blood flow to the brain and skeletal tissues (AACN & Hartjes 2022).

Cyanosis

Cyanosis is a bluish discolouration of the skin and mucous membranes due to inadequate oxygenation, and can be either peripheral or central. Peripheral cyanosis results in local vasoconstriction and is usually visible in the nail beds and the lips. Central cyanosis is the result of more severe hypoxia and affects all body organs. It is most visible in highly vascular areas such as the lips, nail beds, tip of the nose, the external ear and the underside of the tongue. In people with naturally dark brown or black skin, cyanosis is most accurately detected by inspecting the mucosa inside the mouth. Cyanosis appears when haemoglobin oxygen saturation is greatly reduced below 92% (AACN & Hartjes 2022).

Syncope

Syncope (transient loss of consciousness) may result when cardiac dysfunction causes an inadequate flow of blood to the brain. Sudden loss of consciousness due to heart block is known as Stokes-Adams syndrome. Heart block is defined as 'impairment of conduction in heart excitation; often applied specifically to atrioventricular heart block' (Parrillo & Dellinger 2019).

Oedema

Oedema (local or generalised accumulation of fluid in the tissues) may result from certain cardiac diseases. Peripheral or systemic oedema generally develops from right-sided cardiac failure and is first noticed in the lowest, or dependent, parts of the body, such as the legs, fingers, sacral area, periorbital area, in the abdomen (ascites) and intestines (causing constipation) (Parrillo & Dellinger 2019). As venous stasis increases, oedema increases. In left-sided cardiac failure, fluid accumulates in the lungs (pulmonary oedema). In advanced cardiac failure, total body oedema may develop. The severity of the oedema will depend on the degree to which venous return and/or cardiac output are reduced (Parrillo & Dellinger 2019).

Pulse abnormalities

Pulse rate, volume or rhythm may be abnormal in the presence of cardiac dysfunction. Tachycardia may accompany cardiac failure, while heart block commonly results in bradycardia. A low cardiac output, and therefore a reduced pulse volume, is associated with cardiac failure and acute myocardial infarction (Parrillo & Dellinger 2019). Certain cardiac disorders cause arrhythmias accompanied by an irregular pulse.

Manifestations of peripheral blood vessel disorders

Peripheral blood vessel disorders can lead to a range of symptoms and manifestations due to compromised blood flow in the extremities. These disorders affect the arteries, veins, or both and can have significant effects on the affected areas. Some common manifestations of peripheral blood vessel disorders are presented below.

Pale cold extremities

Pale cold extremities indicate impaired blood flow to the limb.

Altered peripheral pulses

Altered peripheral pulses may be present when arterial blood flow is impeded. Examining peripheral pulses is a useful and accurate way to rule out significant peripheral artery disease (Hanna 2022).

Typical claudication

Typical claudication is described as a discomfort, fatigue or weakness in the lower extremities, brought on by exercise but relieved by rest (usually within 10 minutes) (Hanna 2022). The pain is commonly experienced in the calf muscle during walking and is thought to be due to accumulation of lactic acid in the tissues, rather than to ischaemia of the contracting muscle.

Rest pain

Rest pain is described as persistent, unrelenting pain in the lower limbs that occurs without any preceding activity (Gallagher et al 2020). Pain occurs when chronic arterial occlusive disease is advanced, or when a vessel is blocked by a thrombus or embolus. As a result, the blood supply to the surrounding tissues is diminished, causing ischaemic pain (Hanna 2022).

Ulceration

Ulceration in the lower limbs is a common manifestation of peripheral artery disease and usually accompanies claudication and rest pain. Ulcers typically occur at the toe level (Hanna 2022).

Limb ischemia

In more severe cases of peripheral diseases, when the blood flow to the affected limb becomes severely compromised, the condition can progress to limb ischemia. Lower extremity ischemia can present as acute or chronic. Acute limb ischemia is considered an emergency; if unrecognised, it can result in limb loss, and is suggested by the six 'Ps': limb pulselessness, pain, pallor, paraesthesias, paralysis and poikilothermia (also known as cold-bloodedness) (Gallagher et al 2020; Gerhard-Herma & Aday 2020). Wounds or ulcers may develop, and tissue damage can lead to non-healing wounds, infection, and, in extreme cases, gangrene.

Gangrene

Gangrene, which causes death of tissue, may occur as a result of chronic arterial insufficiency and is the consequence of severe and prolonged ischaemia (Hanna 2022).

Manifestations of blood and blood-forming organ disorders

Bruising and bleeding

Bruising and bleeding may occur when there is abnormal thrombocyte production or function or reduced levels of clotting factors in the plasma. The appearance of any bruising or haemorrhagic spots in the absence of injury is suggestive of a blood disorder. Types of bruising and bleeding include:

- Purpura: Haemorrhagic areas under the skin and in the mucous membranes. If the haemorrhages are small, they are termed petechiae; larger purpuric areas are called bruises or ecchymoses.
- Petechiae: Red-brown pinpoint haemorrhages in the skin. Petechiae can occur over any part of the skin but are most common where pressure has been applied to a body part; seen in meningococcal meningitis and anthrax as well as common viral infections.
- Ecchymoses: Haemorrhagic spots larger than petechiae. They may be precipitated by an injury or may occur spontaneously.
- Gastrointestinal bleeding: Appears as haematemesis and/or melaena and may occur in certain disorders of the blood such as thrombocytopenia, but may also occur as a result of liver failure, oesophageal varices, gastrointestinal ulcerations and drug therapies.
- Menorrhagia: May occur in haemorrhagic disorders as well as gynaecological disorders.
- Haematuria: May occur in haemorrhagic disorders as well as renal disorders.
- Neurological changes (e.g. headaches, blurred vision, disorientation or altered consciousness): May occur if there is bleeding within the central nervous system.

Changes in the skin may accompany disorders of the blood or blood-forming organs. Changes that may occur include pallor, rubor, jaundice, pruritus, thickened nails and ulcerations.

Fatigue

Fatigue or weakness are common manifestations of many haematological disorders, such as anaemia and leukaemia. An individual with anaemia may also experience shortness of breath, particularly on exertion.

Enlarged lymph nodes

Enlarged lymph nodes may be present in disorders such as Hodgkin's disease or leukaemia. Pain may be experienced in many haematological disorders. For example, bleeding into a joint may result in joint pain, and bone pain can occur in leukaemia or lymphoma.

SPECIFIC DISORDERS OF THE CIRCULATORY SYSTEM

Globally, deaths from cardiovascular disease are increasing, particularly in low- and middle-income countries (Braunwald et al 2021). Understanding the conditions and factors that affect the cardiovascular system is imperative to assist with reducing the burden to healthcare cardiovascular diseases are causing.

Disorders of the circulatory system may be congenital or due to multiple causes, pathogens or chemicals, or they may be drug-related, neoplastic, obstructive, degenerative or the result of trauma. It is beyond the scope of this text to provide in-depth information on the various conditions related to the circulatory system. Listed below are some examples of circulatory system conditions.

Congenital disorders

Congenital disorders are conditions that exist at birth (Mars 2020). These disorders include ventricular septal defect; atrial septal defect; coarctation of the aorta; patent ductus arteriosus; tetralogy of Fallot; transposition of the great vessels; thalassaemias (sickle-cell anaemia); and bleeding disorders (haemophilia A, haemophilia B, von Willebrand disease).

Disorders of multiple cause

It is beyond the scope of this text to provide in-depth information on the various conditions related to the disorders of multiple causes; only a few of the most common conditions are briefly discussed here.

Hypertension

Over the last century, hypertension has been one of the most studied topics in healthcare and has been one of the most significant comorbidities contributing to the development of stroke, myocardial infarction, heart failure and renal failure (Iqbal & Jamal 2019).

Hypertension is frequently asymptomatic until the individual experiences a major problem such as cerebral haemorrhage, renal failure or myocardial infarction. Symptoms that may be due to hypertension include dizziness, chest pain, palpitations, epistaxis, headaches and brief episodes of memory loss (transient ischaemic attacks).

Hypertension should not be diagnosed from one single blood pressure measurement, but rather it should be based on multiple blood pressure measurements taken on several separate occasions (National Heart Foundation of Australia 2016). There is increasing evidence supporting ambulatory blood pressure monitoring (ABPM) for diagnosing hypertension (National Heart Foundation of Australia 2016).

High arterial blood pressure over 135/85 mmHg is generally classified as either primary ('essential') or secondary hypertension. Primary hypertension is the most common form and, while the cause is often unknown, many factors have been implicated as contributing to its development, including high sodium intake, obesity, diabetes, hypercholesterolaemia, genetic factors, alcohol, cigarette smoking and psychosocial factors. Antihypertensive drug therapy may be prescribed to hypertensive persons and evidence shows that these therapies should be implemented in a stepped care approach until target blood pressure levels are achieved (Donald et al 2019).

Secondary hypertension is caused by either disease or certain medications. Diseases that result in secondary hypertension include those in which renal, vascular, endocrine or neurological mechanisms are involved, such as renal artery stenosis or intercranial lesions. Medications that may lead to secondary hypertension include oral contraceptives, corticosteroids and monoamine oxidase inhibitors. If secondary hypertension is suspected, a specialist referral should be considered (National Heart Foundation of Australia 2016).

Malignant hypertension is the term used to describe primary hypertension when there is a rapid rise of blood pressure to a very high level, such as 250/150 mmHg. It is accompanied by severe headache, visual disturbances and oliguria. If untreated, death may occur rapidly from cardiac or renal failure or cerebrovascular accident.

CRITICAL THINKING EXERCISE 25.2

Mr Davis, 68 years old, has a history of chronic hypertension. His hypertension management plan includes a daily dose of 40 mg of Lasix (furosemide) to promote diuresis and restrict his daily fluid intake. However, Mr Davis is struggling to adhere to his fluid restriction and he consistently reports feeling excessively thirsty. During your assessment, you observe that he has developed oedema in his lower extremities. Consider what nursing interventions could be implemented to assist Mr Davis.

Coronary artery disease

Coronary artery disease is a disorder in which the arteries that supply blood to the heart muscle become diseased and fail to supply the heart with sufficient oxygen-rich blood (Mars 2020).

Arteriosclerosis is the most common cause of coronary artery disease, leading to disturbances of blood flow within the coronary arteries that give rise to altered myocardial perfusion and disruption of the electrical cycle controlling heart rhythm. Atherosclerosis is one type of arteriosclerosis in which narrowing of the arteries occurs as a result of deposits of lipids in and around the smooth muscle, roughening of the endothelial lining and loss of elasticity, with fibrosis and calcification (Mars 2020). Eventually, the artery becomes occluded, inelastic and incapable of dilating.

Although the precise cause of arteriosclerosis and coronary artery disease is unclear, there is general agreement that many factors contribute to its development, including genetic influences, gender (males are more commonly affected), hypertension, lack of exercise, cigarette smoking, stress, metabolic or endocrine disorders, obesity, diabetes mellitus, hypercholesterolaemia and dietary factors. The dietary factors that are considered to contribute to coronary artery disease are salt, saturated fats and lack of dietary fibre. Coronary artery disease may be asymptomatic until the individual experiences angina or a myocardial infarction, which may result in sudden death (Valchanov et al 2019).

Acute coronary syndrome

Acute coronary syndrome is a term used to describe a range of conditions resulting from reduced blood flow to the heart muscle due to the narrowing or blockage of coronary arteries (ANZCOR 2023). It is a medical emergency that requires immediate attention and intervention.

Clinically, acute coronary syndrome is divided into three syndromes that are characterised by the presence or absence of ST elevation on the ECG; these syndromes are referred to as:

i. STEMI: This is the most severe form of ACS. It occurs when there is a complete blockage of a coronary artery, leading to a significant portion of the heart muscle being deprived of oxygen and nutrients. This can result in irreversible damage to the heart muscle if not treated promptly.
ii. NSTEMI: In this, there is a partial blockage of a coronary artery that leads to reduced blood flow and damage to a portion of the heart muscle. While it is not as severe as a full STEMI, NSTEMI still requires urgent medical attention.
iii. Unstable angina is characterised by chest pain or discomfort that is new, occurs at rest, or is more severe, prolonged or frequent than the individual's usual angina pattern. It signifies that there is a significant blockage in a coronary artery, but there is no permanent damage to the heart muscle.

Blood flow to the myocardium may be obstructed by arteriosclerosis (narrowing or clogging of arteries with deposits of fat, cholesterol and other substances) or by thrombus formation within an atheromatous coronary artery (ANZCOR 2023). The most common site of infarction is the anterior surface of the left ventricle, resulting from occlusion of the left coronary artery. An infarction may affect some or all of the layers of the heart.

The major complications of a myocardial infarction are left ventricular failure, pericarditis and arrhythmias, which together account for a large percentage of deaths following myocardial infarction. It is generally recognised that the risk of death is greatest in the first few hours after myocardial infarction, with the risk decreasing after that time.

A myocardial infarction may be asymptomatic (a silent myocardial infarction). More commonly, it may manifest with pain in the centre of the chest, arms, neck, jaw or back lasting longer than 5 minutes, pallor, sweating, anxiety, shortness of breath, nausea or vomiting or sudden collapse (Parrillo & Dellinger 2019). Early and accurate identification as to whether the chest pain is a myocardial infarction event is essential to ensure emergency reperfusion therapy is provided (Parrillo & Dellinger 2019).

Other disorders of multiple cause include arrhythmias, valvular heart disease, heart failure, cardiogenic shock, cardiac arrest, Raynaud's disease, disseminated intravascular coagulation, idiopathic thrombocytopenic purpura, agranulocytosis and Buerger's disease.

Heart failure

Heart failure is a complex syndrome that affects approximately 38 million people worldwide (NHFA CSANZ Heart Failure Guidelines Working Group 2018). Causes of heart failure include myocyte damage or loss (such as ischaemia, inflammation, toxic damage, genetic abnormalities), abnormal loading condition (such as hypertension, valvular dysfunction) and arrhythmias (NHFA CSANZ Heart Failure Guidelines Working Group 2018). Signs and symptoms of heart failure generally occur on exertion but may occur at rest. Common symptoms include dyspnoea, orthopnoea and fatigue, and less common symptoms include wheeze, nocturnal cough, palpitation and dizziness (NHFA CSANZ Heart Failure Guidelines Working Group 2018). Heart failure is diagnosed clinically and the extent of the heart failure is diagnosed according to the classification of the left ventricular ejection fraction (LVEF) (NHFA CSANZ Heart Failure Guidelines Working Group 2018). Treatment of heart failure is focused on prevention and management (Case Study 25.2).

Anaemias

Anaemias are a group of disorders characterised by reduced oxygen-carrying capacity of the blood. Causes of anaemia are numerous and are related to the altered production or destruction of erythrocytes, and to blood loss. Anaemias can thus be classified as due to haematopoietic, haemolytic or haemorrhagic causes.

Aplastic anaemia is caused by injury or destruction of the haematopoietic cells in bone marrow, resulting in reduced or abnormal erythrocyte production. In this disorder, the normal haematopoietic tissue is replaced by fatty bone marrow. Aplastic anaemia may be idiopathic or it may be caused by medications, toxic agents, radiation or immunological factors. Manifestations of aplastic anaemia are related to pancytopenia (abnormal depression of the cellular components of blood). They include pallor, tiredness, repeated infections and bleeding tendencies. Bleeding may present as petechiae, ecchymoses, haemorrhage from the mucous membranes (such as the gums) or gastrointestinal haemorrhage.

Pernicious anaemia is characterised by a metabolic defect involving the absence of intrinsic factor, which is secreted by the parietal cells of the gastric mucosa and is essential for vitamin B absorption in the terminal ileum. Pernicious anaemia is thought to result from an autosomal dominant defect. Other causes include gastric cancer, gastrectomy and malabsorption disorders involving the ileum. Manifestations of pernicious anaemia include pallor, tiredness, sore tongue and numbness and tingling in the extremities. Because of vitamin B deficiency, demyelination of nerves and degeneration of nerve tissue occurs, producing neurological effects such as ataxia, altered vision, poor memory, depression and paralysis.

Iron-deficiency anaemia is characterised by small and pale erythrocytes because of reduced haemoglobin concentration. The two most common causes of iron-deficiency anaemia are chronic blood loss and an inadequate dietary intake of iron. Manifestations include pagophagia (craving for ice), pallor, chronic tiredness, tachycardia and shortness of breath on exertion.

Folate deficiency anaemia results from an inadequate dietary intake of folate, a disorder of the small intestine, where folate is absorbed, or from altered metabolism. Manifestations are similar to those associated with pernicious anaemia.

Acute blood-loss anaemia is a condition that results from sudden loss of erythrocytes and, consequently, depletion of haemoglobin and iron. Acute blood-loss anaemia may result from severe trauma, postoperative haemorrhage, invasive neoplasm, ruptured peptic ulcer, ruptured aneurysm or coagulation defects. Acute blood loss itself produces features associated with hypovolaemia and hypoxia, such as pallor, faintness, restlessness, anxiety, hypotension and a weak rapid pulse.

If anaemia is persistent and the individual's haemoglobin levels decrease, the individual may require a transfusion of blood.

CASE STUDY 25.2

Margaret, an 81-year-old female, has been admitted to the hospital due to atrial fibrillation. She has a history of ischemic heart disease, chronic obstructive pulmonary disease (COPD), and hypertension. This morning, she had managed to walk to the bathroom for her morning routine but is now complaining of increasing shortness of breath. Her respirations have increased, and she is speaking in short, 1–2 word sentences. Margaret's ankles are swollen, and her heart rate is elevated.

1. What are your first actions?
2. Who would you notify?
3. What test may be undertaken to assist with the management plan of this individual?

Neoplastic and obstructive disorders

Tumours may occur in any of the chambers of the heart and may affect one or all of the layers of the heart. Secondary metastatic tumours that infiltrate the heart are more common than primary cardiac tumours. Manifestations are related to which part of the heart is affected, and include signs of heart failure, arrhythmias, angina, heart block and infarction. It is beyond the scope of this text to provide in-depth information on the various conditions related to neoplastic and obstructive disorders and only a few of the most common conditions are briefly discussed here.

Leukaemia

Leukaemia is a neoplastic disorder characterised by an accumulation and proliferation of abnormal cells in the bone marrow. Cells fail to develop and are unable to function normally, and the accumulation of leukaemic cells in the bone marrow prevents normal haematopoiesis. The precise cause of leukaemia is unknown but several factors have been implicated in its development including chromosome abnormality, exposure to radiation from power lines, viruses or chemicals, such as certain weedkillers or insecticides. Leukaemia occurs either in acute forms, which involve the proliferation of immature cells, or in chronic forms, which involve the proliferation of mature cells. The four most common forms of leukaemia are acute myeloid, chronic myeloid, acute lymphocytic and chronic lymphocytic.

Although manifestations of leukaemia vary according to the particular form of the disorder, there is a similarity in the signs and symptoms, which are related to the lack of normal haematopoiesis in the bone marrow. Bone marrow dysfunction results in:

- anaemia, which may present as pallor, lethargy and shortness of breath
- thrombocytopenia, which commonly manifests as petechiae, easy bruising, bleeding gums and haemorrhage (e.g. as occult haematuria)
- leucopenia, which renders the individual susceptible to recurrent infections. There is generally splenic enlargement, lymphadenopathy and bone pain.

Central nervous system involvement may be present in any of the leukaemias, giving rise to symptoms such as nausea and vomiting, irritability, headache and blurred vision.

Hodgkin's disease

Hodgkin's disease is a malignant disorder of the lymph node macrophages, characterised by painless and progressive enlargement of the lymph nodes, spleen and other lymphoid tissue. Untreated, Hodgkin's disease metastasises via the lymphatics to sites outside the lymphatic system. The precise cause of the disorder is unknown, but both genetic and environmental factors seem to be implicated in its development. Manifestations of Hodgkin's disease are painless enlargement of the lymph nodes, especially the cervical nodes, pruritus, night sweats, malaise and weight loss. Other symptoms depend on the degree and location of systemic involvement.

Other conditions related to neoplastic and obstructive disorders include arteriosclerosis obliterans, acute arterial obstruction, thrombophlebitis, chronic venous insufficiency, Burkitt's lymphoma, multiple myeloma and malignant lymphomas.

Degenerative disorders

Cardiomyopathy

Cardiomyopathy results from extensive damage to the myocardial muscle fibres, causing hypertrophy of the entire heart, especially of the septum. Although the heart is enlarged, the ventricular chambers are small and are resistant to filling during diastole. Cardiomyopathy leads to congestive cardiac failure, arrhythmias and, frequently, sudden death.

The cause of most cardiomyopathies is unknown but the condition is thought to be genetically transmitted. Some forms of cardiomyopathy result from hypertension, congenital defects and myocardial destruction by toxic, infectious or metabolic agents. The most common manifestation of cardiomyopathy is dyspnoea, as a result of congestive cardiac failure. As cardiac failure progresses, peripheral cyanosis, oedema, liver enlargement and jugular venous distension become evident.

Aortic aneurysm

Aortic aneurysm is a dilation of the wall of the aorta. There are several types of aneurysm:

- saccular: an outpouching of one side of the arterial wall
- fusiform: a spindle-shaped enlargement of the entire circumference of the artery
- dissecting: a haemorrhagic separation between the medial and internal layers of the artery.

The most common cause of an aneurysm is arteriosclerosis, which weakens the aortic wall and gradually distends the lumen at the weakened area (Parrillo & Dellinger 2019). Other causative factors include congenital defects, infection, hypertension and trauma.

Manifestations of an aortic aneurysm depend on its location, and may not develop until enlargement of the aneurysm exerts pressure on nearby structures. Depending on the location, an aortic aneurysm may manifest as dyspnoea; chest pain; dysphagia; dilated superficial veins on the chest, neck and arms; prominent abdominal pulsation; or dull abdominal or low back pain. A dissecting aneurysm may produce a sudden 'tearing' pain accompanied by pallor, shortness of breath, sweating and syncope. The main complication of an aortic aneurysm is rupture and, without immediate surgical intervention, the individual may bleed to death (Parrillo & Dellinger 2019).

Varicose veins

Varicose veins are dilated, tortuous branches of the saphenous veins. They result from incompetent valves, which cause a backflow of venous blood. Varicose veins may result from congenital weakness of the valves, from injury or thrombophlebitis, or from conditions that produce venous stasis, such as pregnancy or occupations that necessitate standing for long periods. Superficial varicose veins may be unsightly but produce no symptoms. Deeper varicose veins may produce mild to severe leg symptoms, such as a feeling of heaviness, cramps, dull aching and discomfort that increases with prolonged standing. Over time, dilation of the veins results in venous stasis, with oedema and changes in skin pigmentation. Visible and palpable protrusions frequently occur along the veins, resulting in disfigurement of the leg(s) (Carlson 2018).

Infectious and inflammatory disorders

Pericarditis

Pericarditis (inflammation of the pericardium) may be an acute or chronic condition. Acute pericarditis may be accompanied by a purulent, serous or haemorrhagic exudate, which can produce further complications (Parrillo & Dellinger 2019). Chronic pericarditis is characterised by fibrous pericardial thickening. As well as being caused by infection, pericarditis may result from trauma, radiation, neoplasms, cardiac surgery or myocardial infarction. The prime manifestation is chest pain that increases with deep inhalation, and decreases when the person sits up and leans forward. Other manifestations include dyspnoea and the signs of a systemic infection (Parrillo & Dellinger 2019).

Myocarditis

Myocarditis (inflammation of the myocardium) may be an acute or chronic condition. Myocarditis may result from viral or bacterial infections, radiation, chemicals or metabolic disorders (Parrillo & Dellinger 2019). Infective myocarditis usually causes non-specific symptoms that reflect a systemic infection. Myocarditis sometimes produces manifestations of severe congestive cardiac failure (Parrillo & Dellinger 2019).

Endocarditis

Endocarditis (inflammation or infection of the endocardium) may result from invasion by microorganisms or from non-infective injury to the lining of the heart, or via intravenous (IV) cannulas, dental surgery or any other invasive procedure. Infective endocarditis involves the endocardium of the heart valves more frequently than the endocardium lining the heart chambers. The microorganisms stimulate the deposit of fibrin around them, producing vegetative growth on the endocardium.

Early manifestations are commonly non-specific, and the symptoms of acute endocarditis resemble those associated with influenza: pyrexia, sweats, anorexia, headaches and musculoskeletal aches (Parrillo & Dellinger 2019). If a heart murmur develops, the pulse rate may be rapid and, if vegetative growths become dislodged, there may be manifestations of embolisation, producing the features of splenic, renal, cerebral, pulmonary or peripheral vascular occlusion.

Rheumatic heart disease

Rheumatic heart disease refers to the cardiac manifestations of rheumatic fever and includes pericarditis, myocarditis, endocarditis and chronic valvular disease (Watkins et al 2018). Rheumatic fever is associated with the type A beta-haemolytic streptococcus and is thought to be immunological in origin. It may be as long as 10 years after an attack of rheumatic fever before signs of heart valve disease become evident (Watkins et al 2018). The end result of the disease progression is stenosis of a heart valve, inability of the valve to close properly, or valve incompetence, which leads to regurgitation of blood through the valve during systole. Manifestations of rheumatic heart valve disease depend on the valve affected and on the degree of valve dysfunction. There may be signs of reduced cardiac output, pulmonary congestion, cardiac enlargement, heart failure and the presence of heart murmurs (Watkins et al 2018).

Lymphangitis

Lymphangitis is an acute or chronic inflammation of the lymphatic vessels, which generally results from a streptococcal infection of an extremity. The accompanying lymph node enlargement (lymphadenopathy) may be localised or generalised. Lymphangitis is characterised by red, warm, tender streaks spreading up a limb from a focal point of infection. The regional lymph nodes become enlarged and tender, and the individual experiences pyrexia and malaise.

RESPIRATORY DIAGNOSTIC TESTS

Certain tests may be used to assist or confirm the diagnosis and severity of respiratory disorders.

Pulmonary function studies

These studies are used to determine the presence and degree of respiratory dysfunction and are a measure of the functional ability of the lungs. Spirometry or plethysmography is used to assess the individual's lung volume by measuring and recording the volume of inhaled and exhaled air. The values are then compared with the normal values against predicted values for an individual of the same sex, weight, height and age. Table 25.2 lists types of pulmonary function tests and the normal expected values.

Polysomnography

This test is used to measure upper obstruction and pattern of respirations during sleep, using various pieces of equipment.

Chest X-ray

A chest X-ray is one of the most common procedures used to evaluate the lungs, and generally involves posterior, anterior and lateral views. Abnormal findings that may be evident on a chest X-ray include areas of density, presence of a mass or accumulation of fluid.

Ventilation/perfusion scan

A ventilation/perfusion scan involves the administration of a radioactive gas. The radioactive particles are distributed and trapped in the pulmonary capillary bed, and the lung scan produces a visual image of pulmonary blood flow. Tissue that does not pick up the radionuclide will show as a light-coloured area, indicating lack of adequate lung perfusion. Conditions such as pulmonary oedema, lung cancer or COPD may cause abnormal perfusion.

Cultures

A specimen of secretions is obtained, for example, via a nose swab or nasopharyngeal aspirate or throat swab. Care must be taken to ensure that only the back of the throat is swabbed, which represents microorganisms in the respiratory tract. Samples are sent to the laboratory so that any microorganisms present can be identified by use of a special growth medium (the culture). Sensitivity studies

TABLE 25.2 | Pulmonary function tests

Tests	Explanation	Normal value
Tidal volume	Amount of air inhaled or exhaled during normal breathing	500 mL
Total lung capacity	Total volume of the lungs when maximally inflated	6000 mL
Vital capacity	Total volume of air that can be forcibly exhaled after a maximum inhalation	3000–6000 mL
Functional residual capacity	Amount of air remaining in the lungs after normal exhalation	2400 mL
Inspiratory capacity	Amount of air that can be inhaled after normal exhalation	3600 mL
Expiratory reserve volume	Amount of air that can be exhaled after normal exhalation	1200 mL
Forced expiratory volume (in one second [FEV_1])	Maximal amount of air that can be forcibly exhaled, in 1 second, after full inhalation	3000–5000 mL
Residual volume	Amount of air remaining in the lungs after a maximal forced exhalation	1200 mL

(Hartley 2018)

may then be conducted to determine which drug is effective against the specific microorganism.

Sputum cytology

A specimen of sputum is obtained and sent to the laboratory, where it is examined to detect the presence of pus, pathogenic microorganisms or malignant cells. See Clinical Skill 25.3 and Chapter 18.

Skin tests

A common skin test performed is the Mantoux test, used in the detection of tuberculosis (TB). A medical officer or Registered Nurse (RN) qualified in intradermal administration injects intradermally 0.1 mL of solution containing old tuberculin. A positive reaction may be defined as an area of redness or induration of at least 5 mm in diameter appearing within 48–72 hours. The greater the reaction size, the greater the exposure to antibodies to the tubercle bacillus.

Bronchoscopy

Bronchoscopy involves the direct viewing of the trachea and bronchi by means of an instrument called a bronchoscope. A bronchoscopy is used in the diagnosis of respiratory tract disorders and may be used to remove foreign bodies or flush out secretions in the airways and to obtain a specimen of secretions or tissue for microscopic examination (Valchanov et al 2019).

Thoracentesis

In thoracentesis, the thoracic wall is punctured with a needle to obtain a specimen of pleural fluid for analysis. The procedure may also be performed to relieve pulmonary compression caused by a pleural effusion. A local anaesthetic is injected into the skin before the needle is inserted.

Arterial blood gas analysis

Blood gas analysis shows how well an individual's lungs are delivering oxygen to the bloodstream and eliminating carbon dioxide. Blood is collected for analysis of pH, $PaCO_2$, PaO_2, bicarbonate and base levels (AACN & Hartjes 2022).

Capillary acid–base balance

Capillary acid–base balance analysis is performed by a finger prick. Blood is collected in a glass capillary tube to analyse the acid–base balance and PCO_2.

Other tests

Blood microscopy and culture or viral tests may also be carried out to detect and identify the source of bacterial or viral infections. Other diagnostic tests that may be performed include fluoroscopy, tomography, bronchography and pulmonary angiography (Parrillo & Dellinger 2019).

CRITICAL THINKING EXERCISE 25.3

Mr Anderson visits a nearby clinic, reporting he has been feeling unwell for the past 2 weeks. He describes his symptoms as profound fatigue, a persistent dry cough, and unintentional weight loss. Consider the relevant inquiries to include when conducting the nursing history.

CARDIOVASCULAR DIAGNOSTIC TESTS

Assessment of the individual with a suspected circulatory system disorder, or evaluation of the progress of a disorder, requires that certain cardiovascular tests be performed.

Assessment of cardiac function

Electrocardiography (ECG)

Electrocardiography (ECG) (Figure 25.20) is a diagnostic test that records the electrical activity of the heart over a specific period of time. It is a valuable tool in evaluating the heart's rhythm and detecting any abnormalities in its electrical signals (Urden et al 2022; Valchanov et al 2019). The ECG is performed using a machine called an electrocardiograph, which consists of electrodes attached to the person's skin in specific locations across the chest, arms and legs.

During an ECG, the electrodes detect and amplify the small electrical signals generated by the heart's electrical system as it contracts and relaxes. These signals are then displayed on a graph, known as the ECG tracing. The tracing consists of a series of waves and intervals that represent different phases of the cardiac cycle.

Here is a breakdown of the key components of an ECG tracing:

- P wave: Represents the depolarisation (contraction) of the atria, the upper chambers of the heart. It is a small upward deflection on the ECG.
- QRS complex: Represents the depolarisation of the ventricles, the lower chambers of the heart. It consists of a Q wave (initial downward deflection), an R wave (upward deflection) and an S wave (downward deflection).
- T wave: Represents the repolarisation (recovery) of the ventricles. It is a slightly rounded upward deflection.
- ST segment: The interval between the end of the QRS complex and the beginning of the T wave. Changes in the ST segment can indicate certain heart conditions, such as myocardial infarction (heart attack).
- QT interval: Represents the total time for ventricular depolarisation and repolarisation. Prolonged QT intervals can be associated with certain arrhythmias.
- U wave: A small wave that may sometimes appear after the T wave, typically not always present or easily noticeable. Its significance is not fully understood.

(Urden et al 2022)

By analysing the patterns and intervals in the ECG tracing, healthcare professionals can determine a variety of information about the heart's functioning, including:

- heart rate: the number of heart beats per minute
- rhythm: whether the heart's rhythm is regular or irregular

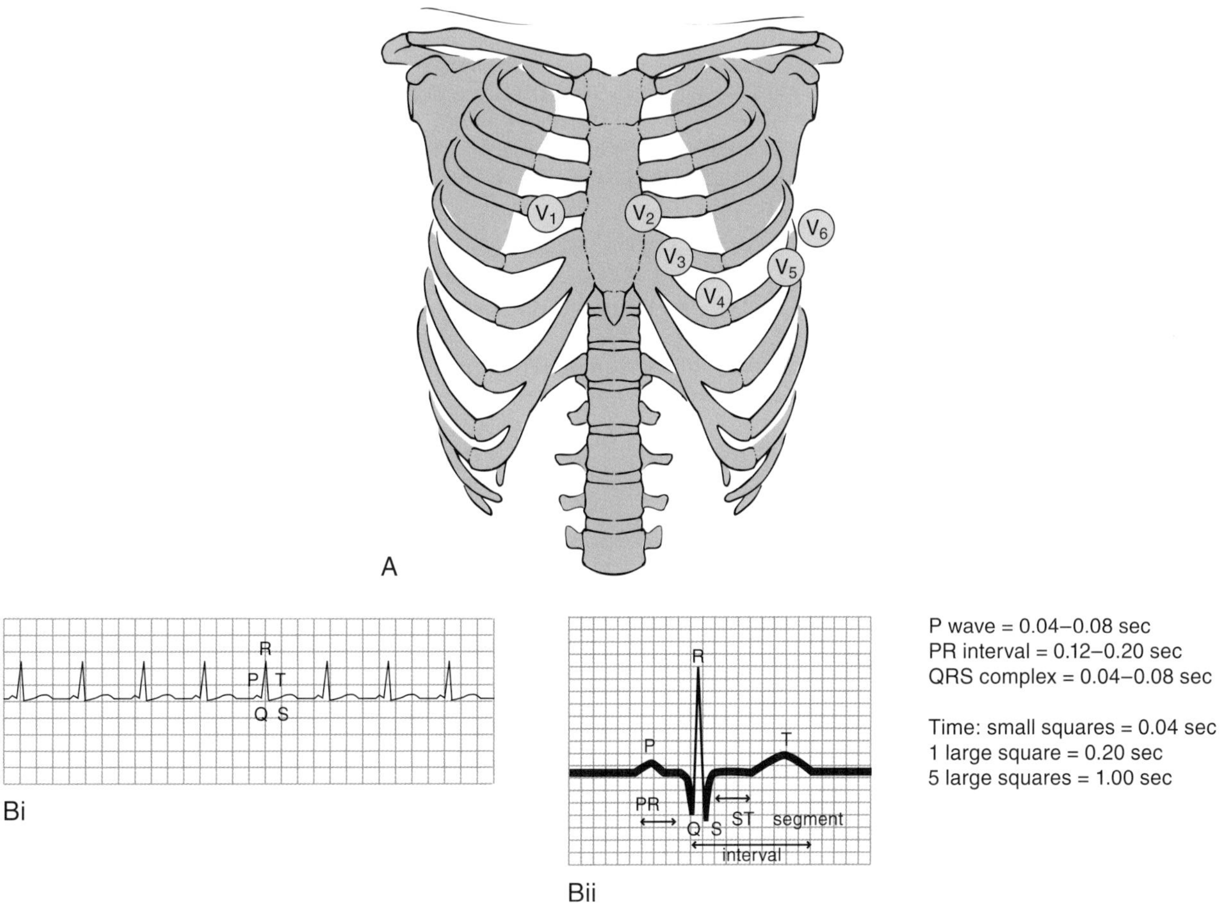

Figure 25.20 Electrocardiogram (ECG)

A: Placement of the chest leads, **B:** A normal ECG, **(i)** Regular sinus rhythm, **(ii)** Detail of an ECG.

(Lewis et al 2014)

- conduction abnormalities: any disruptions in the electrical pathways of the heart
- enlargement or hypertrophy: abnormalities in the size and structure of the heart chambers
- ischemia or infarction: indications of reduced blood supply to parts of the heart muscle.

Interpreting an ECG requires knowledge and expertise, often performed by trained medical professionals like cardiologists. The ECG is a fundamental tool for diagnosing and monitoring various heart conditions and is commonly used in routine medical check-ups, emergency situations, and pre-operative assessments. See Clinical Skill 25.1 for performing an ECG.

Echocardiography

Echocardiography is a painless non-invasive test that directs ultra-high-frequency soundwaves through the chest wall into the heart, which then reflects those waves to a transducer and a recording device (Valchanov et al 2019). As the sound transects the various heart structures, echoes are produced and recorded. Echocardiography evaluates cardiac structure and function and can reveal valve deformities, septal defects, cardiomyopathy and pericardial effusion.

Exercise stress test

An exercise stress test, or exercise tolerance test, is used to test a person's cardiac response to exercise (Kucia & Jones 2022). During a stress test, the individual exercises on a treadmill or stationary bike while their heart activity is monitored. It helps evaluate the heart's response to physical stress and can diagnose conditions like coronary artery disease (Kucia & Jones 2022).

CLINICAL SKILL 25.1 Performing an ECG

Please adhere to the policy and procedures of the facility/organisation prior to undertaking the skill. Ensure this skill is in your scope of practice.

NMBA Decision-making Framework considerations (refer to NMBA Decision-making framework for nursing and midwifery 2020): 1. Am I educated? 2. Am I authorised? 3. Am I competent? If you answer 'no' to any of these, do not perform that activity. Seek guidance and support from your teacher/a nurse team leader/clinical facilitator/educator.	**Equipment:** ECG machine Electrodes Gauze squares/tissues Razor/hair clippers Conduction gel Covering to maintain privacy/modesty

PREPARE FOR THE SKILL

(Please refer to the Standard Steps on pp. xviii–xx for related rationales.)
Mentally review the steps of the skill.
Discuss the skill with your instructor/supervisor/team leader, if required.
Confirm correct facility/organisation policy/safe operating procedures.
Validate the order in the individual's record.
Identify indication and rationale for performing the activity.
Assess for any contraindications.
Locate and gather equipment.
Perform hand hygiene.
Ensure therapeutic interaction.
Identify the individual using three individual identifiers.
Gain the individual's consent.
Assess for pain relief.
Prepare the environment.
Provide and maintain privacy.
Assist the individual to assume an appropriate position of comfort.

Skill activity	Rationale
Position in supine position, head supported. Make note if the person has chest pain. Loosen or remove clothing above the waistline. Remove jewellery (including piercings). **Note:** If the individual has breathing difficulties position in the semi-Fowler's position.	Ensures an accurate ECG can be taken, and helps reduce the amount of artefact.

CLINICAL SKILL 25.1 Performing an ECG—cont'd

PERFORM THE SKILL

(Please refer to the Standard Steps on pp. xviii–xx for related rationales.)
Perform hand hygiene.
Apply PPE: gloves, eyewear, mask and gown as appropriate.
Ensure the individual's safety and comfort throughout skill.
Promote independence and involvement of the individual if possible and/or appropriate.
Assess the individual's tolerance to the skill throughout.
Dispose of used supplies, equipment, waste and sharps appropriately.
Remove PPE and discard or store appropriately.
Perform hand hygiene.

Skill activity	Rationale
Attach limb leads to clean, hair-free sites on arms and legs.	Area chosen should be over fleshy, not bony, tissue. Skin needs to be clean to ensure the best conduction of electrical impulses. If skin is unclean or wet, use an alcohol swab or soap and water to clean and dry the sites for electrode placement. Excess hair is removed as it prevents adequate contact with the skin.
Determine chest sites and attach electrodes to clean, dry, hair-free sites. V_1—4th intercostal space, right sternal border V_2—4th intercostal space, left sternal border V_3—5th intercostal space, left sternal border V_4—5th intercostal space, left mid-clavicular line V_5—5th intercostal space, left anterior axillary line V_6—5th intercostal space, left mid-axillary line	**Note:** Care must be taken that the electrodes are accurately placed, since errors in diagnosis can occur if the electrodes are incorrectly placed. If the individual has large breasts, place under the breasts.
Attach lead wires to all electrodes.	Attaching the electrodes to the leads ensures the electrical activity is conducted to the ECG machine.
Follow manufacturer's instructions for calibrating and preparing the ECG machine.	Machines may be single channel or multichannel. Familiarity with the machine will increase accuracy of recording and decrease individual and nurse stress.
Ask the individual to relax, refrain from moving and breathe normally. Record ECG and provide to RN for review.	Lack of experience and ability in interpreting an ECG recording might lead the nurse to overlook changes that are significant. RN can also compare ECG to any previous ECGs.
Remove electrodes and conduction gel.	Increases comfort.

AFTER THE SKILL

(Please refer to the Standard Steps on pp. xviii–xx for related rationales.)
Communicate outcome to the individual, any ongoing care and to report any complications.
Restore the environment.
Report, record and document assessment findings, details of the skill performed and the individual's response.
Report, record and document any abnormalities and/or inability to perform the skill.
Reassess the individual to ensure there are no adverse effects/events from the skill.

Skill activity	Rationale
Document on ECG—actual recording, noting name, medical record number, doctor, date and time. Some machines have the ability to program this information so that it is printed out on the ECG recording. Document if individual was pain free or had chest pain during procedure.	Medicolegal requirement. Allows for the planning and implementation of care.

(Aitken et al 2019; Menzies-Gow 2018; Perry et al 2022; Rebeiro et al 2021)

Cardiac catheterisation and angiography

Cardiac catheterisation involves the insertion of a catheter into the heart's blood vessels to inject contrast dye, making the blood vessels visible on X-rays. It helps identify blockages or abnormalities in the coronary arteries and assesses blood flow. The catheter is inserted through a vein in the arm or the groin (in recent years, there has been an increased use in the radial access and a decline in the femoral approach) and advanced into the vena cava; the passage of the catheter is observed on a fluorescent screen and X-ray films are taken (Valchanov et al 2019). A contrast medium may be injected through the catheter and X-ray films taken (angiography). For coronary angiography, the catheter is advanced into the aortic arch and positioned into a coronary artery; a contrast medium is then injected to outline the coronary arteries as a series of X-ray films is taken (Valchanov et al 2019).

Magnetic resonance imaging (MRI)

Cardiac magnetic resonance imaging (MRI) is a non-invasive test that provides detailed images of the heart's structure and function using a powerful magnetic field, radio waves and a computer to produce detailed images (Kucia & Jones 2022). It can assess heart muscle damage, tumours and other conditions.

Nuclear cardiology

A nuclear stress test, also known as myocardial nuclear perfusion imaging, is a diagnostic procedure used to assess the blood flow to the heart muscle. Cardiovascular abnormalities can be viewed, recorded and evaluated using radioactive tracer substances. It provides valuable information about the heart's performance during rest and exercise. These studies are useful for detecting myocardial infarction (MI) and decreased myocardial blood flow and for evaluating left ventricular ejection (Ignatavicius et al 2021). An IV injection, for example of the radioisotope thallium-201, is administered to the individual while they are exercising and a scan performed to detect thallium uptake. Healthy myocardial tissue absorbs the radioisotope, but ischaemic or necrotic tissue does not (Ignatavicius et al 2021).

Central venous pressure

The central venous pressure test measures the functioning of the right atrium. A catheter, which is threaded through the subclavian or jugular vein into or near the right atrium, is connected to a manometer (Valchanov et al 2019). This procedure enables accurate determination of right atrial blood pressure, which reflects right ventricular pressure. This test is also used to assess blood volume.

Intracardiac pressure monitoring

This test involves the insertion of a balloon-tipped flow-directed catheter, such as the Swan–Ganz catheter, into a large vein and then advancing it until it reaches the right atrium. Once the balloon is inflated, the flow of blood carries the catheter into the pulmonary artery. The procedure permits measurement of both pulmonary artery pressure (PAP) and pulmonary artery wedge pressure (PAWP) (Valchanov et al 2019). In addition, this procedure evaluates pulmonary vascular resistance and tissue oxygenation.

Blood tests

Blood tests are important for three reasons: (1) assisting with diagnosis, (2) providing information to tailor treatment and management of the condition and (3) providing a baseline against which health status can be tracked and monitored (Kucia & Jones 2022). Several blood tests are important for assessing cardiac disease (e.g. electrolytes, renal function). Cardiac biomarkers like troponin and creatine kinase-MB are measured to assess if heart muscle damage (myocardial infarction) has occurred (Kucia & Jones 2022).

Assessment of peripheral blood vessels

Skin temperature studies

Skin temperature studies may be performed to evaluate skin temperature of the extremities, which helps determine adequacy of blood circulation in arterial disease. Direct skin temperature readings are taken; in arterial disease the temperature in the extremities may be lower than in other body areas. The cold stimulation test may be used to demonstrate Raynaud's syndrome by recording temperature changes in the individual's fingers before and after their submersion in ice water. Normally, digital temperature returns to pre-test level within 15 minutes, but with Raynaud's syndrome return to pre-test level takes longer than 20 minutes.

Doppler ultrasonography

Doppler ultrasonography involves the transmission of soundwaves through the skin, which are reflected from moving blood cells in underlying blood vessels. This test evaluates blood flow in the major veins and arteries in the limbs, and helps to detect peripheral vascular aneurysms and deep vein thrombosis (DVT).

Arteriography

Arteriography (angiography) is the radiographic examination of one or more arteries after injection of a contrast medium into a major artery, usually the femoral artery. Arteriography can demonstrate blood flow status, collateral circulation, vascular anomaly and tumour and aneurysm formation (Valchanov et al 2019).

Lower limb venography

Lower limb venography is the radiographic examination of a vein after an injection of contrast medium and is often used to assess the condition of deep leg veins. Venography is the definitive test for DVT but may also be used to distinguish clot formation from other forms of venous obstruction or to locate a suitable vein for arterial bypass grafting.

Impedance plethysmography

Impedance plethysmography is a non-invasive test for measuring venous flow in the limbs and is helpful for detecting DVT. Electrodes are applied to the leg to measure changes in electrical resistance that result from blood volume variations.

Assessment of haematological status

Red blood cell count

Red blood cell (RBC) (erythrocyte) count is the measurement of the number of erythrocytes found in a microlitre of blood. Together with haematocrit and haemoglobin determinations, this test is most often used to calculate mean corpuscular volume, mean corpuscular haemoglobin and mean corpuscular haemoglobin concentration (Carlson 2018).

Haematocrit

Haematocrit is a blood test used to measure the percentage of a given volume of blood occupied by erythrocytes.

Erythrocyte indices

Erythrocyte indices involve examination of the size, weight and haemoglobin content of the average erythrocyte (mean corpuscular haemoglobin and mean corpuscular haemoglobin concentration).

Total haemoglobin

Total haemoglobin measures the grams of haemoglobin (Hb) in 100 mL of whole blood.

Stained red cell examination

Stained red cell examination determines abnormalities in the size, shape or structure of erythrocytes.

Reticulocyte count

Reticulocyte count measures the number of reticulocytes present in a sample of blood, which is then expressed as a percentage of the total RBC count. (Reticulocytes are immature erythrocytes.)

Erythrocyte sedimentation rate (ESR)

ESR measures the time required for erythrocytes, in a sample of whole blood, to settle to the bottom of a vertical tube.

Erythrocyte osmotic fragility

Erythrocyte osmotic fragility measures red cell resistance to haemolysis when exposed to a hypotonic solution.

White blood cell (WBC) count

White blood cell (WBC) (leucocyte) count is the measurement of the number of white cells found in a microlitre of whole blood. A differential WBC count determines the distribution and morphology of the various WBCs and provides more information about the immune system than the WBC count (Carlson 2018).

Coagulation

Coagulation function is measured by a wide variety of tests, including:

- Platelet count, which measures the number of circulating thrombocytes (platelets).
- Bleeding time, which measures the duration of bleeding after a standardised skin incision, commonly two small punctures made on the forearm.
- Capillary fragility test, which measures the ability of capillaries to remain intact under increased intracapillary pressure. A blood pressure cuff is placed around the upper arm and inflated to midway between the systolic and diastolic pressures. After 5 minutes of sustained pressure, the number of petechiae on a selected area of the forearm are counted.
- Clot retraction test, which estimates the quantity and quality of thrombocytes and fibrinogen.
- Prothrombin time (PT), which measures the time required for a fibrin clot to form in a citrated plasma sample.
- Partial thromboplastin time (PTT), which evaluates the entire coagulation system with the exception of factors VII and XIII.
- Factor VIII activity test, which measures the amount of factor VIII in the blood and identifies a deficiency of that factor (e.g. as in haemophilia).

Immunoglobulin studies

Immunoglobulin studies evaluate the amount and types of immunoglobulins present.

Serum ferritin

Serum ferritin measurements evaluate the amount of iron stored in body tissues.

Total iron-binding capacity (TIBC)

Total iron-binding capacity (TIBC) measures the amount of available transferrin (a protein that binds with iron) in the blood.

Sickle-cell test

Sickle-cell test detects the presence of haemoglobin S in suspected sickle-cell anaemia.

Gastric fluid analysis

Gastric fluid analysis involves measuring the acidity of secretions in the stomach and is used in the diagnosis of pernicious anaemia.

Bone marrow examination

Bone marrow examination provides information about the character, integrity and production of erythrocytes, leucocytes and thrombocytes in the marrow. Bone marrow can be removed by aspiration or needle biopsy. Aspiration of bone marrow involves the removal of a small amount of bone marrow, generally less than 5 mL. Biopsy, performed under local anaesthesia, is performed when a larger amount of bone marrow is required. A needle is inserted through the skin and tissue (e.g. over the iliac crest, until it reaches bone). The needle is then directed into the marrow cavity, and a sample of bone marrow is withdrawn.

Assessment of the lymphatic system

Lymphangiography is the radiographic examination of the lymphatic system after the injection of a contrast medium into a lymphatic vessel in each foot. X-ray films are taken to demonstrate the filling of the lymphatic vessels and, 24 hours later, to visualise the lymph nodes. Clinical Interest Box 25.4 outlines additional nursing assessment of oxygenation status.

NURSING AN INDIVIDUAL WITH A RESPIRATORY AND/OR CARDIAC SYSTEM DISORDER

A holistic approach to nursing care should be delivered to individuals with a respiratory or cardiac system disorder. Specific nursing actions and medical management will vary depending on the disorder; however, the main aims of nursing care are to:

- Maintain airway patency.
- Maintain fluid and nutritional status.
- Facilitate normal and effective breathing.
- Promote efficient gas exchange.
- Promote comfort and relieve pain.
- Provide psychological support.

CLINICAL INTEREST BOX 25.4 Nursing assessment—oxygenation status

- Pulse oximetry is the non-invasive measurement used to measure oxygen saturation and is indicated in individuals who have an unstable oxygen status or at risk of impaired gas exchange.
- An assessment for risk factors that may cause a decreased oxygen saturation level should be undertaken (e.g. acute or chronic respiratory conditions, chest wall injury, recovery from anaesthesia).
- An assessment for factors that may influence the measurement should be performed (e.g. oxygen therapy, haemoglobin level, nail polish).
- A senior healthcare professional should be notified immediately of any readings lowers than SpO_2 of 95% or values specific to the person.

(Perry et al 2022)

- Maintain skin integrity.
- Promote and maintain mobility.
- Prevent infection.
- Administer prescribed medication.
- Provide care before, during and after a diagnostic test.

(AACN & Hartjes 2022)

An individual with a respiratory system disorder will commonly experience problems such as a change in breathing pattern and discomfort associated with breathing. Individuals with cardiac disorders may experience multi-system problems associated with circulation, including pain or discomfort with exercise, difficulty breathing, palpitations and fatigue. Nursing activities include alleviating discomforts associated with exercise and breathing, administering oxygen, positioning, monitoring the individual and their vital signs and helping the individual with cardiovascular and breathing exercises. As well as planning care to meet specific needs, nurses must also consider the individual's other needs, such as nutrition, fluid intake, skin integrity, elimination and the need for comfort (AACN & Hartjes 2022).

Promoting a clear airway

One of the most important aspects of care is the maintenance or restoration of a clear airway, which includes measures directed at removing secretions. Commonly, an inflammatory respiratory tract disorder results in the production of excessive secretions, made more tenacious by dehydration caused by tachypnoea, mouth breathing and pyrexia. Nursing interventions that promote a clear airway and mobilisation of pulmonary secretions help the individual achieve and maintain a clear airway and help promote lung expansion and gas exchange (Crisp et al 2021).

Adequate hydration

Dehydration can make secretions more viscous and difficult to expectorate, so an adequate fluid input is important (Pinsky et al 2019). Unless contraindicated, the individual should be encouraged to drink at least 2–3 L a day. In certain conditions, such as cardiac failure, fluid may need to be restricted to 1500 mL or less. The nurse should assess fluid balance by measuring fluid input and output and by observing for signs of oedema. Weighing the individual (e.g. each day) is another way of assessing their fluid status. If they are unable to tolerate sufficient fluids orally because of dyspnoea, nausea and/or vomiting, or the presence of an oxygen mask that can make drinking more difficult, alternative fluids may be administered by the IV route if necessary (Pinsky et al 2019).

Maintaining nutritional status

Commonly, an individual with a cardiovascular disorder will be prescribed a diet that aims to reduce serum cholesterol and triglyceride levels. Sodium intake may also be reduced (e.g. in the control and prevention of hypertension). If the individual with either a respiratory or a cardiovascular disorder is obese, a weight-reduction diet is generally prescribed. The diet generally should be low in total fat content, particularly saturated fats, and low in sodium. Kilojoules may be reduced to correct or prevent obesity, and alcohol should be restricted since it can raise kilojoule intake and serum lipid levels. Beverages and foods containing caffeine should be restricted since caffeine is a metabolic stimulant that can worsen tachycardia, hypoxaemia and arrhythmias.

In specific blood disorders, the individual may be prescribed a diet high in one or more nutrients (e.g. a diet high in iron is generally prescribed in the treatment of iron-deficiency anaemia). When a specific diet is prescribed the dietitian consults with the individual to plan the diet and to ensure that they understand any dietary modifications or restrictions.

It is important that nurses are aware of the type of diet that has been prescribed and ensure that the individual receives the correct tray at mealtimes. Nurses encourage the individual to follow the diet and may need to assist at mealtimes (e.g. if the individual is unable to eat meals/independently). (Information on assisting at mealtime is provided in Chapter 30.)

Cessation of smoking

If the individual is a smoker, they should be encouraged to stop smoking. Cigarette smoke impairs function of the cilia, and smoking generally aggravates any existing respiratory and cardiac disorder. Nurses play a crucial role in smoking cessation for individuals. Their involvement can greatly enhance the success of quitting smoking and improving overall health through intensive behavioural support, telephone counselling, and mobile tobacco cessation (mTobacco) interventions (Terzi et al 2023).

Nebulisation and humidification

As well as drinking adequate fluid, additional fluid may be administered directly into the airways by means of humidifiers, inhalations or nebulisers. Nebulisation or humidification reduces the viscosity of secretions, facilitating easy expectoration. Physiotherapy may be used concurrently. (Information on the use of humidifiers and nebulisers is provided later in this chapter.)

Positioning

If an individual with a respiratory condition experiences dyspnoea, they should be assisted into a more upright position. This facilitates alveolar expansion since gravity allows more blood to perfuse the bases of the lung, improving the ventilation/perfusion (V/Q) ratio. Nurses should ensure that sufficient pillows are placed so that the individual's back, neck, head and arms are well supported, or that the head of the bed is elevated (Pinsky et al 2019).

Medication

Medications may be prescribed to reduce pain, loosen secretions, relieve bronchospasm, increase cilia beating speed, combat infection, increase or decrease coughing, relieve pulmonary oedema, alter blood pressure and cholesterol levels or correct arrhythmias. Medications may be given by inhalation, orally or by intramuscular or IV routes. The types of medications prescribed may include analgesics, decongestants, antihistamines, antibiotics, bronchodilators or expectorants.

Oronasopharyngeal suction

If coughing is ineffective in removing secretions, suction may be necessary. Oronasopharyngeal suction removes secretions from the pharynx by means of a suction catheter inserted through the mouth or nostril. This technique is used to maintain a patent airway and is indicated for an individual who is unable to clear their airway effectively with coughing and expectoration (Pinsky et al 2019).

Chest physiotherapy

Chest physiotherapy assists the individual to mobilise and eliminate secretions, re-expand airways and alveoli and promotes the efficient use of the muscles of ventilation. Chest physiotherapy includes postural drainage, chest percussion and vibration, coughing and deep-breathing exercises (Pinsky et al 2019).

Postural drainage

Postural drainage (Figure 25.21) encourages pulmonary secretions to empty by gravity into the bronchioles, bronchi or trachea, so that they may be expectorated (Pinsky et al 2019). The individual with a respiratory disorder is assisted to assume positions that promote drainage from the affected parts of the lungs. Effectiveness of the technique largely depends on positioning that allows drainage by gravity. Postural drainage should be avoided immediately before or after meals, to prevent nausea and aspiration of food or vomitus (Pinsky et al 2019).

Percussion and vibration

Percussion and vibration are employed to help loosen respiratory secretions and are commonly used in conjunction with postural drainage (Pinsky et al 2019). Percussion is performed by rhythmic tapping using cupped hands over the affected segments of the lungs (Pinsky et al 2019). Care should be afforded to individuals with osteoporosis, fractures or recent surgery. Vibration is performed by placing the hands over the affected area and shaking, so that the chest wall is vibrated while the individual is forcibly exhaling. To ensure sufficient force is being used, the individual can be asked to vocalise and a vocal fremitus should be heard.

After postural drainage, percussion and vibration, the individual should be asked to cough to remove the loosened secretions. This is performed by a physiotherapist or allied health assistant. Oral hygiene should be attended to after the procedure because the expectorated secretions may have an offensive taste or odour.

LUNG SEGMENT	POSITION OF PATIENT	LUNG SEGMENT	POSITION OF PATIENT
Adult			
Bilateral 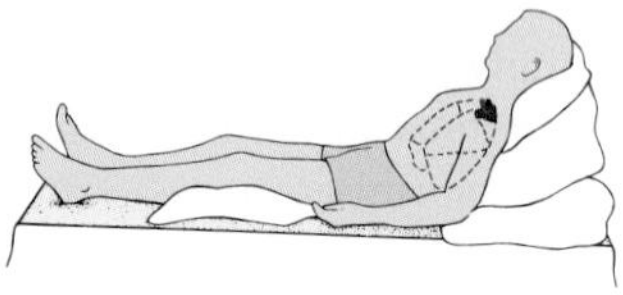	High Fowler's	Left lower lobe—lateral segment 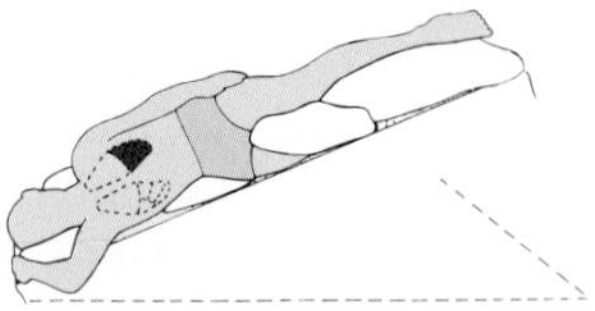	Right side-lying in Trendelenburg's position
Apical segments	Sitting on side of bed	Right lower lobe—lateral segment 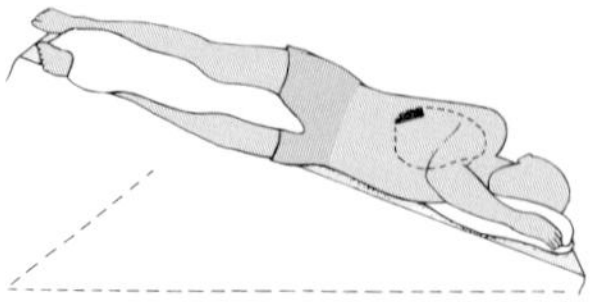	Left side-lying in Trendelenburg's position
Right upper lobe—anterior segment 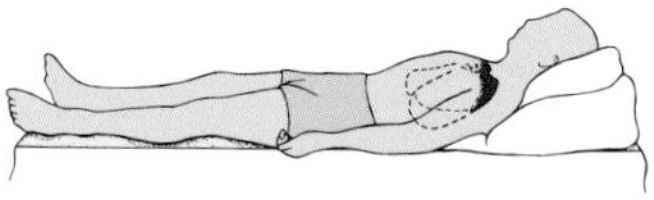	Supine with head elevated	Right lower lobe—posterior segment 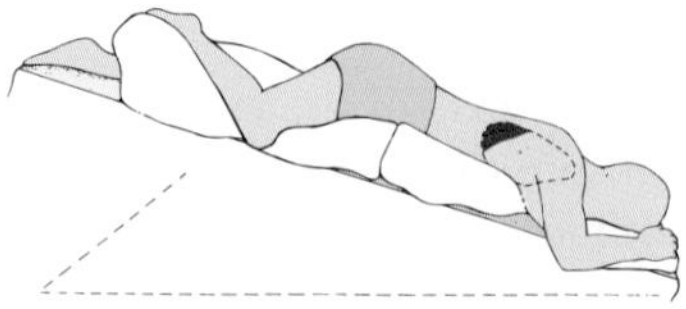	Prone with right side of chest elevated in Trendelenburg's position
Left upper lobe—anterior segment 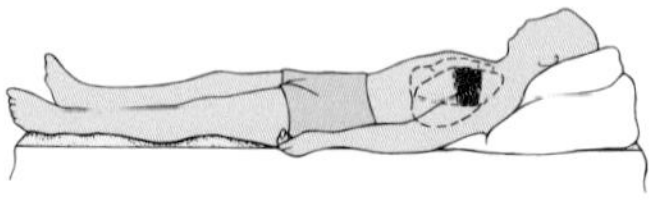	Supine with head elevated	Right middle lobe—posterior segment 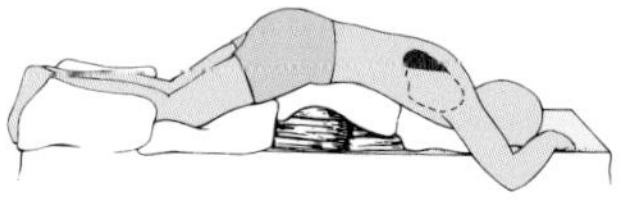	Prone with thorax and abdomen elevated
Right upper lobe—posterior segment 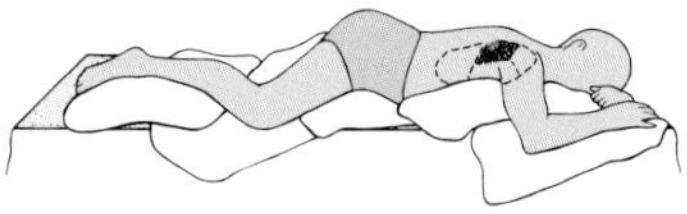	Side-lying with right side of chest elevated on pillows	Both lower lobes—anterior segments 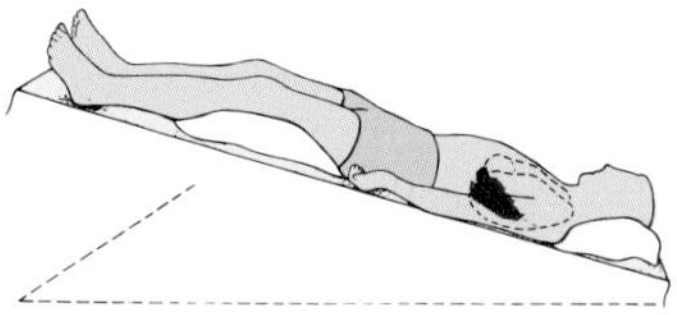	Supine in Trendelenburg's position
Left upper lobe—posterior segment 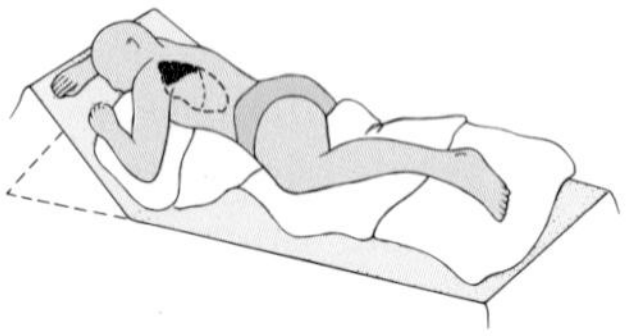	Side-lying with left side of chest elevated on pillows	Both lower lobes—posterior segments 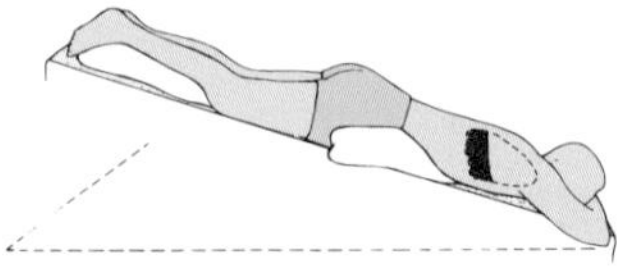	Prone in Trendelenburg's position
Right middle lobe—anterior segment 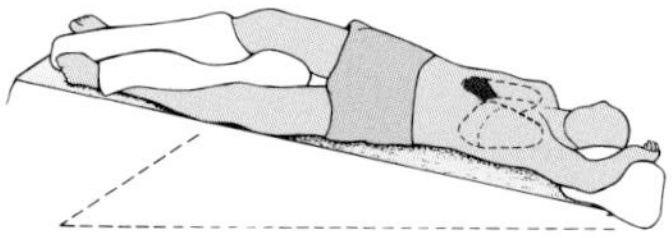	Three-quarters supine position with dependent lung in Trendelenburg's position		
Child			
Bilateral—apical segments 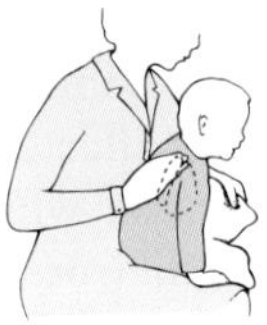	Sitting on nurse's lap, leaning slightly forwards flexed over pillow	Bilateral lobes—anterior segments 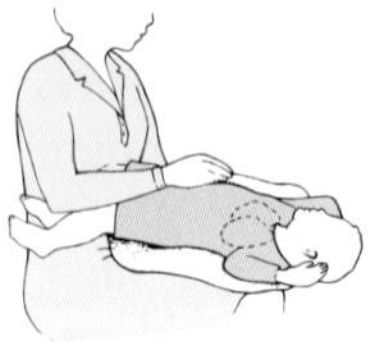	Lying supine on nurse's lap, back supported with pillow
Bilateral—middle anterior segments 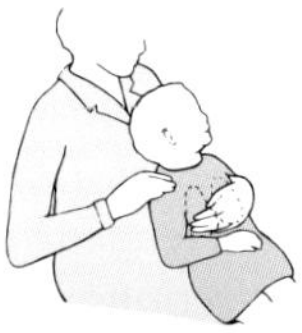	Sitting on nurse's lap, leaning against nurse		

Figure 25.21 Postural drainage

(Potter et al 2023)

Promoting comfort and relieving pain

In many disorders of the circulatory system, the aim is to increase the individual's activity progressively without pain. Comfort is promoted if the individual is provided with a bed made to meet their specific needs.

The individual may experience pain (e.g. as a result of myocardial infarction or peripheral vascular dysfunction), so relief of pain is an important aspect in the promotion of comfort. In certain respiratory conditions, such as pleurisy, severe pain may increase on inspiration. The presence of indwelling tubes, wires or cannulas all contribute to further discomfort. Pain-relieving measures, such as the administration of adequate analgesic medication, are implemented so that the individual is able to rest comfortably, sleep without discomfort and perform the activities of daily living without experiencing pain or significant side effects of the medication. The individual is also advised on what precautions to take to avoid pain, which includes identifying any precipitating factors such as physical exertion or emotional stress. The incidence of pain can generally be reduced by careful planning of activity, modifying risk factors and use of prophylactic measures (Pinsky et al 2019).

Providing psychological support

Anxiety and fear are common responses to hospitalisation. An individual who is experiencing a major respiratory or cardiovascular dysfunction, such as myocardial infarction, pneumonia or blood dyscrasias, often becomes extremely anxious, apprehensive and depressed about dyspnoea, pain, disability, loss of independence and dying. The individual and their significant others may experience great concern about the alterations in lifestyle imposed by their disorder. Nurses provide psychological support by establishing and maintaining a trusting relationship with the individual and their significant others and by encouraging them to express their feelings and concerns. They should be encouraged to discuss any lifestyle adjustments that may be necessary and they should be offered guidance on how to cope with change (Pinsky et al 2019).

Stress and anxiety can be reduced if the individual's symptoms, such as pain or dyspnoea, are alleviated, and the nurse should try to provide an environment that is as stress-free as possible. The individual should be provided with sufficient information about their illness because knowledge helps to diminish anxiety and apprehension and assists them to develop effective coping skills. All procedures, treatments and monitoring techniques being implemented are explained so that the individual understands the treatment. The individual should be encouraged to participate in their care as much as possible and, when appropriate, to gradually assume responsibility for self-care to prevent loss of independence. The individual should be informed about support groups and community resources, such as rehabilitation classes, which may be helpful after they are discharged from hospital.

Maintaining skin integrity

An individual with a respiratory, cardiac, peripheral vascular, blood or lymphatic disorder is at risk of impaired skin integrity. Decreased peripheral perfusion and oxygenation can result in skin breakdown. With poor arterial circulation, the tissues lack adequate oxygen and nutrients and this can lead to cellulitis, ulcers, poor wound healing and necrosis. Maintenance of skin integrity includes:

- assessing the skin for any signs of breakdown
- keeping the skin clean and dry
- protecting the extremities from exposure to extremes of temperature and from trauma
- position changes to avoid prolonged pressure on the skin
- the use of accessories (e.g. a sheepskin) to reduce pressure
- promoting mobility.

(Pinsky et al 2019)

Preventing skin breakdown includes keeping the feet clean and dry, avoiding rough drying movements, using creams or lotions that prevent drying and cracking, avoiding scratching itchy areas on the legs or feet, providing nail care by a podiatrist and protecting the feet with socks, slippers or well-fitting shoes.

Promoting and maintaining mobility

Maintenance of mobility is necessary to prevent the complications of immobility, such as decubitus ulcers, venous stasis and pulmonary complications. Problems of immobility should be counteracted with position changes, range-of-motion (ROM) exercises, and coughing and deep-breathing exercises. Ambulation of the individual as soon as possible is important to prevent the complications of immobility (Pinsky et al 2019).

In the initial stages of illness, such as immediately after myocardial infarction, the individual's level of activity may be reduced to a minimum. As their tolerance increases, their level of physical activity gradually increases. The individual should understand the importance of adequate physical exercise, which provides the necessary muscle contraction for movement of arterial blood and lymph to and from the peripheral areas of the body. Exercise or activity programs are generally implemented gradually, and the individual is encouraged to rest after the exercise periods. As the individual's condition improves, moderate exercise is encouraged as long as pain is not induced.

Preventing infection

An individual with any of the disorders mentioned previously may be susceptible to infection as a result of nosocomial infections, altered nutritional status, medications such as steroids, invasive procedures and changes in immune status. Measures to prevent infection must be implemented, such as good handwashing techniques, and aseptic techniques for any procedure. Precautions must be taken to prevent damage to the skin or mucous membranes, as injured tissues create a portal for bacterial invasion. If the individual's WBC count is low (leucopenia), it may be necessary to use protective isolation techniques to protect them against infection. The individual must be monitored closely to detect the early manifestations of infection so that appropriate treatment can be prescribed (Pinsky et al 2019).

Promoting effective breathing and aeration

In addition to the measures employed to promote a clear airway, other measures may be necessary to maintain adequate ventilation. Breathing exercises may be used by the individual to promote and maintain optimal pulmonary ventilation, and oxygen may be prescribed to supplement that being obtained from the atmosphere.

Breathing exercises

When respiratory system disorders produce ineffective breathing patterns and inadequate ventilation, the individual may be educated to perform deep-breathing exercises or airway clearance techniques (Pinsky et al 2019).

Deep breathing

Deep, or diaphragmatic, breathing uses the diaphragm and abdominal muscles to fully ventilate the lungs. The individual should be assisted into a sitting position to promote optimal alveolar expansion. One hand is placed on the chest and the other hand is placed on the abdomen. If the individual is breathing correctly, the hand on the abdomen should rise with inhalation and fall with exhalation; the hand on the chest should remain still. The individual is educated to inhale deeply and slowly, pushing the abdomen out, to promote optimal distribution of air to the alveoli. Individuals may also be educated to exhale through pursed lips, while contracting their abdomen. Exhalation through pursed lips improves ventilation pressures and encourages a slow deep-breathing pattern. Abdominal contraction pushes the diaphragm upwards, exerts pressure on the lungs and helps to empty them.

Breathing exercises are performed according to the individual's condition (e.g. short sessions may be indicated if the individual becomes fatigued easily). The duration and frequency with which deep-breathing exercises are performed vary; they may, for example, be performed for 1 minute, with gradual progression to a 10-minute exercise period four times daily (Pinsky et al 2019).

Incentive spirometry/peak flow

Incentive spirometry (Figure 25.22) uses a breathing device to encourage the individual to achieve maximal ventilation. The device measures peak respiratory flow or respiratory volume, and requires the individual to take a deep, slow breath and hold it for several seconds; this allows the alveolar to hyperinflate. The exercise is inexpensive, simple to use and does not require supervision once the individual is trained (Toor et al 2021). See Clinical Skill 25.2 for incentive spirometry/peak flow.

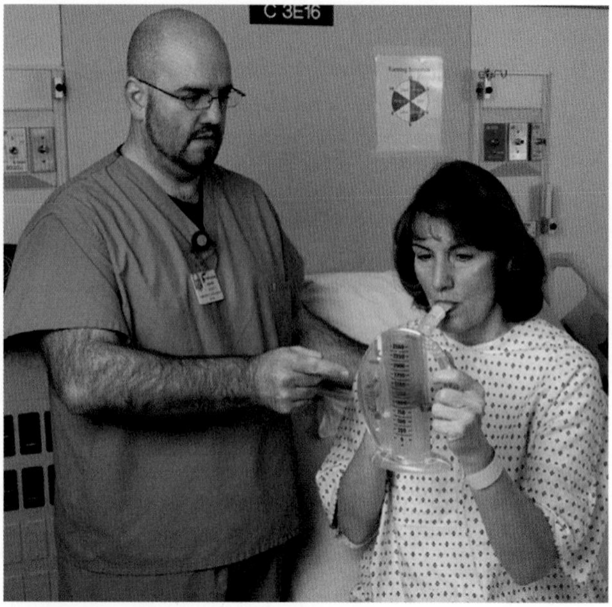

Figure 25.22 Spirometry

(Potter et al 2013)

Oxygen therapy

An individual with a respiratory system disorder may be prescribed supplemental oxygen to be administered intermittently or continuously. The administration of oxygen is discussed in more detail later in this chapter.

Promoting efficient gas exchange

Any disorder of the respiratory system may result in impaired gas exchange (AACN & Hartjes 2022). Depending on the extent to which it interferes with ventilation and perfusion, hypercapnia, **hypocapnia** and/or hypoxaemia may develop. The aim of management of these conditions is to maintain adequate oxygenation and removal of carbon dioxide (AACN & Hartjes 2022). In addition to the measures already described, which promote a clear airway and effective breathing, other measures may be necessary, including the insertion of an artificial airway and/or mechanical ventilation. (Information on both these topics is provided later in this chapter.) The nurse must observe the individual for the signs and symptoms of impaired gas exchange (see Table 25.3). Clinical Interest Box 25.5 outlines cardiopulmonary health promotion for young to older adults.

Specific interventions

Specific nursing interventions relevant to caring for an individual with a respiratory system disorder include:

- collecting specimens of sputum
- obtaining nasal or throat swabs
- administering oxygen
- suction via the oral, nasal or tracheal routes
- inhalation therapy.

(Pinsky et al 2019)

CLINICAL SKILL 25.2 Incentive spirometry

Please adhere to the policy and procedures of the facility/organisation prior to undertaking the skill. Ensure this skill is in your scope of practice.

NMBA Decision-making Framework considerations (refer to NMBA Decision-making framework for nursing and midwifery 2020):	Equipment:
1. Am I educated? 2. Am I authorised? 3. Am I competent? If you answer 'no' to any of these, do not perform that activity. Seek guidance and support from your teacher/a nurse team leader/clinical facilitator/educator.	Incentive spirometer Disposable mouthpiece/tube

PREPARE FOR THE SKILL

(Please refer to the Standard Steps on pp. xviii–xx for related rationales.)
Mentally review the steps of the skill.
Discuss the skill with your instructor/supervisor/team leader, if required.
Confirm correct facility/organisation policy/safe operating procedures.
Validate the order in the individual's record.
Identify indication and rationale for performing the activity.
Assess for any contraindications.
Locate and gather equipment.
Perform hand hygiene.
Ensure therapeutic interaction.
Identify the individual using three individual identifiers.
Gain the individual's consent.
Assess for pain relief.
Prepare the environment.
Provide and maintain privacy.
Assist the individual to assume an appropriate position of comfort.

Skill activity	Rationale
Sit individual into an upright position (if able) and lean forwards either on side of the bed or in a chair.	Facilitates breathing and lung expansion.

PERFORM THE SKILL

(Please refer to the Standard Steps on pp. xviii–xx for related rationales.)
Perform hand hygiene.
Apply PPE: gloves, eyewear, mask and gown as appropriate.
Ensure the individual's safety and comfort throughout skill.
Promote independence and involvement of the individual if possible and/or appropriate.
Assess the individual's tolerance to the skill throughout.
Dispose of used supplies, equipment, waste and sharps appropriately.
Remove PPE and discard or store appropriately.

Skill activity	Rationale
Instruct the individual to practise inhaling and exhaling three times, letting all of their last breath out. Ask them to place their lips over the mouthpiece of the spirometer.	Enables the person to practise inhaling and exhaling. Allows for more accurate results.
Instruct the individual to inhale slowly (elevating the balls or cylinder) and hold their breath for 2–3 seconds, then exhale slowly.	Slow breathing prevents or minimises pain from sudden pressure change in the chest. Holding their breath and slowing exhalation helps to maintain maximal inspiration and reduces the risk of progressive collapse of individual alveoli. Prevents anxiety.

Continued

CLINICAL SKILL 25.2 Incentive spirometry—cont'd

Ask the person to remove the mouthpiece, and relax and breathe slowly for a few seconds.	Alleviates anxiety and relaxes chest.
Repeat for a total of 10 times every hour or as indicated by the doctor/physiotherapist If they feel light-headed or dizzy, ask the individual to slow down their breathing and wait longer intervals between cycles. Once 10 cycles have been completed ask the individual to cough up and expectorate any sputum.	Allows for chest clearance and proper expansion of the lungs and prevents atelectasis. Coughing can facilitate removal of any secretions. Feeling light-headed and dizzy is a normal reaction; provide reassurance to alleviate anxiety.

AFTER THE SKILL

(Please refer to the Standard Steps on pp. xviii–xx for related rationales.)
Communicate outcome to the individual, any ongoing care and to report any complications.
Restore the environment.
Report, record and document assessment findings, details of the skill performed and the individual's response.
Report, record and document any abnormalities and/or inability to perform the skill.
Reassess the individual to ensure there are no adverse effects/events from the skill.

(Crisp et al 2021; Perry et al 2022)

TABLE 25.3 | Impaired gas exchange

Condition	Possible cause	Manifestations
Respiratory acidosis (hypercapnia)	Hypoventilation as a result of chronic obstructive pulmonary disease, pneumonia, drugs or trauma	Flushed warm skin, hypertension, tachycardia, headaches, drowsiness, confusion, irritability, coma
Respiratory alkalosis (hypocapnia)	Hyperventilation as a result of acute asthma, cerebral trauma or congestive cardiac failure	Diaphoresis, pallor, tachypnoea, tingling and numbness in the limbs, or around the mouth, carpopedal spasm (tetany) and convulsions
Hypoxia	Obstructive lung diseases, and restrictive lung diseases (e.g. chronic bronchitis, emphysema, sarcoidosis)	Pallor or cyanosis, tachypnoea, tachycardia, breathlessness, headaches, irritability, confusion

Collecting sputum

Sputum is a mucus secretion produced by the mucous membranes that line the respiratory tract. Mucus secretion increases in response to inflammation, infection or congestion. Laboratory examination of sputum may be necessary to determine whether any microorganisms, blood or malignant cells are present. The nurse should observe the sputum, noting the amount, consistency, colour and presence of blood or odour. Sputum is normally clear in colour but may turn white if the individual smokes or has a viral infection; yellow, rust-coloured or green to dark-brown sputum may indicate the presence of an infection. It may be tinged with blood or contain streaks of blood that can suggest inflammation, dryness or infection or conditions such as pulmonary oedema or carcinoma. The consistency varies from watery to mucoid to tenacious.

When a specimen of sputum is required, it is best collected early in the morning before any food or fluid is given since this ensures that there is an accumulation of secretions to be obtained. To avoid the risk of cross-infection with airborne microorganisms the nurse should stand beside rather than in front of an individual when collecting the sputum specimen. Sputum for laboratory testing should be free of saliva and food particles (see Clinical Skill 25.3 for collection of sputum) (Pinsky et al 2019).

Nasopharyngeal and throat swabs

Laboratory examination of secretions from the nasopharynx or throat may be necessary to determine the presence of pathogenic microorganisms. Collection of a specimen involves swabbing the inflamed tissues and collecting any exudate with a sterile cottonwool-tipped swab. The

CLINICAL INTEREST BOX 25.5 Cardiopulmonary health promotion for young to older adults

- Maintain ideal body weight.
- Eat a low-fat, low-salt, kilojoule-appropriate diet.
- Monitor cholesterol and triglyceride levels.
- Engage in regular aerobic exercise.
- Use stress-reduction techniques.
- Be smoke free.
- Avoid second-hand smoke and other pollutants.
- Use a filter mask when exposed to occupational hazards.
- Monitor blood pressure.
- Get an annual influenza vaccine if at risk of developing influenza.
- Get a pneumococcal vaccine if appropriate.
- Reduce exposure to secondary infections.

(Crisp et al 2021)

nurse should refer to the healthcare institution's policy manual for information about the type of applicator, culture tube and transport medium to use (see Clinical Skill 25.4 for collecting a nasopharyngeal swab) (Pinsky et al 2019).

Oronasopharyngeal suction

Oronasopharyngeal suction may be required when secretions or foreign substances are causing an obstruction to the individual's airway. Suction is indicated for the individual who is unable to clear the airway effectively with coughing and expectoration, such as the severely debilitated or unconscious individual. The removal of excess secretions and mucus from the airway aids breathing, promotes pulmonary gas exchange and prevents the accumulation of secretions that may cause secondary atelectasis or pneumonia. Suctioning is achieved by means of a catheter, which is introduced through the mouth or nose into the pharynx. The basic equipment consists of:

- wall suction or portable suction apparatus
- collection bottle
- connecting tubing
- water suitable for flushing the catheter and tubing in a small container
- sterile suction catheters
- protective glasses
- disposable gloves
- tongue depressor.

(Pinsky et al 2019)

Suction equipment is usually kept in readiness at the bedside if there is an indication that it may be needed frequently, as an emergency measure or as part of the healthcare institution's policies. In general, the pressure is set at

CLINICAL SKILL 25.3 Collection of sputum

Please adhere to the policy and procedures of the facility/organisation prior to undertaking the skill. Ensure this skill is in your scope of practice.

NMBA Decision-making Framework considerations	Equipment:
NMBA Decision-making Framework considerations (refer to NMBA Decision-making framework for nursing and midwifery 2020): 1. Am I educated? 2. Am I authorised? 3. Am I competent? If you answer 'no' to any of these, do not perform that activity. Seek guidance and support from your teacher/a nurse team leader/clinical facilitator/educator.	**Equipment:** Disposable gloves Sterile specimen container Tissues Biohazard bag Pathology form—completed by the medical officer Mouth care equipment

PREPARE FOR THE SKILL

(Please refer to the Standard Steps on pp. xviii–xx for related rationales.)
Mentally review the steps of the skill.
Discuss the skill with your instructor/supervisor/team leader, if required.
Confirm correct facility/organisation policy/safe operating procedures.
Validate the order in the individual's record.
Identify indication and rationale for performing the activity.
Assess for any contraindications.
Locate and gather equipment. Perform hand hygiene.
Ensure therapeutic interaction.
Identify the individual using three individual identifiers.
Gain the individual's consent.
Assess for pain relief.
Prepare the environment.
Provide and maintain privacy.
Assist the individual to assume an appropriate position of comfort.

Continued

CLINICAL SKILL 25.3 Collection of sputum—cont'd

Skill activity	Rationale
Check the pathology form, ensuring that it is completed, and verify details with the individual.	Ensures need for the procedure and prevents errors. Assist the person to a sitting position.
Offer mouth care/rinse out the mouth with water.	Facilitates coughing and expectoration. Reduces contamination of the specimen with any debris in the mouth.

PERFORM THE SKILL

(Please refer to the Standard Steps on pp. xviii–xx for related rationales.)
Perform hand hygiene.
Apply PPE: gloves, eyewear, mask and gown as appropriate.
Ensure the individual's safety and comfort throughout skill.
Promote independence and involvement of the individual if possible and/or appropriate.
Assess the individual's tolerance to the skill throughout.
Dispose of used supplies, equipment, waste and sharps appropriately.
Remove PPE and discard or store appropriately.
Perform hand hygiene.

Skill activity	Rationale
Ask the person to start deep breathing and coughing to help facilitate sputum expectoration.	Facilitates coughing and expectoration. A normal saline nebuliser (if ordered) may be required to help loosen sputum and facilitate expectoration.
Instruct the person to cough and to expectorate 15–30 mL of sputum into a sterile specimen container.	A sterile container ensures that the specimen is not contaminated.
Place the lid on the container, wipe the outside of the container if contaminated.	Prevents cross-infection.
Ensure that the container is clearly labelled with the relevant information. Specimen container is placed in the zip lock section of the plastic biohazard bag.	Ensures the correct person's sputum is tested to avoid errors.
Pathology request form is checked for the person's details. The pathology request form is placed in the other section of the bag.	Ensures correct form and specimen are sent to pathology department and correct test will be undertaken in the pathology department.
Offer/perform oral hygiene using a mouth swab and/or mouth rinse.	Reduces bad taste or halitosis in mouth. Clears the mouth of residual secretions.

AFTER THE SKILL

(Please refer to the Standard Steps on pp. xviii–xx for related rationales.)
Communicate outcome to the individual, any ongoing care and to report any complications.
Restore the environment.
Report, record and document assessment findings, details of the skill performed and the individual's response.
Report, record and document any abnormalities and/or inability to perform the skill.
Reassess the individual to ensure there are no adverse effects/events from the skill.

Skill activity	Rationale
The specimen should be transported to the laboratory as soon as possible, or stored in a refrigerator until transport can be arranged.	Proliferation of microorganisms occurs if the specimen is not dispatched as soon as possible after collection.

(Carter & Notter 2024; Perry et al 2022)

CLINICAL SKILL 25.4 Collecting a nasopharyngeal (nasal) or nasalpharynx (throat) swab

Please adhere to the policy and procedures of the facility/organisation prior to undertaking the skill. Ensure this skill is in your scope of practice.

NMBA Decision-making Framework considerations (refer to NMBA Decision-making framework for nursing and midwifery 2020):	Equipment:
1. Am I educated? 2. Am I authorised? 3. Am I competent? If you answer 'no' to any of these, do not perform that activity. Seek guidance and support from your teacher/a nurse team leader/clinical facilitator/educator.	Disposable gloves Pathology form completed by medical officer Tissues Biohazard bag Normal saline 0.9% Penlight torch Tongue depressor Throat swab

PREPARE FOR THE SKILL

(Please refer to the Standard Steps on pp. xviii–xx for related rationales.)
Mentally review the steps of the skill.
Discuss the skill with your instructor/supervisor/team leader, if required.
Confirm correct facility/organisation policy/safe operating procedures.
Validate the order in the individual's record.
Identify indication and rationale for performing the activity.
Assess for any contraindications.
Locate and gather equipment.
Perform hand hygiene.
Ensure therapeutic interaction.
Identify the individual using three individual identifiers.
Gain the individual's consent.
Assess for pain relief.
Prepare the environment.
Provide and maintain privacy.
Assist the individual to assume an appropriate position of comfort.

Skill activity	Rationale
Check the pathology form, ensuring that it is completed, and verify details with the individual.	Ensures need for the procedure and prevents errors.
Inform the individual that they may experience the urge to sneeze or gag during the swabbing.	Reduces anxiety/apprehension and gains trust and cooperation. Promotes participation in care and understanding of health status.
Assist the person, if possible, to a sitting position.	Facilitates collection of the specimen.

PERFORM THE SKILL

(Please refer to the Standard Steps on pp. xviii–xx for related rationales.)
Perform hand hygiene.
Apply PPE: gloves, eyewear, mask and gown as appropriate.
Ensure the individual's safety and comfort throughout skill.
Promote independence and involvement of the individual if possible and/or appropriate.
Assess the individual's tolerance to the skill throughout.
Dispose of used supplies, equipment, waste and sharps appropriately.
Remove PPE and discard or store appropriately.
Perform hand hygiene.

Continued

CLINICAL SKILL 25.4 Collecting a nasopharyngeal (nasal) or nasalpharynx (throat) swab—cont'd

Skill activity	Rationale
For a nasopharyngeal (nose) swab: Request the person to blow their nose. If the nasal passage is dry, dip the tip of the swab into the normal saline. Request the individual to tilt their head back. Insert the swab 2 cm into each nostril, rotating against the anterior nasal mucosa.	Clears the nasal passages. Prevents trauma. Normal saline prevents degradation of viruses or bacteria. Facilitates collection of the specimen.
For a swab of the nasopharynx (throat): Request the individual to open their mouth, depress the tongue with a tongue depressor and use a torch to illuminate the throat. If the throat is dry, dip the tip of the swab into normal saline. Ask the person to say 'ah'. Pass the swab over the tonsils, posterior pharyngeal wall and posterior edge of the soft palate.	Gentle insertion prevents tissue damage. Do not force the swab. Facilitates access and visualisation. Prevents trauma and facilitates the collection of microorganisms. Normal saline prevents degradation of viruses or bacteria. Raises the uvula to expose proper site of collection.
Ensure that the container is clearly labelled with the relevant information. Specimen container is placed in the zip lock section of the plastic biohazard bag.	Ensures the correct specimen is tested to avoid errors.
Pathology request form is checked for the person's details. The pathology request form is placed in the other section of the bag.	Ensures correct form and specimen are sent to pathology department and correct test will be undertaken in the pathology department.

AFTER THE SKILL

(Please refer to the Standard Steps on pp. xviii–xx for related rationales.)
Communicate outcome to the individual, any ongoing care and to report any complications.
Restore the environment.
Report, record and document assessment findings, details of the skill performed and the individual's response.
Report, record and document any abnormalities and/or inability to perform the skill.
Reassess the individual to ensure there are no adverse effects/events from the skill.

Skill activity	Rationale
The specimen should be transported to the laboratory as soon as possible.	Proliferation of microorganisms occurs if the specimen is not dispatched as soon as possible after collection.

(Perry et al 2022)

80–120 mmHg for an adult (and considerably lower for a child), depending on the diameter of the catheter and the viscosity of the secretions. The medical officer will prescribe the level of suction to be used. If using the nasal route, suctioning should be alternated between the left and right nostrils to reduce trauma to the one nostril. It may also be necessary to lubricate the tip of the catheter with a sterile water-soluble lubricant before insertion into the nostril. (See Clinical Interest Box 25.6 and Clinical Skill 25.5.)

Inhalation therapy

Various forms of inhalation therapy may be prescribed for an individual with a respiratory disorder, including humidified air or oxygen, and nebulised air or oxygen. These can be administered by aerosol devices, electric nebulisers and humidifiers or an intermittent positive-pressure ventilator.

Electrical humidifiers and nebulisers

Water vapour may be provided by means of a humidity cot, tent or via a mask or tube attached to the individual. Various electrical devices can provide both humidification and nebulisation, depending on the fitting used. The device has water fed by a sterile container to an electrically warmed core that heats up the fluid contained in it as it passes through a chamber. The warmed water vapour is delivered to the individual via large-bore corrugated tubing and the oxygen

CLINICAL INTEREST BOX 25.6 Promote safety and comfort when suctioning

If performed incorrectly, suctioning can cause serious harm. During suctioning, the oxygen supply is disrupted. This action has the potential to result in adverse effects on the respiratory, cardiovascular and nervous systems, ranging from modified respiratory function to life-threatening complications.

(Perry et al 2022)

concentration can be regulated from room air to 100% oxygen by means of an oxygen venturi-type diluter. The individual inhales the vapour through a nebuliser-type mask.

Nebulisation provides a visible mist of large water droplets that are delivered into the airways. Nebulisation is used to treat atelectasis and airway infections and to loosen and decrease the viscosity of secretions to facilitate expectoration. It can be delivered through a mask or tracheotomy tube. Humidification provides water vapour in an almost invisible fine mist of small droplets that can travel further into the airways than by nebulisation by virtue of the droplet size and weight. Humidification is used to provide humidity to prevent stasis of mucus, tissue dehydration and to reduce drying,

CLINICAL SKILL 25.5 Oronasopharyngeal suction

Please adhere to the policy and procedures of the facility/organisation prior to undertaking the skill. Ensure this skill is in your scope of practice.

NMBA Decision-making Framework considerations	Equipment
NMBA Decision-making Framework considerations (refer to NMBA Decision-making framework for nursing and midwifery 2020): 1. Am I educated? 2. Am I authorised? 3. Am I competent? If you answer 'no' to any of these, do not perform that activity. Seek guidance and support from your teacher/a nurse team leader/clinical facilitator/educator.	**Equipment:** Suction catheter Suction apparatus Suction tubing Yankauer suction catheter Disposable gloves Oronasopharyngeal tube Sterile water and infectious waste bag Normal saline 0.9% (if ordered) Waterproof pad Goggles or face shield (if appropriate)

PREPARE FOR THE SKILL

(Please refer to the Standard Steps on pp. xviii–xx for related rationales.)

Mentally review the steps of the skill.
Discuss the skill with your instructor/supervisor/team leader, if required.
Confirm correct facility/organisation policy/safe operating procedures.
Validate the order in the individual's record.
Identify indication and rationale for performing the activity.
Assess for any contraindications.
Locate and gather equipment.
Perform hand hygiene.
Ensure therapeutic interaction.
Identify the individual using three individual identifiers.
Gain the individual's consent.
Assess for pain relief.
Prepare the environment.
Provide and maintain privacy.
Assist the individual to assume an appropriate position of comfort.

Skill activity	Rationale
Perform an assessment of the individual, ensuring their vital signs are stable and their oxygen saturations are adequate to allow for the suctioning. If possible, position the individual in a sitting position or with the neck extended. Place a waterproof pad across individual's chest.	Ensures the individual is stable so as to prevent complications. A burst of oxygen or normal saline nebuliser may be required prior (if ordered) to help loosen secretions and allow for better clearance of mucus during suctioning. Promotes lung expansion and effective coughing.

Continued

CLINICAL SKILL 25.5 Oronasopharyngeal suction—cont'd

PERFORM THE SKILL

(Please refer to the Standard Steps on pp. xviii–xx for related rationales.)
Perform hand hygiene.
Apply PPE: gloves, eyewear, mask and gown as appropriate.
Ensure the individual's safety and comfort throughout skill.
Promote independence and involvement of the individual if possible and/or appropriate.
Assess the individual's tolerance to the skill throughout.
Dispose of used supplies, equipment, waste and sharps appropriately.
Remove PPE and discard or store appropriately.
Perform hand hygiene.

Skill activity	Rationale
Remove oxygen mask or nasal cannulae if in situ.	Facilitates catheter insertion. **Note:** If suctioning required due to a mucus plug this will facilitate better oxygen saturations.
Attach collection bottle to the suction unit, attach connecting tubing, connector and catheter.	Equipment must be assembled and checked for function before the procedure starts.
Turn on the suction and dip the tip of the catheter into sterile water.	Lubricates the catheter to facilitate insertion. Prevents the introduction of microorganisms.
With the suction off (e.g. by using the Y-connector), gently introduce the catheter into the mouth or nostril. If the oral route is used, the individual's tongue may be depressed with a tongue depressor.	Suction during insertion may damage the mucosa. Facilitates insertion of the suction catheter. Do not put the catheter into the nose and then the mouth. Ensure it is cleaned between suctions.
Ensure that suction pressure is below 120 mmHg. Apply suction as the catheter is withdrawn, rotating the catheter as it is being withdrawn.	Pressure above 120 mmHg may damage the mucosa. Rotating motion prevents tissue trauma and obtains maximal volume of secretions. **Note:** Do not force the catheter into the nasal cavity as this can cause trauma. When suctioning neonates, infants or children, ensure correct measurement is obtained of their nasal cavity to ensure the catheter is not inserted too far, which may cause irreversible damage.
Apply suction for a maximum of 5–10-second intervals, or less in the young or critically unwell individual, then remove from the airway. Allow the individual time to rest (30 seconds) between suctioning.	Suctioning for longer than 10 seconds can cause tissue trauma and hypoxia. Allows the individual time to rest and replace oxygen until the next suction.
If secretions are tenacious, dip the tip of the catheter into the sterile water and apply suction. If a specimen is required for virology or bacterial studies, use of normal saline is recommended.	Clears the lumen of catheter. Normal saline prevents degradation of viruses or bacteria.
Repeat the procedure, if necessary, until the mucus obstruction has been removed.	Promotes a clear airway.
After suctioning, instruct the individual (if able) to take several slow deep breaths.	Relieves hypoxia and promotes relaxation. Facilitates coughing.
Dip the catheter into the sterile water and apply suction.	Clears catheter and connecting tubing. Prevents the reintroduction of microorganisms and contamination.

CLINICAL SKILL 25.5 Oronasopharyngeal suction—cont'd

AFTER THE SKILL

(Please refer to the Standard Steps on pp. xviii–xx for related rationales.)
Communicate outcome to the individual, any ongoing care and to report any complications.
Restore the environment.
Report, record and document assessment findings, details of the skill performed and the individual's response.
Report, record and document any abnormalities and/or inability to perform the skill.
Reassess the individual to ensure there are no adverse effects/events from the skill.

(Perry et al 2022; Rebeiro et al 2021)

inflammation and irritation of the air passages. These devices provide precise control of oxygen delivery and protection against cross-contamination by means of a sterile pre-filled container of solution, such as sterile water or normal saline.

Other similar devices are used in positive-pressure ventilators, such as Bird or Bennet ventilators, to deliver humidity or medication to an individual on a ventilator or during intermittent positive-pressure breathing therapy. Nurses should know their role and responsibilities regarding inhalation therapy and administration of medications, and should be familiar with the healthcare facility's infection control guidelines. The nurse should check the devices hourly for leaks, cracks and oxygen concentration. Bedding and clothing are changed as soon as they become damp. Care should also be taken to observe the skin surrounding the mask for signs of breakdown.

Mechanical and electrical nebulisers are used to deliver moisture or medication as a fine mist into the airways of individuals with conditions such as asthma or emphysema. Bronchodilators are commonly prescribed in the management of asthma. The devices operate off mains or 12-volt power and are generally used by individuals at home, commonly in individuals with airways disease due to the hypoxic drive effect. Care must be taken to ensure that the device is placed on a stable surface, and regular maintenance of the filters is required.

Gas-driven nebulisers are used with compressed air or oxygen to deliver nebulised vapour or medication. The prescribed solution is inserted into the nebuliser, either alone or together with a prescribed amount of sterile water or saline, and one end of the oxygen tubing is attached to the nebuliser, which is directly connected to a nebuliser mask. The other end of the tubing is attached to an oxygen regulator and then to the pressurised gas source, which is turned on to check for proper misting. To produce particles of the correct size and to better ensure their arrival at the most distal airways, a flow rate of 6–10 L/min is generally recommended. The individual is instructed to breathe deeply, slowly and evenly through the mouthpiece or mask and to hold their breath for 2–3 seconds at the end of inhalation to receive the full benefit of the medication. The individual should be encouraged to cough and expectorate.

Steam inhalations are not generally used because of the risk of burns and the improved effectiveness in providing fluids by other means.

Mechanical ventilation

Mechanical ventilation is sometimes indicated for an individual with a respiratory system disorder. Mechanical ventilation artificially assists or controls respiration and it is indicated to correct or prevent gas transport abnormalities. To maintain adequate pulmonary blood gas exchange, an endotracheal or tracheostomy tube is inserted (see below) and connected to the ventilator.

A variety of ventilators are available, which may be one of two main types: pressure controlled or volume controlled. With the pressure-controlled ventilator, the gas is delivered to the lungs until a predetermined pressure is reached, then inspiration is terminated. With a volume-controlled ventilator, a set volume of gas is delivered with each inspiration. The ventilation rate may be pre-set, controlled by the individual, or may be a combination of both.

Care of an individual receiving mechanical ventilation should be provided by nursing staff who are qualified and experienced to provide it. An individual who requires mechanical ventilation is generally nursed in an intensive care unit (ICU) since they require constant physical attention and emotional support.

THE INDIVIDUAL WITH AN ARTIFICIAL AIRWAY

The placement of an artificial airway is indicated to relieve obstruction, to facilitate suctioning of the lower respiratory tract, to prevent aspiration or to allow for mechanical ventilation. Artificial airways include the oropharyngeal airway, the endotracheal tube and the tracheostomy tube.

Oropharyngeal airway

An oropharyngeal airway (Figure 25.23) is a curved rubber or plastic device inserted into the mouth to the posterior pharynx to establish or maintain a patent airway (Potter et al 2023). The airway allows air to pass around and through the tube and facilitates oropharyngeal suctioning (Pinsky et al 2019).

It is used for the short term only, such as in the immediate post-anaesthetic period. If an individual requires respiratory assistance for a longer period, an endotracheal or tracheostomy tube is generally used.

Endotracheal tube

An endotracheal tube is a flexible cuffed tube inserted via the mouth or nostril through the larynx into the trachea (Figure 25.24). Endotracheal intubation establishes and maintains a patent airway, prevents aspiration by sealing the trachea off from the digestive tract, facilitates the removal of tracheobronchial secretions and provides a means whereby optimal ventilation can be achieved. Endotracheal intubation may be required in an emergency or for an elective procedure requiring airway securement and oxygenation.

The tube is inserted by a medical officer, who uses a laryngoscope to visualise the trachea and facilitate the passage of the tube. Most endotracheal tubes in adults have a cuff, which is inflated with air to provide a seal that prevents the leakage of air around the tube when the individual is ventilated. Uncuffed tubes are generally used in infants and children unless there is excessive leakage of air past the tube. To avoid inadvertent removal or displacement of the tube, string and tape may be applied to secure the tube in position. Continuous expert care is required after endotracheal intubation to ensure airway patency and to prevent complications. An individual who has been intubated is generally nursed in an ICU and receives constant physical attention and emotional support.

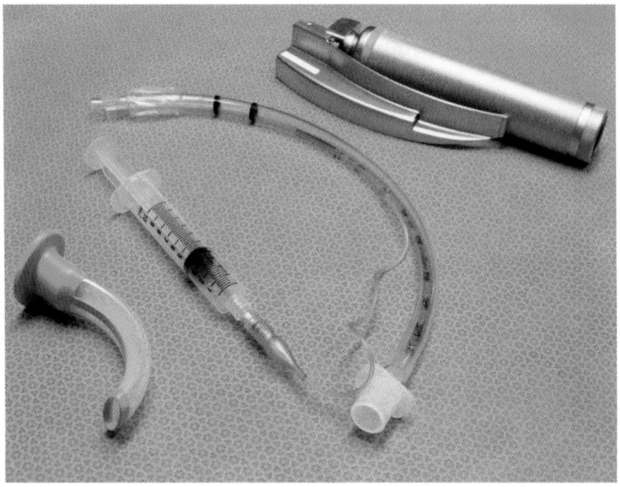

Figure 25.24 Equipment to insert an endotracheal tube (ETT)

Left to right: oropharyngeal airway (bite block), 10-mL syringe to inflate the cuff, cuffed ETT, and laryngoscope.

(Stein & Hollen 2024)

Tracheostomy

A tracheostomy (Figure 25.25) is a surgical creation of an external opening into the trachea, and may be performed as an emergency temporary measure, a permanent measure or during prolonged mechanical ventilation (Deng et al 2021). The insertion of a tracheostomy tube aims to provide a patent airway, prevent aspiration of secretions, allow removal of tracheobronchial secretion by suction and permit the use of a mechanical ventilation device (Flaherty 2020).

A tracheostomy tube is a short curved tube fitted with a flange that assists in stabilising the tube. Tracheostomy tubes are available in a range of styles, materials and sizes and usually have an inner and outer cannula (Flaherty 2020). Some tracheostomy tubes are fitted with an inflatable cuff that forms a seal in the airway to create positive pressure ventilation (Flaherty 2020; Pruitt 2022). The choice of tracheostomy tube is dependent upon clinical factors, such as respiratory status, airway anatomy and pathology, and the clinical setting in which the person is being cared for (Flaherty 2020).

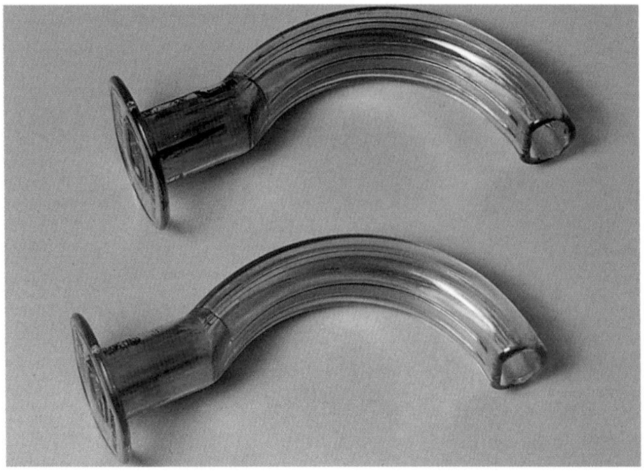

Figure 25.23 Oropharyngeal airway

(Potter et al 2023)

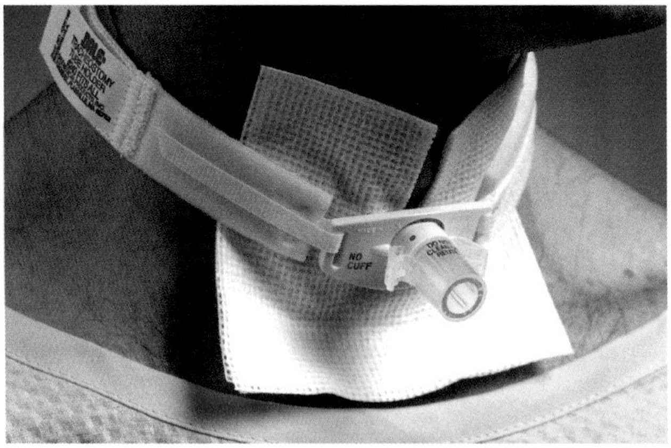

Figure 25.25 Tracheostomy tube

(Ignatavicius et al 2021)

NURSING AN INDIVIDUAL WITH AN ARTIFICIAL AIRWAY

Nurses play an important role in preparing, monitoring and caring for a person before, during and after the insertion of a tracheostomy. The care of an individual with an artificial airway—whether it has been inserted for the short term or long term—involves many physical actions and the provision of emotional support. The main aspects of care include:

- continued assessment of airway status
- maintenance of correct cuff pressure to prevent tissue ischaemia and necrosis
- continued monitoring for complications
- keeping the tube free of mucus to ensure airway patency
- preventing infection
- providing psychological support.

(Aitken et al 2019)

Nursing a person with a tracheostomy

The role of the nurse in caring for a person with a tracheostomy involves eight essential principles (Flaherty 2020) as outlined below. Other aspects essential for care include swallowing, decannulation and tube changes; however, these are often managed by the wider healthcare team.

1. Infection control
2. Humidification
3. Cuff management
4. Suctioning
5. Management of the inner cannula
6. Dressings
7. Oral hygiene
8. Communication

In the event of an emergency, including accidental dislodgement or obstruction of the tube, the following should always be available at the bedside:

- spare sterile tracheostomy tube or inner tube
- tracheal dilator
- scissors
- syringe for a cuffed tube
- manual ventilation bag
- oxygen and sterile 'Y' suction catheters.

(Aitken et al 2019)

A person with an artificial airway will be apprehensive about asphyxiation or choking, which can be further increased by an impaired ability to communicate their needs to others. The individual's ability to effectively remove secretions by coughing may be grossly impaired. When unable to cough or expectorate secretions, suctioning must be performed. In the first few days after the insertion of a tracheostomy tube, the procedure is uncomfortable and frightening, and the individual must be provided with an explanation of the suctioning technique before it is performed. The nurse should be aware of their role in tracheostomy suctioning and also the regulations, procedures and policies of the healthcare facility regarding tracheostomy suctioning. A suggested method of tracheostomy suctioning is outlined in Clinical Skill 25.6. The basic equipment for tracheostomy suctioning is:

- sterile 'Y' suction catheters
- wall or portable suction apparatus
- connecting tubing
- disposable gloves
- container of sterile or tap water for clearing the catheter (depending on the institution's policy)
- bag or container for contaminated catheters.

Tracheostomy care, which is performed using sterile equipment and aseptic technique to prevent infection, involves cleansing of the inner cannula and the area around the stoma. The frequency with which the care is provided may vary depending on the amount of secretions present, and may be as frequent as every half hour to 1 hour or may only be required once every 8 hours.

Some tracheostomy tubes have an inner replaceable tube that can be changed as part of routine daily care (e.g. 4-hourly to daily). It is essential that a spare inner tube is kept close at hand and replaced if the inner tube becomes blocked. The inner tube is cleaned using a suitable solution and dried and made accessible for future use.

Tracheostomy tubes may be cuffed or uncuffed. A cuffed tube creates a seal in the trachea to facilitate positive pressure ventilation and to reduce aspiration or secretions into the lungs. Ensuring the cuff pressure is at the recommended range will prevent tracheal necrosis and stenosis. The frequency of cuff pressure measurement will vary dependent on the situation; however, it is suggested that at a minimum, cuff pressure is measured at least every 8 hours, or when clinically indicated (NSW Agency for Clinical Innovation 2021).

To prevent the trachea or lower airways from drying and bleeding, a humidification connector, a 'Swedish nose', may be applied. This consists of a single or dual barrel that encloses the tube's orifice; humidity is provided by rolled absorptive paper filters pre-moistened with normal saline. If secretions are present on the outside of the suction catheter, additional sterile saline may be required to be instilled into the tracheostomy tube to loosen secretions and maintain the patency of the tracheostomy tube.

Communication is a significant problem for individuals who are conscious. To alleviate anxiety and apprehension, an alternative means of communication should be provided. Communication options include:

- a pad and pencil
- mouthing
- gesturing
- heading movement or an alternative motor activity (e.g. blinking)
- picture and letter boards
- writing and drawing
- use of electrcolarynx
- electronic communication devices (tablets and apps).

(NSW Agency for Clinical Innovation 2021)

CLINICAL SKILL 25.6 Tracheostomy suctioning and tracheal stoma care

Please adhere to the policy and procedures of the facility/organisation prior to undertaking the skill. Ensure this skill is in your scope of practice.

NMBA Decision-making Framework considerations (refer to NMBA Decision-making framework for nursing and midwifery 2020):	Equipment:
1. Am I educated? 2. Am I authorised? 3. Am I competent? If you answer 'no' to any of these, do not perform that activity. Seek guidance and support from your teacher/a nurse team leader/clinical facilitator/educator. Tracheostomy suctioning and tracheal stoma care is an advanced skill for an Enrolled Nurse (EN).	Sterile gloves Disposable gloves Plastic apron Protective eyewear Waterproof pad Sterile dressing pack Sterile gauze squares Sterile cotton tip applicators Normal saline 0.9% Clean tapes cut to the correct length Suction apparatus Suction catheter Sterile water Swedish nose or equivalent humidification filter and inner tube

PREPARE FOR THE SKILL

(Please refer to the Standard Steps on pp. xviii–xx for related rationales.)

Mentally review the steps of the skill.
Discuss the skill with your instructor/supervisor/team leader, if required.
Confirm correct facility/organisation policy/safe operating procedures.
Validate the order in the individual's record.
Identify indication and rationale for performing the activity.
Assess for any contraindications.
Locate and gather equipment.
Perform hand hygiene.
Ensure therapeutic interaction.
Identify the individual using three individual identifiers.
Gain the individual's consent.
Assess for pain relief.
Prepare the environment.
Provide and maintain privacy.
Assist the individual to assume an appropriate position of comfort.

Skill activity	Rationale
Tracheostomy suctioning	
Perform an assessment of the individual, ensuring their vital signs are stable and their oxygen saturations are adequate to allow for the suctioning. The individual should be informed that suctioning may cause transient coughing or gagging.	Ensures the individual is stable so as to prevent complications. A burst of oxygen or normal saline nebuliser may be required prior (if ordered) to help loosen secretions and allow for better clearance of mucus during suctioning. **Note:** If suctioning is required due to a mucus plug, this will facilitate better oxygen saturations.
If possible, position the individual in a sitting position or with the head hyperextended. Place a waterproof pad across individual's chest.	Reduces stimulation of gag reflex, assists secretion drainage. Reduces transmission of microorganisms.

PERFORM THE SKILL

(Please refer to the Standard Steps on pp. xviii–xx for related rationales.)

Perform hand hygiene.
Apply PPE: gloves, eyewear, mask and gown as appropriate.
Ensure the individual's safety and comfort throughout skill.
Promote independence and involvement of the individual if possible and/or appropriate.
Assess the individual's tolerance to the skill throughout.
Dispose of used supplies, equipment, waste and sharps appropriately.
Remove PPE and discard or store appropriately.
Perform hand hygiene.

CLINICAL SKILL 25.6 Tracheostomy suctioning and tracheal stoma care—cont'd

Skill activity	Rationale
Open procedure pack using corners. Assemble the required equipment, using aseptic technique. Drop sterile equipment into sterile field.	Facilitates performance of the procedure and promotes functional body alignment and body mechanics while the procedure is being performed. Prevents contamination of sterile items.
Remove any humidification (or ventilation) device (i.e. Swedish nose). Inner tube may also need to be removed and cleaned prior to suctioning.	Allows access to the tracheostomy tube. Prevents a mucus plug from forming and allows for proper removal of secretions.
Attach the catheter to the suction tubing and set suction pressure to 80–120 mmHg. Catheter size must be smaller than the diameter of the tracheostomy/inner tube.	Pressure above 120 mmHg may damage the tracheal mucosa. Prevents obstruction of airway.
Ask the individual to cough and breathe slowly and deeply.	Coughing helps loosen secretions, and deep breathing helps to minimise hypoxia.
If necessary, or prescribed, the individual's lungs are hyperoxygenated before aspiration.	Helps to prevent hypoxia.
Insert the catheter without suction into the tracheostomy tube just past the correct length of the tracheostomy tube.	Prevents hypoxia and tracheal mucosa trauma. Suctioning to the xiphoid process can cause trauma and permanent damage to the cartilage, especially in neonates, infants and children; it also prevents discomfort.
Apply suction and withdraw the catheter, rotating it gently. Suction for no longer than 5–10 seconds at a time. Allow the individual to take four to five breaths between each aspiration. If secretions are thick, dip the catheter into sterile water and apply suction.	Rotating motion avoids tissue trauma. Short-term suctioning limits the amount of oxygen removed and prevents hypoxia. Helps to clear the lumen of the catheter. **Note:** In neonates and infants do not rotate catheter but simply insert in and out to the required measurement.
Report immediately if there is any difficulty in inserting the catheter into the tube.	The tube may be partially blocked with secretions.
When suctioning is completed, the individual may need to be hyperoxygenated again. Replace any humidification device (unless tracheal stoma care/dressing is to be performed). Reinsert the clean inner tube. Clear suction catheter and tubing with sterile water.	Prevents hypoxia and promotes relaxation. Re-establishes delivery of humidity. Prevents the reintroduction of microorganisms. **Note:** Suction catheters can be used for up to 24 hours prior to disposal if cleaned thoroughly after use.
Tracheal stoma care	
Open procedure pack and prepare equipment using ANTT.	Prevents contamination of sterile items.
Remove and discard the tracheostomy dressing into a suitable waste receptacle. Ensure ties secure around tracheostomy tube.	Correct disposal prevents cross-infection and abides by infection prevention policies and procedures. Prevents dislodgement of tracheostomy tube.
Perform hand hygiene and don sterile gloves. For a newly formed stoma, use a sterile drape around the tracheostomy site.	Prevents cross-infection. Provides a sterile field around the stoma.
Cleanse the skin around the stoma and the flanges of the tube using gauze and normal saline. Take care not to let normal saline or strands of gauze enter the tube or stoma. Use cotton tip applicators dipped in normal saline for hard-to-reach areas of the stoma.	Removes accumulated secretions and crusts. Prevents aspiration and the risk of infection.

Continued

CLINICAL SKILL 25.6 Tracheostomy suctioning and tracheal stoma care—cont'd

Inspect the surrounding area and stoma site for inflammation or skin breakdown. Inspect for the formation of a granuloma, especially in older tracheostomy stoma sites.	Signs of impaired healing or infection require immediate attention. Granulomas are generally a collection of macrophages forming a nodular area around the stoma site. These are quite common, especially in older stomas, and can be treated with silver nitrate.
Apply a sterile tracheostomy dressing using aseptic non-touch technique.	Protects the stoma site and reduces transmission of microorganisms.
Replace the tracheostomy tapes if they are soiled or loose. Two people are required to change the tapes (one must be an RN who has achieved competency; the EN would assist with the procedure).	Tracheostomy tube must be secured in position. Soiled tapes predispose the person to infection. Prevents accidental dislodgement of the tube.
Replace any humidification device (Swedish nose). Change to a new one if the old one soiled.	Re-establishes delivery of humidity and helps filter the air to prevent the introduction of microorganisms.

AFTER THE SKILL

(Please refer to the Standard Steps on pp. xviii–xx for related rationales.)
Communicate outcome to the individual, any ongoing care and to report any complications.
Restore the environment.
Report, record and document assessment findings, details of the skill performed and the individual's response.
Report, record and document any abnormalities and/or inability to perform the skill.
Reassess the individual to ensure there are no adverse effects/events from the skill.

Skill activity	Rationale
Document the time of suctioning, the type and amount of aspirate and the individual's response. Document and report on the dressing change.	Appropriate care can be planned and implemented.

(Berman et al 2020; Carter & Notter 2024; Perry et al 2022; Rebeiro et al 2021)

The individual should be provided with information about their progress and any procedures that are to be performed. They should be encouraged to participate in their own care as much as possible to reduce any sense of dependency, and the significant others should be involved in the care. The individual may be discharged from hospital with a tracheostomy tube in situ. As soon as possible, they and the significant others are educated in self-care so that they feel comfortable and confident about caring for their tracheostomy. The individual should be provided with information about relevant support groups such as tracheostomy associations that they may wish to contact.

Before the permanent removal of a tracheostomy tube, the individual will require sufficient information and emotional support since they may feel that they will not be able to breathe without the tube. The tube may be removed when the individual is able to maintain independent respiratory function, is able to breathe through the upper respiratory tract and has satisfactory protective reflexes, such as the cough reflex.

To prepare the individual for permanent removal of the tracheostomy tube, a fenestrated tube may be inserted. This type of tube has an opening in the outer cannula that allows the individual to breathe around as well as through the tube. Thus, they are able to adjust gradually to removal of the tube. Alternatively, the tube may be occluded, or 'corked', by an adhesive tape to determine the individual's ability to cope without the tube. With uncuffed tubes this is routinely achieved to enhance communication by allowing the individual to occlude the tube with their fingers while speaking. By covering the tube, they may be able to speak, breathe normally through the upper airway and expectorate secretions.

Before the tube is removed, suction is applied to remove tracheal and pharyngeal secretions. The cuff is then deflated and the tube removed. Generally, a dry occlusive dressing is placed over the stoma and the individual closely monitored for the first 24 hours. Healing and reduction in the tracheostomy can take 12 months or longer and care must be taken during this time to prevent aspiration and infections. After a period of time, when the individual's airway is stable, the stoma can be surgically sutured together (see Clinical Skill 25.6 for tracheal stoma care).

Complications of tracheostomy

The insertion of an artificial airway can result in several complications:

- infection due to altered ciliary function or colonisation of the airway with bacteria
- tracheal necrosis and stenosis due to excessive pressure on the trachea from the cuff
- tracheo-oesophageal fistula
- partial or complete airway obstruction (e.g. due to an accumulation of secretions in the tube)
- subcutaneous emphysema
- psychological effects, such as frustration at being unable to communicate as usual.

(AACN & Hartjes 2022)

THE INDIVIDUAL WITH THORACIC DRAINAGE TUBES

The principle of chest drains is to maintain respiratory function and haemodynamic stability (Perry et al 2022). Insertion of chest-drainage tubes (Figure 25.26 and Figure 25.27) permits the drainage of air or fluid from the pleural space which, if not removed, alters intrapleural pressure and causes lung collapse (Parrillo & Dellinger 2019). Ventilation is adversely affected by any disruption of the intrapleural pressure, which may be caused by surgery, trauma or pulmonary disease. Insertion of chest tubes drains the excess air or fluid and enables the lungs to function normally (Parrillo & Dellinger 2019).

Chest-drainage tubes may be inserted at the time of surgery, while an individual is anaesthetised, or they may be inserted using local anaesthetic. Because the procedure is painful, a conscious individual is generally given analgesic medication about 30 minutes before tube insertion. The procedure is performed by a medical officer, using sterile equipment and aseptic technique. The insertion site is selected according to the individual's condition, and one or more tubes may be inserted at the same time (Parrillo & Dellinger 2019). See Clinical Skill 25.7 for care of chest tube/drainage.

Underwater seal drainage

After insertion, the chest tube is connected to a drainage system that permits drainage out of the pleural space and prevents backflow into that space. The tubing leads to a collection system positioned well below the level of the individual's chest. This dependent position facilitates the removal of air or fluid from the pleural cavity and prevents backflow (Parrillo & Dellinger 2019). To prevent the entry of air into the pleural cavity, the distal end of the tubing is submerged underwater. This provides a closed water-seal drainage system. The depth of water that the tube is placed under determines the water pressure used to create a seal (e.g. 5 cm) and is ordered by a medical officer.

Some commercial systems of underwater seal drainage (e.g. the Pleur-evac® system) are available already assembled and are disposed of after use. Other types of thoracic drainage

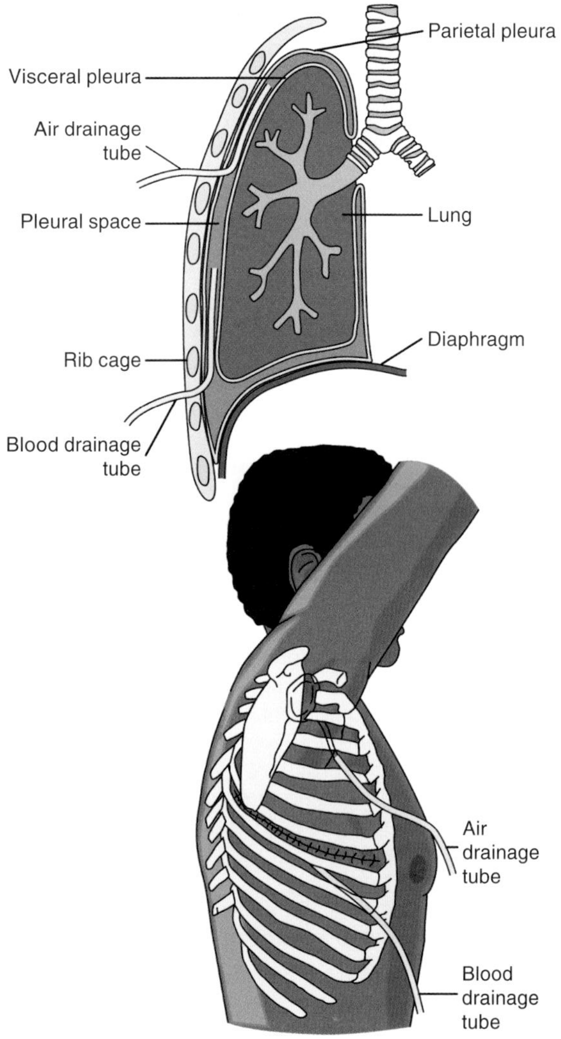

Figure 25.26 Chest tube placement

(Ignatavicius et al 2021)

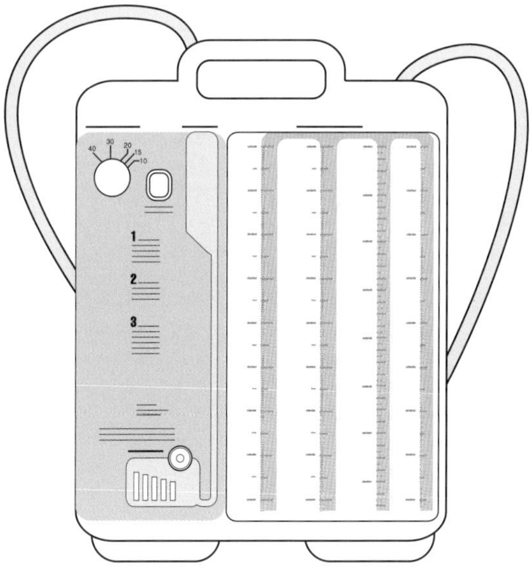

Figure 25.27 Disposable, commercial chest-drainage system

CLINICAL SKILL 25.7 Care of chest tube/drainage and dressing change

Please adhere to the policy and procedures of the facility/organisation prior to undertaking the skill. Ensure this skill is in your scope of practice.

NMBA Decision-making Framework considerations (refer to NMBA Decision-making framework for nursing and midwifery 2020):	**Equipment:**
1. Am I educated? 2. Am I authorised? 3. Am I competent? If you answer 'no' to any of these, do not perform that activity. Seek guidance and support from your teacher/a nurse team leader/clinical facilitator/educator.	Disposable and sterile gloves Sterile dressing pack Approved antiseptic solution (2% chlorhexidine gluconate in 70% isopropyl, 10% povidone-iodine or 70% alcohol) Normal saline 0.9% Split dressing/gauze Occlusive dressing Fluid balance chart or chest drain observation chart Two artery forceps

PREPARE FOR THE SKILL

(Please refer to the Standard Steps on pp. xviii–xx for related rationales.)
Mentally review the steps of the skill.
Discuss the skill with your instructor/supervisor/team leader, if required.
Confirm correct facility/organisation policy/safe operating procedures.
Validate the order in the individual's record.
Identify indication and rationale for performing the activity.
Assess for any contraindications.
Locate and gather equipment.
Perform hand hygiene.
Ensure therapeutic interaction.
Identify the individual using three individual identifiers.
Gain the individual's consent.
Assess for pain relief.
Prepare the environment.
Provide and maintain privacy.
Assist the individual to assume an appropriate position of comfort.

Skill activity	**Rationale**
Care of chest tube/drainage	
Ensure the individual is nursed in a semi-Fowler's or high Fowler's position. Perform an assessment of the individual, ensuring their vital signs are stable and their oxygen saturations are within range as specified by the medical officer. Assess for any pain during inspiration or expiration and/or at the insertion site. Check for bilateral rise and fall of the chest and that there is no respiratory distress.	Allows for adequate chest expansion and better respiration. Semi-Fowler's position is preferred for pneumothorax to evacuate air. High Fowler's is preferred for haemothorax to drain fluid. Reduces anxiety and embarrassment. Ensures individual is stable so as to prevent any complications.
Provide two artery forceps for each chest tube, attached at top of bed with adhesive tape.	Chest tubes are clamped only under specific circumstances and with medical orders. Double-clamp close to the individual's chest for as short a time as possible only in the following circumstances: a. To assess air leak. b. To quickly change the disposable underwater seal drain (UWSD), which should only be performed by a nurse who has received training in this procedure. c. To assess if the individual is ready to have chest tube removed (which is done by medical order); the nurse must monitor for re-accumulation of pneumothorax. d. During drainage of large volumes to reduce shock (on doctor's orders). e. To prepare for removal (on doctor's orders). f. When the system may have to be raised above chest level.

CLINICAL SKILL 25.7 Care of chest tube/drainage and dressing change—cont'd

PERFORM THE SKILL

(Please refer to the Standard Steps on pp. xviii–xx for related rationales.)
Perform hand hygiene.
Apply PPE: gloves, eyewear, mask and gown as appropriate.
Ensure the individual's safety and comfort throughout skill.
Promote independence and involvement of the individual if possible and/or appropriate.
Assess the individual's tolerance to the skill throughout.
Dispose of used supplies, equipment, waste and sharps appropriately.
Remove PPE and discard or store appropriately.

Skill activity	Rationale
Assess the chest tube dressing and insertion site to ensure the dressing is dry and intact and observe for any signs of infection. Report any signs of infection to the RN/medical officer.	Prevents complications from arising and prevents the introduction of microorganisms. Appropriate care can be planned and implemented.
Assess the drain tube and drainage for any bubbling, swing and drainage. Observe the tubing for kinks, clots or dependent loops. Check wall suction and connection to underwater sealed drain (UWSD) is intact Ensure the UWSD is upright and below the level of the chest.	Increased bubbling indicates an air leak, which may mean the connection to the person and the tube is faulty. This can lead to a pneumothorax if not sealed properly. Swing refers to oscillation of the fluid in the tubing. Ensures the tubing is patent. Wall suction should be set at >80 mmHg with the suction on the UWSD unit being set at 20 cmH_2O for adults (5 cmH_2O for neonates and 10–20 cmH_2O for children) or as prescribed by the doctor. Suction helps facilitate the reinflation of the lung. Prevents the introduction of microorganisms. Prevents fluid from flowing back into the pleural cavity.
Chest tube dressing change	
Open procedure pack and prepare equipment using ANTT.	Prevents contamination of sterile items.
Gently remove the old dressing ensuring that there is a little slack on the tube.	Prevents the accidental dislodgement of the tube. Tautness of the tube can cause discomfort and pull on the sutures, causing trauma to the area. **Note:** Chest tubes are usually sutured in place.
Perform hand hygiene and don sterile gloves. Use normal saline 0.9% to cleanse area, ensuring the tubing is also cleaned well.	Prevents cross-infection and the introduction of microorganisms.
Apply approved skin antiseptic solution and allow to dry. 2% chlorhexidine gluconate in 70% isopropyl is the preferred choice, or 10% povidone-iodine or 70% alcohol as the alternative.	Prevents cross-infection and eliminates the introduction of microorganisms.
Apply split gauze around the insertion site and then place a sandwich dressing over the area (two large pieces of occlusive dressing).	Helps collect any exudate. Ensures the insertion site and surrounding skin can be seen readily and secures tubing to prevent irritation.

AFTER THE SKILL

(Please refer to the Standard Steps on pp. xviii–xx for related rationales.)
Communicate outcome to the individual, any ongoing care and to report any complications.
Restore the environment.
Report, record and document assessment findings, details of the skill performed and the individual's response.
Report, record and document any abnormalities and/or inability to perform the skill.
Reassess the individual to ensure there are no adverse effects/events from the skill.

Continued

CLINICAL SKILL 25.7 Care of chest tube/drainage and dressing change—cont'd

Skill activity	Rationale
Document observations, pain, drain tube assessment and drainage hourly or as per policy and procedure on the relevant observation and/or fluid balance chart. Document the respiratory status of the individual, the amount, colour and consistency of drainage, the presence of swinging and bubbling.	Ensures the safety of the individual. Abides by facility/organisation policy. Monitors for any complications and excessive drainage. **Note:** The individual may be on a patient-controlled analgesia (PCA) infusion for analgesia maintenance, which will also need to be documented hourly as per policy.
(Carter & Notter 2024; Knapp 2019; Perry et al 2022; Rebeiro et al 2021)	

systems include the one-, two- or three-bottle systems. The one- and two-bottle systems are primarily gravity systems, which can be provided with suction to facilitate drainage (Parrillo & Dellinger 2019). Such systems provide a water seal and can be connected to suction. A medical officer is required to order the application of suction, which is used to facilitate faster drainage of air or fluids. A low-flow suction regulator device is used to ensure that the suction provides a minimal bubbling effect.

NURSING A PERSON WITH A CHEST DRAIN

The aim of closed-chest underwater seal drainage is to maintain respiratory function and haemodynamic stability by facilitating drainage of air, blood and/or other fluids (Perry et al 2022). Care of the person includes:

- Nursing them in an upright position when possible, to facilitate optimal lung expansion and to promote drainage by gravity.
- Providing adequate explanation and emotional support to reduce anxiety. The individual may tend to restrict their breathing and movement for fear of dislodging the tube, so it is essential to explain that the tube is secured in position with tape and/or sutures.
- Administering adequate analgesic medication to decrease discomfort. It may be necessary to administer analgesic medication 30–45 minutes before physiotherapy, to promote pain relief and relaxation.
- Encouraging the individual to breathe deeply and cough frequently (e.g. hourly) to help drain the pleural space and expand the lungs.
- Regularly assessing the individual's respiratory status. The individual should be observed for discomfort and any difficulty in breathing, and it is important to observe whether their chest is expanding symmetrically. The ventilations are assessed at regular intervals (e.g. hourly) for rate, rhythm and character.
- Maintaining the water seal and preventing air leakage, which is essential to prevent entry of air into the pleural space. The fluid level in the drainage bottle should be checked frequently (e.g. hourly) and sterile water added if necessary to ensure that the distal end of the water seal tube remains submerged at the ordered level.
- Observing and documenting the drain output; usually this will be recorded every 1–4 hours. The sequence of drain behaviour depends upon the reason for drain insertion (whether it is to remove air or fluid). Check for presence of bubbling and amount of fluid output (Millar & Hillman 2018).
- Taking precautions to prevent separation of the connections, such as taping the joints and securing the tube to the individual's clothing. Care must be taken to ensure that the underwater seal system remains below the individual's chest to prevent fluid or air re-entering the pleural cavity, which can cause subsequent pneumothorax or empyema.
- Securing the drainage system to the bed or placing it securely on the floor to protect it from toppling over and from accidental breakage. If the system is accidentally disconnected or broken, air will enter the pleural space and the lungs may collapse. It is general practice to have two chest clamps in plain view at the bedside for any individual with a chest drain; in the event of disconnection, the two clamps are applied immediately to the chest tube, and assistance is summoned immediately. There is some controversy surrounding this emergency measure since some authorities believe that clamping a chest tube could result in a tension pneumothorax. It is essential that the nurse is aware of the healthcare institution's measures to be taken should accidental disconnection of the system occur. If a chest tube is accidentally dislodged or falls out, the individual is asked to exhale forcefully and the opening on the skin surface is sealed with an airtight dressing until the tube can be reinserted.
- Maintaining patency of the drainage system, which is essential to facilitate expansion of the lung. The system must be checked hourly for loose connections and for fluctuation in the water-seal bottle. As the individual inhales, the fluid should rise in the water-seal tube, and as they exhale the level should fall back (this is termed 'swinging').

- Ensuring that, if the system is connected to suction, the fluid line in the water-seal tube remains constant. During exhalation, bubbling is normally present in the water-seal bottle. Gently bubbling in a suction control bottle indicates that the correct level of suction has been achieved.
- Observing the tubing for, and keeping it free from, kinks. Kinking of the tubing will obstruct the flow of air or fluid. To prevent kinking, or dependent loops of tubing, the tubing should be coiled flat on the bed and may be attached to the edge of the bed with tape and a safety pin. The tubing should fall in a straight line from the coil to the drainage bottle, to facilitate flow. The nurse should ensure that the individual is able to move freely without pulling or lying on the tubing.
- Double-clamping the chest tube near the site of insertion when it is necessary to replace a drainage system bottle. The bottle, and, if necessary, the connection tubing, is replaced and the clamps removed. The tubes should not be clamped for longer than 2 minutes since a tension pneumothorax may result when air or fluid is prevented from escaping. As a safety precaution, two nurses should be present whenever a drainage bottle or system is being replaced.
- Protecting the insertion site by an occlusive dressing (e.g. Opsite). Using sterile equipment and aseptic techniques to prevent infection, the dressing is renewed in accordance with the healthcare institution's policy.
- Assessing and documenting the colour, volume and type of drainage. Any alteration in the amount, colour or flow of drainage must be reported immediately. Sudden cessation of flow of drainage may indicate a malfunction of the system or disconnection of the tubing. A gradual reduction in flow may indicate occlusion by blood or proteins, that the tube position has moved in the pleural cavity or that the chest has reinflated.

Removal of a chest drain tube is very painful and individuals require adequate analgesia and preparation time (Carter & Notter 2024). Chest drain removal must be performed by a qualified RN or medical officer. Generally, the tube is clamped for up to 24 hours before removal, and a chest X-ray is performed immediately beforehand to determine lung expansion. If the individual develops respiratory distress or a pneumothorax, the clamps are removed and the tube left in place. Analgesic medication is usually administered 30–45 minutes before tube removal. The tube is removed swiftly and immediately covered with an occlusive dressing to provide an airtight seal. In some cases, the site is closed with purse string sutures that are tightened during removal.

One hour after the removal of the tube, an X-ray is taken to ensure that there has been no ingress of air during or after the removal. The insertion site is checked regularly for sounds of air leakage and the individual is observed for manifestations of pneumothorax, infection, subcutaneous emphysema and respiratory distress (Millar & Hillman 2018; Carter & Notter 2024).

NURSING PRACTICE AND OXYGEN ADMINISTRATION

Nursing staff must be educated to adequately administer oxygen therapy (Crisp et al 2021). Oxygen therapy is the delivery of oxygen to the individual by some device or equipment in concentrations greater than that found in normal room air (room air is 21%). Oxygen therapy is not a cure and does not remove the underlying disease or condition but aims to decrease the workload of the cardiopulmonary system and to protect the individual from tissue hypoxia. Regardless of the mode of delivery the individual must be able to maintain a patent airway, or an artificial airway must be established.

It is important for nursing staff to assess, initiate and monitor oxygen delivery systems within the prescribed parameter (Crisp et al 2021). An exception to this would be in an emergency when no individual should be denied adequate oxygenation. In such cases, oxygen should be given first and documented later.

Assessment

An individual's respiratory status is assessed to ascertain whether they are receiving an adequate supply of oxygen and excreting sufficient carbon dioxide to meet their body's needs. A respiratory assessment should consider the following:

- observing the individual for signs and symptoms of hypoxaemia and respiratory distress
- identifying any deviations from normal and by assessing their ventilations.

Assessing the respiratory status and identifying any actual or potential problems is assisted by obtaining information from the individual regarding:

- allergic reactions such as coughing, watery eyes, sneezing or shortness of breath that may occur as a result of exposure to allergens such as dust mites, pet hair or pollen
- exposure to environmental air pollutants such as chemical wastes, smoke or dust
- history of tobacco and inhaled recreational drugs
- presence of a cough and the volume, quality and quantity of sputum
- chest pain.

(Crisp et al 2021)

Signs and symptoms of hypoxaemia and respiratory distress

The person should be observed for signs and symptoms of hypoxaemia, which is defined as a diminished availability of oxygen to the body tissues. Hypoxaemia may result from disorders that limit the volume of air entering the lungs, or from obstructive lung diseases, such as asthma and emphysema. The signs and symptoms of hypoxia and respiratory distress include:

- cyanosis
- elevated blood pressure and pulse rate

- shortness of breath (dyspnoea), fatigue and intolerance to exercise
- abnormal respiratory rate, depth or rhythm
- sighing, gasping, breath holding
- flaring of the nares
- use of accessory muscles during breathing (e.g. substernal recession, tracheal tugging, shoulder shrugging and intercostal muscles during expiration)
- apprehension, aggression, non-compliance or agitation
- confusion or reduced level of consciousness
- visible or excessive perspiration (diaphoresis).

(Crisp et al 2021)

Assessment of an individual with chronic respiratory disorder

A person with a chronic respiratory disorder should also be assessed for a barrel-shaped chest, which is an increase in the anteroposterior diameter of the chest wall, commonly associated with air trapping, as in atelectasis or chronic obstructive airways disease. Individuals with chronic hypoxaemia may experience the same symptoms as above but may have clubbing of the fingers, where the angle of the nail bed increases to over 85 degrees, caused by an increase in capillary numbers to supply poorly perfused tissue, with subsequent increase in size (AACN & Hartjes 2022).

Meeting an individual's need for oxygen

Breathing is an automatic activity, but rate and depth can be changed voluntarily. Normally, room air at normal atmospheric pressure, such as at sea level, provides sufficient oxygen to meet the metabolic needs of the body. However, admission to hospital, or a respiratory condition, may affect an individual's normal pattern of breathing. For example, if a person has an infection or is apprehensive or anxious, they may experience temporary breathing difficulties. In these instances, measures to promote the return of normal breathing are performed. Nurses provide individuals with adequate information to allay some of the anxiety relating to their condition, investigations and hospitalisation. The nurse should also attempt to ensure that the room is ventilated adequately and at a comfortable temperature (Crisp et al 2021).

Individuals who experience breathing difficulties due to a clinical condition may require assistance to meet any increase in either oxygen demands or carbon dioxide retention. Some methods include, for example, positioning in a more upright position, nebulisation, humidification, physiotherapy (which may include deep-breathing and coughing exercises) and mobilisation. Individuals who suffer from an oxygen deficiency will commonly require administration of oxygen to supplement that being obtained from the atmosphere. (See Clinical Skill 25.8.)

CLINICAL SKILL 25.8 Oxygen therapy—nasal, mask

Please adhere to the policy and procedures of the facility/organisation prior to undertaking the skill. Ensure this skill is in your scope of practice.

NMBA Decision-making Framework considerations (refer to NMBA Decision-making framework for nursing and midwifery 2020):	Equipment:
1. Am I educated? 2. Am I authorised? 3. Am I competent? If you answer 'no' to any of these, do not perform that activity. Seek guidance and support from your teacher/a nurse team leader/clinical facilitator/educator.	Oxygen source (wall outlet, cylinder) Flow meter Humidifier and sterile water (if indicated) Oxygen tubing Oxygen delivery system (if FiO_2 required) Nasal cannula Oxygen mask (or required mask) Pulse oximeter

PREPARE FOR THE SKILL

(Please refer to the Standard Steps on pp. xviii–xx for related rationales.)
Mentally review the steps of the skill.
Discuss the skill with your instructor/supervisor/team leader, if required.
Confirm correct facility/organisation policy/safe operating procedures.
Validate the order in the individual's record.
Identify indication and rationale for performing the activity.
Assess for any contraindications.
Locate and gather equipment.
Perform hand hygiene.
Ensure therapeutic interaction.
Identify the individual using three individual identifiers.
Gain the individual's consent.
Assess for pain relief.
Prepare the environment.
Provide and maintain privacy.
Assist the individual to assume an appropriate position of comfort.

CLINICAL SKILL 25.8 Oxygen therapy—nasal, mask—cont'd

Skill activity	Rationale
Perform an assessment of the person, record their vital signs and oxygen saturations. Assess indications for oxygen requirement: • Dyspnoea, tachypnoea, bradypnoea, apnoea • Pallor, cyanosis • Lethargy or restlessness • Use of accessory muscles: nasal flaring, intercostal or sternal recession, tracheal tug.	Baseline observations attended to assess for initiation of oxygen therapy. Enables safe administration of oxygen therapy.
Sit person into an upright or semi-Fowler's position (if able).	Facilitates breathing and lung expansion.

PERFORM THE SKILL

Please refer to the Standard Steps on pp. xviii–xx for related rationales.)
Perform hand hygiene.
Apply PPE: gloves, eyewear, mask and gown as appropriate.
Ensure the individual's safety and comfort throughout skill.
Promote independence and involvement of the individual if possible and/or appropriate.
Assess the individual's tolerance to the skill throughout.
Dispose of used supplies, equipment, waste and sharps appropriately.
Remove PPE and discard or store appropriately.
Perform hand hygiene.

Skill activity	Rationale
Attach oxygen delivery device to oxygen tubing and attach to oxygen source at prescribed rate. Apply the appropriate delivery device to the individual.	Oxygen delivery devices change the amount and the concentration of oxygen being delivered: **Low-flow delivery devices** • Nasal cannulae: 1–6 L/min (24–44%) • Simple face mask: 6–12 L/min (35–50%) • Reservoir mask (non-rebreathing mask): 10–15 L/min (60–90%) **High-flow delivery devices** • Venturi system (used in high-flow oxygen): FiO_2 and amount of oxygen determined as per dialled amount (24–50%) • High-flow nasal cannula or mask (adjustable FiO_2 (21–100%) with modifiable low flow (up to 60 L/min)) • Continuous positive airway pressure (CPAP) and bilevel positive airway pressure (BiPAP) (21–100%)
Monitor the individual's response to oxygen and their observations as indicated by the medical officer until stable (usually every 15 minutes to hourly). Ensure tubing is not kinked, check mask or cannula stay in correct position.	Prevents complications and ensures treatment is working.
Offer/perform oral hygiene using a mouth swab and/or mouth rinse. Wash face masks daily with warm soapy water. Observe the nares and top of the individual's ears for skin breakdown.	Reduces bad taste or halitosis in mouth. Provides comfort and maintains moist mucosa. Oxygen therapy can dry the nares and the cannula tubing or elastic can cause skin irritation.

Continued

CLINICAL SKILL 25.8 Oxygen therapy—nasal, mask—cont'd

AFTER THE SKILL

(Please refer to the Standard Steps on pp. xviii–xx for related rationales.)
Communicate outcome to the individual, any ongoing care and to report any complications.
Restore the environment.
Report, record and document assessment findings, details of the skill performed and the individual's response.
Report, record and document any abnormalities and/or inability to perform the skill.
Reassess the individual to ensure there are no adverse effects/events from the skill.

(Carter & Notter 2024; Perry et al 2022; Rebeiro et al 2021)

Administering oxygen

To prevent or reverse hypoxia and to improve tissue oxygenation, oxygen may be administered via a number of devices. Oxygen is a drug; it is prescribed by a medical officer who determines the concentration, route and length of time that it is to be administered. To promote the safety and comfort of the individual receiving oxygen therapy, the nurse should be aware of certain principles relevant to the administration of oxygen (Berman et al 2020):

- Hypoxaemia can result from insufficient oxygen flow or delivery. Equipment and connections must be checked at regular intervals (e.g. hourly) to ensure that it is functioning properly. If signs or symptoms of hypoxaemia occur, they must be reported immediately, as adjustment to the concentration being administered may be necessary, or alternative investigations or treatment implemented.
- Although oxygen is not normally combustible, it does support combustion and it is essential to implement safety precautions to reduce the risk of fire. Smoking is prohibited in the vicinity, and measures are taken to prevent sparks, which may be given off by electrical or mechanical items. Inflammable substances such as oil or alcohol should not be used near or on the oxygen equipment.
- Administration of any gas can dry and irritate mucous membranes; this is particularly so with nasal prongs. In some healthcare institutions the gas is humidified by passing it through a sterile water humidification system before administration.
- Oxygen is colourless and odourless, so accurate gauges on gas cylinders and oxygen concentrators are used to indicate the volume of oxygen remaining or rate of flow. An oxygen regulator limits the flow of the gas. Care must be taken to ensure that connections on the regulator are tight, otherwise a reduced volume or concentration will be administered.
- Oxygen toxicity is a hazard with prolonged administration or concentrations over 50%. The individual's capillary, venous or arterial blood gases are commonly measured during oxygen therapy and the concentration of oxygen or method of delivery can be adjusted. Damage and inflammation to airways, blood vessels and nervous tissue may result in acute respiratory distress syndrome (ARDS).
- Nosocomial infections can occur using oxygen therapy, particularly with the use of non-sterile oxygen bubble humidifiers. Masks, tubing, cannulae and catheters are for single individual use and are discarded on discharge. Care must be taken to clean the mask or nebuliser regularly (e.g. every 8 hours).

The nurse must know how to check that the equipment is functioning correctly and that all connections are secure and do not leak. Cleaning and disposal of equipment is done as per the individual healthcare institution's infection control guidelines (Pinsky et al 2019).

Oxygen delivery equipment

Oxygen is often piped to a wall outlet or, less commonly, is supplied via a portable cylinder or oxygen concentrator and may be delivered to the individual via an oxygen regulator using one of several devices. Oxygen is prescribed in litres per minute or in percentage as FiO_2 (fraction of inspired oxygen). The mode chosen for the delivery of oxygen is dependent on the individual's clinical condition, concentration of oxygen required, degree of ventilatory support required and the individual's ability to comply with the therapy (see Table 25.4 for description of oxygen delivery equipment and concentration) (Pinsky et al 2019).

Nasal cannula

A nasal cannula (nasal prongs) (Figure 25.28) is made from a soft plastic material and contains two short prongs that fit into the nostrils. It may be secured in position by an adjustable ring or strap around the back of the head or taped onto the cheeks to prevent dislodgement. Because it does not enclose the nose or mouth, the cannula is comfortable and convenient for the person and there is less risk of aspiration of vomitus than a mask. The cannula is connected to the oxygen supply and the oxygen turned on at a low flow rate, with the flow checked before positioning it in the nares. The prongs are inserted following the natural curve of the nostrils, and the tubes are positioned over each ear and around the back of the head. The ring or strap is adjusted to maintain the position of the prongs, and care is taken to

TABLE 25.4 | Oxygen equipment

Type	Oxygen concentration flow rate	Indication
Nasal cannula/ catheter	FiO_2: 24–38%, flow 1–2 L/min FiO_2: 30–35%, flow 3–4 L/min FiO_2: 38–44%, flow 5–6 L/min	This device is well tolerated by most individuals. The fraction of inspired oxygen varies depending upon the flow of oxygen (L/min) and the rate and depth of the individual's breathing.
Simple face mask	FiO_2: 35–50%, flow 6–12 L/min	High flow of oxygen is required to prevent the rebreathing of carbon dioxide.
Partial and non-rebreather masks	FiO_2: 60–75%, flow 6–11 L/min FiO_2: 60–90%, flow 10–15 L/min	These masks have a reservoir bag but no flaps. For best oxygen delivery, be sure that the bag remains slightly inflated at the end of inspiration. This device allows for a higher FiO_2 to be administered. A valve closes during expiration so that exhaled air does not enter the reservoir bag and be rebreathed. Never remove the one-way valve.
Venturi mask	FiO_2: 60–100%, flow 4–15 L/min	This device is one of the most accurate ways to deliver oxygen without intubation. Different-sized adapters are used to deliver a fixed or predicted FiO_2. It is ideal for CO_2 retainers or hypoxic drive individuals.
Head box	FiO_2: 21–100%, low 0.25–3 L/min	A transparent plastic box that fits over the head or shoulders of an infant. The infant can be observed easily, and high concentrations of oxygen can be administered.

(Ignatavicius et al 2021; Pinsky et al 2019; Potter et al 2023)

ensure that the strap is not too tight. An over-tight strap can cause pressure on the nostrils, the nose, the upper lip and cheeks. When the cannula has been positioned correctly, the flow of oxygen is adjusted to the prescribed rate. Minimum flow is 0.25 L/min to a maximum of 6 L/min, but this will often cause nasal dryness and can be uncomfortable. Flow rates of 1–4 L/min are most commonly used, equating to a concentration of approximately 24–40% oxygen. Higher volumes increase irritation and drying of the nasal mucosa. The oxygen concentration that the individual receives is indeterminable and is reduced if the individual mouth breathes, eats or drinks (Pinsky et al 2019).

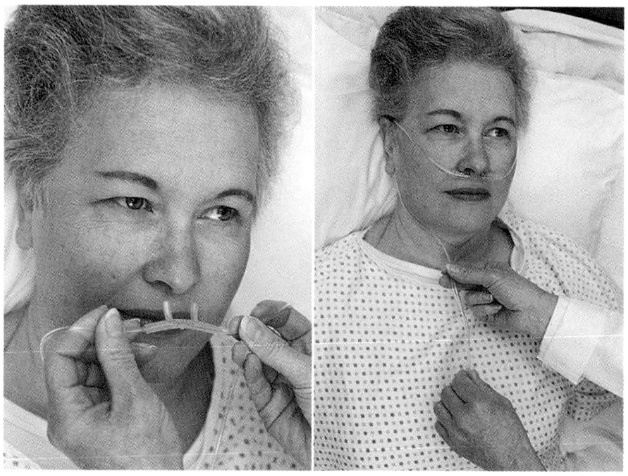

Figure 25.28 Applying a nasal cannula

(Potter et al 2023)

Nasal catheter

An intranasal oxygen catheter is made from a soft plastic material and contains a series of holes at the distal ends. The approximate length to be inserted is estimated by holding the catheter in a straight line from the tip of the individual's nose to their earlobe, and marking the catheter with an indelible pen to ensure that the insertion length can always be seen. The tip of the catheter may be lubricated with sterile water or a water-soluble lubricant to facilitate insertion. Before insertion, the catheter is connected to the oxygen supply and the oxygen turned on at a low flow rate. As with nasal prongs, oxygen concentration varies with factors such as mouth breathing. The catheter can induce gastric distension if forced into the stomach.

The catheter is gently inserted through one nostril into the nasopharynx to the pre-measured length. Using hypoallergenic tape, the catheter may be secured to the nose or cheek, avoiding traction on the nostril, which could cause skin breakdown. When the catheter has been positioned correctly, the flow of oxygen is adjusted to the prescribed rate. Because it is an invasive device, the catheter may cause irritation of the mucosa, so it is usual to remove it after about 8 hours and insert a clean one into the other nostril. Rotating the site reduces the risks of mucous membrane irritation and skin breakdown at the tip of the nose (Pinsky et al 2019).

Face mask

Face masks (Figure 25.29) are available in several styles and sizes. They are made from a lightweight vinyl material and are designed to fit over the nose and mouth and secured in position by an elastic band around the head. As the mask covers both the nose and the mouth, it is confining and impedes activities such as eating, drinking and communication as well as potentiating the risk of aspiration of vomitus.

Minimum flow rate for masks is normally 5 L/min since a lower flow rate is not adequate to clear the mask of exhaled carbon dioxide and can cause hypercapnia (CO_2 retention). Depending on the style, a mask can deliver oxygen from 28% at 4 L/min to 100% concentration at higher flow rates. A mask is commonly used when the individual requires higher concentrations and more accurate amounts of oxygen, such as when the individual is mouth breathing, eating, talking or is able to breathe only through the mouth. Oxygen masks are recognisable by the presence of multiple small holes on the sides of the mask, as opposed to nebuliser masks, which have one large-diameter hole each side.

The style and size of a mask is assessed by measuring from the chin to the top of the nose, and an appropriate size is selected. The mask is connected to the oxygen supply via a flexible plastic tube, and the oxygen turned on to check that there are no leaks at a low flow rate. The mask is placed over the nose, mouth and chin, and the elastic strap secured around the back of the head; some masks have pliable metal straps that can be used to mould the mask to the individual's face shape. The strap is adjusted to ensure that the mask is firmly positioned but not uncomfortable, and the flow of oxygen adjusted to the prescribed rate. It is important that the mask fits closely but is not uncomfortable, and the nurse should ensure that there is no leakage of oxygen from the top of the mask. Leakage of oxygen from the top of the mask can flow across the eyes, causing dryness and irritation of the delicate tissues. Masks can create pressure areas on the skin and can be made more comfortable by applying self-adhesive foam to the edges in contact with skin (Pinsky et al 2019).

Non-rebreather

A non-rebreather mask with an oxygen reservoir bag can be used to deliver high concentrations of oxygen to an individual who can breathe spontaneously. A one-way valve on the mask closes during expiration so that exhaled air does not enter the reservoir bag to be rebreathed. The reservoir bag also helps increase the inspired oxygen concentration by preventing the individual from breathing room air upon inspiration.

Venturi face mask

A venturi face mask device mixes oxygen with room air, delivering a predetermined high-flow enriched oxygen concentration. This device is one of the most accurate ways to deliver oxygen. Different-sized adapters are used to deliver a fixed or predicted FiO_2. It is ideal for CO_2 retainers or hypoxic drive individuals.

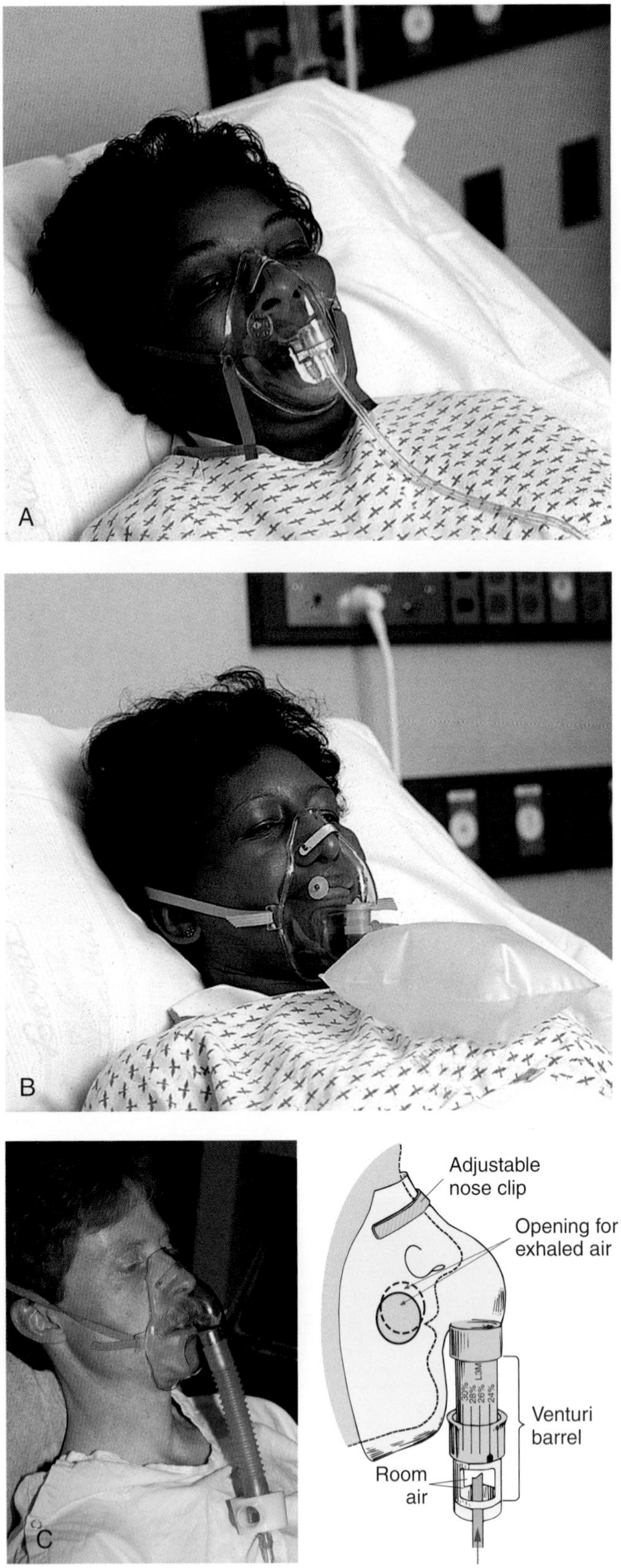

Figure 25.29 Examples of face masks

A: Simple face mask, **B:** Plastic face mask with reservoir bag, **C:** Venturi mask.

(Potter et al 2023)

Head box

A head box may be used to deliver oxygen to an infant and consists of a transparent plastic box that fits over the head or shoulders. The infant can be observed easily, and high concentrations of oxygen can be administered.

The concentration of oxygen to be delivered to the individual will be specified by the medical officer and depends on the delivery device used and the rate at which the oxygen flows. Oxygen can be delivered from concentrations of 21% to 100%, and the flow rate adjusted by oxygen regulators from 0.25 L/min (low flow) to 3 L/min (high flow). The flow rate is adjusted by turning the valve on the flow meter (Figure 25.30) and observing the ball or dial that indicates the number of litres per minute at which the oxygen is flowing.

Whenever oxygen is to be administered, the nurse should refer to the directions that accompany the device, to ensure that the correct concentration of oxygen is delivered to the individual (Pinsky et al 2019).

Mechanical ventilation

Mechanical ventilation is a life-saving measure. Although ventilators are complex machines, the underlying principles on which they work remain the same (Parrillo & Dellinger 2019). Ventilators use electric or compressed power to generate breath and ventilate the lungs (Parrillo & Dellinger 2019). These devices may use either positive or negative pressure.

Positive pressure

Intermittent positive-pressure ventilation (IPPV) devices push atmospheric or oxygen-rich air into the individual's airways to promote adequate lung expansion. Commonly, IPPV is performed via an endotracheal or tracheostomy tube and allows effective control of ventilation and oxygenation. The flow of air to the lungs is set at a predetermined pressure and, as the pressure is attained, the flow is stopped, pressure is released and the person exhales. Types of IPPV devices include:

- Positive end-expiratory pressure (PEEP): Maintains a positive pressure in the lungs at the end of the individual's respiratory cycle, by increasing pressure within airways.
- Continuous positive airway pressure (CPAP): A device that uses a certain amount of pressure to maintain the patency of large and small airways and alveoli. CPAP devices are commonly used in individuals with sleep apnoea. It can be administered with a tight-fitting face mask or over a tracheostomy and is often used to slow or prevent the need for mechanical ventilation.

(Parrillo & Dellinger 2019)

Negative pressure

Negative pressure chambers use a negative pressure to maintain inflation of the lung and can be used to administer high volumes of oxygen. Examples include the iron lung and barochamber.

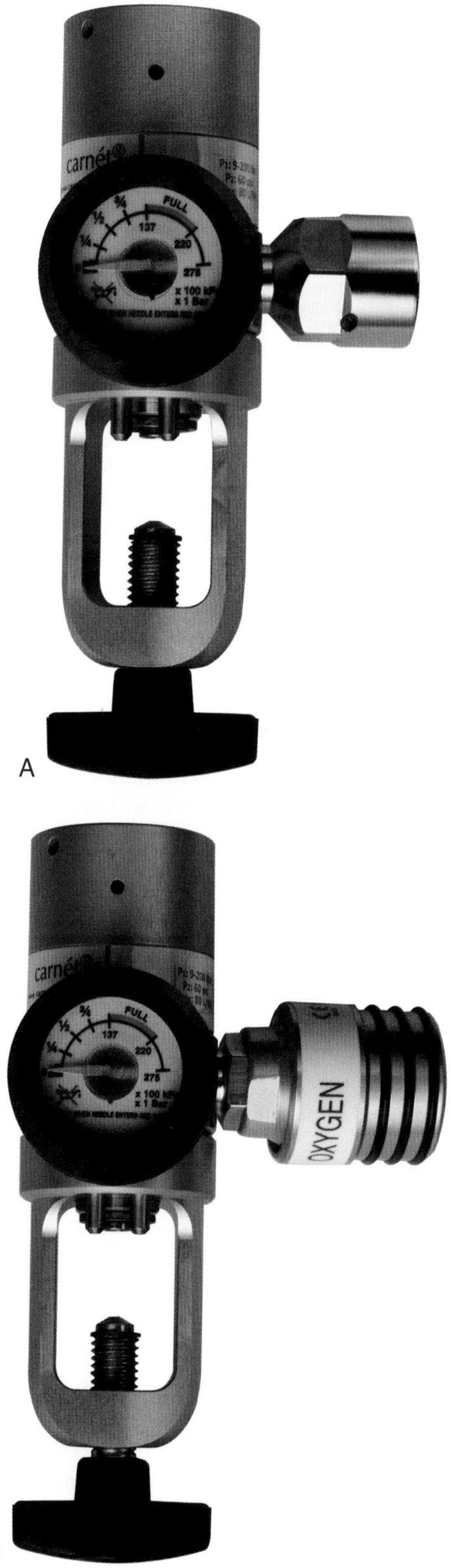

Figure 25.30 Oxygen regulators

A: An example of an Australian standard regulator, **B:** An example of a New Zealand standard regulator.

(Images of Carnét® Oxygen Pressure Regulators (AS and BS) courtesy of BOC Limited, a member of the Linde group)

Measures to promote the comfort and safety of the individual receiving oxygen

There are a number of measures that nurses should consider when caring for an individual receiving oxygen. Such measures include:

- Reducing any anxiety the individual or their significant others experience related to the administration of oxygen. Some people may feel that the administration of oxygen is a sign that the individual's condition is deteriorating, and individuals using face masks may experience anxiety related to having both their nose and their mouth covered. The nurse should explain the purpose of the oxygen and the equipment that is being used. Some people may be educated to use the equipment independently and thus feel they have some control over the situation. Frequent visits to the individual, prompt attention to their needs and efficient handling of the equipment will help to reduce their anxiety.
- Constantly monitoring the equipment to ensure that it is functioning correctly. The nurse should check the flow rate and ensure that the prescribed concentration of oxygen is being delivered to the individual. Connections on regulators, concentrators and humidifiers should be checked to ensure their tightness and that they are free of leaks. Measures should be taken to prevent the oxygen tubing becoming twisted, kinked or disconnected, to facilitate a free flow of oxygen to the individual.
- Informing the individual of the importance of maintaining the delivery device in the correct position, as changing its position may alter the amount of oxygen being delivered.
- Prevention of infection. In the past, oxygen that was delivered by an oxygen mask, nasal cannula or nasal catheter was humidified to prevent drying of the mucous membranes. Normal practice in most healthcare agencies is to use only sterile methods of humidification and dispose of the equipment according to infection control or manufacturer's guidelines to reduce the potential for nosocomial infections. Oxygen masks and cannulas provide sufficient atmospheric water to humidify the oxygen.
- Assisting the individual to meet their hygiene needs. The skin under the tubing, elastic straps or mask should be kept dry to promote comfort and to reduce the risk of skin breakdown caused by humidity or perspiration. Both the individual's face and the face mask should be wiped dry at least every 2 hours, and the skin under the delivery device checked for signs of pressure or irritation. Oral and nasal hygiene needs should be met and a water-based cream or balm may be applied to the lips or nares to prevent dryness and discomfort.
- Replacing the mask with a nasal cannula if necessary, while the individual is eating or having their oral hygiene needs met.
- Measuring the individual's temperature by the tympanic or axillary route rather than the oral route, as placement of the thermometer in the mouth may cause further ventilatory distress.
- Monitoring the individual's condition constantly to assess the effectiveness of the treatment. The individual should be observed for signs of hypoxia or oxygen toxicity. Hypoxia may occur if the oxygen concentration is inadequate or if the equipment is not functioning properly. Oxygen toxicity is more likely to occur if the individual is receiving high concentrations (e.g. over 50%), which can be detrimental to the central nervous system. Manifestations of oxygen toxicity include nausea, muscle twitching, dizziness, restlessness and irritability, convulsive seizures and coma. Prolonged administration of high concentrations of oxygen may also cause damage to the linings of the bronchi and alveoli, resulting in pulmonary congestion or collapse of lung tissue. Any indications of hypoxaemia, hypercapnia (CO_2 retention) or toxicity must be reported immediately since the concentration of oxygen being administered may need to be adjusted. It should also be noted that people with chronic obstructive airways disease, such as emphysema, may have an 'oxygen drive', in which their respiratory rate is controlled by decreasing levels of oxygen, as opposed to the normal regulation of respiratory rate, which is due to an increasing CO_2 level. These individuals are never prescribed high-flow oxygen since it reduces their respiratory drive and rate and increases hypercapnia.
- Observing the individual closely after oxygen therapy has been discontinued since the therapy may need to be resumed if signs of hypoxia become evident.
- Handling the oxygen equipment. The equipment used to deliver oxygen to the person should be cared for in the manner specified in the healthcare institution's policy manual. Most of the delivery devices are disposable, which reduces the risk of cross-infection.

EDUCATION

Planning for an individual's discharge from hospital is of particular importance if their respiratory disorder is chronic or recurrent. The individual must be provided with sufficient information because, by understanding their condition and how to manage the symptoms, they will be better able to cope with chronic respiratory disease. The individual should be encouraged to pursue as normal a lifestyle as possible and should be given information about:

- the importance of avoiding factors that may precipitate or exacerbate their condition, such as extremes of temperature, exposure to allergens or environmental irritants, fatigue or emotional stress

- the importance of avoiding close contact with individuals who have a respiratory tract infection
- the importance of contacting their medical officer at the first sign of a respiratory tract infection
- the nature and correct use of any prescribed medications, nebulisers or aerosol therapy
- public health education about smoking and its relationship to lung cancer and chronic obstructive pulmonary disease; the means of preventing droplet-spread infection; and the effects of air pollutants on the respiratory tract
- immunisation against infections such as pertussis, influenza and TB
- how and when to use oxygen, which an individual may need to have immediate access to at all times
- when to contact their medical officer or go to hospital (e.g. if the measures implemented at home fail to sufficiently control their symptoms).

Progress Note 25.1

01/04/2024 1430 hrs	Nursing: Mr Jones reported shortness of breath and difficulty breathing. Upon assessment, observations were noted to be BP 140/70 mmHg, HR 96 beats/min, RR 22 breaths/min, SaO_2 89% on 4 L/min O_2. Salbutamol administered via spacer with effect. Deep-breathing and coughing exercises performed. Oxygen saturation levels have improved SaO2 to 96% on 4 L/min. Encourage regular fluids as tolerated, administer antibiotics as ordered.
	C Westinghouse (WESTINGHOUSE), *EN*

DECISION-MAKING FRAMEWORK EXERCISE 25.1

You have been employed as an Enrolled Nurse in a cardiovascular surgical ward for 5 years. On the shift with you tonight there is one senior Registered Nurse, one recently Registered Nurse and three Enrolled Nurses. You have been assigned three patients—all are at least 3 days postoperative. During your shift, one of your patients requires a blood transfusion. Using the decision-making framework:

1. Is this within your scope of nursing practice?
2. Are you supported appropriately by other staff members to care for this person?
3. Is this model of care appropriate?
4. What strategies could you consider in this situation?

Summary

The human body requires oxygen and nutrients in order to survive. The circulatory system functions as the mechanism through which every cell in the body receives oxygen and nutrients, while also facilitating the removal of waste products from cells and transporting them to different organs for excretion. This system encompasses two main components: the cardiovascular system and the lymphatic system. The cardiovascular system comprises the heart, blood vessels and blood, whereas the lymphatic system includes lymph, lymphatic capillaries, vessels, nodes and ducts.

Blood, a dense substance, consists of plasma fluid containing three types of formed elements: erythrocytes, leucocytes and platelets, each carrying out distinct functions. Blood's primary roles encompass transporting oxygen, nutrients and other substances to cells, expelling waste materials from cells, safeguarding the body against infections, distributing heat evenly throughout the body, and preventing excessive blood loss through clotting. The heart pumps blood into major arteries, which progressively branch into smaller arteries and arterioles. These arterioles connect to a network of tiny vessels known as capillaries. Subsequently, blood flows into small veins or venules, which merge to form larger veins, ultimately transporting blood back to the heart. Blood continually circulates throughout the body in systemic, pulmonary or portal circulation.

The heart, a hollow muscular organ located in the thoracic cavity, propels deoxygenated blood to the lungs and oxygenated blood to all body parts. Breathing facilitates the exchange of oxygen and carbon dioxide in the lungs, while the cardiovascular system ensures the transportation of these gases to and from cells. Brainstem centres sensitive to CO_2 levels regulate ventilation, while factors like an individual's health condition, diseases, physical activity or emotions impact breathing rate, rhythm and depth. Diffusion is the process by which oxygen and CO_2 molecules move between alveoli and capillaries, and between cells. Diffusion abnormalities may arise from cardiac issues causing pulmonary oedema, respiratory disorders reducing functional lung tissue, or fibrosis of alveolar walls.

Respiratory dysfunction stems from insufficient ventilation, diffusion abnormalities across the pulmonary membrane, or inadequate transport between lungs and tissues. Besides lung or respiratory structure issues, disruptions in other body systems like the cardiac system can affect respiratory function, and vice versa. Common signs of respiratory disorders encompass chest pain, cough, voice changes, dyspnoea, altered breathing patterns,

Continued

Summary—cont'd

hypoxia and chest skeletal anomalies. Respiratory system disorders can be grouped as multifactorial, infection-related, neoplasm-related, obstructive or due to injury. Diagnostic tests include blood exams, electrolyte analysis, ultrasounds, pulmonary function tests, oximetry, chest X-rays, lung scans, blood gas analysis, cultures, sputum cytology, skin tests, bronchoscopy and thoracentesis.

Managing individuals with respiratory system disorders involves ensuring clear airways, promoting local hydration, correct positioning, medication administration, oronasopharyngeal suction, chest physiotherapy and oxygen therapy. Nurses might need to collect sputum specimens for lab tests, obtain nasal or throat swabs, or deliver inhalation therapy. Specific respiratory disorders might necessitate artificial airway insertion or mechanical ventilation. Inserting chest tubes could be required to drain air or fluid from the pleural space. Caring for those with cardiac or lymphatic disorders includes similar measures as respiratory care, along with fluid restrictions, weight monitoring, attention to chest or limb pain, and skin care. Some circulatory disorders may call for surgical intervention.

Some individuals require the administration of oxygen, which can be delivered using one of the various devices available. Whenever oxygen is being administered, the nurse must promote the individual's safety and comfort as part of assisting them to meet their need for oxygen.

Review Questions

1. Name the various parts of the respiratory tract.
2. Discuss the structure and function of the respiratory system.
3. Discuss the structure and function of the cardiovascular system.
4. What are the common causes of upper respiratory problems?
5. What is the significance of respiration?
6. Explain the process of ventilation.
7. How is oxygen transported?
8. What is oxyhaemoglobin and how is it formed?
9. Identify the four blood groups and the Rh factors.
10. List some of the common clinical features of respiratory disease.
11. List some of the most common manifestations of cardiovascular disease.
12. Describe the differences in cardiac pain for angina and myocardial infarction.
13. What are the main aims of nursing care for an individual with a respiratory or cardiovascular disorder?
14. Describe the nursing care for an individual receiving oxygen therapy.
15. Explain the difference between hypoxia and hypoxaemia.
16. Identify the key areas a person with a chronic or recurrent respiratory condition should be educated on when being discharged from hospital.

Evolve® Answer guide for the Review Questions, Critical Thinking Exercises, Decision-making Framework Exercises and Critical Thinking Questions in Case Studies is hosted on Evolve: http://evolve.elsevier.com/AU/Koutoukidis/Tabbner.

References

Abraham, S.E., 2023. Oxygen saturation and the pulse oximeter: This is sometimes considered the "5th" vital sign. *Podiatry Management*, 123–128. Available at: <https://podiatrym.com/pdf/2023/2/Abraham223web.pdf>.

Aitken, L.M., Marshall, A., Chaboyer, W., (eds.) 2019. *Critical care nursing*, 4th ed. Elsevier Australia, Chatswood, NSW.

American Association of Critical Care Nurses (AACN), Hartjes, T. (ed.), 2022. *Core curriculum for high acuity, progressive, and critical care nursing*, 8th ed. Elsevier Health Sciences, London.

Australian and New Zealand Committee on Resuscitation (ANZCOR), 2023. Guideline 14 Acute Coronary syndrome. Available at: <https://www.anzcor.org/assets/anzcor-guidelines/guideline-14-acute-coronary-syndromes-300.pdf>.

Berman, A., Kozier, B., Erb, G.L., 2020. *Kozier and Erb's fundamentals of nursing: Concepts, process and practice*, 5th ed. Pearson Australia, Melbourne.

Boltz, M., (ed.) 2021. *Evidence-based geriatric nursing protocols for best practice*, 6th ed. Springer Publishing Company, New York, New York.

Braunwald, E., Libby, P., Bhatt, D., et al., 2021. *Braunwald's heart disease: A textbook of cardiovascular medicine*. Elsevier.

Broaddus, V., Ernst, J.D., King, T.E., et al., 2021. *Murray & Nadel's textbook of respiratory medicine*, 7th ed. Elsevier Health Sciences, Philadelphia.

Carlson, B., 2018. *The human body: A functional approach to its structure*. Elsevier Science & Technology, St Louis.

Carter, C., Notter, J., 2024. *Handbook for registered nurses*. Elsevier Ltd.

Craft, J., Gordon, C., McCance, K.L., et al., 2023. *Understanding pathophysiology Australia and New Zealand edition*, 4th ed. Elsevier, Chatswood.

Crisp, J., Douglas, C., Rebeiro, G., et al. (eds.), 2021. *Potter and Perry's fundamentals of nursing*, 6th ed. Elsevier, Australia and New Zealand, New South Wales.

Deng, H., Fang, Q., Chen, K., et al., 2021. Early versus late tracheotomy in ICU patients: A meta-analysis of randomized controlled trials. *Medicine (Baltimore)* 100(3), e24329.

Donald, C., Randal, T., Bhalla, V., et al., 2019. 2019 AHA/ACC clinical performance and quality measures for adults with high blood pressure. A report of the American College of Cardiology/American Heart Association Task Force on Performance Measures. Circulation. *Cardiovascular Quality and Outcomes* 12, e000057.

Dover, A.R. (ed.), 2023. *Macleod's clinical examination*, 15th ed. Elsevier, Edinburgh.

Elsherbiny, A., Mazeed, A., Saied, A., et al. 2018. The significance of uvula after palatoplasty: A new technique to improve the aesthetic outcome. *Cleft Palate-Craniofacial Journal* 55(3), 451–455.

Flaherty, C., 2020. Tracheostomy care: The role of the nurse before, during and after insertion. *Nursing Standard* 35(8), 76–82.

Gerhard-Herman, M., Aday, A., 2020. Peripheral artery disease. In: *Manual of vascular medicine*. Springer, Cham.

Gallagher, K.A., Rectenwald, J.E., Froehlich, J.B., Henke, P.K., 2020. Lower extremity ischemia. In: Baliga, R., Eagle, K. (eds.), *Practical cardiology*. Springer, Cham. Available at: <https://doi.org/10.1007/978-3-030-28328-5_28>.

Global Initiative for Asthma (GINA), 2023. Global strategy for asthma management and prevention: updated 2023. Available at: <https://ginasthma.org/reports>.

Hanna, E., 2022. *Practical cardiovascular medicine*. John Wiley & Sons, Ltd, Chichester, UK, pp. 457–475.

Hartley, J., 2018. Respiratory rate 2: Anatomy and physiology of breathing. *Nursing Times* 104(6), 43–44.

Iqbal, A., Jamal, S., 2019. Essential hypertension. In: StatPearls [Internet]. StatPearls Publishing, Treasure Island (FL).

Ignatavicius, D., Workman, M., Rebar, C., et al., 2021. *Medical-surgical nursing: Concepts for interprofessional collaborative care*, 10th ed. Elsevier Inc.

Knapp, R., (ed.), 2019. *Respiratory care made incredibly easy!* 2nd ed. Wolters Kluwer, Philadelphia, Pennsylvania.

Koeppen, B.M., Stanton, B.A., Hall, J.M., Swiatecka-Urban, A., (eds.), 2023. *Berne & Levy physiology*, 8th ed. Elsevier, Philadelphia, PA.

Kucia, A.M., Jones, I.D., 2022. *Cardiac care: A practical guide for nurses*. Wiley.

Le Goff, D., Aerts, N., Odorico, M., et al., 2023. Practical dietary interventions to prevent cardiovascular disease suitable for implementation in primary care: An ADAPTE-guided systematic review of international clinical guidelines. *International Journal of Behavioral Nutrition and Physical Activity* 20(1), 93.

Lewis, S.M., Dirksen, S.R., Heitkemper, M.M., 2014. *Medical–surgical nursing. Assessment and management of clinical problems*, 9th ed. Mosby, St Louis.

Magee, D., 2014. *Orthopedic physical assessment*, 6th ed. Elsevier Inc.

Mars, L., 2020. *Cardiovascular disease handbook and resource guide*. Grey House Publishing, Amenia, NY.

Marieb, E.N., Hoehn, K., 2019. *Human anatomy and physiology*, 11th ed. Pearson, Harlow, England.

Menzies-Gow, E., 2018. How to record a 12-lead electrocardiogram. *Nursing Standard* 33(2), 38–42. doi: 10.7748/ns.2018.e11066.

Millar, F., Hillman, T., 2018. Managing chest drains on medical wards. *British Medical Journal* 363, k4639.

National Heart Foundation of Australia, 2016. Guideline for the diagnosis and management of hypertension in adults. National Heart Foundation of Australia, Melbourne. Available at: <https://www.heartfoundation.org.au/getmedia/c83511ab-835a-4fcf-96f5-88d770582ddc/PRO-167_Hypertension-guideline-2016_WEB.pdf>.

NHFA CSANZ Heart Failure Guidelines Working Group, 2018. National Heart Foundation of Australia and Cardiac Society of Australia and New Zealand: Guidelines for the prevention, detection, and management of heart failure in Australia 2018. *Heart Lung and Circulation* 27(10), 1123–1208. Available at: <https://doi.org/10.1016/j.hlc.2018.06.1042>.

NSW Agency for Clinical Innovation, 2021. Care of adult patients in acute care facilities with a tracheostomy: Clinical practice guide. Sydney. Available at: <https://aci.health.nsw.gov.au/__data/assets/pdf_file/0004/685300/ACI-CPG-Tracheostomy.pdf>.

Nursing and Midwifery Board of Australia (NMBA), 2020. Decision-making framework for nursing and midwifery. Available at: <https://www.nursingmidwiferyboard.gov.au/Codes-Guidelines-Statements/Frameworks.aspx>.

Pahal, P., Avula, A., Sharma, S., 2023. Emphysema. In: StatPearls [Internet]. StatPearls Publishing, Treasure Island (FL).

Parrillo, J., Dellinger, R., (eds.), 2019. *Critical care medicine: Principles of diagnosis and management in the adult*, 5th ed. Elsevier, Philadelphia.

Patel, S., Mohiuddin S., 2019. Physiology, oxygen transport and carbon dioxide dissociation curve. In: StatPearls [Internet]. StatPearls Publishing, Treasure Island (FL).

Patton, K., Thibodeau, G., 2019. *Anatomy and physiology*, Adapted international edition. Elsevier Ltd.

Perry, A.G., Potter, P.A., Ostendorf, W., Laplante, N., 2022. *Nursing interventions and clinical skills*, 10th ed. Elsevier Inc, St Louis.

Pinsky, M., Teboul, J., Vincent J., (eds.), 2019. *Hemodynamic monitoring*. Springer International Publishing, Cham.

Potter, P.A., Perry, A.G., Stockert, P., et al., 2023. *Fundamentals of nursing*, 11th ed. Mosby, St Louis.

Pruitt, B., 2022. Tracheostomy care and the respiratory therapist. *RT: The Journal for Respiratory Care Practitioners* 35(6), 26–30.

Rebeiro, G., Wilson, D., Fuller, S., 2021. *Potter and Perry's fundamentals of nursing workbook*, 4th ed. Elsevier, Chatswood.

Sajadi-Ernazarova, K., Martin, J., Gupta, N., 2022. Acute pneumothorax evaluation and treatment. In: StatPearls [Internet]. StatPearls Publishing, Treasure Island (FL).

Smith, M.L., Leslie, K.O., Wick, M.R., 2024. *Practical pulmonary pathology: A diagnostic approach*, 4th ed. Elsevier, Philadelphia, Pennsylvania.

Smith, R.S., Vanzant, E., Catena, F., 2020. Pneumothorax and hemothorax. In: *Thoracic surgery for the acute care surgeon*. Springer International Publishing, Cham, pp. 159–168.

Stein, L., Hollen, C., 2024. *Concept-based clinical nursing skills: Fundamental to advanced competencies*, 2nd ed. Elsevier Inc.

Terzi, H., Kitiş, Y., Akin, B., 2023. Effectiveness of non-pharmacological community-based nursing interventions for smoking cessation in adults: A systematic review. *Public Health Nursing* 40(1), 195–207.

Thomas, L., 2018. Transport of substances in the body part 2: How oxygen and carbon dioxide are transported in the blood. *AMWA Journal* 33(4), 147–151.

Thomsett, R., Cullen, L., 2018. The assessment and management of chest pain in primary care: A focus on acute coronary syndrome. *Australian Journal of General Practice* 47(5). Available at: <https://www1.racgp.org.au/ajgp/2018/may/chest-pain-in-primary-care>.

Toor, H., Kashyap, S., Yau, A., et al., 2021. Efficacy of incentive spirometer in increasing maximum inspiratory volume in an out-patient setting. *Cureus* 13(10), e18483.

Tortora, G.J., Derrickson, B., Burkett B., et al., 2021. *Principles of anatomy and physiology*, 3rd Asia-Pacific edition. Wiley, Milton, Qld.

Treuting, P., Dintzis, S., Montine, K., 2018. *Comparative anatomy and histology: A mouse, rat, and human atlas*, 2nd ed. Elsevier, London.

Urden, L.D., Stacy, K.M., Lough, M.E., 2022. Diagnosis and management. In: Urden, L.D., Stacy, K.M., Lough, M.E., (eds.), *Critical care nursing*, 9th ed. Elsevier, Amsterdam.

Valchanov, K., Jones, N., Hogue, C. (eds.), 2019. *Core topics in cardiothoracic critical care*, 2nd ed. Cambridge University Press, Cambridge.

Watkins, D., Beaton, A., Carapetis, J., et al., 2018. Rheumatic heart disease worldwide. *Journal of the American College of Cardiology* 72(12), 1397–1416.

World Health Organization (WHO), 2020. A guide to WHO's guidance on COVID-19. WHO, Geneva. Available at: <https://www.who.int/emergencies/diseases/novel-coronavirus-2019/technical-guidance>.

Recommended Reading

Berbenetz, N., Wang, Y., Brown, J., et al., 2019. Non-invasive positive pressure ventilation (CPAP or bilevel NPPV) for cardiogenic pulmonary oedema. *Cochrane Database of Systematic Reviews* 4, CD005351.

Curtis, E., Fernandez, R., Lee, A., 2018. The effect of topical medications on radial artery spasm in patients undergoing transradial coronary procedures: A systematic review. *JBI Database of Systematic Reviews and Implementation Reports* 16(3), 738–751.

NHFA CSANZ Heart Failure Guidelines Working Group, Atherton, J., Sindone, A., et al., 2018. National Heart Foundation of Australia and Cardiac Society of Australia and New Zealand: Guidelines for the prevention, detection, and management of heart failure in Australia 2018. *Heart, Lung & Circulation* 27(10), 1123–1208.

Sabharwal, N., 2017. State of the art in nuclear cardiology. *Heart* 103(10), 790.

Saleh, M., Ambrose, J.A., 2018. Understanding myocardial infarction. *F1000Research* 7, 1378.

Sandra, O., 2016. Practical procedures: Oxygen therapy. *Nursing Times* 112(1–2), 12–14.

Srivasta, A., 2023. *Trauma surgery essentials: A must-know guide to emergency management.* Elsevier Inc.

Stein, L., Hollen, C., 2024. *Concept-based clinical nursing skills: Fundamental to advanced competencies*, 2nd ed. Elsevier Inc.

Stewart, J., Manmathan, G., Wilkinson, P., 2017. Primary prevention of cardiovascular disease: A review of contemporary guidance and literature. *Journal of the Royal Society of Medicine Cardiovascular Disease* 6, 1–9.

Online Resources

American Association for Respiratory Care: <www.aarc.org>.

American Journal of Respiratory and Critical Care Medicine: <www.atsjournals.org/journal/ajrccm>.

Australian and New Zealand Society of Blood Transfusion: <https://anzsbt.org.au/education-research/elearning>.

Australian Red Cross Blood Service: <https://www.redcross.org.au>.

Australian Resuscitation Council: <https://resus.org.au>.

JBI Evidence Synthesis: <https://journals.lww.com/jbisrir/pages/default.aspx>.

JBI EBP Database: <https://www.wolterskluwer.com/en/know/jbi-resources/jbi-ebp-database>. (Database available via OVID; login required, use the search function to find a variety of recommended practices and evidence summaries.)

National Asthma Council Australia: <https://www.nationalasthma.org.au/health-professionals>.

Respiratory Nurses' Interest Group (NSW) Inc: <http://www.rnig.org.au/resources.html>.

CHAPTER
26

Fluids and electrolytes

Kalpana Raghunathan

Key Terms

acid
acidosis
active transport
albumin
aldosterone
alkaline
alkalosis
anions
antidiuretic hormones (ADH)
base
body fluid
buffer
cations
dehydration
diffusion
diuretics
electrolytes
extracellular fluid (ECF)
filtration
fluid balance
fluid volume deficit
fluid volume excess
homeostasis
hydrostatic pressure
hypertonic
hypotonic
ions
insensible losses
interstitial
intracellular fluid (ICF)
intravascular
isotonic
normal range
oedema
osmolality
osmosis
osmotic pressure
pH
phlebitis
sensible losses
solutes
specific gravity (SG)
tonicity
transcellular

Learning Outcomes

At the completion of this chapter and with further reading, learners should be able to:

- Define the key terms, concepts, physiological processes and mechanisms related to fluid and electrolyte distribution, composition, movement and regulation.
- Describe common health problems associated with common fluid, electrolyte and acid–base imbalances.
- Identify interventions utilised in correction of fluid, electrolyte and acid–base imbalances in the clinical environment.
- Apply principles of safe and appropriate person-centred care for individuals receiving intravenous therapy.
- Apply principles of person-centred care in assessment, planning, implementation and evaluation of nursing care related to maintaining fluid, electrolyte and acid–base balance.

CHAPTER FOCUS

This chapter outlines theoretical foundations in the science of fluid and electrolyte homeostasis and acid–base balance. Key physiological processes that regulate the delicate fluid, electrolyte and acid–base balance and pathophysiology of altered homeostasis are discussed. Signs and symptoms indicative of problems as well as predisposing factors are highlighted. Monitoring and maintaining adequate fluid, electrolyte and acid–base balance is an important part of nursing care. Specific evidence-based interventions and management of nursing care related to common disturbances of fluid, electrolyte and acid–base status are described to assist in developing best nursing practice and advance skills in providing comprehensive person-centred care throughout the lifespan. In this chapter, a brief overview of the topic is addressed—additional reading is recommended to enhance your knowledge base.

LIVED EXPERIENCE

As clinicians, understanding the role of fluids and electrolytes and acid–base balance is central to expert patient management. More than half of the human body is made up of water. The organs and functions of the body depend on the circulation of blood and lymphatic fluid for the coordination of metabolism including the carriage of oxygen and hormones, nutritional supply and waste disposal. As such, so many bodily functions depend on maintaining a stable fluid and electrolyte status. Having a thorough knowledge of fluid and electrolyte physiology is essential for effective nursing care and medical management of fluid and electrolyte status in both health and disease. Nurses have a vital role that includes careful observation of a patient's general condition and the accurate measurement of fluid balance with both intake orally and intravenously and output including in urine, sweat and faeces. Daily weighing of the unwell patient and fluid balance charting is an important part of patient monitoring. Accurate clinical assessment data is critical to provide a picture of the patient's overall health status and assists timely and effective interventions by the healthcare team, including prescribing medications and fluid therapy.

Dr Andrew, Physician

INTRODUCTION

The delicate balance of fluids, electrolytes, acids and bases plays a vital role in the maintenance of a healthy internal environment of the human body. The normal value for these variables is a range of values known as the **normal range** (or reference range). For example, the normal range for blood pH is 7.35 and 7.45 and, as such, slight variations could remain within normal levels, with small changes corrected internally to maintain a stable environment (Craft et al 2023). **Homeostasis** is this state of equilibrium or stability in the internal environment of the body, which is naturally maintained by adaptive or compensatory responses at the cellular and local level to promote health survival (Brown et al 2020). However, when significant deviations or alterations outside the reference range occur, it can lead to serious health problems (Williams & Hopper 2019). In the healthcare environment, it is usually the responsibility of the nurse to monitor and maintain fluid balance; therefore, it is critical for nurses to develop a sound understanding of the mechanisms involved in maintaining homeostasis. This knowledge will inform nurses' ability to anticipate fluid, electrolyte and acid–base disturbances and initiate appropriate person-centred nursing assessment and management.

The significance of the nursing role in maintaining and restoring homeostasis can be demonstrated by the multitude of conditions a person presents with that may result in fluid and electrolyte or acid–base disturbances. The person might consume a number of different common medications that can also impact on maintenance of homeostasis. Nursing care includes the early identification of individuals in this group, their assessment and monitoring, and the development of a collaborative plan of care (LeMone et al 2020). Table 26.1 lists common conditions that can affect fluid and electrolyte homeostasis.

Distribution of body fluids

A large proportion of the human body is made up of **body fluid** or water and its **solutes**, which are small particles of dissolved substances. In healthy adults, total body water accounts for 50% of total body mass in women and 60% in men. This value changes quite significantly with age. For example, in a newborn, total body fluid is approximately 70 to 80% and this will gradually decrease as the individual ages (Craft et al 2023). The proportion of body water is dependent on the amount of lean body mass. Since men generally tend to have more lean body mass than women, men naturally have greater body water content than women. Older people have less lean mass and therefore a lower body water volume, rendering them more intolerant to fluid loss. Infants and older people require a particularly astute nursing assessment of their fluid volume status.

TABLE 26.1 | Common factors affecting fluid and electrolyte homeostasis

Fluid loss or shift	Conditions/factors
Skin losses	Excessive sweating, burns, fever
Gastrointestinal losses	Diarrhoea, vomiting, nasogastric suctioning
Renal losses	Diuretics
Osmotic diuresis	Diabetic ketoacidosis (DKA)
Volume loss	Haemorrhage, diabetes insipidus (DI)
Third spacing	Burns, sepsis, bowel obstruction, pancreatitis
Others	IV fluid administration, chronic heart failure, chronic renal failure, crush injuries

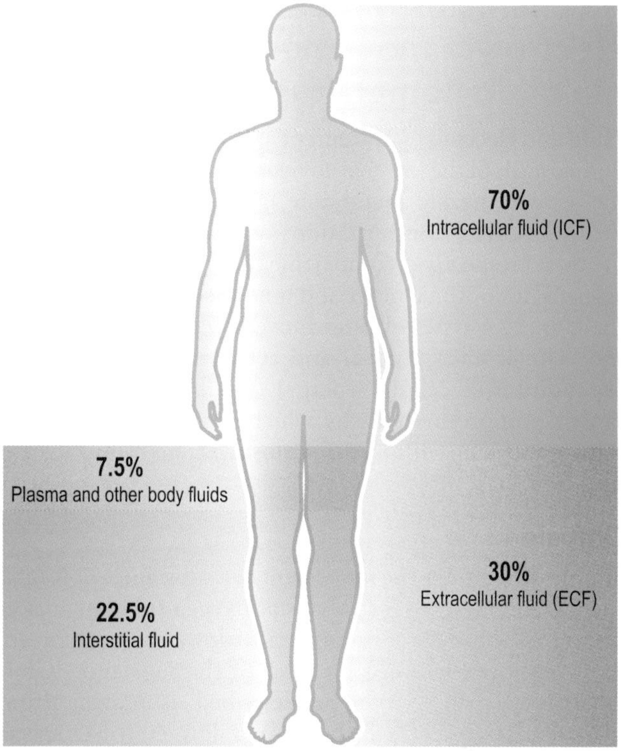

Figure 26.2 Distribution of body water in a 70 kg person

(Waugh & Grant 2023)

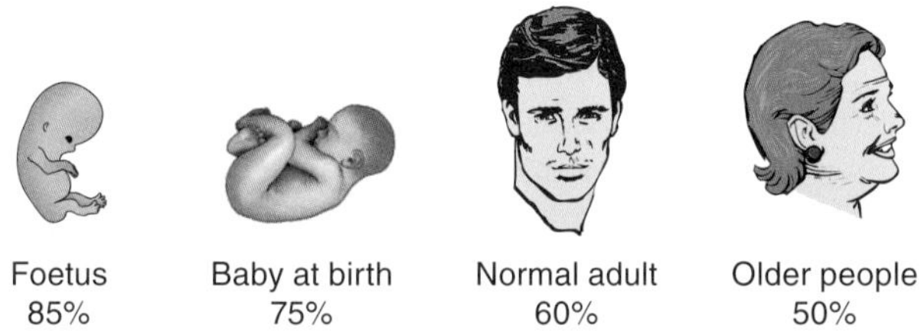

Figure 26.1 Percentage of water in the human body

Fluids and electrolytes are usually discussed simultaneously because body fluid is the mode of transport for electrolytes and other substances. Figure 26.1 illustrates the percentage of water content in the body.

Fluid volume distribution

Body water is distributed between two major compartments, approximately two-thirds in the intracellular space and one-third in the extracellular space (Craft et al 2023). (See Figure 26.2.)

Intracellular fluid (ICF) is the fluid contained inside the cells, which accounts for approximately 40% of total body weight (LeMone et al 2020). Electrolytes contained within the ICF include potassium, phosphorus and magnesium. **Extracellular fluid (ECF)** is located outside the cells and can be further divided into:

- **intravascular**: contained within the blood vessels (plasma) accounting for 5% of body weight
- **interstitial**: the fluid that surrounds cells accounting for approximately 15% of body weight
- **transcellular**: includes fluid in spaces between joints (synovial) and other compartments such as pericardial, pleural, intraocular, cerebrospinal and secretions
- sodium and chloride: the electrolytes found in the extracellular compartment.

(LeMone et al 2020)

The ICF and ECF are separated by two specific membranes: a semipermeable cell membrane and the blood vessel wall including the capillary membrane. Under normal healthy conditions the volume of fluid within each compartment remains relatively unchanged, although fluids and electrolytes move between compartments to maintain their relative compositions (Craft et al 2023). Fluids and electrolytes can move between compartments via the semipermeable membrane, meaning only selected substances can cross it. Water and solutes, depending on their size, solubility, electrical properties and concentration, can pass through the cell membrane (Craft et al 2023). This membrane is an example of a homeostatic mechanism, and it plays an integral role in maintaining fluid, electrolytes and other substances at their optimal levels and in the correct spaces for a healthily functioning body. The pathophysiology of diseases affecting the function of the semipermeable membrane is explored later in this chapter.

Mechanisms of fluid and electrolyte movement to maintain homeostasis

Fluid and electrolyte movement are critical in maintaining homeostasis of the internal environment. Movement across the semipermeable membrane is facilitated to maintain the appropriate concentrations of fluids and electrolytes in their respective compartments; this is particularly essential for optimal nerve and muscle function. Generally, there are two types of fluid movement: passive transport (no cellular energy used) and active transport (requires expenditure of cellular energy) (Craft et al 2023). The most common methods by which electrolytes and other solutes move are diffusion, osmosis, active transport and filtration.

Diffusion

Simple **diffusion** is the movement of a substance, or solute, such as sodium (an electrolyte) or oxygen from an area of greater concentration to an area of lower concentration, resulting in an even distribution of the substance (Craft et al 2023). This could be described as moving from a particularly crowded space to a less crowded space, termed as moving down a concentration gradient. This movement of molecules stops when the concentration reaches equilibrium in both areas. Many substances in the body move by diffusion, such as electrolytes, amino acids and glucose. The diffusion of fluids occurs through a permeable membrane, as in the movement of oxygen from alveoli in the lungs through the capillary membrane into the bloodstream.

Facilitated diffusion occurs when substances need to move but they need a little help to get to their destination. This assistance comes in the form of proteins, which transport substances through specific channels in the cell membrane. As a result of these substances moving down a concentration gradient (to the less crowded area), this process does not require energy (Craft et al 2023). In diffusion through ion channels, the membrane proteins allow the movement of specific electrolytes through the cell membrane. The channels are selective, and some channels are gated, opening only when stimulated to do so, playing an important part in the electrical activity of body cells (Craft et al 2023).

Osmosis

Osmosis is the movement of water through a semipermeable membrane from an area of low substance (high water) concentration to an area of high substance (low water) concentration (Brown et al 2020). This process requires no expenditure of energy, which simply means water will move to where there is a stronger concentration of electrolytes—like adding more water to a strong cup of tea or coffee. Subsequently, this has a dilutional effect on the solution. Osmosis continues until the concentration reaches equilibrium on either side of the membrane, and the membrane is only permeable to water. The rate at which osmosis occurs depends upon several factors, including:

- concentration of electrolytes
- temperature of the solution
- electrical charge of the electrolytes
- difference between the osmotic pressures exerted by the solutions.

See Table 26.2 for a summary of movement mechanisms for water and substances.

Active transport

Active transport is the movement of substances from an area of lower concentration to an area of higher concentration. Unlike diffusion, this process requires substances to move up the concentration gradient (Crisp et al 2021). This process could be described as like swimming against a strong current, therefore requiring more energy. Energy for this process comes in the form of adenosine triphosphate (ATP). The sodium–potassium ATP pump is an example of this type of movement. Concentrations of sodium and potassium are maintained within a tight range in the ECF and ICF, which is essential for optimal nerve conduction. As electrolytes have a tendency to want to reach equilibrium on either side of the membrane, they have to be pumped 'against the current' to maintain their concentrations. The sodium–potassium ATP pump is responsible for maintaining their concentrations and the cell 'charge', providing there is enough ATP available for this process (LeMone et al 2020). If ATP is depleted through disease processes, the consequences of homeostasis breakdown would potentially have a significant impact on the health of the person.

Filtration

Filtration is the movement of water and solutes through a permeable membrane because of pressure from within the capillaries into the interstitial space (Crisp et al 2021). The pressure in the fluid compartments as a result of the movement of fluid and solutes out of the compartment is known as filtration pressure. Hydrostatic and oncotic pressures are involved in this process (Craft et al 2023). In the cardiovascular system, hydrostatic pressure is the blood pressure generated in the vessels when the heart contracts. In the renal system, the proper excretory functioning of the kidneys is dependent on glomeruli filtration, and it is particularly relevant to nurses providing care for individuals with compromised renal function. *Creatinine* clearance in the urine is especially important to know before giving certain medications that are excreted by the kidneys, in order to prevent kidney damage (Berman et al 2020). See Clinical Interest Box 26.1 for examples of medications affecting urine production and elimination.

TABLE 26.2 | Mechanisms of fluid and electrolyte movement

Transport mode	Image	Movement of	Movement summary	Is ATP required?
Osmosis	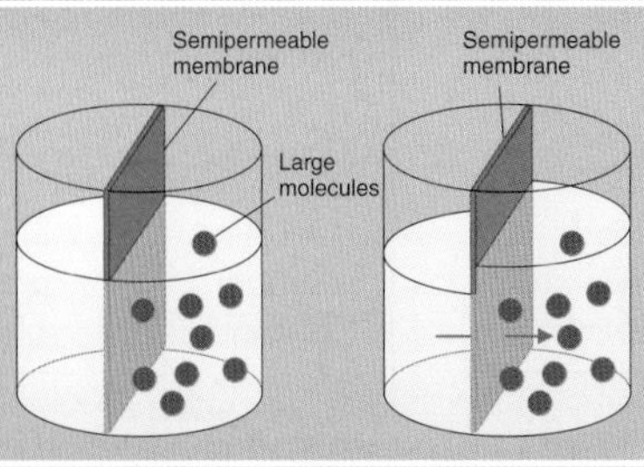	Water	Movement of water from high to low concentration.	No
Simple diffusion	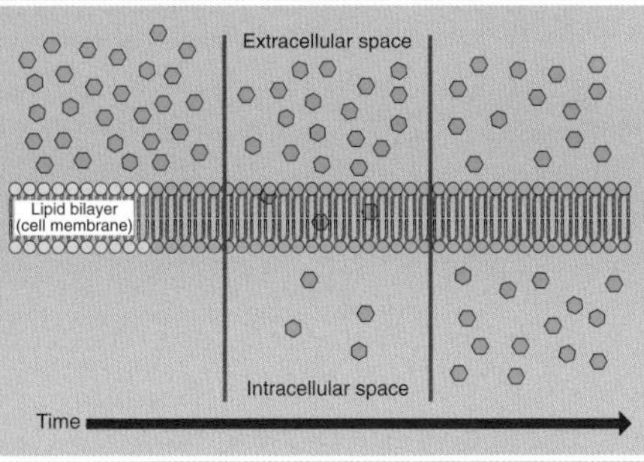	Substances	Movement of substances from a high to low concentration (crowded to less crowded).	No
Facilitated diffusion	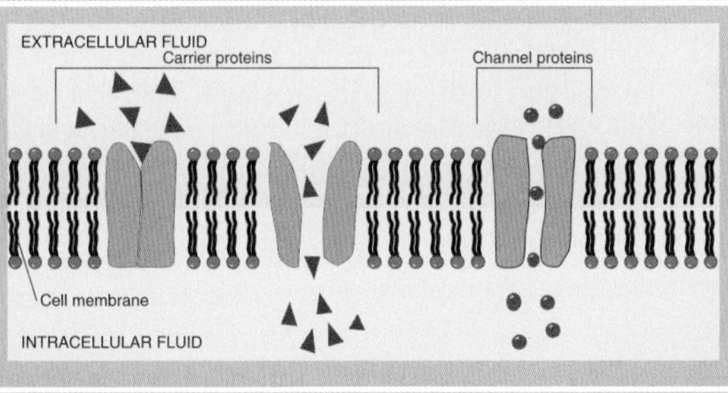	Substances	Proteins assist in movement from a high to low concentration (crowded to less crowded).	No
Active transport	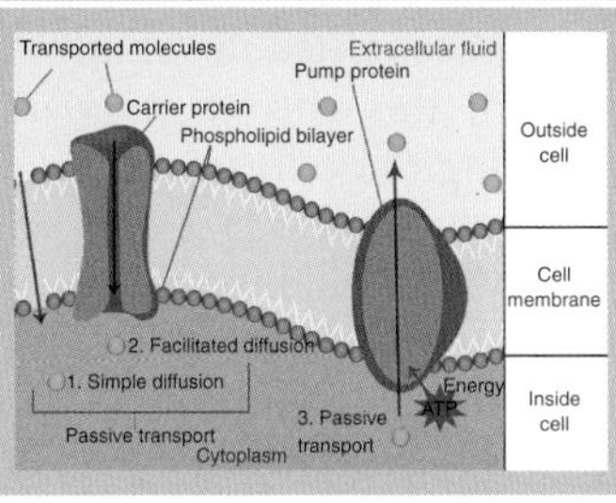	Substances	Movement from low to high concentration (to a crowded space).	Yes

(Adapted from Craft et al 2018. Active transport image © Balint Radu/Fotolia.com)

Osmotic pressure and hydrostatic pressure

Osmotic pressure (also called oncotic pressure) refers to the concentration of molecules in solution, which is expressed as a pressure unit, usually mmHg. Osmotic pressure is the drawing power for water in osmosis (Crisp et al 2021). Movement of water can be affected by differences in osmotic pressure on opposite sides of the membrane. Plasma has a higher concentration of proteins compared with interstitial fluid; these proteins (especially albumin) exert osmotic pressure, causing water to remain in the intravascular space (LeMone et al 2020).

Hydrostatic pressure is the force exerted by water in the fluid compartment and can be described as water-pushing pressure (Williams & Hopper 2019). Movement of water through a membrane can be affected by differences in hydrostatic pressure on either side of the membrane. The process of water moving from an area of high hydrostatic pressure to low hydrostatic pressure is called filtration (LeMone et al 2020). In the cardiovascular system, the blood pressure is the hydrostatic pressure exerted on the blood vessels.

Hydrostatic and osmotic pressures greatly influence the movement of water between the interstitial and intravascular

CLINICAL INTEREST BOX 26.1 Examples of medications affecting urine production and elimination

- Some antibiotics such as gentamicin can be nephrotoxic.
- Abuse of analgesics such as Act-3, Actiprofen, Brufen and Nurofen can be nephrotoxic.
- Diuretics cause moderate to severe increase in production and excretion of urine.
- Cholinergic medications, such as pilocarpine, stimulate urine production.
- Some analgesics and tranquillisers suppress the central nervous system (CNS) and interfere with urination and neural reflex.
- Certain drugs change the colour of the urine (e.g. anticoagulants—red, diuretics—pale yellow, B-complex vitamins—green or blue-green, levodopa—black or brown).

(Hall et al 2022)

compartments. For example, hydrostatic pressure at the arterial end of capillaries pushes water into the interstitial space, until the hydrostatic pressure is finally reduced due to the movement of water. The osmotic pressure at the venous end of the capillary is then greater than hydrostatic pressure and so encourages water to move back into the capillary (LeMone et al 2020). Conditions affecting the integrity of the membrane or the amount of protein in intravascular space will have a profound impact on health. See Figure 26.3 for a visual representation of water movement and capillary hydrostatic and oncotic pressure.

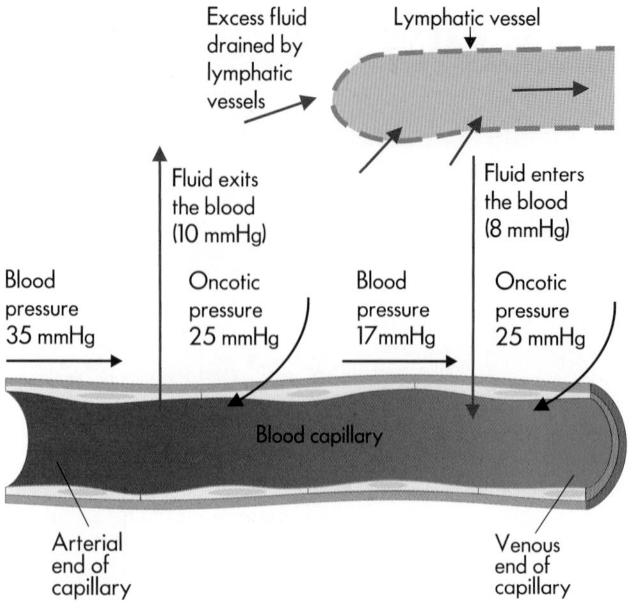

Figure 26.3 Water movement between the plasma and the interstitial space

At the arterial end of the capillary, fluid exits the blood, as the blood pressure in the capillary is greater than the tissue (interstitial) oncotic pressure; this fluid exit results in a small reduction in the blood pressure. There is no net movement of fluid near the midpoint. Net reabsorption occurs near the venous end, as the reduced blood pressure is now lower than the tissue oncotic pressure, which promotes fluid entry into the blood vessel.

(Craft et al 2023)

Tonicity

Tonicity is related to the concentration or osmolality of a solution (Craft et al 2023). The terms 'osmolality' and 'osmolarity' are often used interchangeably to express concentration of a solution. **Osmolality** refers to the measure of solute concentration dissolved in a kilogram of fluid, while osmolarity refers to the solute concentration in a litre of fluid. The tonicity of a solution refers to the concentration of one fluid compared with another, and the effect that the solution's osmotic pressure has on the movement of water across cell membranes. It is measured against the normal osmolality fluid within, which is between 275 and 295 mOsm/kg (LeMone et al 2020). Osmolality is used to measure the concentration of plasma and urine.

Solutions are categorised as isotonic, hypotonic or hypertonic (LeMone et al 2020). An **isotonic** solution has the same tonicity or concentration as body fluid, meaning this solution will not cause water movement into or out of cells if they were placed in this solution. A **hypotonic** solution is less concentrated than body fluid with higher water concentration; therefore, it will encourage water to move into the cell, causing it to swell and perhaps burst (haemolyse) if there is a significant influx of water. **Hypertonic** solution is more concentrated than body fluid with lower water concentration; this encourages water movement out of the cell, causing the cells to shrink. The concept of tonicity is particularly relevant to nurses providing care and ongoing management for individuals receiving treatment with intravenous (IV) fluids to monitor its effects on the person's health. Further discussion of IV fluids follows at a later point in this chapter. See Figure 26.4 for a visual representation of fluid tonicity and water movement.

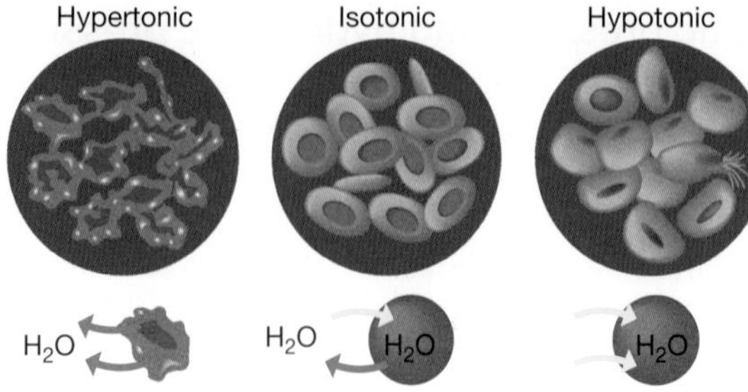

Figure 26.4 Hypertonic, isotonic and hypotonic solutions

(LadyofHats, Wikimedia Commons http://commons.wikimedia.org/wiki/File:Osmotic_pressure_on_blood_cells_diagram.svg.)

FLUID BALANCE

Fluid balance relates to the dynamic balance of fluid input and output required in the body and indicates that the body's required amount of water is present and distributed proportionally (Craft et al 2023; Litchfield et al 2018). Body fluids are regulated by fluid intake, hormonal controls and fluid output. This regulation of body fluids and physiological balance is managed by several feedback mechanisms working together to maintain homeostasis (Crisp et al 2021). (See Figure 26.5.)

In the healthcare environment, nurses are involved in the assessment of individuals in their care and play a vital role in monitoring and managing fluid balance. It is therefore important that nurses have a knowledge of the mechanisms involved in fluid regulation and its impact on health. When caring for young children, older people and acutely ill individuals, it is particularly important to carefully monitor fluid balance. Infants and children have relatively higher fluid requirements compared with adults because of greater body water content (Dixon & Porter 2018; Kear 2017). Older people are less likely to respond to the thirst mechanism with age-related changes and are at risk of inadequate fluid balance (Brown et al 2020). Acute illness is associated with poor appetite and reliance on others for assistance with hydration and nutrition, and physiological effects that may result in fluid loss. Several factors can cause reduced or insufficient fluid intake, which in turn can affect the water balance in the body. (See Clinical Interest Box 26.2.)

Fluid intake

Fluid gain in the body is a homeostatic mechanism triggered by dehydration (Craft et al 2023). Fluid intake is mainly regulated by the sensation of thirst (through the 'thirst response' negative feedback system), which plays an important role in maintaining the body's water balance

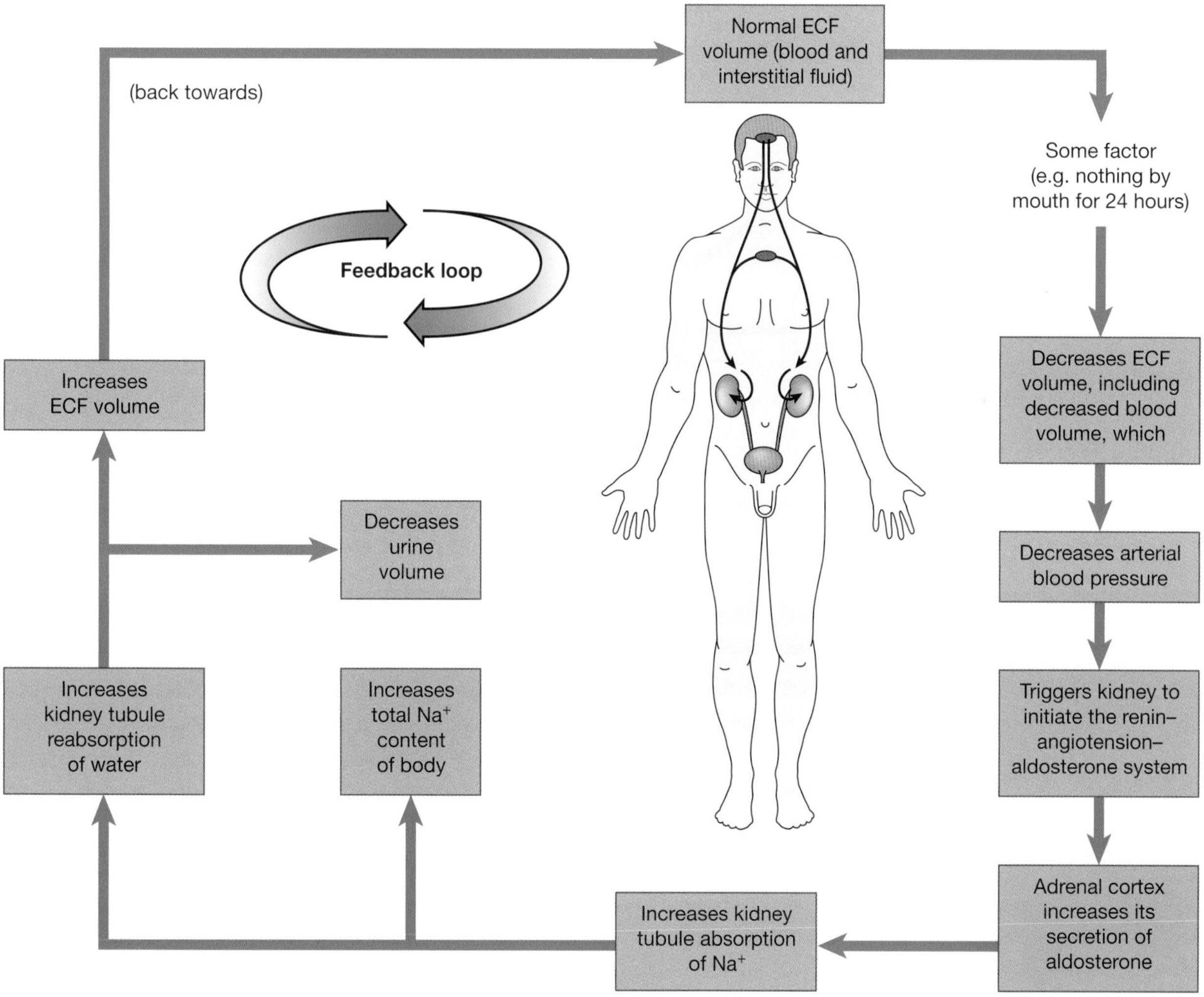

Figure 26.5 Feedback mechanisms for maintaining fluid balance

ECF = extracellular fluid.

(Crisp et al 2021)

CLINICAL INTEREST BOX 26.2 Causes for reduced or inadequate intake of fluids

- Age-related illness and physical disabilities
- Being ill
- Cognitive impairment, dementia, Alzheimer's disease
- Effects of diuretics and laxatives
- Fasting for medical/surgical procedures
- Fluid restrictions for medical conditions such as heart failure and renal disorders
- Refusal to drink fluid for fear of incontinence
- Reduced thirst sensation with ageing
- Physically weak and frail
- Reliance on others for assistance with fluid intake
- Nausea

(LeMone et al 2020; Schub & Oji 2018)

and preventing dehydration (Craft et al 2023). Thirst is described as the conscious desire for water, and it generally controls fluid intake, stimulated by cellular dehydration and a decrease in circulating blood volume (Crisp et al 2021). Figure 26.6 shows triggers stimulating thirst. Fluid intake replaces measurable and insensible fluid losses from the body. The kidneys, on average, produce and filter 1500 mL of urine a day to remove waste products. Therefore, for an adult, the normal daily recommended intake of fluids is between 2000 and 3000 mL to maintain a proper fluid balance (Brown et al 2020). See Table 26.3 for average adult fluid balance. However, hydration requirements for each person are highly individual, depending on the person's age, gender, body mass, sweating, environment and activity or exertion levels, and other types of fluid loss. For example, athletes and people who exercise require a higher fluid intake than someone who is less active. A person living in cold climate environments may not experience thirst as much as someone living in hot or humid locations.

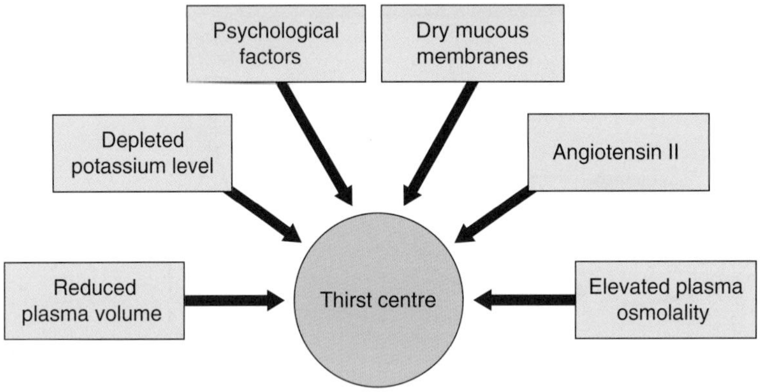

Figure 26.6 Triggers stimulating thirst mechanism

(Adapted from Crisp et al 2021)

TABLE 26.3 | Average adult fluid balance

Input	Amount (mL)
Fluids	1200
Food	1000
Metabolism (breakdown of food/water from oxidation)	300
Total	2500
Output	
Urine	1500
Stools/faeces	100
Breathing and sweating (insensible losses)	900
Total	2500

(Adapted from Brown et al 2020)

Fluid output

Fluid loss from the body and the volume of body water is mainly regulated by the kidneys, determined by the levels of sodium chloride excreted in the urine through hormonal control (Craft et al 2023). Fluid losses are described as sensible or insensible losses. **Sensible losses** are those that can be measured. These losses include urine, faeces, blood, emesis and wound and gastric drainage. In an average adult, under normal circumstances the body loses about 1200–1500 mL of water in urine and about 100–200 mL of water through faeces daily (Kear 2017). Urine output measurements in the clinical setting are calculated in relation to body weight—for an adult, urine output should be at least 0.5 mL/kg/hour (Brown et al 2020).

Insensible losses occur in the form of invisible vaporisation and are difficult to measure. Insensible losses occur through the skin (perspiration) and lungs (respiration), amounting to approximately 800–900 mL daily (Crisp et al 2021). Increased water loss is associated with an accelerated metabolism and several factors can increase fluid loss in the body. (See Clinical Interest Box 26.3.)

CLINICAL INTEREST BOX 26.3 Factors that can increase fluid loss

- High temperature
- High altitude
- High-fibre diet
- High sodium intake
- Humidity
- Increased respiratory rate and depth
- Caffeine and alcohol consumption
- Exercise

CRITICAL THINKING EXERCISE 26.1

Fluid excess

Joan, 80 year old, was admitted to hospital by her GP after presenting with swollen ankles, pitting oedema and shortness of breath. Joan has a medical history of renal impairment and hypertension. Recently, Joan's GP had prescribed new medications and altered some of her previous dosages to improve treatment and management of her condition. Joan became confused with her new medications and dosages and subsequently missed some of her prescribed regular doses. Her symptoms developed progressively over the past week. Considering Joan's symptoms and based on her medical history, what specific medication do you think she may have missed that may have led to her situation?

Antidiuretic hormone (ADH)

Several mechanisms are integral in the maintenance of fluid balance or water balance in the body and homeostasis. See Table 26.4. The **antidiuretic hormone (ADH)** is the primary regulator of water balance. Water balance in the body is controlled by pressure sensors in the vascular system that stimulate or inhibit release of ADH from the pituitary gland (Williams & Hopper 2019). ADH is secreted when plasma concentration is elevated or when blood volume or blood pressure is decreased. When plasma concentration is increased, osmoreceptors in the hypothalamus respond by stimulating the sensation of thirst to encourage fluid intake. Osmoreceptors also signal the posterior pituitary to release ADH, increasing reabsorption of water by the

TABLE 26.4 | A systems approach to fluid balance

Hypothalamus and pituitary	The primary regulator of fluid intake is the thirst mechanism. Thirst can result from fluid loss or an increase in plasma osmolality (an increase in plasma concentration). The thirst centre, located in the hypothalamus, is highly sensitive to changes in the concentration or osmolality of the blood. A change in the blood osmolality or a decrease in blood volume stimulates osmoreceptors in the hypothalamus to trigger the sensation of thirst and the release of the antidiuretic hormone (ADH). ADH is released from the posterior pituitary and acts in the renal tubules, causing water reabsorption. Through these mechanisms, there is an increase in water in the body and a decreased plasma osmolality.
Renal control renin–angiotensin–aldosterone system (see Figure 26.7)	In an average adult, total blood volume is filtered through the kidneys numerous times daily. Most of this filtrate (99%) is reabsorbed, resulting in the production of approximately 1500 mL of urine daily. Fluid and electrolytes are selectively reabsorbed in the renal tubules according to the plasma concentration. The renal tubules are where the ADH and aldosterone perform their actions. Aldosterone secretion can be stimulated by decreased renal perfusion: a person presenting with a low blood pressure, for instance. Aldosterone can retain sodium and excrete potassium. It forms part of the renin–angiotensin system. In response to reduced renal perfusion, renin is released by the kidneys. Angiotensinogen is produced by the liver and is also found in the blood. Renin is an enzyme; it reacts with angiotensinogen to produce angiotensin I, which is converted to angiotensin II by angiotensin-converting enzyme (ACE). Angiotensin II activates the secretion of ADH and aldosterone. Aldosterone works to reabsorb both sodium and water in the renal tubules. The end result is the restoration of plasma volume and concentration.

Continued

TABLE 26.4 | A systems approach to fluid balance—cont'd

Adrenal cortical control	Glucocorticoids and mineralocorticoids are secreted by the adrenal cortex, and both play a role in fluid and electrolyte imbalance. Glucocorticoids have an anti-inflammatory effect and increase glucose levels in the plasma. Cortisol is an example of a glucocorticoid. Mineralocorticoids, such as aldosterone, work by increasing sodium retention and thus water reabsorption, and excretion of potassium. An increase in the secretion of these steroid hormones is associated with physical and psychological stress.
Cardiac control	An elevation in blood volume or blood pressure causes atrial natriuretic peptide hormone (ANP) to be released from cells located in the atria of the heart. ANP inhibits activation of the renin–angiotensin system (RAS), promoting excretion of sodium and water.
Gastrointestinal control	The gastrointestinal tract secretes approximately 800 mL of fluid a day and in a healthy adult most of this is reabsorbed. A small amount of fluid is eliminated in faeces. From this information, it is easy to imagine the impact diarrhoea and vomiting would have on the secretion and absorption of water.

(Brown et al 2020; Craft et al 2023)

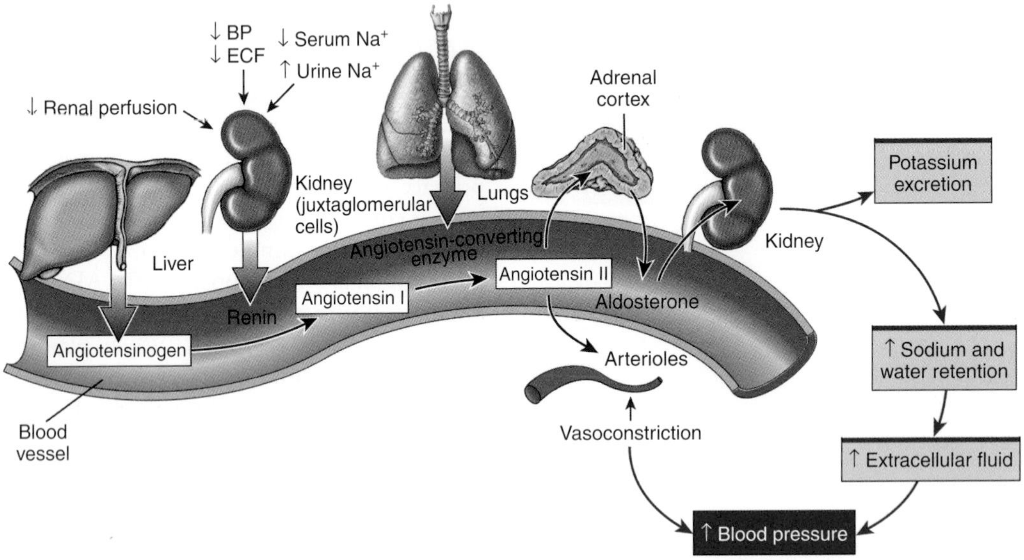

Figure 26.7 The renin–angiotensin–aldosterone system

BP, blood pressure; ECF, extracellular fluid; Na^+, sodium ion.

(Herlihy & Maebius 2011)

kidneys (Figure 26.7). This reduces the amount of water lost in urine, and the reabsorbed water reduces plasma concentration (Craft et al 2023). Clinical Interest Box 26.4 lists other factors that may trigger thirst when fluid volume is normal.

Electrolytes

Electrolytes are also commonly referred to as 'solutes'; the two terms are used interchangeably and carry the same meaning. In this chapter the term 'electrolytes' is used.

CLINICAL INTEREST BOX 26.4 Other factors that can trigger thirst when fluid volume is normal

Factors such as mouth breathing or eating dry or salty foods can be misinterpreted by the body as thirst. Situations such as these can cause additional fluid intake even though the osmolality of the blood or the blood volume is within normal range.

TABLE 26.5 | Cations and anions

Cations	Anions	Major intracellular	Major extracellular
Sodium (Na^+)	Bicarbonate (HCO_3^-)	K^+	Na^+
Magnesium (Mg^+)	Chloride (Cl^-)	PO_4^-	Cl^-
Potassium (K^+)	Phosphate (PO_4^-)	Mg^+	Ca^+ HCO_3^-

(Craft et al 2023; Shrimanker & Bhattarai 2023)

Electrolytes are inorganic substances that dissociate into electrically charged particles called 'ions' when dissolved in water. These can be negatively or positively charged—known as **anions** and **cations**, respectively. Electrolytes have an 'osmotic potential'—their ability to pull water into a compartment. Sodium and dextrose are examples of electrolytes with high osmotic potentials. Movement of these electrolytes can result in major fluid shifts between the ICF and ECF (Craft et al 2023). Table 26.5 lists some familiar anions and cations.

Electrolytes vary in number depending on whether they belong inside or outside the cell (in the ICF or ECF). For example, sodium (Na^+) is the most abundant cation outside the cell (in the ECF), whereas potassium (K^+) is the most predominant cation inside the cell (in the ICF). It is critical for nerve function that electrolytes retain their numbers within relative compartments to maintain a 'charge'. If this charge is lost, it will ultimately impact on the transmission of electrical impulses across the cell membranes of nerve and muscle cells (Craft et al 2023). Fluctuations outside the normal reference ranges in electrolyte balance can impact body functioning and could have a detrimental impact on maintaining health. Electrolyte balance is essential for basic life functioning and sodium, potassium and chloride are the significant electrolytes along with magnesium, calcium, phosphate and bicarbonates. Electrolytes within the body come from food and fluids (Shrimanker & Bhattarai 2023).

Discussion of all the electrolytes is beyond the scope of this chapter. Electrolyte imbalances commonly encountered in the clinical environment are discussed along with a summary of common themes associated with electrolyte imbalances in general. See Table 26.6 for blood values of electrolytes. It is important to note that normal laboratory values for tests may vary and be specific to the population group. For instance, reference ranges for neonates or paediatrics and adults will be different. See Online Resources—Pathology Tests Explained for more information about interpreting test results.

Fluid and electrolyte imbalance

Several factors can disturb the body's fluid and electrolyte balance, resulting in fluid volume deficit or fluid volume excess. Water volume imbalances are usually accompanied by electrolyte imbalances, particularly sodium. It is important to note that the term 'fluid volume deficit' does not carry the same meaning as 'dehydration' (Brown et al 2020). Dehydration usually refers to the loss of pure water alone, without the associated loss of sodium.

Dehydration

Dehydration is the excessive loss of fluid from the body; it can be defined as a sudden loss of $>3\%$ to 4% of the individual's body weight (Schub & Oji 2018). Dehydration is caused by inadequate intake of fluid, excessive fluid

TABLE 26.6 | Adult reference range for electrolyte values

Sodium	Na^+	135–145 mmol/L
Chloride	Cl^-	95–110 mmol/L
Potassium	K^+	3.5–5.2 mmol/L
Calcium	Ca^+	2.1–2.6 mmol/L
Magnesium	Mg^+	0.7–1.1 mmol/L
Phosphate	PO_4^-	0.75–1.5 mmol/L
Bicarbonate	HCO_3^-	22–32 mmol/L

(The Royal College of Pathologists of Australia, nd—online manual)

TABLE 26.7 | Classification of dehydration

Type of dehydration	Underlying cause
Isotonic	There are balanced water and salt losses, caused by osmotic diuresis, fasting, vomiting or diarrhoea.
Hypotonic (hyponatraemic) dehydration	Salt losses exceed water losses, caused by overuse of diuretics, salt-wasting renal disease, trauma, burns, surgery, reduced salt and water intake, or excessive vomiting and diarrhoea.
Hypertonic (hypernatraemic) dehydration	Water loss is greater than salt loss, through renal tubular disease, osmotic glucose effects, vasopressin resistance, insensible losses, fever and rapid respiration.

(Schub & Oji 2018)

output or a combination of the two (Schub & Oji 2018). When sensible and insensible fluid losses exceed fluid intake over a period, dehydration occurs. It is an underlying cause for many common problems including urinary tract infections, constipation, malnutrition, pressure ulcers and confusion. Left untreated, dehydration can lead to electrolyte imbalances and life-threatening conditions, such as cardiac arrhythmias, acute renal failure and death in some cases. Clinical assessment of dehydration is classified as isotonic, hypotonic or hypertonic dehydration. (See Table 26.7.) Serum osmolality is considered as the most accurate test for dehydration. (See Clinical Interest Box 26.5 for biochemical indictors of dehydration.)

People considered to be at a higher risk for dehydration include young children, the older person, people with increased insensible fluid loss, confused and immobile individuals, someone with trauma or surgical wounds, and individuals being treated with medications that alter electrolyte balance. Infants and children have a greater proportion of body surface area to body mass and are therefore more prone to dehydration (Dixon & Porter 2018). Age-related factors, health issues and social factors can increase risk for dehydration in older people (Bellman 2022; Schub & Oji 2018). Dehydration is a common clinical presentation among older people and children. Older adults are more likely to be admitted to hospital for dehydration, while dehydration in children is considered a leading cause of morbidity and mortality worldwide.

Special considerations associated with dehydration assessment for older people include:
- loss of appetite and thirst sensation
- physical changes resulting in loss of independence
- biochemical effects of ageing
- cognitive impairment.

Comorbidities can also have a profound effect on hydration. For example, individuals experiencing incontinence will frequently reduce their fluid intake; this can cause other problems and predispose the person to urinary tract infections. Dehydration in acutely ill individuals causes decreased blood circulation volume, seriously affecting cardiovascular and renal functions. (See Clinical Interest Box 26.6 for signs of dehydration.)

The opposite of dehydration is over-hydration. Over-hydration (fluid overload) can have a serious effect on people with underlying pathological conditions such as renal failure and heart failure. It can cause low sodium levels (hyponatraemia), increasing the risk for arrhythmias, kidney damage, water intoxication and death. Complications of severe and rapid onset of hyponatraemia include confusion, vomiting, seizures, coma and irreversible neurological damage (Brown et al 2020). Fluid overload occurs when the body is unable to deal with the excess water simply by increasing urine output, resulting in fluid retention. Excess fluid leaks into the surrounding tissue and is drawn into the cells causing them to swell (oedema). In the lungs, fluid leaks through the capillaries, resulting in fluid accumulation (pulmonary oedema) and breathing difficulty (dyspnoea). Symptomatic water intoxication and pulmonary oedema are a medical emergency. (See Clinical Interest Box 26.7 for signs of over-hydration.)

CLINICAL INTEREST BOX 26.5 Biochemical indicators of dehydration

Biochemical signs of dehydration in the presence of clinical signs of dehydration:
- raised serum or urine osmolality
- raised serum sodium (hypernatremia)
- raised urea/creatinine ratio
- raised haematocrit
- raised serum lactate
- raised urine specific gravity
- reduced estimated glomerular filtration rate (eGFR)
- metabolic acidosis
- negative base excess.

(Ashraf & Rea 2017; Brown et al 2020; Crisp et al 2021)

CLINICAL INTEREST BOX 26.6 Signs and symptoms of dehydration

Early signs of dehydration include:
- thirst sensation (although often absent in older people)
- dry mouth
- headaches
- reduced concentration
- dark and concentrated urine.

Moderate dehydration in acutely ill individuals:
- decreased and concentrated urine output (darker in colour and stronger odour)
- low-grade fever and dizziness
- poor cognition and confusion
- reduced activity levels or lethargy
- headache and fatigue
- reduced skin turgor/elasticity
- sunken and dry eyes
- dry lips and oral mucosa.

If dehydration persists, the individual will develop:
- reduced blood pressure and tachycardia
- reduced cardiac output, rapid and thready pulse
- increased respiratory rate
- prolonged capillary refill time
- vasoconstriction and cold extremities
- agitation and confusion or sleepiness and reduced responsiveness
- reduced consciousness level
- oliguria.

(Banasik 2022; Brown et al 2020; Crisp et al 2021)

CRITICAL THINKING EXERCISE 26.2

Dehydration

A 30-year-old male was admitted to hospital. He became lost bushwalking before being found after 3 days by the local community search and rescue group. Data on admission: blood glucose level (BGL) (3.0 mmol/L), dehydrated and hungry. Urea and electrolyte results: Na^+ and K^+ slightly elevated; urea −30 mmol/L, creatinine −200 mmol/L. Explain the clinical presentation. What is the collaborative treatment and management?

Fluid volume deficit

Fluid volume deficit is also called hypovolaemia and refers to abnormal loss of both body fluid and electrolytes in similar proportions from the ECF (Berman et al 2020). Causes for fluid volume deficit can include:
- decreased fluid intake as a result of unavailability of fluids, or secondary to other conditions (e.g. unconsciousness)
- increased fluid output secondary to other conditions (e.g. diarrhoea, vomiting, excessive urine output, hyperventilation, excessive perspiration, diabetes insipidus, prolonged fever, haemorrhage or inadequate replacement of aspirated or drained fluids)
- increased electrolyte load secondary to other conditions (e.g. hyperglycaemia associated with uncontrolled diabetes mellitus, excessive IV infusion of hyperosmotic or concentrated solutions of glucose or sodium bicarbonate).

Fluid volume deficit can also occur when fluid shifts abnormally from plasma (intravascular space) to the interstitial space between cells (Kear 2017). In the clinical environment, this is commonly referred to as 'third-space fluid shifts'. There is not an absolute loss of fluid, it has simply moved to another compartment, resulting in decreased vascular fluid to support normal physiological processes. (See Figure 26.8.) Either disease process causing this shift creates an imbalance in hydrostatic and oncotic pressure and/or there is destruction of the semipermeable membrane that usually contains fluids within their compartments. (See Clinical Interest Box 26.8.) The pleural, peritoneal, abdominal and pericardial cavities are the most common sites within the body for third spacing.

Signs and symptoms of fluid deficit include:
- thirst
- reduced urine output and increased urine concentration
- drier mucous membranes and sunken eyes
- decreased skin and tongue turgor
- dizziness, syncope, headache and confusion
- weak and thready pulse, and increased capillary refill time
- reduced blood pressure and rapid shallow breathing
- decreased weight in rapid fluid loss
- orthostatic hypotension.

(Brown et al 2020; Kear 2017)

CLINICAL INTEREST BOX 26.7 Signs and symptoms of over-hydration (fluid overload)

- Weight gain
- Pitting oedema, peripheral oedema, generalised oedema, dependent oedema
- Engorged varicose veins, peripheral and neck vein distension
- Elevated central venous pressure
- Hypertension, tachycardia with full bounding pulse
- Muscle weakness, headache
- Tachypnea with or without dyspnoea, orthopnoea
- Productive cough and crackles on chest auscultation
- Pale and cool skin

(Brown et al 2020; Kear 2017)

Fluid volume excess

Fluid volume excess, also referred to as hypervolaemia, is a condition whereby the body retains both water and sodium

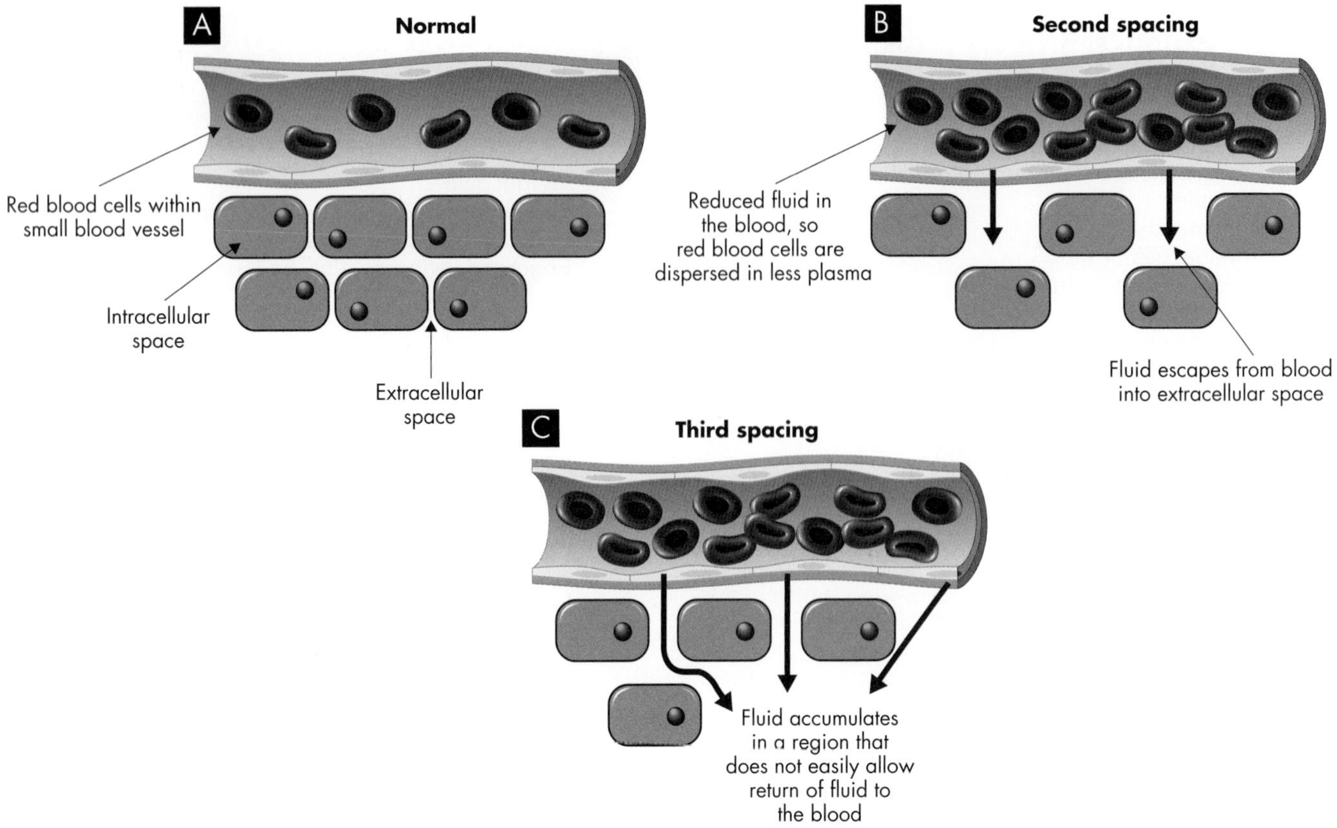

Figure 26.8 Fluid movements in third spacing

A: In normal tissue, the amount of fluid in the extracellular space is normal, **B:** In second spacing, excess fluid moves into the extracellular space, such as during oedema, although it is possible to correct this, **C:** However, in third spacing, a significant increase in volume within a specific region of the extracellular space creates abnormal localisation of fluid, which is difficult to treat.

(Craft et al 2023)

CLINICAL INTEREST BOX 26.8 Pathological processes related to third spacing

- Trauma
- Surgery
- Burns
- Gastrointestinal obstruction
- Pancreatitis
- Ascites
- Sepsis

(Kear 2017)

in similar proportions to the normal ECF (Berman et al 2020). This could be as a result of excess intake or due to disease processes that result in an imbalance in hydrostatic and oncotic pressures causing fluid to shift into the vascular compartment or shift into the interstitial space. The latter exhibits signs such as oedema. Although the overall volume of the ECF does not change, it does affect the volume of fluid in the intravascular space. Fluid volume excess can be caused by a number of factors including impaired homeostatic mechanisms and over-administration of IV fluids. (See Clinical Interest Box 26.9.)

Symptoms of fluid retention vary depending on the severity of fluid overload. In the case of acute fluid overload, there may be sudden onset of acute dyspnoea as a result of fluid in the lungs. A person with a chronic history of fluid overload may show signs of fatigue, dyspnoea and pitting oedema. This can be seen in individuals with uncontrolled chronic heart failure.

Signs and symptoms of fluid volume excess include:

- weight gain
- peripheral or generalised oedema
- headache, confusion, lethargy
- crackles, dyspnoea, orthopnoea, cough
- bounding pulse, elevated blood pressure, elevated central venous pressure
- jugular venous distension, engorged carotid vessels
- polyuria.

(Brown et al 2020; Kear 2017)

CLINICAL INTEREST BOX 26.9 Factors contributing to fluid volume excess

- Excessive administration of intravenous fluids or hypotonic solutions
- Compromised homeostatic mechanisms (kidney, cardiac or liver failure)
- Long-term use of steroids
- High sodium diets and drugs or preparations rich in sodium leading to fluid retention and fluid volume excess
- Primary polydipsia
- Inappropriate ADH secretion due to cerebral infections, head injury or increased intracranial pressure

(Brown et al 2020; Kear 2017)

CRITICAL THINKING EXERCISE 26.3

Fluid balance

A 78-year-old man was having multiple IV antibiotics throughout the day. Each dose was administered with 100 mL 0.9% sodium chloride six times a day. Nursing care included 6-hourly vital signs observations to be recorded, daily weight, fluid balance chart, total fluid restriction of 1200 mL daily and a low-salt diet. The person has renal impairment. After 24 hours, the individual is exhibiting signs of swollen ankles and shortness of breath. The fluid balance chart shows oral intake is 1200 mL and output is 800 mL over 24 hours. What has caused the person's symptoms and fluid retention in this case? What is the critical issue with the fluid balance charting for this person?

Oedema

Oedema (swelling) occurs due to accumulation of fluid in the interstitial spaces (Craft et al 2023). Causes of oedema include increased capillary hydrostatic pressure, where fluid from the vascular space is forced into the interstitial spaces. This can occur in individuals with heart failure. A lowered plasma oncotic pressure also causes fluid to shift into the interstitial spaces; this can occur in a person with a low albumin level. Increased capillary permeability affects the ability of the capillary membranes to maintain fluid within the vascular compartment, resulting in fluid shift to the interstitial space. Examples of conditions with increased capillary permeability include burns and systemic inflammatory response syndrome (SIRS). Figure 26.3 shows capillary hydrostatic and oncotic pressure.

ELECTROLYTE IMBALANCES

Electrolyte imbalance involves either a deficit or an excess of electrolytes such as sodium, potassium, calcium, magnesium or phosphate. Sodium and potassium imbalances are two of the most common presentations associated with fluid and electrolyte imbalances (Craft et al 2023). Sodium and potassium are discussed in this chapter; further reading is required in relation to the other electrolytes. (See Table 26.8.)

Sodium (Na^+)

Normal plasma value: 135–145 mmol/L. Sodium imbalance is one of the most prevalent electrolyte imbalances encountered in the clinical environment. Sodium plays an integral role in the maintenance of irritability and conduction of nerve and muscle tissue. It is the most important electrolyte in ECF. It affects volume and concentration of ECF, maintains acid–base balance and influences levels of other electrolytes such as potassium and chloride.

TABLE 26.8 | Serum electrolyte imbalances

Sodium	Low serum Na^+	Hyponatraemia
	High serum Na^+	Hypernatraemia
Potassium	Low serum K^+	Hypokalaemia
	High serum K^+	Hyperkalaemia
Calcium	Low serum Ca^+	Hypocalcaemia
	High serum Ca^+	Hypercalcaemia
Phosphate	Low serum PO_4^-	Hypophosphataemia
	High serum PO_4^-	Hyperphosphataemia
Magnesium	Low serum Mg^+	Hypomagnesaemia
	High serum Mg^+	Hypermagnesaemia

(Data from Shrimanker & Bhattarai 2023)

Sodium homeostasis

The kidneys are the primary organs responsible for regulating the plasma concentration (ECF) of sodium within the tightly controlled limits of 135–145 mmol/L. Sodium balance is regulated by the hormone **aldosterone**, which is secreted by the adrenal cortex (Craft et al 2023). If plasma sodium levels are decreased, aldosterone is secreted to increase sodium reabsorption in kidney tubules and, as a result, plasma sodium level will rise.

Sodium imbalances are referred to as being either hyponatraemia or hypernatraemia. Hyponatraemia refers to sodium deficit—a low concentration of sodium in ECF caused either by loss of sodium or by gaining more water. It is the most frequent form of electrolyte disorders (Shrimanker & Bhattarai 2023). Hyponatraemia can be caused by impaired renal function, fluid loss related to burns, impaired ADH secretion, sodium loss associated with diuretics or hyperglycaemia (Craft et al 2023). Decreased sodium causes fluid to move by osmosis from the less concentrated ECF compartment to the ICF space, resulting in a fluid shift. This fluid shift can lead to swelling of the cells and cerebral oedema. Severe hyponatraemia has neurological manifestations and can cause seizures and neurological damage (Hall et al 2022; Shrimanker & Bhattarai 2023). Hypernatraemia is the opposite—it refers to an excess of sodium in the ECF as a result of water loss or an overall surplus of sodium. Hypernatraemia can occur as a result of excessive consumption of salt in the diet, prolonged diarrhoea and vomiting or dehydration. Symptoms of hypernatraemia include an intense thirst, hypertension, oedema, agitation and convulsions (Craft et al 2023). See Table 26.9 for a list of conditions and signs and symptoms associated with hypernatraemia and hyponatraemia. These will be dependent on whether there is an associated hypervolaemic or hypovolaemic state. Refer to the Online Resources—Nutrient Reference Values from the National Health and Medical Research Council for information about specific electrolyte values.

TABLE 26.9 | Causes, signs and symptoms associated with hypo/hypernatraemia

Causes of hyponatraemia	Associated signs and symptoms
Water retention (dilutional): chronic heart failure, renal failure, liver failure Na^+ in excess of water: diuretics, diarrhoea, vomiting, hyperglycaemia, nasogastric (NG) suctioning, third-space losses	Cramps Muscle weakness Headache Anorexia Nausea Confusion Seizures Ataxia Respiratory depression Coma
Causes of hypernatraemia	**Associated signs and symptoms**
Dehydration: pure water loss caused by insensible losses: sweat, burns, hyperventilation, GIT losses, diabetes insipidus (DI), hyperglycaemia, excessive Na^+ intake, IV fluids	Hypovolaemic signs: tachycardia, thready pulse, hypotension Thirst Dry mucous membranes Cool extremities Muscle weakness Lethargy Confusion Seizures Coma

CRITICAL THINKING EXERCISE 26.4

Electrolyte imbalance

Nathan is a participant in a local marathon. He was admitted to the emergency department by ambulance after collapsing at the event. During the run, Nathan had only been drinking water. His results show BP 95/55 mmHg, HR 60 beats/minute, BGL 3 mmol/L, sodium 126 mmol/L, potassium 3.5 mmol/L and he is unable to pass urine. Consider his results. What has happened to Nathan?

Potassium (K^+)

Normal plasma value: 3.5–5.0 mmol/L. Potassium is the chief intracellular cation and has a major role in the concentration of intracellular fluid and neural function. It is particularly essential for the neuronal function of cardiac, musculoskeletal and smooth muscles. Because of this, imbalances in potassium levels in the intracellular or extracellular environment can be potentially life-threatening and often present as a medical emergency (Craft et al 2023). Clinical Interest Box 26.10 outlines nursing considerations for an individual taking potassium.

Potassium homeostasis

Potassium is regulated by the kidneys. It is filtered by the nephrons, reabsorbed back into the blood and secreted according to bodily requirements and functioning. An alteration in the flow of urine also influences secretion of potassium. For a person taking **diuretics** (substances that increase excretion of water), the urine flow will be increased, resulting in increased levels of potassium in urine. Aldosterone also increases secretion of potassium when levels are high. Potassium balance is also affected by acid–base disturbances. For example, an increase in hydrogen ions (H^+) will cause potassium to shift outside the cell in exchange for H^+ ions to maintain a balance of cations on either side of the cell.

Potassium imbalances are referred to as being either hypokalaemia or hyperkalaemia and associated with cardiac

CLINICAL INTEREST BOX 26.10 Nursing considerations for potassium

- Foods rich in potassium may need to be restricted in individuals with chronic renal failure. Such foods include dates and bananas.
- Potassium is a high-risk medicine, and the clinical protocol for intravenous administration and monitoring must be carefully followed.
- IV K^+ administration can be painful, so infusion rate and intravenous access (PIVC or central) should be carefully considered.
- Consider oral route of administration if appropriate to the clinical situation.
- Preparations such as Resonium exchange K^+ for calcium (Ca^+) in the gut and have a long-lasting effect.
- Administration of blood products can cause hyperkalaemia and hypocalcaemia.
- K^+ levels are usually kept in the high/normal range for individuals with cardiac complaints (i.e. >4.0).
- Digoxin is a medication commonly encountered in the clinical environment. Therapeutic levels of this drug are influenced by serum K^+ levels.

arrhythmias (Shrimanker & Bhattarai 2023). Hypokalaemia refers to potassium deficit in the ECF. It can be caused by excess fluid loss, dehydration, decreased levels of potassium intake, renal impairment, overuse of laxatives, some diuretics and prolonged diarrhoea and vomiting. Symptoms include thirst, muscle weakness, cramps, increased urine output and confusion. Low potassium can have an effect on cardiac cell activity and cause arrhythmias in severe cases (Craft et al 2023). Hyperkalaemia is the excess of potassium in ECF. It can be caused by high potassium intake, tissue trauma caused by burns or accidents and renal failure inhibiting potassium excretion. Symptoms include skeletal muscle weakness, paralysis, irritability, nausea and vomiting. High potassium levels can have a serious effect on the cardiac muscle function and cause arrhythmias and even cardiac arrest if untreated (Craft et al 2023). Hyperkalaemia is a critical electrolyte disturbance; it requires immediate treatment to lower serum potassium levels and prevent reoccurrence (Craft et al 2023). Table 26.10 outlines conditions and signs and symptoms associated with hyper/hypokalaemia.

NURSING ASSESSMENT OF INDIVIDUALS WITH FLUID AND ELECTROLYTE NEEDS

In the healthcare environment, nurses are usually responsible for accurate assessment and adequate fluid management for

TABLE 26.10 | Causes, signs and symptoms associated with hypo/hyperkalaemia

Causes of hyperkalaemia	Associated signs and symptoms
Renal failure Acidosis IV K^+ administration Blood products K^+ sparing diuretics Trauma Burns	Lethargy Confusion Muscle weakness Calf pain ECG changes Arrhythmias
Causes of hypokalaemia	**Associated signs and symptoms**
Diuretics Nasogastric (NG) suction Diarrhoea and vomiting Starvation Alkalosis	Fatigue Muscle weakness/cramps Nausea/vomiting Arrhythmias Digoxin toxicity

individuals in their care. Poor fluid management and record keeping can contribute to worsening of a person's health condition. The nursing process is integral to the provision of person-centred care for individuals in healthcare settings. The process encompasses the following:

- assessment
- nursing diagnosis
- planning
- implementation
- evaluation.

The nursing process is not merely a series of steps; it involves a critical thinking approach, with analyses at each stage along with updates or changes to plans according to an individual's needs (Crisp et al 2021). (Read Chapter 6 and Chapter 7 for further information on critical thinking in nursing practice and the nursing process.)

The assessment phase refers to the collection, validation, organisation and documentation of data retrieved from the individual (Berman et al 2020). During this phase, the nurse will gather information about the person's health status. The use of a model to promote systematic data collection to prevent the omission of important relevant data is recommended. This data will include subjective and objective information, both of which are essential. This will provide the nurse with a holistic overview of the individual's health status to inform the provision of person-centred care. Also see Progress Note 26.1 for an example of a person admitted with fluid and electrolyte needs and monitoring.

With specific reference to fluid and electrolyte needs, obtaining an initial health history would be an appropriate starting point. This could include questioning the person about their present illness, condition or complaint and their past history, including family history where relevant. Subjective data collection should include questioning the person about their lifestyle habits and psychosocial status. For assessment of fluid and electrolyte needs it is particularly important to gather data on:

- past medical history: any conditions associated with fluid/electrolyte disturbances
- medications: any medications associated with fluid/electrolyte disturbances
- diet: any specific requirements/restrictions, eating habits, supplements, factors limiting access to adequate nutrition/fluid intake
- exercise: how often, type of exercise and the conditions; whether there are specific nutritional/fluid requirements associated with it
- other personal habits: alcohol consumption, sports drinks
- social data: cultural affiliation (some religious practices include fasting during certain periods)
- psychological: mental health history (e.g. eating disorders; anxiety, stress).

(Berman et al 2020)

Table 26.11 outlines assessment findings associated with fluid volume deficit or excess.

Gathering objective data will include a thorough physical assessment of the person, frequently performed using a systems approach to facilitate comprehensive systematic data collection. These physical findings will be dependent on the associated disease process the person is experiencing. For example, a person with acute pulmonary oedema may be agitated and confused due to hypoxaemia caused by reduced ability of oxygen to diffuse into the pulmonary capillaries.

CRITICAL THINKING EXERCISE 26.5

Assessing fluid status

You are handed over two individuals with different presentations:

- An 89-year-old woman with ischaemic cardiomyopathy. Presentation: Shortness of breath, ankle oedema, crepitation at base of chest on auscultation, wheezy when speaking, elevated jugular venous pressure (JVP), lethargic. Blood pressure normal, pulse irregular.
- A 15-year-old boy admitted with severe diarrhoea and vomiting. Presentation dry mouth, decreased skin turgor, confused, low blood pressure, pulse weak and rapid.

Consider the presentation for each person. Is each person in fluid volume excess or fluid volume deficit?

Urine

Urine volume and concentration is a helpful clinical assessment about a person's fluid, electrolyte and acid balance status (Hall et al 2022). It is important to also be aware that when assessing urine there are no absolutes. Urine tests may not be reliable, especially in individuals with medical conditions such as renal or heart failure or people taking diuretics. Diuretics are prescribed to manage conditions associated with excessive fluid retention and therefore need to be taken into consideration when assessing urine and urinary output (Brown et al 2020).

Urine **specific gravity (SG)** refers to the density of urine compared with water. Osmolality refers to the concentration of the urine. Urine SG can be measured with a dipstick using a fresh urine sample or through laboratory tests. Normal urine SG is between 1.003 and 1.030, and osmolality between 300 and 1300 mOsm/kg (Brown et al 2020). In states of volume deficit, urine SG can be elevated and the osmolality high, usually accompanied by a decrease in urine output (except in diabetic ketoacidosis). In volume excess, urine tends to be dilute with a low SG and osmolality. See Clinical Interest Box 26.11 and Clinical Interest Box 26.12 for more tips on undertaking a physical assessment and additional information to consider when assessing fluid needs of individuals. (See also Chapter 31.)

Paediatric assessment

There are some important issues to consider in paediatric assessment. These issues will obviously depend on the age of the child. A detailed account is beyond the scope of this chapter. However, an overview of questions to consider includes:

- Feeding regimen—are there problems with feeding? (e.g. lethargy, poor sucking, regurgitation, colic, irritability)
- What is the typical intake over 24 hours?
- Type of formula?
- Type of fluids?
- Number of wet nappies?
- Bowel movement—any vomiting/diarrhoea?
- Any weight gain/loss?
- Allergies?

Important aspects of physical assessment include:

- obtaining age-appropriate vital signs
- assessment of state of alertness (how interactive is the child?)
- sunken eyes, pallor, reduced tears, dry arm creases, dry mucous membranes or depressed fontanelle (age appropriate) may suggest dehydration
- weight.

If the child's current weight and pre-morbid weight are available, this information can be the most reliable indicator of the fluid volume deficit (refer to the Online Resources the Royal Children's Hospital Melbourne, Clinical practice guidelines: Intravenous fluids). In addition, there are also physical signs frequently exhibited with varying degrees of fluid volume deficit. Volume loss in children is commonly expressed as a percentage of body weight. For example, a 10 kg child who is 5% dehydrated would have a fluid deficit of approximately 500 mL. See Table 26.12 for clinical signs of dehydration that might be observed in children less than 12 years old, depending on the severity of fluid loss. See Clinical Interest Box 26.13 for further details on estimating volume loss in children.

TABLE 26.11 | Assessment findings associated with fluid volume deficit or excess

Body system	Physical assessment findings—fluid volume excess	Physical assessment findings—fluid volume deficit
Central nervous system	Agitation Confusion Numbness, tingling, seizures with associated electrolyte losses	Headache Irritability/agitation Confusion/delirium Dizziness Lethargy Numbness, tingling, seizures with associated electrolyte losses
Respiratory	Increased work of breathing: use of accessory muscles Dyspnoea Orthopnoea Adventitious breath sounds: crackles, wheezes Hypoxaemia	Non-specific findings Increased work of breathing related to disease process
Cardiovascular	Bounding pulse Distended neck veins Third heart sound Oedema Hypertension	Tachycardia Thready pulse Orthostatic blood pressure changes Hypotension Decreased capillary refill Flat neck veins Arrhythmias associated with electrolyte imbalances
Renal	Oliguria or anuria Diuresis	Oliguria or anuria Increased urine specific gravity
Gastrointestinal	Distended abdomen	Abdominal cramps Diarrhoea/vomiting Sunken or distended abdomen Hyperactive bowel sounds
Skin	Non-specific	Cracked lips Tongue furrows Dry mucous membranes Decreased skin turgor (not reliable in older adults) Decreased sweat Reduced or increased body temperature Flushed or pale skin

CLINICAL INTEREST BOX 26.11 Physical assessment tips for nurses when assessing fluid needs of individuals

- Physical examination is a critical element for assessing and treating disorders of fluid balance.
- It is often more reliable than data obtained by invasive monitoring.
- Weight gain is the most consistent sign of volume excess.
- Gravity-dependent oedema is an important finding; not usually apparent until 2–4 kg of fluid have been retained.

CLINICAL INTEREST BOX 26.12 Important nursing considerations when assessing fluid needs

- **F**luid/dietary restrictions.
- **L**oss of fluid: What is the source, what is the fluid and electrolyte imbalance associated with this?
- **U**nderlying disease processes.
- **I**V fluids: What treatment is the person receiving and why?
- **D**rugs, digoxin, diuretics.
- **S**ystems assessment.

TABLE 26.12 | Characteristics of dehydration according to severity for children

	Mild	Moderate	Severe
Level of dehydration	1–5%	5–10%	>10%
Breathing	Normal	Increased respiratory rate	Increased respiratory rate
Pulse	Normal	Increased heart rate	Rapid, weak
Systolic BP	Normal	Normal, low	Decreased, very low
Urine output	Decreased	Decreased	Oliguria
Buccal mucosa	Slightly dry	Dry	Parched
Anterior fontanelle	Normal	Sunken	Markedly sunken
Eyes	Normal	Sunken	Markedly sunken
Skin turgor/capillary refill time	Normal	Decreased	Markedly decreased
Skin	Normal	Cool	Cool, mottling

(Children's Health Queensland Hospital and Health Service 2023; Knight & Waseem 2023)

CRITICAL THINKING EXERCISE 26.6

Paediatric assessment

A 2-year-old child is admitted for gastroenteritis and is 7% dehydrated. The child has been refusing all oral rehydration fluids. What clinical signs would you expect to find in your assessment of the child and the reasons for your findings?

Care planning and intervention

Data gathered from comprehensive person-centred assessments will identify actual or potential issues, and assist subsequent planning of care and nursing interventions. However, formulation of actual or potential issues requires critical thinking skills to be utilised by the nurse (Crisp et al 2021). Diagnostic statements should be specific, including a 'qualifier' in the statement. These qualifiers include:

- deficient
- impaired
- decreased
- ineffective
- compromised.

The statement should also include the causative factors.

Healthcare organisations generally utilise criteria-based, preset standardised care plans. However, an integral component of person-centred care is that the plan must be individually relevant to the particular individual's needs. Care plans essentially incorporate the following key components:

- actual or potential issues
- desired outcomes/goals
- nursing interventions
- rationales
- evaluation.

(See Nursing Care Plan 26.1 for a sample of a plan of care for a person with fluid and electrolyte needs.)

Some important general aspects of care to assist an individual who requires encouragement with their usual fluid intake, or requires assistance in meeting a higher than usual intake, include:

- providing assistance to individuals who experience difficulty in pouring fluid or holding a cup or glass
- explaining the importance of consuming a normal or increased fluid volume
- providing the individual's preferred types of fluid if not contraindicated
- ensuring that all fluids are presented attractively and at the correct temperature.

CLINICAL INTEREST BOX 26.13 Assessment of dehydration in children

An evaluation of dehydration is based on clinical signs and the degree of dehydration. The degree of dehydration is based on recent loss of body weight.

- Mild dehydration: Less than 5%, generally no clinical signs
- Moderate dehydration: 5–10%, with some clinical signs
- Severe dehydration: More than 15%, with multiple pronounced clinical signs
- Minimal dehydration: Loss of less than 3% of body weight

(Knight & Waseem 2023)

NURSING CARE PLAN 26.1

Assessment: Fluid balance and hydration
Issue/s to be addressed: At risk of acute dehydration
Goal/s: Prevent dehydration through:

- maintaining fluid balance—input and output
- maintaining urine output at 0.5 mL/kg/hour (or as per criteria stated in individual's care plan)
- maintaining urine specific gravity (SG) 1.003 and 1.030
- monitoring current weight
- maintaining serum Na^+ levels within the normal range
- maintaining moist mucous membranes.

Care/actions	Rationale
Monitor fluid intake and output on a fluid balance chart and communicate imbalances with medical staff.	To identify fluid volume deficit/excess early and prevent complications.
Administer and monitor intravenous therapy (IVT) as prescribed and record on the fluid balance chart.	IV therapy is an important adjunct in maintaining hydration in a person when unable to tolerate oral fluids.
Perform urinalysis to assess SG.	Urine SG is an indicator of increased or decreased serum osmolality.
Daily weights.	Weight loss or gain is a reliable indicator of fluid loss/gain.
Monitor serum Na^+ levels.	Serum Na^+ levels are strongly associated with fluid loss/gain.
Observe all mucous membranes and provide necessary care to maintain integrity.	Mucous membranes are a reliable indicator of hydration status and they may be at risk of breakdown.
Document findings and liaise with interdisciplinary team accordingly.	Alterations may require prompt medical management.

Evaluation:
Assessment and monitoring of individual to include:

- fluid intake and output on a fluid balance chart
- status of IV site, IV cannula and dressing
- check IVT flow rate
- mobility and comfort level with IVT
- urinalysis
- daily weight
- serum Na^+ levels
- observation of skin integrity and mucous membranes
- vital signs (temp, BP, HR, RR).

- encouraging smaller amounts of fluid at more frequent intervals
- ensuring that about 75% of the total volume of fluid is taken by early evening so that sleep is undisturbed
- ensuring that toilet facilities are easily accessible
- documenting input and output to assess and maintain the person's fluid and electrolyte balance.

On the other hand, some people may have restrictions on their fluid intake for medical reasons (e.g. individuals with renal failure). Basic nursing actions to assist individuals in this group might include:

- Explaining to the person and significant others the importance of consuming only the volume ordered.
- Planning to distribute fluid evenly throughout the day, including fluid to swallow medications.
- Encouraging small amounts at regular intervals to avoid thirst.
- Providing thirst-quenching fluids (e.g. water) and avoiding sweetened drinks that increase thirst.
- Notifying ancillary staff (e.g. dietitians and kitchen staff) of changes.
- Ensuring that the person's mouth does not become dry, and ensuring regular attention to oral hygiene.
- If not contraindicated, the person may be permitted sweets or sugar-free gum to stimulate production of saliva to keep the mouth moist.

Fluid balance charts and weighing

Clinical assessment of individuals, accurate intake and output measurements on fluid balance charts and monitoring blood chemistry are key elements for assessing fluid balance and hydration. Fluid balance charts (Table 26.13) are commonly utilised in clinical practice and are an important aspect of nursing care documentation. Fluid balance charts are a record of fluid input and output, documented hourly over a 24-hour period, indicating if the person is in fluid balance, deficit or overload (Crisp et al 2021). Fluid balance charts are a non-invasive method of monitoring input and output. They are used by clinicians to make decisions supporting prescription of IV fluids and medications, for timely identification and reporting of abnormalities in fluid status, to determine existence of any underlying life-threatening

TABLE 26.13 | Sample fluid balance chart

FLUID BALANCE CHART												IDENTIFICATION LABEL
Date	**Input**						**Output**					
										OTHER		
Time	**Oral**	**Enteral**	**IV**	**IV**	**IV**	**Total input**	**Time**	**Urine**	**Faeces**	**Gas asp**	**Wound**	**Total output**
0700	Water 150 mL		N/S 0.9% 1 L/10 hours			150 mL		400 mL				400 mL
0800			100 mL			250 mL						
0900												
1000	Tea 150 mL		100 mL			500 mL			150 mL (loose)			550 mL
1100	Water 150 mL		100 mL			750 mL		350 mL				900 mL
1200			100 mL			850 mL						
1300	Water 150 mL		100 mL			1100 mL		150 mL				1050 mL
1400	Tea 150 mL		100 mL			1350 mL						
1500			100 mL			1450 mL			100 mL (loose)			1150 mL

conditions affecting fluid and electrolyte homeostasis, and to identify potential risks and complications in order to plan appropriate preventative care (Liaw & Goh 2018; Simpson & McIntosh 2021).

In practice, fluid balance charts should be used concurrently with the person's daily weight to assess hydration status. The use of fluid balance charts alone to accurately monitor a person's fluid balance status can be problematic because of issues related to inaccurate records and cumulative fluid balance, inconsistency with standardised body weight measurements, omission or duplication of information, inappropriate chart design and arithmetical errors (Sivapuram 2022). Factors associated with poor quality fluid balance charting include lack of time and lack of proper education or training among nursing staff (Crisp et al 2021; Liaw & Goh 2018). Inconsistencies, errors, incomplete and poor documentation affect accurate assessment of fluid status of the person and can result in delayed interventions. Maintaining fluid balance charts is the responsibility of nurses in the clinical environment. It is therefore important that nurses accurately complete fluid balance charting. Accurate documentation provides quality assessment data to assist clinical decision-making and timely interventions. Moreover, this data supports not just nursing care, but it is also important for other members of the multidisciplinary healthcare team to assist planning and appropriate healthcare delivery.

Best clinical practice evidence currently recommends the use of daily weights without the use of fluid balance charts (JBI 2022); however, fluid balance charts continue to be used in many healthcare facilities to monitor the hydration status. If the decision is made to use a fluid balance chart, best practice evidence strongly supports the individual's involvement in completing the chart to achieve more accurate charting (Sivapuram 2022; Liaw & Goh 2018). Involving the person in their own care by prompting them to monitor their own intake will provide a more accurate record of input and output for the day. It is also important to record fluid balance hourly, because this will provide accurate and real-time fluid status (Simpson & McIntosh 2021).

Monitoring weight changes is considered a more accurate method than fluid balance charting for assessing hydration status. Assessment of weight loss or weight gain can indicate fluid volume deficit or fluid overload or retention. However, obtaining weight in individuals who are acutely ill or immobile can be difficult daily (Crisp et al 2021; Davies et al 2019). For individuals with heart failure and renal failure, measuring daily weight is critical to monitor their health status (Crisp et al 2021). The person should be weighed daily at the same time, wearing the same type of clothing and using the same set of scales. Weight can be measured with a standing scale or chair or bed scale, and measurements should be recorded on the designated observation form. An individual's weight can be affected by bowel and urine elimination patterns and this should be taken into account. Table 26.14 outlines the key aspects of care for a person with fluid imbalance. See Clinical Skill 26.1 for the correct steps in completing a fluid balance chart.

FLUID AND ELECTROLYTE REPLACEMENT

All fluid and electrolyte imbalances require correction of the underlying problem to maintain therapeutic range. The kidneys, important hormones such as ADH, and the renin–angiotensin–aldosterone system play a sentinel role in maintaining homeostasis (Craft et al 2023). However, when a person is acutely ill, homeostatic disturbances are common and the body's natural biological correction mechanisms are disrupted. Interventions such as fluid restriction or oral fluid and electrolyte replacement may not be appropriate or adequate to treat the problem in situations that require rapid fluid and electrolyte corrections (Crisp et al 2021). For mild to moderate deficits, oral medications and oral supplements can be given. In cases of more severe deficits or fluctuations, and for individuals unable to take oral fluids, parenteral replacement of fluid and electrolytes is necessary to address the problem. Parenteral administration is infusion of fluid and electrolytes directly into the bloodstream. It includes administration of total parenteral nutrition (TPN), and IV fluid and electrolyte therapy, volume expanders, blood and blood products (Crisp et al 2021).

INTRAVENOUS THERAPY

Intravenous therapy (IVT) is the administration of medications or fluids directly into the bloodstream via a catheter or cannula. Medications and fluids delivered via this route are faster acting, allow for rapid delivery of fluids and medications in an emergency, and can be given as bolus or intermittent or continuous infusions based on planned outcomes of the treatment (Williams & Hopper 2019). Administration of IV fluid and electrolyte therapy is an integral part of nursing care and it is the responsibility of nurses to assess and monitor individuals receiving IV therapy. Read Chapter 20 for clinical skills and procedures for IV administration.

Based on indications, as well as the type and duration of infusion, IV infusions are administered through vascular access devices placed into larger central veins, or through peripherally inserted catheters, which are the most commonly

TABLE 26.14 | Key aspects of care for individuals with fluid imbalance

Fluid volume deficit	Fluid volume overload
Administer pharmacological interventions (within scope of practice) as prescribed: • Antiemetics. • Medications for the treatment of diarrhoea. • Paracetamol for fever if appropriate. • IV fluids. • Electrolyte replacement as ordered, monitor for effects and consider a 12-lead ECG and continuous cardiac monitoring. • Rehydration via nasogastric or gastrostomy tube (if this is the person's usual method of fluid intake). A nasogastric tube may need to be inserted for rehydration—more commonly used in the paediatric setting as a non-invasive method of fluid administration. • Continuous nursing assessment and evaluation of response to management. • Monitor vital signs—frequency according to the acuity of the person's condition. • Infection control measures for individuals with suspected gastroenteritis. • Comfort measures—fans, blankets as appropriate. • Monitor serum electrolytes and urine SG. • Monitor input/output on a chart. • Maintain skin integrity and attend to hygiene needs.	Administer pharmacological interventions (within scope of practice) as prescribed: • Treatment of the underlying condition may require management with diuretics. • Monitor associated electrolyte imbalances and replace as required/prescribed. Consider a 12-lead ECG and continuous cardiac monitoring. • Continuous nursing assessment and evaluation of response to management. • Monitor vital signs—frequency according to the acuity of the person's condition. • Record fluid balance. • Daily or twice-daily weighing. • Care of oedematous limbs: increased risk of skin breakdown. Also, reduced healing capabilities due to reduced blood supply. • Elevation where appropriate and comfortable. • Adhere to dietary/fluid restrictions.

CLINICAL SKILL 26.1 Fluid balance charting

Please adhere to the policy and procedures of the facility/organisation prior to undertaking the skill. Ensure this skill is in your scope of practice.

An accurate fluid balance chart (FBC) should be completed using the correct equipment listed below. Charting should be completed immediately post meals; it includes oral intake, nasogastric, percutaneous endoscopic gastrostomy (PEG) and liquid medicines. Intravenous (IV) fluid should be recorded hourly and any IV medications and accompanying flush should be recorded on the FBC. All sensible (measurable) losses (urine, faeces, emesis, nasogastric aspirates/drainage and drain tubes) should be recorded. Accurate measurements of urine, drainage and aspirates should be recorded. Fluid input and output is measured and recorded hourly over a 24-hour period. Six-hourly subtotals should be recorded, which will enable an individual's accurate fluid status assessment. The cumulative balance is the 24-hour total, which is usually obtained at midnight. It is important that the healthcare facility's policy and procedure regarding recording of FBCs is adhered to.

NMBA Decision-making Framework considerations (refer to NMBA Decision-making framework for nursing and midwifery 2020):

1. Am I educated?
2. Am I authorised?
3. Am I competent?

If you answer 'no' to any of these, do not perform that activity. Seek guidance and support from your teacher/a nurse team leader/clinical facilitator/educator.

Equipment:

Fluid balance chart (either in EMR or physical form)
Weigh scale (calibrated)
Calculator
Bedpan and/or urinal if the person does not have an IDC
Measuring jug/containers for each type of output
Appropriate PPE

PREPARE FOR THE SKILL

(Please refer to the Standard Steps on pp. xviii–xx for related rationales.)

Mentally review the steps of the skill.
Discuss the skill with your instructor/supervisor/team leader, if required.
Confirm correct facility/organisation policy/safe operating procedures.
Validate the order in the individual's record.
Identify indication and rationale for performing the activity.
Assess for any contraindications.
Locate and gather equipment.
Perform hand hygiene.
Ensure therapeutic interaction.
Identify the individual using three individual identifiers.
Gain the individual's consent.
Assess for pain relief.
Prepare the environment.
Provide and maintain privacy.
Assist the individual to assume an appropriate position of comfort.

Skill activity	Rationale
Establish the reason for the commencement of a fluid balance chart (FBC): • fluid restriction • IV fluid administration • critically ill/haemodynamically unstable • prevention of fluid overload • actual or potential fluid imbalance • dehydration • electrolyte replacement • multiple infusions • blood product administration • indwelling catheter (IDC)/urinary retention • IV medication administration.	Ensures correct use of FBC.

CLINICAL SKILL 26.1 Fluid balance charting—cont'd

PERFORM THE SKILL

(Please refer to the Standard Steps on pp. xviii–xx for related rationales.)
Perform hand hygiene.
Apply PPE: gloves, eyewear, mask and gown as appropriate.
Ensure the individual's safety and comfort throughout skill.
Promote independence and involvement of the individual if possible and/or appropriate.
Assess the individual's tolerance to the skill throughout.
Dispose of used supplies, equipment, waste and sharps appropriately.
Remove PPE and discard or store appropriately.
Perform hand hygiene.

Skill activity	Rationale
Ensure a list of the correct amount of millilitres per container of fluid (intake) is available. Ensure all IV fluid administration is via an IV pump (where possible).	Ensures accuracy of individual's intake.
Ensure urinal, bedpan or plastic urinal female toilet available for the individual to urinate into, or that an IDC is in situ if haemodynamically unstable. Ensure all wound drainage, vomitus, loose bowel actions and gastric fluid is also recorded on the individual's output.	Ensures accuracy of individual's output.
Separate input and output routes in the columns on the FBC. Maintain and monitor hourly input and output over the 24-hour period. Calculate 6-hourly subtotals (or more frequently if indicated and as per organisation's guidelines). Obtain a cumulative 24-hour total at midnight (or as per healthcare organisation's guidelines). Subtract the difference between total input and output for the 24-hour period. Observe for any signs of under- or over-hydration.	Provides quantity or measurement via each input and output route/type. Establishes an accurate positive or negative balance to determine the individual's fluid status so that intervention may be prompt. Prevents circulatory overload and complications.

AFTER THE SKILL

(Please refer to the Standard Steps on pp. xviii–xx for related rationales.)
Communicate outcome to the individual, any ongoing care and to report any complications.
Restore the environment.
Report, record and document assessment findings, details of the skill performed and the individual's response.
Report, record and document any abnormalities and/or inability to perform the skill.
Reassess the individual to ensure there are no adverse effects/events from the skill.

(Berman et al 2020; Crisp et al 2021; Simpson & McIntosh 2021)

used access for short-term IV therapy. Central venous access devices (CVAD) are effective for delivering medications and solutions that are irritating to veins and for long-term IV therapy. CVADs include central venous catheters (CVC), peripherally inserted central catheters (PICCs) and implanted infusion ports (Crisp et al 2021). Nurses must undertake further education and training and follow their workplace guidelines for care and management of these central devices. This chapter primarily focuses on peripherally inserted cannulas.

General care and management of individuals receiving IVT incorporates:

- monitoring the IV site and cannula patency
- maintenance of IVT equipment
- preparing IV fluids and medications for administration
- prevention of complications occurring during and after completion of IV infusions
- educating the individual
- assistance with mobility needs
- continuous assessment.

Peripheral intravenous cannula (PIVC) is the most common venous access route, providing quick and direct access to the bloodstream to implement fluid and electrolyte replacement interventions. Refer to Quality Statement 3 of the Australian Commission for Safety and Quality in Health Care's Management of Peripheral Intravenous Catheters Clinical Care Standard for guidance regarding competency in relation to PIVCs. The purpose of this quality statement states 'To minimise trauma to the patient by ensuring that PIVCs are inserted and/or maintained by appropriately skilled members of the healthcare team' (ACSQHC 2021, p. 17). Insertion of an IV cannula is routinely performed by a medical officer or a Registered Nurse (RN) who is certified in IV cannulation within their scope of practice. Specialty and extended practice Enrolled Nurses who are certified in IV cannulation may also be able to insert PIVCs within their scope of practice in some settings. Prior to the insertion of a cannula the most appropriate site is selected, which depends on several factors, including the condition of the person's veins—avoiding areas that are oedematous, infected or otherwise impaired and general comfort considerations (see Figure 26.9). (See Clinical Interest Box 26.14.)

Other site determinants include:

- A vein in the non-dominant arm is preferable.
- The initial site should be in the most distal part of the vein to allow more proximal replacement in the same vein in the event of cannula blockage, infiltration or **phlebitis**.
- A commonly selected site is one of the superficial veins on the dorsum of the hand.
- If the site chosen is near a joint, extension and splinting of the limb may be necessary.

Peripheral cannula insertion is an invasive clinical procedure. Complications associated with PIVCs include local infections, necrosis, phlebitis and more serious catheter-related bloodstream infections (Gorski 2023; Swe 2022; Porritt 2021). Healthcare facilities will have individual policies and guidelines pertaining to the management and insertion of IV cannulas. One such example is the following guideline: *Peripheral Intravenous Cannulation (PIVC) Insertion, Care and Removal (Adults)* (SESLHD 2022). Essentially, IV cannulas should be inserted by competent, accredited healthcare professionals. They are an invasive medical device and should be inserted, accessed and removed using an aseptic technique. Documentation should include the time, anatomical placement and reason for insertion of the PIVC. The insertion site is often labelled with the corresponding date/time.

Nursing care involves regular monitoring of the PIVC site. Phlebitis or inflammation of the vein can occur from cannulation trauma or from administration of medications and fluids that irritate the vein. A critical aspect of care is monitoring and documenting the condition of the insertion site each shift for complications such as tenderness, pain, redness and swelling. The recommended risk assessment tool is the Visual Infusion Phlebitis Score (VIPS) (Swe 2022). A site that is suspicious for infection should be reported and managed immediately. IV cannulas should be reviewed daily for ongoing need and removed if no longer required, when malfunctioning, or when complications develop (ACSQHC 2021). If a medical officer requests that a PIVC remains in situ past the usual dwell time, the reason and plan must be documented in the clinical notes, including the date to review the cannula; for example, the next day. Infections from IV sites can have potentially serious complications for individuals and preventing them is integral to hospital quality and risk programs. For more information on VIPS, refer to Chapter 20 and the Online Resources at the end of this chapter. For more information on PIVC management, refer to Chapter 20 and the ACSQHC Clinical Care Standard (ACSQHC 2021).

INTRAVENOUS FLUIDS

Nurses caring for individuals receiving IV therapy have the responsibility of ensuring that the person's care is within their scope of practice. Prescription of IV fluids depends

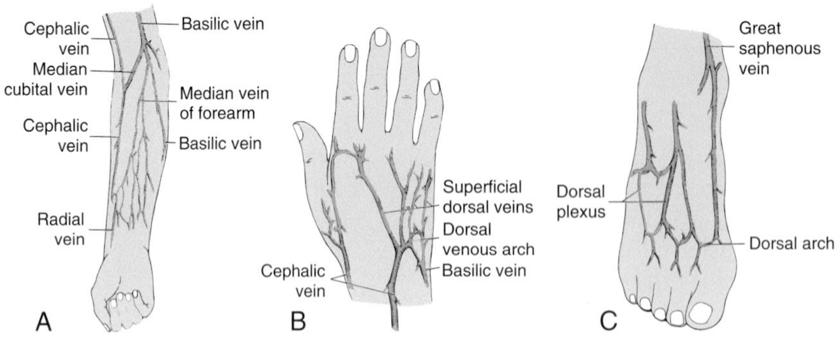

Figure 26.9

Common intravenous sites

A: Inner arm, **B:** Dorsal surface of the hand, **C:** Dorsal surface of the foot (infants and children)

(Potter & Perry 2021)

CLINICAL INTEREST BOX 26.14 Consideration for vein selection in intravenous therapy

- The age of the person
- The availability of sites for cannulation
- Size of the cannula to be used
- Purpose of the infusion therapy
- Osmolarity and pH of the infusion solution
- The volume, rate and duration of infusion
- The degree of mobility desired during the infusion

(ACSQHC 2021; Williams & Hopper 2019)

on the desired treatment outcome for the individual. Fluid tonicity and osmolarity (previously discussed) is an extremely important concept relevant to the administration of IV fluids. There are three basic types of IV solutions:

- Isotonic solution: Has the same tonicity or concentration of solutes as the internal environment of the body—it has approximately the same amount of Na^+ concentration. Therefore, the administration of this type of fluid is used to increase the circulating fluid volume or simply used for fluid/hydration maintenance. 0.9% sodium chloride is an example.
- Hypotonic solution: Has a lower tonicity or solute concentration than the internal environment. This type of solution will attract water into the cell—causing cells to swell. It is used for individuals who are very dehydrated, individuals with an elevated Na^+ (depending on the cause) or increased serum osmolality. An example of a hypotonic solution is 5% dextrose. The dextrose is metabolised (used by the body for energy) so it leaves behind water.
- Hypertonic solution: Has an increased tonicity or greater solute concentration compared to the internal environment. Therefore, it draws water out of the cells and into the vascular space. An example is 20% albumin. **Albumin** is an important protein in the maintenance of plasma oncotic pressure and so assists with attracting fluid into the vascular compartment.

Most commonly used fluids for IV therapy are dextrose and sodium solutions, which are known as crystalloid solutions (see Table 26.15). Other solutions used in fluid and electrolyte replacement are Ringer's solution and Hartmann's solution, which balance electrolyte solutions and have the same tonicity as body fluids (Williams & Davidson 2019).

TABLE 26.15 | Commonly used intravenous solutions

Solution	Concentration/tonicity
Dextrose in water solutions (glucose)	
5% in water	Isotonic
10% in water	Hypertonic
Saline (sodium chloride) solutions	
0.45%	Hypotonic
0.9%	Isotonic
3–5%	Hypertonic
Dextrose in saline solutions (glucose)	
5% in 0.9%	Hypertonic
5% in 0.45%	Hypertonic
Multiple electrolyte solutions	
Hartmann's solution	Isotonic
Ringer's solution	Isotonic

Care of individuals with an intravenous infusion

As previously stated within this chapter, nurses have a professional accountability and responsibility to be aware of the scope of their role in relation to the management of IV infusions. The scope of practice and responsibilities for care and management of IV infusions vary in nursing practice in different clinical settings. Enrolled Nurses must ensure that they practise within their scope and educational level in relation to IV infusions. See the Nursing and Midwifery Board of Australia's (2022) *Enrolled nurses and medicines administration* for specific information about IV administration.

Of prime importance is careful observation of the individual and the IV equipment used during the infusion, and accurate reporting of the person's assessment and vital signs. Nurses tasked with IV administration must be knowledgeable about IV-therapy-related complications and how to prevent, recognise and manage the problem. Complications that may occur when a person has an IV infusion, and which must be recognised and reported immediately, are:

- a flow rate that is too slow or too fast, or cessation of flow
- infection, pain or infiltration at the insertion site
- phlebitis of the vein being used for the infusion
- circulatory overload
- air embolism.

Nurses also have a responsibility to promote the general comfort of the individual along with ensuring that the infusion is administered as prescribed and to observe for and prevent complications. Complications associated with peripheral IV therapy are either local or systemic problems (see Table 26.16). (See also Chapter 20.)

TABLE 26.16 | Complications of peripheral intravenous therapy

Local complications
Haematoma
Thrombosis
Phlebitis
Infiltration/extravasation
Local infection at the site
Venous spasm
Systemic complications
Septicaemia
Circulatory overload
Venous air embolism
Speed shock

(Williams & Hopper 2019)

Key aspects related to the care of a person with an IV infusion include the following:

- Checking that the flow rate is set as prescribed and adjusted when necessary to deliver the correct amount of fluid within the prescribed time.
- Utilising a calibrated burette (e.g. macrodrip or microdrip volume control set) with the infusion system, particularly if an electronic infusion pump is not available. Such devices enable very small or precise amounts of fluid to be administered and can also be used for administering IV medications. (See Chapter 20 for formula to calculate the flow rate or drops per minute using gravity feed IV delivery set.)
- When calculating the rate, it is essential to know the calibration of the drip rate for each manufacturer's product, as these vary from 10 drops/mL to 60 drops/mL.
- The flow rate should be checked every 15 minutes (if an electronic infusion pump is not been used) to ensure that the drip rate is stable, then every hour or at the set time intervals specified in the institution's policy on IV infusions.
- Check the level of solution to determine the volume of fluid remaining in the flask. It is important to ensure that a flask does not empty completely since this can interfere with the flow rate and permit air to enter the tubing, which could lead to an air embolism. Air emboli can result in sudden decrease in blood pressure, rapid weak pulse, cyanosis and loss of consciousness.
- Check the cannula insertion site at least once per shift (or eight hours) and more frequently if required, including if the individual raises concerns. Check for signs of infection, inflammation or infiltration. Infection at the insertion site is indicated by redness, warmth, swelling and tenderness. The vein may become injured or irritated and phlebitis may occur. Signs and symptoms that indicate phlebitis are pain, swelling and inflammation along the course of the vein; the vein may also feel hard and warm to touch. Infiltration occurs if the needle becomes displaced, causing IV solution to flow into the surrounding tissues. Signs and symptoms of infiltration are cool skin in the site area, swelling and discomfort at the site, oedema of the limb, sluggish flow rate and absence of blood in the tubing when it is lowered.
- Observe the person for signs of over-hydration or circulatory overload, caused by excessive or too rapid fluid administration. Signs and symptoms of circulatory overload include elevated blood pressure, venous dilation (especially of the neck veins), coughing, tachypnoea and shortness of breath.
- Check the information on the flask label when each new flask is started and at the start of each shift. It is essential that the person receives the prescribed solution; the nurse should therefore follow the facility protocol regarding checking of IV solutions.
- The type, volume and expiry date of the solution is checked. Glass containers are inspected for chips and cracks and the seal over the opening is observed to ascertain if it is intact. Plastic containers should be squeezed gently to detect leaks. The solution is examined for particles, abnormal discolouration and cloudiness. The container is not to be used if any doubt exists, and the intact container is retained for further investigation.
- Throughout the course of the infusion, document details of the flow rate, the type and amount of fluid and additives being administered as well as the person's fluid input from other sources and fluid output. Vital signs (temperature, pulse, respirations and blood pressure) are also measured regularly and documented.

(See Case Study 26.1.)

There are also several equally important safety and quality initiatives around IV therapy that must be adhered to in order to prevent risk of infections. Prior to using the IV line, it is important that the IV access port is vigorously cleaned with a single-use alcohol swab and allowed to dry before each use. Sterile single-use devices must be used for intermittent medication administration through the IV access ports. Where possible, it is also recommended that continuous IV fluids should be administered to promote patency of the line and maintain asepsis. Disconnecting and reconnecting lines for intermittent infusions increases the risk of infection. Health facilities will have specific guidelines with details for care of IV lines. As an example, refer to *Peripheral Intravenous Catheter (PIVC) Guideline* (Western Australia Country Health Service 2022).

CASE STUDY 26.1

Administering intravenous fluids

Jean, an 80-year-old female, is admitted to the medical ward. Jean lives at a residential aged-care home. Jean had become increasingly confused and developed a fever of 38.2°C. Medical diagnosis on admission: urinary tract infection, dehydration and fever. Medical history of stroke affecting her ability to self-care, atrial fibrillation and myo-congestive failure. Treatment and management plan were for slow rehydration (intravenous Hartmann's solution, 12-hourly rate), oral intake as tolerated, intravenous antibiotics stat order (1 g Ceftriaxone) while waiting for urine and blood culture sensitivities. Vital signs 4-hourly, monitor BP, urine output and daily weight. Referral to dietitian, physio and occupational therapist.

1. What risk factors could have contributed to Jean's dehydration?
2. What risk factors could have contributed to Jean developing a urinary tract infection?
3. What are some possible nursing diagnoses for Jean?
4. How will you manage Jean's infusion of IV fluid? What are some important considerations?
5. What will your ongoing assessment of Jean consist of and what potential complications will you be monitoring Jean for?
6. Why is Jean prescribed Hartmann's solution at the 12-hourly rate to treat and manage dehydration?

Electrolyte replacement

Maintaining normal electrolyte levels is vital for basic body functioning and having high or low levels of electrolytes (imbalance) can disrupt normal bodily functions and can even lead to serious life-threatening complications. Nurses should be especially cautious when administering IV solutions containing electrolytes or fluids that have had electrolytes added to them. Rapid correction of electrolyte imbalances and sudden increase or decrease in electrolyte levels can lead to serious consequences (Shrimanker & Bhattarai 2023).

Potassium (K^+) is a classified high-risk medication in IV replacement therapy and may require the person to be cardiac monitored along with blood tests to check electrolytes. It is important for nurses to be aware of and to monitor serum K^+ levels because of its narrow reference range. Even a slight increase or decrease outside the therapeutic range can cause serious problems related to cardiac arrhythmias. A common side effect associated with administration of IV potassium is significant pain at the IV site and sometimes to the whole limb. This is usually associated with larger doses and shorter administration times. Cold packs can be applied, but it might be necessary to liaise with the medical team for further problem resolution. For more information about medication safety, high-risk medicine resources, and APINCHS classification of high-risk medicines, refer to Chapter 20 and the Australian Commission on Safety and Quality in Health Care (ACSQHC) Online Resources at the end of this chapter. (See Case Study 26.2.)

CASE STUDY 26.2

Fluid and electrolyte disturbance

John, a 26-year-old man, presents to the emergency department with a 5-day history of severe vomiting and diarrhoea. John returned from an overseas trip. He was admitted to the ward for treatment and management of his condition.

1. What are some electrolyte disturbances you might expect to see in John and why?
2. What clinical symptoms are associated with these electrolyte disturbances?
3. What type of IV fluids might be initiated for John and why?
4. What is the reason for caution when administering IV solutions containing electrolytes or fluids that have had electrolytes added to them?
5. What would you expect John's urine SG and osmolality to be and why?

Intravenous fluid administration in paediatrics

Intravenous fluid therapy is less commonly used in children and is indicated only in emergency situations. Wherever possible, the enteral route (usually via a nasogastric tube) should be used in paediatric settings. If the enteral route is not suitable, then IV fluid administration can be used. Nurses need to exercise caution prior to and during the administration of IV fluids in children and should ensure that it is within their scope of practice. Accurate prescribing of the fluid and careful monitoring is critical for IV fluid administration in children. Strict measurement of input and output is important in infants and children receiving IV therapy to prevent over-hydration. Input and output monitoring is also vital to detect any existing underlying life-threatening conditions affecting the ability of the kidney to properly regulate fluid and electrolyte balance (Simpson & McIntosh 2021). If a nurse is uncertain of the fluid order for any reason, liaising with the prescribing medical officer is critical and safe practice. Healthcare facilities will have specific guidelines pertaining to managing IV fluid administration in paediatric settings. As an example, see the Sydney Children's Hospital Network's (SCHN) *Intravenous Fluid and Electrolyte Therapy—SCH, Practice Guideline* (SCHN 2017).

In a child with normal fluid volume status and not consuming oral fluids, maintenance fluid will usually be

TABLE 26.17 | Fluid requirements in paediatric settings

Child's weight	mL/day	mL/hour
3–10 kg	100 × wt	4 × wt
10–20 kg	1000 plus 50 × (wt − 10)	40 plus 2 × (wt − 10)
>20 kg	1500 plus 20 × (wt − 20)	60 plus 1 × (wt − 20)

wt = weight in kg
(Adapted from SCHN 2017)

administered. It is termed 'maintenance' because it replaces generally expected insensible losses. A child's maintenance fluid requirement decreases proportionately with increasing age (and weight). The calculations in Table 26.17 approximate the maintenance fluid requirements of well children according to weight in kilograms.

Choice of IV fluid will depend on the clinical situation. A commonly used maintenance fluid is 0.45% NaCl with 5% glucose, although it may not be appropriate in all situations.

If a child presents with dehydration, then initial replacement of the fluid loss is essential. The formula for this is 10–20 mL/kg administered as boluses until the desired clinical outcome is achieved. The fluid of choice in this situation is usually 0.9% sodium chloride.

The Royal Children's Hospital Melbourne outlines the following recommendations in its guidelines (refer to the Online Resources the Royal Children's Hospital Melbourne, *Clinical practice guideline: Intravenous fluids*).

Monitoring of children receiving treatment with IV fluids should include the following:

- Obtaining a weight from the child prior to commencement and then 6–8-hourly after fluid has been commenced. Daily weights should then continue.
- Electrolytes and glucose should be checked prior to fluid administration and within 24 hours.

Clinical Interest Box 26.15 outlines the treatment of gastroenteritis in children.

ACID–BASE BALANCE

Acids and bases

Acids and bases are formed as a natural part of the metabolic processes of the human body and require maintenance within a narrow range to achieve homeostasis (Williams & Hopper 2019). Maintaining acid–base balance is essential to normal functioning of the body; even slight fluctuations in acid–base homeostasis can significantly alter the body's physiological processes at the tissue and cellular levels (Craft et al 2023). Nurses require a sound understanding of mechanisms that regulate acid–base homeostasis and the normal values and be able to recognise signs and symptoms of imbalance to ensure timely interventions are implemented.

An **acid** is any substance that releases hydrogen **ions** (H^+) when dissolved in water and the stronger the acid the greater the number of hydrogen ions released. Acids have chemical properties which are essentially opposite to those of bases. Examples of acids found in the body include hydrochloric, lactic, pyruvic, carbonic, citric, folic and fatty acids. A **base** is any substance that binds or accepts hydrogen ions in chemical reactions. Alkalis are bases that are soluble in water. Examples of bases found in the body include hydrogen bicarbonate and sodium hydroxide (Craft et al 2023).

CLINICAL INTEREST BOX 26.15 Paediatric gastroenteritis

Treatment of gastroenteritis in the young individual requires special attention to fluid and electrolyte balance. Fluids such as flat lemonade and mineral water are often used for rehydration. This treatment has potential life-threatening consequences. Lemonade has a high sugar content, and sugar acts as an osmotic agent, drawing water into the gastrointestinal tract (GIT) from the body's fluid compartments. This fluid loss results in increased diarrhoea and dehydration. Sugar is also utilised by bacteria in the gastrointestinal tract as a form of nutrition, resulting in increased gas production by the bacteria, causing gaseous distension and abdominal pain.

Hydration in the young needs to be assessed by a medical officer. The person often requires rehydration with products such as Gastrolyte, by oral or nasogastric administration and, in more severe cases, intravenous therapy may be required.

The meaning of pH

The **pH** scale is used to express the concentration of hydrogen ions (H^+) in acids or bases. The 'p' stands for potential or power, and the 'H' stands for hydrogen. Therefore, pH represents the potential, or power, of hydrogen ions present in body fluids, and pH of a solution is determined by measuring the amount of H^+ present. (See Figure 26.10.) The scale is numbered from 0–14; the lower the number on the scale, the more H^+ present, and the more acidic the solution. A pH of 7 indicates a neutral solution, while a pH above 7 is termed basic, or alkaline, and a solution below 7 is acidic.

Essentially, the acidity or alkalinity of a fluid is dependent on the concentration of H^+ in the solution (Brown et al 2020). Each integral step in the pH scale (i.e. 14, 13, 12 ... to 0 pH) represents a tenfold increase in H^+ ion concentration; thus, the pH scale is an inverse logarithmic scale of the amount of hydrogen ions present.

ACID–BASE REGULATION

In order to maintain optimal cellular function, the hydrogen ion (H^+) concentration of body fluid is maintained within a narrow range (LeMone et al 2020). The pH of body

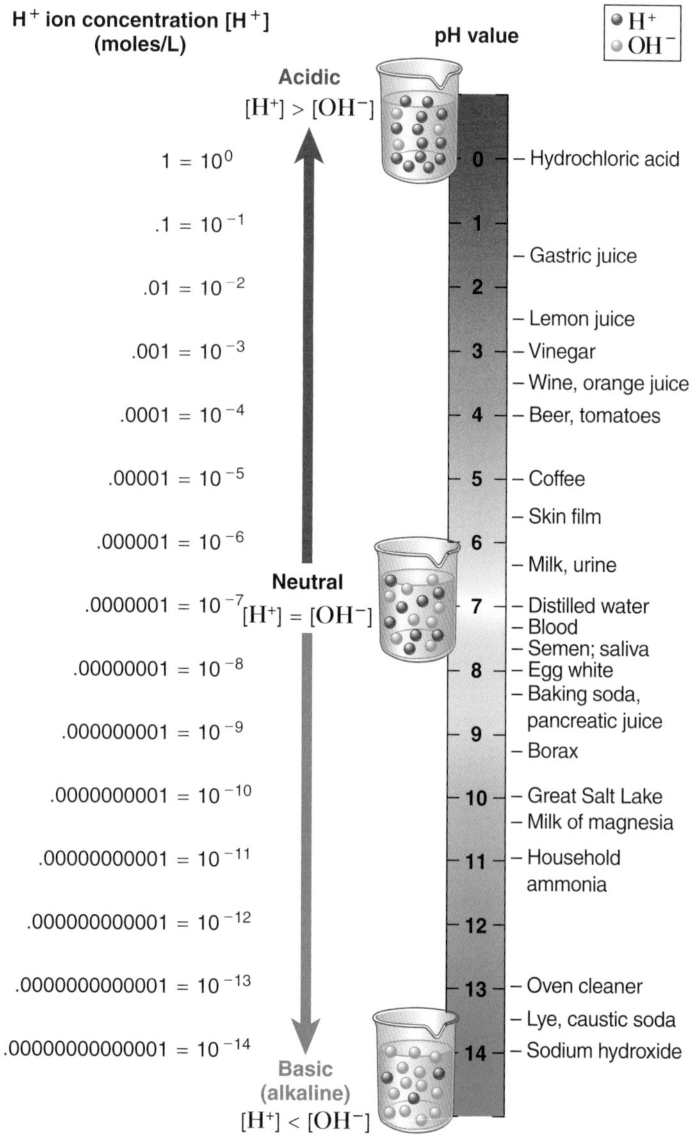

Figure 26.10 The pH range

The overall pH range is expressed numerically on what is called a logarithmic scale of 0–14. This means that a change of 1 pH unit represents a tenfold difference in actual concentration of hydrogen ions. Note that as the concentration of H+ increases, the solution becomes increasingly acidic and the pH value decreases. As OH^- concentration increases, the pH value also increases, and the solution becomes more and more basic, or alkaline. A pH of 7 is neutral, a pH of 2 is very acidic, and a pH of 13 is very basic.
(Patton et al 2024)

fluid is maintained between 7.35 and 7.45; this means it is slightly basic (**alkaline**) as neutral is a pH of 7. A number of buffering systems are required to maintain a normal pH; this is because the normal cellular metabolism of nutrients in the human body continuously produces acids (LeMone et al 2020).

The body's capacity to form, excrete and 'buffer' acids and bases is known as the acid–base balance. Acid–base imbalances are classified as either respiratory or metabolic depending on the underlying cause (Berman et al 2020). The acid–base balance is critical to the survival of the human body. Variations outside the normal arterial range of a pH of 7.35–7.45 indicate serious dysfunction in the body and can become life-threatening. The normal metabolism of nutrients by cells produces large amounts of H^+ that form acids. This concentration of H^+ in the cells and tissues must, however, be kept low to prevent cellular damage. To maintain pH within normal limits, the body excretes acids at the same rate that they are produced and buffers any excess hydrogen ion (Craft et al 2023).

In the clinical environment, arterial blood gas (ABG) analysis is the test used to accurately measure acid–base status. Interpretation of ABG values assists in assessing respiratory and metabolic status and determines the acid–base disorders and the underlying causes (Crisp et al 2021). ABG analysis measures pH levels, serum oxygen and carbon dioxide levels in arterial blood. (See Table 26.18 for ABG and venous blood gas reference ranges.) Note that reference values will be different in arterial and venous blood gas measurements.

TABLE 26.18 | Adult reference range for blood gas values

Arterial blood gas values	
pH	7.36–7.44
$PaCO_2$	35–45 mmHg
HCO_3^- (bicarbonate)	22–32 mmol/L
PaO_2	80–100 mmHg
SaO_2	>95%
Base excess	±3.0 mmol/L
Venous blood gas values	
pH	7.32–7.43
$PvCO_2$	42–50 mmHg
PvO_2	37–42 mmHg
HCO_3^- (bicarbonate)	22–26 mmol/L

(The Royal College of Pathologists of Australia, nd—online manual)

CRITICAL THINKING EXERCISE 26.7

Acid–base disturbance

Tom is 16 years old. He has been complaining of excessive thirst and passing a lot of urine. His breath smells, and he is deep breathing. His results show BGL 21 mmol/L and pH 7.1. What could be the problem in this case?

Buffer systems

A **buffer** is a chemical substance that resists changes in the pH of solutions by either removing or releasing hydrogen ions (LeMone et al 2020). Examples of buffers are proteins, haemoglobin, bicarbonate and phosphates (Williams & Hopper 2019). When bodily fluid is too acidic, buffers bind with hydrogen ions to keep the pH within the homeostatic range. When body fluid is alkaline, buffers release hydrogen ions, again returning the pH to normal (LeMone et al 2020). Two important chemical buffers that react to acid–base imbalances in seconds are *bicarbonate buffer* and *carbonic acid system.* (See Figure 26.11.)

For example, CO_2 is a product of cellular metabolism and when combined with water, forms carbonic acid ($CO_2 + H_2O = H_2CO_3$), which drains back into the circulation. Excess carbonic acid in the blood is rapidly decomposed into carbon dioxide and water ($H_2CO_3 = CO_2 + H_2O$) and the CO_2 is excreted by the lungs to maintain the pH at normal physiological levels. Conversely, if water is lost from the blood, it is replaced by the ionisation of carbonic acid, and a rise in pH is prevented. Thus, carbonic acid acts as a buffer in the blood. An example of the buffering action of bicarbonate ion is its reaction with lactic acid. Lactic acid is produced from glucose during muscle contraction, and the dissociation of lactic acid tends to lower the pH. Since lactic acid is stronger than carbonic acid, its conjugate base (lactic ion) is weaker. The stronger base (bicarbonate ion) combines

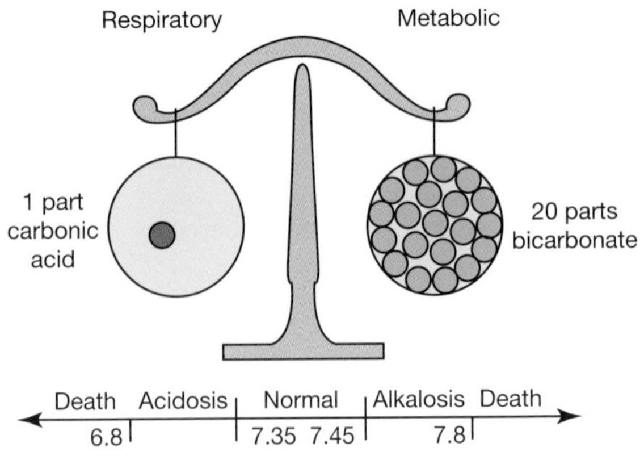

Figure 26.11 Carbonic acid-bicarbonate ratio and pH

(Crisp et al 2021)

with the hydrogen from lactic acid, forming dissociated carbonic acid (Craft et al 2023).

The three mechanisms involved in the control of acid–base fluctuations are the protein or cellular buffering system, the respiratory system and the renal system, with each mechanism responding or reacting at different points (Craft et al 2023; Williams & Hopper 2019). When the acid–base balance is disturbed, as an immediate response at the first level the buffering system attempts to restore the pH to the normal range involving substances present in the blood that act to provide short-term adjustments. Then the lungs, as the second level of defence, assist to restore pH through the respiratory process. The lungs react to remove acid, related to carbon dioxide levels in the blood, within minutes. Finally, the kidneys, which are responsible for long-term regulation of acid–base balance, respond to changes in pH levels in hours or days and remove excess acid or base from the body fluid. The kidneys are the slowest to respond to serum pH changes, assisting with compensation and regulating the amount of base in the body. The lungs and kidneys are the two major organs involved in the regulation of acid–base balance. Adjustments to pH fluctuations through the respiratory and renal system are known as compensation (Craft et al 2023). Changes in pH are compensated by the respiratory system by retaining or eliminating carbon dioxide level through ventilation, whereas the renal system compensates by producing more acidic or alkaline urine. A pH correction is said to occur when values for both carbonic acid and bicarbonate return to normal levels (Craft et al 2023).

Acid–base imbalances

Acidosis is a condition in which the blood becomes acidic (pH <7.35) due to an increase in hydrogen ion concentration as a result of accumulation of an acid, or the loss of a base. **Alkalosis** is a condition characterised by an increased pH, above 7.45, due to a decrease in hydrogen ion concentration as a result of a loss of acids or the accumulation of a base.

An acid–base imbalance occurs when there is a deficit or excess of carbonic acid or base bicarbonate. In some situations, in which a person cannot efficiently excrete enough CO_2—for example, in an individual with pneumonia—the buffer system may be unable to keep the pH within the normal range. In this situation, the excess CO_2 will make the blood more acidic, reducing pH levels. If the pH falls below 7.35, the condition is termed acidosis; if the pH rises above 7.45, the condition is termed alkalosis. Normally the body can absorb or neutralise acids as they are formed (buffering), which is done through:

- Blood: Initial buffering of acids occurs in tissue, blood cells and the plasma.
- Lungs: Rapidly altering blood pH by increasing or decreasing the respiratory rate, increasing the removal of carbon dioxide.
- Kidneys: Excreting additional acids that cannot be excreted by any other method; they also reabsorb bicarbonate back into the bloodstream after acids have been excreted.

A pH above or below the normal pH of arterial blood (7.35–7.45) may result in severe dysfunction and potential death. See Table 26.19 for interpreting ABG values.

Causes of pH disturbances

As noted earlier in this section, the pH is maintained within a narrow range in the body by many regulatory mechanisms. Just as deviations in fluid and electrolytes can cause serious health complications, acid–base disturbances can also lead to serious health problems. Untreated, they can be potentially life-threatening. Alterations in pH can occur due to respiratory or metabolic problems, or they may be of mixed origin.

Respiratory causes

Respiratory acidosis occurs as a result of alveolar hypoventilation and accumulation of CO_2. The body is unable to ventilate enough CO_2 out of the lungs, which may be due to airway obstruction, emphysema, asthma or opiate overdose. (The kidneys compensate, for example, by retaining bicarbonate.) Respiratory acidosis can be classified as either acute or chronic (Sommers 2023). Acute respiratory acidosis is linked to sudden ventilation failure. In chronic respiratory acidosis, which is seen in individuals with chronic lung disease, long-term hypoventilation leads to chronic elevated levels of CO_2 (hypercapnia), and low oxygen level (hypoxemia) becomes the major drive for respiration.

TABLE 26.19 | Interpreting arterial blood gas values

Acid–base imbalance	pH	$PaCO_2$	HCO_3^-
Respiratory acidosis	↓	↑	↑ (compensated) or normal (uncompensated)
Respiratory alkalosis	↑	↓	↓ (compensated) or normal (uncompensated)
Metabolic acidosis	↓	↓ (compensated) or normal (uncompensated)	↓
Metabolic alkalosis	↑	↑ (compensated) or normal (uncompensated)	↑

(Craft et al 2023)

Respiratory alkalosis occurs with hyperventilation, when rapid respirations blow off too much carbon dioxide, resulting in alkalosis of a respiratory nature, such as in panic attacks. (The kidneys compensate, for example, by excreting more bicarbonate.) The primary cause for this form of acid–base imbalance is deep and rapid breathing (Craft et al 2023). Respiratory alkalosis is the most frequently occurring form of acid–base imbalance in the clinical environment (Sommers 2023).

CRITICAL THINKING EXERCISE 26.8

Acid–base respiratory imbalance

A 28-year-old homeless male was admitted to hospital. Presentation: Temperature 39°C, short of breath, trouble breathing, chest pain on respiration, cough (productive green sputum).

Tests:

- chest X-ray—right lower lobe pneumonia
- blood cultures—*Streptococcus pneumoniae*
- sputum cultures—high white cell count, *S. pneumoniae*, sensitive to penicillin
- blood gases—pH 7.30, PaO_2 78 mmHg, $PaCO_2$ 48 mmHg, HCO_3^- 30 mmol/L, SaO_2 83%.

Are the blood gas values within reference range? What is the collaborative care?

Metabolic causes

Metabolic acidosis occurs when the body is unable to excrete enough acids because of a problem with malabsorption (such as diarrhoea) or metabolism (e.g. diabetic ketoacidosis) (see Clinical Interest Box 26.16 and Chapter 36) or organ failure (such as kidney failure). There is an excess of acids over bases. (The lungs compensate, for example, by increasing ventilation and increasing excretion of acidifying CO_2.). Bicarbonate levels are driven by acid–base status of the blood and imbalances can lead to either metabolic acidosis or alkalosis (Shrimanker & Bhattarai 2023).

Metabolic alkalosis is an excess of bases over acids. It occurs as a result of two altered states: an excess of bases or when too much acid is lost (e.g. by prolonged vomiting, nasogastric drainage or use of some diuretics). (The lungs compensate, for example, by decreasing ventilation and decreasing excretion of acidifying CO_2.) Individuals at higher risk for this form of acid–base imbalance are people with a history of congestive heart failure and hypertension on sodium-restricted diets and diuretic therapy (Sommers 2023).

Although acid–base imbalances are discussed individually, they can also present as mixed disorders. Mixed acid–base alterations, for instance, may occur in the form of respiratory acidosis and metabolic alkalosis, or respiratory alkalosis and metabolic acidosis in certain conditions. (See Table 26.20 for common causes and Table 26.21 for signs and symptoms for acid–base disorders.)

CLINICAL INTEREST BOX 26.16 Diabetic ketoacidosis

Individuals with diabetes who have not been administered enough insulin or are unwell, or those with undiagnosed diabetes, are at risk of developing diabetic ketoacidosis. Without adequate insulin, the body uses its muscle and fat for metabolism, producing ketone acids. To rid the body of acids, emesis and later hyperemesis occurs, resulting in a loss not only of acid but also of fluid and other electrolytes. The ketone acids can severely affect the pH of the blood, causing a metabolic acidosis. The body tries to compensate by excreting acid by the lungs (compensatory respiratory alkalosis), kidneys and skin.

Hyperglycaemia causes an osmotic-induced polyuria and a subsequent fluid and electrolyte imbalance and may result in severe dehydration. If insulin is not administered and the correct rehydration therapy instigated, in severe cases the condition can result in cerebral oedema, coma and death.

CRITICAL THINKING EXERCISE 26.9

Acid–base imbalance metabolic

A 17-year-old schoolgirl is seen by the admitting medical officer; she has been well previously. Presentation: Confused, acting irrationally, passing urine frequently, thirsty, breath smells, lost 5 kg in 8 weeks, performing poorly at school, uncharacteristically.

Assessment data: Decreased skin turgor, blood pressure 90/65, afebrile, breathing deeply, dehydrated.

Tests:

- urine presence of ketones, no white cells
- full blood examination normal, slightly raised eGFR
- BGL 16 mmol/L
- blood gases: pH 7.25, PaO_2 97 mmHg, $PaCO_2$ 30 mmHg, HCO_3^- 20 mmol/L, SaO_2 96%.

What is the suspected problem? Are the blood gas values within reference ranges?

Compensation

A change in pH by one system of the body will tend to cause an opposite compensatory change in pH, known as respiratory or metabolic compensation. The system tries to return pH level to normal, or near normal, through compensation. If respiratory acidosis exists, the body will compensate by producing a metabolic alkalosis. If metabolic alkalosis exists, the body will compensate by producing a respiratory acidosis. It is important to note that overcompensation will not occur. As pH returns to normal levels, the drivers for the compensation mechanism cease. (See Table 26.19 and Case Study 26.3.)

TABLE 26.20 | Common causes of acid–base problems

Acid–base imbalance	Common causes
Respiratory acidosis	Chronic obstructive pulmonary disease (COPD), airway obstructive respiratory conditions resulting in decreased lung function Sedative opiates, barbiturates, anaesthetics that depress breathing Neurological problems that depress breathing Chest wall disorders, respiratory muscle disorders Abdominal distension
Respiratory alkalosis	Hyperventilation from hypoxia, pulmonary disease, hypotension, high altitudes, acute asthma, pneumonia Stimulated central respiratory centre due to pain, anxiety, fever, infection, head trauma, central nervous system disease Mechanical hyperventilation
Metabolic acidosis	Renal failure Shock, fever Cardiopulmonary arrest, strenuous exercise Diabetic ketoacidosis, alcoholic ketoacidosis Ingestion of drugs and chemicals Pancreatitis, gastrointestinal problems Starvation, severe diarrhoea
Metabolic alkalosis	Severe vomiting, excessive nasogastric suctioning Overuse of antacids, baking soda, ingestion of bicarbonates and other bases Diuretic therapy, hypokalaemia, excessive mineralocorticoid
Mixed respiratory/ metabolic disturbances	Respiratory acidosis and metabolic alkalosis: A person with COPD with diuretics for concomitant heart failure Respiratory alkalosis and metabolic acidosis: Large amounts of salicylate ingestion, a person with chronic renal failure hyperventilating secondary to anxiety Metabolic acidosis and respiratory acidosis: A person with acute pulmonary oedema after an acute myocardial infarction

TABLE 26.21 | Signs and symptoms of acid–base disorders

Respiratory acidosis (carbonic acid excess)	Metabolic acidosis (bicarbonate deficit)
Confusion, impaired judgment, restlessness, dizziness, impaired motor coordination, headache, blurred vision, lethargy Dysrhythmias, warm flushed skin, low blood pressure, increased heart rate	Confusion, dizziness, headache, weakness, fatigue Dysrhythmias, warm flushed skin, low blood pressure, increased heart rate, warm flushed skin Rapid and deep breathing (Kussmaul's respiration) Abdominal cramps, nausea, vomiting, dehydration
Respiratory alkalosis (carbonic acid deficit)	**Metabolic alkalosis (bicarbonate excess)**
Light-headedness, anxiety, confusion, poor concentration Muscle cramps, spasms, numbness and tingling of extremities, tetany, convulsions Nausea, vomiting, epigastric pain Hyperventilation, increased heart rate, arrhythmias	Light-headedness, agitation Muscle weakness, cramping, numbness and tingling of extremities, tetany Anorexia, nausea, vomiting

Implementing nursing care for individuals with acid–base imbalances involves monitoring, prevention and correction of the imbalance. Treatment and care of individuals in these situations is directed towards reversal or correction of the acid–base disorder and may include modification of dietary and fluid intake, administration of medications, IVT and the administration of blood, blood products or TPN (Hall et al 2022). See Clinical Interest Box 26.17. Acid–base imbalances can be caused by several factors and individuals across the lifespan are at risk for acid–base disorders. They can significantly affect people with acute illness and chronic health conditions. (See Clinical Interest Box 26.18.)

CASE STUDY 26.3

Acid–base disturbances

A 75-year-old former underground miner and chain smoker in the past (more than 20 cigarettes per day) is complaining of shortness of breath. Presentation: Physically wasted, pink-faced, heavy breathing, bent over, supporting his chest with his hands on his knee.

Tests: Chest X-ray—hyperinflated lung fields, flattened diaphragm, diagnosing emphysema. Blood gases—pH 7.50, PaO_2 80 mmHg, $PaCO_2$ 29 mmHg, HCO_3^- 18 mmol/L, SaO_2 82%.

1. Consider the presentation and test results. Is there a link with the acid–base imbalance?
2. Interpret the ABG values. Is there compensation?
3. What is the collaborative care?

CLINICAL INTEREST BOX 26.17 Collaborative management in acid–base imbalances

Respiratory acidosis

- Oxygen therapy, if indicated (caution in COPD, CO_2 retention)
- Pharmacological interventions based on the underlying cause (sodium bicarbonate, bronchodilators, antibiotics)
- Chest physio, if indicated

Respiratory alkalosis

- Reassurance, sedation, rebreather mask/paper bag
- Oxygen therapy if indicated
- Pharmacological interventions based on the underlying cause (anti-anxiety medications, potassium supplements)
- Adjustments to mechanical ventilator setting

Metabolic acidosis

- Pharmacological interventions based on the underlying cause (sodium bicarbonate)

Metabolic alkalosis

- Pharmacological interventions based on underlying cause (IV saline solutions, potassium supplements, histamine antagonists, carbonic anhydrase inhibitors)

CLINICAL INTEREST BOX 26.18 Genetic, gender and lifespan considerations in acid–base imbalances

Metabolic imbalances

- Inherited genetic conditions linked to impaired salt reabsorption disorders, inborn metabolism errors.

Metabolic acidosis risks

- Diabetes mellitus and chronic renal failure regardless of age.
- Severe diarrhoea and associated fluid imbalances (children and older adults at greater risk).
- Popular fad diets of starvation (young women at greater risk).

Metabolic alkalosis risks

- Metabolic alkalosis is the most common acid–base disorder in hospitalised individuals
- Delicate fluid and electrolyte status of older people.
- Self-induced vomiting associated with bulimia nervosa (young women at greater risk).
- Chronic hypercapnia respiratory failure treated with mechanical ventilation, steroids or antacids (middle-aged men and women).

Respiratory acidosis

- Injury or illness resulting in alveolar hypoventilation regardless of age.
- Electrolyte and fluid imbalances leading to respiratory depression (older adults at greater risk).
- People with chronic obstructive pulmonary disease (highest risk).

Respiratory alkalosis

- Large doses of salicylate ingestion (older children and adults).
- High incidence of pulmonary disorders, especially pneumonia (older adult).

(Sommers 2023)

Progress Note 26.1

20 February 2024 1530 hours	Nursing: Jean, an 80-year-old female, admitted with diagnosis of UTI, dehydrated and a fever of 38.2°C. Medical history of stroke, atrial fibrillation and myo-congestive failure. Seen by RMO on admission to ward. Prescribed IV fluids (Hartmann's solution 12-hourly rate commenced at 1330 hours) and IV antibiotics Ceftriaxone 1 g stat order. Oral intake as tolerated. Waiting for urine and blood culture sensitivities. For blood tests, FBE and U&E. Nursing care, 4-hourly vital signs observations, BP monitoring, daily weight, fluid balance chart. Referral to dietitian, physio and occupational therapist. *JJ Sanders* (SANDERS), *EN*

DECISION-MAKING FRAMEWORK EXERCISE 26.1

Sophia is an 83-year-old woman with heart failure. She has a medical history of ischaemic heart disease, including a myocardial infarction 3 years ago. Sophia is admitted to your ward with swollen ankles and shortness of breath, suggesting fluid overload. She is on a small dose of furosemide (20 mg), weighs 76 kg and is 155 cm tall. Her urea and electrolyte blood tests come back showing a sodium low of 133 mmol/L and a reduced potassium of 3.1 mmol/L. Blood glucose is elevated (12 mmol/L). Sophia has been ordered IV furosemide and insulin (subcutaneous) by the admitting medical officer.

How should you (as her nurse) respond to this situation in accordance with clinical practice standards and the decision-making framework for nurses?

Summary

This chapter provides an overview of the key physiological concepts associated with fluid, electrolyte and acid–base homeostasis within the body. Water is distributed within both intracellular and extracellular compartments. This fluid provides a transport medium for electrolytes and other substances. Movement of fluids and electrolytes is dynamic and constant and is essential for a healthily functioning body. Osmosis is the mechanism of movement for water; diffusion and active transport are mechanisms facilitating the movement of other substances. The semipermeable membrane is a critical structure in the regulation of intracellular and extracellular fluid composition and in the maintenance of electrolytes within optimal levels in their respective compartments. Damage to the semipermeable membrane through disease processes, such as burns and infections/sepsis, can result in fluid and electrolyte shifts detrimental to healthy function.

It is natural for the body to lose water through both sensible and insensible mechanisms. Key systems for these mechanisms of action are the neural system (hypothalamus and pituitary), the renal system (RAS—aldosterone) and the gastrointestinal tract (GIT). Major cations and anions have been discussed with reference to their significance in maintaining nerve and muscle function. Electrolyte imbalance rarely occurs in isolation; there is usually more than one imbalance involved. Sodium (Na^+) is associated with water imbalance, and it is important for the clinician to establish whether there has been a loss of sodium, for example, or an increase in water volume. Potassium (K^+) is an extremely important electrolyte in the maintenance of an optimally functioning cardiac conduction system. It should be monitored closely and administered with caution since it is associated with potentially lethal complications. Maintenance of blood pH within a closely regulated range is critical to survival. Maintenance is achieved through both renal and respiratory buffering capabilities. However, these buffering mechanisms can be overwhelmed by disease processes.

Individuals undergoing treatment with IV fluids must be monitored appropriately and continuously reassessed. It is vital for the nurse to understand the clinical reason for IV fluid administration so effects of the prescribed treatment can be evaluated accordingly. (See Chapter 20 and Table 20.5.)

Because this knowledge informs and promotes high-quality, safe, evidence-based, person-centred care, developing an understanding of these theoretical underpinnings is critical for nurses. To consolidate learning, further reading and completion of the review and critical thinking exercises is highly recommended.

Review Questions

1. List five common conditions that can affect fluid and electrolyte homeostasis.
2. Briefly describe what constitutes extracellular fluid.
3. How is the active transport method of moving electrolytes and other solutes different from diffusion and osmosis?
4. Explain osmotic and hydrostatic pressures.
5. Differentiate between isotonic, hypotonic and hypertonic.
6. Why is monitoring fluid balance particularly important in infants, children and older people?
7. What is the daily recommended fluid intake and average fluid input and output balance for an adult?
8. What are sensible and insensible fluid losses?
9. What are the symptoms associated with a chronic history of fluid overload?
10. What are the signs and symptoms associated with dehydration?
11. Draw a table. In the first column, name the electrolytes that play an important role in fluid and electrolyte homeostasis. In the second column, write the serum reference intervals for these electrolytes. In the third column, write the terms used to describe the electrolyte imbalance (high and low).
12. Refer to the fluid balance chart provided as a sample in Table 26.13 and, as a practice exercise, complete a fluid balance chart for an 8-hour shift based on the following information:
    - Shift AM. Volume of cup is 100 mL.
    - Individual has had two glasses of water since 0700 hrs (0800, 1300).

- The person has also had a cup of tea at 1030 hrs.
- Urine output 0830 hrs is 200 mL, 1100 hrs is 150 mL, 1330 hrs is 150 mL.

13. Draw a table with three columns. Title the first column 'Fluids' and list the fluids below in that column. Title the second column 'Tonicity of the fluid' and the third 'Indications for use'. Complete the table.
    - 0.9% sodium chloride
    - 5% glucose
    - 4% glucose and 0.18% sodium chloride
    - Hartmann's solution/lactated Ringer's solution
    - 0.45% sodium chloride
    - IV therapy 0.9% sodium chloride 1 L bag running at a 24-hourly rate, commenced at 0700 hrs
14. List common local complications associated with peripheral IV therapy.
15. What is phlebitis and how is it caused?
16. Describe acids and bases.
17. What is the meaning of pH and what is the normal reference interval?
18. What is meant by acid–base balance and how is acid–base imbalance classified?
19. How is acid–base status measured? What is measured?
20. How does the body correct acid–base fluctuations?
21. Explain acidosis and alkalosis.
22. Interpret these ABG levels: pH 7.23, $PaCO_2$ 30 mmHg, HCO_3 19 mmol/L.

Evolve® Answer guide for the Review Questions, Critical Thinking Exercises, Decision-making Framework Exercises and Critical Thinking Questions in Case Studies is hosted on Evolve: http://evolve.elsevier.com/AU/Koutoukidis/Tabbner.

References

Ashraf, M., Rea, R., 2017. Effect of dehydration on blood tests. *Practical Diabetes* 34(5), 169–171. Available at: <https://doi.org/10.1002/pdi.2111>.

Australian Commission for Safety and Quality in Health Care (ACSQHC), 2021. Management of peripheral intravenous catheters clinical care standard. Available at: <https://www.safetyandquality.gov.au/standards/clinical-care-standards/management-peripheral-intravenous-catheters-clinical-care-standard>.

Banasik, J., 2022. *Pathophysiology*, 7th ed. Elsevier, St Louis.

Bellman, S., 2022. Dehydration in older adults: Assessment and diagnosis. Evidence summaries. (JBI20302.) JBI Evidence Based Practice Database. Available at: <http://ovidsp.ovid.com/ovidweb.cgi?T=JS&PAGE=reference&D=jbi&NEWS=N&AN=JBI19998>.

Berman, A., Frandsen, G., Snyder, S., et al., 2020. *Kozier and Erb's fundamentals of nursing*, 5th ed. Pearson, Melbourne.

Brown, D., Edwards, H., Buckley, T., et al., 2020. *Lewis's medical–surgical nursing: Assessment and management of clinical problems*, 5th ed. Elsevier, Sydney.

Children's Health Queensland Hospital and Health Service, 2023. Queensland paediatric emergency care: Skill sheets. CHQ-NSS-51004 Hydration Assessment v2.0 Developed by the State-wide Emergency Care of Children Working Group. Queensland Government. Available at: <https://www.childrens.health.qld.gov.au/wp-content/uploads/PDF/qpec/nursing-skill-sheets/hydration-assessment.pdf>.

Craft, A.J., Gordon, C.J., Huether, S.E., et al., 2023. *Understanding pathophysiology*, 4th ed. Elsevier, Sydney.

Crisp, J., Douglas, C., Rebeiro, G., et al. (eds.), 2021. *Potter & Perry's fundamentals of nursing*, 6th ed. Elsevier, Chatswood.

Davies, H., Leslie, G., Morgan, D., Jacob, E., 2019. Estimation of body fluid status fluid balance and body weight in critically ill adult patients: A systematic review. *Worldviews on Evidence-Based Nursing* 16(6), 470–477.

Dixon, S., Porter, L., 2018. Dehydration: Infant. Quick lesson CINAHL Information System: Division of EBSCO Information Services. Available at: <https://www.ebscohost.com/assets-sample-content/NUTRRC-Infant-Dehydration-Quick-Lesson.pdf>.

Gorski, L., 2023. *Phillip's manual of IV therapeutics: Evidence-based practice for infusion therapy*, 8th ed. F.A. Davis Company, Philadelphia.

Hall, H., Glew, P., Rhodes, J., 2022. *Fundamentals of nursing and midwifery: A person-centred approach to* care, 4th ANZ ed. Lippincott Williams & Wilkins, Sydney.

Herlihy, B., Maebius, N., 2011. *The human body in health and disease*, 4th ed. Saunders, Philadelphia.

JBI, 2022. Fluid balance: Monitoring. Recommended practices. (JBI2003.) Available at: <http://ovidsp.ovid.com/ovidweb.cgi?T=JS&PAGE=reference&D=jbi&NEWS=N&AN=JBI2003>.

Kear, T.M., 2017. Fluid and electrolyte management across the age continuum. *Nephrology Nursing Journal* 44(6), 491–497.

Knight, B.P, Waseem, M., 2023. Pediatric fluid management. In: StatPearls [Internet]. Treasure Island (FL): StatPearls Publishing. Available at: <https://www.ncbi.nlm.nih.gov/books/NBK560540>.

LeMone, P., Bauldoff, G., Gubrud-Howe, P., et al., 2020. *Medical–surgical nursing: Critical thinking in person-centred care,* 4th ed. Pearson, Melbourne.

Liaw, Y.Q., Goh, M.L., 2018. Improving the accuracy of fluid intake charting through patient involvement in an adult surgical ward: A best practice implementation project. Systematic Reviews and Implementation Reports. *JBI Database of Systematic Reviews and Implementation Reports* 16(8), 1709–1719. doi: 10.11124/JBISRIR-2017-003683.

Litchfield, I., Magill, L., Flint, G., 2018. A qualitative study exploring staff attitudes to maintaining hydration in neurosurgery patients. *Nursing Open* 5(3), 422–430. Available at: <https://doi.org/10.1002/nop2.154>.

Nursing and Midwifery Board of Australia (NMBA), 2020. Decision-making framework for nursing and midwifery. Available at: <https://www.nursingmidwiferyboard.gov.au/Codes-Guidelines-Statements/Frameworks.aspx>.

Nursing and Midwifery Board of Australia (NMBA), 2022. Fact sheet: Enrolled nurses and medicine administration. Available at: <https://www.nursingmidwiferyboard.gov.au/Codes-Guidelines-Statements/FAQ/Enrolled-nurses-and-medicine-administration.aspx>.

Patton, K.T., Williamson, P., Thompson, T., et al., 2024. *The human body in health & disease,* 8th ed. Elsevier.

Porritt, K., 2021. Peripheral intravenous cannula (PIVC): General care and catheter lumen patency. Evidence summaries. (JBI20302.) JBI Evidence Based Practice Database. Available at: <http://ovidsp.ovid.com/ovidweb.cgi?T=JS&PAGE=reference&D=jbi&NEWS=N&AN=JBI20302>.

Potter, P.A., Perry, A.G., 2021. *Fundamentals of nursing*, 10th ed. St. Louis, Mosby.

Schub, T., Oji, O., 2018. Hydration: Maintaining oral hydration in older adults. CINAHL Nursing Guide. Evidence-Based Care Sheet, T700987.

Shrimanker, I., Bhattarai, S., 2023. Electrolytes. In: StatPearls [Internet]. Treasure Island (FL): StatPearls Publishing. Available at: <https://www.ncbi.nlm.nih.gov/books/NBK541123>.

Simpson, D., McIntosh, R., 2021. Measuring and monitoring fluid balance. *British Journal of Nursing* 20(12), 706–710.

Sivapuram, M., 2022. Fluid balance charts: Documentation. Evidence summaries. (JBI183.) JBI. Available at: <http://ovidsp.ovid.com/ovidweb.cgi?T=JS&PAGE=reference&D=jbi&NEWS=N&AN=JBI183>.

Sommers, M.S., 2023. *Davis's diseases and disorders: A nursing therapeutics manual*, 7th ed. F.A. Davis Company, Philadelphia.

South Eastern Sydney Local Health District (SESLHD), 2022. Peripheral intravenous cannulation (PIVC) insertion, care and removal (adults). NSW Ministry of Health. Available at: <https://www.seslhd.health.nsw.gov.au/sites/default/files/documents/SESLHDPR%20577%20-%20Peripheral%20Intravenous%20Cannulation%20%28PIVC%29%20Insertion%2C%20Care%20and%20Removal%20%28Adults%29.pdf>.

Swe, K.K., 2022. Phlebitis: Risk assessment. Evidence summaries. (JBI15427.) JBI Evidence Based Practice Database. Available at: <http://ovidsp.ovid.com/ovidweb.cgi?T=JS&PAGE=reference&D=jbi&NEWS=N&AN=JBI5427>.

Sydney Children's Hospital Network (SCHN), 2017. Intravenous fluid and electrolyte therapy—SCH practice guideline. Available at: <https://www.schn.health.nsw.gov.au/_policies/pdf/2013-7033.pdf>.

Waugh, A., Grant, A., 2023. *Ross & Wilson anatomy and physiology in health and illness*, 14th ed. Elsevier.

Western Australia (WA) Country Health Service, 2022. Peripheral intravenous catheter (PIVC) Guideline. Government of Western Australia, WA Country Health Service. Available at: <https://www.wacountry.health.wa.gov.au/,/media/WACHS/Documents/About-us/Policies/Peripheral-Intravenous-Cannula-PIVC-Guideline.pdf?thn=0s Cannula (PIVC) Guideline (health.wa.gov.au)>.

Williams, L.S., Hopper, P.D., 2019. *Understanding medical surgical nursing*, 6th ed. F.A. Davis Company, Philadelphia.

Recommended Reading

Campbell, N., 2014. Recognising and preventing dehydration among patients. *Nursing Times* 110(46), 20–21.

Coulter, K., 2016. Successful infusion therapy in older adults. *Journal of Infusion Nursing* 39(6), 352–358.

Georgiades, D., 2016. A balancing act: Maintaining accurate fluid balance charting. *Australian Nursing and Midwifery Journal* 24(6), 28–31.

Kaufman, G., 2014. Diuretics: How they work, cautions and contraindications. *Nursing and Residential Care* 16(2), 83–86.

Larkin, B.G., Zimmanck, R.J., 2015. Interpreting arterial blood gases successfully. *Association of Perioperative Registered Nurses (AORN) Journal* 2, 342–357. Available at: <http://dx.doi.org/10.1016/j.aorn.2015.08.002>.

Masco, N., 2016. Acid-base homeostasis: Overview for infusion nurses. *Journal of Infusion Nursing* 39(5), 288–295.

McGloin, S., 2015. The ins and outs of fluid balance in the acutely ill patient. *British Journal of Nursing* 24(1), 14–18.

McLafferty, E., Johnstone, C., Hendry, C., et al., 2014. Fluid and electrolyte balance. *Nursing Standard* 28(29), 42–47.

Pinnington, S., Ingleby, S., Hanumapura, P., et al., 2016. Assessing and documenting fluid balance. *Nursing Standard* 31(15), 46–54.

Shells, R., Morrell-Scott, N., 2018. Prevention of dehydration in hospital patients. *British Journal of Nursing* 27(10), 565–569.

State of Victoria, 2022. Dehydration: Standardised care process. Department of Health and Human Services, Melbourne. Available at: <https://www2.health.vic.gov.au/ageing-and-aged-care/residential-aged-care/safety-and-quality/improving-resident-care/standardised-care-processes>.

Walker, M., 2016. Fluid and electrolyte imbalances: Interpretation and assessment. *Journal of Infusion Nursing* 39(6), 382–386.

Online Resources

Acid–base terminology: <www.acid-base.com/terminology.php>.

Australian Commission on Safety and Quality in Health Care (ACSQHC), 2021. NSQHS Standards. Recognising and responding to acute deterioration standard: Standard 8: <https://www.safetyandquality.gov.au/standards/nsqhs-standards>.

Australian Commission on Safety and Quality in Health Care (ACSQHC), nd. High risk medicines resources: <https://www.safetyandquality.gov.au/our-work/medication-safety/high-risk-medicines/high-risk-medicines-resources>.

Australian Commission on Safety and Quality in Health Care (ACSQHC), nd. APINCHS classification of high risk medicines: <https://www.safetyandquality.gov.au/our-work/medication-safety/high-risk-medicines/apinchs-classification-high-risk-medicines>.

Infusion Nurses Society: <https://www.ins1.org/default.aspx>.

IVTEAM VIP Score: <https://www.ivteam.com/vip-score>.

National Health and Medical Research Council (NHMRC). Nutrient reference values for Australia and New Zealand: <https://www.nrv.gov.au/nutrients>.

Pathology Tests Explained (PTEx): <https://pathologytestsexplained.org.au>.

The Royal Children's Hospital Melbourne, Australia. Clinical practice guidelines: Intravenous fluids: <https://www.rch.org.au/clinicalguide/guideline_index/Intravenous_Fluids>.

Victorian Department of Health. Older people in hospital: <https://www2.health.vic.gov.au/hospitals-and-health-services/patient-care/older-people>.

The Royal College of Pathologists of Australia, nd. RCPA Manual—Online. ISSN 1449-8219: <https://www.rcpa.edu.au/Manuals/RCPA-Manual>.

CHAPTER 27

Rest and sleep

Nicole Dillon

Key Terms

central sleep apnoea (CSA)
circadian rhythm
insomnia
narcolepsy
non-rapid eye movement (NREM)
obstructive sleep apnoea (OSA)
parasomnias
polysomnography (PSG)
rapid eye movement (REM)
rest
restorative sleep
reticular activating system (RAS)
shift work sleep disorder (SWSD)
sleep
sleep apnoea
sleep cycle
sleep disorder
sleep disturbance
sleep hygiene
sleep–wake cycle
snoring

Learning Outcomes

At the completion of this chapter and with further reading, learners should be able to:

- Define the key terms.
- Describe the importance of rest and sleep to the wellbeing of the individual.
- Explain the functions of sleep.
- Outline and describe the phases of the sleep cycle.
- State factors that may interfere with rest and sleep.
- Describe the supportive nursing measures that may be implemented to promote the individual's need for rest and sleep.
- Demonstrate an awareness of the need to identify a range of sleep disorders and the impact of these disorders on health wellbeing.

CHAPTER FOCUS

Rest and sleep are important factors to enable individuals to achieve and maintain a state of wellbeing. Rest is a state of feeling mentally and physically relaxed, calm and free from worry (Gordon 2021). Sleep is a basic physiological need and relates to a decreased level of consciousness that occurs on a cyclical basis. The state of sleeping enables a period of rest, which is essential for restoration of physiological and psychological processes of the body (Gordon 2021). The amount of sleep an individual requires depends on age, lifestyle, personality, environment and state of health. The need for a required amount of sleep generally becomes less as a person ages.

'Sleep affects all areas of our life; it is a fundamental building block of achieving and maintaining good health along with good nutrition and adequate exercise. Yet it is often overlooked and ignored.'

Commonwealth of Australia 2019

An important nursing responsibility is implementing measures that will promote physical and emotional comfort, thereby assisting the individual to experience sufficient rest and sleep. Factors affecting rest and sleep can result from a variety of physical, environmental or psychosocial reasons (Kulpatcharapong et al 2020). Kulpatcharapong et al (2020) suggest hospitalisation often adversely affects a person's sleep quality, particularly in the first days of admission. Without adequate rest and sleep, the ability to perform the normal activities of daily living may be affected (Gordon 2021). Most people report 'difficulty with sleeping' at some stage in their lives, and for most this is usually a temporary problem. Nurses need to assess the individual's sleep problems and use critical thinking skills to implement measures to promote effective sleep (Gordon 2021).

This chapter explores the promotion of optimal rest and sleep and strategies the nurse can provide to enhance the individual's physical and psychological comfort and wellbeing. The ability to achieve adequate rest and sleep is closely associated with comfort; therefore, the nurse should be aware of the measures necessary to ensure that comfort needs are met. Rest and relaxation can occur only when there is freedom from physical discomfort and emotional tension, and individuals are more likely to sleep well if normal sleep hygiene habits are maintained.

LIVED EXPERIENCE

Maria was admitted to hospital following a rupture of her medial collateral ligament (MCL), playing touch football. She was in a great deal of pain, with a pain score of 7–8/10. Despite pain relief, she could not settle, and was looking forward to lights out, when things would quieten down. Unfortunately, it was a busy night on the ward, with many postoperative patients. Lights went on and off, IV pump alarms were going off, buzzers were going all night. Maria describes her night in hospital as exhausting. The pain, anxiety about her upcoming operation, clinical observations and the noise of the ward kept her awake most of the night. She was almost relieved to go to theatre to get some peace and quiet.

Marie, 42 years old

INTRODUCTION

Rest is a state where the individual assumes a comfortable position and is relaxed for a period of time, allowing the individual to feel refreshed and rejuvenated, ready to continue with daily activities (Gordon 2021). Individuals at rest are considered free from any physical or mental exertion (Cooper & Gosnell 2022). Lamp et al (2019) suggest waking rest 'is a period of quiet, reflective thought that allows the brain time to consider and process whatever arises spontaneously' and encourage waking-rest to promote beneficial effects on mental health and overall physical wellbeing. Individuals who are confined to bed for physical reasons may not always feel rested since psychological issues may impact on the ability to completely rest (Gordon 2021). Individuals have different methods of achieving adequate rest and this may be disrupted when admitted to a healthcare facility (Cooper & Gosnell 2022).

PHYSIOLOGY OF SLEEP

Sleep can be defined as a period of reduced conscious awareness of the environmental surroundings from which individuals can be easily woken (Harding et al 2023). Certain stimuli (e.g. a sudden loud noise) will usually rouse the individual, although not necessarily to full alertness. Kulpatcharapong et al (2020) suggest light, sound and nurse disturbance were identified as the most frequent issues affecting a patient's sleep pattern when hospitalised. The **sleep–wake cycle** is a process that promotes sleep and maintains wakefulness (Cooper & Gosnell 2022).

Sleep regulation

The control and regulation of the sleep–wake cycle depends on the interrelationship between structures in the brainstem, hypothalamus and thalamus (Harding et al 2023). The sleep–wake cycle is controlled by the brain's higher centres, where one mechanism causes wakefulness, while the other causes sleep (Gordon 2021). The **reticular activating system (RAS)** is located in the upper brainstem and is believed to contain special cells that maintain alertness and wakefulness (Gordon 2021). The RAS is activated when it receives visual, auditory, pain and tactile sensory stimuli, as well as thoughts and emotions. When a person tries to sleep in a darkened room they become relaxed, and stimuli to the RAS is decreased (Gordon 2021). In addition, the hypothalamus releases neurotransmitters and peptides, which promote sleep by inhibiting the RAS (Harding et al 2023). The pineal gland also plays a part in the sleep–wake cycle by releasing melatonin as the environment gets darker, inducing sleep. With light exposure, from natural or artificial light, melatonin release is suppressed and the individual awakens (Harding et al 2023).

Circadian rhythm

The concept of circadian rhythm (derived from the Latin: *circa*—about and *dies*—day) refers to the cyclical measures that are part of our everyday life (Gordon 2021). **Circadian rhythms** are physical, mental and behavioural changes that follow roughly a 24-hour cycle, responding primarily to light in the environment (Harding et al 2023). Circadian rhythms are produced by natural factors within the body, but they are also affected by environmental signals such as television, mobile phone or computer usage (Serin & Acar 2019). The circadian rhythm influences many biological processes in the body including hormone secretion, metabolism, cardiovascular health, regulation of body temperature, glucose homeostasis, and mood and sensory awareness (Gordon 2021; Serin & Acar 2019). It appears that the 24-hour cycle to which the human body synchronises is highly individualised, allowing variations, with some people distinctly described as 'morning people', while others fit well into the 'night-owl' category. Any disruption to a person's circadian rhythm can cause discomfort and manifest in a disturbed sleep pattern (Gordon 2021). Short-term disruptions to a person's circadian rhythm can lead to impaired wellness, fatigue and lack of concentration (Serin & Acar 2019). Long-term disruptions, however, have more serious consequences, such as premature death, and increase the risk of obesity, impaired glucose tolerance, diabetes, mental health disorders and cancer (Serin & Acar 2019).

An example of the consequences of a disrupted circadian rhythm is the state known as 'jet lag'. This condition occurs when a person's circadian rhythm is disrupted by travel across several time zones in a relatively short timeframe. It is characterised by fatigue, insomnia and sluggish physical and mental function. Individuals who are ill in hospital may also experience sleep disruptions where quantity and quality of sleep are affected (Lopez et al 2018). A person who engages in shift work may experience symptoms similar to jet lag since the body attempts to adapt to changes in the 24-hour biological clock. Working on night shift removes sleeping from the normal night-time routine and renders it out of order with the body's normal circadian rhythm (Cooper & Gosnell 2022).

Stages of sleep

Sleep is a complex process that includes **non-rapid eye movement (NREM)** or quiet sleep, and **rapid eye movement (REM)** or active sleep (Gordon 2021). It is generally recognised that each **sleep cycle** consists of five stages. NREM sleep consists of the first four stages where light sleep occurs in stages 1 and 2 and progresses through to a deeper sleep in stages 3 and 4 (Cooper & Gosnell 2022). The reverse then occurs, where the person will progress from stage 4 back to stage 2, ending with the fifth stage of sleep, REM (see Figure 27.1). This process takes about 90 minutes and continues with the person going through 4–6 of these cycles of sleep per night, with the REM stage increasing in length and the NREM stages shortening with each cycle (Gordon 2021). If the person wakes fully on occasions during sleep, the sleep cycle needs to restart at stage 1; if this occurs, the total time spent in deep sleep may be lessened. Infants spend a greater proportion of time in REM sleep than adults, with about 40% of total sleep time being REM sleep. With adults, about 20% of total sleep time is REM sleep. See Clinical Interest Box 27.1 for details of the five stages of sleep and Clinical Interest Box 27.2 for physiological changes during NREM and REM sleep.

Dreams

Dreams occur during both the NREM and the REM sleep stages. Dreams are more vivid and elaborate in the REM sleep period, which is also believed to contribute to the consolidation of long-term memory (Gordon 2021). Through each REM period, dreams may progress in content, including current events to emotional dreams from childhood, or events and experiences that have occurred in the past. Dreams often relate to experiences that may have occurred over the day, or incidents that have caused stress, such as relationships and work (Gordon 2021). Many dreams are forgotten and not recalled; therefore, people do

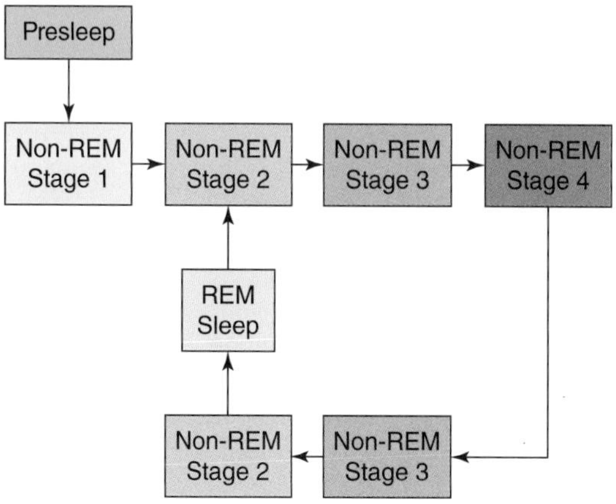

Figure 27.1 Adult sleep cycle

(Webb & Scott 2023)

CLINICAL INTEREST BOX 27.1 Sleep cycle stages

Stage 1: NREM

Stage 1 sleep is light sleep. It can be considered a transition from awake to sleeping, an experience of drifting in and out of sleep. It lasts only a few minutes (1–7 minutes). Aspects of this stage include:
- Easily woken.
- Eye movement and body movements slow down.
- May experience sudden jerky movement of legs or other muscles.
- Easily awoken and, if awoken, may not feel like having been asleep.

Stage 2: NREM

Stage 2 lasts for approximately 10–25 minutes. Relaxation progresses. Aspects of this stage include:
- More difficult to rouse.
- Body temperature starts to decrease.
- Heart rate begins to slow.

Stage 3: NREM

Stage 3 is the first stage or transitional phase to deep sleep. Muscles are completely relaxed. It lasts a few minutes. Aspects of this stage include:
- Very difficult to wake.
- If woken during this stage, may feel groggy and disoriented for several minutes.
- Vital signs decrease but remain regular.

Stage 4: NREM

Stage 4 sleep is the second stage of deep sleep. It lasts 20–40 minutes. Aspects of this stage include:
- Very difficult to wake up.
- Both stages of deep sleep are important for feeling refreshed in the morning.
- If these stages are too short, sleep will not feel satisfying.
- Sleepwalking and enuresis may occur.

Stage 5: REM sleep

Lasts 5–30 minutes, begins about 90 minutes after falling asleep. Aspects of this stage include:
- The sleep stage in which dreaming occurs, but will usually not be remembered unless person briefly rouses
- Breathing becomes fast, irregular and shallow.
- Brain becomes highly active.
- Difficult to rouse.
- Distinctive eye movement occurs; voluntary loss of muscle tone and reflexes; men may develop an erection.
- The REM period of first sleep cycle is usually shorter than subsequent REM periods.
- REM sleep is not fully understood. What is known is that REM sleep is important in the creation of long-term memory.

The full sleep cycle usually lasts 90–110 minutes.

(Adapted from Berman et al 2020; Cooper & Gosnell 2022; Gordon 2021)

CLINICAL INTEREST BOX 27.2 Physiological changes during NREM sleep

- Arterial blood pressure falls.
- Pulse rate decreases.
- Peripheral blood vessels dilate.
- Cardiac output decreases.
- Skeletal muscles relax.
- Basal metabolic rate decreases.
- Growth hormone levels peak.
- Intracranial pressure decreases.

(Adapted from Cooper & Gosnell 2022; Gordon 2021)

not believe they have dreamt at all. Remembering a dream requires a person to consciously think about their dream upon waking. Recall of vivid dreams usually occurs if the person has woken just after a period of REM sleep (Gordon 2021).

Quality of sleep

The quality of sleep is a subjective experience where the amount of restfulness, depth of sleep, number of times woken and amount of sleep impact on the individual's perception of quality of sleep. The quality of sleep is equally as important as the quantity of sleep achieved. The amount of sleep a person reports that they need to feel refreshed is both subjective and individualised (Rogers 2023). It is also reported that quality of sleep decreases with age, although many middle-aged individuals will report a change in sleep quality, and sleep disorders may be diagnosed during this period of the lifespan (Gordon 2021). The length of lighter stages of sleep (especially stage 1) is often increased in older people and stages 3 and 4 often decrease. This may explain why many older adults often report the quality of their sleep as poor and feeling less rested even after being observed to have slept soundly.

Sleep patterns across the lifespan

There are many variations in the optimal amount of sleep each individual requires. The range of 7–9 hours per night is the average required for an adult, meaning that about one-third of the day and, consequently, one-third of an individual's life is spent sleeping (Gordon 2021). Sleep patterns change throughout the lifespan and as a person ages, the amount of time spent sleeping at night is usually less than earlier in life. The quantity of sleep diminishes from about 20 hours a day in infancy to about 8–12 hours a day in adolescence, to perhaps as little as 6–8 hours of sleep at night in adulthood. In older adulthood, the amount of sleep achieved at night will often decrease; however, older adults often report 'napping' during the day. Daytime napping may occur due to poor night-time sleep, early wakening and/or changes in the central nervous system's (CNS) regulation of sleep and circadian rhythm. In addition, many older adults will wake more often during the night and report an inability to return to sleep after rousing (Gordon 2021). Clinical Interest Box 27.3 outlines the sleep requirements across the lifespan.

There are several theories about the purpose of sleep, with the most frequently accepted concept being that sleep contributes to physiological and psychological restoration, influencing and regulating body functions and behavioural responses (Rogers 2023). It appears that the level of circulating hormones, such as human growth hormone and those secreted by the adrenal glands, vary during sleep. The levels of these hormones circulating during sleep is thought to facilitate cell growth and repair (Berman et al 2020). Sleep is also a time that allows for conservation of energy, prevention of fatigue and provision of organ respite, with the relaxation of skeletal muscles and the lowering of basal metabolic rate (Rogers 2023). Alternatively, cerebral function during periods of sleep is increased, with important cognitive restoration and the filtering and storage of the day's activities (Gordon 2021). It is therefore of particular importance that the person who is ill or hospitalised can benefit from the rest and healing nature of sleep (Lopez et al 2018). **Restorative sleep** allows a person to wake feeling refreshed. Restorative theory of sleep suggests sleep provides time for the body to replenish itself (Brinkman, Reddy & Sharma 2023). Non-restorative sleep (NRS) is where sleep is disturbed, is of poor quality or the person wakes feeling unrefreshed. NRS can lead to psychological disorders including depression and is linked to metabolic syndrome which includes obesity, type 2 diabetes mellitus, cardiovascular disorders and hypercholesterolemia (Otsuka et al 2023).

CLINICAL INTEREST BOX 27.3 Sleep requirements across the lifespan

- Newborns: 16–18 hours/day
- Infants: 14–15 hours/day
- Toddlers: 12–14 hours/day
- Preschoolers: 11–13 hours/day
- School-age children: 10–11 hours/day
- Adolescents: 9–10 hours/day
- Adults: 7–9 hours/day
- Older adults: 7–9 hours (with more difficulty)

(Adapted from Berman et al 2020)

Sleep disturbances

Any interruptions to sleep may have an impact on a person's ability to carry out their usual daily activities. **Sleep disturbance** is a generalised term which provides a broad definition for poor sleep quality from any number of factors (Harding et al 2023). A person who experiences a sleep disturbance may exhibit changes in behaviour response and performance, and may show signs of irritability, lack of energy and fatigue (Harding et al 2023). According to a 2018–2019 Australian parliamentary study into Australian sleep health awareness, the Royal Australasian College of Physicians (RACP) stated that approximately 33–45% of Australian adults experience inadequate sleep (Commonwealth of Australia 2019). Sleep-pattern disturbances include difficulty in falling asleep, periods of wakefulness during the night, waking earlier than usual and not feeling rested after sleep (see Clinical Interest Box 27.4

CLINICAL INTEREST BOX 27.4 Conditions for proper rest

- Physical comfort.
- Eliminate sources of physical irritation and pain.
- Control room temperature and provide adequate ventilation.
- Maintain proper alignment and anatomical position.
- Remove environmental distractions.
- Freedom from worry.
- Have knowledge of health problems and their implications.
- Make own decisions.
- Participate in personal healthcare.
- Practise restful and relaxing activities frequently.
- Know that environment is safe.
- Sufficient sleep.
- Know and obtain the hours of sleep that are needed to feel refreshed.
- Follow good sleep hygiene habits.

(Cooper & Gosnell 2022; Gordon 2021)

CLINICAL INTEREST BOX 27.5 Cultural aspects of sleep

- Practices and patterns of sleep and rest differ between cultures.
- Many cultures favour daytime rest and shorter night-time sleep periods.
- Western cultures reinforce autonomy in children sleeping independently, whereas Asian and African cultures favour infants and children co-sleeping for much of their childhood. Even within these cultures, differences now being seen may be due to industrialisation.
- Co-sleeping in which infants sleep with their parents may result in alterations to both parents' and child's sleeping patterns.
- Research continues on the value of touch in inducing rest and sleep, especially in neonatal intensive care situations, and parental bonding and attachment.

(Adapted from Gordon 2021)

for conditions of proper rest and Clinical Interest Box 27.5 for cultural aspects of sleeping).

Some people experience nightmares or sleepwalking. A nightmare is a dream that arouses feelings of intense fear or extreme anxiety and usually wakes the sleeper. Sleepwalking is a state that culminates in the individual walking about but they will have no recollection of the episode. Other disorders that affect sleeping patterns include insomnia, snoring, sleep apnoea, narcolepsy and parasomnias. A person who develops a sleep disorder may require referral to a sleep disorder centre for investigation (Webb & Scott 2023; Robertson 2023).

SLEEP DISORDERS

Individuals may at some stage in their lives experience a **sleep disorder** that results in inadequate sleep. Common sleep disorders include obstructive sleep apnoea (OSA), insomnia, excessive daytime sleepiness (EDS) and restless leg syndrome (Hillman et al 2018). A report written by Deloitte Access Economics and released by the Sleep Health Foundation in 2021 estimates that poor sleep costs Australia $14.4 billion each year in financial costs, with a further $36.6 billion in non-financial costs related to loss of wellbeing. The report calculates productivity losses at $11 billion in 2019–2020. These costs were distributed across three major sleep disorders—obstructive sleep apnoea, insomnia and restless leg syndrome (Sleep Health Foundation & Deloitte Access Economics 2021). Sleep disorders decrease quality of life, causing increased morbidity and mortality (Harding et al 2023), and contribute to workplace incidents and motor vehicle accidents (Hillman et al 2018).

If a sleep disturbance persists, despite the implementation of sound sleep hygiene measures and lifestyle changes, medical advice may be sought. A referral can be made to a sleep physician so that **polysomnography (PSG)** sleep studies can be conducted at a sleep clinic or in the individual's home. Night-time PSG involves attaching monitoring leads to multiple areas of the body. While the person sleeps, data regarding the stages of sleep are recorded, as well as night-time wakefulness, to detect any sleep abnormalities (Gordon 2021). This process usually involves an overnight admission in a sleep disorder unit or an in-home PSG, where sleeping patterns are monitored. Prior to the PSG test occurring, a specialised nurse or technician obtains a thorough sleep history from the individual, which includes information of both past and current sleep problems. Specific information collected in relation to sleep includes the time of settling and waking, the number of times sleep is disturbed, physical illnesses, medications, diet, any aids or techniques that the person is currently using to achieve sleep and an environmental assessment (Douglas et al 2017).

Sleep deprivation

Many individuals experience disturbed sleep and sleep deprivation as a result of hospitalisation (Delaney et al 2018). This results in decreased amount, quality and consistency of sleep due to sleep being interrupted or fragmented. This causes changes in the normal sequence of sleep stages, and the normal cycles cannot be completed (Gordon 2021). Gradually, cumulative sleep deprivation occurs (see Clinical Interest Box 27.6). Chronic sleep deprivation is linked to several common health problems, many related to metabolic syndrome, such as cardiovascular disease, weight gain, type 2 diabetes, poor memory, depression, digestive problems and even links to cancer (Harding et al 2023).

CLINICAL INTEREST BOX 27.6 Signs and symptoms of sleep deprivation

Physiological symptoms

- Ptosis, blurred vision
- Fine motor clumsiness
- Decreased reflexes
- Slowed response time
- Decreased reasoning and judgment
- Decreased auditory and visual alertness
- Cardiac arrhythmias

Psychological symptoms

- Stress and anxiety
- Confusion and disorientation
- Increased sensitivity to pain
- Irritable, withdrawn, apathetic
- Agitation
- Hyperactivity
- Decreased motivation
- Excessive sleepiness

(Gordon 2021)

The severity of symptoms is often related to the duration of sleep deprivation. The most effective treatment for sleep deprivation in any environment is eliminating or correcting the factors that lead to disruption of sleep (Gordon 2021).

Insomnia

Insomnia is the most common sleep disorder experienced and is characterised by difficulty falling asleep or staying asleep, occurring more than three times a week (Harding et al 2023). The individual may complain of trouble falling asleep or staying asleep, early awakening and feeling unrefreshed upon awakening (Harding et al 2023). This results in insufficient quantity and quality of sleep, which may lead to excessive daytime sleepiness (EDS). Acute insomnia is the most common of the insomnias and is often in relation to one or several factors that are associated with sleep disorders (illness, stress or change in sleeping environment) (Gordon 2021). This type of insomnia will usually subside once the acute event or causative factor has passed or been eliminated. In the short term, having less sleep than normal usually causes no harmful effects. Often lifestyle and environmental conditions can be easily modified, such as by reducing alcohol and caffeine intake before bed, not napping through the day and use of stress-modifying techniques. Teaching individuals about the factors influencing sleep and sleep routine (sleep hygiene) may help in improving sleep quality in the individual suffering insomnia.

Chronic insomnia consists of the same symptoms as acute insomnia; however, it lasts for more than a month or longer (Harding et al 2023). It may be the result of an underlying medical, behavioural or psychiatric problem. Depression can often cause insomnia. Chronic insomnia usually requires investigation as to its cause, and treatment usually requires more than simple lifestyle and environmental assessment and modifications (Gordon 2021). The fear of not being able to sleep can be enough to cause wakefulness, thus potentiating the underlying feelings of sleep deprivation, and daytime sleepiness, fatigue, depression and anxiety (Rogers 2023).

Snoring

Snoring is defined as breathing during sleep accompanied by harsh sounds and is caused by any obstruction of the air passages at the back of the mouth and nose. Poor muscle tone, excessive tissue or deformities such as a deviated septum may cause snoring. Obstructed airways due to colds or allergies can also cause snoring. Snoring can also be a symptom of sleep apnoea. The mild snorer should exercise to develop good muscle tone and lose weight if needed (Williams 2023).

Sleep apnoea

Sleep apnoea is a disorder characterised by the lack of airflow through the nose and mouth for periods of 10 seconds or more. There are three types of sleep apnoea: obstructive sleep apnoea (OSA), central sleep apnoea (CSA) and mixed sleep apnoea, with OSA being the most common (Gordon 2021).

Obstructive sleep apnoea

Obstructive sleep apnoea (OSA) occurs when the upper airway closes repetitively during sleep, causing a partial or full obstruction. OSA may occur numerous times during the sleep cycle and obstruction may last up to 1 minute in duration (Australian Institute of Health and Welfare [AIHW] 2021). According to the Australasian Sleep Association (2022), OSA is the most common form of respiratory disorder during sleep. Structures in the upper airway collapse during sleep, which may involve the tongue and soft palate falling backwards, causing air entry to cease from anywhere between 15 and 90 seconds (Harding et al 2023). The individual may be seen to be attempting to breathe with the rise and fall of the chest or abdominal wall, but since the airway is obstructed there is no air entry (Rogers 2023). The decrease in oxygen to the brain causes the person to rouse slightly, often snorting and gasping, causing the soft palate and tongue to move forwards, allowing the airway to open (Harding et al 2023). Often the person will not become consciously aware that they are rousing and will continue to sleep, with further apnoeic cycles occurring. The individual fails to maintain the deep sleep period required for a restful sleep (Gordon 2021). Nurses monitoring hospitalised individuals during sleep may observe apnoeic episodes and will need to document the findings and report to the medical officer for further assessment. (See Progress Note 27.1.)

In 2019, an average of 133,000 people attended a sleep study service. Between 2018–2019 the AIHW identified nearly 40,000 admissions to hospital with a principal diagnosis of OSA. Males constituted the most prevalent presentation, with approximately 8.3 per 1000 population, compared to 5.2 per 1000 for women (AIHW 2021).

Given that the major modifiable risk factor for OSA is obesity, the prevalence of OSA is increasing (Rogers 2023). OSA is a serious and potentially life-threatening condition. The body's organ systems may begin to function abnormally and possibly contribute to other disorders such as hypertension, heart attack and stroke (Gordon 2021; AIHW 2021). It also commonly leads to excessive daytime sleepiness, which is the most common presenting complaint of individuals suffering sleep apnoea, leading to poor concentration, potentially causing many workplace and road accidents (Rogers 2023).

Treatment options typically begin with lifestyle changes, if these are indicated, such as weight loss and a decrease in alcohol intake (Gordon 2021). The Australasian Sleep Association (2022) recommends following guidelines developed by the National Centre for Sleep Health Services Research using evidence-based information for the ongoing care of a person with OSA. The guidelines provide steps in the assessment and management of OSA for general practitioners and supporting healthcare workers. Based on the individual's history and presentation, a referral may need to be made to an ear, nose and throat (ENT) surgeon to assess whether airway obstruction could be caused by mechanical factors. A dental splint may be utilised in mild cases of OSA to hold the jaw in a forced-forward position, keeping the airway open. Non-invasive ventilation (NIV) delivers mechanical ventilatory support to the individual who is breathing spontaneously and is able to protect their airway. A well-fitting mask over the face or nose is used to provide either continuous positive airway pressure (CPAP) or bilevel support (BiPAP), which assists both the inspiratory and expiratory phases of breathing. CPAP provides the same amount of positive pressure via a mask throughout the respiratory cycle (i.e. on inhalation and exhalation). While CPAP delivers one pressure, BiPAP delivers two pressures. These two pressures are known as inhalation positive airway pressure (IPAP) and exhalation positive airway pressure (EPAP). A higher pressure is delivered on inspiration. BiPAP is often used with individuals who need extra respiratory support.

Moderate to severe sleep apnoea usually requires the long-term use of an NIV device while sleeping (Harding et al 2023). Individuals require education and support to adapt to the use of an NIV device because non-compliance is considered to be high; however, in the long term, OSA can be managed, and effective restorative sleep achieved (Harding et al 2023). (See Clinical Interest Box 27.7.)

Central sleep apnoea

Central sleep apnoea (CSA) is similar to OSA, where breathing periodically ceases. However, there is no obstruction in the upper airways. CSA occurs because signals fail to reach the respiratory muscles, and therefore there is no respiratory effort. When breathing slows during sleep, the respiratory control centres in the brain do not respond fast enough to the changes in oxygen and carbon dioxide levels in the blood (Sleep Disorders Australia 2022a). When the signal eventually does come through, breathing is quietly resumed, without the snorts and jerks associated with obstructive apnoea. This condition is commonly seen in people with congestive heart failure. Other disorders, like stroke or a weakened diaphragm, can also contribute to CSA (Sleep Disorders Australia 2022a). CSA is managed with CPAP therapy, at low pressure, providing a positive impact on the quality of sleep achieved. Individuals requiring high levels of CPAP pressure are often more comfortable using BiPAP.

CLINICAL INTEREST BOX 27.7 CPAP

Continuous positive airway pressure (CPAP) is a device used for obstructive sleep apnoea, consisting of a mask that is worn at night, either only over the nose or over both the nose and mouth. The pressure generated by the CPAP machine is tailored to each individual's needs. CPAP causes a continuous backward pressure in the airway, keeping it open and allowing effective airflow and oxygen into the lungs. The therapeutic effects of CPAP therapy may be noticed immediately since improved oxygenation overnight assists in decreasing the daytime symptoms such as tiredness (Sleep Disorders Australia 2022b). Some CPAP devices have humidification and heat settings. The humidification chamber needs to be refilled with water each night.

Care of the device requires that the mask is cleaned daily and condensation is emptied from the wide-bore tubing because this is an ideal environment for bacteria to grow.

Narcolepsy

Narcolepsy is a chronic sleep disorder characterised by an abnormality in the sleep–wake area of the brain resulting in persistent EDS (Harding et al 2023). An overwhelming urge to sleep overcomes the individual during hours of wakefulness and brief periods of sleep occur, lasting from seconds to several minutes (Harding et al 2023). Individuals with narcolepsy may experience symptoms of EDS, loss of muscle tone, hallucinations and disrupted sleep at night and may be unaware of their actions (Mattice 2019). The individual will often fall straight into the REM period of sleep (Harding et al 2023). Narcolepsy often occurs in individuals in their teens or early 20s and research suggests the prevalence is increased if family members have narcolepsy (Mattice 2019). There is no cure, but narcolepsy may be managed with medication (i.e. amphetamines), changes in lifestyle, counselling and support (Gordon 2021). Narcolepsy is usually diagnosed by conducting a daytime sleep study measuring the individual's tendency to fall asleep.

Parasomnias

Parasomnias are sleep disorders that include a range of physical and behavioural occurrences, such as sleep walking, nightmares, enuresis (bed wetting) and bruxism (tooth grinding), which occur more commonly in children than in adults (Gordon 2021). These can occur during REM or NREM periods of sleep. Sudden infant death syndrome (SIDS) is also considered a parasomnia and is thought to be an autonomic nervous system abnormality causing apnoea, hypoxia and cardiac arrhythmias during sleep (Rogers 2023). It is recommended that infants are placed in the supine position during sleep (see Chapter 45). There are specific treatments recommended for parasomnia disorders that vary according to the sleep disturbance. Safety is paramount when providing education and treatment to support the individual with their disorder (Gordon 2021).

FACTORS AFFECTING SLEEP

Frequently a number of factors affect the quantity and quality of sleep, rather than one individual factor (Gordon 2021). Clinical Interest Box 27.8 outlines the factors that affect sleep. Some of these factors are often transient; however, the individual may seek advice about a sleeping problem. Many stressors associated with daily living, and particularly with illness, may have a detrimental effect on a person's ability to rest and sleep, and this will further impact on their general wellbeing. It is vital that the nurse is aware of the factors that affect a person's ability to sleep in order to assist in alleviating or minimising these factors.

CLINICAL INTEREST BOX 27.8 Factors affecting sleep

Physical illness: Pain and discomfort may interfere with falling asleep, or disrupt the sleep pattern. The impact of a plaster cast, traction, a brace or splint will physically limit movement and position when sleeping.
Pain: Chronic pain can increase feelings of fatigue, and intensity may be increased at night.
Nocturia: Getting up at night to urinate will disrupt sleep, and difficulty in falling back to sleep may be experienced.
Dyspnoea: The position that must be assumed to sleep and to ease difficulty breathing may be different or difficult for the individual to adjust to without disruption to sleep cycle. Fear of increasing difficulty in breathing is often experienced at night, particularly in cardiac disease when individuals may awaken with dyspnoea.
Hypertension: Individuals may experience increased fatigue and early morning awakening.
Drugs and substances: See Clinical Interest Box 27.11.
Lifestyle: Work shifts (especially rotating shifts) disrupt sleep patterns. It may take several weeks for the body to adjust to shifts, such as night duty, with the change in exposure to light and activity levels (refer to 'circadian rhythm').
Exercise and fatigue: Physical activity that results in individuals feeling tired may actually increase quality of sleep. However, fatigue and feelings of exhaustion often result in difficulty falling asleep.
Nutrition: Changes in body weight can influence sleep patterns, with weight gain causing longer sleep periods, and weight loss sometimes causing a reduction in sleep continuity. The timing and type of meals (e.g. a heavy or spicy meal close to the time of sleeping) may interfere with falling asleep and the ability to achieve restorative sleep, as the digestive system will be engaged in activity during sleep periods.
Stress and emotional state: Worry over personal problems, health or work issues can disrupt sleep. Emotional problems cause tension, both physically and psychologically, and can interfere with the relaxation and calm required to fall asleep. Individuals may become frustrated at not being able to fall asleep, may wake frequently because of their emotional state or may oversleep as a result of sleep-pattern disturbances.
Grief: Also a realistic cause of sleep disturbance, not just in relation to death of a loved one, but also in relation to loss of position in society (such as retirement) or in relocation, such as moving home.
Environment: Simple factors such as heating/cooling, lighting, comfort and familiarity of bed and bedding, noise (such as that experienced in hospitals or residential care facilities) may all impact on the ability to fall asleep and/or remain asleep.

(Cooper & Gosnell 2022; Gordon 2021)

Shift work

Approximately 15–16% of the Australian workforce report being shift workers (Australian Bureau of Statistics [ABS] 2022). Shift work can affect an individual's normal circadian rhythms, resulting in altered sleep patterns and quality of sleep (Commonwealth of Australia 2019). **Shift work sleep disorder (SWSD)** can occur when the individual's circadian rhythm is desynchronised, resulting in difficulty sleeping when they want or need to and daytime sleepiness (Australasian Sleep Association nd). Shift work causes disruption to the body's circadian rhythm, affecting physical and psychological wellbeing (Jenkins 2019). Altered sleep patterns caused by shift work can lead to fatigue, resulting in slower reaction times, impaired alertness and inability to make appropriate decisions in the workplace, contributing to workplace injuries and even death (Work Safe Australia 2022). Shift workers have increased physical health risks for cardiovascular disease and type 2 diabetes mellitus, obesity and cancer (Commonwealth of Australia 2019). Shift work is a necessary and inherent part of the nursing profession. Nurses rotate through day, afternoon and night shifts, all of which may occur over a working week. Work Safe Australia (2022) recommends that shift workers are educated on the impact of fatigue and take responsibility for their own safety and health, as well as ensuring the health and safety of others are not adversely affected by acts or omissions due to fatigue. (See Clinical Interest Box 27.9.)

CRITICAL THINKING EXERCISE 27.1

Care of the nurse and shift work

You are rostered to work a late/early on the medical ward after finishing two night shifts. You already feel tired from working the night shifts and were not able to sleep in the daytime following your last shift. You completed your evening shift and commence the AM shift with only 5 hours of sleep in-between, and now feel fatigued. The handover from the night shift RN reported that it had been quite a busy night shift. There are a few palliative individuals requiring specialised care to manage their pain and comfort levels. There is also a long-term individual who has high acuity needs after suffering a stroke.
What strategies can you put in place to manage shift work and care for yourself?

ASSESSING REST AND SLEEP PATTERNS

Assessment of rest and sleep patterns plays an important role in assisting individuals and their caregivers to identify habits and factors that contribute to poor sleep (Harding et al 2023). The information gathered can allow the nurse to identify strategies and incorporate them into the nursing care provided (Gordon 2021).

CLINICAL INTEREST BOX 27.9 Ways to manage shift work

Managing your sleep hygiene routine during shift work can be difficult; however, the following tips may assist:

- Make time to sleep. Let friends and family know you are on rotating roster and schedule events around your roster. Let them know you are not available.
- Set yourself bedtime schedules based on your shifts (e.g. day shift in bed by 10 pm, evening shift in bed within 30 minutes of arriving home, night shift within 30 minutes of getting home and set an alarm for at least 7 hours sleep). A rest or nap before heading to night shift may help.
- Invest in ear plugs and eye mask, and a good quality pillow.
- Darken your room—this may mean heavy curtains or light restricting curtains.
- Avoid caffeine, alcohol, nicotine and sleeping tablets before going to bed.
- Use your regular relaxation techniques—bath or shower, soft music, mindfulness or meditation.
- Engage in regular exercise.
- Do what works best for you.

(Sleep Health Foundation 2023)

CLINICAL INTEREST BOX 27.10 Questions to assess sleep patterns

- What time do you usually go to sleep?
- How quickly do you fall asleep?
- What is the average number of hours you sleep during the night?
- How many times do you wake at night?
- Do you know what wakes you at night?
- When do you usually wake in the morning?
- Do you rise once you wake or do you stay in bed?
- How do you feel physically after awakening in the morning?

(Cooper & Gosnell 2022; Gordon 2021)

Sleep pattern

When assessing an individual's status in relation to comfort, rest and sleep, the nurse should obtain information of the individual's usual periods of rest and sleep behaviour, such as periods of rest during the day and the time normally gone to sleep, the quality of sleep and the time of waking (Gordon 2021). (See Clinical Interest Box 27.10.) It is helpful to know the individual's sleep hygiene routine (e.g. if they normally have a hot drink before bedtime, or if they require medication to help them sleep). (See Clinical Interest Box 27.11.)

CLINICAL INTEREST BOX 27.11 Effects of medications on sleep

Alcohol

- Speeds onset of sleep
- Reduces REM sleep
- Awakens person during night and causes difficulty returning to sleep

Anticonvulsants

- Decrease REM sleep time
- Cause daytime drowsiness

Antidepressants and stimulants

- Suppress REM sleep
- Decrease total sleep time

Beta-adrenergic blockers

- Cause nightmares
- Cause insomnia
- Cause awakening from sleep

Benzodiazepines

- Alter REM sleep
- Increase sleep time
- Increase daytime sleepiness

Caffeine

- Prevents person from falling asleep
- Causes person to awaken during night
- Interferes with REM sleep

Corticosteroids

- Lead to vivid dreams and nightmares
- Cause anxiety
- Impair ability to fall asleep
- Cause fluid retention and weight gain
- Increase blood glucose levels

Diuretics

- Night-time awakenings caused by nocturia

Hypnotics

- Interfere with reaching deeper sleep stages
- Provide only temporary (1 week) increase in quantity of sleep
- Eventually cause 'hangover' during day; excess drowsiness, confusion, decreased energy
- Sometimes worsen sleep apnoea in older adults

Narcotics

- Suppress REM sleep
- Cause increased daytime drowsiness

(Cooper & Gosnell 2022; Gordon 2021; Tiziani 2022)

Physiological factors

The nurse should also assess whether there is any discomfort that may disturb rest and sleep, such as nausea, difficulty breathing, or any acute or chronic pain related to the illness. Pain is associated with chronic poor sleep. Individuals undergoing surgical procedures often have disrupted sleep due to pain, restricted movement and discomfort (Magowan & Lynass 2020). Postoperative effects of anaesthesia can include hypoxia and hypercapnia that can affect the CNS response and alter sleep patterns with decreases in REM and sleep disturbance including reduced time asleep. The inflammatory response following surgery can also cause neuroinflammation that may affect the CNS (Rampes et al 2020). Opioids may also affect sleep patterns, causing disrupted REM and reduction in sleep time. Postoperative sleep disturbances can also lead to increased pain due to tiredness and alterations in coping strategies and pain perception (Rampes et al 2020). (See Case Study 27.1.)

Nursing assessment of individuals with chronic illness is important so that the sleeping environment can be modified, or referral for further assessment can be initiated, to assist in achieving adequate rest and sleep. Individuals with chronic lung disease or congestive heart failure are often short of breath when lying flat and may require two or more pillows or bed head elevated to assist sleep. They may be woken during the night due to congestion or shortness of breath (Gordon 2021). Nocturnal chest pain (nocturnal angina) is common in the early hours of the morning in people with coronary artery disease and thought to be related to the REM period of sleep and when dreams occur (Rogers 2023). Hypertension also causes early morning waking and fatigue (Gordon 2021).

Nocturia disturbs sleep due to the frequent waking to void or when incontinence occurs. Nocturia may be caused by diabetes where high blood sugars cause polyuria; loss of bladder tone causing incontinence or frequent urination; congestive heart failure where elevating legs in bed results in increased venous return and the filtering of increased blood volume creates more urine; or prostatic enlargement resulting in frequent urination overnight (Gordon 2021).

CASE STUDY 27.1

Mr Andrews is an 85-year-old retiree who experienced a right-sided stroke 3 weeks ago. He has been left with a dense left hemiplegia and is totally dependent for all his activities of daily living (ADLs). Mr Andrews has also developed chronic regional pain syndrome, which is causing spasms and pain in his left leg and arm. The pain is more prevalent at night and he is finding it difficult to sleep. You can see that he becomes quite distressed when his pain is not well controlled. He also tells you he feels helpless and anxious about his wife having to manage his care and normal household activities.

1. Identify complementary therapies to decrease stress and anxiety for Mr Andrews.
2. Formulate a sleep hygiene routine to assist Mr Andrews in promoting sleep.
3. What non-pharmacological pain management strategies could you put in place to promote comfort, rest and sleep for Mr Andrews?

Musculoskeletal issues affecting sleep include inability to reposition self when uncomfortable or in pain; restless leg syndrome where deep muscles become aching, throbbing, itchy or creeping sensation, and the only relief is by moving them; and muscle cramps due to poor circulation in the legs causing pain and the person to wake suddenly (Gordon 2021).

Gulia and Kumar (2018) noted that as part of the normal ageing process sleep patterns are altered. Although the same amount of sleep is required across the lifespan, many elderly people struggle to get the required amount of 8 hours of sleep in one block. They frequently have difficulty falling asleep and wake several times throughout the night (Gulia & Kumar 2018).

Emotional factors

It is important also to assess for psychological and emotional factors (which may not be visible) that may be impacting on the individual's ability to relax and achieve a state of calm to facilitate rest and sleep. Worry or stress about an illness state or the impact of the illness on an individual's lifestyle can result in poor sleep habits (Gordon 2021).

Environmental factors

The sleep patterns of hospitalised individuals may be affected by illness or the hospital environment and routines (Gordon 2021). The normal pattern and quality of sleep deteriorates greatly when a person is in a hospital environment (Delaney et al 2018). There is a correlation between disruptions to sleep and noise levels. Delaney et al (2018) identified that hospitalised individuals perceived that one of the main causes of noise levels that affected their sleep was nursing staff talking either at the nursing station or in providing clinical care. Repeated environmental stimuli such as strange noises from equipment, frequent monitoring and care given by nurses and doctors, ever-present lights and lack of colour stimulation can lead to sleep deprivation (Gordon 2021). Assessment of environmental factors affecting a person's ability to maintain sleep is important in being able to modify the environment to promote sleep and rest. This may be as simple as turning down the volume of the volumetric pump or dimming lights. Nurses also need to be aware of the noises they make in conversations and activities that may impact on the rest and sleep of individuals in hospital and other care settings.

Review Case Study 27.2 in relation to changes in sleep patterns due to hospitalisation.

Medication factors

Assessment of the individual's medication regimen is important to determine if the side effects of particular prescribed medications are contributing to daytime sleepiness or drowsiness (Gordon 2021) or night-time wakefulness (e.g. prednisolone taken at night causes insomnia and nightmares, which is why it should be prescribed as a daily morning dose). If so, the ability to achieve an adequate night's sleep may be affected. An individual may need the assistance of medications to fall asleep and maintain sleep

CASE STUDY 27.2

Mrs Walsh is a 75-year-old woman diagnosed with bowel cancer, who has been admitted to the surgical ward preoperatively for an anterior bowel resection with the possibility of the formation of a colostomy. She has been admitted for preoperative bowel preparation. On admission, Mrs Walsh tells you that she dreads coming into hospital because she finds it difficult to sleep, and when she gets home it takes her ages to catch up on all the sleep she has lost.

1. What steps will you undertake to develop a sleep plan to assist Mrs Walsh to improve her expected sleep pattern in hospital? What strategies might she use to regain her previous sleep quality once home?
2. Identify factors that may impact on Mrs Walsh's ability to sleep post-surgery. Develop a brief care plan to meet postop rest and sleep needs.
3. What do you believe individuals should expect to achieve in terms of quality sleep while in hospital and how would you implement nursing strategies that could improve quality of sleep?

CLINICAL INTEREST BOX 27.12 Controlling noise in the hospital setting

- Close doors to individual's room when possible.
- Keep doors to work areas of unit closed when in use.
- Reduce volume of nearby telephone and paging equipment.
- Wear rubber-soled shoes. Avoid clogs.
- Turn off bedside oxygen and other equipment that is not in use.
- Turn down alarms and beeps on bedside monitoring equipment.
- Turn off room TV and radio unless individual prefers soft music.
- Avoid abrupt loud noise such as flushing a toilet or moving a bed.
- Keep necessary conversations at low levels, particularly at night.
- Conduct conversations and reports in a private area away from individuals' rooms.

(Gordon 2021)

but these are indicated for short-term management only (Knights et al 2023).

The information obtained, together with observation of the individual, provides the nurse with a foundation on which to plan and implement nursing actions to promote comfort, rest and sleep. When possible, the person's usual sleep hygiene routine should be maintained, and the immediate environment arranged so that it is conducive to comfort, rest and sleep.

Hospitalisation/residential care

In addition to environmental factors affecting rest and sleep in hospitalised individuals, Delaney et al (2018) identified frequent disturbances from staff for clinical care interventions, the presence of another person's television noise and snoring in the room as major disturbances to sleep (Delaney et al 2018).

Both short- or long-stay hospitalisation can cause sleep deprivation, leading to negative health outcomes. Adequate rest and restorative sleep is crucial for optimal recovery from illness (Delaney et al 2018; Lopez et al 2018). The need to promote adequate rest is an important aspect of nursing care since, without it, individuals may experience fatigue and irritability, as well as having a decreased ability to deal with stressors (Cooper & Gosnell 2022). Nursing interventions should therefore be aimed at improving the quality of rest and sleep to promote health (Gordon 2021).

Many of the causes of sleep deprivation in hospitalised individuals are environmental, and the nurse needs to ensure duty of care and focus on reducing these effects, by modifying the environment (Delaney et al 2018). An individual in hospital may be subjected to sensory stimulation notnormally experienced in the home environment (see Clinical Interest Box 27.12). During the night, nurses continue to observe individuals and perform certain procedures or treatments as required. Nurses can control the ward environment to optimise sleep by avoiding waking individuals for non-essential activities, and timing them so they are completed when the individuals are awake (Gordon 2021). However, as part of the nurse's responsibility and accountability in delivering care, it is at times unavoidable to disturb individuals from their sleep to perform nursing observations and activities required to ensure an individual's safety and wellbeing. For example, an individual on hourly neurological observations may appear to be having a restful sleep but has deteriorated neurologically. A critical error can be made if the individual is not woken up for the hourly assessment and the changes in neurological status are not detected.

It is optimal to achieve at least 90 minutes of continuous sleep as this gives the individual at least one full REM cycle needed to experience restorative sleep (Pachecho & Singh 2023). Clarke and Mills (2017) reported that hospitalised individuals identified strategies, such as closing the door and blinds, dimming the lights and providing a warm blanket, which nurses could implement to promote rest and sleep. If the individual is woken and experiences difficulty resettling, measures such as a change of position, adjustment to the bedding or a warm drink may help with resuming sleep. It should be noted if an individual does not resettle after these supportive measures have been implemented, the nurse on night duty must ensure that the individual's comfort and safety are promoted.

CRITICAL THINKING EXERCISE 27.2

Effects of medication on sleep

Derek is a 58-year-old man who suffers from infective bronchial asthma each winter. When this occurs, he has weeks of episodes of persistent coughing, which wakes him up frequently in the night. He works full time as a manager of independent living units in residential aged care. His work routine consists of ensuring the residents have the care and services they need on a daily basis. This involves walking around to each of the resident's units, in the cold and wet weather. He was admitted to the ward for IV antibiotics and 100 mg of IV prednisolone QID. He is ready for discharge and has been prescribed an oral corticosteroid, prednisolone 50 mg on a reducing dose, as well as his usual preventer and reliever inhalers.

Identify factors that may affect his ability to sleep, and briefly describe nursing interventions that may assist him to rest to facilitate his recovery.

Continuity of care is essential and, since there are usually fewer staff working at night, the nurse's observational skills are vital in detecting any change in an individual's condition or comfort levels. The nurse is also in a position to observe any specific physiological problems related to sleep, including pain, discomfort, excessive restlessness, snoring or airway obstruction. Referrals may also need to be made to a sleep study centre, pain management team, social worker, counsellor or psychologist to address the sleep disturbance issue.

Stressors or psychological issues associated with illness or hospitalisation may cause difficulty in maintaining usual sleep pattern (Gordon 2021). Being in hospital involves a variety of potential stressors; the nurse should therefore implement measures to provide as stress-free an environment as possible. Anxiety related to illness, and its consequences, may prevent relaxation and interrupt sleep. Emotional tension may be reduced by providing individuals with adequate information before any treatment or procedure starts. See Nursing Care Plan 27.1 on sleep alteration. To provide opportunities for

NURSING CARE PLAN 27.1

Assessment: Mr Andrews is an 85-year-old retiree who experienced a right-sided stroke 3 weeks ago. He has been left with a dense left hemiplegia and is totally dependent for all his ADLs. Mr Andrews has also developed chronic regional pain syndrome, which is causing spasms and pain in his left leg and arm. The pain is more prevalent at night and he is finding it difficult to sleep. You can see that he becomes quite distressed when his pain is not well controlled. He also tells you he feels helpless and anxious about his wife having to manage his care and normal household activities.
Issue/s to be addressed: Disturbed sleep pattern related to pain in left leg and arm and stress.
Goal/s: Mr Andrews will be able to have improved quality of sleep within 2 weeks.
Mr Andrews will achieve a normal sleep pattern within 2 weeks.

Care/actions	Rationale
Assess and manage pain levels prior to sleep.	To prevent pain waking Mr Andrews.
Refer Mr Andrews to pain management team.	To provide adequate treatment to optimise pain relief measures, allowing optimal sleep.
Commence a sleep chart.	To monitor sleep patterns and identify variations from normal sleep patterns.
Complete or cluster nursing interventions prior to sleep time.	To ensure Mr Andrews is not disturbed frequently during sleep time.
Adjust the environment to minimise the noise levels; close door, darken room or play soft music.	A quiet, darkened environment promotes sleep and soft music masks environmental noises that may keep a person awake while hospitalised.
Encourage Mr Andrews to verbalise concerns to decrease stress prior to sleep.	Excess worry or stress prior to sleep may stimulate wakefulness.
Refer family situation to a social worker to enable Mr Andrews to discuss concerns.	To decrease worry and concern, which may relax Mr Andrews, enabling him to sleep.
Promote relaxation techniques to promote sleep.	Relaxation techniques may promote sleep by decreasing thought processes and reducing stress.
Provide aids to promote comfort; air mattress to cushion body against pressure.	Falling asleep only occurs if a person feels relaxed and comfortable.
Correct body alignment supported with pillows to promote comfort.	

Evaluation:
Discuss with Mr Andrews his perception of quality of sleep.
Discuss with Mr Andrews if pain management is effective.
Observe amount of night-time wakefulness and daytime sleepiness.
Review sleep chart to ascertain if Mr Andrews' sleep is disturbed.

(Flynn Makic & Martinez-Kratz 2022; Carpineto 2022; Gordon 2021)

questions to be asked and answered, the nurse should promote a climate that is conducive to communication by spending time with the individual and their significant others.

Sleep disorders are higher in individuals in residential aged-care homes, which is largely attributed to the ageing process, comorbidities, decreased melatonin levels and altered circadian rhythms. In addition, environmental noises within the home, loss of autonomy in own sleep patterns and nursing interventions disturb sleep (Smyth 2021; Gilsenan 2023). Alzheimer's disease and other dementias can cause sleep disturbances, including night-time waking or wandering, sleep fragmentation and sleepiness during the day (Webb & Scott 2023).

Some healthcare facilities have regulations and specified visiting hours, which are designed to provide rest periods and avoid overtiring hospitalised individuals. Throughout the rest periods, visitors to, and activities in, the ward are kept to a minimum to provide a quiet relaxed environment where individuals should be encouraged to try to sleep or to engage in some relaxing non-stressful activity. To facilitate rest and relaxation, an individual's physical comfort should be promoted since it is difficult to rest in the presence of discomfort such as pain, a full bladder or an uncomfortable position. (See Clinical Interest Box 27.13.)

CLINICAL INTEREST BOX 27.13 Promoting rest and sleep in hospitalised adults

- Follow regular sleep hygiene routines.
- Encourage individuals to wear loose-fitting nightwear.
- Remove any irritants against the individual's skin, such as moist or wrinkled sheets or drainage tubing.
- Position and support body parts to protect pressure areas and aid muscle relaxation.
- Administer necessary personal hygiene measures.
- Keep linen clean and dry.
- Encourage the individual to void before going to sleep.
- Administer any analgesics or sedatives about 30 minutes before bedtime.
- Provide a quiet environment.

(Gordon 2021)

CRITICAL THINKING EXERCISE 27.3

Effects of hospitalisation on sleep

Mr Robert Waters is a 72-year-old man who had a hip replacement with a spinal anaesthetic 2 days ago. He went into urinary retention 6 hours after surgery and now has an IDC in situ. You are working on the night shift, and find him awake at 0100 hours. He tells you that he has been having trouble sleeping since his surgery and after having the IDC inserted. He states he normally sleeps well at home.

What strategies could you implement to assist Mr Waters to have optimal sleep?

SLEEP-PROMOTION MEASURES

Sleep is influenced by a variety of factors that may be described as physical, psychological or environmental. Establishing and maintaining a regular **sleep hygiene** routine prior to bedtime assists the body in recognising it is time for sleep (Sleep Foundation 2023). Sleep hygiene is the routines and habits an individual performs prior to sleep to maximise the effectiveness of sleep. Effective sleep may also be facilitated by a range of natural/non-pharmacological measures, which include:

- Ensuring enough exposure to daylight during the day and that at night the room is quiet, darkened and at a comfortable temperature (coolness or warmth), and has sufficient fresh air or ventilation.
- Engaging in physical exercise/activity during the day to promote rest at night.
- Limiting daytime naps to less than 30 minutes.
- Spending some time relaxing and unwinding before going to bed. Sleep may also be more easily achieved if the person is calm and has been able to resolve any problems prior to going to bed.
- Resisting stimulants such as tea, coffee or cocoa, or heavy foods immediately before going to bed. Individuals may find it easier to sleep if they avoid going to bed feeling hungry or overfull.
- Adopting a sleep hygiene routine (e.g. similar time each night, warm bath or shower, warm drink and some peaceful music or relaxing reading).

(Sleep Foundation 2023)

CRITICAL THINKING EXERCISE 27.4

Lifestyle effects on sleep

Mr Alexander is a 58-year-old fly in, fly out worker. He is on a 4 weeks on, 2 weeks off work cycle and flies to and from Western Australia on the 'red-eye flight'. He works shift work when onsite. He eats mostly take-away meals. He gets home at all hours of the day and night; therefore, there is no regularity to his sleep pattern. When he gets home from a big trip, he likes to watch TV and have a few beers before going to bed. He said he often falls asleep in his chair and wakes up a few hours later, when he takes himself off to bed. You perform a sleep assessment on Mr Alexander's sleep habits and history.

How could you assist Mr Alexander to develop effective sleep hygiene habits that will improve his sleep patterns?

Meeting sleep needs/sleep hygiene

Good sleep hygiene practices promote quality sleep and increase daytime alertness, both of which are essential for physical and psychological health (Sleep Foundation 2023). Hospitalised individuals should be encouraged to maintain their usual pre-sleep routine (Gordon 2021). (See Clinical Interest Box 27.14.) In hospital, the nurse should assist a person in preparation for sleep by ensuring that the following key physiological and psychological needs are met.

CLINICAL INTEREST BOX 27.14
Sleep hygiene

- Bedtime routines and sleeping environment
- Use of sleep and other prescription medications, and over-the-counter drugs
- Pattern of dietary intake and amount of substances that influence sleep
- Symptoms experienced during waking hours
- Physical illness
- Recent life events
- Current emotional and mental status

(Adapted from Gordon 2021)

Hygiene needs

When required, the individual should be assisted to meet all hygiene needs, such as washing face and hands and cleaning teeth. An ambulant individual may like to have a warm shower or bath before settling to sleep. A non-ambulant individual may require repositioning and turning.

Nutritional and fluid needs

Large spicy meals, caffeine and alcohol must be reduced or avoided prior to retiring to bed since they can disturb sleep (Gordon 2021). A warm drink and snack could be offered to the individual, unless this is contraindicated. An individual may prefer a non-stimulating milk-based drink rather than tea or coffee, which can have a stimulating effect. In addition, oral fluids that can be consumed during the night, if desired, should also be provided.

Elimination needs

Individuals should be provided with toilet facilities before settling for sleep. The nurse may need to provide assistance with the appropriate toileting aids and facilities. Urinary drainage equipment should be checked, and the collection bag emptied if necessary.

Comfort needs

Preparing the individual's room includes ensuring that there is adequate ventilation, the room is a comfortable temperature and that lighting is reduced to a minimum (Gordon 2021). The individual's nurse call bell and any other items that may be required during the night need to be placed within easy reach. Nursing measures include ensuring that the individual is positioned comfortably and that the bedclothes and pillows are arranged to meet the individual's needs. The bottom sheets should be free of wrinkles or creases, supplementary items such as a pressure-relieving device or bed cradle may be used to enhance comfort and to prevent the risk of pressure on skin and bony prominences. Whenever possible, treatments and procedures are completed before the individual settles for sleep. For example, any splints or dressings should be checked and, if necessary, adjusted or changed (Gordon 2021). (See Chapter 19.)

Protection and safety needs

The National Safety and Quality Health Service (NSQHS) (ACSQHC 2021) Standards on preventing and managing pressure injuries, and preventing falls and harm from falls, need to be considered in the protection and safety needs of hospitalised individuals (see Chapter 15). Extended bed rest from illness and immobility can lead to pressure injuries and can occur in individuals with risk factors including poor nutrition, skin integrity and pressure points, or can be age-related (ACSQHC 2021). The intention of the NSQHS Standard regarding pressure injuries is to prevent the occurrence of pressure injuries. The nurse needs to perform a risk assessment on admission to provide the appropriate interventions when assisting the individual with rest and sleep needs.

The NSQHS Standard regarding falls prevention aims to prevent falls or minimise the harm from falls. Measures need to be taken to promote the individual's safety during sleep. If a person is restless (but not confused or disoriented), the use of bed rails (one or both) may be indicated, but a comprehensive falls risk assessment must be completed with appropriate consent and documentation undertaken. An individualised falls prevention plan then must be implemented (ACSQHC 2021). For a confused individual, it is usually more appropriate to adjust the height of the bed to its lowest level. As an alternative safety measure, 'hi-lo' beds, which can be situated at floor level, may be appropriate for an individual who is disoriented and inclined to get out of bed and wander. The risks to a confused or disoriented individual are greatly increased in raising bed rails since the feeling of being enclosed or limited in activity may result in them climbing over the rails, thus causing an unnecessary injury. Confused or disoriented individuals need frequent monitoring and measures that limit the risk of injury. Adequate lighting should be provided, perhaps via a night light, particularly if the individual needs to mobilise during the night.

Other safety measures include regular monitoring throughout the night to assess an individual's health status and ensure that any equipment such as intravenous infusion apparatus, monitoring leads, indwelling catheters, drain tubes or any assistive devices are in place and functioning appropriately.

Physiological needs

It is the role of the nurse to assess an individual for any physiological disturbances that may impact on adequate sleep and to promote comfort conducive for rest and sleep (Gordon 2021). This includes interventions such as alleviating pain, attending to hygiene or any distressing symptoms, such as difficulty breathing, which may affect adequate rest and sleep (Gordon 2021). In collaboration with other members of the multidisciplinary team, measures (either non-pharmacological or pharmacological) should be undertaken to alleviate these factors (as much as possible).

Psychological needs

Hospitalised individuals may feel stressed and anxious, which can interfere with effective sleep. If an individual is anxious or worried, the nurse should try to ascertain the reason and provide appropriate support. For example, a person may be concerned about some aspect of treatment, such as forthcoming surgery, and providing them with more information (as appropriate within scope of practice) may help to alleviate some of their anxiety (Gordon 2021). Reassurance that a nurse will be available to respond to needs may also be helpful.

Pharmacological measures

In the short term, and particularly while hospitalised, an individual may be prescribed medication by a medical officer to promote sleep (e.g. a sedative). Long-term use of sedatives can be detrimental to sleep routines. Therefore, alternative measures to assist a person to improve sleep patterns are important (Gordon 2021). Natural sleep hygiene measures to promote settling should be undertaken first but, if difficulty getting to sleep persists, mild sedation may be considered by the medical team to be appropriate (Centre for Clinical Interventions 2020). After a sedative medication has been administered, the individual should be encouraged to relax and allow it to take effect. In most cases, light sedatives assist individuals to fall asleep, but do not have an impact on keeping the individual asleep; therefore, once the individual has settled, activity, noise and light should be reduced to a minimum. The response to, and effects of, such medication must be noted and recorded (Gordon 2021).

Stress reduction

A range of techniques are available for reducing stress and promoting relaxation, all of which aim to help the individual control reactions to stress. A calm relaxed person is likely to fall asleep quickly and sleep soundly through the night. Relaxation techniques should initially be learnt in a quiet restful environment and, with practice, may then be used in most situations to reduce stress. Physical and psychological relaxation is the aim of relaxation techniques, reducing the body's physical tension as well as interrupting constant thoughts that prevent sleep. Some individuals benefit from utilising relaxation techniques and do sleep longer; however, not all people respond to relaxation techniques. Individuals should be encouraged to pursue activities that reduce stress (Potter et al 2023).

Management of weight

Individuals who are overweight tend to sleep longer and have fewer interruptions than an individual who is underweight, who will have more interruptions and wake earlier (Cooper & Gosnell 2022). Discussion with a dietitian should be made to assist in formulating a dietary plan to manage weight issues to promote health and wellbeing and reduce the risk of diet-related conditions and chronic diseases (Australian Dietary Guidelines 2015).

Complementary and alternative therapies

Individuals are increasingly turning to complementary therapies to use alongside traditional medical treatments to enhance health and wellbeing (Cooper & Gosnell 2022). A range of complementary therapies can assist with promoting rest and sleep. Some of these may include meditation techniques, relaxation, exercise, creative therapies, religious activities, acupuncture, biofeedback, massage, reflexology, aromatherapy and herbal treatments (Cooper & Gosnell 2022). They are known as alternative therapies when the complementary therapy becomes the main form of treatment, replacing medical treatment. It is important to discuss all herbal treatments with the treating physician and/ or pharmacist to ensure compatibility with any prescribed medications.

Yoga, mindfulness, meditation and tai chi

Yoga, meditation and tai chi are forms of relaxation and exercise that are helpful to many people and, while they have degrees of difficulty, can be performed by many age groups and people of varying degrees of wellness. Mindfulness is a form of self-awareness meditation that may improve both medical and psychological outcomes, including the quality of sleep (Greeson et al 2018). Yoga is a safe, non-intrusive way of promoting relaxation and sleep quality. It is important that techniques for alternative therapies are taught by people with expertise in these methods (Better Health Channel 2021).

Relaxation breathing

This technique consists of controlled breathing, performed while the individual assumes a comfortable position. The person is encouraged to concentrate on their breathing and may find it helpful to visualise each breath as providing muscles with energy-giving oxygen. The person is encouraged to take a deep breath, hold it briefly and then exhale slowly. With each exhalation the person is encouraged to say 'relax' and, as the technique is repeated, should feel progressively more relaxed (Beyond Blue 2022).

Progressive muscular relaxation

The theory behind this technique is that a relaxed body leads to a relaxed mind. The technique consists of consciously tensing and relaxing the major muscles of the body in sequence. The individual is encouraged to tense one or a group of muscles for approximately 10 seconds, feel the tension and then slowly ease the tension by relaxing the muscles (Beyond Blue 2022). As the technique is repeated there should be an awareness of the sensation of relaxation in the muscles.

Massage

Massage therapy releases chemical neurotransmitters (endorphins) that contribute to a feeling of wellbeing, and decreases the levels of stress hormones, adrenaline, cortisol and noradrenaline. Muscles contract and become tense in stressful situations, and massage can be an effective method of promoting muscle relaxation (Salvo 2023). There are many types of massage and, while most are relatively easy to learn, instructors with experience can teach caregivers simple relaxation massage techniques to assist others to relax.

Although a massage can be beneficial, some people may not feel comfortable about being massaged. Also, an individual's physical condition may contraindicate the use of massage. In older individuals, with age-related skin changes, extreme care must be taken to ensure that massage is gentle and light to avoid disruption of the epidermal–dermal junction, which becomes weaker with age (Salvo 2023). In older individuals, the risk of skin tears is greatly increased because of this junction weakness, and massage should be limited to small areas of the hands, feet or shoulders as tolerated. In the right situation, however, massage, particularly of the neck and back, can be relaxing and promote rest (Salvo 2023).

Exercise

Exercise can be useful in sleep promotion; however, it is recommended that it be performed at least 2 hours prior to bedtime to allow the body to relax (Gordon 2021). In relation to older adults who may have age-related changes or chronic ill-health, or those who are experiencing episodes of illness or changes to health status (such as surgery or treatment), the degree of physical activity that may be undertaken may be limited, but simple activity such as sitting out of bed or gentle ambulation several times a day may meet the same activity level for an individual with health limitations that regular exercise has for a person in a state of wellbeing (Cooper & Gosnell 2022). Exercise is not always practical, especially if the person is unwell; therefore, relaxation techniques may be used instead (Cooper & Gosnell 2022). Clinical Interest Box 27.15 outlines some ways in which sleep and rest can be promoted at home.

CLINICAL INTEREST BOX 27.15 Promoting rest and sleep at home

Sleep pattern

- Establish a regular bedtime and waking time for all days of the week. Eliminate lengthy naps during the day. Limit naps to only 30 minutes a day.
- Exercise adequately during the day. Avoid physical exertion 2 hours before bedtime.
- Avoid dealing with work or family problems before bedtime.
- Establish a regular sleep hygiene routine before sleep (e.g. reading, listening to music).
- When unable to sleep, pursue a relaxing activity until you feel drowsy.
- If having trouble falling asleep, get up until you feel sleepy.
- Use the bed mainly for sleep; avoid activities like watching TV.

Environment

- Ensure appropriate lighting, temperature and environment.
- Keep noise to a minimum.

Diet

- Avoid heavy meals in the 3 hours before bedtime.
- Avoid alcohol- and caffeine-containing foods and beverages at least 4 hours before bedtime.
- Decrease fluid intake 2–4 hours before sleep.
- If a bedtime snack is necessary, consume only a light snack or a warm milk drink.

Medications

- Use sleeping medications only as a last resort.
- Take analgesics 30 minutes before bedtime to relieve aches and pains.
- Consult with a healthcare provider about adjusting other medications that may cause insomnia.

(Adapted from Berman et al 2020)

Progress Note 27.1

15/02/24 0630 hrs	Nursing: Mr Adams was admitted to the medical ward at 2230 hrs for overnight observation and review by the cardiac physician in the morning. He was brought in by the ambulance to the emergency department with chest pain 9/10 at 1400 hrs. His chest pain was relieved with 600 microg of Anginine × 3 and 2.5 mg of IV morphine given by the ambulance officers. He has a past history of angina and a stent to his left main coronary artery. On arrival to the ward, he was pain free, and admission ECG and vital signs were within normal parameters. Refer to medication chart for medications commenced. At 0200 hrs, Mr Adams was observed to have an apnoeic period. He struggled for breath, awoke slightly snorting and then resumed a normal breathing pattern. Vital signs were performed and no alterations from previous observations were noted. The oxygen saturation probe was left in situ. The oxygen saturation machine alarmed approximately every 15–30 minutes with varied desaturations down to SpO_2 of 7%. Mr Adams was reviewed overnight by the night resident medical officer as per the medical emergency team (MET) call criteria. Appointment to be made upon discharge for the sleep study clinic.

Heather Andrews (ANDREWS), *EN*

DECISION-MAKING FRAMEWORK EXERCISE 27.1

You are looking after Mr Adams on night shift. You attend to his vital signs at 0200 hours and notice that he does not appear to be breathing normally. When you touch his arm and speak to him he rouses and starts to snort. You ask him if he has had any sleep issues at home. He tells you that he is not aware of any, although his wife reports she hears him stop breathing at home sometimes and usually gives him a nudge, which makes him start breathing again. You apply the SpO_2 saturation probe to his finger and leave it in situ. Not long after that Mr Adams falls back to sleep and the SpO_2 machine alarms. You enter the room and his SpO_2 is at 79%.

1. What is your responsibility in regard to the nursing care for Mr Adams?
2. Using the decision-making framework, what is your role in reporting Mr Adams' low saturations?

Summary

Comfort is necessary for relaxation, rest and sleep. A person's ability to relax and achieve comfort, and therefore to receive sufficient rest and sleep, may be disrupted during illness or hospitalisation. Measures that can be implemented to promote rest may include certain techniques that facilitate relaxation. Sleep can also be promoted by allowing the hospitalised individual to maintain their normal pre-sleep routine, and by ensuring that the person's safety and comfort are promoted during the night, as at any other time. Sleep behaviours and patterns can be assessed by the nurse, and simple measures to promote effective sleep may be taught and implemented. Assisting individuals and self to meet comfort, rest and sleep needs is essential in the promotion of individual physical and psychological wellbeing.

Review Questions

1. Describe the importance of rest and sleep to a person's wellbeing.
2. Briefly describe the five stages of the sleep cycle.
3. List the factors that may interfere with the process of rest and sleep.
4. What is the circadian rhythm?
5. Describe the supportive nursing measures that may be implemented to promote the individual's need for rest and sleep.
6. Briefly describe why individuals have difficulty achieving restful sleep while hospitalised.
7. Identify factors across the lifespan that may impact on an individual's perception of their quality of sleep.
8. What measures can be implemented by nurses to assist an older individual to re-establish their sleep pattern when they have changed their living environment (such as moving to a new home or aged-care home)?

Evolve® Answer guide for the Review Questions, Critical Thinking Exercises, Decision-making Framework Exercises and Critical Thinking Questions in Case Studies is hosted on Evolve: http://evolve.elsevier.com/AU/Koutoukidis/Tabbner.

References

Australian Bureau of Statistics, 2022. Working arrangements. Available at: <https://www.abs.gov.au/statistics/labour/earnings-and-working-conditions/working-arrangements/latest-release>.

Australian Institute of Health and Welfare (AIHW), 2021. Sleep-related breathing disorders with a focus on obstructive sleep apnoea. Available at: <https://www.aihw.gov.au/reports/chronic-respiratory-conditions/sleep-related-breathing-disorders/summary>.

Australasian Sleep Association, 2022. New GP Guideline on obstructive sleep apnoea and insomnia. Available at: <https://www.sleep.org.au/Public/Public/Resource-Centre/GP-guideline.aspx?hkey=d89fcffc-1dbb-4361-aea3-f1f7dbc1b600>.

Australasian Sleep Association, nd. Shift work sleep disorder – on the spot management information for health professionals. Available at: <https://sleep.org.au/common/Uploaded%20files/Public%20Files/Professional%20resources/Adult%20resources/Shiftwork%20Disorder_0617.pdf>.

Australian Commission on Safety and Quality in Health Care (ACSQHC), 2021. *National safety and quality health service standards*, 2nd ed. ACSQHC, Sydney.

Australian Dietary Guidelines, 2015. About the Australian dietary guidelines. Available at: <https://www.eatforhealth.gov.au>.

Berman, A., Snyder, S.J., Levett-Jones, T., et al., 2020. *Kozier and Erb's fundamentals of nursing*, 5th ed. Pearson, Melbourne.

Better Health Channel, 2021. Yoga – health benefits. Available at: <https://www.betterhealth.vic.gov.au/yoga-health-benefits>.

Beyond Blue, 2022. Relaxation exercises. Available at: <https://www.beyondblue.org.au/get-support/staying-well/relaxation-exercises>.

Brinkman, J., Reddy, V., Sharma, S., 2023. *Physiology of sleep*. National Library of Medicine. Available at: <https://www.ncbi.nlm.nih.gov/books/NBK482512/#:~:text=The%20restorative%20theory%20states%20that,depleted%20throughout%20an%20awake%20day>.

Knights, K., Rowland, A., Darraoch, H., et al., 2023. *Pharmacology for health professionals*, 6th ed. Elsevier, Chatswood.

Carpineto, L.J., 2022. *Handbook of nursing diagnosis: Application to clinical practice*, 16th ed. Lippincott Williams & Wilkins, Philadelphia.

Centre for Clinical Interventions, 2020. Sleep hygiene. Available at: <https://www.cci.health.wa.gov.au/Resources/Looking-After-Yourself/Sleep>.

Clarke, A., Mills, M., 2017. Can a sleep menu enhance the quality of sleep for the hospitalized patient? *MEDSURG Nursing* 26(4) 253–257.

Commonwealth of Australia, 2019. Bedtime reading. Inquiry into sleep health awareness in Australia. Available at: <www.aph.gov.au/Parliamentary_Business/Committees/House/Health_Aged_Care_and_Sport/SleepHealthAwareness/Report>.

Cooper, K., Gosnell, K., 2022. *Foundations and adult nursing*, 9th ed. Elsevier, St Louis.

Delaney, L.J., Currie, M.J., Huang, H.-C.C., et al., 2018. 'They can rest at home': An observational study of patients' quality of sleep in an Australian hospital. *BMC Health Services Research* 18(524). Available at: <https://bmchealthservres.biomedcentral.com/articles/10.1186/s12913-018-3201-z>.

Douglas, J.A., Chai-Coetzer, C.L., McEvoy, D., et al, 2017. Guidelines for sleep studies in adults – a position statement of the Australasian Sleep Association. *Sleep Medicine* 36(1), S2–22. Elsevier. Available at: <https://doi.org/10.1016/j.sleep.2017.03.019>.

Flynn Makic, M.B., Martinez-Kratz, M.R., 2022. *Ackley and Ladwig's nursing diagnosis handbook*, 13th ed. Elsevier Ltd.

Gilsenan, I., 2023. Sleep and rest – hospital or institutional admission. In: Ross, F., *Redfern's nursing older people*, 5th ed. Elsevier Limited.

Gordon, C., 2021. Fostering sleep. In: Crisp, J., Douglas, C., Rebeiro, G., et al. (eds.), *Potter and Perry's fundamentals of nursing*, 6th ed. Elsevier, Chatswood.

Greeson, J.M., Zarrin, H., Smoski, M.J., et al., 2018. Mindfulness meditation targets transdiagnostic symptoms implicated in stress-related disorders: Understanding relationships between changes in mindfulness, sleep quality, and physical symptoms. *Evidence-Based Complementary and Alternative Medicine*, Article ID 4505191. doi: org/10.1155/2018/4505191.

Gulia, K.K., Kumar, V.M., 2018. Sleep disorders in the elderly: A growing challenge. *Psychogeriatrics* 18(3), 155–165.

Harding, M., Kwong, J., Hagler, D., 2023. *Lewis's medical–surgical nursing*, 12th ed. Elsevier, Missouri.

Hillman, D., Mitchell, S., Streatfeild, J., et al., 2018. The economic cost of inadequate sleep. *Sleep* 41(8), 1–13. Available at: <https://academic.oup.com/sleep/article/41/8/zsy083/5025924>.

Jenkins, J., 2019. Sleeping. In: Holland, K., *Applying the Roper-Logan-Tierney model in practice*, 3rd ed. Elsevier Limited.

Kulpatcharapong, S., Chewcharat, P., Ruxrungtham, K., et al., 2020. Sleep quality of hospitalized patients, contributing factors, and prevalence of associated disorders. *Sleep Disorders*, 8518396.

Lamp, A., Cook, M., Soriano Smith, R.N., Belenky, G., 2019. Exercise, nutrition, sleep, and waking rest? *Sleep* 42(10), zsz138. doi: 10.1093/sleep/zsz138. PMID: 31562740; PMCID: PMC6783897.

Lopez, M., Blackburn, L., Springer, C., 2018. Minimizing sleep disturbances to improve patient outcomes. *MED-SURG Nursing* 27(6), 368–371.

Magowan, R., Lynass, M., 2020. Nursing the patient undergoing surgery. In: Peate, I., *Alexander's nursing practice: Hospital and home*, 5th ed. Elsevier Ltd.

Mattice, C., 2019. Narcolepsy. In: Mattice, C., Brooks, C., Lee-Chiong T.I. (eds.), *Fundamentals of sleep technology workbook*, 3rd ed. Lippincott, Williams & Wilkins, China.

Otsuka,Y., Kaneita,Y., Tanaka, K., et al, 2023. Nonrestorative sleep is a risk factor for metabolic syndrome in the general Japanese population. *Diabetology & Metabolic Syndrome* 15(26). Available at: <https://doi.org/10.1186/s13098-023-00999-x>.

Pachecho, D., Singh, A., 2023. Deep sleep: How much do you need. Available at: <https://www.sleepfoundation.org/stages-of-sleep/deep-sleep>.

Potter, P.A., Perry, A.G., Stockert, P., et al., 2023. *Fundamentals of nursing*, 11th ed. Elsevier, St Louis.

Rampes, S., Ma, K., Divecha, Y.A., et al., 2020. Postoperative sleep disorders and their potential impacts on surgical outcomes. *Journal of Biomedical Research* 34(4), 271–280. Available at: <https://doi.org/10.7555/JBR.33.20190054>.

Robertson, J., 2023. Depressants – types and stages of sleep. In: McCuistion, L. *Pharmacology: A patient centred nursing process approach*, 11th ed. Elsevier Inc.

Rogers, J., 2023. *McCane & Huether's pathophysiology*, 9th ed. Elsevier, Sydney.

Salvo, S.G., 2023. *Massage therapy: Principles and practice*, 6th ed. Elsevier, St Louis.

Serin, Y., Acar, T.N., 2019. Effect of circadian rhythm on metabolic processes and the regulation of energy balance. *Annals of Nutrition and Metabolism* 74, 322–330. Available at: <https://doi.org/10.1159/000500071>.

Sleep Disorders Australia, 2022a. Central sleep apnoea. Available at: <https://www.sleepoz.org.au/_files/ugd/a1218b_85cb6bb4e43c4ba1824b07a04ed2f9e9.pdf>.

Sleep Disorders Australia, 2022b. Fact sheets: CPAP – Continuous positive airway pressure. Available at: <https://www.sleepoz.org.au/_files/ugd/a1218b_5abcda411f84439b879a709ddfea9493.pdf>.

Sleep Foundation, 2023. Sleep hygiene. Available at: <https://www.sleepfoundation.org/articles/sleep-hygiene>.

Sleep Health Foundation & Deloitte Access Economics, 2021. Rise and try to shine: The social and economic cost of sleep disorders in Australia. Available at: <https://www.sleephealthfoundation.org.au/files/Special_reports/Final_report_-_Cost_of_sleep_disorders_-_14042021.pdf>.

Sleep Health Foundation, 2023. Shiftwork. Available at: <https://www.sleephealthfoundation.org.au/shiftwork.html>.

Smyth, A., 2021. Sleep disorders in older people – sleep and nursing care. In: Vafeas, C., *Gerontological nursing*. Elsevier Australia.

Tiziani, A., 2022. *Harvard's nursing guide to drugs*, 11th ed. Elsevier, Sydney.

Webb, M., Scott, K., 2023. Promoting and maintaining health and wellness. In: Scott, K., *Long-term caring*, 5th ed. Elsevier Australia.

Williams, P.A., 2023. *deWit's fundamental concepts and skills for nursing*, 6th ed. Elsevier Saunders, Philadelphia.

Work Safe Australia, 2022. Fatigue. Available at: <https://www.safeworkaustralia.gov.au/safety-topic/hazards/fatigue/overview>.

Recommended Reading

America Psychological Association, 2019. Why sleep is important and what happens when you don't get enough. Available at: <http://www.apa.org/topics/sleep/why.aspx>.

Chen, L., Bell, J.S., Visvanathan, R., et al, 2016. The association between benzodiazepine use and sleep quality in residential aged care facilities: A cross-sectional study. *BMC Geriatrics* 16, 196. Available at: <https://doi.org/10.1186/s12877-016-0363-6>.

Drake, C.L., Hays, R.D., Morlock, R., 2015. Development and evaluation of a measure to assess restorative sleep. *Journal of Clinical Sleep Medicine* 10(7), 733–741. doi: 10.5664/jcsm.3860.

Dzierzewski, J.M., Mitchell, M., Rodriguez, J.C., et al., 2015. Patterns and predictors of sleep quality before, during, and after hospitalization in older adults. *Journal of Clinical Sleep Medicine* 11(1), 45–51.

Fillary, J., Chaplin, H., Jones, G., et al., 2015. Noise at night in hospital general wards: A mapping of the literature. *British Journal of Nursing* 24(10), 536–540.

Hamilton, G.S., Joosten, S.A., 2017. Obstructive sleep apnoea and obesity. *Australian Family Physician* 46(7), 460–463.

Muza, R.T., 2017. Central sleep apnoea: A clinical review. *Journal of Thoracic Disease* 7(5), 930–937. doi: 10.3978/j.issn.2072-1439.2015.04.45.

National Sleep Foundation, 2023. Shift worker disorder. Available at: <https://www.sleepfoundation.org/shift-work-disorder/what-shift-work-disorder/facts-about-shift-work-disorder>.

Pryce, C., 2016. Impact of shift work on critical care nurses. *Canadian Journal of Critical Care Nursing* 27(4), 17–21.

Salzmann-Erikson, M., Lagerqvist, L., Pousette, S., 2016. Keep calm and have a good night: Nurses' strategies to promote inpatients' sleep in the hospital environment. *Scandinavian Journal of Caring Science* 30, 356–364.

Sleep Disorders Australia, 2022a. Narcolepsy. Available at: <https://www.sleepoz.org.au/_files/ugd/a1218b_21bfc69744fc4076a6536d5d68ff5da7.pdf>.

Sleep Disorders Australia, 2022b. Sleep apnoea. Available at: <https://www.sleepoz.org.au/_files/ugd/a1218b_5a154d757f734442b20c23675919c66d.pdf>.

Sleep Health Foundation, 2019. Facts about sleep. Available at: <https://www.sleephealthfoundation.org.au/facts-about-sleep.html>.

Online Resources

Australasian Sleep Association: <https://www.sleep.org.au>.

National Sleep Foundation: <https://www.thensf.org>.

Sleep Disorders Australia: <https://www.sleepoz.org.au>.

Sleep Foundation: <https://www.sleepfoundation.org>.

Sleep Health Foundation: <https://www.sleephealthfoundation.org.au>.

CHAPTER 28

Movement and exercise

Heather Wakefield

Key Terms

active
ankylosis
body mechanics
contractures
dangling
deep vein thrombosis (DVT)
dislocation
dynapenia
embolus
fracture
gait
haematopoiesis
hypoxaemia
isokinetic exercise
isometric exercise
isotonic exercise
muscle atrophy
muscular dystrophy
myasthenia gravis
orthostatic or postural hypotension
osteoarthritis
osteoblasts
osteoclasts
osteogenic sarcoma
osteomalacia
osteomyelitis
osteopenia
osteoporosis
plantar flexion (foot drop)
pressure injuries
PRICE: prevention, rest, ice, compression and elevation
pursed-lip breathing
range-of-movement (ROM)
sarcopenia
sedentary
sprain
strain

Learning Outcomes

At the completion of this chapter and with further reading, learners should be able to:

- Define the key terms.
- Describe and implement the principles of good posture and body mechanics.
- Describe the role of the musculoskeletal system in the regulation of movement.
- Describe how joints are involved in movement.
- State differences between isotonic, isometric, isokinetic exercise, passive and active exercises.
- Describe and define range-of-movement (ROM).
- Identify and demonstrate joint movements involved in ROM exercises.
- Describe the benefit of exercise across the lifespan.
- Identify and describe the complications associated with immobility and formulate appropriate preventative measures.
- State the influences and effects associated with disorders of the musculoskeletal system.
- Identify the major musculoskeletal system disorders that impact movement and exercise.
- Briefly describe the specific disorders of the musculoskeletal system outlined in this chapter.
- Define the diagnostic tests that may be used to assess musculoskeletal function.
- Assess individuals for impaired mobility and activity intolerance.
- Assist in planning and implementing nursing care plans for individuals with a musculoskeletal disorder.
- According to specified role and function, perform the nursing activities described in this chapter safely and accurately in the clinical environment.

CHAPTER FOCUS

Exercise and physical activity are integral to health and wellbeing. Movement and exercise are essential components for restoring, maintaining and enhancing physical and psychosocial health, and regular exercise promotes health and feelings of wellbeing and prevents illness throughout the lifespan. Studies are showing that increasingly sedentary lifestyles in younger and older populations contribute to ageing, disease processes and morbidity. Government and health agency research suggests that despite the rising trend in health conditions related to obesity and immobility, the commencement of an exercise program can delay and even reverse the progression of conditions such as osteoporosis, heart disease, diabetes mellitus and the effects of ageing.

The human body is ideally suited to movement and this is made possible by the muscular, skeletal and nervous systems. These interconnected systems work together to make movement possible and, for most human movement, they must function effectively for optimal physical performance. Disease processes that disable one or more of these systems may inhibit or restrict mobility. To ensure mobility and exercise are maximised and maintained, medical, nursing and allied health teams should devise care plans to meet individual needs and abilities based on the specific strengths and disabilities of each individual in their care.

Healthcare workers are in a unique position to educate and support people to make lifestyle changes for improvement in health and prevention of disease. Effective and timely health promotion can significantly contribute to the long-term physical and mental health of a person and potentially reduce disease progression and hospital readmission. For those with recurring mobility issues, nurses and allied health professionals can support the transition to mobility aids and promote independence and quality of life on discharge to home or an assisted facility. Nurses who promote and encourage mobility and movement play a significant role in the individual's healthcare experience, which can have a lasting impact on a person's recovery and rehabilitation, and benefit society with its positive outcomes.

LIVED EXPERIENCE

I wasn't particularly active in my younger years, but during COVID-19 lockdown, my arthritis played up and I found my joints were very stiff. I started making myself walk every day with my neighbour and found the stiffness got better, my mood was better and now I walk twice a day, every day.

Jesinda, 72 years old

INTRODUCTION

The skeletal system

The skeletal system is the internal framework that supports, shapes, protects and moves the human body. The bones that form the skeleton serve many functions. These functions include support of body shape, protection of organs, movement, storage of fat and minerals and **haematopoiesis** or blood cell formation in bone marrow. In order to understand the importance of the skeletal system, imagine performing a task such as running or throwing. If the bones required in this movement are disabled due to damage or pain, this activity becomes more challenging, if not impossible, to perform (Patton & Thibodeau 2019).

The muscular system

The muscular system enables body movement, joint stabilisation and maintenance of posture. The function of muscle is to contract or shorten (see Clinical Interest Box 28.1). Skeletal muscle attaches to bone and can rapidly contract to exert great power or fine movement under voluntary control. Muscles are supported by a network of connective tissue and tendons that anchor muscle to bone for strength and support. Skeletal muscle is classified by the kind of movement it makes. For example, flexors allow joints to bend or flex, while abductors allow shortening so

CLINICAL INTEREST BOX 28.1 Muscle coordination

The muscular system plays a vital role in maintaining correct body posture by means of good muscle tone and coordinated activity. Most skeletal muscles work in pairs or groups, with one pair or group antagonising the action of another pair or group to achieve controlled movement. For example, during elbow flexion, the triceps muscle relaxes to allow the forearm to be pulled up when the biceps muscle contracts. Extension of the arm is made possible by the relaxation of the biceps, as the triceps contracts and pulls on the arm. The erect position of the trunk is maintained as a result of coordination of groups of muscles.

(Marieb & Keller 2022; Patton & Thibodeau 2019)

that joints are straightened or abducted (moved away from the body). When muscle contracts it pulls on a bone or bones and produces movement at a joint, where two bones meet. As joints are weak points in the skeleton, synovial fluid, cartilage, ligaments and tendons add protection and support (Patton & Thibodeau 2019).

The nervous system

Muscle movements occur as a result of stimulation by a motor or efferent nerve. These nerves activate muscles to respond to voluntary signals, such as grasping an object or towel drying hair. Muscle can respond to voluntary control, those movements controlled by human thought, or to involuntary control through the autonomic nervous system (Marieb & Keller 2022). Transmission of the impulse from the nervous system to the musculoskeletal system requires a chemical transmitter to cross the myoneural junction. Acetylcholine transfers the electric impulse from the nerve to the muscle to stimulate muscle and initiate movement (Crisp et al 2021). An imbalance in this chemical neurotransmitter can result in impeded nerve transfer, which delays the potential for coordinated or rapid musculoskeletal response.

The co-dependent relationship between the skeletal, muscle and nervous system in body movement can be demonstrated in a person with a spinal cord injury. A lesion in the spinal cord inhibits nerve transmission beyond the point of injury. With no nerve impulse to contract or react, muscle lays dormant. While still providing shape and connection with the underlying bones, the posture cannot be supported and the bones are unable to mobilise due to absence of muscle contraction and voluntary stimulation (Marieb & Keller 2022).

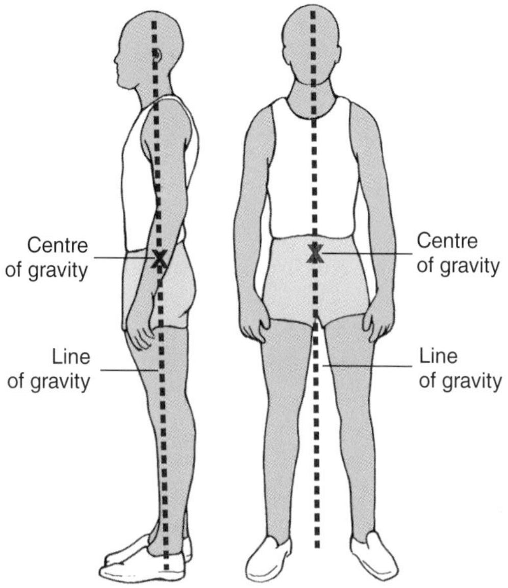

Figure 28.1 Body mechanics: Correct standing posture

(Crisp et al 2021)

BODY MECHANICS

Fatigue, muscle strain and injury can result from improper use or positioning of the body during activity or rest. Good posture is achieved when all parts of the body are in correct alignment when sitting, lying, standing or moving. Normal spinal curves should be maintained and the joints should be supported in their normal positions. Good posture and alignment reduces strain on all muscles and enables internal organs to function without interference (Figure 28.1). **Body mechanics** is the term used to describe the physical coordination of all parts of the body to promote correct posture and balanced effective movement. The practice of correct body mechanics results in less fatigue and reduces the risk of muscle and joint injury (Marieb & Keller 2022).

Protection of the musculoskeletal system is essential to ensure continuing ability to undertake activities of daily living (ADLs). Everyday activities including walking, showering, cooking and employment are dependent on a functioning and healthy body support system. Nurses, in their own activities and during instruction of an individual, must familiarise themselves with the mechanics of movement to protect themselves and assist the individual in movement and recovery.

The Australian Bureau of Statistics (ABS) National Health Survey 2017–2018 revealed that about 4 million Australians (16% of the population) have back problems (Australian Institute of Health and Welfare [AIHW] 2023). Backache may be a symptom of various health conditions, yet up to 80% of cases result from weak muscles in the abdominal, back and hip regions. These muscles reinforce spinal posture, and weakened or damaged muscles through inactivity or poor lifting techniques can result in pain, discomfort and even disability. To maintain a healthy back for optimal posture and mobility, weight control, daily exercise and correct alignment should be practised (Marieb & Keller 2022). (See Clinical Interest Box 28.2.)

CLINICAL INTEREST BOX 28.2 Protecting the back through correct body alignment

- Pull abdominal muscles inwards to support your back and counterbalance weight.
- Avoid high-heeled shoes because they change spinal alignment and increase stress on abdominal and back muscles.
- Stand straight with head and back aligned.
- Practise safe lifting techniques—wide stance with bent knees, hold load close to the body.
- Face the direction of movement, avoid twisting.
- Use other methods to move things, such as rolling, turning or pivoting.
- Include periods of rest into activities.
- Avoid sitting for long periods of time.
- Stretch for 10 minutes a day to strengthen abdominal muscles and stretch and loosen skeletal muscles.

(Adapted from Marieb & Keller 2022)

DISEASE PROCESSES THAT INFLUENCE BODY MECHANICS

Diseases of the bones and skeletal system

Osteoporosis

Osteoporosis is a condition in which the amount of bone tissue is reduced because the rate of bone deposition lags behind the rate of resorption. It may be progressive, temporary or permanent. Cancellous bone is usually affected before compact bone. Osteoporosis may be localised or occur throughout the skeleton. Bones become brittle and are susceptible to fractures. The factors that contribute to excessive bone loss include diminished oestrogen levels, immobility and lack of exercise, nutritional deficiencies and certain endocrine disorders. Manifestations include low back pain, kyphosis (rounded back) and spontaneous or pathological fractures from minor injuries (Cooper & Gosnell 2023).

Osteomalacia

Osteomalacia (also known as Paget's disease) is a metabolic disease of inadequate or delayed bone mineralisation. This results in bones becoming soft, bowed and prone to fractures. Paget's disease is found in people over 40 years of age. The disease is of unknown origin and characterised by hyperactivity of **osteoblasts** (bone forming cells) and **osteoclasts** (bone absorbing cells), with rapid turnover of bone tissue. Bones are soft, thick and enlarged and may 'bow'. Usually, the pelvis, long bones, lumbar vertebrae and skull are affected.

Tumours

Tumours of the bone may be benign, primary malignant or metastatic. **Benign tumours** may be single or multiple, or of several types. The most common benign form is giant-cell tumour, which is composed of multinucleate giant cells or osteoclasts. Individuals complain of pain and tenderness, with localised swelling. **Osteogenic sarcoma** is the most common primary malignant bone tumour. The areas most often affected are the ends of long bones, especially the distal femur or proximal tibia, and metastases may occur most commonly in the lungs. Bone tumours are characterised by the gradual onset of pain in a limb, or the sudden onset of pain after a minor injury to the limb, with a localised mass, swelling and limp in weight-bearing limbs. Fatigue is a common symptom. **Metastatic bone tumours** occur when cells of a malignant primary tumour in another part of the body enter the blood or lymph and are spread to the bone (Cooper & Gosnell 2023).

Osteomyelitis

Osteomyelitis is an acute or chronic infection involving bone, bone marrow and surrounding soft tissues. Acute osteomyelitis is characterised by rapid onset of severe pain in the involved bone, with local heat, swelling and inflammation as well as pyrexia, tachycardia, nausea and malaise. Chronic osteomyelitis is characterised by slight pyrexia, pain and persistent drainage of purulent material from a sinus tract injury (Cooper & Gosnell 2023; Marieb & Keller 2022).

Disorders of the joints and tendons

Rheumatoid arthritis

Rheumatoid arthritis (RA) is a chronic, systemic disease characterised by symmetrical inflammation of the synovial joint linings, with periods of remission and exacerbation. Joints most commonly affected are those of the wrists, hands and feet, but can affect hips, knees and elbows also. Primary signs and symptoms of RA are joint stiffness and swelling, pain and palpable warmth progressing to joint deformities due to joint capsule and surrounding connective tissue weakening. Systemic signs and symptoms include fever, fatigue and weight loss. Factors associated with poor outcomes in RA include older age, cigarette smoking, alcohol, diagnosis and treatment delays (Firestein et al 2021).

Osteoarthritis

Osteoarthritis is a degradative, non-infectious disease that causes pain and restricted movement (stiffness) of affected joints (Figure 28.2 A & B). Characterised by degeneration of joint cartilage, marginal bone hypertrophy and inflammatory changes within the joint capsule, osteoarthritis may be classified as primary (no predisposing cause) or secondary (caused by trauma or metabolic conditions for example). Risk factors predisposing an individual to development of the disease include age (older age), obesity, joint location (commonly weight-bearing joints), joint malalignment and trauma, genetic predisposition and sex (twice as likely to develop in women than men) (Firestein et al 2021).

Gout

Gout is a metabolic condition characterised by joint inflammation due to accumulation of sodium urate crystals in joints and tendons. Causes include a metabolic defect responsible for urate overproduction and decreased renal excretion of uric acid. Additionally, ingestion of purine rich foods (seafood and red meat), fructose and alcohol contribute to elevated serum urate levels. Commonly affected is the first metatarsophalangeal joint (big toe), which may result in tenderness, inflammation and development of a tophi (accumulation of uric acid crystals) (Firestein et al 2021).

Diseases of the muscles

Myasthenia gravis

Myasthenia gravis is an autoimmune disease of unknown origin. Defective muscle stimulation is caused by the development of antibodies that damage receptors in the neuromuscular junction, blocking impulses to muscle fibres. Progressive and extensive muscle weakness occurs,

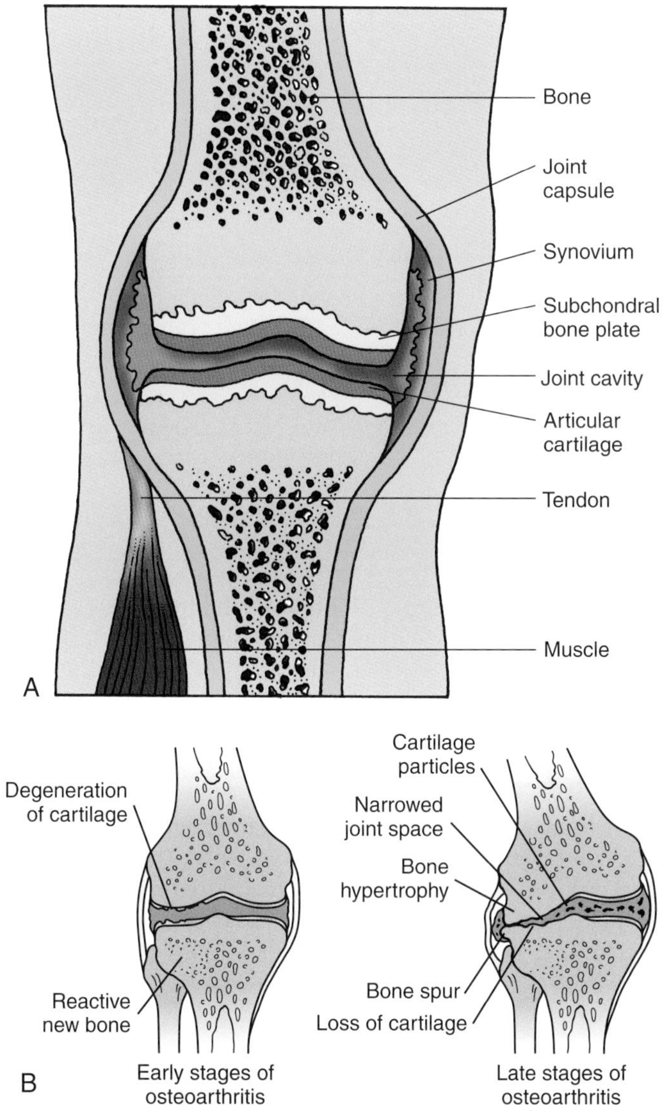

Figure 28.2 Pathological changes in osteoarthritis
A: Normal synovial joint, **B:** Deterioration of articular cartilage and new bone formation—smooth cartilage softens and loses its elasticity, progressing to complete wearing away of cartilage, reduced joint space and bone on bone contact.
(McHugh Pendleton & Schultz-Krohn 2018)

worsening over the day related to repeated muscle work. Muscle weakness differs amongst different muscle groups and individual muscles. Most frequently affected are extraocular muscles, muscles innervated by the cranial nerves and proximal muscles of the extremities. Remissions and relapses are precipitated by repeated or sustained exertion and fatigue, infections, emotional disturbances and pregnancy (Crisp et al 2021; Gilhus et al 2019).

Muscular dystrophies

Progressive **muscular dystrophies** are an inherited group of diseases in which there is severe, progressive degeneration of groups of muscles. The major differences between these types of conditions are age of onset, rate of progression and groups of muscles involved. For example, the Duchenne type is gender-linked (predominantly affecting males) and can present at age 2–3 years old as difficulty climbing stairs and frequent falls, escalating to the need for a wheelchair at age 10–12 years and ventilatory assistance at age 20 years (Crisp et al 2021; Duan et al 2021).

Diseases of the nervous system

Multiple sclerosis, Parkinson's disease and Huntington's disease are progressive neurological disorders that affect neurotransmission along motor pathways. With varying aetiology and signs and symptoms, these diseases affect voluntary and involuntary muscle groups and have long-term effects on gait, mobility and ability to independently undertake and complete ADLs (Cooper & Gosnell 2023; Crisp et al 2021; Marieb & Keller 2022).

DEVELOPMENT OF MOVEMENT AND EXERCISE THROUGH THE LIFESPAN

The provision of holistic care must consider individuals within the context of their life and development. A well-structured nursing care plan will incorporate growth and developmental changes, family and social support, and cultural, spiritual and ethnic influences that give a person's life meaning and purpose (Crisp et al 2021). To achieve this goal, nurses gather subjective and objective data. Identification of disorders of movement and mobility through systematic assessment of the individual contributes to the formulation of goals of care for the individual. The Comprehensive Care Standard (Australian Commission on Safety and Quality in Health Care [ACSQHC] 2021) aims to protect the public from harm and to improve the quality of health service provision. Nurses and allied health staff assess and identify existing conditions and formulate and deliver safe care based on a comprehensive care plan. The standard especially relates to pressure injuries and falls prevention, which are consequences of musculoskeletal disorders. Care is planned and implemented based on identified nursing diagnoses and development of goals that can be measured, achievable and relevant to human stages of development.

The body changes throughout the lifespan (see Table 28.1). Nurses encounter people in all stages and are in a perfect position to promote health and wellbeing to assist optimal performance, regardless of an individual's age, ability or co-existing medical conditions. The role of exercise in health and wellbeing has been found to have benefits for both people and society and should be practised by all. Not only can physical activity improve cardiorespiratory and muscular fitness but also promote emotional and mental health. Yet, resistance to movement and physical exertion is a well-documented phenomenon and has been proven to

TABLE 28.1 | Stages of development

Stage	Physical development
Infant	Flexible musculoskeletal system that matures to allow for movement from rolling to crawling and standing when lumbar spine matures.
Toddler	Swayback and protruding abdomen gives awkward appearance as legs and feet are splayed apart for balance when walking.
Preschool to adolescent	Greater coordination, skeletal growth and improved balance continue to adolescence when periods of rapid growth, sexual organ maturation and muscle development predominate.
Adult	Period of greatest strength, coordination and muscle/posture changes related to pregnancy.
Older adult	Bone density reduction related to inactivity, hormonal changes and bone tissue absorption result in weakening skeletal system with risk of fracture, injury and falls.

(Adapted from Hockenberry et al 2022)

contribute to low grade systemic inflammation and fat deposition, and has a negative effect on the management of chronic diseases such as diabetes mellitus, and cardiovascular disease (Cerasola et al 2022).

Regular physical activity is essential for health across the lifespan and research has proven that there is a relationship between parents and children's physical activity. Active parents can role model physical activity, either directly or indirectly, to their children, enhancing the child's own physical activity. Physical activity is also affected by neighbourhood environment, access to play spaces, parents' type of jobs and preferred sport (Matos et al 2021). (See Figure 28.3.)

Community strategies to improve children's health and wellbeing propose that environments support physical activity, and access to healthy food options be made available. Settings such as schools and hospitals should remove unhealthy food products and increase accessibility to healthy alternatives. Government initiatives should disincentivise unhealthy food and beverages, while making healthy options more affordable. Infrastructure to promote sport and recreation, such as bike and walking paths, sportsgrounds and facilities, encourages and allows children to participate in planned and incidental physical activity (Roberts et al 2018). (See Figure 28.4.)

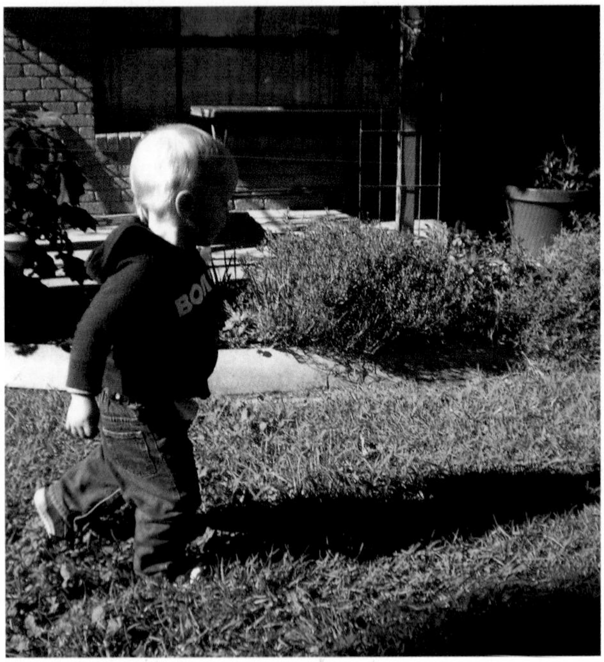

Figure 28.3 Toddler development and activity

(© Christine Ingram)

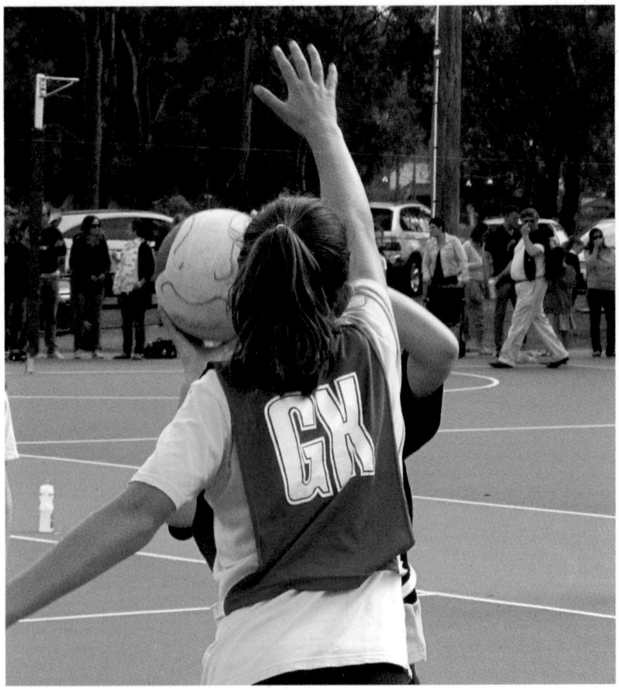

Figure 28.4 Child playing team sport

CRITICAL THINKING EXERCISE 28.1

The physical education teacher from the local secondary school is concerned about the number of overweight 13–15-year-old adolescents at the school who do not play sport regularly. He seeks your advice on how to engage these teenagers in participating in physical activity. As an Enrolled Nurse what strategies might you recommend?

The challenge to keep children active into adulthood may be lost post secondary school because a downward trend towards inactivity occurs (Crisp et al 2021). While community and government initiatives support increased activity, the stresses of work, family, money and time constraints can sometimes make participation a challenge. The World Health Organization (WHO 2022a) suggests that worldwide, one in four adults are not active enough and that insufficient physical activity contributes significantly to death worldwide.

The AIHW (2018) indicates that people over the age of 65 years spend less time on physical activity, and more time sitting, than those under the age of 65 years. These findings demonstrate that older Australians need to increase their activity and movement levels. Not only because of the immediate benefits, but because of the associated health issues that **sedentary** behaviour intensifies. Sitting or lying down for reasons other than sleeping are considered sedentary behaviours (Department of Health & Aged Care 2021b). Surprisingly, a Commonwealth Scientific and Industrial Research Organisation (CSIRO) study revealed that Australians' diet score increases above average in the 71+ age bracket, considering physical activity declines (CSIRO 2022). A score closer to 100 reflects better compliance with CSIRO dietary guidelines and a higher-quality diet. Physical inactivity increases the risk of a range of diseases, such as cardiovascular disease, type 2 diabetes mellitus and some cancers (AIHW 2017).

OVERWEIGHT AND OBESITY IN AUSTRALIA

In 2014–2015, over 63% of Australians aged 18 years and over were considered overweight or obese (ABS 2018a). **Overweight** and **obesity** are defined as abnormal or excessive fat accumulation that may impair health (WHO 2021). In 2016, 39% of people aged 18 years and over were overweight, and 13% were obese (WHO 2021).

Childhood obesity is of particular concern because of its predisposition to weight-related diseases. In 2014–2015, around one in four (27.4%) children aged 5–17 years were overweight or obese (ABS 2018b). Overweight children are more likely to develop disorders such as sleep apnoea, breathlessness, hypertension and type 2 diabetes mellitus, and are more likely to become overweight or obese in adult life. Parents have influence over their child's dietary behaviours and physical activity levels. Nurses need to be aware of the impact of poor dietary behaviours and inactivity, and work in conjunction with the individual and their family to rectify them (Crisp et al 2021). Clinical Interest Box 28.3 provides an outline of some self-care behaviours and exercises.

CLINICAL INTEREST BOX 28.3 Self-care behaviours and exercise

- Make the most of opportunities for exercise—use stairs, park a kilometre away from work or walk to work once or twice a week, walk faster and use lunchtimes for exercise.
- Choose an enjoyable physical activity and participate regularly.
- Plan three to four exercise activities per week.
- Before starting exercise sessions, ensure medical clearance if in a high-risk group.
- Alternate different types of exercise to keep interest up (e.g. Pilates followed by weight-training sessions then walking or bike riding).
- Invite a friend to walk or join a health club or gym.
- Build up exercise sessions gradually to avoid over-exertion.
- Keep it simple—gradually increase your exercise time and activity.

(Adapted from Goldman & Schafer 2019)

Fit versus fat

Obesity and fitness may be considered polar opposites, but can an individual be fit and 'fat'? A recent study by Lassale et al (2018) hypothesised that an individual could be metabolically healthy and obese. Results from the study showed that metabolically unhealthy individuals have a higher risk of cardiovascular disease than healthy individuals *and*, regardless of metabolic health, overweight and obese individuals have a higher risk than lean individuals of cardiovascular disease (Lassale et al 2018).

THE BENEFITS OF PHYSICAL ACTIVITY

Participation in regular exercise can enhance the life of individuals, families, community groups and society. (See Figure 28.5.) At least 30 minutes of moderate exercise (or 150–300 minutes per week) is recommended and provides considerable health benefits (Department of Health & Aged Care 2021a).

Physical activity has been proven to have many positive effects on the physiology of ageing. Lack of exercise has been linked to cardiovascular diseases including coronary artery disease, metabolic syndrome (obesity/hypertension/

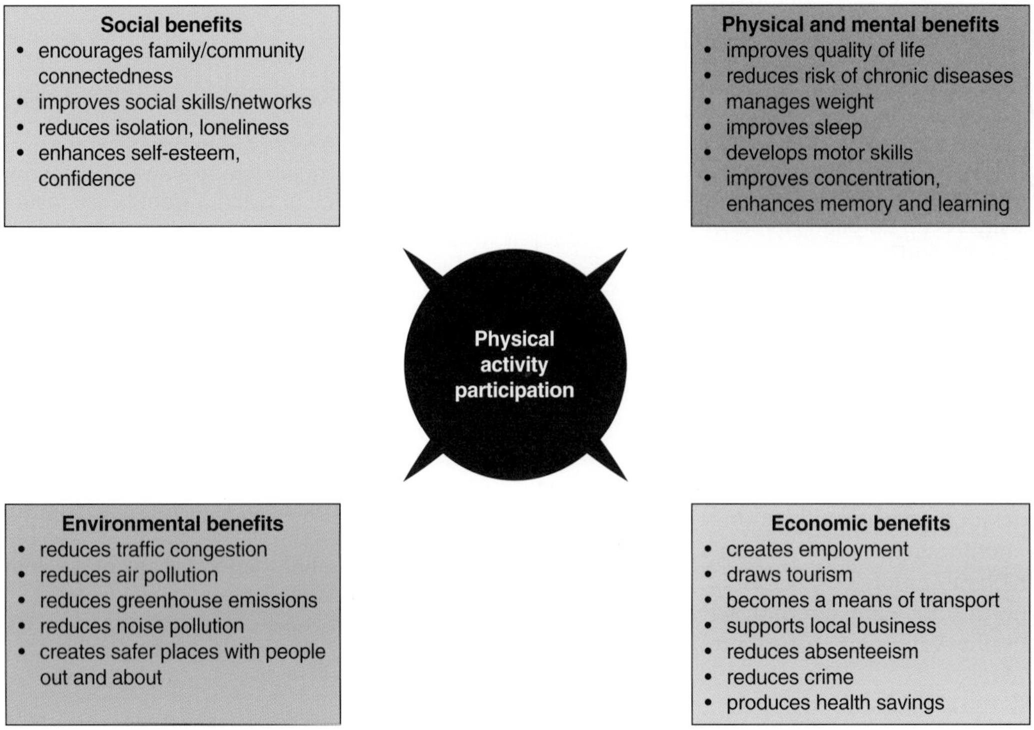

Social benefits
• encourages family/community connectedness
• improves social skills/networks
• reduces isolation, loneliness
• enhances self-esteem, confidence
Physical and mental benefits
• improves quality of life
• reduces risk of chronic diseases
• manages weight
• improves sleep
• develops motor skills
• improves concentration, enhances memory and learning
Physical activity participation
Environmental benefits
• reduces traffic congestion
• reduces air pollution
• reduces greenhouse emissions
• reduces noise pollution
• creates safer places with people out and about
Economic benefits
• creates employment
• draws tourism
• becomes a means of transport
• supports local business
• reduces absenteeism
• reduces crime
• produces health savings

Figure 28.5 Benefits of physical activity

(© The State of Queensland [Queensland Health] 1996–2016)

hyperglycaemia/hyperlipidaemia/low high density lipoproteins), loss of muscle mass (**sarcopenia**), muscle strength (**dynapenia**) and low bone mineral density (**osteopenia**). Exercise contributes to cognitive performance and mood, reduces stress, anger and anxiety and improves overall physical performance (Xiao 2020).

Exercise and the older adult

Exercise is linked to many and varied health benefits including cardiac and respiratory health; increased bone and muscle health; increased resistance to type 2 diabetes mellitus, cancer and depression; and improved cognitive function (Lachman et al 2018). Exercise improves cardiopulmonary fitness, strength, coordination, mental health, motor control and cognitive function. Improved flexibility, balance and muscle tone can help prevent falls (Figure 28.6).

Physical activity is important across all ages and can be integrated into everyday activities. Physical activity can be considered formal, such as structured exercise (walking, cycling, dance) or informal (such as cleaning, carrying, lifting). Individuals benefit from regular physical activity to maintain not only physical, social and mental health, and an active society reduces fossil fuel usage and promotes safer roads and cleaner air (WHO 2018).

Falls risk

Individuals who are at greatest risk for falls are those who may be frail, confused, be in an unfamiliar environment, have comorbidities (such as arthritis, dementia or cardiovascular conditions), have a visual impairment, urinary incontinence and known mobility problems. Other factors that determine whether an individual is at risk for a fall are whether they have a history of falls, polypharmacy and issues such as a cluttered environment or inappropriate footwear.

Individuals should be assessed for falls risk upon admission to a healthcare facility, daily as part of a care plan and after a fall or change in health status. Several falls assessment tools exist, and the best preventative measure to reduce the risk of a fall is to comprehensively assess an individual, minimise intrinsic and extrinsic factors that may contribute to one and involve other members of the multidisciplinary healthcare team (Flynn & Mercer 2018). (See also Chapter 15.)

Physical inactivity and Aboriginal and Torres Strait Islander communities

Physical inactivity is one of the six risk factors that contributes to disease burden in Aboriginal and Torres Strait Islander Peoples. Even considering the evidence that exercise protects against diseases such as obesity, cardiovascular disease and diabetes mellitus, physical inactivity in Aboriginal and Torres Strait Islander populations contributes to a reduced life expectancy of 8.4% in comparison to the non-Aboriginal and Torres Strait Islander population (Dahlberg et al 2018).

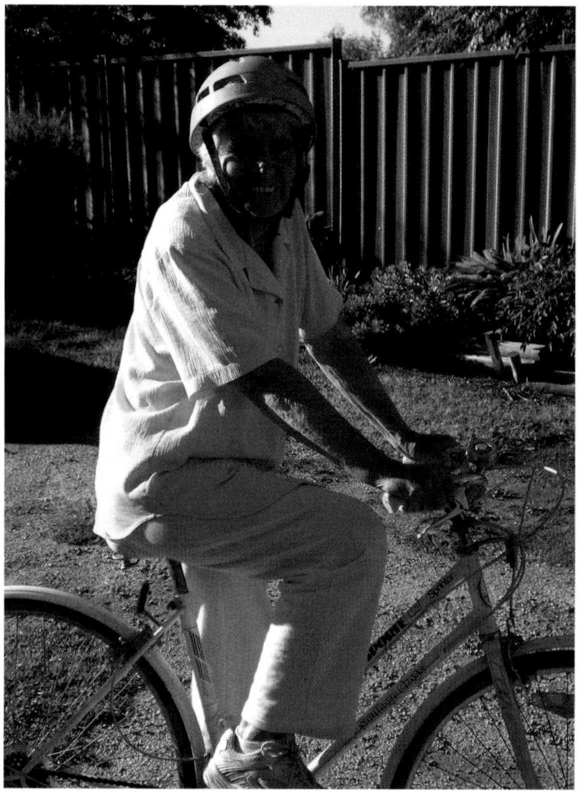

Figure 28.6 Regular activity creates a sense of health and wellbeing

(© Dorothy Lanyon)

Finding exercise to suit the individual

Like any activity that humans undertake, exercise must be enjoyable or rewarding if commitment is to be assured. While some are motivated by weight loss or muscle definition, others may be encouraged by improvement in mood, freedom of movement or cardiovascular fitness.

New Australian physical activity guidelines recommend that doing any physical activity is better than doing none. Guidelines recommend 150–300 minutes per week of moderate physical activity (e.g. brisk walking or swimming) or 75–150 minutes per week of vigorous physical activity (e.g. jogging or aerobics), or an equivalent combination of both. Guidelines also suggest an individual be active most days, perform muscle strengthening activities at least 2 days per week and minimise prolonged sitting time (Department of Health & Aged Care 2021a). (See Figure 28.7.)

Movement and exercise should form part of any treatment program for individuals with neurological disorders. **Parkinson's disease** is a progressive neurodegenerative disease caused by dopamine depletion in the brain (Buttaro et al 2020). Characteristic motor symptoms of Parkinson's disease include risk of falling due to loss of balance and freezing of gait. Strength training and task-specific exercise can improve mobility, strength and balance in individuals with Parkinson's disease. Specifically, a combination of strategy (interventions that may enhance stability), strength training and behavioural modification (i.e. ensuring correct

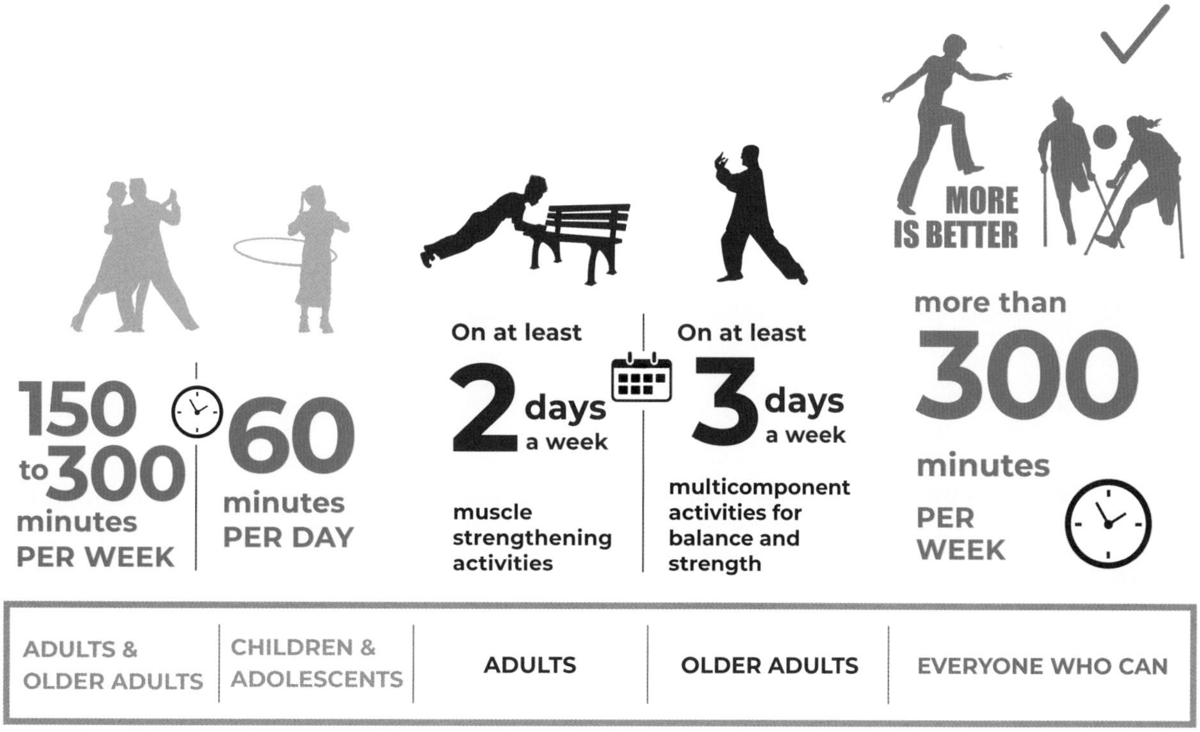

Figure 28.7 Recommended physical activity

(© WHO 2022b)

footwear) can reduce the risk of falling in individuals prone to falling and increase fitness as well (Lennon et al 2018).

Benefits of physical activity in the older adult include increased motor fitness and independence, social engagement, cognitive stimulation and prevention of disease. However, normal ageing is often accompanied with deterioration in motor and functional skills. The ability to engage in physical activity may be impacted by intrinsic (related to health problems, attitude, lack of motivation) and/or extrinsic (lack of transport, availability of physical activity program, culture) factors (Buckinx et al 2022; Cordes et al 2019). In an aged-care home, lifestyle is often sedentary and many individuals are incapable of participating in active exercise due to increased risk of fall, lack of expert staff and appropriate equipment and the individual's inability to move. Bed rest leads to the development of cardiovascular disease due to decreased hydrostatic pressure, reduction in plasma volume and reduction of blood flow to the organs and limbs. The use of passive exercise (such as passive knee flexion and extension) has been found to improve blood flow and stimulate vasculature, thus preventing complications from stasis and vascular disease (Pedrinolla et al 2022). (See Case Study 28.1 and Clinical Interest Box 28.4.)

CRITICAL THINKING EXERCISE 28.2

Working as an Enrolled Nurse in an aged-care home, you are concerned that one of the new residents is becoming less active since moving into the facility. Outline the steps you could take to facilitate the resident attending a scheduled exercise class.

PRINCIPLES OF MUSCLE MOVEMENT IN EXERCISE

Isotonic exercise

Isotonic exercise involves muscle shortening and active contraction and relaxation of muscles. Isotonic activity occurs with movement, such as carrying out ADLs, independent **range-of-movement (ROM)** flexing exercises, swimming, walking, running, cycling or jogging.

CASE STUDY 28.1

Lorenzo Durutto is an 87-year-old man with limited English. He has dense right hemiplegia and requires a shower after an incontinent episode. The care plan states he requires transferring using a hoist. You are an agency nurse, unfamiliar with the hoists used in this aged-care home; however, Lorenzo is becoming increasingly impatient and upset.

1. State what nursing care is priority at this time.
2. Outline how you will transfer this individual to a commode chair.
3. List other assessments you will make of Lorenzo while transferring and attending to his hygiene.

CLINICAL INTEREST BOX 28.4 To facilitate chair-based exercises

- Ensure person goes to the toilet before the exercise session.
- Administer analgesia prior to or after an exercise session.
- Plan exercise into daily activities.
- Educate the person about the benefits of the exercise and what is to be expected.
- Dress the individual appropriately for exercise.
- Ensure the individual is positioned safely to exercise and that there is no risk of falling.
- Use a variety of techniques to teach the exercise, such as repetition, demonstration and one-on-one assistance.
- Ensure the individual can see and/or hear the exercise instructor.

(Adapted from Crisp et al 2021)

Isometric exercise

Isometric exercise involves muscle contraction without shortening of the muscle length. These exercises build muscle bulk and are a popular muscle activity for bodybuilders (e.g. lifting weights).

Isokinetic exercise

Isokinetic exercise causes muscle contraction, shortening and relaxation at an even speed. Isokinetic movement occurs during swimming as arms move evenly through water resistance (Marieb & Keller 2022).

CRITICAL THINKING EXERCISE 28.3

Jenny is preparing for discharge post foot surgery and is concerned that the prescribed restriction in activity may cause a decline in her overall health and wellbeing. Using the above principles of exercise, create a simple program for Jenny to follow.

Encouraging maintenance and restoration of muscle strength

As communities become increasingly sedentary, the cost is reflected in the calibre of individuals in the healthcare system. With increasing numbers of cases of osteoporosis and arthritis requiring in-hospital care, nurses may frequently find themselves caring for immobilised or physically disabled people. To aid return to mobility after the acute care phase, provision of movement activities is essential to prevent long-term complications sustained during immobility. Until this stage, nurses should undertake muscle and joint movement. Using the principles of muscle movement, a range of exercises can be incorporated into everyday situations to enhance the individual's health and recovery (Crisp et al 2021):

- Isotonic bed exercises: These exercises have visible joint movement, constant weight and variable speed. Examples of isotonic exercise are pushing or pulling against a stationary object, using a trapeze to lift the body off the bed, lifting the buttocks off the bed by pushing with the hands against the mattress and pushing the body to a sitting position.
- Isometric bed exercises: Isometric exercise generates muscle force with no visible joint movement (such as a quadriceps extension: push knee into mattress while attempting to lift heel off bed to strengthen thigh muscles). Other examples may include lifting of hand weights and gripping of tennis ball to aid arm strength and mobility. Benefits of isotonic and isometric exercise include increase in muscle tone, mass and strength, improved joint mobility, increased circulation and osteoblastic activity.
- Isokinetic bed exercises: Isokinetic exercise has visible joint movement, variable external resistance and constant speed. Examples include rehabilitative exercises for knee and elbow injuries. In this case, isokinetic devices are used to take muscles and joints through a complete ROM without stopping, with resistance at each point. Mechanical devices are available for specific joints, which place these joints through continuous passive ROM, encouraging maintenance of joint mobility.

Joints are capable of a wide ROM or motion (Figure 28.8). ROM or motion exercises are either **active**, when the individual is able to move the joints themselves, or **passive**, when the nurse moves the individual's joints within the normal ROM, noting joint flexibility and/or limitations of movement. Joints that are not moved regularly can develop contractures (shortening of a muscle and, eventually, ligaments and tendons, with eventual loss of function). It must be remembered that when a nurse performs passive ROM exercises in which a person's muscles do not exert effort, some of the potential benefits are reduced in favour of improved joint mobility and circulation (Cooper & Gosnell 2023; Cuccurullo et al 2021).

The frequency with which ROM exercises are performed depends on the individual's condition and medical and nursing management, but they are commonly performed at least twice daily. However, it is important not to overtire the person partaking in the exercises. ROM exercises may be performed independently or with assistance. Using appropriate movements, all joints are exercised in a logical sequence. Exercise routines are normally individually designed and the intensity and frequency depend upon a person's general condition, level of fitness and capabilities (Crisp et al 2021).

ASSESSMENT OF MOVEMENT, MOBILITY AND THE MUSCULOSKELETAL SYSTEM

Undertaking a systematic assessment of an individual will identify issues of movement and mobility. After prioritising care by applying first aid and pain management measures prior to examination, the nurse should obtain a musculoskeletal medical history that includes:

- activity and exercise level prior to hospital presentation
- past history of muscle and joint pain or injury
- current treatment for existing muscle and joint pain or injury, including medications, physiotherapy, osteopathy, chiropractic or other complementary therapies
- presenting problem including details of injury, cause of injury, symptoms, duration and treatment received (if hospital presentation is due to a musculoskeletal condition)
- recent changes in mobility or movement unrelated to current hospital presentation
- use of aids for mobility.

On completion of verbal data collection, a physical examination should be undertaken to provide a baseline for ongoing assessment and completion of a management or care plan. Identifying current and potential movement and mobility issues will tailor treatment needs and identify potential discharge issues. A physical assessment will incorporate observation of gait and posture, pain and nerve changes, limb deformities, neurovascular assessment and spinal conditions including congenital and acquired pain or abnormalities (Crisp et al 2021).

See Clinical Skill 28.1 for information and guidelines on assisting with transfer.

Gait

Gait describes the manner of walking and, while varying from one person to another, there is normally a certain rhythm to a person's walk. Gait abnormalities may occur when there is a disorder of the musculoskeletal or nervous system (e.g. unilateral hip dislocation produces a distinct 'waddle' with each step). A staggering, or ataxic, gait may be caused by a lesion in the brain or spinal cord, and a 'scissors' gait is one in which the legs cross each other in progression. An abnormal gait may also result from pain or discomfort due to a lesion on the foot, such as a corn, or from ill-fitting and uncomfortable shoes (Crisp et al 2021).

Pain and nerve (sensory) changes

Pain is a common symptom of musculoskeletal disorders, as a result of trauma, inflammation, haematoma formation, tissue anoxia, tissue degeneration and pressure. People may describe the pain as mild, aching, severe, burning or throbbing, and it may be localised or generalised, depending on the specific disorder. Pain may increase with movement, be exacerbated by changes in external temperature and relieved by rest. It may be worse at certain times (e.g. joint

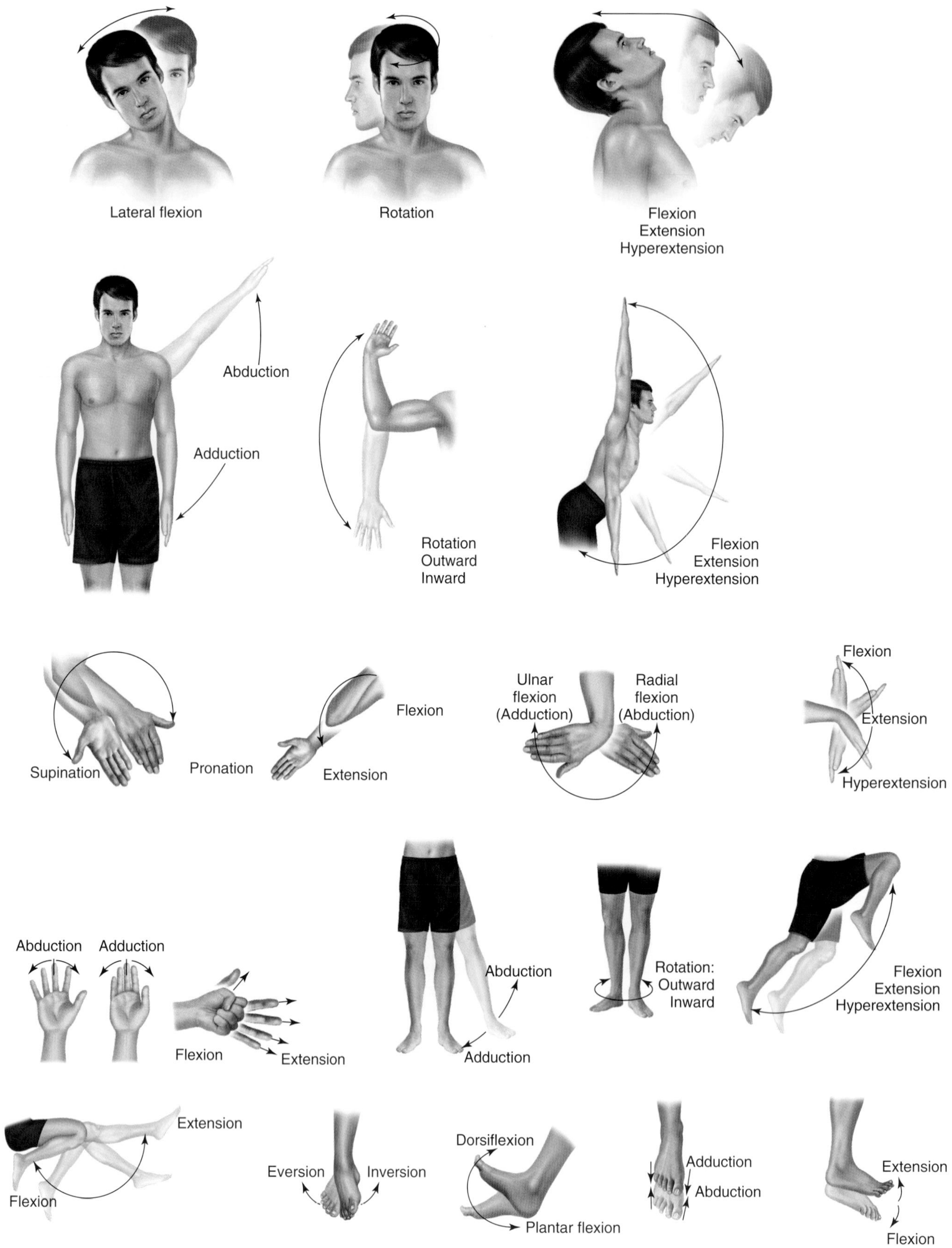

Figure 28.8 Range of joint movement

(Fig. 28.4 from Yoost & Crawford 2019)

CLINICAL SKILL 28.1 Assisting with transfer

Please adhere to the policy and procedures of the facility/organisation prior to undertaking the skill. Ensure this skill is in your scope of practice.

NMBA Decision-making Framework considerations (refer to NMBA Decision-making framework for nursing and midwifery 2020):	Equipment (as needed):
1. Am I educated? 2. Am I authorised? 3. Am I competent? If you answer 'no' to any of these, do not perform that activity. Seek guidance and support from your teacher/a nurse team leader/clinical facilitator/educator.	Transfer belt Sling Lap board Slide sheet Mechanical/hydraulic lift

PREPARE FOR THE SKILL

(Please refer to the Standard Steps on pp. xviii–xx for related rationales.)
Mentally review the steps of the skill.
Discuss the skill with your instructor/supervisor/team leader, if required.
Confirm correct facility/organisation policy/safe operating procedures.
Validate the order in the individual's record.
Identify indication and rationale for performing the activity.
Assess for any contraindications.
Locate and gather equipment.
Perform hand hygiene.
Ensure therapeutic interaction.
Identify the individual using three individual identifiers.
Gain the individual's consent.
Assess for pain relief.
Prepare the environment.
Provide and maintain privacy.
Assist the individual to assume an appropriate position of comfort.

Skill activity	Rationale
Assess the individual for: • joint mobility • presence of paralysis or paresis • activity tolerance • orthostatic blood pressure • level of consciousness • pain level • ability to follow instructions.	Provides information regarding the individual's ability to transfer and the number of people required to assist.

PERFORM THE SKILL

(Please refer to the Standard Steps on pp. xviii–xx for related rationales.)
Perform hand hygiene.
Apply PPE: gloves, eyewear, mask and gown as appropriate.
Ensure the individual's safety and comfort throughout skill.
Promote independence and involvement of the individual if possible and/or appropriate.
Assess the individual's tolerance to the skill throughout.
Dispose of used supplies, equipment, waste and sharps appropriately.
Remove PPE and discard or store appropriately.
Perform hand hygiene.

Skill activity	Rationale
Assisting individual into sitting position on side of bed	
With the individual in a supine position, raise the head of bed to 30 degrees.	Decreases amount of work required by the individual and nurse to raise person to a sitting position.

Continued

CLINICAL SKILL 28.1 Assisting with transfer—cont'd	
Where possible, the individual should be encouraged to move into the position themselves.	Decreases amount of work needed by individual and nurse to raise person to a sitting position.
Turn the individual to the side, facing nurse on the side of bed on which the individual will be sitting.	Prepares the individual to move to the side of bed and protects the individual from falling.
Stand opposite to the individual's hips and turn diagonally to face the individual and the far corner of foot of bed.	Places nurse's centre of gravity near to individual. Reduces twisting.
Place feet apart with foot closer to head of bed in front of other foot.	Increases balance and allows nurse to transfer weight as individual is brought to sitting position on side of bed.
Place arm nearer head of bed under individual's shoulder, supporting head and neck.	Maintains alignment of head and neck as nurse brings individual to sitting position.
Place other arm over individual's thighs.	Supports hip and prevents individual from falling backwards during procedure.
Move individual's lower legs and feet over side of bed. Pivot towards rear leg, allowing the individual's upper legs to swing downwards.	Decreases friction and resistance. Weight of individual's legs when off bed provides gravity to lower legs, and weight of leg helps pull upper body into a sitting position.
At same time, shift weight to rear leg and elevate individual.	Allows nurse to transfer weight in direction of motion.
Remain in front of the individual until they regain balance.	Reduces risk of falling.
Transfer individual from bed to chair	
Adjust the bed so that it is slightly higher than the chair. Assist the individual to a sitting position on side of the bed. Have chair in position at 45-degree angle to the bed and ensure the brakes are on.	Positions chair within easy access for transfer.
Apply transfer belt or other transfer aids if required.	Reduces risk of falling.
Ensure individual has stable, non-skid shoes. Weight-bearing or stronger leg is placed forwards with weaker foot back.	Decreases risk of slipping. Bare feet increases risk of falls.
Spread feet apart.	Ensures balance with wide base of support.
Flex hips and knees, aligning feet and knees with individual's feet.	Flexion of knees and hips lowers nurse's centre of gravity to object to be raised; aligning knees with individual allows for stabilisation of knees when individual stands.
Grasp transfer belt from underneath, if used, or reach through individual's axillae and place hands on individual's scapulae.	Transferring individual with hands on scapulae reduces pressure on axillae and maintains the individual's stability. Transfer belt is grasped at each side to provide movement of individual at centre of gravity.
Rock individual up to standing position on count of three while straightening hips and legs and keeping knees slightly flexed. Individual is instructed to use hands to push up if possible.	Rocking motion gives individual body momentum and requires less muscular effort to transfer individual.
Maintain stability of individual's weak or paralysed leg with knee.	Ability to stand can often be maintained in paralysed or weak limb with support of knee to stabilise.
Pivot on foot further from chair.	Maintains support of individual while allowing adequate space for individual to move.
Instruct the individual to use armrests on chair for support and ease themselves into chair.	Increases individual's stability.

CLINICAL SKILL 28.1 Assisting with transfer—cont'd

Flex hips and knees while lowering individual into chair.	Prevents injury to nurse from poor body mechanics.
Assess the individual for proper alignment for sitting position. Provide support for paralysed extremities. Lap board or sling will support flaccid arm. Stabilise leg with bath blanket or pillow.	Prevents injury to individual from poor body alignment.
Praise individual's progress, effort and performance.	Continued support and encouragement provides incentive for individuals.
Use mechanical/hydraulic lift to transfer individual from bed to chair (two nurses)	
Assess the individual's mobility and strength.	To determine whether the individual can offer help during transfer.
Bring lift to bedside. Before using lift, be familiar with its operation. Check hoist sling, straps, hooks and chains in safe working order.	Prepares environment for safe use of lift and subsequent transfer.
Position chair near bed and allow adequate space to manoeuvre hoist.	Prepares environment for safe use of lift and subsequent transfer.
Raise bed to safe working height with mattress flat. Lower side rails.	Allows nurse to use proper body mechanics.
Roll the individual towards one nurse.	Positions individual for use of lift sling.
Place sling evenly under individual's back (follow manufacturer's guidelines) and roll individual to opposite side to position sling.	Places sling under individual's centre of gravity and greatest portion of body weight.
Roll individual supine on sling and position hoist over individual. Lower boom and attach sling to frame with the head end attached first. Raise individual's knees and feed the leg sections of the sling under the thighs and attach to frame.	Sling should extend from shoulders to knees to support individual's body weight equally.
Elevate head of bed.	Positions individual in sitting position.
Ask or assist the individual to fold arms over the chest.	To prevent injury during transfer.
Pump hydraulic handle using long, slow, even strokes, or activate electronic hoist until individual is raised off bed ensuring the head is supported.	
Using steering handle to move, lift from bed and manoeuvre to the chair. Slowly lower the individual onto chair.	Moves individual from bed to chair.
Detach sling from frame and remove hoist. Pull leg straps to the side, tilt the individual forwards to slide out the sling.	Safely guides individual into back of chair as seat descends.
Reposition the individual to a comfortable and safe position.	

AFTER THE SKILL

(Please refer to the Standard Steps on pp. xviii–xx for related rationales.)
Communicate outcome to the individual, any ongoing care and to report any complications .
Restore the environment.
Report, record and document assessment findings, details of the skill performed and the individual's response.
Report, record and document any abnormalities and/or inability to perform the skill.
Reassess the individual to ensure there are no adverse effects/events from the skill.

(Crisp et al 2021; Rebeiro et al 2021; Tollefson & Hillman 2022)

discomfort from degenerative disease is often worse in the evenings). Numbness, tingling and lack of sensation are other sensory changes. Swelling from injury or tumours may cause pressure on nerves, resulting in loss of sensation (LeMone et al 2020).

Swelling, deformity and impaired mobility

Swelling of an affected area may be the result of the formation of inflammatory exudate in response to injury from physical trauma, chemicals or infection. Swelling will also occur when blood is lost from the circulation into surrounding tissues (haematoma) (e.g. after a fracture). A joint may become swollen if there is an increase in the amount of synovial fluid or if blood or purulent discharge is present in the joint capsule. Deformity may be the result of growths, fractures, dislocations, abnormal curvature of the spine or contractures. The effects of a deformity include changes in range of joint motion, posture and gait. Mobility may be impaired to such an extent that the individual is unable to move without pain or unable to carry out ADLs, or it may only restrict mobility at certain times, such as after activity, or be related to certain positions. (See Figure 28.9.)

Sprains

A **sprain** is a stretch and/or tear injury to a ligament, caused when a joint is forced beyond its normal ROM. A ligament may be stretched or torn partially or completely and local bleeding and bruising present with restricted movement and/or joint instability. Sprains commonly occur in the wrist and ankle. Treatment is aimed at resting, elevating and supporting the area and reducing pain and inflammation with anti-inflammatory medications (LeMone et al 2020).

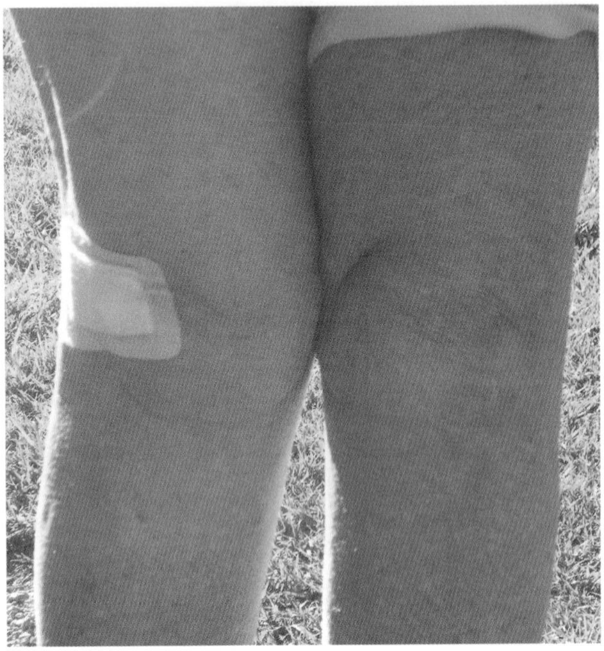

Figure 28.9 Knee joint deformity caused by osteoarthritis

(© Dorothy Lanyon)

Strains

A **strain** is a stretching injury to a muscle and/or a tendon, resulting from excessive physical effort. Both sprains and strains cause pain, limited motion and swelling, but strains may cause muscle spasm as well. Nurses can suffer strain injuries from incorrect manual handling techniques such as lifting (Cooper & Gosnell 2023; Crisp et al 2021).

Fractures

A **fracture** is a broken bone, often with nearby soft tissue, blood vessel and nerve damage. A stress fracture occurs when a bone is subjected to repeated or prolonged stress such as jogging. A pathological fracture may occur in weakened bone as a result of osteoporosis. Fractures are classified as open or closed, simple or complicated. Open (or compound) fractures are those in which the bone breaks through the skin, while closed fractures are those where the skin is intact. In a simple fracture only the bone is involved, while in complicated fractures nearby blood vessels, nerves or organs are affected. Table 28.2 and Figure 28.10 demonstrate and

TABLE 28.2 | Types of fractures

Type	Description
Greenstick	The fracture is incomplete and does not extend through the bone. The bone bends, and splits or cracks on one side.
Transverse	The fracture line is straight across the bone.
Oblique	The fracture line is at an angle across the bone.
Spiral	The fracture line coils around the bone. This type of fracture generally results from twisting of the limb.
Impacted	The fragments of broken bone are pushed (telescoped) into each other.
Comminuted	The bone is broken into a number of fragments.
Depressed	The broken edges are pushed below the level of the rest of the bone. This type of injury may occur when the skull is fractured.
Avulsion	A fragment of bone, connected to a ligament, breaks off from the rest of the bone.
Intracapsular	The fracture is within the joint capsule.
Extracapsular	The fracture is close to a joint, but is outside the joint capsule.

(Adapted from Crisp et al 2021; Marieb & Keller 2022; Patton & Thibodeau 2019)

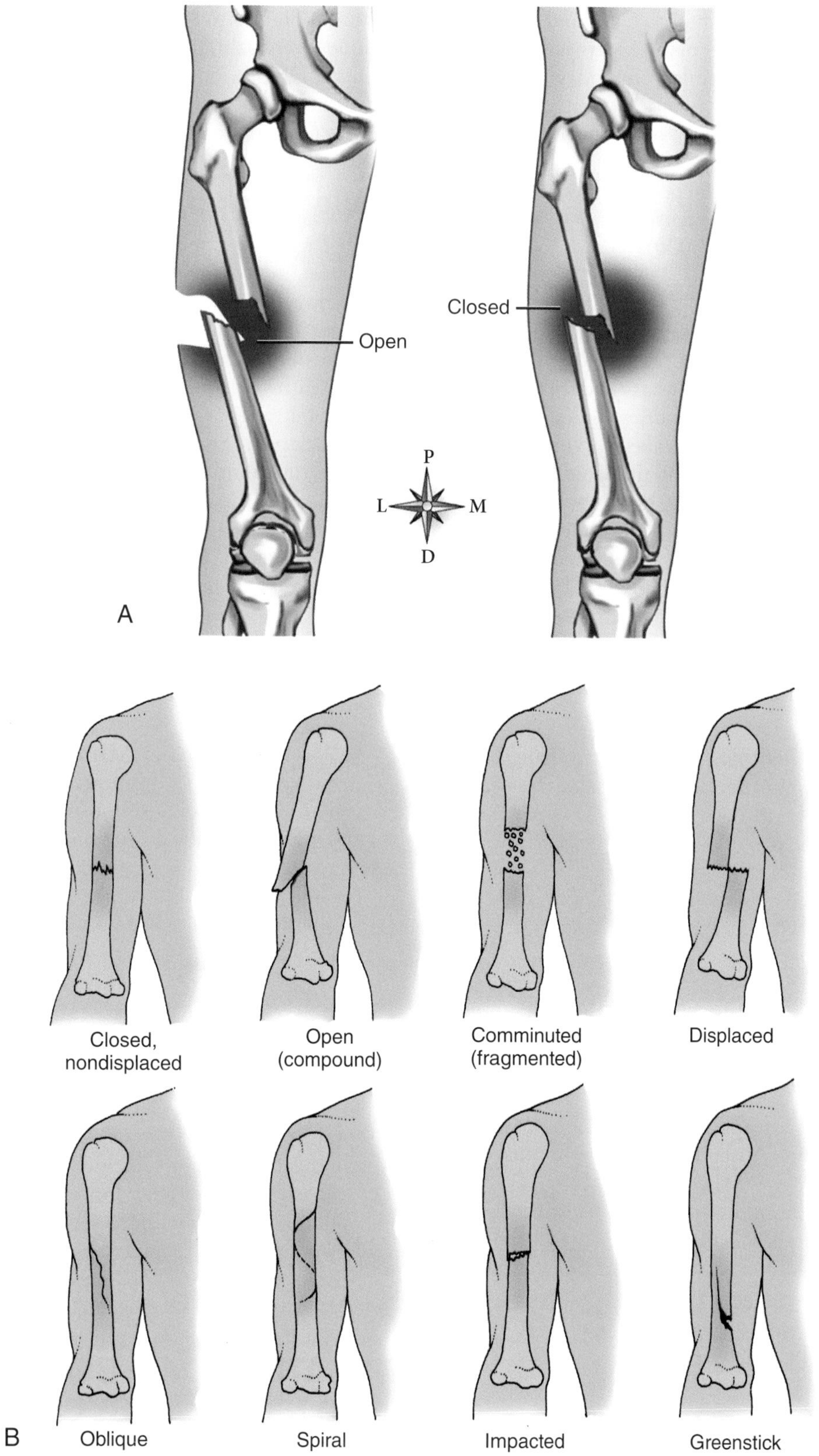

Figure 28.10 Types of fractures

A: Open and closed fracture, **B:** Common types of fractures.

*(**A:** Williamson et al 2024 **B:** Cooper & Gosnell 2023)*

describe the various types of fractures. Signs and symptoms vary but usually encompass pain/tenderness, swelling, muscle spasm, bruising, deformity, numbness, guarding, abnormal mobility and loss of function. Crepitus (grating caused by bone fragments rubbing together or entrance of air into an open fracture) may be heard on examination or experienced and described by the person. Shock may occur as a result of haemorrhage or extensive damage (Patton & Thibodeau 2019; LeMone et al 2020).

Neurovascular assessment

A neurovascular assessment is performed on people who have experienced a fracture, have been fitted with a cast, have undertaken vascular surgery or have had spinal surgery. Neurovascular protocols vary depending on the individual's diagnosis and treatment undertaken. Nurses should familiarise themselves with neurovascular guidelines within their place of work. For example, a person with a fracture should have neurovascular observations undertaken every hour for 24 hours, then every 4–8 hours if fitted with a cast. The 5 Ps (pain, paraesthesia, pallor, pulses and paresis) may indicate neurovascular deterioration (Berman et al 2020; LeMone et al 2020).

Assessment must be undertaken by the primary care nurse at the commencement and throughout the shift to identify early changes that can indicate a pathological deterioration. Inability to recognise significant changes in a timely manner may influence an individual's potential for recovery and rehabilitation. A neurovascular assessment should include inspection of:

- *Skin:* Inspect area distal to the injury; inspect for skin discolouration and palpate skin temperature with the back of the hand and compare with the opposite extremity or site.
- *Movement:* Have the person move the area distal to the injury, or move it passively; there should be no discomfort.
- *Sensation:* Enquire about feelings of numbness or tingling; check sensation with a paper clip and compare bilaterally—sensation should be the same.
- *Pulses:* Palpate pulses distal to the injury; compare bilaterally.
- *Capillary refill*: Check this in the nail beds distal to the injury. Capillary refill should occur within 3 seconds and within 5 seconds in the older adult.
- *Pain:* Enquire about the degree, location, nature and frequency of pain, noting any increase in intensity or change in the type of pain.

(Williams 2021)

(See Chapter 35.)

Dislocation

Dislocation is complete displacement and subluxation is partial displacement of a joint's articulating surfaces; both processes damage surrounding soft tissue structures. Joint effusion is the accumulation of synovial fluid in a joint and occurs if blood vessels in the synovium are damaged. Joint effusions may result from severe sprains, dislocations or fractures. Signs and symptoms of dislocation and effusion include severe pain, limited movement, joint deformity and swelling. Dislocations may affect fingers, elbows, shoulders, hips, knees and ankles and are often caused by sporting injuries or pressure on the affected area after a fall (Marieb & Keller 2022).

Lower back pain

Lower back pain is a common symptom that has a variety of causes including poor posture, injury, inflammatory conditions, obesity, metabolic bone disorders, degenerative processes and intervertebral disc disease. Discomfort or pain may be mild, severe, continuous or intermittent and be aggravated by certain movements or posture; it may radiate into the buttocks or down the back of the legs. People with lower back pain should not sit for more than 30 minutes at any one time, and frequent stretching (thrusting the hips forwards while the upper body leans back) is recommended. Most lower back pain can be safely and effectively treated after an examination by an orthopaedic surgeon and a prescribed period of activity modification and medication to relieve the pain and diminish the inflammation. Although a brief period of rest may be helpful, most studies show that light activity speeds healing and recovery. It may not be necessary to discontinue all activities, including work. Instead, people may adjust their activity under the guidance of medical officers or physiotherapists (Marieb & Keller 2022).

Exercise therapy has been proven to be beneficial in the treatment and rehabilitation of low back pain. ROM exercises, stretching, core stabilisation and general conditioning can contribute to short-term pain relief and functional improvement. Other studies suggest that individuals who are physically fit experience less low back pain than those who are physically inactive (Buttaro et al 2020; Crisp et al 2021).

DIAGNOSIS OF A MUSCULOSKELETAL DISORDER

Diagnosis of musculoskeletal disorder will be confirmed by:

- presenting history of injury, disorder or change in ROM
- physical examination including observation, palpation and assessment of joint movement
- radiological examinations including plain X-ray, arthrogram, arthrography, bone scan, arthroscopy, biopsy, ultrasound, MRI and CT scan.

(Marieb & Keller 2022) (See Figure 28.11 and Table 28.3.)

TREATMENT OF BONE INJURIES AND MUSCULOSKELETAL DISORDERS

Individuals with a bone injury

Bone fractures can take weeks or months to heal, and healing occurs in stages:

- Stage 1: The formation of a haematoma between the two ends of the bones.

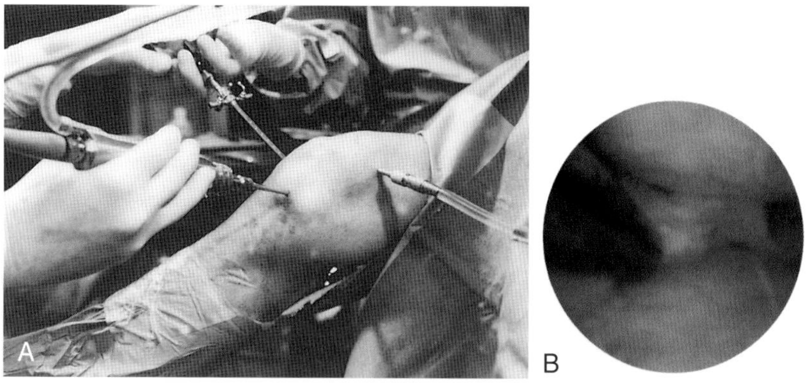

Figure 28.11 Arthroscopy of knee

A: Insertion of a fibreoptic light source into joint, **B:** Internal view of joint.

(Courtesy of Lanny L Johnson, MD, East Lansing, MI. Used with permission)

TABLE 28.3 | Musculoskeletal diagnostic tests

Type	Description
Plain X-ray	Standard X-ray of bones and joints that detects abnormalities in shape and alignment.
Arthrogram	Outlines soft tissue (e.g. meniscus) that is not usually visualised on X-ray.
Arthroscopy	Visual examination of a joint with a fibreoptic endoscope. Commonly performed on the knee to remove loose fragments, view suspected damage or obtain a biopsy.
Biopsy	May be performed on bone, muscle or synovial membrane. Takes blood and tissue samples to test for tumours, enzymes, antibodies and antigens, erythrocyte sedimentation rate (ESR) and calcium, phosphorus and uric acid levels.
Arthrocentesis	Aspiration of synovial fluid for analysis of infection and inflammation.
Bone scan	Provides imaging of the skeleton after intravenous injection of a radioactive isotope that collects in bone tissue at sites where there is increased activity (i.e. at the site of a tumour) and lesions can be detected earlier.
Ultrasound	2D examination of soft tissue for signs of bleeding, haematoma and fluid collection.
Magnetic resonance imaging (MRI)	Magnetism and radio waves form cross-sections and images to detect pathological abnormalities in soft tissue and blood vessels.
Computerised axial tomography (CT or CAT scan)	3D cross-sections that provide detail about injuries to ligaments, tendons, tumours and fractures difficult to determine on plain X-ray. May use iodine contrast medium for greater clarity of affected area to be examined.

(Adapted from Crisp et al 2021; Marieb & Keller 2022; Patton & Thibodeau 2019)

- Stage 2: Inflammation and accumulation of white cells to break down (phagocytose) the haematoma (this takes approximately 5 days).
- Stage 3: The development of granulation tissue and new blood vessels is followed by the development of a callus (calcified osteoblasts) and shaping of new bone by osteoclasts, which remove excess callus. (See Figure 28.12.)

Bone healing is individualised. For most, healing takes place within a standardised timeframe; however, some healing is delayed and can be influenced by the following factors:

- infection from contamination at time of injury or as a result of surgery
- fat emboli (from the bone marrow) enter the blood-stream and travel to the lungs, kidneys, brain and other organs, blocking small blood vessels and causing ischaemia
- splinters of dead bone/fragments not removed by phagocytosis

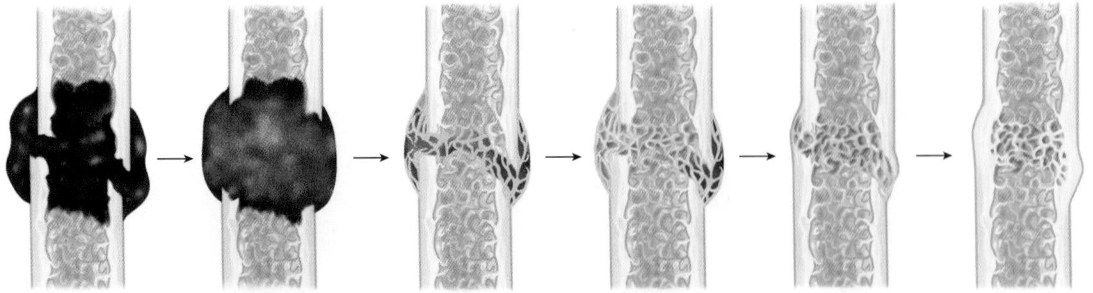

Figure 28.12 Stages in bone healing

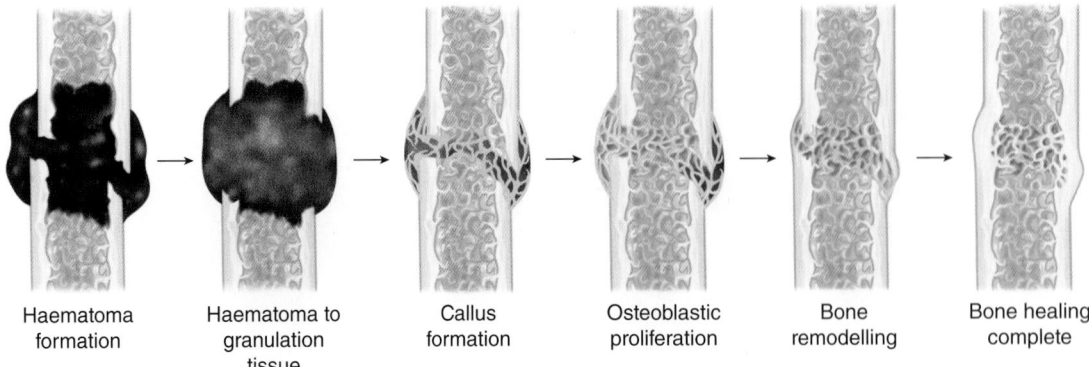

A: Bleeding at fractured ends of the bone with subsequent haematoma formation, **B:** Organisation of haematoma into fibrous network, **C:** Invasion of osteoblasts, lengthening of collagen strands and deposition of calcium, **D:** Callus formation: new bone is built up as osteoclasts destroy dead bone, **E:** Remodelling is accomplished as excess callus is reabsorbed and trabecular bone is laid down.

(Silvestri & Silvestri 2023)

- ischaemia (the neck of the femur is vulnerable since it has a poor blood supply)
- delayed union related to inadequate nutrition, inadequate immobilisation, immunosuppression, infection, necrosis, age
- reflex sympathetic dystrophy (post-traumatic pain, hyperaesthesia, decreased motion, changes in temperature and skin colour).

(Marieb & Keller 2022; LeMone et al 2020)

Surgical repair

For some bone and joint disorders, surgical repair of the affected area is essential to restore alignment, control pain and enhance rehabilitation for full joint mobility. Simple fractures require return of bone fragments to their original position and may be achieved by surgical review and realignment with an internal or external fixture. Compound fractures require surgical debridement to remove dirt, foreign material and necrotic bone fragments (Cooper & Gosnell 2023; Patton & Thibodeau 2019).

A closed fracture may be reduced using closed reduction manipulation, where bony fragments are repositioned into normal alignment by applying pressure and traction distal to the fracture. An open reduction and internal fixation (ORIF) requires subsequent assessment of the wound (colour, approximation of edges, odour, drainage, temperature) and pain and neurovascular status (LeMone et al 2020).

Skeletal fixation devices such as casts, metal pins, braces, skeletal and skin traction are used to hold bone and bone fragments in a normal position. Internal fixation is a surgical procedure in which pins, screws, plates and rods fix bony fragments into normal alignment. This procedure is called an open reduction with internal fixation (ORIF) (Cooper & Gosnell 2023).

External fixation involves the insertion of pins directly into the long axis of a bone, above and below a fracture to immobilise the bone. The pins are then attached to an external frame, which is adjusted to achieve bone alignment. While external fixation allows for early ambulation and/or limb mobility, the pins require frequent assessment for infection (redness, drainage, tenderness) (LeMone et al 2020).

Traction

Skeletal traction may be applied to the bone via the skeletal fixation device. Traction aids reduction and immobilisation of fractures, as well as being used to treat muscle spasms or correct or prevent deformities and relieve pressure on a nerve. A steady pull in opposite directions keeps the bone in place. Weights, ropes and pulleys are used to create the pull required to stabilise the limb. Traction can be applied to the neck, arms, legs or pelvis. Skin traction is applied directly to adhesive materials attached to the skin below the site of the fracture. Weights are attached to the pulley system and to a boot, splint or elastic bandage (Cooper & Gosnell 2023). (See Figure 28.13.)

Casts

Casts are immobilisation devices used to relieve pain, to stabilise a fracture and to immobilise a fracture to promote healing. Casts are made of plaster or fibreglass and may be complete (circumferential) or partial (backslab) (Hockenberry et al 2022). Backslabs are applied longitudinally to the affected limb to splint the injury and are bandaged into place while still soft. Indications for a backslab include an acute fracture with swelling.

Application of a cast may cause pain, and the individual may experience a hot sensation as part of the chemical reaction of the product.

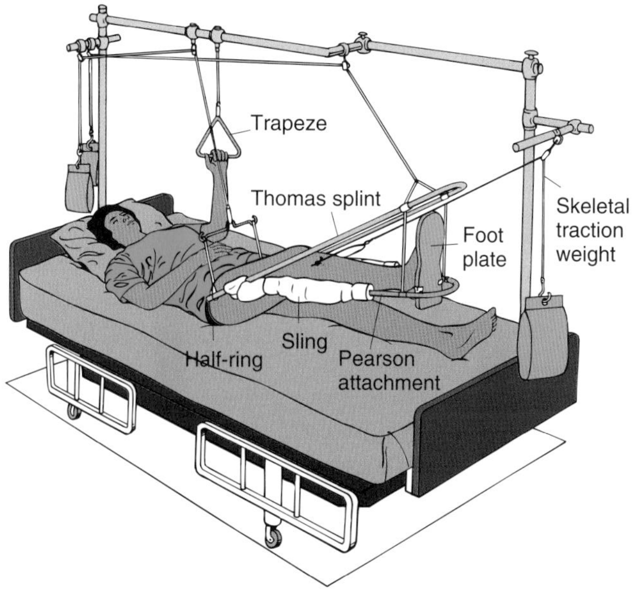

Figure 28.13 Common type of traction

(Fig 17.8 from Perry et al 2019)

Tight or ill-fitting casts cause complications such as neurovascular compromise (Curtis et al 2019).

A person with a fracture should have neurovascular observations undertaken every 1–2 hours for 24 hours, then every 4–8 hours if fitted with a cast (or per facility protocol) (Berman et al 2020). As stated previously, the neurovascular assessment should include skin colour, sensation, presence of pulses distal to the injury, movement of the limb distal to the injury, capillary refill and pain presence and characteristics (LeMone et al 2020; Williams 2021).

People discharged home wearing a cast should have their cast inspected for rough edges and signs of bleeding or drainage, and be educated to seek medical advice if they notice their cast is cracked, moist or emitting an offensive odour. A cast may take up to 48 hours to dry and, following that, must be kept dry (plastic bag to cover if bathing or outside in rain). Scratching or inserting foreign objects inside the cast should be avoided, as both may cause skin breakdown and infection. Blowing cool air under the cast from a hair dryer on a cool setting relieves itchiness (LeMone et al 2020). The limb should be kept elevated to reduce swelling and advice sought if the limb becomes cool, swollen, increasingly painful or changes colour. Casts may remain in place for several weeks to some months, depending on the bone or joint requiring immobilisation (Berman et al 2020; Williams 2021).

Compartment syndrome is a condition of progressive arterial vessel compression and decreased blood supply to an extremity. Factors predisposing to development of compartment syndrome are fractures of the tibia or forearm resulting in muscle oedema, and too-tight casts or dressings (Cooper & Gosnell 2023). If a developing compartment syndrome is suspected, the affected limb should be placed at heart level (not elevated). Maintaining the limb at heart level maximises perfusion and minimises swelling. To alleviate pressure, the cast should be removed and if the pressure is internal, a fasciotomy performed (surgical intervention in which muscle fascia is cut to relieve pressure) (LeMone et al 2020).

NURSING CARE OF THE INDIVIDUAL WITH A MUSCULOSKELETAL DISORDER

While medical management and nursing care will depend on the specific disorder, the general aims of care of an individual with a musculoskeletal disorder are to:

- Promote rest and relieve pain.
- Prevent complications of inactivity and promote movement when possible.
- Maintain skin integrity.
- Maintain or improve nutritional status.
- Prevent and recognise potential psychosocial problems.
- Promote remobilisation and rehabilitation.

(Berman et al 2020; Crisp et al 2021)

Promoting rest

Rest helps minimise pain and swelling, promotes healing of injured tissues, relieves muscle spasms and prevents further tissue destruction in inflammatory conditions. Rest may be classified as general, when the individual is confined to bed (e.g. if several joints are inflamed) or local, when a specific body part is immobilised, such as a limb in a splint or cast. General care during the rest phase involves:

- providing a suitable chair or bed with a firm mattress, pillows and pressure relieving devices such as sheepskins to promote comfort
- assisting the individual to perform ADLs through use of assistive devices such as long handled tongs or special eating utensils
- preventing complications associated with immobility by performing ROM exercises and change of position at least every 2 hours
- maintaining correct posture and body alignment.

(LeMone et al 2020; Williams 2021)

Maintaining joint movement

Some joints require movement rather than immobilisation post repair. The continuous passive movement (CPM) device provides gentle forward and backward joint movement after total knee replacement surgery (arthroplasty). Used on people who are resting in bed, the joint is strapped into the device and moved continuously while the person is immobilised. This movement ensures the joint remains mobile, resulting in reduced pain, swelling and eventual immobility (Crisp et al 2021). Because the patella is not disrupted in partial knee replacement surgery, the individual usually may resume walking 3–4 hours after surgery.

Mobilisation of the affected joint after hip replacement surgery (arthroplasty) is dependent on the prostheses used and treating medical officer. Physiotherapists may start mobilisation (weight-bearing or non-weight-bearing) day 1 post surgery per the medical officer's orders. Exercises may be passive or active involving straight leg raising, flexion and extension to all joints, including the replaced joint (Cooper & Gosnell 2023).

Maintaining skin integrity

Individuals who are immobilised for prolonged periods are at high risk of developing pressure injuries. Skin must be maintained in good condition and protected from irritation, friction and prolonged pressure (Crisp et al 2021). General care of the skin and prevention of pressure injuries are described in Chapter 29.

Positioning techniques

People with musculoskeletal disorders who are immobilised require help from nurses to ensure proper body alignment and comfort. Aids to comfort in bed, such as pillows, foot boards, trochanter rolls, trapeze bars, sandbags and slippery-type sheets for ease of movement in bed, are all useful to ensure that an immobilised person is comfortable (Crisp et al 2021). See Clinical Skill 28.2 for more information and guidelines on positioning individuals in bed.

Various positions and proper positioning are discussed in Chapter 19.

CLINICAL SKILL 28.2 Positioning individuals in bed

Please adhere to the policy and procedures of the facility/organisation prior to undertaking the skill. Ensure this skill is in your scope of practice.

NMBA Decision-making Framework considerations (refer to NMBA Decision-making framework for nursing and midwifery 2020):	**Equipment:**
1. Am I educated? 2. Am I authorised? 3. Am I competent? If you answer 'no' to any of these, do not perform that activity. Seek guidance and support from your teacher/a nurse team leader/clinical facilitator/educator.	Slide sheet/slip sheet Pillows Lifting device, if required

PREPARE FOR THE SKILL

(Please refer to the Standard Steps on pp. xviii–xx for related rationales.)

Mentally review the steps of the skill.
Discuss the skill with your instructor/supervisor/team leader, if required.
Confirm correct facility/organisation policy/safe operating procedures.
Validate the order in the individual's record.
Identify indication and rationale for performing the activity.
Assess for any contraindications.
Locate and gather equipment.
Perform hand hygiene.
Ensure therapeutic interaction.
Identify the individual using three individual identifiers.
Gain the individual's consent.
Assess for pain relief.
Prepare the environment.
Provide and maintain privacy.
Assist the individual to assume an appropriate position of comfort.

Skill activity	Rationale
Assess the individual's physical ability to help with moving and positioning.	Ensures individual's independence is maintained. Determines need for additional assistance. Ensures safety.
Account for all tubing, drains and attached equipment.	Prevents spillage and dislodgement if equipment catches on bed frame or mattress.

CLINICAL SKILL 28.2 Positioning individuals in bed—cont'd

Place the individual in supine position with head of the bed flat and remove the pillows, place pillow at the head of the bed.	Enables nurse to assess body alignment. Reduces gravity's pull on individual's upper body. Prevents striking the individual's head against head of the bed.
Assess the need for extra help.	Ensures the individual's and nurse's safety.

PERFORM THE SKILL

(Please refer to the Standard Steps on pp. xviii–xx for related rationales.)
Perform hand hygiene.
Apply PPE: gloves, eyewear, mask and gown as appropriate.
Ensure the individual's safety and comfort throughout skill.
Promote independence and involvement of the individual if possible and/or appropriate.
Assess the individual's tolerance to the skill throughout.
Dispose of used supplies, equipment, waste and sharps appropriately.
Remove PPE and discard or store appropriately.
Perform hand hygiene.

Skill activity	Rationale
Determine the most appropriate position for the individual.	Various conditions and diseases preclude moving individuals into some positions.
Utilise principles of efficient body mechanics.	To protect the nurse's back.
Perform pressure area care. Wash and dry area. Apply moisturiser, if appropriate. Change linen.	Prevents skin breakdown. Maintains skin integrity.
Move and position individual appropriately using appropriate friction-reducing device (such as slide sheet). Ensure pressure is relieved by positioning in a different position. Pressure-relieving devices may be utilised.	Promotes individual's comfort.
The body must be supported to maintain its natural contours, symmetry and alignment.	Maintains and helps to restore body functioning and helps to prevent the complications with bed rest and immobility.
Assess the skin.	Ongoing assessment of the skin is necessary to detect early signs of pressure damage.

AFTER THE SKILL

(Please refer to the Standard Steps on pp. xviii–xx for related rationales.)
Communicate outcome to the individual, any ongoing care and to report any complications.
Restore the environment.
Report, record and document assessment findings, details of the skill performed and the individual's response.
Report, record and document any abnormalities and/or inability to perform the skill.
Reassess the individual to ensure there are no adverse effects/events from the skill.

(Perry et al 2019; Rebeiro et al 2021; Tollefson & Hillman 2022)

Maintaining or improving nutritional status

Nutrition for individuals with a musculoskeletal disorder includes a well-balanced diet and maintenance of recommended body weight. The diet should contain adequate amounts of protein, calcium and vitamin D to promote healing and maintenance of the musculoskeletal system. Adequate fibre and fluids aid elimination. If a person is overweight, a weight-reduction diet is recommended to prevent stress on inflamed or diseased joints (Berman et al 2020; Crisp et al 2021). (See also Chapter 30.)

Relieving pain

While the general approaches to pain management described in Chapter 33 are relevant to people with musculoskeletal disorders, specific measures may also be indicated. A person may experience acute or chronic pain, depending on the specific disorder, and general measures to promote comfort and minimise pain should be implemented; that is, changing position, massage, handling a painful limb gently and rest. If not contraindicated, elevating the limb may relieve discomfort and pain. Specific measures include checking to ensure that splints, casts or dressings are not too tight or rubbing against the skin. Hot or cold packs or treatments may be used to provide relief and increase ROM. Heat is sometimes used in chronic joint disorders since it relaxes muscles, relieves stiffness and provides analgesia, and is often applied before exercise and massage. Applying a cold pack to a limb or area is useful for acute pain or acutely inflamed joints. When these treatments are used, caution is necessary to prevent tissue damage. Analgesia may be prescribed and administered in accordance with nursing regulations and the institution's policy (Crisp et al 2021).

CRITICAL THINKING EXERCISE 28.4

You are caring for an individual who is recovering from a motor vehicle accident. The individual sustained a fractured left tibia and fibula and a fractured left humerus, both of which are in a full cast. Outline the strategies you will employ to ensure this individual mobilises comfortably and safely.

Prevention of psychological problems

Management of a musculoskeletal disorder may require a person to be confined to bed, and possibly hospital, for an extended time, and often leads to boredom, frustration or depression. Ongoing psychological deterioration may affect the individual's pain tolerance, immune system and general health. To prevent such problems, the individual should be encouraged to express their feelings and be allowed to participate in making decisions about their care. Communication should be open, honest and individuals treated with respect, kindness and dignity. Active involvement in all aspects of care and self-care techniques are taught, as this allows the individual to take responsibility for some of their care and can help to reduce problems associated with dependence and immobilisation. Regular programs of activity developed with the individual and other allied health professionals need to be incorporated into the nursing care plan. Participation in group physiotherapy or rehabilitation sessions promotes social interaction with others in similar situations (Crisp et al 2021; Jester et al 2021).

Promoting remobilisation and rehabilitation

Because the musculoskeletal system is crucial to activity, a routine of exercise and rehabilitation is developed and implemented. Goals of rehabilitation are to restore the affected individual to their functional maximum potential, while meeting psychological, social and physical needs.

The overall aim of rehabilitation is to limit the effects of a disability and increase independence in ADLs. Rehabilitation requires a comprehensive assessment of the individual, setting of realistic and achievable goals, collaboration within the multidisciplinary care team and regular evaluation of the individual's progress. The rehabilitation team includes many health professionals, such as medical officers, nurses, social workers, physical and occupational therapists, speech therapists and even members of the individual's own family (Jester et al 2021). Preparation for discharge should begin as soon as possible and includes assessment and determination of a suitable discharge destination, collaboration with the individual and family, provision of verbal and written information regarding medications, ongoing exercise regimens, future appointments and signs and symptoms of complications (Jester et al 2021). Information on rehabilitation is provided in Chapter 40.

GENERAL TREATMENT OF MUSCULOSKELETAL DISORDERS

Nursing care of the older person requiring prolonged bed rest

Older people are more prone to problems associated with prolonged bed rest. These individuals need careful planning and enactment of care to minimise these potential problems. (See Nursing Care Plan 28.1, Case Study 28.2 and Case Study 28.3.)

General treatment for exercise-related injuries

Exercise can be the cause of injuries that are mostly orthopaedic in nature and caused by irritation of bones, tendons and ligaments and/or muscle tissue. Injury may be as a result of weight-bearing stress or collision. Nurses can teach individuals the acronym **PRICE**: **prevention**, **rest**, **ice**, **compression** and **elevation**, and advise of the need for a medical officer to diagnose the injury. Basic principles for managing injuries include to avoid unnecessary handling, immobilise the injury, dress wounds with clean dressings, control bleeding and check for pain, pulselessness, paraesthesia, pallor and paralysis distal to the injury (Baca 2018; Cooper & Gosnell 2023).

Meeting movement and exercise needs

To determine what the individual can and cannot do without assistance, the clinician must assess the individual

NURSING CARE PLAN 28.1

Assessment: Post amputation right forefoot, has diabetes mellitus, faecally incontinent, older-aged person.
Issue/s to be addressed: Potential for pressure area injury related to reduced mobility, unstable blood glucose and incontinence.
Goal/s: The individual's areas of dependence will remain intact with no signs of pressure injury (redness, excoriation or pain) during the period of reduced mobility.

Care/actions	Rationale
Reposition the individual every 2 hours while sitting or resting in bed.	Repositioning relieves pressure on dependent tissues and enables the nurse to visualise and assess sacral areas for changes in skin condition.
Clean, dry and moisturise sacral skin three times a day or as indicated by incontinence.	To reduce friction caused by moisture of body fluids and to enable the nurse to visualise and assess the sacral area.
Manage incontinence using incontinence aids such as absorbent pads.	To prevent maceration and irritation of the skin from contact with urine and faeces.
Use slide sheets and lifting devices to change the person's position.	To reduce friction and shearing caused by dragging the person across surfaces.
Apply pressure-relieving devices, such as an air mattress, pressure-reducing foam mattress or pressure-reducing mattress overlay, under the individual.	To reduce pressure points on dependent tissues and promote rest and sleep.
Assess areas of dependence when changing person's position and assisting with hygiene/toileting.	To monitor for deterioration of skin and implement strategies to protect in a timely manner.
Monitor individuals BGL QID or as directed by medical team.	Elevated glucose levels cause micro and macrovascular complications that affect wound healing.

Evaluation: During the period of reduced mobility the individual's dependent skin areas remained intact with no signs or symptoms of redness, excoriation or pain.
(Adapted from ACSQHC 2021; Crisp et al 2021; Gulanick & Myers 2022)

CASE STUDY 28.2

Harold Chin is an 85-year-old, non-English speaking resident of an aged-care home. Up until Harold fractured his left hip 6 months ago, he was ambulant and quite active. As Harold's nurse, you would like him to start participating in the 'passive exercises' exercise program that the facility offers.

1. You are having difficulty communicating with Harold due to the language barrier, but would like to explain your proposed plan and the benefits of exercise to him. Outline three ways you could communicate effectively with Harold.
2. In educating Harold, outline five benefits of exercise for the older individual.
3. Outline how you would plan for Harold to attend the exercise classes, including overcoming physical and psychological barriers to participating in exercise.
4. Describe exercise appropriate for an 85-year-old man with limited mobility.

CASE STUDY 28.3

Jonathon Deary is an 84-year-old man recovering from a fractured pelvis, after falling off a ladder. Jonathon is to be placed on strict bed rest, and has a past history of angina and right-side heart failure.

1. Identify and give rationale for the potential problems of immobility that Jonathon may experience.
2. Because of Jonathon's history of angina and heart failure, outline some strategies to prevent formation of a deep vein thrombosis (DVT).
3. List the assessments you would perform on an individual with a musculoskeletal disorder.

in how cognitive and physical deficits cause disabilities. The nurse assists the health professional team by providing subjective and objective data about the individual, and facilitating rehabilitation activities and exercises (Jankovic et al 2021).

It is important to identify potential problems that may affect a person's ability to exercise. Impaired mobility may result from:

- a decrease in the individual's strength
- presence of pain or discomfort
- impaired cognition or perception, such as dementia, severe anxiety or depression
- impaired neuromuscular or skeletal function
- imposed restrictions such as bed rest.

NURSING CARE PLAN 28.2

Assessment: Individual day 2 post ORIF compound leg fracture partial weight-bearing, ambulate with supervision using axillary crutches, with pain score of 5/10 at rest.
Issue/s to be addressed: Decreased mobility related to injury and surgical pain.
Goal/s: To increase mobility (walk 25 metres with crutches, three times a day) by end of the shift.

Care/actions	Rationale
Assess pain characteristics (quality, severity, location, onset, duration, causing and relieving factors) every 4 hours.	To map and evaluate the pain in the individual.
Administer analgesics as prescribed, at regular intervals when pain present and/or prior to pain-inducing activities (i.e. exercise).	To maintain therapeutic analgesic serum levels within the person.
Apply non-pharmacological therapies to reduce pain, such as heat/cold packs, relaxation exercises, position change, massage.	To provide adjunct therapy to reduce pain experience, a combination of pharmacological and non-pharmacological is most effective in pain management.
Encourage passive exercises every hour while resting in bed.	Passive exercises promote circulation, relieve pressure and can prevent complications such as DVT due to immobility.
Encourage rest between activity.	Rest and relaxation promote better pain management and recovery.
Encourage and supervise ambulation TDS. To provide support and supervision while ambulating.	To increase and maintain muscle strength and tone.

Evaluation: By the end of the shift, the individual ambulated three times, a distance of 25 metres with minimal pain or discomfort (pain score 3/10).

(Adapted from Crisp et al 2021; Gulanick & Myers 2022; Touhy & Jett 2019)

Being in hospital is likely to alter a person's normal movement and exercise routine and, although there is often a degree of restriction in activities and ability to ambulate, they should be encouraged to do so, while those who are immobilised may require assistance to move. Nurses promote safety and comfort while encouraging, when possible, a return to independent function (Crisp et al 2021).

When planning care to meet an individual's need for movement and exercise the nurse must consider factors such as:

- maintaining and promoting normal mobility
- assisting those with restricted mobility
- providing and assisting with use of equipment to aid mobility
- preventing and alleviating discomfort associated with reduced mobility.

A sample nursing care plan is shown in Nursing Care Plan 28.2.

CRITICAL THINKING EXERCISE 28.5

An individual's post neurological injury has varying degrees of mobility. Select one form of paralysis resulting from a spinal cord injury. When planning care to meet an individual's needs for movement and exercise after a neurological injury that has resulted in a loss of mobility, what factors must the nurse consider?

AMBULATION AFTER PROLONGED IMMOBILISATION

'Dangling' before ambulating

Ambulating, or walking, is encouraged and facilitated to prevent the complications associated with short-term—but especially with long-term—periods of immobility. Certain individuals may need to relearn how to walk. For example, after a cerebrovascular accident or leg surgery, an individual may need the assistance of aids such as a walking stick, crutches or walking frame. After an extended period of immobility, nurses need to instruct the individual to mobilise progressively. A bedridden person who is able to raise each leg 4–6 cm straight up from the bed usually possesses enough strength to walk, provided that they are mentally alert.

Due to blood pressure dropping when an individual stands up, a technique called '**dangling**' is implemented to stimulate circulation prior to ambulation. The individual is assisted to sit on the edge of the bed and move their legs back and forth in a circular motion for 1–5 minutes. If tolerated, the individual may progress to transferring to a chair or gentle ambulation. Thromboembolic stockings also aid venous return and therefore maintenance of blood pressure (Sorrentino & Remmert 2021). (See Progress Note 28.1.)

When the nurse assists an individual who has a one-sided weakness, or hemiplegia, it is important to decide which walking aid or technique has been recommended.

Although the method used to assist is individualised, most people require assistance and support on the affected side. When assisting a person to walk, it is helpful if they remain close to a railed wall and are able to rest on a chair before beginning the return walk. If an ambulant person has an intravenous infusion or urinary or wound-drainage bag, the nurse ensures that therapy or drainage is not affected, by checking tubing or drainage bags in case they have become dislodged after exercise.

Well-fitting, supportive, non-slip footwear should always be worn, the floor should be clean and dry and the environment cleared of obstacles. The individual should not be allowed to walk barefoot or with just socks or slippery footwear (e.g. women with nylon hose) on the feet. Each individual is encouraged to walk at their own pace and resting points established along the way should the individual become tired, dizzy or unsteady. If the individual begins to fall, the nurse should assume a wide stance and guide the person to the floor, protecting their head as they do (Crisp et al 2021).

WALKING AIDS

Walking aids broaden the base of support and increase stability, thus providing the individual with improved mobility and independence. The type of aid appropriate for an individual depends on the following:

- cognitive function
- goal for mobility
- functional ability
- health status
- home environment
- ability to afford the equipment.

An individual is commonly instructed in the use of walking aids by a physiotherapist; however, it is important for nurses to know the principles involved in the use of walking aids. Walking aids that may be required on a temporary or permanent basis include crutches, walking sticks or canes, and walking frames (Sehgal et al 2021). Callipers, leg braces or splints may be used to provide extra support for a weak leg, to prevent or correct deformities or prevent joint movement.

Crutches

Crutches enable a person to ambulate by taking higher levels of weight of the body off one or both legs. Successful use of crutches requires balance, stability, upper body strength and the use of both hands. Selection of crutches and particular type of gait depends on individual needs, but must be appropriate to be safe and effective. The three types commonly used are the underarm (axillary), platform and forearm crutches. (See Figure 28.15.)

Underarm crutches are often used by people with a lower limb injury or fracture. Underarm crutches must be measured so that the person's weight is carried on their wrists and palms and not on the axillae. Body weight should not be applied to the axillary pad; therefore, the axilla bar should be 4–5 cm below the axilla, and the hand bar positioned to permit 15–30-degree flexion of the elbow at rest.

Forearm crutches are easily adjustable, lightweight and allow better hand freedom but require trunk balance and higher levels of upper body strength. The height of the handpiece should be set so the elbow is at 15–30-degree flexion at rest.

Platform crutches allow for weight-bearing by having an axillary crutch with an attached forearm pad. These crutches are ideal for the individual with a weak handgrip and are more stable than a standard axillary crutch.

Before crutches are used, they should be assessed for safety, ensuring that all screws and bolts are tightened and rubber tips are in good repair. It is important to ascertain the amount of weight-bearing allowed on the affected leg(s) (i.e. partial or none) (Berman et al 2020; Crisp et al 2021; Sehgal et al 2021). (See Figure 28.14, Figure 28.15, Figure 28.16.)

Crutch-walking gaits

Individuals are instructed in one of several crutch-walking gaits, according to need. The most common is the three-point gait, in which weight is borne on the unaffected leg, and the crutches moved forwards first, followed by the unaffected leg, then the affected leg follows in a swinging movement because it is raised from the ground. This gait is used when a person is unable to bear weight on one leg. The two-point and four-point gaits are used when both feet can bear some weight (i.e. partial weight-bearing). The two-point gait requires the individual to advance one crutch

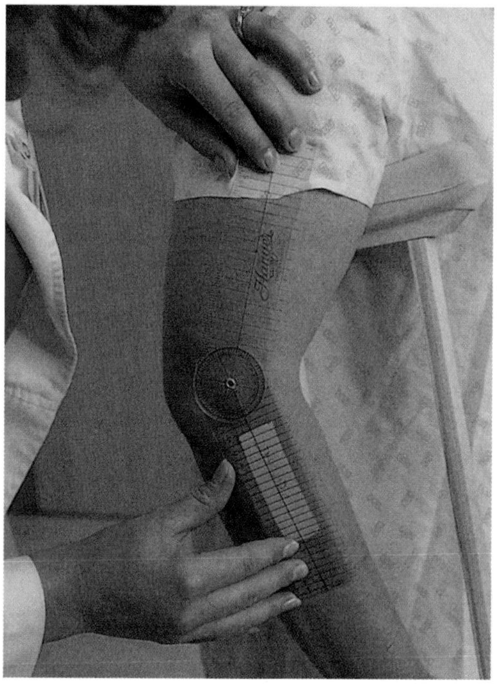

Figure 28.14 Using the goniometer to verify correct degree of elbow flexion for crutch use

(Potter et al 2023)

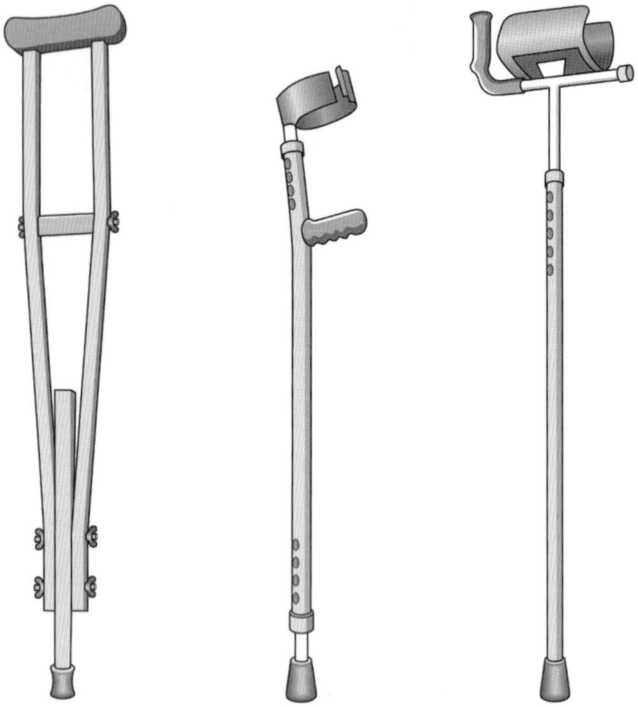

Figure 28.15 Types of crutches: axillary (left), forearm (centre) and forearm (right)

(Richards et al 2023)

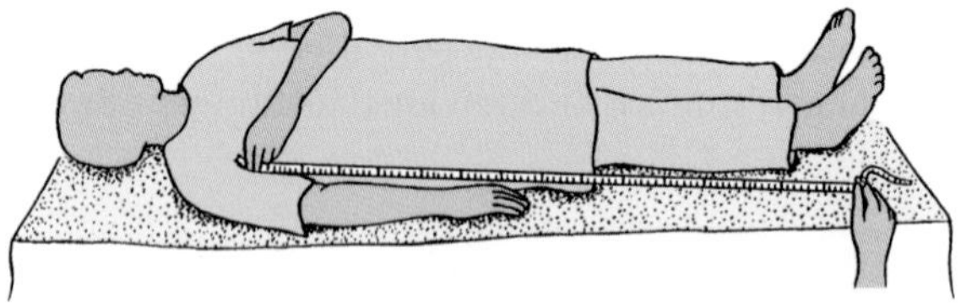

Figure 28.16 Measuring crutch length

(Potter et al 2023)

and the opposite leg together, followed by the other crutch and leg. The four-point gait requires greater coordination but provides more stability since there are always three points on the floor as each leg is moved alternately with the opposite crutch.

The swing-through gait is used when a person has no use of the lower body (i.e. in paraplegia) and both crutches are advanced simultaneously. The person swings both legs either parallel with or beyond the crutches, the pelvis moving first, followed by the shoulders and head in order to maintain balance.

When rising from a chair the individual is taught to hold both crutches in one hand, opposite the affected leg, tips resting firmly on the floor, and to push up with their free hand, using the crutches for support. The individual supports their body weight on the unaffected leg and the crutches. To sit down, the process is reversed, the person supports themselves with the crutches in one hand, holds the arm of the chair with a free hand and lowers into the chair. When mobilising up stairs, the individual steps the uninjured limb onto the upper step, and pushes through the crutches to raise the injured limb up onto the same step. The crutches then follow. To mobilise down stairs, the individual puts the crutches down onto the lower step, steps the uninjured limb down and then follows with the injured limb (Crisp et al 2021).

Walking sticks

A walking stick or cane may be used for people with hemiparesis or injury, occasional loss of balance, mild ataxia or to reduce weight-bearing on a lower limb. The use of a walking stick requires upper body strength, and dexterity and sufficient balance, to provide balance and support for walking, reduce fatigue and strain on weight-bearing joints and improve standing tolerance. Walking sticks should extend from the individual's greater trochanter to the floor, and be fitted with a rubber tip to prevent slippage. Sticks may be standard (single tipped), offset (single tipped but offset angle of the handle) or tripod or quadripod. The stick should permit 15–30-degree flexion of the elbow and be positioned as vertical as possible. Three- and four-point sticks provide a broad base and greater stability, and are more appropriate for the person with poor balance or one-sided weakness. (See Figure 28.17.)

To use a stick, the individual holds it close to the body on the opposite side to the affected lower limb, taking the weight off the affected leg. The person then moves the stick and the affected leg simultaneously, followed by the unaffected leg. Individuals are encouraged to keep the stride of each leg, and the timing of each step, equal. While a person is learning to use the stick, the nurse stands behind them to support them if they become unsteady. When going up stairs the stick should be held in one hand and the person encouraged to hold the stair rail, leading with the unaffected leg; when going down stairs the affected leg leads (Seghal et al 2021).

Walking frames

Walking frames consist of an adjustable metal frame with hand grips, four legs and one open side. (See Figure 28.18.) A frame may be used by an older adult since it provides greater support and sense of security than a stick and is useful for those with an unsteady gait, or when partial weight-bearing is recommended. Walking frames, however, require upper body strength, the ability to at least partially weight-bear and can be difficult to manoeuvre. The height is selected to allow 15–30-degree flexion of the elbows when the hand grips are held. Attachments such as baskets and trays are available to meet specific needs and to promote greater independence.

Standard walkers have four rubber-tipped legs and must be completely lifted by the individual for any movement, thus slowing the individual's gait. Rolling walking frames (two wheels) are easier to manoeuvre, allowing a more normal gait. Four wheel walking frames are the least stable type of frame and best suited to individuals who need no weight-bearing support. (See Figure 28.19.)

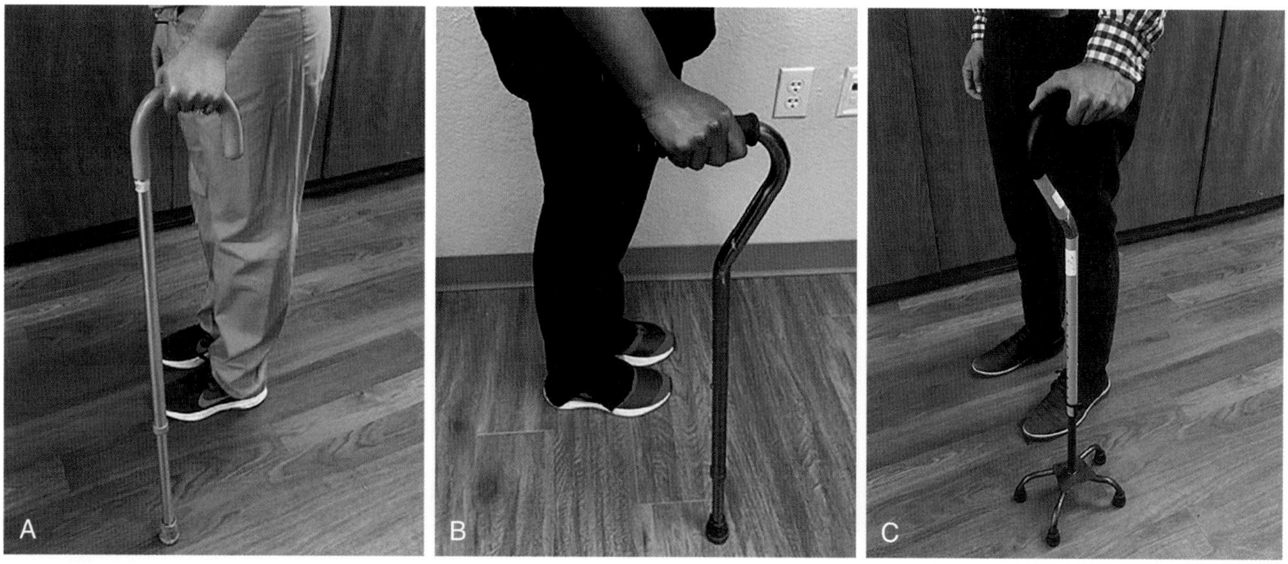

Figure 28.17 Types of walking sticks

(Sehgal et al 2021)

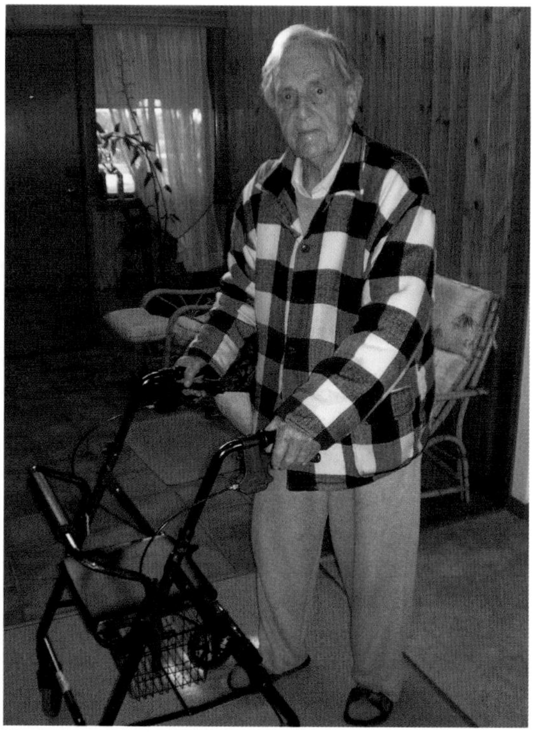

Figure 28.18 Walking frame

(© Norman Lanyon)

When an individual is learning to use a frame, the nurse stands behind them to support the hips and encourages the person to stand upright and look straight ahead. To safely rise from a chair, the frame is placed in front of the person, who then inches forwards in the seat of the chair and, with both feet firmly on the ground and both hands on the arms of the chair, pushes with their arms to stand and, when standing, grasps the frame. Commonly, the individual picks the frame up and moves it 15–20 cm forward, then moves one foot, followed by the other, up to the frame. If an individual has a one-sided weakness, the affected leg is moved first. To sit down, the person stands with the back of their knees against the front of the chair, then reaches behind to securely grip the armrests, bending their arms to lower themselves into the chair. When a walking aid is employed, the person is assisted until they are confident in the use of the aid (Crisp et al 2021; Seghal et al 2021).

COMPLICATIONS ASSOCIATED WITH REDUCED MOBILITY

The body works more efficiently when people are active, so when a person is confined to bed or immobilised, each system can be negatively affected. Depending on age, health status and length and degree of immobility, inactivity can cause both short- and long-term complications. Disuse of muscles leads to degeneration and subsequent loss of function and it is important that individuals receive some form of exercise to prevent **muscle atrophy**. Muscle atrophy is defined as a wasting or decrease in size of muscle mass due to physical inactivity (Harris et al 2019). Atrophy begins almost as soon as muscles are immobilised. Individuals also experience a limitation in their endurance, which makes ADLs difficult. Restoring muscle strength and tone in people who have been immobilised for any length of time is a slow process.

systemic effects of immobility include:

- pressure injuries
- contractures
- cardiovascular and pulmonary stasis
- urinary stasis
- constipation
- depression, anxiety or boredom.

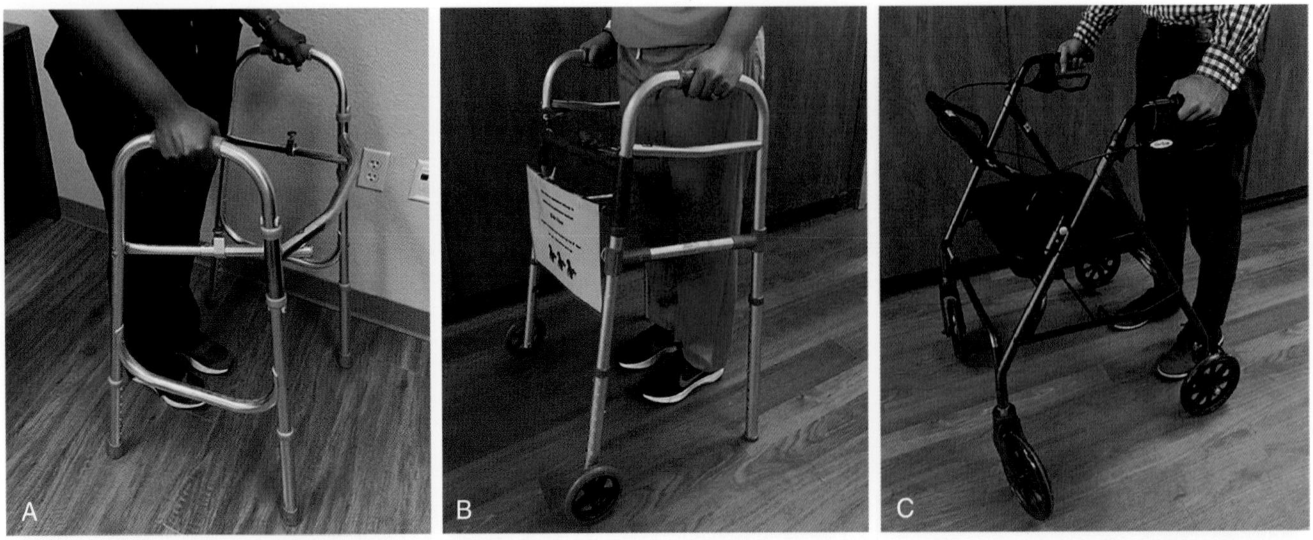

Figure 28.19 Types of walking frames

(Sehgal et al 2021)

Monitoring of individuals with disorders of movement and mobility promotes early identification of acute physiological deterioration and prompts implementation of actions to prevent further deterioration. Nursing and allied health staff should utilise the National Safety and Quality Health Service (NSQHS) Standard 'Recognising and Responding to Acute Deterioration' to ensure that acute deterioration in a person's cognitive, physical or mental condition is recognised as soon as possible and appropriate action is taken. The standard suggests vigilant monitoring and documentation of vital signs and reporting of discrepancies as strategies for identifying problems so that comprehensive care plans can be implemented (ACSQHC 2021).

Pressure injuries

Pressure injuries are localised damage to the skin and underlying tissue caused by pressure, shear or friction (for a bedridden person, shear or amount of friction increases as their head is elevated). Pressure, especially on bony prominences, results in poor circulation, so that the area is deprived of essential nutrients and oxygen, and cellular death may occur. A pressure injury risk assessment such as the Braden Scale, should be performed on any individual with:

- limited mobility or prior history of pressure injury
- oxygenation and/or circulation deficits
- impaired nutritional status
- impaired cognition
- extremes in age
- moist skin from incontinence or diaphoresis
- immobility related to surgery, injury or critical illness.

Pressure injuries remain a significant problem in hospitals and residential care settings despite being largely preventable (Crisp et al 2021; Overall 2022). See Chapter 29 for factors that affect skin integrity and Chapter 15 for pressure injury risk assessment.

Effects of immobility upon the musculoskeletal system

Effects of immobility are evident after even short periods of inactivity. People who attempt to walk after several days of bed rest are surprised at how weak their leg muscles have become. Immobilisation and the resultant disuse of muscles lead to decreased joint mobility, bone demineralisation and atrophy of muscles with decreased size, strength and tone.

Contractures and ankylosis

Contractures are abnormal conditions of a joint characterised by flexion and fixation and caused by atrophy and shortening of muscle fibres. The term 'acquired deforming hypertonia' has been proposed to replace the term 'contracture' since it more precisely describes it as joint deformity with increased resistance to passive movement and decreased range of movement. **Ankylosis** is joint consolidation and immobilisation. Contractures may result from improper support or positioning of a joint, or as a result of inadequate joint movement. For example, if a joint is allowed to remain in one position for an extended length of time, the muscle fibres that normally provide movement shorten to accommodate that position, and lose the ability to contract and relax. Weight-bearing activity stimulates bone formation and balance; however, during immobilisation, bone formation slows, while breakdown of bone increases. With the subsequent loss of bone calcium, phosphorus and matrix, disuse osteoporosis results, and the brittle demineralised bones fracture easily.

Joint contractures in upper limbs may lead to a reduced ability to groom, dress and eat independently. Contractures of the lower limbs may result in inability to walk, instability and increased risk of confinement to bed. Overall, joint contractures may lead to physical discomfort, functional impairment, loss of independence, social isolation and increased care demands. Principles of therapy include regular periods of standing and/or walking; passive stretching of the individual's muscles and joints; positioning of the individual's limbs to encourage extension and flexion; and splinting (Berman et al 2020; Crisp et al 2021; Dehail et al 2019; du Toit 2018).

Foot drop

Foot drop is another term for **plantar flexion**, which is caused by damage to the nerve supply of the muscle responsible for dorsiflexion of the foot. (See Figure 28.20.) If an individual's feet are allowed to assume plantar flexion for long periods, they become fixed in that position so that, when that individual attempts to stand or walk, they will be unable to place their heels on the floor and walk normally.

Prevention includes using a foot board or firm pillow in the bed to maintain the feet in proper alignment, or dorsiflexion, as if in a standing position (if not contraindicated) (i.e. at a 90-degree angle). Devices and techniques to keep pressure off the feet should be used, such as a bed cradle or foot pleat in the upper bedclothes. The person's feet should be exercised through their ROM, either actively or passively. If foot drop occurs, management includes use of an orthopaedic brace, intensive physiotherapy or surgical intervention (Crisp et al 2021).

Effects on the cardiovascular and pulmonary systems

The primary negative effects of immobility on the cardiovascular system are increased cardiac workload, postural hypotension and venous thrombosis. An increase in the workload on the heart may be due to less resistance by blood vessels and changes in blood distribution. Heart rate increases and cardiac output falls after prolonged rest. A significant drop in blood pressure on standing (25 mmHg systolic and 10 mmHg diastolic) is termed **orthostatic or postural hypotension**, and is due to a decrease in neurovascular reflexes and muscle tone. In addition, stasis of blood may precipitate clot formation. A lack of muscular activity that would normally help move blood towards the heart results in calcium exiting the bones to enter the systemic circulation. This action influences clot formation. If a clot or thrombus detaches from the vessel wall and is transported in the bloodstream, it is called an **embolus**. Emboli that lodge in the pulmonary artery tree are referred to as pulmonary emboli. Depending on the size of the embolus, consequences may be serious (Berman et al 2020; Marieb & Keller 2022).

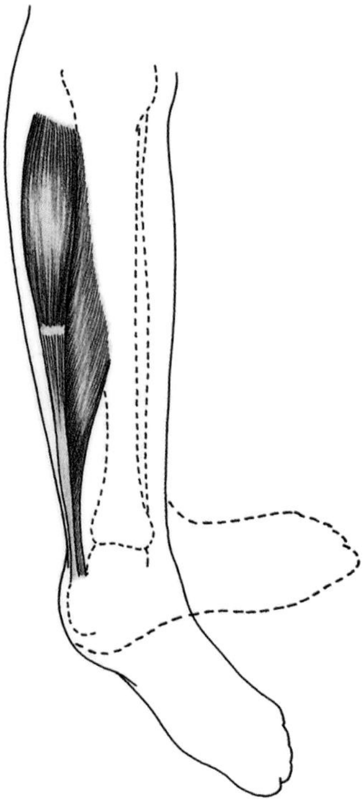

Figure 28.20 Foot drop

(Potter et al 2023)

Prevention of venous thromboembolism

Prevention of venous thromboembolism (VTE) begins with questioning individuals about previous or current clotting and bleeding disorders. Active prevention includes educating about and encouraging the individual to perform active (early ambulation if possible) or passive 2-hourly exercises to stimulate venous circulation in the legs. Individuals are advised not to cross their legs while lying in bed or sitting or use bed rolls or pillows that can constrict vessels under the knee. See Chapter 15 for venous thromboembolism assessment.

Anti-embolic elastic stockings may be prescribed to facilitate venous return from the lower extremities, prevent venous stasis and venous thrombosis and reduce peripheral oedema. The stockings expose the toes but cover the foot and extend up the leg to the knee or groin. They give firm support to superficial veins in the leg, maintaining adequate venous pressure and reducing the incidence of thrombi. The individual's leg(s) are measured to ensure correct fit, then the stockings applied by rolling them slowly from the foot up the leg. Firm, even pressure is essential, and the toes are exposed to check that they remain warm and pink and blood supply is not impeded by the stockings.

An alternative or adjunct therapy to prevent VTE is sequential compression device (SCD) therapy. These fabric or vinyl leg sleeves use alternating compression and relaxation to mimic skeletal muscle activity, preventing venous stasis and clotting in deep veins of the leg. SCDs are indicated in individuals undergoing general anaesthesia and extremes of positioning intraoperatively. SCD is contraindicated in individuals with **deep vein thrombosis (DVT)**, compartment syndrome, extremity deformities and open wounds of the extremities. SCDs may be applied directly onto the legs or over thromboembolic prevention stockings (Potter et al 2023).

For people requiring surgery, additional preventative measures may include antithrombotic agents preoperatively and postoperatively (Berman et al 2020; Crisp et al 2021).

See Clinical Skill 28.3 for more information and guidelines on the application of anti-embolic stockings.

CLINICAL SKILL 28.3 Application of anti-embolic stockings

Please adhere to the policy and procedures of the facility/organisation prior to undertaking the skill. Ensure this skill is in your scope of practice.

NMBA Decision-making Framework considerations (refer to NMBA Decision-making framework for nursing and midwifery 2020):	Equipment:
1. Am I educated? 2. Am I authorised? 3. Am I competent? If you answer 'no' to any of these, do not perform that activity. Seek guidance and support from your teacher/a nurse team leader/clinical facilitator/educator.	Tape measure Correct size of anti-embolic elastic stockings Talcum powder (optional)

PREPARE FOR THE SKILL

(Please refer to the Standard Steps on pp. xviii–xx for related rationales.)
Mentally review the steps of the skill.
Discuss the skill with your instructor/supervisor/team leader, if required.
Confirm correct facility/organisation policy/safe operating procedures.
Validate the order in the individual's record.
Identify indication and rationale for performing the activity.
Assess for any contraindications.
Locate and gather equipment.
Perform hand hygiene.
Ensure therapeutic interaction.
Identify the individual using three individual identifiers.
Gain the individual's consent.
Assess for pain relief.
Prepare the environment.
Provide and maintain privacy.
Assist the individual to assume an appropriate position of comfort.

Skill activity	Rationale
Observe for signs and symptoms and conditions that might contraindicate the use of anti-embolic elastic stockings: • dermatitis • skin grafts • size of things • peripheral vascular disease.	Anti-embolic elastic stockings may aggravate skin conditions. Continuous pressure is necessary to keep graft adherent to recipient bed, but pressure should not be so firm as to cause death of the graft. Anti-embolic elastic stockings that do not fit correctly due to larger thighs may cause excessive pressure and constriction around the thighs, which could then lead to reduced venous return. Circulation may be further reduced in conditions of altered circulation.

PERFORM THE SKILL

(Please refer to the Standard Steps on pp. xviii–xx for related rationales.)
Perform hand hygiene.
Apply PPE: gloves, eyewear, mask and gown as appropriate.
Ensure the individual's safety and comfort throughout skill.
Promote independence and involvement of the individual if possible and/or appropriate.
Assess the individual's tolerance to the skill throughout.
Dispose of used supplies, equipment, waste and sharps appropriately.
Remove PPE and discard or store appropriately.
Perform hand hygiene.

CLINICAL SKILL 28.3 Application of anti-embolic stockings—cont'd

Skill activity	Rationale
Assess individual's skin, colouration and circulation of legs.	Identifies a baseline of skin condition and quality of pedal pulses.
Use tape measure to measure individual's legs to determine correct stocking size.	Stockings must be measured as per the instructions on the packaging. The length of the stockings will be determined by the medical orders and the individual's condition. If stockings are too large, they will not support the extremities adequately. If stockings are too small, circulation may be impeded.
Position individual in supine position.	Ensures good body mechanics for the nurse and enables ease of application. Stockings should be applied before standing to prevent stagnation of blood in lower extremities.
Ensure the individual's legs are clean and dry and apply a small amount of talcum powder.	Allows for easier application and reduces friction.
Stockings are applied by rolling them slowly from the foot up the leg. Ensure the foot fits into toe and heel position of the stocking. Ensure the stocking is completely extended up the leg. Ensure it is smooth and no creases are present. Ensure toes are able to be exposed to check they remain warm and pink and blood supply is not impeded by the stockings.	Creases in stockings can impede circulation to lower region of extremities.
Inspect stockings to make sure there are no creases or binding at the top.	Can lead to increased pressure and alter circulation.
Ensure individual is aware not to adjust stockings or roll them down. Note individual's reaction to stockings.	Rolling down of stockings can have a constricting effect and impede venous return. Ensure the individual is adapting to stockings and is not experiencing discomfort.
Ensure individual wears shoes/slippers over stockings to ambulate.	Slip/fall prevention strategy.
Remove stocking once per shift.	Ensure they remain in the correct position. Ensures skin intact. Ensures adequate circulation. Identifies any complications.

AFTER THE SKILL

(Please refer to the Standard Steps on pp. xviii–xx for related rationales.)
Communicate outcome to the individual, any ongoing care and to report any complications.
Restore the environment.
Report, record and document assessment findings, details of the skill performed and the individual's response.
Report, record and document any abnormalities and/or inability to perform the skill.
Reassess the individual to ensure there are no adverse effects/events from the skill.

Skill activity	Rationale
Document size and length of stockings that were applied. Record skin condition and circulatory assessment.	Informs healthcare professionals and assists with planning and implementing care.

(Crisp et al 2021; Rebeiro et al 2021)

Prevention of postural hypotension

Prevention involves the gradual reintroduction of ambulation and allowing time to adjust to changes such as moving from a lying to a sitting or standing position (see 'dangling technique' earlier in this chapter).

Development and management of pulmonary embolus

Management of emboli in the pulmonary system includes administration of oxygen, analgesia and anticoagulant therapy. When immobilised, a person's pulmonary system declines in function and effects are related to a decrease in the rate and depth of breathing and effort, as well as an increase in bronchial secretions. Lung expansion decreases and breathing deeply is inhibited. In addition, secretions pool in the bronchial tract, which predisposes a person to respiratory tract congestion and infection. Hypostatic pneumonia may result and the risk increases when a person is dehydrated or is given medication that causes respiratory depression, such as morphine.

Atelectasis, or collapse of the lung, may occur and inhibits gaseous exchange at the alveoli. This results in **hypoxaemia**, which is reduced levels of oxygen in arterial blood (Harris et al 2019). Signs and symptoms of lung congestion include a cough and production of sputum, rattling, distressed or painful breathing and increased body temperature (Berman et al 2020; Crisp et al 2021; Kennedy-Malone et al 2018).

Prevention of pulmonary stasis

Preventing pulmonary stasis includes nursing an individual sitting up when possible and encouraging coughing and deep breathing. Deep-breathing exercises are performed with the person in a sitting position. The nurse places one hand on the chest and the other on the abdomen just below the ribs. The person is instructed to inhale slowly and deeply, pushing the abdomen out to promote optimal distribution of air to the alveoli, then breathe out through pursed lips while contracting their abdomen, which forces air out of the lungs. **Pursed-lip breathing** improves oxygen diffusion, encourages a slow deep-breathing pattern and puts positive back-pressure on the airways so that they stay open longer and expel greater amounts of stale air. Abdominal contraction pushes the diaphragm upwards, exerts pressure on the lungs and helps to empty them. Deep breathing and coughing (DB&C) involves incorporating deep-breathing exercises with voluntary coughing. Deep breathing before coughing stimulates the cough reflex. The nurse instructs the individual to take a deep slow breath and exhale slowly (and repeated several times). The individual then takes a short breath and coughs from deep inside the lungs. Analgesia may need to be administered prior to DB&C to facilitate effective results (Hinkle et al 2021).

Additional chest physiotherapy, such as postural drainage and chest percussion and vibration, may be added. Fluids should be increased (provided there are no contraindications) to help liquefy secretions and facilitate coughing up secretions or phlegm. Oxygen therapy may be necessary, and medications such as antibiotics may be prescribed if infection is present. Analgesia is offered before chest physiotherapy begins. Nebulisation using normal saline can loosen secretions for ease of expectoration (Berman et al 2020; Crisp et al 2021; Potter et al 2023).

Urinary stasis

Immobility can lead to retention of urine, urinary tract infection or renal calculi. Difficulty in using the pan or bottle in bed can result in incomplete bladder emptying and stasis of urine. Immobility reduces the amount of circulating lactic acid, which leads to alkaline urine (i.e. high urinary pH values) and, together with excess blood calcium (which is excreted by the kidneys), may result in kidney stones.

Prevention and management of urinary stasis

To prevent stasis of urine, nurses promote an adequate intake of fluids (unless contraindicated) and ensure that the person understands the importance of not postponing urination and of the need to empty the bladder completely. Management depends on the cause and includes increasing fluids and treating any infection (Berman et al 2020; Crisp et al 2021; Potter et al 2023). Information on elimination of urine and disorders affecting the urinary system is provided in Chapter 31.

Constipation

Constipation may occur as a result of decreased intestinal peristalsis due to reduced mobility or as a result of difficulty in using the bedpan in bed. Preventing and managing constipation includes promoting adequate fluids, exercise and fibre, as well as the appropriate aperient or suppository when required. Individuals are encouraged to maintain as normal a routine as possible to promote normal bowel function. Information on bowel elimination is provided in Chapter 32.

Psychological effects of reduced mobility

Psychological stress, anxiety, depression or boredom can occur when a person is immobilised. Loss of independence occurs when people have to rely on other people or aids to carry out ADLs. It interferes with all aspects of living, and people become bored by the lack of stimulation or variety. A change in the level of independence and physical impairment or isolation from family and friends results in feelings of depression, and people may also be anxious and feel worthless, irritable, apathetic and restless. Nurses need to try to improve the person's self-esteem.

Individuals are encouraged to participate in decisions regarding care, which allows some control over their life. Changes of environment may be beneficial (e.g. some time spent in the day room or outside, reading, exploring the internet, using the radio, TV or telephone may prevent boredom). Encourage the individual to pursue hobbies or studies, or an occupational therapist may be able to provide alternative activities. A social worker may assist with any problems about finance or the home situation. Flexible visiting hours are important, as well as communication with the person showing concern, respect and empathy, active listening, and providing information about care and treatment. It is important that people are allowed to express their emotions (Berman et al 2020; Crisp et al 2021).

Progress Note 28.1

30/05/2025 1500 hrs	Nursing—CNS: Individual alert and orientated. Equal strength and movement upper limbs, noted weakness right leg compared to left. PEARL. Reporting pain 4/10 in right hip, paracetamol 1000 mg PO given with lunch. Pain now reported to be 1/10. CVS: Peripherally warm to touch, pedal pulses present. Oedema observed to both feet. TED stockings applied and feet elevated at rest. HR 84 beats/min and regular. BP 130/80 mmHg. ECG taken as per orders doctor, awaiting results. Respiratory: Equal air entry auscultated right and left lungs. RR 22 breaths/min, SpO_2 92% room air—reported to Dr Jones, apply O_2 2 L/min nasal prongs applied as per Dr Jones' orders. Nil cough. GIT: Tolerating light ward diet. Abdomen soft, bowels open twice this morning. Auscultated bowel sounds +++. Renal: Urinalysis SG 1.010, fluids encouraged. Continent of urine. FBC commenced. Musculoskeletal: Ambulant with walking stick, right-sided limp observed. Integumentary: Skin intact, no signs of pressure injury observed. 2-hourly pressure care enforced. *K Adams* (ADAMS), *EN*

DECISION-MAKING FRAMEWORK EXERCISE 28.1

You are caring for an individual who returned from theatre 3 hours ago after having a plate removed from a previous surgery for a fractured leg. Postoperative orders state strict rest in bed for 4 hours. The individual is demanding to get up to go to the toilet because he needs to defecate.

How should you respond to this situation in accordance with legal and ethical aspects of nursing, and the decision-making framework for nurses?

Refer to the Decision-making framework summary: Nursing (NMBA 2020) for steps to guide actions in this situation.

The steps are:

1. Identify potential risks/hazards associated with mobilising this patient.
2. Reflect on whether they have the necessary educational preparation, experience, capacity, confidence and competence to safely perform the activity.
3. Decide whether there is a justifiable, evidence-based reason to perform the activity.
4. Identify strategies to meet the patient needs without compromising their safety.

Summary

Knowledge of the musculoskeletal system gives the nurse insight into how the body functions during exercise and movement and the way in which exercise can improve health and wellbeing. Pathological changes in the musculoskeletal system can result from inflammation, infection, degeneration, nutritional influences, neoplasms or trauma. Major manifestations of pathological changes include pain, sensory changes, swelling, deformity and loss of movement. Disorders of the musculoskeletal system may be classified as congenital, degenerative, infectious or inflammatory, immunological, metabolic, neoplastic, traumatic or from multiple causes.

Movement and exercise are proven to promote and maintain joint mobility, muscle strength and tone. Systemic benefits of movement and exercise include cardiopulmonary efficiency, improved psychological state and reduced risk of chronic disease.

All individuals should be assessed for their ability to participate in physical activity. Nurses have a duty of care to identify, plan and implement safe, appropriate nursing interventions to promote movement. By implementing simple nursing measures, movement and exercise can be promoted and complications from immobility prevented. Any technique or aid used to assist a person should be one that promotes safety, comfort and independence.

Goals of care for individuals with musculoskeletal disorders include promoting rest, preventing complications of immobility, maintaining skin integrity, relieving pain, preventing psychosocial problems, remobilisation, regaining independence and rehabilitation. Nurses need

Continued

Summary—cont'd

to facilitate correct body alignment and positioning of the immobilised individual. Nursing care needs to include management of devices and interventions to restore musculoskeletal health, such as internal and external fixation.

Exercise has many physical and psychological benefits that greatly enhance wellbeing. Healthy attitudes towards regular exercise can mean a population that ages well and values exercise to prevent disease and illness.

Review Questions

1. What are the principles of good posture and body mechanics?
2. Describe the benefits of exercise on the human body.
3. What is the difference between isotonic, isometric and isokinetic exercise?
4. Describe the range-of-movement (ROM) exercises used to maintain joint mobility in the immobilised person.
5. Outline how physical activity can be promoted in adolescents and children.
6. Describe the benefits of exercise on health, fitness and the older person.
7. What are the complications associated with bed rest and immobility?
8. List interventions to prevent complications of bed rest and immobility.
9. Outline the components of a neurovascular assessment.
10. List factors that may contribute to delayed healing of a person with a neuromuscular disorder.
11. Outline the subjective and objective data that should be collected from the individual with a neuromuscular disorder.
12. Describe aspects of care for the individual with a cast.

Evolve® Answer guide for the Review Questions, Critical Thinking Exercises, Decision-making Framework Exercises and Critical Thinking Questions in Case Studies is hosted on Evolve: http://evolve.elsevier.com/AU/Koutoukidis/Tabbner.

References

Australian Bureau Statistics (ABS), 2018a. Overweight and obesity. Available at: <https://www.abs.gov.au/statistics/health/health-conditions-and-risks/overweight-and-obesity/latest-release#cite-window1>.

Australian Bureau Statistics (ABS), 2018b, Children's risk factors. Available at: <https://www.abs.gov.au/statistics/health/health-conditions-and-risks/childrens-risk-factors/latest-release#cite-window1>.

Australian Commission on Safety and Quality in Health Care (ACSQHC), 2021. National safety and quality health service standards, 2nd ed. ACSQHC, Sydney. Available at: <https://www.safetyandquality.gov.au/publications-and-resources/resource-library/national-safety-and-quality-health-service-standards-second-edition>.

Australian Institute of Health and Welfare (AIHW), 2017. Impact of physical inactivity as a risk factor for chronic conditions: Australian burden of disease. Available at: <https://www.aihw.gov.au/reports/burden-of-disease/impact-of-physical-inactivity-chronic-conditions/contents/summary>.

Australian Institute of Health and Welfare (AIHW), 2018. Physical activity across the life stages. Available at: <https://www.aihw.gov.au/reports/physical-activity/physical-activity-across-the-life-stages/contents/table-of-contents>.

Australian Institute of Health and Welfare (AIHW), 2023. Back problems. Cat. no. PHE 231. AIHW, Canberra. Available at: <https://www.aihw.gov.au/reports/chronic-musculoskeletal-conditions/back-problems>.

Baca, A., 2018. *Musculoskeletal and soft tissue trauma*, 5th ed. ASTNA Patient transport. Elsevier, St Louis.

Berman, A., Frandsen, G., Snyder, S.J., et al., 2020. *Kozier and Erb's fundamentals of nursing*, 5th ed. Pearson Australia, Melbourne.

Buckinx, F., Maton, L., Dalimier, V., et al., 2022. Development and validation of new exercises to promote physical activity in nursing home settings. *Geriatrics (Basel)* 7(5), 100. Available at: <https://pubmed.ncbi.nlm.nih.gov/36136809>.

Buttaro, T.M., Polgar-Bailey, P., Sandberg-Cook, J., Trybulski, J., 2020. *Primary* care, 6th ed. Elsevier, St Louis.

Cerasola, D., Argano, C., Corrao, S., 2022. Lessons from COVID-19: Physical exercise can improve and optimize health status. *Frontiers in Medicine*, 9.

Commonwealth Scientific and Industrial Research Organisation (CSIRO), 2022. CSIRO Healthy diet score 2022. Available at: <https://www.totalwellbeingdiet.com/media/1194/2016-csiro-healthy-diet-score.pdf>. <https://www.csiro.au/en/research/health-medical/diets/csiro-healthy-diet-score>.

Cooper, K., Gosnell, K., 2023. *Adult health nursing*, 9th ed. Mosby Elsevier, St Louis.

Cordes, T., Bischoff, L.L., Schoene, D., et al., 2019. A multi-component exercise intervention to improve physical functioning, cognition and psychosocial well-being in elderly nursing home residents: a study protocol of a randomized controlled trial in the PROCARE (prevention and occupational health in long-term care) project. *BMC Geriatrics* 19(1), 369–369.

Crisp, J., Douglas, C., Rebeiro, G., Waters, D., 2021. *Potter & Perry's fundamentals of nursing*, Australian version, 6th ed. Elsevier, Sydney.

Cuccurullo, S.J., Joki, J., Luke, O., 2021. *Introduction to physical medicine and rehabilitation.* In: *Firestein & Kelly's textbook of rheumatology*, 11th ed. Elsevier, Philadelphia.

Curtis, K., Ramsden, C., Shaban, R.Z., et al., 2019. *Emergency and trauma care for nurses and paramedics*, 23rd ed. Elsevier, Chatswood

Dahlberg, E.E., Hamilton, S.J., Hamid, F., et al., 2018. Indigenous Australians' perceptions of physical activity: a qualitative systematic review. *International Journal of Environmental Research Public Health* 15(7), 1492. Available at: <https://doi.org/10.3390/ijerph15071492>.

Dehail, Patrick, Nathaly Gaudreault, Haodong Zhou, et al., 2019. "Joint Contractures and Acquired Deforming Hypertonia in Older People: Which Determinants?" *Annals of Physical and Rehabilitation Medicine* (formerly *Annales de réadaptation et de médecine physique*) 62(6), 435–441.

Department of Health and Aged Care, 2021a. Australia's physical activity and sedentary behaviour guidelines. Available at: <https://www.health.gov.au/topics/physical-activity-and-exercise/physical-activity-and-exercise-guidelines-for-all-australians/for-adults-18-to-64-years>.

Department of Health and Aged Care, 2021b. Sedentary behaviour. Available at: < <https://www.health.gov.au/topics/physical-activity-and-exercise/physical-activity-and-exercise-guidelines-for-all-australians?utm_source=health.gov.au&utm_medium=callout-auto-custom&utm_campaign=digital_transformation>.

Duan, D., et al., 2021. Duchenne muscular dystrophy. *Nature Reviews Disease Primers* 7(1), 13–13. Available at: <https://doi.org/10.1038/s41572-021-00248-3>.

du Toit, M., 2018. Prevention of contractures in older people living in long term care settings. *Nursing Older People* 30(4), 24–30.

Firestein, G.S., Budd, R.C., Gabriel, S.E., et al., 2021. *Firestein & Kelly's textbook of rheumatology*, 11th ed. Elsevier, Philadelphia.

Flynn, M., Mercer, D., 2018. *Oxford handbook of adult nursing*. Oxford University Press, Oxford.

Gilhus, N.E., Tzartos, S., Evoli, A., et al., 2019. Myasthenia gravis. *Nature Reviews Disease Primers* 5(1), 30–30. Available at: <https://doi.org/10.1038/s41572-019-0079-y>.

Goldman, L., Schafer, A.I., 2019. *Goldman-Cecil medicine*, 26th ed. Elsevier Saunders, New York.

Gulanick, M., Myers, J. L., 2022. *Nursing care plans: Diagnoses, interventions, and outcomes*, 10th ed. Elsevier Mosby, St Louis.

Harris, P., Nagy, S., Vardaxis, N., 2019. *Mosby's Dictionary of medicine, nursing and health professions*, 3rd ed. Elsevier, Chatswood.

Hinkle, J.L., Cheever, K.H., Overbaugh, K., 2021. *Brunner and Suddarth's textbook of medical-surgical nursing*, 15th ed. Lippincott, Williams & Wilkins, Philadelphia.

Hockenberry, M.J., Wilson, D., Rodgers, C.C., 2022. *Wong's essentials of paediatric nursing*, 11th ed. Elsevier, St Louis.

Jankovic, J., Mazziotta, J., Pomeroy, S., et al., *2021. Bradley's neurology in clinical practice*, 8th ed. Elsevier, Philadelphia.

Jester, R., Santy-Tomlinson, J., Rogers, J., 2021. *Oxford handbook of trauma and orthopaedic nursing*, 2nd ed. Oxford University Press, Oxford

Kennedy-Malone, L., Martin-Plank, L., Duffy, E.G., 2018. *Advanced practice nursing in the care of older adults*, 2nd ed. F.A. Davis Company, Philadelphia.

Lachman, M.E., Lipsitz, L., Castaneda-Sceppa, C., et al., 2018. When adults don't exercise: Behavioral strategies to increase physical activity in sedentary middle-aged and older adults. *Innovation in Aging* 2(1), 1–12. Available at: <https://academic.oup.com/innovateage/article/2/1/igy007/4962182>.

Lassale, C., Tzoulaki, I., Moons, K.G.M., et al., 2018. Separate and combined associations of obesity and metabolic health with coronary heart disease: A pan-European case-cohort analysis. *European Heart Journal* 39(5), 397–406.

LeMone, P., Bauldoff, G., Gubrud-Howe, P., et al., 2020. *Medical–surgical nursing: critical thinking in person-centred care*, 4th ed. Pearson, Melbourne.

Lennon, S., Ramdharry, G., Verheyden, G., 2018. *Physical management for neurological conditions*. Elsevier, Amsterdam.

Marieb, E.N., Keller, S.M., 2022. *Essentials of human anatomy & physiology*, 13th ed. Pearson, New York.

Matos, R., Monteiro, D., Amaro, N., Antunes, R., et al, 2021. Parents' and Children's (6-12 Years Old) Physical Activity Association: A systematic review from 2001 to 2020. *International Journal of Environmental Research and Public Health* 18(23).

Nursing and Midwifery Board of Australia (NMBA), 2020. Decision-making framework for nursing and midwifery. Available at: <https://www.nursingmidwiferyboard.gov.au/Codes-Guidelines-Statements/Frameworks.aspx>.

Overall, B., 2022. Pressure injury prevention strategies (adults): Risk assessment. Available at: <http://ovidsp.ovid.com/ovidweb.cgi?T=JS&PAGE=reference&D=jbi&NEWS=N&AN=JBI1553>.

Patton, K.T., Thibodeau, G.A., 2019. *Anatomy and physiology*, 10th ed. Mosby Elsevier, St Louis.

Pedrinolla, A., Magliozzi, R., Colosio, A.L., et al., 2022. Repeated passive mobilization to stimulate vascular function in individuals of advanced age who are chronically bedridden: A randomized controlled trial. *The Journals of Gerontology*. Series A, *Biological Sciences and Medical Sciences* 77(3), 588–596.

Perry, A.G., Potter, P.A., Ostendorf, W.R., 2019. *Nursing interventions & clinical skills*, 7th ed. Elsevier, St Louis.

Potter, P.A., Perry, A.G., Stockert, P.A., et al., 2023. *Fundamentals of nursing*, 11th ed. Elsevier/Mosby, St Louis.

Rebeiro, G., Wilson, D., Fuller, S. 2021. *Fundamentals of nursing: Clinical skills workbook*, 4th ed. Elsevier, Chatswood.

Richards, J., Whittle, M., Levine, D., 2023. *Whittle's gait analysis*, 6th ed, Elsevier, St Louis.

Roberts, N., et al., 2018. Can the target set for reducing childhood overweight and obesity be met? A system dynamics modelling study in New South Wales, Australia. Available at: <https://onlinelibrary.wiley.com/doi/full/10.1002/sres.2555>.

Sehgal, M., Jacobs, J., Biggs, W. S., 2021. Mobility assistive device use in older adults. *American Family Physician* 103(12), 737–744.

Silvestri, A., Silvestri, L., 2023, *Saunders comprehensive review for the NCLEX-RN Examination*, 9th ed, Elsevier, St Louis.

Sorrentino, S.A., Remmert, L.N., 2021. *Mosby's textbook for nursing assistants*, 10th ed. Elsevier, St Louis.

Tollefson, J., Hillman, E., 2022. *Clinical psychomotor skills: Assessment tools for nursing students*, 8th ed. Cengage Learning Australia, South Melbourne.

Touhy, T.A., Jett, K., 2019. *Ebersole & Hess' toward healthy aging*, 10th ed. Elsevier, St Louis.

Williams, P., 2021. *Fundamental concepts and skills for nursing*, 6th ed. Saunders Elsevier, Philadelphia.

Williamson, P., Thompson, T., Bell, F., Patton. K., 2024. *The human body in health & disease*, 8th ed. Elsevier, St Louis

World Health Organization (WHO), 2018. Global action plan on physical activity 2018–2030: More active people for a healthier world. Available at: <https://apps.who.int/iris/bitstream/handle/10665/272722/9789241514187-eng.pdf>.

World Health Organization (WHO), 2021. Obesity and overweight. Available at: <https://www.who.int/news-room/fact-sheets/detail/obesity-and-overweight>.

World Health Organization (WHO), 2022a. Physical activity. Available at: <https://www.who.int/news-room/fact-sheets/detail/physical-activity>.

World Health Organization (WHO), 2022b. Global status report on physical activity 2022, World Health Organization. Available at: <https://www.who.int/publications/i/item/9789240059153>.

Xiao, J., 2020. *Physical exercise for human health*. Springer, Singapore.

Recommended Reading

Easy moves for active ageing. Active Ageing. Available at: <https://activeageing.org.au/stay-active-resources/how-to-keep-active>.

Harding, M., Kwong, J., Hagler, D., Reinisch, C. 2023. *Lewis's medical-surgical nursing*, 12th ed. Elsevier, St Louis.

How to start exercising. Health Direct. Available at: <https://www.healthdirect.gov.au/tips-for-getting-active>.

Fitness and exercise. Health Direct. Available at: < https://www.healthdirect.gov.au/fitness-and-exercise>.

Online Resources

Ageing & aged care: <https://www.health.vic.gov.au/ageing-and-aged-care>.

Australian Bureau of Statistics: <https://www.abs.gov.au>.

Walk Easy Inc: <https://walkeasy.com/explore/crutch-gaits.php>.

CHAPTER 29

Skin integrity and wound care

Jing Wan (Persephone Wan)

Key Terms

acute wound
biofilm
burn injuries
chronic wound
compression therapy
debridement
dermis
epidermis
epithelialising
granulating
haemoserous
haemostasis
HEIDI
inflammation phase
integumentary system
leg ulcers
macerated
multiple organ dysfunction syndrome (MODS)
pressure injuries
primary intention
proliferation phase
purulent
remodelling phase
risk factors
sanguineous
secondary intention
serous
skin tears
slough
surgical wound
tertiary intention
TIME
wound assessment
wound bed preparation
wound infection

Learning Outcomes

At the completion of this chapter and with further reading, learners should be able to:

- Define the key terms.
- Describe the structure of the skin.
- Describe the functions of the skin.
- Identify the risk factors for loss of skin integrity.
- Discuss the wound-healing process.
- Describe the different wound-healing intentions.
- Describe the classifications of wound types.
- Identify the principles of wound management.
- Identify nutritional needs to promote wound healing.
- Describe the differences between acute and chronic wounds.
- Describe the procedures related to care of surgical wounds.
- Describe the care required to prevent and manage pressure injuries.
- Discuss the differences between arterial and venous leg ulcers.
- Describe the care required to prevent and manage skin tears.
- Describe the management of loss of skin integrity related to burns.
- Describe the major manifestations of skin disorders.
- Complete an assessment for an individual with impaired skin integrity.
- Assist in planning and implementing nursing care for the individual with a loss of skin integrity.
- Identify the purpose of commonly used wound dressings.
- List appropriate nursing interventions for the individual with impaired skin integrity.

CHAPTER FOCUS

The skin, or integumentary system, is the largest organ of the body, with primary functions of protecting the body against infection, physical trauma and ultraviolet radiation. Any disorder that disrupts normal skin function will affect the efficiency with which it carries out its functions and may place the physiological integrity of the individual at risk. Effects that skin disorders may have on the individual range from minor or temporary to major and life-threatening. Skin disorders can affect an individual's self-esteem and body image, dependent on location of injury, age, gender and cultural background. Protecting skin integrity and wound management are major aspects of the role of the nurse. It is important that all nurses understand normal wound healing and the variances that can occur with ageing and disease processes. There is an abundance of literature on wound management and a vast array of wound-care products. The aim of this chapter is to assist the nurse to increase their knowledge in this rapidly changing area.

LIVED EXPERIENCE

I had been struggling with a leg ulcer for almost a year. It was very painful and really limited my walking and daily life. Every time I thought it was healing, it got worse again. My GP referred me to a wound clinic. The nurses there did series of tests. They also involved my doctor and other health professionals like the physiotherapist, occupational therapist, dietitian and social worker in my care. I had to have frequent dressing changes and wear layers of compression bandages. The clinic organised nurses to visit me every third day to check my wound and reapply my bandages until it eventually healed. The physiotherapist provided me a walker so that I could still walk around safely. The dietitian provided me more information on what I should and should not eat to promote healing and the social worker organised community services for me since I live on my own.

It has been a long journey, but with all the support I received I'm so grateful the ulcer has finally healed. Now I just need to keep wearing compression stockings every day, but I can continue my life without the pain and wound in my leg. I really appreciate all the effort those wonderful nurses and other health professionals have put in to help me have a normal life.

Dorothy, 75 years old

INTRODUCTION

The **integumentary system** consists of the skin and its appendages: the hair, nails and sweat and sebaceous glands. The skin (or integument) is the largest organ of the body, covering about 7500 cm^2 of surface area in an average adult (Figure 29.1). It is a protective barrier to the outside world, plays a vital role in homeostasis and thermoregulation and provides a means of communication through touch and sensation. The appendages of the skin, hair, nails and sweat glands arise from the epidermis but are present in the dermis (Carville 2023; Patton & Thibodeau 2019; Scanlon & Sanders 2019).

Structure of the skin

The skin comprises two basic layers: the **epidermis** and **dermis**. Under the dermis is a layer of adipose tissue called subcutaneous tissue. While this layer is not considered to be part of the skin, subcutaneous tissue does protect and insulate the deeper tissues and is composed primarily of fat and connective tissue (Scanlon & Sanders 2019).

The epidermis

The epidermis is the thin outermost layer and is composed of epithelial cells arranged in layers of stratified epithelium. The number of layers varies dependent on the use and exposure experienced (e.g. there are many more layers on the soles of the feet and the palms of the hands than there are between the toes and the fingers) (Carville 2023).

The epidermis is divided into two layers. The horny layer (stratum corneum) is the uppermost layer, and consists of about 30 layers of dead, flattened, keratinised cells. These keratinocytes contain a waterproof hard protein substance called keratin (Scanlon & Sanders 2019). Keratin's waterproofing properties protect the body and prevent the escape of fluid from the deeper tissues. Keratin is also responsible for the formation of hair and nails. The germinative layer (stratum germinativum) is the deeper layer of the epidermis. It is here that new cells are constantly being formed and pushed upwards to replace cells that die and shed. Millions of new cells are produced daily and are pushed up away from the source of nutrition, to become part of the outermost layer.

Melanocytes are present in the germinative layer. Their function is to produce a brown pigment called melanin. Melanin gives colour to the skin and protects the body against the damaging effects of ultraviolet rays in sunlight. Skin tone is determined by the amount of melanin produced: dark-toned skin results when large amounts of melanin are produced, whereas light-toned skin results

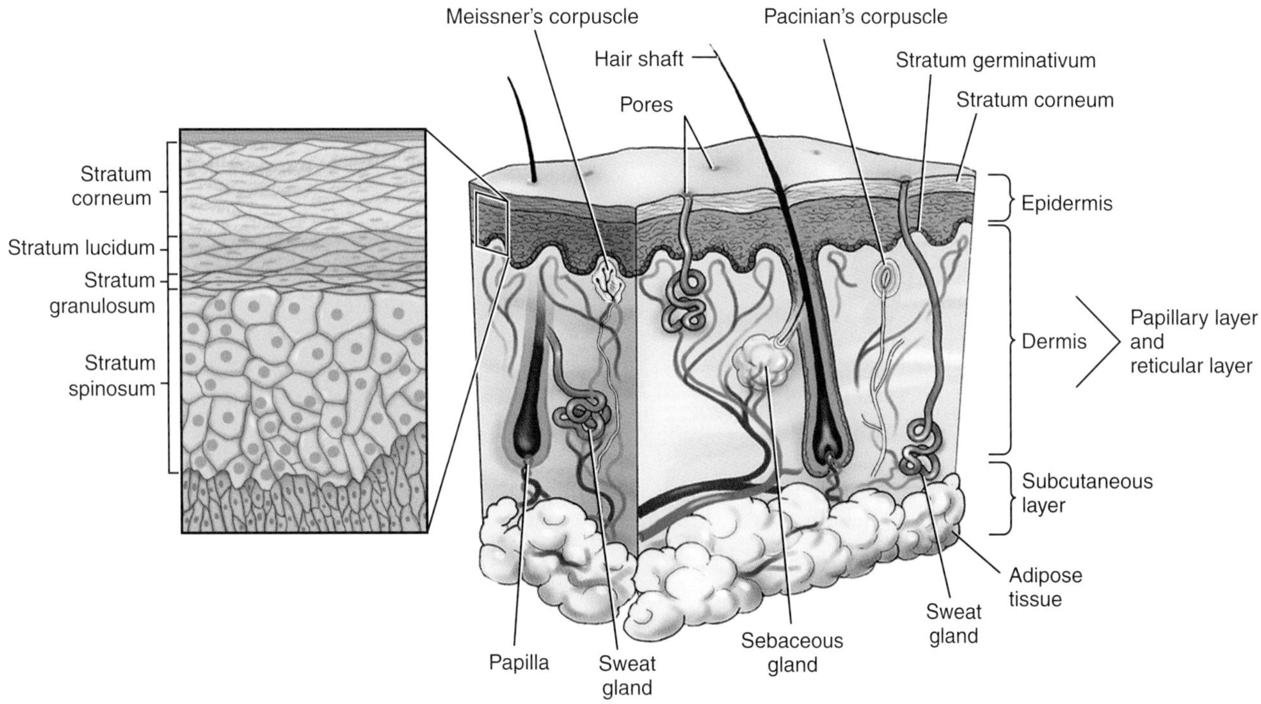

Figure 29.1 Diagram of the skin
(Zenith 2018)

when the body produces less melanin (Patton & Thibodeau 2019; Scanlon & Sanders 2019).

The epidermis does not contain any blood vessels but receives its essential nourishment from fluid that is diffused from the blood supply of underlying structures. As cells are pushed towards the surface, away from the source of nutrition, they die and are eventually shed. This process usually takes place between 28 and 35 days (Peate & Stephens 2020).

The patterns of lines and ridges in the epidermis are due to projections in the dermis called papillae. On the fingertips, these patterns are the fingerprints, which are different in every individual. For this reason, fingerprints are useful for purposes of identification. Nails are formed from the stratum corneum and are composed of modified epithelium (Patton & Thibodeau 2019).

The dermis

The dermis lies beneath the epidermis and consists of collagen, reticular fibres and elastic tissue. The dermis contains blood capillaries, nerve endings, sweat glands, hair follicles and other structures. Elasticity of the skin allows for essential strength, flexibility and protection. As a natural consequence of ageing, the fibres become less elastic, causing wrinkles and folds to appear in the skin and an increased risk of skin injury.

The following structures are contained in the dermis:

- network of blood vessels
- nerve endings
- hair follicles and hair
- arrector pili muscles.

(Kapp & Tomkins 2020)

Network of blood vessels

The blood vessels transport blood containing oxygen and nutrients to the dermis and transport blood containing wastes such as carbon dioxide away from the dermis. The blood vessels also play a role in regulating body temperature. If the body temperature is elevated, the dermal capillaries become engorged with blood, which allows loss of body heat from the skin surface through radiation. If the environmental temperature is low, blood vessels in the skin constrict, conserving body heat by reducing radiation from the body (Carville 2023; Patton & Thibodeau 2019; Scanlon & Sanders 2019).

Nerve endings

The dermis has a rich nerve supply consisting of several types of nerve endings. Each type of nerve ending reacts to a different stimulus, such as pain, touch, pressure and temperature. Impulses are transmitted from the nerve endings to the brain for interpretation (Patton & Thibodeau 2019).

Hair follicles and hairs

Hairs grow from hair follicles, which are deep pouch-like cavities in the skin. Although hair follicles are present in most areas of the skin, they are not found on the palms of the hands, lips or the soles of the feet. Hair is composed of modified epithelium and grows from roots deep in the follicles. The part of a hair projecting above the epidermis is called the shaft. Hair colour reflects the amount of pigment, generally melanin, in the epidermis. Hair is a protection from the elements and from trauma. For example, the scalp hair and eyebrows are barriers against sunlight, and the nasal hairs filter inhaled air (Carville 2023; Patton & Thibodeau 2019; Scanlon & Sanders 2019).

Hair growth is influenced by the sex hormones oestrogen and testosterone. An excessive growth of hair is called hirsutism. Like other cells that compose the skin, the hair cells also become keratinised. The hair that we wash, brush or comb and style is a collection of dead keratinised cells. Hair colour is genetically controlled and is determined by the type and amount of melanin (Carville 2023). The absence of melanin produces white hair. Grey hair is due to a mixture of pigmented and non-pigmented hairs. Red hair is due to a modified type of melanin that contains iron. Hair is important cosmetically. Hair loss can be very distressing for some people. The most common type of hair loss is male-pattern baldness. It is a hereditary condition characterised by a gradual loss of hair with ageing (Patton & Thibodeau 2019).

Arrector pili muscles

The arrector pili muscles are minute involuntary muscles, with one end attached to a hair follicle and the other end to the dermis. When these muscles contract (e.g. during fear or exposure to cold), the follicles and hairs become erect. Contraction of the muscles also causes some elevation of the skin around the hairs, giving rise to the 'goose bump/pimple' appearance. The contraction of the arrector pili muscles increases heat production. This response is called shivering (Patton & Thibodeau 2019).

Skin glands

Two major types of glands are associated with the skin: sebaceous glands and sweat glands (Carville 2023; Patton & Thibodeau 2019; Scanlon & Sanders 2019).

Sebaceous glands

Sebaceous glands are small glands, most of which open into hair follicles. The glands produce sebum, which is an oily substance and a lubricant that keeps the skin soft and moist and prevents the hair from becoming brittle. Combined with sweat, sebum forms a moist, oily acidic film that is mildly antibacterial. During periods of increased hormonal activity, such as adolescence, sebaceous glands become very active and the skin becomes oilier. Sebaceous glands are present on all areas of the skin except for the palms of hands and soles of feet, and are most abundant on the face, scalp and upper chest and back.

Sweat glands

Sweat glands, which are widely distributed, are either eccrine or apocrine. Eccrine glands are present all over the body and produce a clear perspiration. Apocrine glands are found mainly in the axillary and genital areas and secrete sweat that has a strong characteristic odour. Sweat glands are coiled in appearance, with a straight duct that releases sweat onto the surface of the skin through an opening called a pore.

Sweat glands play a part in regulating body temperature. They excrete large amounts of sweat when the external (or body) temperature is high. When sweat evaporates off the skin's surface, it carries large amounts of body heat with it. Sweat consists of water that contains sodium chloride, phosphates, urea, ammonia and other waste products. Under normal circumstances, the amount of sweat secreted by an individual is about 700 mL/day. Under some conditions, such as strenuous physical exertion or pyrexia, the amount can be increased to as much as 1500 mL/day. Much of the water lost through the skin evaporates immediately, so it is not noticeable and is called insensible perspiration. Sweat that makes the skin damp and is noticeable is called sensible perspiration.

Functions of the skin

The major functions in which the skin and its appendages play a role are protection, thermoregulation, metabolism and sensory perception (Carville 2023; Patton & Thibodeau 2019; Scanlon & Sanders 2019).

Protection

The skin is the first line of defence against the external environment. It provides a barrier to a variety of harmful agents, such as microorganisms, radiant energy and chemical substances. The skin acts as a barrier to harmful agents only as long as it remains intact. The waterproof quality of the outer layer prevents excess water absorption and abnormal loss of body fluids. The skin contains nerve endings that are sensitive to painful stimuli. The nerve endings transmit impulses to the brain that alert the individual that damage is occurring.

Thermoregulation

The skin plays a major role in the maintenance of constant body temperature. Blood conducts heat from internal structures to the skin for dissipation. The skin dissipates excess body heat by radiation, conduction, convection and evaporative cooling. Body temperature is controlled by the hypothalamus, which is the heat-regulating centre in the brain. This centre is sensitive to the temperature of the blood passing through it and receives sensory stimuli from nerve endings in the skin that react to heat and cold (thermoreceptors). The hypothalamus in turn relays impulses requiring vasodilation and activation of the sweat glands (for cooling), or vasoconstriction and inhibition of sweat glands (for heat retention). Thus, the hypothalamus acts like a thermostat that initiates heat-losing activities when the body temperature begins to rise and heat-retaining activities when the body temperature starts to fall (Scanlon & Sanders 2019).

Metabolism

The skin assists in the regulation of fluid and electrolyte balance by eliminating water and small amounts of sodium chloride through the sweat glands. Sweat consists of 99.4% water, 0.2% salts and 0.4% urea and other wastes. In the presence of sunlight or ultraviolet radiation, the skin begins the process of forming vitamin D (calciferol), a substance required for absorbing calcium and phosphates from food.

Sensory perception

Through perception of a painful stimulus, the skin causes an avoidance reaction, while other receptors perceive sensations of pressure and touch. The skin is therefore an agent of communication between the outside environment and the body, as the activity of sensory nerve endings informs the individual of what is happening outside the body.

Factors that affect skin integrity

Factors affecting skin integrity include the following (but the list is not exhaustive):

- age
- neurological disorders
- malnutrition and poor hydration status
- altered systemic and local circulation and oxygenation disorders
- medications (e.g. polypharmacy, steroid use)
- obesity
- smoking
- incontinence
- sedentary lifestyle
- inappropriate or ill-fitting prostheses and footwear
- exposure to pressure, friction, shearing forces or moisture
- exposure to chemicals, radiation or ultraviolet light
- diseases (e.g. diabetes mellitus)
- infection
- trauma from falls, accidents or burns
- surgical intervention
- psychological status: depression, anxiety
- skin disorders (e.g. genetic factors, idiopathic causes, hypersensitivity rashes).

WOUND HEALING

Wound healing is a dynamic and complex process. Tissue replacement involves two main mechanisms: repair and regeneration. In humans, the mechanism of repair for any wound is determined by the tissue layers involved and their capacity for regeneration (Carter et al 2023; Guillamat-Prats 2021; Tang & Marshall 2017). See Table 29.1 for definitions of repair and regeneration.

The wound-healing process consists of four stages: haemostasis, the inflammation stage, the reconstruction phase and maturation/remodelling phase (Figure 29.2). The process of wound healing begins at the time of injury and follow a natural cascade that may continue for some years (Carville 2023; Peate & Stephens 2020).

Haemostasis

The first stage of wound healing is **haemostasis**, which has three components: vasoconstriction, platelet response and the biochemical response. Vasoconstriction occurs when the bleeding in the wound is arrested by spasm in the arteries, arterioles and capillaries.

The platelet response is commonly described as the formation of the platelet plug. When platelets come into contact with parts of a damaged blood vessel, such as collagen or endothelium, their characteristics change. They become larger and irregular in shape and stick to the collagen fibres in the wall of the vessels and to each other. The platelets release various chemicals: serotonin, prostaglandins, phospholipids and adenosine diphosphate (ADP) that attract more platelets, which stick to the original platelets and form the plug. This platelet plug is very effective in preventing blood loss in a small vessel.

The biochemical component is the formation of a blood clot through the processes of the intrinsic and extrinsic clotting pathways, clot retraction and fibrinolysis. This is a complex process involving different clotting factors that are released from the damaged tissue. A clot is developed and retraction of the wound takes place.

The next stage of the healing process is termed tissue repair. This stage also has three phases: inflammation, reconstruction and maturation, which overlap each other and have varying time intervals.

The inflammation phase

The **inflammation phase** begins the moment that injury is incurred. The capillaries contract and thrombose to facilitate

TABLE 29.1 | Definition of repair and regeneration

Healing properties	Definition	Tissue types
Repair	The process of producing connective tissue to fill the defect or knit tissues back together, which can result in scarring and functional impairment.	Deep dermal structures (e.g. hair follicles, sebaceous glands, sweat glands), subcutaneous tissue, muscle, tendons, ligaments and bone lack the capacity to regenerate.
Regeneration	When damaged cells and tissue are replaced by proliferation of similar cells so that the normal tissue function can be restored.	Wounds that are confined to the epidermal and superficial dermal layers heal by regeneration because epithelial, endothelial and connective tissue can be reproduced.

(Paul & Sharma 2021; Wu et al 2023)

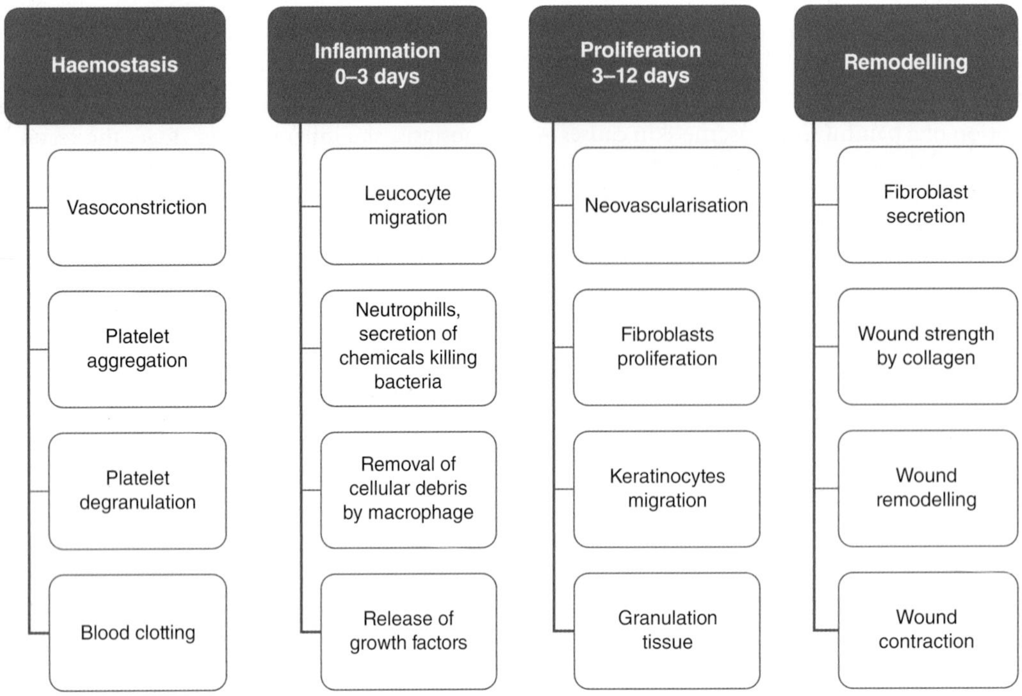

Figure 29.2 Phases/events related to wound-healing process
(Singh et al 2024)

haemostasis. Vasodilation of the surrounding tissues occurs in response to the release of histamine and other vasoactive chemicals. This process causes increased blood flow to the surrounding tissue, which produces erythema, swelling, heat and discomfort, such as throbbing. A variety of white blood cells called polymorphonuclear leucocytes arrives at the site of the wound as a defence response and is involved in the immune response to fight infection. Polymorphs, macrophages and their associated growth factors produce various local and systemic effects. This phase continues for about 3 days.

The reconstruction/proliferation phase

The reconstruction/**proliferation phase** is a time of cleaning and temporary replacement of tissue. The polymorphs kill bacteria, and the phagocytic macrophages digest the dead bacteria and debris to clean up the wound. Dermal repair is necessary if the wound is one of full thickness. New blood capillaries are developed (angiogenesis) and granulation tissue, which consists largely of collagen, is laid down. Epithelial cells migrate over the granulation tissue from the surrounding wound edges, hair follicles, sweat or sebaceous glands in the wound. These cells are very fragile. When the wound is covered, the epithelium begins to thicken to four to five layers, forming the epidermis. Wound contraction then occurs, reducing the overall size of the wound. This phase can continue for 2–24 days.

The maturation/remodelling phase

This is commonly known as the **remodelling phase**. The matrix of collagen cells is reorganised and strengthened. This phase can continue for about 24 days and up to 1 year. The skin matures to approximately 80% of the original tensile strength. The wound is still at risk during this phase and should continue to be protected.

Types of healing

Healing by **primary intention** occurs when wound edges are brought together by sutures, clips/staples, adhesive strips or adhesive tissue glue (Figure 29.3). Surgical wounds where there is minimal tissue loss and the wound bed is not exposed heal by primary intention. Hence, granulation tissue is not obvious. Healing by **secondary intention** occurs when wound edges cannot be brought together, as with an open wound (Carville 2023). Granulation tissue fills in the wound until re-epithelialisation takes place and a large scar results. **Tertiary intention** (delayed primary intention) healing occurs when wound closure is delayed for a few days so that an infected or contaminated wound can be debrided (dirt, foreign objects, damaged tissue and cellular debris are removed from a wound or burn to prevent infection and promote wound healing). Closure of contaminated wounds is usually delayed until all layers of wound tissue show no signs of infection, usually within 4–10 days. At other times, some wounds need surgical intervention, such as the application of skin grafts or flaps, to speed the healing process and reduce the risk of infection. Clinical Interest Box 29.1 provides details on skin grafts.

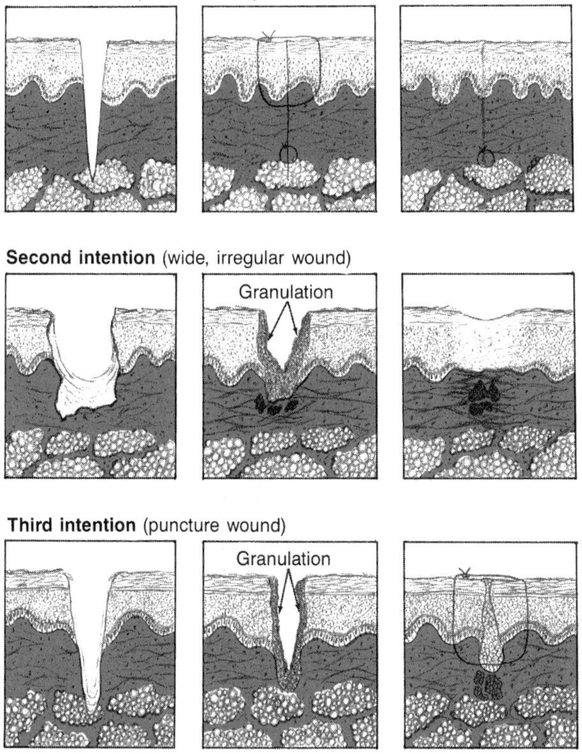

Figure 29.3 Types of wound healing
(Hockenberry et al 2024)

CLINICAL INTEREST BOX 29.1 Skin grafts

Skin grafts speed up the healing process and reduce the risk of infection. Grafts may be partial or full thickness. Skin grafts are classified as:

- Autograft: A surgical relocation of skin (split thickness or full thickness) to the wound from another site of the same individual. A second wound results and is known as the donor site.
- Allograft: A donor graft of skin between allogenic individuals, such as from one person to another.
- Xenograft: A donor graft of tissue transplanted between different species, such as tissue of porcine origin transplanted to a human being.
- Cultured: The cultivation of epidermis from a small number of epithelial cells taken from the donor or recipient's body and cultivated under laboratory conditions to form epidermis, before being transplanted back to the individual.

(Ahangar et al 2018; Wu et al 2023)

WOUND MANAGEMENT

Wound management employs the principles of moist wound healing—that is, keeping the wound bed moist enough to facilitate the movement of new epitheliums across the granulation tissue (Nuutila & Eriksson 2021).

The benefits of moist wound healing are:

- thermoregulation
- less pain
- less injury and damage to cells on removal of the dressing
- more efficient autolytic debridement of necrotic tissue
- less risk of transmission of microorganisms
- fewer dressing changes and therefore less disturbance of the wound bed, resulting in reduced costs in dressing consumables and reduced workload for care staff
- less interruption to the individual's lifestyle and with most dressings the individual can continue to shower as usual.

Wound assessment

An initial holistic assessment of the individual includes a comprehensive health history, demographics, nutritional status, psychosocial status, medication, mobility and activity, vascularity and current health status (Carville 2023; Docherty 2020; Sibbald et al 2021). **Wound assessment** identifies the wound characteristics, cause of the wound (e.g. traumatic, surgical), appearance of the wound bed (tissue type), exudate (amount, characteristics), wound edge and peri-wound skin condition, type of wound (skin tear, pressure injury), location, size of the wound and its chronicity. A wound management history should be obtained to determine previously effective or non-effective treatments. Presence of infection is assessed to be local or systemic. Pain management is a vital aspect of care that impacts on the wound-healing process and the quality of life for the individual with a wound. Clinical Interest Box 29.2 outlines the principles of wound management.

Assessment tools capture essential components of the individual and wound and include medical/surgical history of the individual, clinical history of the wound, relevant investigations to assist diagnosis of aetiology and local wound characteristics. Consistency in the information collected can be obtained in tools such as the mnemonic tool **HEIDI**: **h**istory (H), **e**xamination (E), **i**nvestigation (I), **d**iagnosis (D) and **i**ndicators (I) (Harding et al 2007). There are various specialised assessment tools available for pressure injuries and skin tears, such as National Pressure Injury Advisory Panel (NPIAP)/Agency for Health Care Policy and Research

CLINICAL INTEREST BOX 29.2 Principles of wound management

- Assess and define aetiology.
- Control or correct causative factors (e.g. smoking, nutrition, friction, moisture, infection).
- Set goals of care.
- Optimise wound bed and peri-wound area.
- Perform wound cleansing.
- Prevent wound-related infection.
- Select an appropriate dressing product.
- Optimise wound-related quality of life (e.g. pain, odour).

(Haesler & Carville 2023)

(AHCPR) staging system (European Pressure Ulcer Advisory Panel (EPUAP) et al 2019) and International Skin Tear Advisory Panel (ISTAP) Skin Tear Classification (LeBlanc et al 2018). Any of these relevant assessment tools must be used under the supervision of the Registered Nurse (RN).

Description of wounds

Colour

Wounds may be described by the colour of the wound bed:

- Black or dark brown: Necrotic tissue (dead or devitalised tissue) can be dry or moist.
- Yellow, brown and/or grey black: Usually indicates **slough**, a fibrous material with dead white cells, bacteria in the wound; can be moist or dry.
- Bright red or pink: Healthy **granulating** or **epithelialising** wound.

Degree/depth of injury

- Superficial: Wounds affecting the epidermis.
- Partial thickness: Wounds affecting the epidermis and the dermis.
- Full thickness: Wounds that have affected the epidermis, dermis and the subcutaneous tissue. The muscle, tendon and bone may also be involved.

Wound location

Anatomical description (e.g. lower left lateral leg, upper posterior right arm). This allows consistency in assessment and accurate communication and documentation.

Wound size measurement

- Area
- Depth, at deepest area
- Length, at longest measure in head-to-toe direction
- Width at widest measure from side-to-side direction (Figure 29.4)
- Examples of measurement methods available include simple disposable paper rulers for measuring length and width perpendicular to each other, probes or Q-tip for measuring depth, tracing grids and photography

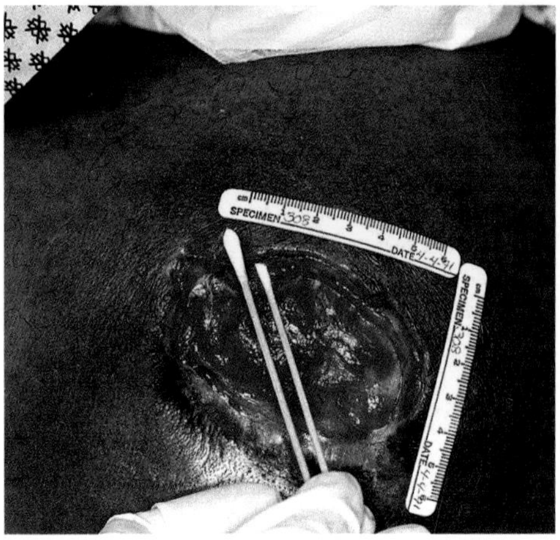

Figure 29.4 The size and depth of the wound are measured by nurse

(Potter 2013)

Exudate

- Type, colour and consistency:
  - **Serous**—clear to clear pale yellow, thin/watery consistency.
  - **Haemoserous**/serosanguineous—slight blood-stained serous fluid, pink or light red in colour, thin/watery consistency.
  - **Sanguineous**—frank bleeding or heavily blood-stained, thin/watery consistency.
  - **Purulent**—containing pus, yellow, tan or green, thick and opaque (Figure 29.5).
- Amount:
  - None/nil—no exudate.
  - Small/scant—exudate can be managed with low absorbent dressing and dressing can be in place for up to 7 days.
  - Moderate—exudate can be managed with absorbent dressing and frequency of dressing is usually every 2–3 days.
  - Large/copious—excessive amount of exudate which may require daily change of absorbent dressing.
- Colour:
  - Clinical indicator for stage of healing or complication. For example, both serous (clear/light colour) and haemoserous (light red to pink) are normal during inflammatory and proliferative/reconstruction phases of healing, while seropurulent and purulent are yellow to tan or green in colour and signify the suspicion of wound infection.

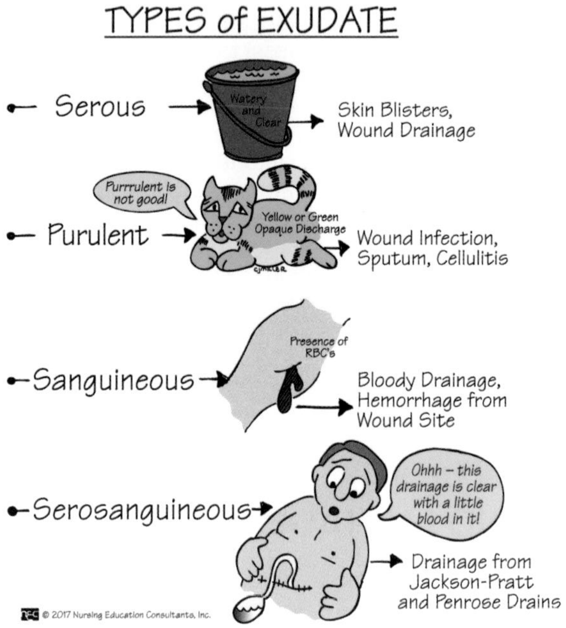
TYPES of EXUDATE
Serous
Watery and Clear
Skin Blisters, Wound Drainage
Purrulent is not good!
Purulent
Yellow or Green Opaque Discharge
Wound Infection, Sputum, Cellulitis
Sanguineous
Presence of RBC's
Bloody Drainage, Hemorrhage from Wound Site
Serosanguineous
Ohhh – this drainage is clear with a little blood in it!
Drainage from Jackson-Pratt and Penrose Drains
© 2017 Nursing Education Consultants, Inc.

Figure 29.5 Types of exudate

(Zerwekh 2017)

- Consistency:
  - Dependent on type of exudate: Thin/watery, thick.
- Odour:
  - Indicates infection or contamination.
  - Sign of non-viable tissue breakdown.
  - Drainage of body fluids such as faeces from a fistula.

Wound edge and peri-wound skin condition

- Wound edge:
  - Indistinct—difficult to differentiate wound bed and wound edge, a sign of re-epithelialisation.
  - Well defined—wound edge easily identifiable. Punched out wound edge is usually seen in arterial or vasculitic ulcers.
  - Rolled—suggestive of malignancy; may be caused by basal cell carcinoma.
  - Everted—suggestive of malignancy from squamous cell carcinoma.
  - Raised—suggestive of malignancy from squamous cell carcinoma, infection or hypergranulation.
  - **Macerated**—white, waxy appearance caused by excess exudate due to dressing not absorbent enough and/or inappropriate intervals between dressing changes.
  - Undermining present/absent. If present, the depth of the undermining, tunnelling, and sinus tracts and the direction/extent by using clock face are to be assessed and documented.
- Peri-wound skin:
  - Red—may indicate cellulitis, contact dermatitis, vasculitis.
  - Macerated—prolonged exposure to the excess amount of exudate, may indicate moisture associated dermatitis.
  - Purplish skin colour—may indicate haematoma, ischemia or vasculitis.
  - Inflamed—may suggest fungal or yeast infection or other conditions.
  - Overall skin colour, warmth, capillary return and any abnormality such as oedema.

Pain

- Identify and manage underlying cause of pain; local or systemic.
- Assess the wound pain for its severity, onset, duration, characteristics, factors affecting the pain.
- Implement appropriate pharmacological and non-pharmacological pain management strategies.
- Document the pain assessment findings, the interventions provided and the effectiveness.

Wound infection

- Monitor for signs and symptoms of infection; local or systemic.
- Infection delays healing.
- Report and manage locally with dressing product or systemically with prescribed pharmacological management.

Psychosocial

- Individual person-focused outcomes are the foundations of care.
- Quality of life/wellbeing.
- Engage consumers, provide education and support to promote wound management and healing.

Wound healing and nutrition

The role of nutrition in wound healing is vital; nurses are expected to provide education and ensure adequate nutritional intake. Whereas good nutrition facilitates healing, malnutrition delays, inhibits and complicates the process. Micronutrients, such as vitamins, minerals and amino acids, play various roles during the healing process (Almadani et al 2021; Bishop et al 2018). For example, vitamin A promotes angiogenesis and collagen synthesis during the reconstructive phase of healing, while zinc facilitates the collagen synthesis. Macronutrients, like carbohydrate, fatty acids and especially protein, provide the energy source for wound repair (Almadani et al 2021; Bishop et al 2018). Therefore, it is vital to assess and promote nutrition as a part of the wound assessment and management process. In other words, the individual's body mass index (BMI) and the risk of malnutrition are to be included as part of the holistic assessment (Bishop et al 2018). There are various nutritional screening tools available, among which the Malnutrition Screening Tool (MST) and Malnutrition Universal Screening Tool (MUST) are more commonly seen in community and hospital settings (Australian Commission on Safety and Quality in Health Care [ACSQHC] 2018; Cortes et al 2020). (See also Chapter 30.)

Nutrition for chronic wounds needs to be assessed on an individual basis; some types of wounds, such as pressure injuries or multiple wounds, place high demand for nutrients on the body. See Table 29.2 for a detailed review of nutrition and wound healing.

The use of arginine-enriched oral nutritional supplements may have a positive effect on the healing of chronic wounds (Schneider & Yahia 2019). Nutrition is a key element in the prevention and treatment of chronic wounds and must be incorporated into the wound management plan (Dent et al 2017; EPUAP et al 2019).

Wound bed preparation

Wound bed preparation is 'the management of the wound to accelerate endogenous healing or to facilitate the effectiveness of other therapeutic measures' (Shamsian 2021). Wound bed preparation uses an algorithm called the TIME principle. These principles identify four key areas of the chronic non-healing wound, though the principles can also be applied to acute wounds. All chronic wounds start as acute wounds but fail to progress and get trapped in the inflammatory phase of healing with bacterial and biochemical imbalance (Shamsian 2021). **TIME** provides a systematic approach to wound care. The four elements are **T** (tissue deficient or viability), **I** (infection or inflammation), **M** (moisture imbalance) and

TABLE 29.2 | Macronutrients and micronutrients and wound healing

Nutrient	Function	Dietary sources
Fat	Energy source, contributes to anti-inflammatory response, involved in cell membrane synthesis, assists in construction of the intracellular matrix.	Butter, margarine, other spreading fats, oils, cream, full-fat milk, cheese, oily fish, nuts, seeds.
Carbohydrate	Major source of calories for cell metabolism; its availability is essential to prevent other nutrients (i.e. protein) from being converted into energy.	Wholegrain cereals, bread, potatoes, rice, pasta.
Protein	Necessary for tissue synthesis and repair and immune system. Deficiency can inhibit wound remodelling and may increase oedema. This will further impair delivery of oxygen and nutrients to the wound.	Beef, chicken, fish, eggs, cheese, milk, yoghurt, celery, wheat, nuts, brussels sprouts, parsley, spinach. Vegetarians and vegans should consume pulses for their protein intake.
Vitamin A	Increases the inflammatory response in wounds, stimulating collagen synthesis. Low levels can result in delayed wound healing and susceptibility to infection.	Milk, cheese, eggs, fish, dark green vegetables, oranges, red fruits and vegetables.
Vitamin C	Involved in collagen synthesis and subsequent cross-linking, as well as the formation of new blood vessels. Adequate levels help strengthen the healing wound. Has important antioxidant properties that help the immune system; increases absorption of iron.	Found mostly in citrus fruits (e.g. orange), green vegetables and potatoes.
Vitamin B	Supports metabolic rate and promotes cell proliferation. Helps with production of energy from glucose, amino acids and fats. Vitamin B6 is important for maintaining cellular immunity and forming red blood cells. Thiamine and riboflavin are needed for adequate cross-linking and collagenation.	Wholegrains, breakfast cereals, milk and milk products, meat, fish, liver.
Vitamin E	Reduces inflammation by controlling excessive free radicals, stabilises cell walls.	Vegetable oil, egg yolk, nuts, seeds.
Vitamin K	Blood clotting.	Liver, green vegetables, avocado, meat and dairy products.
Selenium	An essential element with antioxidant properties that supports reproduction, thyroid hormone metabolism, DNA synthesis, and protects against cell damage and infection.	Poultry, lean meats, shellfish, nuts, seeds, bread and cereals.
Copper	A trace element required for the synthesis of protein and collagen.	Meat, vegetables, cereals, tea, coffee.
Magnesium	Often a cofactor to promote collagen synthesis by increasing fibroblasts and the production of DNA and protein. Component of enzymes needed for tissue regeneration.	Tea, widely distributed in various foods.
Zinc	A mineral that regulates immune responses. A cofactor for protein and collagen synthesis and in tissue growth and healing.	Best sources include red meat, liver, nuts, milk products, cereals.
Iron	Optimises tissue perfusion by forming haemoglobin, assists in collagen synthesis.	Iron absorption from non-meat sources can be enhanced with vitamin C. Best sources are red meat, liver, fortified cereals, pulses, green leafy vegetables.

(Bishop et al 2018; Ahuja & Lio 2023)

E (edge of wound non-advancing or undermining epidermal margin) (Atkin 2019). The wound bed preparation concept has gained international recognition as a framework that provides a structured approach to wound care, which supports nursing practice.

Tissue viability

Viable tissue, such as granulating and epithelialising tissue, is the healthy wound healing-tissue requiring a protective dressing. Non-viable tissue can be necrotic (black/brown, dry thick tissue with leathery consistency) dead tissue or slough (moist, loose, yellow, stringy/dead tissue), which impairs the growth of new tissue, obscures the true depth of a wound and is a haven for bacterial growth, preventing wound healing. Non-viable tissue also increases the risk of wound infection. Serial debridement is required to remove the tissue to promote a healthy wound bed (Atkin 2019).

Infection/inflammation

All wounds contain bacteria at some level often without harmful effects. Early detection and management are necessary to prevent deterioration and improve health outcomes. **Wound infection** results from an imbalance of the host's (the individual) immune system and its ability to combat bacteria (host resistance), and the virulence of the microorganism: some bacteria have greater disease-producing ability than others (Figure 29.6). Table 29.3 provides the differences between inflammatory response and infection.

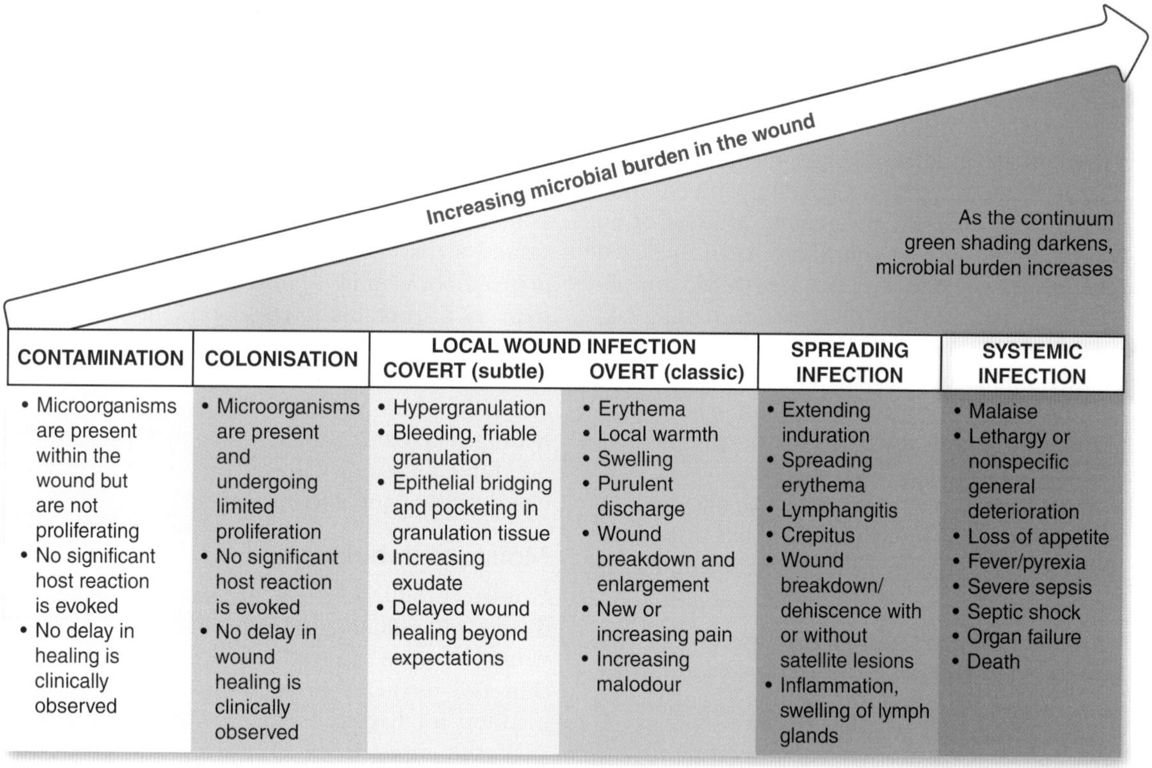

Figure 29.6 Wound infection continuum
(International Wound Infection Institute 2022)

TABLE 29.3 | The differences between inflammatory response and infection

Inflammation	Infection
• Localised redness • Pain • Heat • Swelling	• Erythema (spreading redness) • New onset of or increase in local wound pain • Change in the appearance of the wound tissue • Increase in the amount of wound exudate • Purulent or very malodorous exudate • Induration (hardness of the surrounding tissue) • Systemic signs and symptoms (such as fever, severe sepsis, septic shock, organ failure)

(International Wound Infection Institute [IWII] 2022)

Failure to control bioburden can lead to infection especially in the immune-compromised individual. Chronic wounds are likely to be colonised with bacterial or fungal microorganisms due to the nature of the open wound and tend to be polymicrobial. The presence of slough and necrotic tissue provides an environment for bacterial growth. It is when these bacteria interfere with wound healing that intervention is required.

Infection in acute or surgical wounds is relatively easy to recognise—spreading redness, local pain and swelling (erythema), peri-wound area warm to the touch. Infection in the chronic wound might be less obvious. Delayed healing can be an indicator of infection common to most wounds. Other signs of infection can be an increase or change in wound size and exudate, malodour, or discolouration of the granulation tissue depending on the cause of the wound (Healy & Freedman 2022) (see Clinical Interest Box 29.3). The risk of infection increases when 'any factor debilitates the individual, impairs immune resistance or reduces tissue perfusion' (International Wound Infection Institute [IWII] 2022). Comorbidities such as diabetes mellitus, arterial, cardiovascular or respiratory disease, renal impairment, malignancy, malnutrition, obesity, rheumatoid arthritis or an immune-compromised state all contribute to an increased risk of wound infection and further risk of systemic complications. Certain medications also affect wound healing and increase the risk of infection, such as corticosteroids, cytotoxic drugs and immunosuppressants (Docherty 2020). In a surgical wound, the level of contamination, the type and the length of procedure can all influence the development of postoperative wound infection (IWII 2022).

Furthermore, bacteria can cause prolonged inflammation by stimulating a continuing influx of neutrophils that release cytotoxic enzymes, free oxygen radicals and inflammatory mediators inducing a cycle of continuing tissue damage. Biofilms are increasingly thought to play a role in prolonging inflammation and delaying healing (Atkin 2019). See below for further information on biofilms.

CLINICAL INTEREST BOX 29.3 Identifying signs of wound infection

- New or increasing/spreading erythema
- New local or increasing warmth
- New or worsening swelling
- New purulent and/or increasing discharge
- New or increasing pain
- New or increasing malodour
- Delayed healing
- Wound breakdown
- Enlarged lymph glands
- Hyper- and/or friable granulation
- Epithelial bridging and pocketing in granulation tissue
- New or deterioration systemically (e.g. malaise, lethargy or nonspecific general deterioration, loss of appetite, fever/pyrexia, severe sepsis, septic shock, organ[s] failure)

(IWII 2022)

Biofilms in wounds

It is theorised that biofilms play a role in the delayed healing of chronic wounds. A **biofilm** is composed of multiple bacteria that attach to surfaces or each other to form highly complex communities embedded in a matrix that can be difficult to remove as the matrix offers protection from antimicrobials and the host immune system (Carville 2023; Goswami et al 2023). There is an increasing awareness that microorganisms colonising a wound may be present as a biofilm. Acute bacterial infections are considered to result from growth of planktonic cells (single free-floating bacteria) while many chronic bacterial infections involve biofilms. 80–100% of chronic wounds were anticipated to have evidence that biofilms exist in wounds, such as pressure injuries, diabetic foot ulcers and venous leg ulcers. If the wound fails to progress, reasonable assumption of biofilm presence and further laboratory investigation such as tissue biopsy becomes essential. Biofilms also challenge wound management. Therefore, as part of the wound bed preparation, wound cleansing and debridement are pivotal steps to disrupt biofilm and prevent it from re-forming (IWII 2022). Surfactant-containing antiseptics or pH-balanced solutions are usually recommended, while highly cytotoxic solutions such as those with povidone-iodine and hydrogen peroxide should be avoided (Murphy et al 2020). See Table 29.4 and Clinical Interest Box 29.4 for further description of antimicrobial agents.

Moisture imbalance

Exudate production is a normal part of wound healing during inflammatory and proliferative phases. Excessive wound exudate can lead to maceration of the peri-wound skin and further skin breakdown as well as providing a medium for bacterial growth. Absorbent dressings assist with the removal of excessive exudate to re-establish moisture balance. Too little moisture in a wound desiccates the cells and, in this situation, additional moisture (e.g. a hydrogel dressing) can help provide a moist wound bed. Chronic wound fluid differs from acute wound fluid. Chronic wound fluid contains high levels of tissue enzymes known as matrix metalloproteinases (MMPs) that are destructive to new tissue growth (Carville 2023; Wounds International 2019).

Edge of wound non-advancing or undermined

Failure to address the above three elements of TIME will result in non-migrating keratinocytes and a non-responsive wound (Wounds UK 2017).

Pain

Pain is a significant factor affecting an individual's psychoemotional wellbeing as well as the quality of life

TABLE 29.4 | Examples of topical antimicrobial dressings*

Dressing name (manufacturer)	Content	Rationale and benefits	Consideration
Enzyme alginogel	A gel with the combination of enzymes that has broad-spectrum antibacterial properties and alginate.	• Autolytic debridement. • Moisture balance. • Effective against MRSA, VREF, *Escherichia coli* and *Pseudomonas*. • No bacterial resistance reported. • Non-cytotoxic to tissue cells. • Dressing can stay in situ up to 4 days (exudate level dependent).	• Avoid near eyes or in contact with eyes. • Contraindicated with nanocrystalline silver products. • Secondary dressing required. • Flaminal® Hydro is recommended for dry to moderately exudating wounds. • Flaminal® Forte is recommended for heavy exudating wounds. • Discard product as instructed by the manufacturer.
Iodine (povidone, cadexomer)	Made up of starch micro-beads that contain 0.9% iodine.	• Broad-spectrum antimicrobial effect and is effective against MRSA and biofilm based organisms. • Reduced selection for bacterial resistance. • Absorbent. • Reduces malodour. • Two to three times dressing change a week.	• Contraindicated for people with sensitivity to iodine or with Hashimoto's thyroiditis, Graves' disease or very large wounds. • Not recommended for pregnant women, lactating mothers or children under 12 years of age. • Maximum single application—50 g and not to exceed 150 g a week. • Short-term use (no longer than 3 months in any single course of treatment). • Requires a secondary dressing.
Medical-grade honey	Derived from selected *Leptospermum* or *Eucalyptus marginata* and *Santalum spicatum* species of plants.	• Antimicrobial effect, especially effective against *Pseudomonas* and *Staphylococcus aureus*. • Controls malodour.	• Requires a secondary dressing. • Could lead to maceration to wound edge. • May experience some initial stinging sensation. • To be stored at <30°C and avoid exposure to light.
Silver (Ag)	Contains silver cations with different mechanisms of delivery.	• Broad-spectrum antimicrobial agent. • Effective against MRSA and VRE. • Impregnated in range of mediums (e.g. foam, calcium alginate, gelling fibre).	• Use with caution due to the risk of increased resistance. • Follow manufacturer's instructions for any specific use of silver dressing. • Contraindicated for people with sensitivity to silver, wounds with large surface areas. • Short-term use. • Discontinue if no signs of improvement.

Continued

TABLE 29.4 | Examples of topical antimicrobial dressings—cont'd

Dressing name (manufacturer)	Content	Rationale and benefits	Consideration
Dialykylcarbamoyl chloride impregnated dressing (DACC)	Dressing surface contains hydrophobic acetate which binds with most pathogenic microorganisms.	• Can be used to treat a broad range of microorganisms including: *Staphylococcus aureus*, *Pseudomonas aeruginosa* and *Candida albicans*. • Binds and absorbs pathogens without the risk of resistance to antimicrobial agents.	• The green surface of Sorbact™ is to be in direct contact with the wound. • Dressing change frequency can be from daily to twice a week (exudate dependent).
Polyhexamethylene biguanide (PHMB) Prontosan™	A cationic polymeric biguanide similar to Chlorhexidine.	• Broad-spectrum antibacterial. • Effective against MRSA, VRE, *Candida albicans*. • PHMB solution with betaine is effective to debride non-viable tissue and biofilms. • Non-cytotoxic or non-irritant.	• Contraindicated for people with sensitivity to biguanide products. • Fixative and/or secondary dressing required. Do not combine with other wound cleanser or ointments. • Solution to be warmed to body temperature to soak gauze, then apply to wound and leave in contact for 10 minutes.

**List is not exhaustive. Refer to manufacturer for product information. All trademarks acknowledged.*
(Carville 2023; IWII 2022)

CLINICAL INTEREST BOX 29.4 Definition of antimicrobial agents: Disinfectants, antibiotics and antiseptics

Disinfectants: Non-selective agents recommended by the manufacturer for application to an inert surface to remove or kill microorganisms. Not intended for human tissue.

Antibiotics: Act selectively to inhibit or kill microorganisms. They may be administered systemically (oral or intravenous) or in topical preparations (not commonly recommended). Increasing antibiotic resistance is a major global health concern among healthcare practitioners; hence, antimicrobial stewardship (AMS) must be followed.

Antiseptics: Non-selective agents that are applied topically to inhibit multiplication (bacteriostatic) of or kill microorganisms (bactericidal). They may have a toxic effect on human cells. Development of resistance to antiseptics is uncommon.

(Adapted from IWII 2022; ACSQHC 2023)

for a person with wounds (Brown 2023). Causes of pain vary and include procedural, incident and aetiology of the wound (Brown 2023; Jenkins 2020). Assessment of pain occurs with an initial history taking and is performed before, during and after wound care and documented in the person's medical records. The goal is to minimise pain and optimise comfort level through comprehensive assessment and management in collaboration with the multidisciplinary team. Pain assessment can indicate how the wound is progressing. Worsening pain is usually an indication for a sign of infection. Visual or numerical scales can be used to assist in the assessment of pain. Providing adequate and effective analgesia is vital in controlling pain, especially at dressing changes, and can include oral and topical analgesia (Carville 2023).

Dressing selection can affect wound pain. Dressings that provide a moist wound environment and can stay in place for several days, and therefore require less frequent dressing changes, reduce the risk of trauma to the wound and surrounding skin. Soft silicone dressings facilitate non-traumatic removal and can be considered to reduce pain at dressing changes. To lessen pain experienced by the person, avoid unnecessary changing of the dressing, support the peri-wound upon dressing removal, and use skin barrier product and/or adhesive removal to protect the peri-wound from painful excoriation and painful stripping of the wound and peri-wound (Brown 2023). Accurate documentation on all products used and other interventions (pharmacological and non-pharmacological strategies) can ensure the consistency of care for those experiencing pain from their wound.

Wound debridement

Wound **debridement** refers to the removal of devitalised tissue from a wound to promote wound healing. There are several debridement modalities available in clinical practice. Each debridement method has its own clinical indications, benefits, limitations, precautions, contraindications and requirements for equipment, knowledge and skill. Healthcare professionals are bound by both professional and ethical codes of conduct and regulated by the boundaries of their individual scope of practice. It is imperative that the healthcare professional ensures that they have reviewed local policy regarding debridement, gained appropriate education and training to perform debridement and undertaken risk assessment as part of their clinical decision-making process. The risk assessment for debridement must include the person, their wound, the healthcare practitioner, the health setting and available resources (Sibbald et al 2021).

Mechanical debridement

Wet-to-dry

Wet-to-dry dressings are one of the oldest methods of mechanical wound debridement. Wet (damp) gauze dressings are applied to the wound. The non-viable tissues in the wound bed adhere to the gauze as it dries and will then be physically removed during the dressing change. This non-selective mechanical debridement traumatises the healthy granulating tissues adhered to the gauze upon removal and causes bleeding and pain. Therefore, wet-to-dry is not generally recommended in current wound management (Carville 2023; Thomas et al 2021).

Hydro-surgical debridement

Hydro-surgical debridement is a form of mechanical debridement albeit under more controlled conditions. Hydro-surgical debridement uses a high-pressure water jet pushed through a suitable hose to the tip of a procedure-specific hand piece. This method is fast and precise in the hands of a skilled operator, such as an advanced practice wound specialist, for excising unwanted tissue. Its use in practice is mostly in burn injuries and vascular leg ulcers (Thomas et al 2021).

Low-frequency ultrasound debridement

Low-frequency ultrasound debridement (LFUD) uses lower frequencies than are used in imaging or other forms of therapy. Soundwaves produce energy, which is transferred to the wound via a hand piece using continuous movement and fluid (normal saline). This causes cavitation and acoustic streaming, which in turn break down devitalised tissue promoting wound debridement. This type of debridement promotes efficient wound bed preparation and offers an alternative to surgical/sharp debridement. Specialised equipment, training and skills in advanced practice are required to undertake LFUD, along with adequate local anaesthetic and pre-emptive analgesia to prevent and minimise discomfort during and post procedure (Carville 2023; Thomas et al 2021).

Autolytic debridement

Autolytic debridement occurs spontaneously in most wounds as macrophages and proteolytic enzymes liquefy and separate non-viable tissue and slough, promoting granulation tissue. Dressings that create or maintain a moist wound environment will assist autolysis. Hydrogel is very high in water content and rehydrates the necrotic tissue or dry fibrin slough; while hydrocolloids are moisture retaining and used for low exuding wounds to promote debridement. Film dressings are permeable to water vapour but impermeable to water, bacteria and microorganisms and help to create and maintain a moist wound environment (Carville 2023).

Enzymatic debridement

Enzymatic debridement is a less common method of debridement, which requires the topical application of the enzymatic agents to the wound to facilitate the removal of the non-viable tissue. They need to be replaced frequently to maintain effectiveness as well as to monitor for any maceration or irritation to the wound edge and peri-wound. Several enzyme agents such as collagenase and bromelain are available but not in all countries. Collagenase is often used when autolytic or surgical debridement is not available (Eriksson et al 2022; Sibbald et al 2021).

Biological (larval therapy) debridement

In the biological debridement method, sterile maggots are applied to a wound, covered with a sterile semipermeable dressing for 2–3 days before being removed. The secretion from the maggots (proteolytic enzymes) breaks down the non-viable tissue, while the continuous movement from the maggots in the wound stimulates granulation. The maggots also ingest bacteria, which is beneficial in managing antibiotic-resistant wounds such as methicillin-resistant *Staphylococcus aureus* (MRSA). The procedure is painless though not aesthetically agreeable to all individuals and nurses (King 2020).

Surgical and conservative sharp wound debridement

Surgical sharp debridement is the fastest and most effective method of debridement and is performed by a surgeon in an operating theatre under general or local anaesthesia. It is considered when the presence of non-viable tissue is extensive (Carville 2023). With this method, all non-viable tissue and slough is removed until a clean, healthy wound bed is exposed. Conservative sharp wound debridement (CSWD) is the removal of loose avascular tissue without (or with very minimal) pain or bleeding. It is appropriate when there is a moderate amount of non-viable tissue. Sterile sharp equipment (e.g. scissors, scalpels, forceps and curettes) can be used to remove dead tissues by experienced trained clinicians in an aseptic clinical setting subject to their scope of practice and workplace policies and procedures (Carville 2023).

Managing wound infection

The adverse effects on healing of infection in wounds is well recognised. Effectively managing wound infection requires optimising the host (person) response, minimising risk factors where possible, reducing bacterial load and managing signs and symptoms such as fever and pain. Regular re-evaluation of the individual and the wound and adjustment in treatment is necessary to assess and optimise the effectiveness of treatment. A systemic antibiotic should be carefully considered for locally infected wounds and spreading infection in a wound. Assessment for local or systemic infection should be made before administering antibiotics in consideration of adherence to antimicrobial stewardship practice (IWII 2022).

Managing bioburden (removal of non-viable tissue, preventing and controlling infection and maintaining moisture balance) is essential for wounds to progress to healing. Appropriate observation and reporting are an important aspect of wound management. This should be directed by the clinical response of the tissue and individual to the treatment and not dictated by strict times (e.g. 2 weeks of antibiotic therapy or the length of time an antimicrobial dressing is used). This means adjusting therapy to the clinical signs and symptoms of infection with the use of topical antimicrobial agents. For example, if the wound is progressing after a week of topical antimicrobial therapy, then the therapy may be stopped. See Table 29.4 and Clinical Interest Box 29.4 for definition of antimicrobial agents. If the wound is unchanged after the introduction of therapy, then reassessment and alternative topical therapies need to be used (IWII 2022). Gaining early control requires detection of subtle changes, especially in the chronic wound, such as a reduction in wound odour and reduction in pain. Wound infection requires prompt management to prevent the spread of infection systemically.

Diagnosing wound infection is a combination of clinical signs and symptoms (see Clinical Interest Box 29.3), holistic assessment (including a health history), medications and environment. Microbiological analysis can be used to assist diagnosis. This is achieved by wound swab, wound tissue biopsy or wound fluid aspiration. Wound swabbing is mostly requested and performed after wound cleansing to detect the causative microorganisms but can also be misleading since it will detect only surface microorganisms, not those in the deeper tissue. Therefore, tissue biopsy is the preferred method to identify microbes and their virulence (IWII 2022). It has been reported that the Levine technique is the recommended sampling method. This technique uses a swab that is rotated over a 1 cm^2 area of the wound surface with enough pressure to squeeze fluid from within the wound tissue (IWII 2022). See Clinical Skill 29.1 for performing a wound swab. (See also Chapter 18.)

CLINICAL SKILL 29.1 Wound swab

Please adhere to the policy and procedures of the facility/organisation prior to undertaking the skill. Ensure this skill is in your scope of practice.

NMBA Decision-making Framework considerations	Equipment:
(refer to NMBA Decision-making framework for nursing and midwifery 2020): 1. Am I educated? 2. Am I authorised? 3. Am I competent? If you answer 'no' to any of these, do not perform that activity. Seek guidance and support from your teacher/a nurse team leader/clinical facilitator/educator.	Disposable gloves Wound swab kit Sterile dressing pack Sterile normal saline 0.9% Biohazard specimen transport bag Laboratory request form (signed by a medical practitioner or Nurse Practitioner—may be an electronic document) Dressing trolley Disinfectant wipes/solution Waste receptacle

PREPARE FOR THE SKILL

(Please refer to the Standard Steps on pp. xviii–xx for related rationales.)
Mentally review the steps of the skill.
Discuss the skill with your instructor/supervisor/team leader, if required.
Confirm correct facility/organisation policy/safe operating procedures.
Validate the order in the individual's record.

CLINICAL SKILL 29.1 Wound swab—cont'd

Identify indication and rationale for performing the activity.
Assess for any contraindications.
Locate and gather equipment.
Perform hand hygiene.
Ensure therapeutic interaction.
Identify the individual using three individual identifiers.
Gain the individual's consent.
Assess for pain relief.
Prepare the environment.
Provide and maintain privacy.
Assist the individual to assume an appropriate position of comfort.

Skill activity	Rationale
Wound swabs are often taken at the time of wound dressing changes. These are taken when the wound is suspected of containing microorganisms. Identification of the microorganism will enable correct treatment regimens to be implemented.	
Assess the individual's record to determine previous appearance of wound and any previous dressings.	Determines requirements for equipment and dressing requirements.

PERFORM THE SKILL

(Please refer to the Standard Steps on pp. xviii–xx for related rationales.)
Perform hand hygiene.
Apply PPE: gloves, eyewear, mask and gown as appropriate.
Ensure the individual's safety and comfort throughout skill.
Promote independence and involvement of the individual if possible and/or appropriate.
Assess the individual's tolerance to the skill throughout.
Dispose of used supplies, equipment, waste and sharps appropriately.
Remove PPE and discard or store appropriately.
Perform hand hygiene.

Skill activity	Rationale
Create the aseptic field by using the sterile dressing pack and adding sterile equipment including 0.9% sodium chloride to the field. Open sterile dressing pack by using corners. Open the sterile dressing products away from the aseptic field and add into the field.	Prevents contamination of sterile items and Key-Parts.
Loosen and remove the existing wound dressing and assess wound for suspected clinical signs and symptoms of infection, including the type and amount of exudate on the removed dressing and peri-wound condition. Dispose of wound dressing and the used gloves.	Assesses for signs and symptoms of wound infection (e.g. redness, swelling, warmth, exudate amount and type). Prevents spread of microorganisms.
Position sterile dressing drape below or near the wound.	Protects wound from environmental contamination.
Cleanse the wound with sterile 0.9% sodium chloride.	Removes excessive debris and any dressing residue. Prevents swab from becoming contaminated, which could lead to false positive swab results. If the wound is dry, the swab may be moistened with sterile normal saline; if the wound is moist, the dry swab can be used dry.
Remove wound swab from the swab container and perform Levine technique (rotate swab over a 1 cm^2 area with sufficient pressure to express fluid from tissue) from the cleanest part of the wound bed.	Obtains causative pathogen from both superficial and deep in the wound bed (aerobic and anaerobic bacteria from the wound fluid).

Continued

CLINICAL SKILL 29.1 Wound swab—cont'd

Return the wound swab back to the transport medium. Place used wound swab kit(s) on the lower shelf of the dressing trolley or a clean surface. Repeat with another wound swab if required.	Do not swab pus or exudate since these surface organisms may contain contaminants that are different from those causing the wound infection. Minimises the risk of obtaining contaminated wound swab leading to false positive result.
Apply an appropriate sterile wound dressing (if required) using ANTT and secure. (See Clinical Skill 29.2 for dressing a wound.)	Covers wound and prevents spread of microorganisms.
Label specimen container with the person's name, date of birth, hospital or patient number and the date, time and site of the specimen collection. Add collector's signature/initial.	Ensures that the correct specimen is sent for testing and that it is for the correct person.
Specimen is placed in the zip lock section of the plastic biohazard bag.	Standard infection control precaution.
Pathology request form is checked for the person's details. The pathology request form is placed in the other section of the bag.	Ensures correct form and specimen are sent to pathology department and correct test will be undertaken in the pathology department.

AFTER THE SKILL

(Please refer to the Standard Steps on pp. xviii–xx for related rationales.)
Communicate outcome to the individual, any ongoing care and report any complications.
Restore the environment.
Report, record and document assessment findings, details of the skill performed and the individual's response.
Report, record and document any abnormalities and/or inability to perform the skill.
Reassess the individual to ensure there are no adverse effects/events from the skill.

Skill activity	Rationale
The specimen should be transported to the laboratory as soon as possible, or stored in a refrigerator until transport can be arranged.	Decomposition and cell growth occur if specimen is left standing, and may provide an inaccurate result.

(Adapted from ACIPC 2015; LeMone et al 2020; Berman et al 2020; IWII 2022; Lynn 2022; The-ASAP 2019)

To prevent further wound contamination or cross-contamination, infection control procedures should be used to protect the individual and the wound. This includes thorough hand hygiene, bare below the elbows, and the use of appropriate personal protective equipment (PPE) in addition to gloves at dressing changes. Furthermore, aseptic non-touch technique (ANTT) provides the guiding principles for wound dressing procedures to prevent the spread of infection and cross-contamination (IWII 2022). This has been previously discussed in Chapter 18.

Topical antimicrobial dressings/agents

Topical antimicrobial dressings contain agents that are capable of killing pathogens found in wounds. These agents are impregnated into various wound dressing materials and include silver, iodine, honey, chlorhexidine, polyhexamethylene biguanide (PHMB) and glucose oxidase enzyme systems. As previously described, systemic antibiotic use should be carefully considered in suspected wound infection. Topical antibiotics can be cautiously used to manage wounds that display signs and symptoms of local wound infection and if biofilm is suspected or confirmed (IWII 2022).

Examples of these dressings are listed in Table 29.4, and Clinical Interest Box 29.4 outlines the difference between disinfectants, antibiotics and antiseptics.

Wound dressings

There are many different types of wound dressings available from numerous manufacturers; therefore, the clinician involved in wound care requires a sound clinical knowledge of how the main groups of dressings perform. Dressings alone do not heal wounds, but appropriately selected dressings implemented in consultation with RNs can enhance the body's ability to heal. Maintaining a moist wound bed provides the optimum environment for healing (Nuutila & Eriksson 2021) and forms the foundation for contemporary wound care practice. See Clinical Skill 29.2 for dressing a wound.

CLINICAL SKILL 29.2 Dressing a wound

Please adhere to the policy and procedures of the facility/organisation prior to undertaking the skill. Ensure this skill is in your scope of practice.

NMBA Decision-making Framework considerations	Equipment
NMBA Decision-making Framework considerations (refer to NMBA Decision-making framework for nursing and midwifery 2020): 1. Am I educated? 2. Am I authorised? 3. Am I competent? If you answer 'no' to any of these, do not perform that activity. Seek guidance and support from your teacher/a nurse team leader/clinical facilitator/educator.	**Equipment:** Sterile dressing pack Sterile dressing materials Sterile 0.9% sodium chloride Additional light source (if required) Disposable gloves Waste receptacle Dressing trolley Disinfectant wipes/solution

PREPARE FOR THE SKILL

(Please refer to the Standard Steps on pp. xviii–xx for related rationales.)
Mentally review the steps of the skill.
Discuss the skill with your instructor/supervisor/team leader, if required.
Confirm correct facility/organisation policy/safe operating procedures.
Validate the order in the individual's record.
Identify indication and rationale for performing the activity.
Assess for any contraindications.
Locate and gather equipment.
Perform hand hygiene.
Ensure therapeutic interaction.
Identify the individual using three individual identifiers.
Gain the individual's consent.
Assess for pain relief.
Prepare the environment.
Provide and maintain privacy.
Assist the individual to assume an appropriate position of comfort.

Skill activity	Rationale
Wound dressings are undertaken to provide a moist cover for the wound to prevent the introduction of microorganisms and to promote healing. They also absorb exudate.	
Assess the individual's record to determine previous appearance of wound and any previous dressings.	Determines requirements for equipment and dressing requirements.

PERFORM THE SKILL

(Please refer to the Standard Steps on pp. xviii–xx for related rationales.)
Perform hand hygiene.
Apply PPE: gloves, eyewear, mask and gown as appropriate.
Ensure the individual's safety and comfort throughout skill.
Promote independence and involvement of the individual if possible and/or appropriate.
Assess the individual's tolerance to the skill throughout.
Dispose of used supplies, equipment, waste and sharps appropriately.
Remove PPE and discard or store appropriately.
Perform hand hygiene.

Skill activity	Rationale
Create the aseptic field by using the sterile dressing pack and adding sterile equipment including 0.9% sodium chloride to the field. Open sterile dressing pack by using corners.	Prevents contamination of sterile items and Key-Parts.

Continued

CLINICAL SKILL 29.2 Dressing a wound—cont'd

Open the sterile dressing products away from the aseptic field and add into the field.	
Loosen and remove the existing wound dressing and assess wound for suspected clinical signs and symptoms of infection, including the type and amount of exudate on the removed dressing and peri-wound condition. Dispose of wound dressing and the used gloves.	Assesses for signs and symptoms of wound infection (e.g. redness, swelling, warmth, exudate amount and type). Prevents spread of microorganisms.
Rearrange and assemble the required sterile dressing and equipment in the aseptic field using ANTT without contaminating the Key-Parts.	Maintains ANTT to protect the wound from environmental contamination. Prevents contamination of the Key-Parts.
Position sterile dressing drape below or near the wound.	Protects wound from environmental contamination.
Cleanse the wound with sterile 0.9% sodium chloride. Clean from top to bottom and from a clean area towards a less clean area, usually an outward direction.	Removes debris from the wound bed. Avoids transferring wound exudate and normal flora from the surrounding skin into the wound. Prevents wound contamination.
Assess the wound size, type(s) of tissue in the wound bed and the quantity of each tissue type in percentage (%), signs of infection, type and amount of exudate, odour, inflammation and healing. Assess for pain.	Evaluates condition of the wound, the peri-wound condition, and the stage of healing.
Apply sterile wound dressing using ANTT and secure. If ordered, wound may be left exposed to the air.	Provides a moist wound environment. Facilitates healing, absorbs exudate, protects the wound from infection and irritation (e.g. from clothing).

AFTER THE SKILL

(Please refer to the Standard Steps on pp. xviii–xx for related rationales.)
Communicate outcome to the individual, any ongoing care and report any complications.
Restore the environment.
Report, record and document assessment findings, details of the skill performed and the individual's response.
Report, record and document any abnormalities and/or inability to perform the skill.
Reassess the individual to ensure there are no adverse effects/events from the skill.

(Adapted from ACIPC 2015; LeMone et al 2020; Berman et al 2020; IWWII 2022; Lynn 2022; The-ASAP 2019)

The ideal dressing will have many of the attributes listed below:

- maintains a moist wound environment
- allows for gaseous exchange
- provides an effective bacterial barrier
- protects wound and surrounding tissues
- promotes comfort and reduces pain
- maintains an optimal wound temperature and pH
- controls and prevents odour
- manages exudate
- assists to prevent or manage clinical infection
- covers wound from view of individual and/or significant others
- does not shed damaging substances into the wound
- is easy to apply and comfortable to wear
- produces minimal pain on application and removal
- is accessible and cost effective.

(Carville 2023)

Dressings are generally categorised by mode of action or material. Holistic assessment and individual-focused outcomes identify the characteristics that determine the specific ideal dressing. The criteria listed above will be available in a dressing product, which can be selected to meet the needs of the wound—to promote healing and achieve the desired individual-focused outcomes. Table 29.5 gives some examples of dressings and their actions.

Wound dressings can be classified into three main types:

1. wound hydration products
2. moisture-retentive dressings
3. exudate-management products.

Wound hydration products

Wound hydration products provide additional moisture to dry wounds or wounds with necrotic (dead) or sloughy tissue and are usually in the form of a gel. These products

TABLE 29.5 | Examples and action of wound dressings*

Dressing	Characteristics
Alginates	• Natural polysaccharide from seaweed • Reduces pain by protecting nerve endings (moisture) • Active ion exchange at wound surface forms soluble sodium alginate (gel) to provide moist wound environment • Low allergenic • Biodegradable • Available as flat sheet, ribbons or ropes • Ribbon or rope may be used to pack cavities when wound bed is visible • Absorbent • Reduces wound-associated pain by keeping nerve endings moist • Alginates derived from calcium have haemostatic properties • Use as primary dressing • Requires a secondary dressing
Cadexomer iodine (iodophors)	• Composes three-dimensional starch lattice formed into spherical microbeads that contain 0.9% iodine • Iodine is progressively released into the wound • Absorbs exudate • Reduces malodour • Effective against biofilm • Available as paste, powder or sheet • May feel burning or stinging on application • Requires a secondary dressing • Contraindicated for people with allergies to iodine, thyroid disease, pregnant, lactating or children
Dialkylcarbamoly chloride impregnated (DACC)	• Antimicrobial effect by binding pathogenic microorganisms to a hydrophobic acetate or cotton wound dressing surface • Binds with a range of bacteria including *Staphylococcus aureus* and MRSA • Available as acetate fabric, cotton gauze or in combination with hydrogel
Enzyme alginogel (Flaminal Hydro™ Flaminal Forte™)	• A combination of enzymes (glucose oxidase and lactoperoxidase) and alginate in a gel • Broad-spectrum antibacterial properties • Facilitates autolytic debridement • Absorbs exudate • Requires a secondary dressing
Foam dressings	• Adherent or non-adherent variants • Sheets or cavity-filling shapes • Some incorporate a semipermeable, waterproof, adhesive layer as an outer layer of the dressing • Suitable for moderate to high exudating wounds • Provides protection and conforms to uneven body surfaces • Facilitates a moist wound environment, but may *not* be sufficient to promote autolysis of sloughy tissue • Use as a primary or secondary dressing
Gelling (cellulose) fibre (Hydrofibre™ is a trademark term)	• Made from sodium carboxymethylcellulose (CMC) that form into a moist gel when in contact with the exudate • Suitable for low to heavy amounts of exudate • Absorbs moisture vertically to prevent wound edge maceration • Action similar to alginate but with no haemostatic property • Available as ropes, ribbons or flat sheets • Use as a primary dressing • Requires a secondary dressing • No need to be cut into the size of the wound • Moistening prior to application not required • Promotes a moist wound environment • Promotes non-traumatic dressing removal

Continued

TABLE 29.5 | Examples and action of wound dressings—cont'd

Dressing	Characteristics
Hydrocolloids	• Moisture-retentive • Adhesive • Semi-occlusive or occlusive • Water repellent • Reduces pain by keeping nerve endings moist • Promotes autolytic debridement • Available in various sizes and in transparent and opaque forms • Available as sheets, paste and powder • *Not* to be used on infected wounds
Hydrogels	• Provides moisture to nil or low exudating wounds • Promotes autolytic debridement • Reduces pain and keeps nerve endings moist • Available as amorphous gels or sheets • Use as primary dressing • Requires a secondary dressing • *Not* to be used on infected wounds
Island dressings	• Waterproof • Non-adherent wound contact layer • Suitable for low amounts of exudate • Use as primary dressing
Medicated/medical-grade honey	• Derived from selected Leptospermum or *Eucalyptus marginata* and *Santalum spicatum* species of plants • Has anti-inflammatory properties • Promotes moist wound healing • Promotes autolytic debridement • Antibacterial effect through the slow release of low level of hydrogen peroxide • Antibacterial effect varies depending on the source • Effective against antibiotic resistant bacteria • Especially effective against *Pseudomonas* and *Staphylococcus aureus* • Controls malodour • Available as an ointment, gel, or impregnated into a knitted viscose mesh and alginates • Requires a secondary dressing • Cautions with allergies to honey or bee sting • Not suitable for moderate to heavy levels of exudate
Negative pressure wound therapy (NPWT)	• Topical negative pressure devices • Provides a moist wound environment • Reduces bacterial colonisation • Promotes localised blood flow • Reduces localised oedema • Reduces dead space in wound by the use of gauze or foam • Promotes granulation and epithelialisation • Facilitates collection of wound exudate
Odour absorbing	• Incorporates activated charcoal • Absorbs bacteria • Eliminates odour • Absorbs exudate • May be used as a primary or as a secondary dressing
Polyhexamethylene biguanide (PHMB)	• Has broad-spectrum antibacterial properties • Effective against MRSA, VRE and *Candida albicans* • Non-cytotoxic or non-irritant • Available as a wound irrigation solution, gel, or impregnated in wound dressing • Effective against biofilm

TABLE 29.5 | Examples and action of wound dressings—cont'd

Dressing	Characteristics
Semipermeable film	• Semipermeable • Adhesive • Transparent for wound monitoring without removing dressing • Suitable for nil to low amounts of exudate • Use as a primary or secondary dressing
Silicone dressings	• A soft silicone contact layer or primary layer attached to another dressing • Minimises wound trauma on removal • Conforms to different anatomical shapes • Extended wear time • Requires a secondary dressing for the silicone contact layer
Silver dressing	• Silver is a broad-spectrum antimicrobial agent • Silver comes in a range of dressings: foams, calcium alginate, hydrofibre and synthetic fabric • Not all dressings release silver into the wound bed

**List is not exhaustive. Please refer to manufacturer for product information. All trademarks acknowledged.*
(Adapted from Carville 2023; Gibb 2023; IWII 2022)

are composed of mostly water, bound together by cross-linked polymers. They can be used as cavity fillers in smaller wounds with minimal exudate. These dressings require a secondary dressing to hold the gel in the wound and daily to third-daily changing depending on how quickly the gel is utilised by the wound. These dressings are not suitable for wounds with high amounts of exudate and should be applied in measured amounts to prevent complications from excessive moisture.

Moisture-retentive dressings

Moisture-retentive dressings keep the wound bed moist, assisting keratinocytes to migrate across the surface of the wound (e.g. hydrocolloids). These dressings are used on light-to-moderately exuding wounds. They generally have a waterproof outer layer and are composed of hydrophilic particles (cellulose) and come in various thicknesses, shapes and sizes. They retain the current moisture level to promote autolytic debridement and to stimulate granulation and epithelialisation. Due to their waterproof backing and adhesive border, a secondary dressing is not required. They can be left in position for several days, and are impermeable to microorganisms and water. Some of the dressings are slightly thinner to allow visual inspection of the wound. These dressings are comfortable for the individual and alleviate pain because they protect exposed cutaneous nerve endings.

Exudate-management dressings

Exudate-management products absorb exudate from the wound surface and hold it within the dressing as well as transpiring fluid. These dressings are calcium alginates, which are composed of polysaccharides derived from seaweed; polyurethane or silicone foam dressings; gelling cellulous fibrous dressings, which are made from sodium carboxymethylcellulose; and the combination dressings, which marry the technologies of hydrocolloids and the absorption capacity of polymers.

Negative pressure wound therapy

Negative pressure wound therapy (NPWT) is the application of sub-atmospheric pressure to a wide variety of wounds. This therapy has increased in use over the past 2–3 decades and is now a regular aspect of wound care, undertaken under supervision of RNs, with several versions available. It is used to enhance healing and reduce frequency of dressing changes, nursing time and costs and improve quality of life. Clinical outcomes include exudate management, moist environment, reduction of oedema, mechanical stimulation of wound bed, wound edge contraction, promoted granulation tissue growth, angiogenesis and improved tissue perfusion (Carville 2023; Torbrand et al 2018; Wang et al 2023). It can be used on a variety of wound types: dehiscence, diabetic foot ulcers, burns, venous leg ulcers, surgical infections, skin grafts, traumatic wounds (Wang et al 2023). It is considered when the wound is not healing in the expected timeframe, the wound is in an awkward location or of a difficult size to dress, or a reduction in wound size is required before surgical closure (Carville 2023).

NPWT is a closed suction and drainage system, which consists of a wound filler (foam or gauze), an adhesive film wound dressing sealer with a drainage tube connected to a vacuum pump that has an attached fluid collection canister. These devices are portable, allowing the individual to mobilise and to be managed in the community. Pressure settings vary from −80 mmHg to −125 mmHg and depend on the wound type and individual tolerance (Carville 2023; Kirsner et al 2021; Peate & Stephens 2020; Wang et al 2023).

For example, a thin skin graft will require less pressure than an abdominal wound dehiscence. Negative pressure can be applied continuously or intermittently, though continuous suction is more common, especially for wounds with large volumes of exudate.

Two types of wound filler for the NPWT are used: gauze and foam. Both allow for pressure to be evenly distributed over the wound bed. Foam tends to produce a thicker granulation tissue and subsequent wound edge contraction, with gauze producing a less thick but denser granulation tissue (Carville 2023). Use of either depends on various factors. For example, foam may be used in areas of large tissue loss where contraction of tissue is required before closure. Gauze may be more beneficial when the wound surface is irregular and cosmetic outcome is important. A wound contact layer is often placed under the foam interface when there is concern there may be complications, or there is exposure of vulnerable structures (Mattox 2017). Tissue growth into the foam interface has been reported in the published literature (Mattox 2017), which is also why a wound contact layer is placed under the foam.

A newer and smaller device is available that does not rely on a fluid canister for exudate collection, making it extremely portable. This type of device, such as PICO™ from Smith & Nephew Australia Pty Ltd, has a specialised dressing that absorbs and transpires exudate. The dressing has a tube connection to a small pump that delivers a fixed negative pressure (−80 mmHg). As the technology becomes increasingly used, easy, lightweight and manual systems are becoming available (Carville 2023).

NPWT offers several benefits:

- stimulates new tissue growth (granulation)
- reduces tissue oedema and manages wound exudate
- increases the rate of wound healing reducing the wound area
- helps control bacterial burden (removes exudate that contains bacteria)
- maintains a moist wound environment
- causes a reduction in pain
- removes slough
- reduces frequency of dressing changes required.

Considered before applying NPWT:

- effective management of the individual's symptoms
- dimensions of the wound and ease of application
- placement of tubing
- care setting (e.g. home, hospital) and who will care for therapy
- effective debridement of wound bed
- ability of the individual to give consent to treatment.

Contraindications for NPWT:

- untreated osteomyelitis
- necrotic tissue in the wound
- exposed organs or blood vessels
- malignancy in the wound bed (except in palliative care cases)
- unexplored fistulas.

(Adapted from Carville 2023)

Therapy should be stopped when there is uniform granulation tissue in the wound and the wound's depth has decreased.

See Table 29.6 and Clinical Interest Box 29.5 and Clinical Interest Box 29.6 for discussion on the right dressings for the right wound, an outline of the basic factors to consider when selecting a dressing and using tap water compared with normal saline for cleansing wounds in adults, respectively.

TABLE 29.6 | The right dressing to promote wound healing

Modern wound dressings improve healing time, reduce pain, reduce the time required to dress the wound and require less frequent changes. It is important to use the most appropriate dressing for the wound at the appropriate stage of healing. One dressing will not suit the entire wound-healing process. Match the action of the dressing to the aim of the treatment.

Condition of wound bed	Aim of treatment	Examples of dressings
Non-viable tissue (black, hard, dehydrated, necrotic, eschar)	Rehydrate, debride non-viable tissue (if adequate micro-circulation evident), promote granulation tissue	Hydrogels Hydrocolloid Alginogel (Flaminal™ Hydro) Potential to benefit from sharp or surgical debridement
Slough (soft, yellow, creamy or fibrous)	To encourage autolytic debridement of slough, promote granulation, absorb excess exudate	Hydrocolloids (low to moderate exudate with no local wound infection only) Hydrogel Alginogel (Flaminal™ Hydro or Flaminal™ Forte) Sharp debridement by advanced practitioner Larvae
Granulating (red, moist)	Retain moisture, promote and protect granulation tissue and epithelialisation	Foams Low absorbent Low- or non-adherent

TABLE 29.6 | The right dressing to promote wound healing—cont'd

Condition of wound bed	Aim of treatment	Examples of dressings
Epithelialising (pink wound, evidence of epithelial growth on surface)	Retain moisture, promote and protect epithelialisation	Foams Hydrocolloid Non-adherent dressings Transparent semipermeable film
Infected (local or spreading)	Treat infection with systemic antibiotics (spreading infection), topical antimicrobial dressings, absorb excess exudate, debride slough	Silver-impregnated dressings Cadexomer-iodine Medical-grade honey PHMB-impregnated dressings and gel Hydrophobic antimicrobial dressing (i.e. DACC)
Dry	To restore moisture	Hydrogel Alginogel
Moist (low to moderate level of exudate)	To maintain current level of moisture	Low absorbent Hydrocolloid Foam
Wet (moderate level of exudate)	To absorb excess moisture	Foam Alginate Gelling fibrous dressing
Heavy exudate	To absorb excess moisture	Alginate Gelling fibrous dressing Super absorbent pad The combination of alginate/gelling fibrous dressing and super absorbent pad

(Adapted from Carville 2023; Edwards et al 2019)

CLINICAL INTEREST BOX 29.5 Factors to consider when selecting a dressing

- Wound type: Superficial, full thickness, cavity
- Wound description: Granulating, epithelialising, necrotic, sloughy, infected
- Wound characteristics: Dry, moist, heavily exuding, malodorous, excessively painful, difficult to dress, bleeds easily
- Bacterial profile: Sterile, colonised, infected, infected and potential source of cross-infection
- Dressing to achieve optimum wound bed preparation and healing

(Carville 2023; IWII 2022)

CLINICAL INTEREST BOX 29.6 Using tap water compared with normal saline or potable water for cleansing wounds in adult

Studies indicate that tap water has no significant influence on wound healing or infection rates compared to normal saline or potable water (water of a quality suitable for drinking, cooking and personal bathing). Despite that, contrary opinions exist with regards to its safety, such as fear of wound colonisation by *Pseudomonas* spp. found in plumbing systems of healthcare facilities or damage to the wound bed. The decision to use tap water to cleanse wounds should be based on clinical judgment and take into account the quality of water, the nature of the wound and the individual's general condition. It is recommended that tap water not be used if it is not suitable for drinking, cooking and personal bathing.

(Holman 2023; Sibbald et al 2021; Weir & Swanson 2019)

TYPES OF WOUNDS

Acute and chronic wounds

Acute wounds

An **acute wound** may be caused by traumatic (accidental or unintentional) or surgical intervention (intentional). A **surgical wound** occurs as a result of planned or unplanned surgery. Acute surgical wounds are those that heal by primary intention, proceed through an orderly and timely reparative process, heal fairly quickly (usually within 14 days), without complications and with limited interventions (Carville 2023; Crisp et al 2021). Examples of acute wounds are those made by surgical incision or traumatic injury expected to heal within 2–4 weeks. (See Clinical Interest Box 29.7.)

CLINICAL INTEREST BOX 29.7 Skin flaps

A flap is a surgical relocation of tissue from one part of the body to another part to reconstruct a primary defect. This creates a secondary defect that will require skin grafting or primary closure.

Types of flaps

Skin, or cutaneous, flaps are grafts of tissue consisting of skin and superficial fascia. Composite tissue flaps are described according to the type of tissue they are composed of (e.g. fasciocutaneous flap).

Flaps can be classified as free, pedicle and rotational flaps. A free flap is the relocation of skin and subcutaneous tissue as a complete segment, with an anastomosis of the segment's blood supply to vessels at the affected site. A pedicle flap is the surgical transfer of skin and subcutaneous tissue to another body site. Blood supply to the flap is maintained via a vascular pedicle attached to the body donor site. A rotational flap is a Z-plasty incision to maintain the blood supply at its original site while rotating the tissue to cover an adjacent defect.

(Carville 2023)

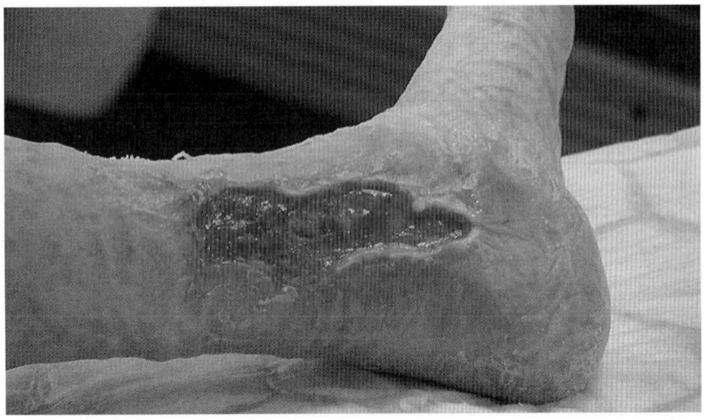

Figure 29.7 Chronic venous ulcer
(Fillit 2017)

Chronic wounds

A **chronic wound** occurs when the reparative process does not proceed through an orderly and timely process as anticipated, and healing is complicated and delayed by intrinsic and extrinsic factors that impact on the person, their wound or their environment (Carville 2023). A chronic wound usually heals by secondary intention. There are four categories of chronic wounds, each with differing aetiologies: arterial ulcers, diabetic foot ulcers, venous leg ulcers (see Figure 29.7) and pressure injuries (McCosker et al 2019).

CRITICAL THINKING EXERCISE 29.1

What factors do you consider in terms of selecting an appropriate dressing product for a given wound type?

PATHOPHYSIOLOGICAL EFFECTS AND MAJOR MANIFESTATIONS OF SKIN DISORDERS

Pathophysiological influences and effects

The major factors that affect normal structure and functions of the skin can generally be classified into six categories:

1. genetic factors
2. idiopathic causes
3. hypersensitivity
4. trauma
5. neoplasia
6. infections and infestations.

Genetic factors

Genetic factors determine skin colour and the amount and distribution of hair. Congenital skin disorders include birthmarks, hypopigmentation (albinism) and a condition called ichthyosis, which involves excessive scaling or thickening of the outermost skin layer. Heredity also plays a role in predisposition to the development of acne and atopic dermatitis.

Idiopathic causes

Many skin disorders have no one known cause (such as vitiligo and psoriasis). Other skin disorders may be associated with emotional or physical stress but there does not seem to be any one identifiable cause.

Hypersensitivity

Some individuals tend to react adversely to contact with various substances (e.g. when a substance is inhaled, ingested or comes in contact with the skin). Some allergic reactions are manifested in alterations in the skin (e.g. reddening and itching of the skin may be side effects of certain medications).

Neoplasia

Any abnormal growth of new tissue, whether benign or malignant, is called a neoplasm. Examples include calluses, which can develop on the toes from friction and chronic pressure, or keloid scarring, which can result after injury to the skin. Benign or malignant neoplasms may develop from any type of cell in the skin, but the melanocytes and keratinocytes are the cells most frequently involved. A mole (naevus) is a common type of benign skin tumour. Some benign epithelial cell lesions may develop into malignant neoplasms.

Infections and infestations

If the skin is broken and pathogenic microorganisms gain entry, infection may result.

Primary skin infections are commonly caused by bacteria, fungi and viruses. Secondary skin infections may occur in conditions such as stasis dermatitis, in which impaired circulation damages skin cells of the lower limbs.

Systemic infections, such as measles, chickenpox and some sexually transmitted infections, also result in manifestations on the skin. Skin infestations occur when parasites such as lice or mites invade and subsist on the skin.

Major manifestations of skin disorders

Various structural and functional changes accompany skin disorders.

Pruritus

Pruritus (itching) is one of the more common and distressing symptoms of a skin disorder. Pruritus is thought to result from a disruption in the skin nerve endings. Scratching to relieve pruritus can result in tissue damage and infection, thereby causing further discomfort.

Lesions

Depending on the type of skin disorder, one or a variety of lesions may be present. Observation of the individual includes assessing any lesions to determine their shape, size and distribution. Table 29.7 lists and describes the various types of skin lesions. Some types of lesions may discharge fluid, referred to as exudate.

Alterations in sensation

In addition to pruritus, the individual may experience other abnormal skin sensations such as numbness, tingling, burning or pain.

Alterations in skin colour

Disorders of the skin may be accompanied by darkened areas of skin (hyperpigmentation), patches of pale skin (hypopigmentation) or inflammation. Burned skin may be reddened, blanched or charred, depending on the extent of the burn. Cold injuries can result in red areas, as in chilblains, or in extreme pallor, as in frostbite.

TABLE 29.7 | Skin lesions

Term	Description	Examples
Atrophy	Loss of tissue.	Striae
Bulla	Elevated, filled with clear fluid. Similar to a vesicle, but larger.	Pemphigus vulgaris, drug eruptions, partial-thickness burns
Comedone	A plug of secretion contained in a follicle.	Acne
Crust	A superficial mass caused by dried blood or exudate.	Scab
Cyst	Encapsulated mass in the dermis or subcutaneous layer. May be raised or flat, and contain fluid or solid material.	Sebaceous cyst
Erosion	Moist, red, depressed break in the epidermis. Follows rupture of a vesicle or bulla.	Chickenpox
Excoriation	Superficial break in the skin, exposing the dermis.	Scratches, abrasions
Fissure	Deep, linear, red crack or break exposing the dermis.	Tinea pedis
Macule	Small, circumscribed discolouration (e.g. red, white, tan or brown).	Freckle, rubella, scarlet fever
Nodule	Circumscribed, elevated area—usually 1–2 cm in diameter.	Ganglion, acne
Papule	Circumscribed, elevated, firm palpable area (<1 cm in diameter).	Mole, wart, pimple
Patch	Macules larger than 1 cm.	Vitiligo
Plaque	Large, elevated, rough, flat-topped areas.	Plaque caused by friction
Pustule	A vesicle or bulla containing pus.	Acne, furuncle, folliculitis, impetigo

Continued

TABLE 29.7 | Skin lesions—cont'd

Term	Description	Examples
Scale	Mass of exfoliated epidermis.	Dandruff, psoriasis
Scar (cicatrix)	Ranges from a thin line to thick, irregular fibrous tissue. May be white, pink or red.	Healed surgical incision or wound
Tumour	Elevated, solid formation.	Lipoma, melanoma, fibroma
Ulcer	Depressed circumscribed area involving loss of the epidermis, exposing the dermis, and may involve subcutaneous tissue.	Pressure injury
Vesicle	Circumscribed, elevated superficial area filled with clear fluid (<1 cm).	Blister, herpes simplex infection, contact dermatitis
Wheal	Transitory, elevated, irregular-shaped swelling of the epidermis.	Medication sensitive hives

(Adapted from Gawkrodger & Arden-Jones 2021; Patton & Thibodeau 2019)

Alterations in skin temperature

In certain skin disorders such as bacterial infection the skin may feel hot to touch, whereas in other conditions, such as frostbite, the skin is cool to touch.

Alterations in texture

Abnormalities of texture (e.g. roughness or hardness) may result from the presence of certain types of lesions such as scabs or papules. Scaling may occur, or the skin may be thick, wrinkled or atrophied. Some skin disorders may result in areas of oedema (e.g. injuries from heat or cold).

Presence of an odour

Certain skin disorders, particularly those that are accompanied by draining lesions, may give rise to an offensive odour.

Systemic manifestations

Certain skin disorders, such as acute contact dermatitis or carbuncles, may be accompanied by systemic effects such as fatigue, nausea, headache and an elevated body temperature.

SPECIFIC DISORDERS OF THE SKIN

Genetic disorders

Genetic disorders of the skin are those that are present at birth, become evident soon after birth or those that may be passed on to the next generation.

Acne vulgaris is a chronic inflammatory condition involving the sebaceous glands and the pilosebaceous follicles, particularly of the face. A blackhead forms and blocks the opening of a sebaceous gland, which becomes infected. Later, a pustule forms. This condition is most often present in adolescents and young adults. Familial tendencies are thought to contribute to the cause or exacerbation of acne. Other causative factors include endocrine imbalances, use of oral contraceptives, hormone therapy, emotional stress and lack of personal hygiene.

Ichthyosis is any one of several inherited conditions in which the skin is dry, hyperkeratotic and fissured, resembling fish scales. It usually appears at, or shortly after, birth. Ichthyosis vulgaris is the most common type and the least severe.

Idiopathic disorders

Idiopathic disorders of the skin are those in which no definite cause can be identified.

Psoriasis is a chronic skin disorder characterised by red patches covered by thick, dry, silvery scales. The lesions may be present on any part of the body but are more common on the extensor surfaces of the elbows and knees, and on the scalp. Psoriasis can be exacerbated by trauma, infection, stress and the use of specific systemic medications.

Pityriasis rosea is thought to be caused by a virus, and is characterised by a scaling, pink macular rash that spreads over the trunk and other parts of the body. The condition is self-limiting and usually disappears within 4–6 weeks.

Vitiligo is a benign disorder consisting of irregular patches of skin totally lacking in pigment.

Seborrhoeic dermatitis is a chronic inflammatory condition characterised by dry or moist, red scaly eruptions. Common sites are the scalp, eyelids, face and trunk. The scales have a greasy feel and yellow crusts. Cradle cap is one form of seborrhoeic dermatitis.

Hypersensitivity disorders

Hypersensitivity disorders of the skin result from an immediate or delayed reaction after exposure to a certain substance.

Contact dermatitis is caused by an irritant substance that comes into direct contact with the skin, such as detergents, hair dye, metals, preservatives, perfumes or specific fabrics. The resultant inflammation and skin rash may be mild or severe, depending on the individual's response. Chronic exposure to an irritant may result in the skin becoming reddened, scaly or cracked.

Atopic dermatitis usually occurs when there is a history of asthma and/or hay fever. The condition is characterised by pruritus, redness of the skin, papules and thickening of the skin. Common sites are the face and neck, behind the knees and in the cubital fossae and on the back of the hands.

Urticaria is a pruritic skin eruption characterised by transient weals with well-defined red margins and pale centres. Urticaria (hives) is most frequently caused by foods, insect bites and inhalants. Specific types of urticaria are associated with systemic diseases. Pruritus associated with urticaria is frequently intense and is commonly accompanied by stinging, numbness or prickling sensations. Urticaria may also be a manifestation of an adverse reaction to a drug, and the skin lesions may appear almost immediately or several days after the drug has been absorbed. Drugs responsible for such adverse reactions include acetylsalicylic acid, penicillin and codeine.

Pemphigus vulgaris is an uncommon disorder of the skin and mucous membranes, characterised by the formation of large bullae containing clear fluid. The disorder is thought to result from an autoimmune response and may be fatal if untreated. The bullae erupt, ooze and bleed readily, and death is often due to a secondary bacterial infection or loss of blood protein.

Trauma

A traumatic injury that involves damage to the skin can result from exposure to extremes of temperature, prolonged pressure on the skin or physical injuries resulting in lacerations, punctures or abrasions.

Erythrocyanosis (chilblains) is redness and swelling of the skin, a result of excessive exposure to cold. Burning, itching, blistering and ulceration may occur; areas most commonly affected are the toes, fingers, nose and ears.

Frostbite is the traumatic effect of extreme cold on the skin and subcutaneous tissues, characterised by pallor of the exposed areas, such as the nose, ears, fingers and toes. Vasoconstriction and damage to blood vessels impair local circulation, resulting in oedema, anoxia and necrosis.

Immersion (trench) foot is a condition of the skin on the feet that develops from continued exposure to wetness and coldness, such as prolonged immersion in cold water. The feet appear pale, cold and swollen, and the individual experiences tingling followed by loss of sensation.

Burns are injuries to the body tissues caused by heat, electricity or chemicals. Thermal burns include injuries caused by flame, steam or hot liquids. Electrical burns result from contact with an electrical current, and chemical burns most often result from contact with caustic substances. A burn may be minor or major, and the degree of local effects and systemic consequences depend on many factors, including the severity of the burn and the age of the individual. (More information on burns and the care of individuals with burns is provided later in this chapter.)

Neoplasia

A *keloid* is a benign overgrowth of fibrous tissue at the site of a wound to the skin. The new tissue is elevated, thickened and reddened. Most keloids flatten and become less noticeable over a period of years. Keloids are more likely to develop if a wound has been infected or if the edges of a wound have been poorly aligned during healing.

Sebaceous cysts are one type of epithelial cyst and consist of a capsule containing a soft yellow–white material. These benign cysts are elevated and firm and range in size from about 0.2–5.0 cm.

A *lipoma* is a common benign tumour composed of adipose tissue, which is generally encapsulated in the subcutaneous layer of the skin. Lipomas vary in size and most frequently occur on the neck, back, thighs or forearms.

Neurofibromatosis is a congenital condition characterised by:

- numerous neurofibromas of the skin and nerves
- café-au-lait spots on the skin
- in some presentations by abnormalities of the muscles, bones and internal organs.

Many large, pedunculated soft-tissue tumours may develop.

Basal cell carcinoma is a malignant lesion characterised by a shallow ulcer surrounded by a raised well-defined edge. Basal cell carcinomas may also be referred to as rodent ulcers. The most common site is the face, particularly the nose, eyelids and cheeks. Basal cell carcinomas usually occur in people aged over 40 and, since metastasis is rare, the prognosis is favourable.

Squamous cell carcinoma is a malignant lesion characterised by a firm, elevated painless nodule. The most common sites are areas of the body most often exposed to ultraviolet rays. Squamous cell carcinoma is most frequently seen in men over age 55 and, as metastasis is probable, this neoplasm has a higher mortality rate than basal cell carcinoma.

A *melanoma* is a malignant tumour that arises from melanocytes. The incidence of melanoma seems to be related to prolonged exposure to the sun, particularly by fair-skinned people. Because metastatic dissemination is relatively common, the mortality rate is high. In its premalignant stage, a melanoma appears as a flat, irregularly pigmented macule. Colour changes appear as the melanoma becomes malignant and invasive, with the colour ranging from red, brown and blue to black. Melanoma can occur on any part of the body but most frequently occurs in areas of the skin exposed to sunlight. There are many types of melanoma and, because of its invasive nature, the nodular type is the most serious. Australians have the highest rate of malignant melanoma in the world, and the incidence is particularly high in Queensland and other tropical regions.

Infections and infestations

Because the surface of the body is constantly exposed to large numbers of pathogenic microorganisms, the skin is a potential area for infection. In addition, dermatological problems are often the result of infestation by parasites. Many factors increase a person's vulnerability to a skin infection, including ill-health, poor standard of hygiene or a break in the continuity of the skin. Bacterial skin infections include carbuncles, erysipelas, folliculitis, furuncles (boils), impetigo and paronychia.

A *carbuncle* is a cluster of staphylococcal abscesses or boils containing purulent matter. Eventually, pus discharges to the skin surface through numerous openings.

Erysipelas is an acute streptococcal inflammatory infection involving subcutaneous tissue. The skin of the affected area is bright red and oedematous, with a sharply defined border. The area may develop vesicles and the individual commonly experiences pain and an elevated body temperature.

Folliculitis is a common infection of the hair follicles, caused by staphylococci. Superficial or deep pustules are evident, and the most common site is the face.

A *furuncle (boil)* is an infection caused by either staphylococci or streptococci. A furuncle starts as a painful, hard, deep follicular abscess, and the overlying skin is hot to touch. The area becomes soft and opens to discharge a core of tissue and pus.

Impetigo is an acute contagious disorder of the superficial layers of the skin, caused by either staphylococci or streptococci. The condition begins as local erythema and progresses to pruritic vesicles which ooze, with the exudate from the lesion forming a yellow-coloured crust. Lesions usually form on the face and spread locally.

Paronychia is a painful inflammatory infection of the tissue around the nails.

Viral skin infections include herpes simplex and herpes zoster infections, and verrucae.

Herpes simplex virus (HSV) has an affinity for the skin and usually produces small irritating or painful fluid-filled blisters on the skin and mucous membranes. HSV-1 infections tend to occur in the facial area, particularly around the mouth and nose, whereas HSV-2 infections are usually limited to the genital region. The blisters erupt and thin yellow crusts form as the lesions begin to heal.

Acute infection with herpes zoster, or varicella-zoster virus (V-ZV), is characterised by the development of very painful vesicular skin eruptions that follow the underlying route of cranial or spinal nerves inflamed by the virus. After about 1 week, the vesicles develop crusts, and the condition may last several weeks. The pain may last for much longer.

A *verruca (wart)* is caused by the human papilloma virus and presents as a firm skin lesion with a rough surface. Different types of verrucae include those that commonly affect the hands, fingers or knees and those that affect the genito-anal region.

Fungal skin infections include candidiasis and tinea. Candidiasis is any infection caused by a species of *Candida*, usually *Candida albicans*, characterised by pruritus, a white exudate, peeling and easy bleeding. Oral or vaginal thrush are common topical manifestations of candidiasis, as are red eroded patches in the genito-anal region.

Tinea (ringworm) is a group of fungal skin diseases caused by dermatophytes of several kinds. It is characterised by itching, scaling and painful lesions. Types of tinea include tinea capitis (affecting the scalp), tinea pedis (affecting the feet) and tinea corporis (affecting non-hairy, smooth skin on the body).

Infestations of the skin by parasites include scabies and pediculosis. *Scabies* is a condition caused by a mite, *Sarcoptes scabiei*, and characterised by a papular rash, intense pruritus and excoriation of the skin from scratching. The sites most commonly affected are the thin-skinned areas between the fingers, flexor surfaces of the wrists and the inner aspect of the thigh. The mite burrows into the outer layers of the skin, where the female lays eggs. Small, thread-like red streaks appear where the mite has burrowed into the skin.

Pediculosis is infestation by blood-sucking lice, which causes intense pruritus, often resulting in excoriation from scratching. Different varieties of pediculi affect the hair on the scalp, the body or the pubic area. The lice can be seen with the naked eye, and their eggs (nits) can be seen as small pear-shaped bodies attached to the hairs.

Diagnostic tests

To diagnose specific disorders of the skin a variety of tests may be performed, as follows:

- direct physical examination and inspection
- skin biopsy
- microscopic examination
- skin testing.

Direct physical examination and inspection

A lesion may be examined using a magnifying lens, or a Wood's lamp may be used to determine the presence of fungal infections. Fungal infections such as ringworm show a characteristic fluorescence under black light.

Skin biopsy

The medical officer obtains a sample of skin or part of a lesion for pathological examination. Certain lesions may be surgically excised to provide sufficient tissue for histological diagnosis.

Microscopic examination

Specimens for microscopic examination may be obtained by gently scraping the scales or crusts of lesions. Exudate from oozing lesions may also be obtained for microscopic examination.

Skin testing

Skin testing may be performed to determine which substance or substances cause a hypersensitive reaction. Patch testing provides a means for assessing contact sensitivity. One or more suspected allergens are placed on a hairless part of the body. The test site is later examined for a visible reaction.

CARE OF THE INDIVIDUAL WITH A SKIN DISORDER

Although nursing care is planned to meet the individual's needs, according to their specific skin disorder, the nursing care of a person with any dermatosis generally involves the following aspects.

Relief of pruritus

Itching, which can be a source of considerable distress, is a feature of many skin disorders. The natural response to pruritus is to scratch, and scratching can cause further discomfort and may lead to tissue damage and infection. While medical therapy is aimed at resolving the problem responsible for the pruritus, certain nursing measures can be employed to provide some relief:

- Since heat tends to aggravate itching, the room should be maintained at a moderate and comfortable temperature. The bedclothes and personal clothing should be light, loose and cool.
- Soothing tepid baths may be helpful in alleviating the itching.
- Diversions that are of interest to the individual, such as reading or watching television, may be helpful.

Topical applications

The application of local soothing preparations or topical medications may be prescribed. The most common mediums used to apply medications to the skin are creams, lotions, powders or ointments and pastes. Medications that are mixed with the appropriate medium for topical application include anti-inflammatory drugs such as corticosteroids, antipruritic agents such as tar or corticosteroids, antiseptics such as phenol, and antibiotics such as neomycin. Specific substances to be added to the bath water may also be prescribed. For example, oatmeal, bath oils or coal-tar preparations may be prescribed when large areas of the body surface are affected. The nurse must ensure that the bath water is at a comfortable temperature and should be aware that many skin disorders result in changes in sensory perception, so it is essential that the water is not too hot.

Whenever topical applications have been prescribed, the nurse must know the level of responsibilities and the regulations regarding administration of medications in the healthcare facility and geographical area in which they work. Each type of topical medication requires proper application, and the nurse must know the amount to use, whether gloves are required during application and the signs of any adverse effects of the medication. A thin layer on application is recommended to avoid excess moisture or use of mediums. The correct administration of medication is required as with any medication. (Please refer to Chapter 20 for further detail.)

In addition to topical applications, systemic medications may be prescribed for symptom management such as analgesics to relieve pain, antihistamines for itching, antibiotics to combat infection or mild sedatives to promote adequate rest.

Dressings may be prescribed as part of the local treatment of skin disorders. Moist dressings may be used in the management of acute inflammatory skin disorders. Any solution that is used to soak the dressing should be warmed to body temperature. Occlusive dressings may be applied over a topical medication to promote penetration of the drug into the epidermis.

Maintenance of fluid and nutritional balance

Fluid and electrolyte balance may be disrupted because of loss of fluid in exudate from skin lesions. It is important to ensure that adequate fluid replacement is provided to compensate for any abnormal fluid loss.

A diet that is rich in protein may be prescribed to replenish losses and to promote healing. It is important to ascertain whether the individual is allergic to any specific foods since skin disorders can be caused or aggravated by food allergies. Any known allergens must be eliminated from the diet.

Preventing infection

Any disruption to the integrity of the skin increases the risk of infection, so measures such as the following should be implemented to protect the skin:

- After bathing or showering, the skin should be gently patted dry. Brisk rubbing could cause damage to already tender skin.
- The nails should be kept short and clean to prevent damage from scratching, and the person should be encouraged to resist scratching. It is important to explain that scratching increases the risk of skin trauma and infection. For some people, such as a young child or a disoriented person, mittens may be placed over the hands to reduce skin damage by scratching.
- All dressings and applications of topical substances must be performed aseptically.
- If the skin disorder is contagious, additional precautions and isolation may be implemented to prevent the spread of infection to others.

Providing psychological support

A severe skin disorder may cause distress and embarrassment to the person who has it. They may be self-conscious about their appearance, and their body image may be severely impaired. If the person feels that other people will avoid contact because of their unsightly appearance, they may experience anxiety or depression, both of which may be exacerbated if the disorder is likely to result in permanent disfigurement. To assist the individual with a skin disorder, the nurse should be careful not to demonstrate any distaste or repugnance. It is important that the individual and their significant others are kept well informed about the disorder and its likely outcome. The individual should be given the opportunity to express their emotions and fears, such as the fear of disfigurement or alienation from their loved ones.

PRESSURE INJURIES

Pressure injuries are defined as 'localised damage to the skin and/or underlying tissue, as a result of pressure or pressure in combination with shear' (EPUAP et al 2019). Pressure injuries usually occur over a bony prominence but may also be related to a medical device or other object. Pressure injuries have previously been referred to as pressure ulcers/areas, decubitus ulcers, trophic ulcers and bedsores. Pressure injuries are preventable, yet the prevalence of pressure injuries in Australia and New Zealand remains high, at 12.9% of all overnight hospital admissions in 2020, despite the implementation of guidelines and interventions to reduce their occurrence (Rodgers et al 2021). Australian prevalence rates in residential care have been reported at between 6.4% and 11.7% with an estimated cost of $13.61 million (Wilson et al 2019). In Australian public hospitals, based on data for 2018–2019, there were nearly 2700 hospital-acquired pressure injuries. These cases cost $56,000 per person on average (ACSQHC 2020). Consequences of hospital-acquired pressure injuries include extended length of stay, impact on individuals and families, increased cost to the healthcare system and, most crucially, pain and discomfort to the individual (ACSQHC 2021).

Pressure injury aetiology

Pressure injuries result from ischaemic hypoxia of the tissues owing to prolonged pressure on the area when it is over a hard surface, such as a mattress or chair. Impaired mobility or activity and impaired sensory perception of the individual affects the ability of the individual to recognise when there is pain and to change position. Clinical Interest Box 29.8 lists conditions in which individuals may be at increased risk of pressure injury.

Pressure impairs blood circulation and the area is deprived of essential nutrients and oxygen, causing cellular death. The major factors contributing to loss of local capillary blood supply are perpendicular pressure and parallel/tangential shearing forces. However, these can be exacerbated by predisposing factors classed as either intrinsic (e.g. advanced age, impaired mobility, malnutrition and medical situation) and/or extrinsic (e.g. moisture, pressure, shear and friction). A combination of these factors increases the risk of pressure injury. Pressure on the skin over bony prominences can distort the blood vessels to such an extent that the blood flow is interrupted. Pressure can also occlude lymphatic vessels, and the consequent accumulation of toxic substances can contribute to cell damage.

Pressure injuries form in a few hours but may take many months to heal; preventing them is therefore of prime importance. Ensuring adequate blood supply to pressure areas is critical since altered blood supply is the primary cause of pressure injuries. Blood supply to promote tissue healing is dependent on adequate circulation that brings antibodies and leucocytes to combat infection, as well as nutrients and oxygen for regeneration of tissues (Carville 2023).

CLINICAL INTEREST BOX 29.8
Individuals with increased risk of exposure to pressure injury

- Spinal cord injury
- Neurological disorders (e.g. stroke, multiple sclerosis)
- Trauma (e.g. fracture)
- Critically ill
- Obesity
- Chronic disease (e.g. diabetes [neuropathy]), pulmonary, vascular
- Older adults
- Medication use (e.g. sedatives, hypnotics, analgesics)
- Surgery
- Paediatric and newborns
- Palliative care

(Adapted from EPUAP et al 2019)

Pressure injuries can develop on body areas when they are subjected to prolonged or excessive pressure (Figure 29.8). The two most frequently reported locations are the sacrum and heels (EPUAP et al 2019). Two impacts of pathophysiology determine pressure injury development: superficial lesions of the epidermis present as non-blanchable redness progressing to severe injuries and are defined by the European Pressure Ulcer Advisory Panel categories as stages I–IV (EPUAP et al 2019), and an initial injury caused by muscle necrosis that results in deep tissue injury (Scheel-Sailer et al 2017), identified as temporary categories.

Classification of pressure injuries

Pressure injuries are categorised into four stages with an additional two temporary categories (EPUAP et al 2019). See Figure 29.9 for images and full descriptions of all the stages. The current standards for pressure injury staging are identified in the *Prevention and Treatment of Pressure Ulcers/Injuries: Clinical Practice Guidelines (The International Guidelines)* (EPUAP et al 2019).

Stages I and II are generally considered partial-thickness wounds (though the skin remains intact in a stage I pressure injury) and stages III and IV are considered full-thickness injuries. Tissue destruction can continue through the layers of tissue unless measures are taken early to relieve pressure and increase local tissue perfusion (see Case Study 29.1).

Stage I: Non-blanchable erythema. Intact skin with non-blanchable redness of a localised area, usually over a bony prominence. Darkly pigmented skin may not have visible blanching; its colour may differ from the surrounding area.

Stage II: Partial-thickness skin loss. Partial-thickness loss of dermis presenting as a shallow, open ulcer with a red-pink

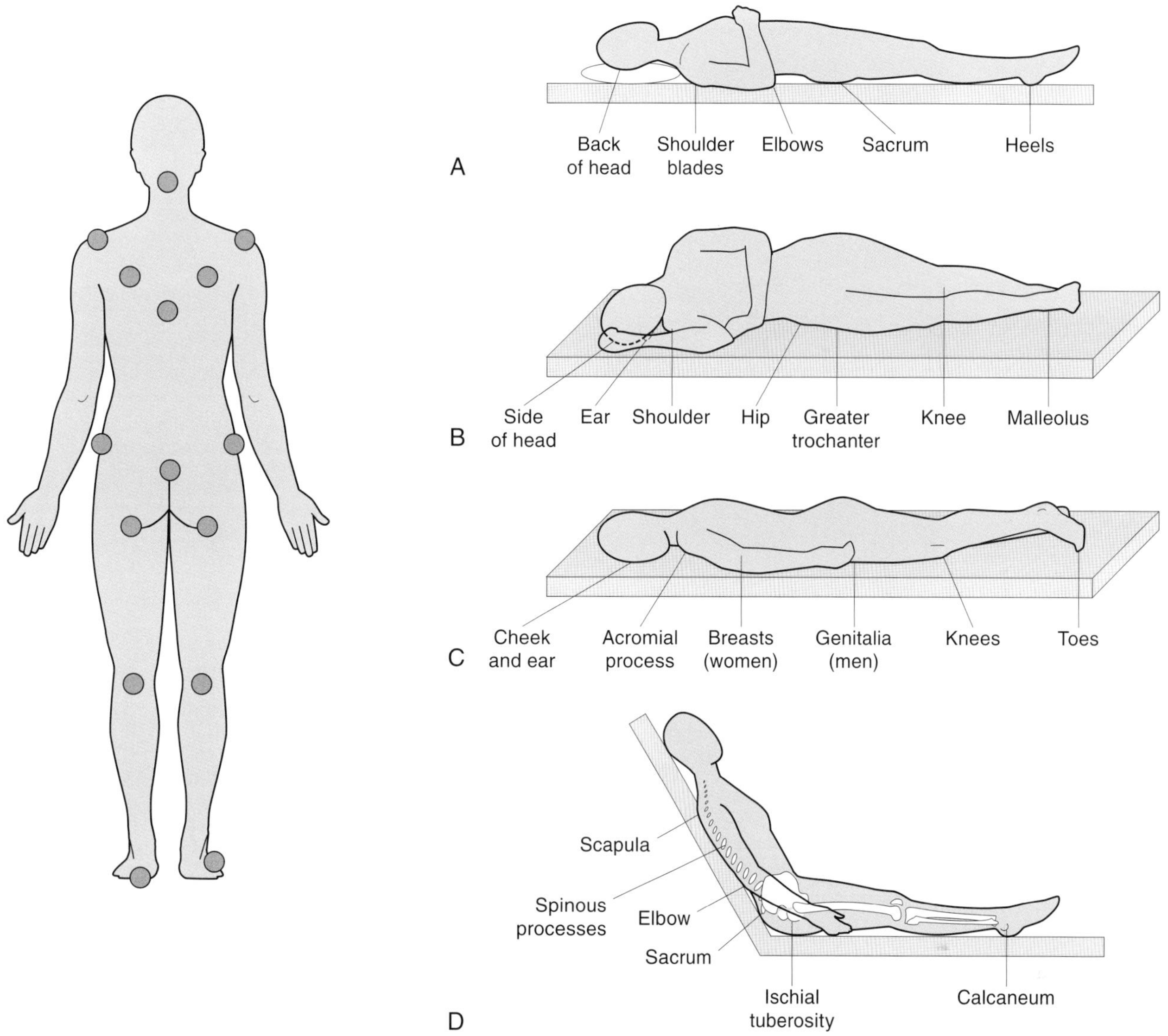

Figure 29.8 Pressure injury sites

A: In the supine position, **B:** In the lateral position, **C:** In the prone position, **D:** In the sitting position.

wound bed, without slough. May also present as an intact or open/ruptured serum-filled blister.

Stage III pressure injury: Full-thickness skin loss. Pressure injury presenting as full-thickness tissue loss in which subcutaneous fat may be visible, but bone, tendon or muscle are not exposed. Slough may be present but does not obscure the depth of tissue loss.

Stage IV pressure injury: Full-thickness tissue loss. Pressure injury presenting as full-thickness tissue loss with exposed bone, tendon or muscle. Slough or eschar may be present on some parts of the wound bed. Often includes undermining and tunnelling.

Temporary categories

Unstageable: Depth unknown; full-thickness tissue loss in which the base of the ulcer is covered by slough (yellow, tan, grey, green or brown) and/or eschar (tan, brown or black) in wound bed. Until enough slough and/or eschar is removed to expose the base of the wound, the true depth, and therefore stage, cannot be determined.

Suspected deep tissue injury (SDTI): Depth unknown; purple or maroon localised area or discoloured, intact skin or blood-filled blister due to damage of underlying soft tissue from pressure and/or shear. The area may be preceded by tissue that is painful, firm, mushy, boggy, warmer or cooler as compared to adjacent tissue.

Review Case Study 29.1, which explores pressure injuries.

Intrinsic factors

Intrinsic factors are characteristics specific to an individual. These factors reduce the skin's tolerance to pressure by affecting the vasculature, lymphatic system and supporting

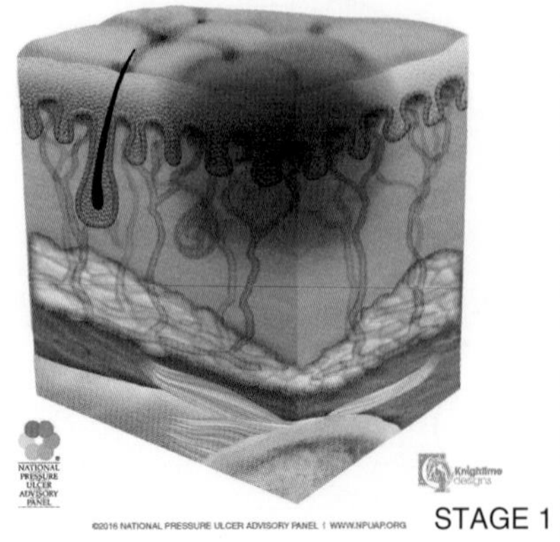	**Stage 1 pressure injury: Non-blanchable erythema of intact skin** Intact skin with a localised area of non-blanchable erythema, which may appear differently in darkly pigmented skin. Presence of blanchable erythema or changes in sensation, temperature or firmness may precede visual changes. Colour changes do not include purple or maroon discolouration; these may indicate deep tissue pressure injury.
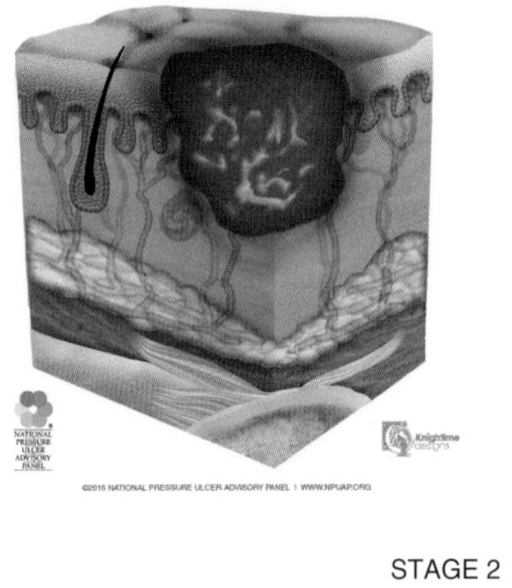	**Stage 2 pressure injury: Partial-thickness skin loss with exposed dermis** The wound bed is viable, pink or red, moist, and may also present as an intact or ruptured serum-filled blister. Adipose (fat) is not visible and deeper tissues are not visible. Granulation tissue, slough and eschar are not present. These injuries commonly result from adverse microclimate and shear in the skin over the pelvis and shear in the heel. This stage should not be used to describe moisture-associated skin damage (MASD) including incontinence-associated dermatitis (IAD), intertriginous dermatitis (ITD), medical adhesive-related skin injury (MARSI) or traumatic wounds (skin tears, burns, abrasions).
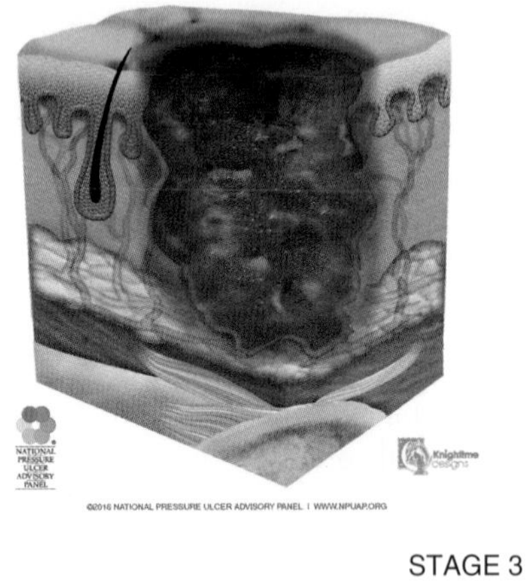	**Stage 3 pressure injury: Full-thickness skin loss** Full-thickness loss of skin, in which adipose (fat) is visible in the ulcer and granulation tissue and epibole (rolled wound edges) are often present. Slough and/or eschar may be visible. The depth of tissue damage varies by anatomical location; areas of significant adiposity can develop deep wounds. Undermining and tunnelling may occur. Fascia, muscle, tendon, ligament, cartilage and/or bone are not exposed. If slough or eschar obscures the extent of tissue loss, this is an unstageable pressure injury.

Figure 29.9 Pressure injury classification system

(EPUAP et al 2019)

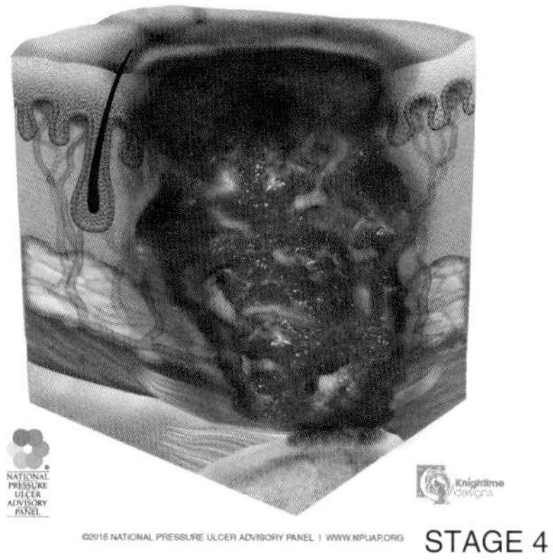

Stage 4 Pressure injury: Full-thickness skin and tissue loss
Full-thickness skin and tissue loss with exposed or directly palpable fascia, muscle, tendon, ligament, cartilage or bone in the ulcer. Slough and/or eschar may be visible. Epibole (rolled edges), undermining and/or tunnelling often occur. Depth varies by anatomical location. If slough or eschar obscures the extent of tissue loss this is an unstageable pressure injury.

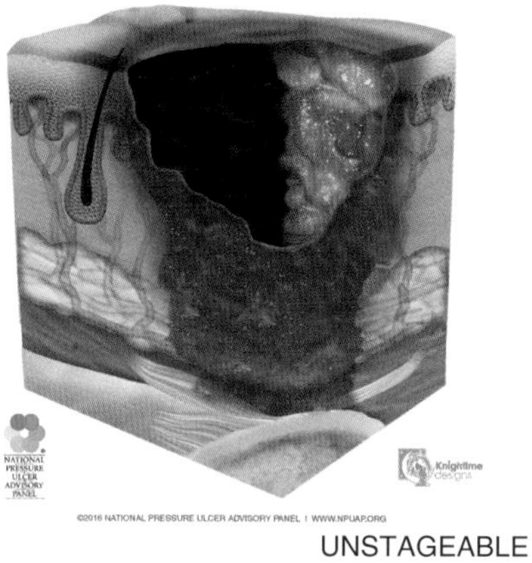

Unstageable pressure injury: Obscured full-thickness skin and tissue loss
Full-thickness skin and tissue loss in which the extent of tissue damage within the ulcer cannot be confirmed because it is obscured by slough or eschar. If slough or eschar is removed, a stage 3 or stage 4 pressure injury will be revealed. Stable eschar (i.e. dry, adherent, intact without erythema or fluctuance) on an ischaemic limb or the heel(s) should not be removed.

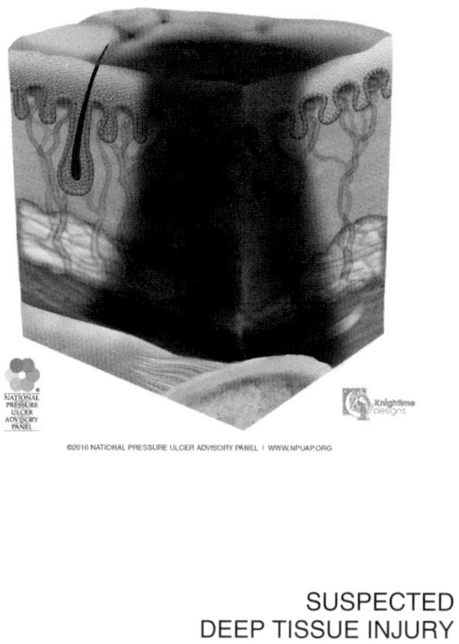

Deep tissue pressure injury: Persistent non-blanchable deep red, maroon or purple discolouration
Intact or non-intact skin with localised area of persistent non-blanchable deep red, maroon, purple discolouration or epidermal separation revealing a dark wound bed or blood-filled blister.
Pain and temperature change often precede skin colour changes.
Discolouration may appear differently in darkly pigmented skin. This injury results from intense and/or prolonged pressure and shear forces at the bone–muscle interface. The wound may evolve rapidly to reveal the actual extent of tissue injury or may resolve without tissue loss. If necrotic tissue, subcutaneous tissue, granulation tissue, fascia, muscle or other underlying structures are visible, this indicates a full-thickness pressure injury (unstageable, stage 3 or stage 4). Do not use DTPI to describe vascular, traumatic, neuropathic or dermatological conditions.

Figure 29.9—cont'd

CASE STUDY 29.1

Pressure injury

Mrs Green, 82 years old, was discharged from hospital following a brief admission for a urinary tract infection. She lives alone and has no family nearby as they either live interstate or overseas. Mrs Green was taken home with an escort by hospital transport. Two days later, a community nurse attended a home visit. On arrival, the nurse found Mrs Green sitting in the lounge chair. The living environment appeared messy with an unpleasant smell. Mrs Green was incontinent to both urine and faeces and stated that she had not been moving round in the room much at all for the past 2 days. Mrs Green gave poor eye contact and had difficulty answering questions appropriately. Mrs Green had hardly eaten or drunk anything and her medications remained in the bag of belongings she was sent home with.

An ambulance transport is initiated for medical review of Mrs Green's current condition. While assisting Mrs Green, the nurse noted a large wound to her sacrum, which is to be reported to the emergency department staff by the paramedics. On assessment in the acute care facility, surgical debridement took place, identifying a stage IV pressure injury on her sacrum.

See Nursing Care Plan 29.1 for the general nursing care recommended for prevention and management of pressure injuries.

1. Describe a pressure injury risk assessment that could inform prevention care for Mrs Green.
2. Explain the reasons referral is made to specific allied health professionals to care for Mrs Green.
3. What considerations for a wound dressing regimen will Mrs Green require?
4. What discharge planning actions could have improved the care outcomes for Mrs Green?

structures. Factors include age, mobility, circulation, nutrition, comorbidities and mobility. Chronic illnesses, particularly those affecting tissue perfusion and oxygen delivery (e.g. peripheral vascular disease) and sensation, also contribute to an increased risk of pressure injury development.

Age

People aged over 65 years are at greatest risk of pressure injuries with the risk increasing over 75 years of age (EPUAP et al 2019).

Nutritional status

Inadequate nutrition prevents efficient cellular growth and repair and renders the tissues more vulnerable to damage. A poorly nourished person may have less protection over the bony prominences and be more vulnerable to the effects of prolonged pressure. Likewise, an overweight or obese person may have poor nutrition and be at risk of pressure injuries (Carville 2023).

Body type

As the sites of maximum skin compression are located over bony prominences, a thin person is more at risk. Conversely, an obese person may be at risk due to shearing forces and added pressure caused by body weight pressing on risk areas, increased risk of intertriginous dermatitis and impairment of vascular and lymphatic systems (Haesler 2018).

Mobility

Altered mobility and activity restricts an individual's ability to redistribute pressure on weight-bearing areas, and consequently impairs the arterial supply to and venous return from the affected area(s), resulting in oedema, hypoxia, ischemia and eventually necrosis.

Health conditions

Reduced sensitivity to pressure or pain may occur in certain disease states, such as spinal cord injury, paralysis, multiple sclerosis or diabetes mellitus. Transmission of impulses from receptors in the skin or to the muscles may be impaired, so that the person does not receive the 'message' to change position regularly, a normal body defence mechanism. Furthermore, the use of epidural analgesia reduces this protection mechanism. Other factors such as carcinoma, peripheral arterial disease (PAD), cardiopulmonary disease, lymphatic issues, renal and hepatic impairment/failure, hypotension and anaemia can also predispose the individual to pressure injuries (EPUAP et al 2019).

Extrinsic factors

Extrinsic factors are those derived from the individual's environment. The main identified factors are pressure (discussed above), shear, friction and moisture; all impact on the ability of the skin to tolerate pressure.

Shearing forces and friction

When pressure is applied to the skin at an angle, movement of the layers of the skin over one another may cause distortion of the tissue. The mechanical shearing forces involved distort and occlude the dermal capillaries, resulting in thrombosis and capillary occlusion, and tissue necrosis. Friction is also a mechanical force between the skin and another surface, such as bed linen, which creates resistance between the two surfaces. Friction immobilises the epidermis while the deeper layers move and is an important factor in an individual whose skin is fragile and at risk.

Moisture

Moisture on the skin can be from incontinence (urinary and faecal), wound exudate, perspiration, mucus or saliva. Prolonged exposure to moisture causes maceration, which weakens the connective fibres of the skin and alters the

NURSING CARE PLAN 29.1

Assessment: Skin assessment and pressure injury risk assessment
Issue/s to be addressed: Risk of pressure injury
Risk factors: Factors related to the individual, such as impaired nutrition, poor oxygen delivery, very young and advanced age, gender, the use of high-risk medicines (i.e. non-steroidal anti-inflammatories), the presence of chronic diseases, impaired mobility
Environmental factors, such as moisture (e.g. incontinence), shear or friction forces acting on the skin, and the use of medical device(s) such as nasal prong and oxygen mask
Goal/s: The individual's skin remains intact, as evidenced by no redness over bony prominences and capillary refill <3 seconds over areas of redness.

Care/actions	Rationale
Identify risk factors for pressure injuries using an agreed screening tool within 8 hours of admission.	Risk-assessment tools can be effective in assisting clinicians to screen for pressure injury risk; this should be combined with clinical judgment.
Undertake a comprehensive skin inspection and clinical assessment.	Healthy skin varies from individual to individual, but should have good turgor (an indication of moisture), feel warm and dry to the touch, be free of impairment (scratches, bruises, excoriation, rashes) and have quick capillary refill (less than 6 seconds). This should be conducted on admission to the healthcare facility or at first visit in community settings as indicated by clinical judgment.
Update risk and skin assessment daily, as well as when the individual's condition changes, on transfer to another department or facility and prior to discharge in alignment with local procedures.	Ongoing assessment is necessary to detect early signs of pressure damage, especially over bony prominences.
Assess the individual's nutritional status.	Nutritional screening is the process used to identify individuals who require a comprehensive nutrition assessment. This should be conducted on admission to the healthcare facility or at first visit in community settings.
Assess skin over bony prominences (sacrum, trochanters, scapulae, elbows, heels, inner and outer malleolus); do not position individual on site of skin impairment.	Areas where skin is stretched over bony prominences are at higher risk for breakdown because the possibility of ischaemia to skin is high as a result of compression of skin capillaries between a hard surface and the bone.
Assess the individual's awareness of the sensation of pressure.	Normally, individuals shift their weight off pressure areas every few minutes; this occurs automatically, even during sleep. People with decreased sensation are unaware of unpleasant stimuli (pressure) and do not shift weight. This results in prolonged pressure on skin capillaries and, ultimately, skin ischaemia.
Assess for faecal and/or urinary incontinence and any environmental moisture; if the person is incontinent, implement an incontinence management plan to prevent exposure to chemicals in urine and stool that can strip or erode the skin.	Keeping skin clean and dry and the use of emollients promote healthy skin that will be resilient to any insults from irritants and shear and pressure. It is important to remember that skin damage from moisture increases the risk of pressure injury or ulceration. The urea in urine turns into ammonia within minutes and is caustic to the skin. Stool may contain enzymes that cause skin breakdown.

Continued

NURSING CARE PLAN 29.1—cont'd

Assess amount of shear and friction on the person's skin.	A common cause of shear is elevating the head of the person's bed; the body's weight is shifted downwards onto the individual's sacrum. Individuals should be positioned and supported to prevent sliding down in bed and creating shear forces. Limit head-of-bed elevation to 30 degrees. Using the knee brake on the bed will also help minimise the person's body slipping downwards in the bed. Common causes of friction include the person rubbing heels or elbows against bed linen and moving the individual up in bed without the use of a lift sheet.
Assess the individual's ability to move (shift weight while sitting, turn over in bed, move from bed to chair).	Immobility is the greatest risk factor in skin breakdown.
Assess surface that the individual spends majority of time on (mattress, cushion).	Individuals who spend the majority of time on one surface benefit from a pressure reduction or pressure relief device to distribute pressure more evenly and lessen the risk for breakdown.
Implement measures to prevent tissue breakdown associated with decreased mobility: • Position the individual properly; use high-specification mattress or pressure redistributing support surface if indicated. • Instruct the individual to use overhead trapeze/monkey bar to lift self and shift weight at least every 30 minutes. • Lift and move the individual carefully using safe manual handling (e.g. a turn sheet and adequate assistance). • Change the individual's position when in bed at least every 2 hours, 24 hours a day.	Repositioning of an individual is undertaken to reduce the duration and magnitude of pressure over vulnerable areas of the body and to contribute to comfort, hygiene, dignity and functional ability. Regular positioning is not possible for some individuals because of their medical condition, and an alternative prevention strategy such as providing a high-specification mattress or bed may need to be considered. The timing of repositioning of the individual is determined by the individual's tissue tolerance, level of activity and mobility, general medical condition, overall treatment objectives, skin condition and comfort.
Referral to other health professionals as clinically indicated for assessment and treatment.	Other interprofessional team members (i.e. physician, nurse, dietitian, podiatrist, speech pathologist, occupational therapist, physical therapist) should develop and document an individualised intervention plan based on the individual's clinical needs.
Education—teach the individual and caregiver the cause(s) of pressure injury development: • Pressure in skin, especially over bony prominences • Incontinence • Poor nutrition • Shearing or friction against skin.	Information should initially be provided to the person and their family/carer at the time of assessment and care planning, and throughout the episode of care. This ensures they understand the importance of this prevention plan. Reinforce the importance of pressure injury prevention and management benefits of adherence to nutritional intake, mobility, turning or ambulation in prevention of pressure injury.

Evaluation: The individual's skin remained intact with nil erythema present. Interventions for care were evaluated as effective in preventing skin breakdown. The individual was able to describe and demonstrate understanding of pressure injury prevention actions and consequences.

(Adapted from ACSQHC 2020; EPUAP et al 2019)

resilience of the epidermis to external forces (EPUAP et al 2019). Abrasions are more likely to form from friction between the skin and the surface under the individual, making shearing forces more severe. Actions such as excessive washing with soap, unsafe manual handling or rubbing can also damage the skin's integrity. Incontinence of urine or liquid faeces can result in incontinence-associated dermatitis from moisture, which can be inaccurately described as a pressure injury. It is important to be able to clinically distinguish between pressure damage and incontinence-associated skin damage for appropriate management and accurate documentation (Francis 2019). Incontinence-associated skin damage creates an added risk of exposure to bacterial and faecal enzymes that alter the normal acidic pH of the skin and may lead to an increased risk of skin infection.

Pressure injury risk assessment

Assessing the potential of an individual for pressure injury development is a combination of the use of a recognised risk-assessment tool, skin and nutritional assessment and clinical judgment. Although the use of a risk-assessment tool can assist management and provide a structured approach to an individual's care plan it should not be used in isolation. A head-to-toe skin assessment is made on admission to a facility, including those entering an emergency department, and at regular intervals throughout their stay. Any change in the individual's clinical and psychological condition also requires skin integrity reassessment.

Risk assessment

It is important to identify individuals at risk of pressure injuries and various assessment tools have been designed to assist healthcare professionals. Implementation of a valid and reliable risk-assessment tool is considered best practice and is used as a guide to identify an individual at risk of pressure injury development. The tools are intended as a measure of criteria to facilitate the implementation of a rational preventative regimen. Several risk-assessment tools have been developed, with the common ones cited in the published literature being the Braden Scale for Predicting Pressure Sore Risk (Braden Scale) (Table 29.8), the Norton Scale and the Waterlow Score. Most encompass a scale or scoring system and include clinical **risk factors** such as mobility, nutrition, mental condition, activity, incontinence, sensory perception, friction and shear. A cumulative score is reached, which is used to inform the development of an individualised care plan in conjunction with clinical judgment for ongoing care. A recommended additional tool for assessment of critically ill persons is the Acute Physiological and Chronic Health Evaluation (APACHE II) score (EPUAP et al 2019). It is important for all healthcare workers, when assessing individuals utilising

TABLE 29.8 | The Braden Scale for predicting pressure sore risk

Patient's name ______________ **Evaluator's name** ______________
Date of assessment ______________

Sensory perception Ability to respond meaningfully to pressure-related discomfort	1. *Completely limited* Unresponsive (does not moan, flinch or grasp) to painful stimuli caused by diminished level of consciousness or sedation. OR Limited ability to feel pain over most of body surface.	2. *Very limited* Responds only to painful stimuli. Cannot communicate discomfort except by moaning or restlessness. OR Has sensory impairment that limits the ability to feel pain or discomfort over half of body.	3. *Slightly limited* Responds to verbal commands but cannot always communicate discomfort or need to be turned. OR Has some sensory impairment that limits ability to feel pain or discomfort in one or two extremities.	4. *No impairment* Responds to verbal commands. Has no sensory deficit that would limit ability to feel or voice pain or discomfort.
Moisture Degree to which skin is exposed to moisture	1. *Constantly moist* Skin kept moist almost constantly by perspiration, urine etc. Dampness detected every time patient is moved or turned.	2. *Moist* Skin often, but not always, moist. Necessary to change linen at least once a shift.	3. *Occasionally moist* Skin occasionally moist, requiring an extra linen change approximately once a day.	4. *Rarely moist* Skin usually dry. Require linen changing only at routine intervals.
Activity Degree of physical activity	1. *Bedfast* Confined to bed.	2. *Chairfast* Ability to walk severely limited or non-existent. Cannot bear own weight and/or must be assisted into chair or wheelchair.	3. *Walks occasionally* Walks occasionally during day but for very short distances, with or without assistance. Spends majority of each shift in bed or chair.	4. *Walks frequently* Walks outside room at least twice a day and inside room at least once every 2 hours during waking hours.

Continued

TABLE 29.8 | The Braden Scale for predicting pressure sore risk—cont'd

Mobility Ability to change and control body position	1. *Completely immobile* Does not make even slight changes in body or extremity position without assistance.	2. *Very limited* Makes occasional slight changes in body or extremity position but unable to make frequent or significant changes independently.	3. *Slightly limited* Makes frequent, although slight, changes in body or extremity position independently.	4. *No limitations* Makes major and frequent changes in position without assistance.
Nutrition Usual food intake pattern	1. *Very poor* Never eats a complete meal; rarely eats more than a third of any food offered; eats 2 servings or less of protein (meat or dairy products) per day. Takes fluids poorly; does not take a liquid dietary supplement. OR Is NPO and/or maintained on clear liquids or IVs for more than 5 days.	2. *Probably inadequate* Rarely eats a complete meal and generally eats only about half of any food offered. Protein intake includes only 3 servings of meat or dairy products per day; occasionally takes a dietary supplement. OR Receives less than optimum amount of liquid diet or tube feeding.	3. *Adequate* Eats over half of most meals; eats a total of 4 servings of protein (meat, dairy products) each day. Occasionally refuses a meal, but usually takes a supplement if offered. OR Is on a tube feeding or total parenteral nutrition regimen that probably meets most of nutritional needs.	4. *Excellent* Eats most of every meal; never refuses a meal; usually eats a total of 4 or more servings of meat and dairy products. Occasionally eats between meals. Does not require supplementation.
Friction and shear	1. *Problem* Requires moderate-to-maximum assistance in moving; complete lifting without sliding against sheets impossible. Frequently slides down in bed or chair, requiring frequent repositioning with maximum assistance. Spasticity, contractures or agitation leads to almost constant friction.	2. *Potential problem* Moves feebly or requires minimum assistance; during a move skin probably slides to some extent against sheets, chair, restraints or other devices. Maintains relatively good position in chair or bed most of the time but occasionally slides down.	3. *No apparent problem* Moves in bed and in chair independently and has sufficient muscle strength to lift up completely during move. Maintains good position in bed or chair at all times.	
				TOTAL SCORE

any risk-assessment tools, to use their clinical judgment to ensure that the risk-prevention plan is appropriate for the individual person and not based solely on the risk-assessment tool measures (EPUAP et al 2019). (See also Chapter 15.)

Nutritional assessment

Nutritional screening identifies malnutrition, dehydration and comorbidities and allows for appropriate interventions. Vulnerable people such as older adults, neonates, those who are critically unwell and/or those with obesity are at risk of malnutrition and pressure injuries. Therefore, nutritional screening and a comprehensive nutritional assessment and individualised nutritional care plan are also highly recommended in the clinical practice guideline (Munoz et al 2022). The Mini Nutritional Assessment Short Form (MNA-SF) is an example of a validated nutritional assessment tool that can be used for older adults with pressure injuries (Dent et al 2017). Assessment includes weight, height and BMI, food intake, dental and oral health, drugs that can

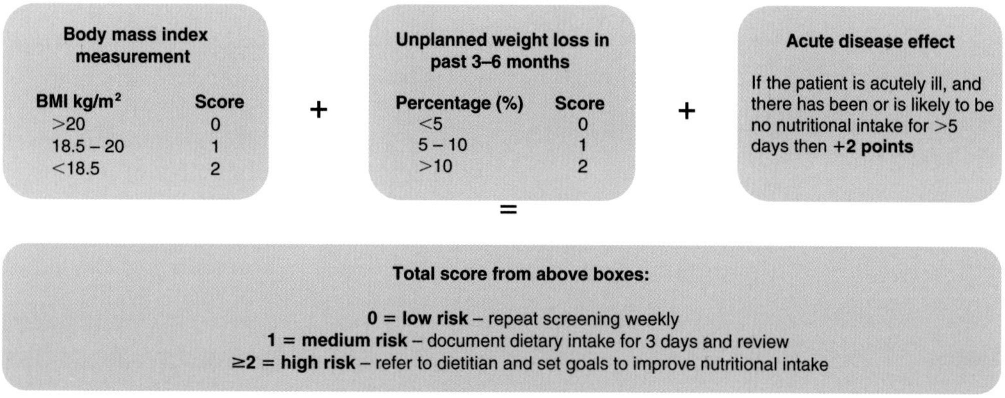

Figure 29.10 Malnutrition Universal Screening Tool (MUST)

(Deans & Paterson 2024)

interfere with appetite, swallowing difficulties and biochemical investigations to detect anaemia, haemoglobin and serum albumin levels. The Malnutrition Universal Screening Tool (MUST) (Figure 29.10) is another recommended for assessing the risk of nutrition deficiency (EPUAP et al 2019). Individuals found to be at risk of nutritional deficit must be referred to a dietitian for assessment and to other specialist healthcare practitioners (e.g. speech and occupational therapists) where appropriate (EPUAP et al 2019). Individual nutrition care plans are important to prevent, or improve healing of, pressure injuries (EPUAP et al 2019). See also Chapter 15 and Chapter 30.

Skin assessment

The International Guideline discusses the importance of skin and tissue assessment in pressure injury prevention, classification, diagnosis and treatment (EPUAP et al 2019). The condition of skin and underlying tissue can serve as an indicator of early signs of pressure damage; therefore, routine skin and tissue assessments provide an opportunity for early identification and treatment of skin damage (EPUAP et al 2019). The 'Comprehensive Care Standard' of the National Safety & Quality Health Service Standards (ACSQHC 2021) outlines the importance of carrying out comprehensive skin inspections for individuals on admission. *The International Guideline* states that a comprehensive skin assessment should be undertaken within 8 hours of admission or on the first visit in the community setting (EPUAP et al 2019). Skin is assessed for erythema, blanching response, moisture damage, infection (e.g. fungal infection), oedema, induration (hardness), localised heat and any sign of loss of integrity (e.g. dry skin). It is important to include observation for pressure damage from medical devices such as oxygen tubing, catheters and drain tubes. It is also important for the nurse to consider the differences of darker skin tones when undertaking a skin inspection for pressure injury risk or incident (Oozageer Gunowa et al 2018).

Psychosocial assessment

As part of a risk-assessment tool, mental or cognitive status is assessed since an impaired status can affect the individual's ability to adhere with treatment (e.g. identify when to change position, unplanned removal of devices due to confusion). Healthcare clinicians need to provide person-focused education in the prevention and management of pressure injuries (EPUAP et al 2019). This should include assessment of social history, previous disease experience, social support, individual preferences and access for the type of care to be received, culture and ethnicity, financial support, quality of life and goals of care.

Wound assessment

Pressure injuries should be assessed by their size, depth, location and degree of tissue (and bony) loss or necrosis. They are classified on the degree of tissue loss (see Figure 29.9). The classifications are useful for documentation of the degree of injury and when considering treatment options, especially for debridement. Undermining and tunnelling are included as part of the assessment for stage III and stage IV pressure injuries when there is extension of the wound under the skin, such that the wound cavity is larger than the skin opening. Documentation of the assessment findings and stage of pressure injury in the individual's medical records is necessary to provide a comparative review with future assessments and to guide treatment interventions to assess progress of wound healing. A hypothetical case of a pressure injury with additional complications, as well as ongoing documentation following the case, have been outlined in Progress Note 29.1 and Progress Note 29.2, respectively.

Specific pressure injury assessment tools, such as the pressure ulcer scale for healing (PUSH) Tool (EPUAP et al 2019), monitor changes in a pressure injury. The PUSH Tool measures three parameters: size of the wound (length × width), amount of exudate and tissue type (e.g. necrotic, slough, granulating, epithelialising). Like a risk-assessment tool, it gives a score for each parameter with the sum giving a total score. It is designed to provide a quick reference to whether the wound is healing.

Prevention and management of pressure injuries

Consideration of psychosocial issues, pain, altered body image and effects on activities of daily living are necessary to provide individual care. Diligent frequent skin checks can be achieved during all aspects of care.

Skin protection

Protection from pressure, friction and shear forces is identified as the most important measure to reduce the risk of pressure injuries. Appropriate positioning, use of pressure redistribution surfaces, skin hygiene and adequate nutrition all play a role. Local measures include appropriate manual handling techniques when transferring and changing the position of an individual (e.g. using transfer devices) that can lift the individual off the bed to avoid friction and shearing. It is not advisable and cannot be recommended to massage or vigorously rub the individual's skin as part of a pressure injury protocol and is contraindicated where there is acute inflammation and where there is the possibility of damaged blood vessels or fragile skin (EPUAP et al 2019). Water-based and pH neutral skin cleansers and creams are suggested to maintain skin hydration. Barrier creams help to maintain hydration and prevent maceration.

Nutrition

Wound healing increases the energy demands on the body. The nutritional requirements of a stage I pressure injury will differ from those of an individual with a stage IV injury and will be affected by the volume of exudate leaking from the wound. As the wound heals, nutritional requirements will also change. Australian and New Zealand dietary guidelines suggest increased protein intake (or the inclusion of protein building blocks such as arginine supplements in the diet) and inclusion of vitamin and mineral supplements to the individual's usual diet (EPUAP et al 2019). These guidelines also offer recommendations based on the probable risk of healing due to nutritional issues. If a person is unable to tolerate oral food or fluids, an alternative method of meeting nutritional needs, such as gastric tube or total parenteral nutrition (intravenous) feeding, may be necessary. *The International Guideline* identifies the importance of nutrition screening using a valid and reliable screening tool on admission, at each significant change in clinical condition and when the pressure injury is failing to heal (EPUAP et al 2019). A registered dietitian, in consultation with the interprofessional team, should develop an individualised nutrition plan that ensures adequate energy intake. The addition of fortified foods and high-protein oral nutritional supplements between meals can be used to meet increased dietary intake needs.

Support surfaces

Specialised support surfaces aim to reduce the interface pressure between the skin and the surface on which the individual is placed, such as the mattress on a bed, trolley, operating table or chair. Support surfaces work by increasing the amount of the body's surface area in contact with the surface or alternating the contact with the surface. Consideration is given to the person's size, weight, mobility, severity and number of pressure injuries and risk factors (EPUAP et al 2019). Using support surfaces does not remove the need for regular skin inspection and basic care and regular repositioning of the individual. Selection is based on mobility of the individual in the bed, comfort, the microclimate and the care setting. Various types of pressure redistribution devices are available and they fall into two main categories: reactive support surfaces and active support surfaces. Reactive devices can be powered (e.g. low air loss mattress/beds) or non-powered (e.g. foam/gel/air/combination mattresses). An active support surface is a powered device that produces alternating pressure through mechanical means and the ability to change its load distribution properties with or without an applied load (EPUAP et al 2019). Mattresses should be checked for correct settings, effectiveness and function such as 'bottoming out'. This means there must be at least 5 cm between the individual's lowest bony prominence and the mattress when the individual is lying supine. Heel protection should place the heel completely off the bed and distribute weight along the calf, avoiding additional pressure on the Achilles tendon. Synthetic sheepskins, fluid-filled gloves, doughnut devices or cut-outs are not recommended and should be avoided since they shift the pressure to another body surface area (EPUAP et al 2019).

Repositioning

Repositioning is an essential component of pressure injury prevention and care. Repositioning of the individual is designed to relieve or redistribute pressure points. It provides an opportunity to observe the skin condition and offer basic nursing care such as food or fluids and interaction with the individual. Repositioning regimens such as frequency, position and evaluation of the regimen must be documented in the individual's care plan or medical records. When lying in bed, individuals should be placed in a 30-degree tilted side-lying position (right side, back, left side) or 30-degree inclined recumbent position. The reduction of pressure and shear at the heel is important. The posterior prominence of the heel sustains intense pressure, even when a pressure redistribution surface is used (EPUAP et al 2019). Because the heel is covered with a small amount of subcutaneous tissue, any pressure is transferred at an angle to the bone, increasing the tissue pressure (EPUAP et al 2019). It is challenging to off-load pressure shear and friction for heels—the use of appropriate equipment to elevate and ensure 100% pressure off-load from the heel is recommended.

When head-of-bed elevation is required avoid a slouched position, which places extra pressure on the sacrum and coccyx. The EPUAP et al (2019) guidelines recommend using a 30-degree lying position in preference to the 90-degree angle. Use aids such as pillows to support the upper body and prevent the individual slipping towards the foot of the bed. An overhead handgrip may be used to lift and relieve pressure from the buttocks and sacral area. More frequent and smaller repositioning may be necessary for some individuals who are intolerant of major changes (e.g. post-surgery pain). The individual sitting in a chair is encouraged to lift from the seat frequently while sitting, to relieve pressure and facilitate tissue perfusion in the buttocks and sacral area. The person is assisted in this action if unable to lift independently. Avoid positioning the individual on medical devices such as drainage tubes; these can create areas of localised pressure. Splints, plaster casts, braces and bandages should be checked and adjusted regularly to relieve pressure. Individual factors are to be evaluated if effective in preventing prolonged pressure on any area. Using correct manual handling techniques can also avoid shearing when repositioning an individual. The person must be moved safely, avoiding dragging the skin along any surface, and surfaces such as bed linen must be kept smooth and dry. In healthcare, annual mandatory competency in use of aids and positioning is recommended and sometimes mandated to maintain best contemporary practice.

CRITICAL THINKING EXERCISE 29.2

After changing an individual's position, you observe redness over the bony prominences. What type of assessment must you perform to obtain correct information regarding pressure injury risk?

Pain assessment and treatment

Pressure injuries are painful. The pain caused by pressure injuries can be constant, severe, and may be the most distressing pressure injury symptom (EPUAP et al 2019). Pain may be the first indicator of a pressure injury related to ongoing pressure, friction and/or shear, damaged nerve endings, inflammation, infection, procedures or treatments, or excoriation from incontinence-associated dermatitis and muscle spasm (EPUAP et al 2019). Assess all individuals for pain related to a pressure injury before and during wound care. Appropriate pain management pharmacologically (e.g. analgesia) and non-pharmacologically (e.g. reposition, pressure offloading equipment) is to be planned and implemented for their quality of life. The increase in intensity of pain may also indicate the deterioration of the wound condition and possible wound infection. There are many different pain assessment tools, such as visual analog scale (VAS) and Wong-Baker FACES®. The individual's developmental stage and cognitive function are to be taken into consideration when assessing pressure injury related pain. (See Chapter 33.)

Wound care including infection management

Wound bed preparation is used as the tool to guide pressure injury wound care. Debridement of non-viable tissue after vascular assessment maximises the healing ability of the wound. In large pressure injuries, therapies such as NPWT may be beneficial to reduce the size of the wound and manage large volumes of exudate. Local wound infection is managed aggressively to avoid spreading infection and speed the healing process. More information on this issue can be found in the wound management section of this chapter.

CRITICAL THINKING EXERCISE 29.3

Murray, 77 years old, is admitted to the acute care hospital for a right total knee replacement. He has been fairly immobile for some time because of deterioration in his right knee. Murray also has type 2 diabetes mellitus and is obese. Murray's postoperative recovery has been complicated by sepsis secondary to the surgical site infection and pain. His hospital stay has consequently been extended for a length of time. Murray developed a stage III pressure injury to his right heel while in hospital. What measures could have been taken to prevent Murray from developing a pressure injury?

Skin tears

Skin tears are injuries caused by a variety of mechanical forces, such as shearing, friction or blunt trauma, falls, manual handling, contact with equipment or adherent dressings. The skin injury can present as a laceration or skin flap, with separation of epidermis and/or dermis. The most vulnerable people who are susceptible to skin tears are older adults due to the increasing skin fragility as ageing takes place and neonates because of their skin immaturity. These events cause pain and distress to individuals and their families, and can often be difficult to heal for some.

In a 2018 review of best practice recommendations for skin tear prevention and management, the International Skin Tear Advisory Panel (ISTAP) defined skin tears as 'a traumatic wound caused by mechanical forces, including removal of adhesives. Severity may vary by depth (not extending through the subcutaneous layer)' (LeBlanc et al 2018).

Prevalence

As part of a study on skin tear prevalence and characteristics, Miles et al (2022) undertook a review of the literature from six relatively old studies published between 2004 and 2014 and found that internationally the occurrence of skin tears in hospital settings was noted to be between 3.3% and 22% and between 3.0% and 20.8% in long-term aged-care settings. The data collected from hospital settings included two from Australia. In the most extensive study conducted in Australia by Santamaria et al (2009) involving 5801 patients, the occurrence of skin tears was recorded at 7.9% and 10.8% in two successive years. Notably, skin tears accounted for 11.9% to 16.7% of all wounds acquired in hospitals and comprised the largest category of wounds within the aged-care population. Based on other international studies, skin tear prevalence was 2.57% in a Wales hospital (Clark et al 2017) and 1.2% in nine Chinese hospitals (Feng et al 2018).

The study by Miles et al (2022) spanning a 10-year period in a tertiary acute care hospital in Queensland reviewed data from 3626 patients. The overall pooled prevalence of skin tears was found to be 8.9%, with a hospital-acquired pooled prevalence of 5.5%. Among the 616 reported skin tears, 60.7% were acquired in the hospital. Nearly 39% of patients had multiple skin tears, and a vast majority (84.8%) of those with skin tears were aged 70 years or older. The largest proportion of skin tears (40.1%) are without a skin flap. Falls or collisions were the primary documented causes, suggesting the strategies addressing both skin tear and fall prevention could be effective (Miles et al 2022).

Risk factors

The risk factors for skin tear can be subdivided into intrinsic and extrinsic risk factors (LeBlanc et al 2018). Intrinsic risk factors refer to the physiological changes to the skin, which increase the susceptibility to any mechanical forces. The extrinsic (or environmental) risk factors of the mechanical forces (e.g. removal of the adhesive tape, scraping from long nails/jewellery/furniture during activities of daily living like hygiene and mobility) are usually combined with the intrinsic risks. Risk factors for skin tears in older adults can be further complicated by dehydration, poor nutritional status, cognitive impairment, impaired vision, altered mobility and decreased sensation. Some examples of the identified risks include:

- extremes of age
- a history of skin tears
- stiffness and spasticity
- dry, fragile skin
- polypharmacy, especially the long-term use of steroid medication that thins the skin
- presence of ecchymosis (bleeding into the subcutaneous tissue)
- dependence for activities of daily living, such as use of assistive devices
- mechanical trauma, such as applying and removing stockings, removal of adhesives
- impaired mobility requiring assistance of repositioning and/or transfers
- cardiac, respiratory or vascular comorbidities.

(Dowsett et al 2020; Idensohn et al 2019)

Research is currently in progress into development of a risk-assessment tool for the prevention of skin tears (Newall et al 2017). Nevertheless, the ISTAP skin tear risk assessment protocol is available to support early recognition and early prevention of those who are at risk of skin tears so that the incidents can be minimised (LeBlanc et al 2018).

Classification for skin tears

The first recognised skin tear classification system was developed and titled the Payne Martin Classification for Skin Tears (Payne & Martin 1993). This system was later revised to include sub-classifications of three main categories and five types of skin tears (Payne & Martin 1993).

Based on the Payne and Martin instrument, Carville et al (2007) developed a skin tear classification system, the STAR skin tear classification system, which is used in Australia and Japan. This system uses five categories depending on the degree of skin loss:

- category 1a, where the edges can be realigned to the normal anatomical position (without undue stretching) and the skin or flap colour is not pale, dusky or darkened
- category 1b, where the edges can be realigned to the normal anatomical position (without undue stretching) and the skin or flap colour is pale, dusky or darkened
- category 2a, where the edges cannot be realigned to the normal anatomical position and the skin or flap colour is not pale, dusky or darkened
- category 2b, where the edges cannot be realigned to the normal anatomical position and the skin or flap colour is pale, dusky or darkened
- category 3, where the skin flap is completely absent.

A simplified version of the skin tear classification has been developed by the Internal Skin Tear Advisory Panel (ISTAP) and validated internationally to standardise skin tear assessment (Idensohn et al 2019). Flap is currently defined by ISTAP as 'a portion of the skin (epidermis/dermis) that is unintentionally separated (partially or fully) from its original place due to shear, friction, and/or blunt force' (Idensohn et al 2019). The ISTAP system uses a simple method to classify skin tears, categorising them as either Type 1, Type 2 or Type 3.

- Type 1—no skin loss where the skin flap can be repositioned to cover the wound bed
- Type 2—partial flap loss where the flap cannot be repositioned to completely cover the wound bed
- Type 3—total flap loss where the wound bed is totally exposed

(LeBlanc 2018)

(See Figure 29.11.)

Skin tear prevention

The majority of skin tears occur during routine care and activities of daily living. Management plans should include strategies that can be adopted by healthcare workers to prevent skin tears from developing and/or prevent further trauma (Campbell et al 2018). Preventing skin tears should start with early identification of those at risk and encompass the following identified risk reduction strategies:

- Assess for risk factors.
- Practise skin hygiene and responsible bathing: avoid the use of soap; use pH neutral cleansers.
- Apply emollients to hydrate the skin and increase suppleness (see Clinical Interest Box 29.9).
- Where adhesive products are used, consider the use of silicone-based adhesives or dressings that have a silicone wound contact layer.

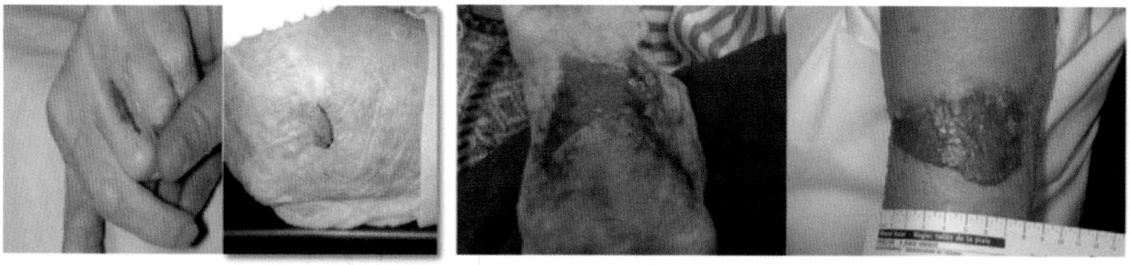
Type 1: No skin loss
Type 2: Partial flap loss
Type 3: Total flap loss
Linear or flap tear that can be repositioned to cover the wound bed
Partial flap loss that cannot be repositioned to cover the wound bed
Total flap loss exposing entire wound bed

Figure 29.11 ISTAP skin tear classification

(LeBlanc et al 2013)

CLINICAL INTEREST BOX 29.9 Skin tear research

Skin tears are traumatic wounds that often occur in older adults regardless of the clinical setting. The skin becomes thinner, drier, more fragile and susceptible to any friction or shearing injuries. Once a skin tear is sustained, it takes longer to heal due to the ageing skin condition and comorbidities that could impede the healing process. Skin tears can often lead to chronic wounds such as leg ulcers, which are painful and debilitating. Interestingly, the upper limbs are the most common sites for skin tear (55.14%) compared to the lower extremities (37.84%). Finch et al (2018) undertook a study with hospitalised people aged 65 years or older who were invited to apply pH-friendly, non-perfumed moisturiser to the extremities twice-daily. The primary outcome measure was the average monthly incidence of skin tears. The results were compared to historical controls and indicated that skin tear rates were significantly lower in older adults who applied twice-daily moisturiser.

(Finch et al 2018)

- Remove the dressing in the direction indicated/marked to prevent reopening the flap (if adhesive dressing is used).
- Avoid using adhesive tapes for dressing security. Alternatively, bandages can be considered.
- Use safe clothing that is easy to apply and remove and is protective.
- Address environmental risk factors by padding surfaces, removing falls risks and providing uncluttered areas and adequate lighting.
- Use correct manual handling techniques for turning, transferring and positioning.
- Provide appropriate nutrition and hydration.
- Use caution when removing any adhesive product. Products to facilitate the removal of the adhesive dressing can be used to minimise further risk of sustaining a skin tear.
- Trim the individual's nails and the carer's fingernails (Campbell et al 2018).
- Clinicians adhere to bare-below-the-elbow practice (e.g. no jewellery or watches).

Assessment

Assessment of a skin tear is the same as for other wound types. The cause of the skin tear must be established, if possible, to implement preventative measures. Holistic assessment, which includes age, gender, medical and surgical history, comorbidities, medications and general health and nutritional status, will determine the potential for wound healing.

Other factors to consider are:

- anatomical location
- wound dimensions (length, width and depth)
- exudate—type and amount
- size and depth of skin and skin flap
- haematoma formation
- condition of the peri-wound skin (e.g. fragility, oedema)
- associated pain
- signs and symptoms of infection where the skin tear is more than a few days old.

The arms and lower leg are reported to be the most common location for skin tears (Campbell et al 2018; Carville 2023; Dowsett et al 2020).

See Clinical Skill 29.3 for guidelines and information on assessment and management of skin tears.

Management

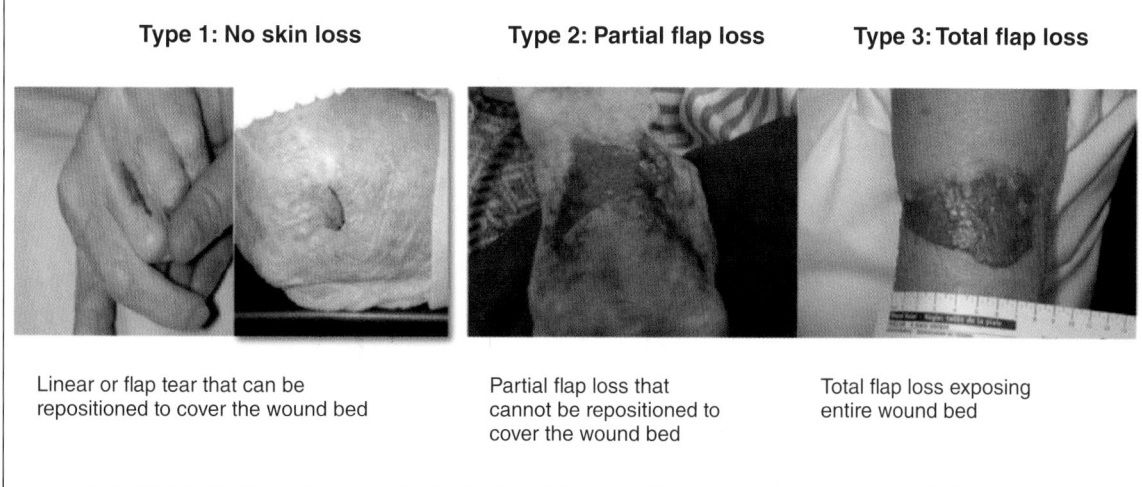

Best practice recommendations have been developed by the ISTAP to ensure evidence-based assessment, classification

CLINICAL SKILL 29.3 Assessment and management of skin tears

Please adhere to the policy and procedures of the facility/organisation prior to undertaking the skill. Ensure this skill is in your scope of practice.

NMBA Decision-making Framework considerations (refer to NMBA Decision-making framework for nursing and midwifery 2020):	Equipment:
1. Am I educated? 2. Am I authorised? 3. Am I competent? If you answer 'no' to any of these, do not perform that activity. Seek guidance and support from your teacher/a nurse team leader/clinical facilitator/educator.	Sterile dressing pack Sterile dressing materials Additional light source (if required) Additional sterile gauze Disposable gloves Sterile 0.9% sodium chloride Waste receptacle Dressing trolley Disinfectant wipes/solution

PREPARE FOR THE SKILL

(Please refer to the Standard Steps on pp. xviii–xx for related rationales.)
Mentally review the steps of the skill.
Discuss the skill with your instructor/supervisor/team leader, if required.
Confirm correct facility/organisation policy/safe operating procedures.
Validate the order in the individual's record.
Identify indication and rationale for performing the activity.
Assess for any contraindications.
Locate and gather equipment.
Perform hand hygiene.
Ensure therapeutic interaction.
Identify the individual using three individual identifiers.
Gain the individual's consent.
Assess for pain relief.
Prepare the environment.
Provide and maintain privacy.
Assist the individual to assume an appropriate position of comfort.

Skill activity	Rationale
Skin tears can result in partial or full separation of the layers of the skin. They may be caused by friction and/or shearing forces and require treatment to prevent wound contamination and infections.	
Assess the skin tear to determine the severity: assess degree of tissue loss and skin or flap colour using ISTAP or STAR classification system.	Severity will depend on the treatment and the type of dressing required.
Assess the size of the wound and surrounding skin for swelling, discolouration or bruising, fragility. Choose appropriate dressing according to skin tear assessment.	Dressing choice will maintain a moist wound-healing environment, control or manage exudate, reduce the risk of infection, and atraumatic removal during dressing change.

PERFORM THE SKILL

(Please refer to the Standard Steps on pp. xviii–xx for related rationales.)
Perform hand hygiene.
Apply PPE: gloves, eyewear, mask and gown as appropriate.
Ensure the individual's safety and comfort throughout skill.
Promote independence and involvement of the individual if possible and/or appropriate.
Assess the individual's tolerance to the skill throughout.
Dispose of used supplies, equipment, waste and sharps appropriately.

CLINICAL SKILL 29.3 Assessment and management of skin tears—cont'd

Skill activity	Rationale
Create the aseptic field by using the sterile dressing pack and add sterile equipment including 0.9% sodium chloride to the field. Open sterile dressing pack by using corners. Open the sterile dressing products away from the aseptic field and add into the field.	Prevents contamination of sterile items and Key-Parts.
Rearrange and assemble the required sterile dressing and equipment in the aseptic field using ANTT without contaminating the Key-Parts.	Maintains ANTT to protect the wound from environmental contamination. Prevents contamination of the Key-Parts.
Position sterile dressing drape below or near the wound.	Protects wound from environmental contamination.
Control bleeding (if required). Cleanse wound with warm 0.9% sodium chloride solution, and remove debris (if required).	Cleans wound, removes debris and prepares for flap realignment. Allows for more accurate wound assessment.
Gently roll out (realign) the skin flap. Avoid stretching and pulling the flap.	Replaces the skin flap into anatomical position. Stretching and pulling may cause the skin flap to be damaged and devitalised or shrink back on itself or it may tear off completely.
Apply an appropriate sterile wound dressing using ANTT and secure. Ensure dressing extends over the wound edge by at least 1.5–2 cm. Date and draw arrow on the dressing in direction of skin flap.	Covers wound and prevents spread of microorganisms. Indicates the direction of dressing removal to reduce the risk of re-trauma to the flap upon removal of dressing as scheduled.

AFTER THE SKILL

(Please refer to the Standard Steps on pp. xviii–xx for related rationales.)
Communicate outcome to the individual, any ongoing care and report any complications.
Restore the environment.
Report, record and document assessment findings, details of the skill performed and the individual's response.
Report, record and document any abnormalities and/or inability to perform the skill.
Reassess the individual to ensure there are no adverse effects/events from the skill.

(Adapted from ACIPC 2015; LeMone et al 2020; Berman et al 2020; IWII 2022; LeBlanc et al 2018; Lynn 2022; The-ASAP 2019)

and treatment is used in the management of skin tears (Campbell et al 2018). The management plan is to be developed based on assessment of the skin tear, wound cleansing, appropriate dressing selection to provide a moist healing environment, pain minimisation upon dressing removal and prevention of potential wound infection. The applied dressing is to be appropriate to the level of exudate from the skin tear and needs to be comfortable and durable (LeBlanc et al 2019). Furthermore, ISTAP advises that sutures, adhesive skin closure strips used for wound closure, films and hydrocolloids are to be avoided based on the potential trauma of stripping the fragile skin upon dressing removal. Iodine-based dressings are also discouraged because these types of products have the tendency to dry out the skin and increase the risk for skin tear (LeBlanc et al 2018). Skin tears may be at risk for infection due to a combination of the wound location and the nature of the injury. Therefore, wound dressings containing antimicrobials can be considered with caution, with the antimicrobial stewardship for use to be taken into consideration as discussed previously in this chapter. In other words, the prophylactic use of antimicrobial dressings is not currently recommended, as early detection and early intervention of wound site infection can potentially prevent complications of deep infection. If wound infection management is indicated for the skin tear, Leptospermum honey and polyhexamethylene biguanide (PHMB) dressings are recommended (LeBlanc et al 2018).

Steps to manage a skin tear

1. Stop the bleeding:
   - Gentle pressure to the affected area is usually sufficient.
   - Where possible, elevate the limb.

2. Clean the wound:
   > Use warm sterile saline or water to clean the surrounding skin.
   > If there is a skin flap gently roll back the flap and flush with warm saline under the flap and the exposed wound.
   > If the skin flap is viable, gently unroll the flap and lay over the open area to cover the wound bed.
   > Avoid physically pulling/stretching the flap.
   > If the skin flap is non-viable, gently trim any non-viable flap (by a skilled clinician).
   > Categorise the skin tear and document on the individual's record.
3. Apply a dressing:
   > Select a dressing based on the assessment of the individual, relevant organisational protocols, the condition of the surrounding skin and any discolouration or bruising.
   > Avoid using skin closure strips.
   > Foam dressings (preferably with silicone contact layer) have been recommended and should be marked with an arrow in the direction of the flap to assist removal and conservation of the skin flap over the wound bed. Dressing selection is to be appropriate to the amount of exudate to re-establish the moisture balance.
   > Leave the dressing in place for several days (usually around 5 days depending on the amount of exudate) to avoid disturbing the wound as per dressing manufacturer's recommendation unless required for additional exudate management.
4. Review and reassess:
   > Gently remove the dressing in the direction of the arrow, without disturbing the skin flap. Consider using adhesive removers to minimise additional trauma of skin stripping.
   > Clean and reassess the skin flap.
   > Assess for signs of infection and non-healing.
   > Re-dress as necessary and document all care given in the individual's records.

(Dowsett et al 2020; Idensohn et al 2019; LeBlanc et al 2018)

Helpful tip: Applying a crepe bandage or a cotton tubular bandage to secure a non-adherent dressing will reduce the risk of further injury from the use of tape and dressing removal. Use of a silicone dressing will also reduce the risk of additional trauma to the skin tear on dressing removal. A formal assessment should be conducted every 14 days. If the skin tear fails to heal, a further assessment and possible referrals for consultation are to be considered (Dowsett et al 2020). (See Case Study 29.2.)

CASE STUDY 29.2

Skin tears

Eleanor Parker is a frail 89-year-old who has been admitted to hospital for functional decline and increased confusion. Her medical history includes hypertension (on twice-daily furosemide), COPD (on a regular inhaler) and rheumatoid arthritis (on disease-modifying anti-rheumatic drugs). She walks with a four-wheelie walker, and her gait has become increasingly unsteady over the past 6 months. She used to cook for herself, but recently has been living on sandwiches and only weighs 42 kgs for her 158 cm height. Upon arrival to the clinical area, a bleeding skin tear is noted on her left leg (pre-tibial region). Eleanor cannot recall how it was sustained. Upon skin assessment, the skin tear is classified as type 2 with partial flap loss according to the ISTAP skin tear classification.

1. In addition to the skin tear classification, what other assessments are required prior to the wound management?
2. What is the required wound care/management for Mrs Parker's skin tear?
3. What preventative measures can be taken for Mrs Parker?

LEG ULCERS

Leg ulcers are of vascular or neuropathic aetiology and are caused by trauma, disease or irritation contributing to a loss of skin integrity (Carville 2023). Most common presentations are described as venous, arterial, mixed venous/arterial and neuropathic.

Venous leg ulcers (VLUs) are frequently occurring long-term wounds on the lower limbs compared to arterial and mixed leg ulcers, prevailing in approximately 1–3% of individuals aged over 65 years of age (Xie et al 2018). Their occurrence differs across countries: in India, around 4.5 per 1000 people develop VLUs annually, while in the UK and Australia, the prevalence stands at 3.5 and 1.1 per 1000 people respectively (Xie et al 2018). This indicates that approximately 57% of chronic leg ulcers are venous ulcers, while the data on the prevalence of arterial leg ulcers in Australia is not as comprehensive. Yet, a cautious estimate suggests that arterial leg ulcers make up roughly half of the remaining chronic leg ulcers identified or approximately 20% of total leg ulcers within the population of 238,000 sample individuals in the metropolitan areas of Australia (Australian Medical Association 2022).

The cost to the Australian healthcare system of managing and treating leg ulcers is substantial, with the average cost per person in 2012–2013 estimated as $8106 (Cheng et al 2018). A report by the Chronic Wounds Solutions Collaborating Group in Australia (Pacella et al 2018) identified the incidence of approximately 40,000 cases of chronic wounds annually, of which 12% were venous and 1% arterial leg ulcers. Leg ulcers incur cost in hospital admissions and in community nursing settings because of the need for frequent home visits (Pacella et al 2018). Leg ulceration is not a disease but rather a symptom of an underlying disease process. Leg ulcers decrease an individual's quality of life, often causing pain, disrupted sleep, limited mobility and activity, frustration, low self-esteem, inconvenience and social isolation, as well as incurring loss of productivity in the workforce. Leg ulcers can take months or years to heal and often recur (Pacella et al 2018). Non-adherence with treatment of VLUs is a common problem and it leads to a failure to heal and recurrence. However, there are several types of leg ulcers and it is important to differentiate between them so that the correct management strategies can be followed. Leg ulcers caused by underlying venous disease are the most common type.

Primary causes

Leg ulcers are classified according to the vasculature involved, as follows:

- arterial, involving arteries and arterioles
- venous, involving veins and venules
- mixed arterial–venous, involving arteries, arterioles, veins and venules
- lymphatic, involving the lymphatic drainage system.

Arterial leg ulcers

The underlying cause of pure arterial ulcers is a lack of arterial blood supply caused by peripheral arterial disease, though this usually presents a more complex problem with coexisting disease such as heart disease or diabetes. A history of cardiovascular disease, stroke or intermittent claudication may indicate underlying arterial disease. Predisposing factors are atherosclerosis, advanced age, diabetes mellitus, hypertension, obesity and smoking. These ulcers are frequently located between toes, at the tip of the toes over phalangeal heads or metatarsal heads, on the side or the sole of the foot, or around the lateral malleolus. Arterial ulcers can present with a well-demarcated edge and a deep, pale wound base. The ulcer may be painful unless diabetic neuropathy is present, and the leg takes on a hairless, thin, shiny appearance with dry skin. The toenails may be thickened and often brittle. The leg is pale when elevated and cool to touch. Pedal pulses are often diminished or absent.

Venous leg ulcers

Ulcers caused by underlying venous disease are referred to as venous ulcers. A venous leg ulcer (VLU) is a breach of the skin integrity in the lower limb with underlying venous disease and fails to heal in 2 weeks (Wound UK 2022). Venous disease can occur for various reasons, such as structural venous incompetency and venous obstruction or functional venous disease (e.g. calf/foot muscle pump failure, inactivity). For example, where a deep vein thrombosis (DVT) damages the valves or walls of the deep veins on the leg (post-thrombotic damage). Where the valves in the large veins (superficial and deep) are damaged, they fail to close properly, allowing venous blood to move up and down the vein. Blood is allowed to flow back down the leg (retrograde flow) and this is known as venous reflux. Additional pressure is created in the veins and fails to fall when the combined actions of the calf muscle pump and foot pumps contract through walking. This is referred to as ambulatory venous hypertension. Over time, the raised pressure in the veins causes fluid to leak into the tissues resulting in oedema (accumulation of fluid in extravascular tissue) and eventual skin ulceration.

These ulcers can take weeks, months or even years to heal and accurate diagnosis of the underlying aetiology is essential to ensure correct management. Compression therapy using bandages or garments is essential to manage the underlying pathophysiology of the VLU and should be initiated as early as possible (Wounds UK 2022). A strong compression system is recommended to aid venous return of blood to the heart (orthograde flow) and a reduction in venous reflux (see 'Compression therapy for venous leg ulcers' below).

In obtaining a diagnosis of venous disease, the person may have a history of:

- venous disease, confirmed by duplex ultrasound
- varicose veins and/or surgery
- family history of leg ulceration
- proven DVT or phlebitis
- surgery/fractures to the affected leg
- episodes of chest pain/pulmonary embolism.

Other predisposing risk factors are:

- pregnancy
- obesity
- history of intravenous drug use.

(Wounds UK 2022)

Leg ulcers with underlying venous disease usually occur on the lower leg. They can be small in the pre-tibial area and anterior to the medial malleolus or larger and circumferential. These ulcers generally have uneven edges and a ruddy granulation tissue and appear to be superficial compared with the arterial ulcer. Discomfort is relieved by elevation of the leg. Venous ulcers are often accompanied by oedema, with fluid seepage and maceration of the surrounding skin. Pruritus and scale formation occurs. The leg can take on a reddish–brown pigmentation caused by haemosiderin, oedema is present and the leg can be quite firm to the touch. There is usually evidence of old healed ulcers, tortuous superficial veins and the limb may be warm to touch. Foot and leg pulses are present. Table 29.9 outlines the difference between venous and arterial ulcers.

Diagnostic tools for the assessment of leg ulcers

- Comprehensive medical and surgical history
- Physical examination including palpation of specific relative pulses
- Doppler ultrasound measurements—ankle/brachial pressure index (ABPI) where appropriate or toe/brachial pressure index (TBPI) if ABPI is too painful
- Photoplethysmography (PPG) measurement of venous refill
- Transcutaneous oxygen perfusion measurements
- Duplex scans
- Arteriography

TABLE 29.9 | Differentiating between venous and arterial ulcers

Indicator	Arterial	Venous
Predisposing factors	Arteriosclerosis Advanced age Diabetes Hypertension Smoking	History of deep vein thrombosis (DVT) Valve incompetence in the deep, superficial or perforating veins Obesity
Associated changes in the leg and skin	Thin, shiny, dry skin Thickened nails Absence of hair growth Pallor on elevation of legs Limb may be cool to touch	Firm ('brawny') oedema Reddish–brown pigmentation Evidence of healed ulcers Dilated and tortuous superficial veins Limb may be warm to touch
Ulcer location	Between toes or at tip of toes Over phalangeal heads Above lateral malleolus (for diabetes or high occlusion), over metatarsal heads, on side or sole of foot	Anterior to medial malleolus Pre-tibia area Generally lower third of leg
Ulcer characteristics	Well-demarcated edges Black or necrotic tissue Dry ulcer bed Deep, pale base	Uneven edges Ruddy granulation tissue Slough in wound bed
Pain	Exceedingly painful Pain at rest, relieved by lowering leg to a dependent position	Moderate to no pain Discomfort relieved by elevation of leg
Surrounding area	May have neuropathy	Leaking exudate can cause maceration and excoriation
Foot/leg pulses	Diminished or absent	Usually normal

(Carville 2023)

Arterial leg ulcer management strategies

The management of arterial leg ulcers is very different from the management of VLUs:

- Consultation with a vascular surgeon is recommended at an early stage.
- Treatment of the underlying disease is important.
- Angiography or angioplasty may be required.
- Chemical sympathectomy may be required.
- Bypass surgery or amputation may be required.

Compression therapy for venous leg ulcers

Early and effective **compression therapy** is essential in the management of VLUs to improve an individual's quality of life with the relief from the lower limb symptoms and pain. The aim of the therapy is to reduce the venous hypertension in the leg and to promote venous return. The application of compression narrows the diameter of the vessels, increases the velocity of flow through the vein, facilitates extracellular fluid returning to the venous system; hence, reducing limb oedema and promoting wound healing. Compression therapy can be applied as bandages, wraps, hosiery or pneumatic compression (dynamic compression). These systems compress the entire lower leg and are contraindicated for individuals with poor arterial circulation since this circulation can be further constricted and compromised. It is recommended that everyone with lower limb oedema/ulceration is assessed for any contraindications (e.g. acute infection, symptoms of sepsis, severe ischemia, suspected DVT and skin cancer) prior to the commencement of the compression therapy (Wounds UK 2023).

Pressure is determined by the tension (stiffness) of the bandage, the circumference of the limb and the width and number of layers applied (Hampton 2018). A recommended pressure of 30–40 mmHg measured at the ankle aims to achieve a reduction in venous hypertension, though it does not account for different limb sizes, bandage application techniques, posture and movement of the limb, condition of the bandage or stocking, the skill of the clinician applying the therapy and the concordance of the individuals. The pressure may decline over a period of time and re-bandaging is required. Pressure beneath the bandage is measured in three main ways: working pressure (when the individual is walking), resting pressure (at rest) and a third factor called the static stiffness index (SSI), which is the increase in pressure per centimetre increase in the circumference of the leg, or the difference in pressure between the supine and standing position. A high SSI (above 10 mmHg) is considered a more inelastic compression system that produces a higher pressure when standing than when lying (Bjork & Ehmann 2019; Carville 2023; Hampton 2018).

Venous and mixed leg ulcers are assessed for suitability before commencing compression therapy; the type and degree of pressure is determined upon completion of investigations and test. An initial trial of bandaging is monitored for increased pain, discolouration of the toes, change of sensation (tingling or loss of sensation) and increased oedema in the toes. If an individual is unable to tolerate compression bandages safely, lower compression levels can be applied to build tolerance. The type of bandage or stocking must also suit the lifestyle and ability of the individual to adhere and self-manage.

Compression bandages

Compression bandages are generally divided into elastic and inelastic bandages. This classification is suitable for a more powerful single layer elastic bandage but does not account for multilayer systems that use two or three layers of weak elastic bandages to achieve compression. Elastic bandages are highly extensible and accommodate changes in the shape of the limb with the contraction of the calf muscle when walking. This gives minimal changes in pressure beneath the bandage and sustained compression at rest. Inelastic bandages have minimal extensibility and greater fluctuations in pressure between walking and resting. Pressure is highest with walking as the expanded calf muscle pushes against the rigid bandage (Hampton 2018; Vowden et al 2020).

Multilayer bandage systems of three or four layers combine inelastic and elastic bandages with a padding layer and/or crepe bandage where each of these components has different functions of protection, padding and retention. Multicomponent systems containing an elastic bandage appear to be more effective than a single-layer system or those composed mainly of inelastic constituents. Two-component bandage systems appear to perform as well as the four-layer bandage (4LB). Individuals receiving the 4LB heal faster than those allocated the short stretch bandaging (SSB) technique. More individuals heal on high-compression stocking systems than with the SSB (Isoherranen et al 2023). Nevertheless, the application of compression bandages requires advanced skills and knowledge to ensure correct application. The manufacturer's instructions for individual brands of compression bandages must be followed (Carville 2023).

Graduated compression stockings (GCS)

Graduated compression stockings (GCS) are used for treating various peripheral venous conditions, such as varicose veins and venous insufficiency. Anti-embolic stockings provide the lowest amount of compression (approximately 16–20 mmHg) compared to the four classes of GCS. Therefore, anti-embolic stockings are generally used to prevent deep vein thrombosis, while the four classes of GCS are prescribed based on the required compression and the manufacturer's guideline (Carville 2023; Hampton 2018). They are generally used for individuals with healed ulcers to prevent recurrence of VLUs. Regular daily garment care and replacement of GCS every 6 months is necessary to maintain compression integrity. Re-measurement is also necessary if the reduction of lower limb oedema is evident (Carville 2023). See Chapter 28 for information on application of anti-embolic stockings.

Pneumatic compression

Pneumatic compression is a device with an inflatable boot attached to a pump to provide compression to legs in a pre-programmed therapy (continuously, intermittently or in sequential cycles). It can be applied in conjunction with the compression therapy or as an alternative for those who are not tolerating the compression bandages or with impaired mobility. Pneumatic compression pumps deliver pressure within 30–50 mmHg. It is worthwhile noting the conditions which are contraindicated for the application of pneumatic compression, such as severe arterial disease, deep vein thrombosis, cellulitis, congestive heart failure and leg injuries (Carville 2023).

Preventing recurrence

VLU recurrence may be prevented with the use of long-term compression therapy tolerated by the individual (Isoherranen et al 2023) to increase adherence. In certain individuals experiencing superficial venous insufficiency, restorative surgery and compression may be more effective than compression on its own (Andriessen et al 2017).

Personalised education and support

Leg ulcer education is centred on prevention of recurrence, skin care, chronic disease management and general health and lifestyle issues such as nutrition and exercise. Self-management, professional monitoring and social supports are recommended activities to prevent recurrence (Australian Medical Association 2022). Further detailed factors including the understanding of the wound management and its rationales, the awareness of the compression therapy and the consequences of non-adherence to the therapy, the associated pain and/or comfort management and cost to the management plan are also important to be addressed as part of health education (Isoherranen et al 2023). Since individuals with chronic wounds commonly contend with other long-term health issues, involving other health professionals especially the allied health team (such as podiatrists, occupational therapists, dietitians, physiotherapists) becomes crucial as part of a holistic approach to care (Australian Medical Association 2022).

Managing leg ulcers often requires long-term complex dressing regimens including packing of the ulcer to aid healing.

(See Clinical Skill 29.4.)

CLINICAL SKILL 29.4 Packing a wound

Please adhere to the policy and procedures of the facility/organisation prior to undertaking the skill. Ensure this skill is in your scope of practice.

NMBA Decision-making Framework considerations (refer to NMBA Decision-making framework for nursing and midwifery 2020): 1. Am I educated? 2. Am I authorised? 3. Am I competent? If you answer 'no' to any of these, do not perform that activity. Seek guidance and support from your teacher/a nurse team leader/clinical facilitator/educator.	**Equipment:** Sterile dressing pack Sterile dressing materials Additional light source (if required) Sterile 0.9% sodium chloride Additional gauze Sterile scissors Sterile gloves Disposable gloves Waste receptacle Dressing trolley Disinfectant wipes/solution

PREPARE FOR THE SKILL

(Please refer to the Standard Steps on pp. xviii–xx for related rationales.)
Mentally review the steps of the skill.
Discuss the skill with your instructor/supervisor/team leader, if required.
Confirm correct facility/organisation policy/safe operating procedures.
Validate the order in the individual's record.
Identify indication and rationale for performing the activity.
Assess for any contraindications.
Locate and gather equipment.
Perform hand hygiene.
Ensure therapeutic interaction.
Identify the individual using three individual identifiers.
Gain the individual's consent.
Assess for pain relief.
Prepare the environment.
Provide and maintain privacy.
Assist the individual to assume an appropriate position of comfort.

Skill activity	Rationale
Wound packing is undertaken to provide a moist cover for the wound to prevent the introduction of microorganisms and to promote healing. Wounds requiring packing heal by secondary intent. The wound packing promotes healing for this type of wound, facilitates mechanical debridement, and minimises dead space. The type of dressing used also absorbs exudate.	
Assess the individual's record to determine previous appearance of wound and previous dressing.	Determines requirements for equipment and dressing requirements.

PERFORM THE SKILL

(Please refer to the Standard Steps on pp. xviii–xx for related rationales.)
Perform hand hygiene.
Apply PPE: gloves, eyewear, mask and gown as appropriate.
Ensure the individual's safety and comfort throughout skill.
Promote independence and involvement of the individual if possible and/or appropriate.
Assess the individual's tolerance to the skill throughout.
Dispose of used supplies, equipment, waste and sharps appropriately.
Remove PPE and discard or store appropriately.
Perform hand hygiene.

CLINICAL SKILL 29.4 Packing a wound—cont'd

Skill activity	Rationale
Create the aseptic field by using the sterile dressing pack and add sterile equipment including 0.9% sodium chloride to the field. Open sterile dressing pack by using corners. Open the sterile dressing products away from the aseptic field and add into the field.	Prevents contamination of sterile items and Key-Parts.
Loosen and remove the existing wound dressing for the visual wound assessment including the type and amount of exudate on the removed dressing and peri-wound condition. Dispose of wound dressing and the used gloves.	Assesses the signs and symptoms of wound infection (e.g. redness, swelling, warmth, exudate amount and type on the dressing). Prevents spread of microorganisms.
Rearrange and assemble the required sterile dressing and equipment in the aseptic field using ANTT without contaminating the Key-Parts.	Maintains ANTT to protect the wound from environmental contamination. Prevents contamination of the Key-Parts.
Position sterile dressing drape below or near the wound.	Protects the wound from environmental contamination.
Remove all existing packing/dressings (irrigate packing if required).	Provides the view for assessing wound bed. Irrigates the existing packing further to minimise pain/discomfort upon removal.
Cleanse the wound with sterile 0.9% sodium chloride. Clean from a clean area towards a less clean area, usually an outward direction.	Removes debris from the wound bed. Avoids transferring wound exudate and normal flora from the surrounding skin into the wound. Prevents wound contamination.
Assess the wound size (including depth), type(s) of tissue in the wound bed and the quantity of each tissue type in percentage (%), signs of infection, type and amount of exudate, odour, and direction and depth of tunnelling (if present). Assess for pain.	Evaluates condition of the wound and the stage of healing.
Gently pack the wound with the required packing materials. (See medical officer's or wound management consultant's orders.) Ribbon or packing gauze is gently placed into the wound cavity.	Do not tightly pack the wound cavity since the dressing will expand as it absorbs exudate and may cause discomfort and pressure to the wound bed. Packing allows for secondary wound healing.
Apply an appropriate sterile wound dressing using ANTT, and secure.	Provides a moist wound environment. Facilitates healing, absorbs exudate, protects the wound from infection and irritation (e.g. from clothing).

AFTER THE SKILL

(Please refer to the Standard Steps on pp. xviii–xx for related rationales.)
Communicate outcome to the individual, any ongoing care and report any complications.
Restore the environment.
Report, record and document assessment findings, details of the skill performed and the individual's response.
Report, record and document any abnormalities and/or inability to perform the skill.
Reassess the individual to ensure there are no adverse effects/events from the skill.

(Adapted from ACIPC 2015; LeMone et al 2020; Berman et al 2020; IWII 2022; Lynn 2022; The-ASAP 2019)

BURN INJURIES

Burns are considered one of the most traumatic injuries for a person to sustain. The physical trauma of a burn goes beyond the damage to the skin. A major burn can cause systemic complications in the short to medium term and physical, emotional and psychological complications in the medium to long term.

Heat, chemicals, electricity, radiation, cold injury and friction can cause **burn injuries**. After a burn injury, intravascular fluid is lost as the capillaries become more permeable. As the intravascular fluid volume decreases, the venous return and cardiac output fall. The clinical signs of 'shock' become apparent and tissue hypoxia threatens internal organs such as the kidneys. Other changes occur in organ function, in electrolyte levels and in metabolic function. Subsequently, complications of major burns can involve any body system because all systems are stressed during the injury and healing phases.

Pathophysiology of burn injuries

While there are many ways a burn injury can be sustained (e.g. thermal, chemical, electrical, friction), all burn injuries cause cell death and tissue ischaemia. The Jackson's Burn Wound Model has been widely used to describe the extent of tissue damage in burns. *Zone of coagulation* (necrosis) is the main area of tissue damage closest to the source of injury with irreversible tissue death; *zone of stasis* (ischaemia) is the medial zone with impaired circulation. With appropriate first aid, ischemia in this zone may be reversed, otherwise this may deteriorate into full necrosis; and *zone of hyperaemia* is the outer zone where the perfusion to tissues increases and erythematous is observed. It usually heals within 7 days unless complicated by concerns such as infection and ongoing oedema. The depth of the burn is related to the amount of thermal energy dissipated in the skin, which is dependent on the temperature and duration of exposure (Carville 2023; Trauma Victoria 2023).

Classification of burns

Burn injuries are classified according to the depth of tissue injury. The classifications reflect the anatomical thickness of the skin layers: epidermal, superficial dermal, mid dermal, deep dermal and full thickness (Table 29.10).

Superficial epidermal burns

In superficial epidermal burns, only the epidermis is involved, with the basal layer of the epithelium remaining intact. The skin is dry, red (erythematous), blanching to pressure, oedematous and hypersensitive. Absence of or delayed mild blistering may be observed. Superficial burns generally heal within 7 days without scarring, and treatment is usually conservative to manage pain, maintain adequate hydration and moisturise the burned area. Epidermal burns are excluded in the assessment of percentage total body surface area (TBSA) burnt (NSW Agency for Clinical Innovation 2018; Trauma Victoria 2023).

Superficial dermal partial-thickness burns

Partial-thickness burns have damage to the epidermis and to the superficial dermis (papillary dermis) and appear pink or red. Moist, thin-walled blisters often form within minutes of the injury as serum is released from injured blood vessels.. They can be tender and very painful, and blanch with pressure. The circulation to the affected area(s) is hyperaemic with brisk capillary return indicating intact blood vessels. When the superficial dermis has been injured, the raw area is resurfaced with epithelium growing from the undamaged walls of the sweat glands and hair follicles. Healing is spontaneous and usually completes within 14 days if there are no complications with minimal scarring, though there may be reduced pigmentation of the skin (NSW Agency for Clinical Innovation 2018; Trauma Victoria 2023).

Mid dermal partial-thickness burns

Mid dermal burns have a zone of damaged non-viable tissue extending into the dermis, with damaged but viable dermal tissue at the base. Compared to a superficial dermal partial-thickness burn, pain is less severe in mid dermal partial-thickness burns because some of the nerve endings remain viable. Blistering may be present and capillary refill is often sluggish. The initial healing trajectory is difficult to predict until the signs of healing or of burn progression are established.

Deep dermal partial-thickness burns

Deep dermal burns leave damage to all layers of the skin but not through the entire dermis. Epidermal appendages are destroyed and there is reduced sensation to the affected area. They are characterised by the early appearance of extensive blisters that usually rupture to expose deep damaged dermis, and diminished capillary refill. Because of the fluid loss from the injury, these burns tend to be dry compared to superficial burns. Scarring will occur and, depending on the anatomical region involved, there may be functional impairment. Surgical intervention and referral to a specialist unit is generally indicated (NSW Agency for Clinical Innovation 2018; Trauma Victoria 2023).

Full-thickness burns

Burns of this depth damage both the epidermal and dermal layers of the skin, and may even involve the underlying structures including subcutaneous fat, fascia, muscles and tendons, vessels and nerves, and even bones and joints. The appearance of the affected area is firm and dry with no blistering, and the tissue appears white, waxy or charred. Sensation and capillary refill are absent due to damage to both sensory nerves and circulation in the dermis. Full-thickness burns do not heal spontaneously, and surgical intervention for dead tissue removal and skin grafting are often indicated. Scarring and complication of contractures will occur to the damaged areas and referral to a specialist unit is required (NSW Agency for Clinical Innovation 2018; Trauma Victoria 2023).

TABLE 29.10 | Burn depth characteristics

	Superficial epidermal (e.g. sunburn) 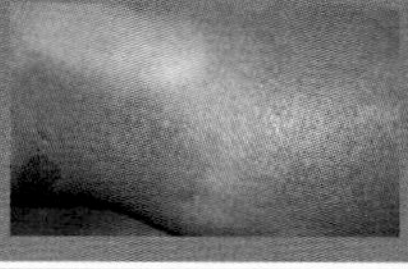	Superficial dermal thickness (partial) 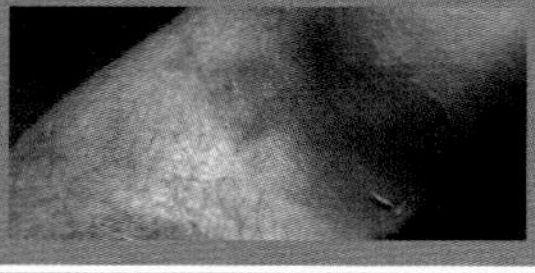	Mid dermal thickness (partial) 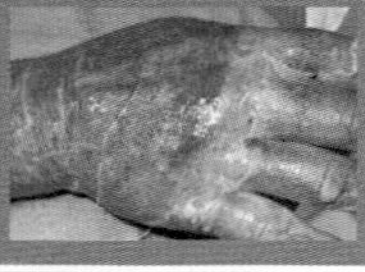	Deep dermal thickness (partial) 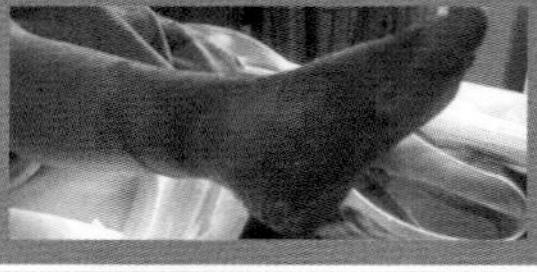	Full thickness 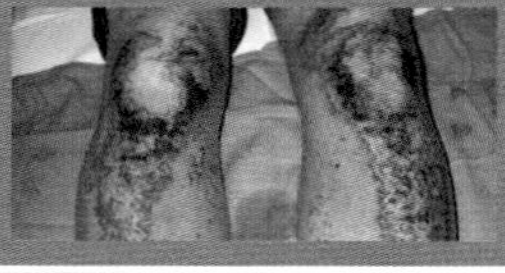
Pathology	Involves epidermis only	Involves epidermis and upper dermis; most adnexal structures intact.	Involves epidermis and mid dermis; adnexal structures may be disrupted.	Involves epidermis and significant part of dermis, with deeper adnexal structures damaged but viable.	Epidermis, dermis and cell adnexal structures destroyed.
Appearance	Dry and red, blanches to pressure. No blisters	Pale pink. Smaller blisters. Wound base blanches with pressure.	Variable pale to dark pink, may have blisters present.	Blotchy red or pale deeper dermis where blisters have ruptured.	White waxy charred. No blisters. No capillary refill.
Sensation	Painful	Increased sensation. Very painful and tender.	Some nerve endings remain viable; pain is present but less severe than pain of superficial burns.	Decreased sensation.	No sensation.
Circulation	Normal, increased	Hyperaemic. Rapid capillary refill.	Capillary return is present but delayed.	Sluggish capillary refill.	Nil.
Colour	Red, warm	Pink.	Pale to dark pink.	White/pale pink/blotchy red.	White/charred/black.
Blisters	None or (days) later or desquamation	Yes (within hours of injury).	Yes, may be present.	Early—usually large blisters that rupture rapidly and slough.	Epidermis and dermis destroyed, no blistering.
Healing time	Within 7 days	7–14 days.	7–28 days.	Over 21 days.	Does not heal spontaneously.
Scarring	No scar	Colour match defect. Low risk of hypertrophic scarring.	Prolonged healing with possible scarring and contracture. Deeper areas or over a joint may need surgical intervention and referral to a specialist unit.	High risk (up to 80%) of hypertrophic scarring.	Wound contraction. Heals by secondary intention.

(Trauma Victoria 2023; Victorian Adult Burns Service 2019)

Assessing burn severity

Burn injuries should be assessed by an experienced burn clinician, especially those requiring admission to hospital. The severity of a burn is largely dependent on its size and depth. Assessing burn depth and size correctly is important since treatment pathways differ depending on the severity of the burn. Furthermore, the greater the severity, the greater the amount of fluid lost from the body, and the greater the degree of shock that ensues. To assess the size of a burn accurately, a chart is used on which the size is expressed as a percentage of the TBSA.

Two methods exist to calculate burn size: the 'rule of nines' and the Lund–Browder method (Figure 29.12). The rule of nines, used for adults only, divides the body into areas that equal 9% which, when totalled, equal 99%, with the genitalia accounting for the remaining 1%. For example, the front and back of each leg is 9%; each arm is 4.5%; the upper and lower torso is 9%. This method is quick and easy, though less accurate than the Lund–Browder method, which is more accurate since it allows for changes in body proportion with age. The numbers on each body portion on the chart indicate the percentage of body surface for that part. Both methods provide a means of determining the extent of the burn or %TBSA. It is worthwhile noting that areas of erythema are not included in these calculations.

Types of burns

Thermal burns

Thermal burns are caused by contact with hot surfaces (such as hot iron), flame (e.g. campfire), scalds (like hot water or oil) and flash injury from an explosion, such as bombing (Carville 2023). The severity of the injury depends on the temperature of the burning agent and the duration of contact time. It is recommended to stop the burning process, cool and cover the affected area(s) and seek medical assistance for further management (Australian & New Zealand Burn Association [ANZBA] 2019).

According to the Burn Registry of Australia & New Zealand (2022) annual report 2020/21, most patients sustained a scald burn (34%) closely followed by flame burn (32%). The top three causes of burn injury (flame burns, scalds and contact burns) accounted for 85% of all injuries. The most common cause of burn injury amongst paediatric patients was scalds (49%), followed by contact (24%), flame (11%) and friction burns (11%). Scalds were the most common cause of injury across all paediatric age groups.

Chemical burns

Chemical burns result from direct contact with a substance or through ingestion or inhalation of acids, alkalis or organic materials occurring most frequently in the

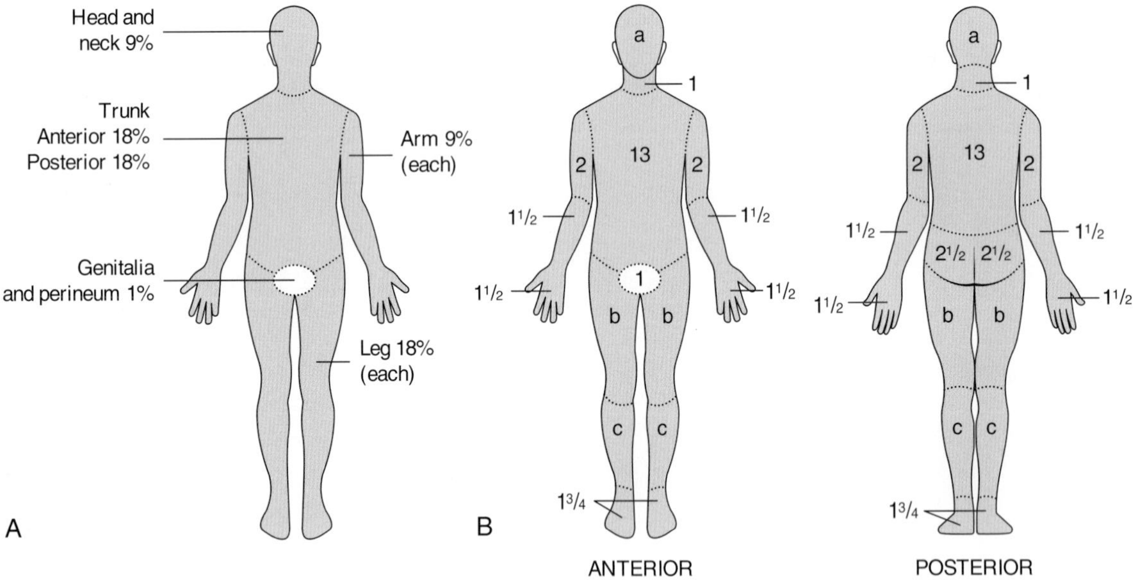

Relative percentage of body surface areas (% BSA) affected by growth

	0 yr	1 yr	5 yr	10 yr	15 yr
a–½ of head	9½	8½	6½	5½	4½
b–½ of 1 thigh	2¾	3¼	4	4¼	4½
c–½ of 1 lower leg	2½	2½	2¾	3	3¼

Figure 29.12 Burn area diagrams

The rule of nines **(A)** and Lund-Browder Burn Estimate and Diagram **(B)** graphically display second- and third-degree burn burden and allow burn formula calculations.

(Curtis & Duane 1965)

industrial workplace (Carville 2023). Individuals with chemical burns should have treatment commenced at the scene of the injury—remove from danger and identify the cause agent where possible. Contaminated clothing should be removed and the area irrigated with large amount of aqueous hypertonic solution if available (Carville 2023). Alternatively, copious amount of water for irrigation can be used (Victorian Adult Burns Service 2019).

Electrical and lightning burns

Faulty electrical wiring, contact with overhead power lines and high-voltage power cables can all be sources of electrical burns. The tissue damage from these burns can be underestimated due to the internal damage that results since it is not always visible on admission and the skin can appear normal yet have muscular tissue destruction beneath it. There will be an exit wound as the electrical current has travelled through the body. Cardiopulmonary function must be assessed in these individuals. Lightning burns can cause cardiac arrest and serious nerve damage. Furthermore, spinal protection is mandatory and thermal burn first aid is to be performed when appropriate (Victorian Adult Burns Service 2019).

Friction or abrasion burns

A friction burn occurs when skin is scraped off by contact with surfaces such as roads, carpets or other hard floor surfaces. It usually is both a scrape (abrasion) and a heat burn. Friction burns are becoming more common, especially in children who injure themselves on exercise machines such as a treadmill or as a result of a road accident on a bicycle, scooter or skateboard. In adults, friction burns result from car and motorbike accidents (road rash) (Carville 2023).

Management of the individual with burn injuries

Management is determined by the depth and size of the burn, the type of burn and the severity. Effective treatment must be in place in the first 24 hours to reduce the damaging effects of inflammation and to avoid burn wound conversion and deeper tissue injury, and it begins with effective first aid. Smaller superficial burns may be managed in the primary health setting. Full-thickness and sub-dermal burns should be hospitalised and managed in a specialist burn centre.

First aid for burn injuries

Adequate and appropriate first aid is vital to the successful management of a burn injury. Applying cool running water for the first 20 minutes within the first 3 hours of a burn injury is considered to be best practice to limit the deepening of the heat damage and ease the pain (Legrand et al 2020; Victorian Adult Burns Service 2019). It can limit the extent of burn depth and the amount of pain and reduce the area of skin affected by the burn. Individuals with larger burns need to be monitored for hypothermia if cool running water is applied for longer periods. Avoid application of lotions, creams, butter, aloe vera, toothpaste and ice as they either mask the full extent of the burn or can interfere with the ongoing management. There is no agreement on the type of burn management a burn-injured individual should receive prior to transfer, and consultation should be with the treating burn surgeon.

When to refer to a specialist burn centre

The Australian & New Zealand Burn Association (ANZBA 2019) provides criteria for referral for specialist treatment:

- burns greater than 10% of TBSA for adults and greater than 5% for children
- full-thickness burns greater than 5% of TBSA
- burns of special areas—face, hands, feet, genitalia, perineum, circumferential limb or chest burns, and major joints
- electrical burns
- chemical burns
- burns with inhalation injury
- burns with pre-existing illness
- burns at the extremes of age—young children and the elderly
- burn injury in pregnant women
- non-accidental burns
- burns associated with major trauma.

Emergency department management

The aim of initial management is to maintain the individual's airway, especially if the individual is exposed to smoke in an enclosed area such as a house fire; assess and monitor breathing and ventilation, particularly if the burn involves circumferential chest wounds since they will restrict ventilation, as well as assess vital signs for any potential changes to circulation as a result of hypovolaemia and/or hypothermal shock. For electrical burns, close cardiac monitoring is essential since cardiac arrest could occur. Furthermore, other health deviations, such as neurological deterioration, are to be assessed and proactively managed. According to ANZBA (2019), fluid resuscitation and pain management are essential for the initial management of severe burns.

Hospital management

Once the individual is stabilised, management will depend on a range of factors with the main aspects of care being:

1. ongoing fluid management
2. burn wound management
   > prevention of infection
   > debridement of dead tissue, blisters, loose skin
   > rapid skin coverage
3. adequate nutrition
4. pain management
5. promotion of mobility
6. scar management
7. psychological support
8. preparation for discharge.

Fluid resuscitation

If the burned area is not too great (e.g. less than 15% in an adult, less than 10% in a child), the body generally compensates adequately for the fluid loss, and only the provision of extra oral fluids is indicated. In more extensive or severe burns, fluid loss is a major cause of shock, so fluid replacement is of prime importance. Fluid resuscitation rates are calculated from the time of injury and are based on the size and depth of the burn, age of the individual and pre-existing illnesses, and other factors such as dehydration. The medical officer calculates the volume of fluid replacement required and prescribes the type of fluid to be administered. There are various resuscitation formulas; however, these should be used only as a guide to fluid replacement. Intravenous fluid administration is through peripheral and central access in large burns. Extensive full-thickness burns may also require blood and/or blood products to compensate for a reduction in erythrocyte and hypoalbuminemia post resuscitation. Intravenous fluid replacement with electrolytes is continually calculated and adjusted according to need. Individuals with electrical and inhalation injuries have higher fluid requirements.

Monitoring techniques that may be performed to assess fluid requirements include insertion of a urinary catheter to enable hourly monitoring of urine output. Hydration aims at maintaining a urine output of 0.5–1.0 mL/kg/hour in an adult and 1 mL/kg/hour in children who are <30 kg in weight (ANZBA 2019).

Wound management

Burn wound management is aimed at preventing infection and providing early skin coverage with dressings or skin grafts. The wound can change in depth and appearance over the first few days and treatment plans should reflect these changes. Wound care consists of regular observation, assessment, cleansing and debridement. Showers and bedside cleansing are used to remove old dressings and loose necrotic skin. Occlusive dressings maintain a moist wound environment, enhance the healing process and reduce the risk of scarring as well as reducing exposure to contamination. These are suitable for superficial dermal burns. Deeper burns require an antimicrobial dressing to decrease microbial load and reduce the risk of infection. Moist wound healing produces better cosmetic outcomes with less scarring. NPWT indications improve wound bed preparation, improve healing when placed over skin grafts to improve graft take of autografts and decrease length of hospital stay. Furthermore, pain management and minimising complications are also essential as part of wound management (Carville 2023).

Infection prevention is a priority and the most serious threat to further tissue necrosis and wound sepsis. Methods of preventing infection include:

- the use of aseptic non-touch technique (ANTT) principles to prevent cross-infection (see Clinical Interest Box 29.10)
- topical antimicrobial dressings (silver dressings or others)
- systemic antibiotic therapy
- enhancing natural defences (e.g. by providing a high protein/kilojoule diet and treating any anaemia).

Prevention of infection

The burn wound provides an ideal culture medium for a range of microorganisms. Preventing infection is achieved by preventing contamination of the wound and preventing invasion of microorganisms into the tissues and bloodstream. There is a lack of established guidelines on prophylactic antibiotic use before surgery and during the intraoperative phase; hence the use of antibacterial agents must be carefully considered (Kim et al 2022; Legrand et al 2020). A specialised burns unit may be available where the air is filtered. The individual is received into a bed prepared with sterile linen and isolation techniques are used to protect against infection. When a specialised unit is not available, the individual is generally nursed in a single room using contact precautions/protective isolation techniques.

Debridement of dead tissue

Early surgical debridement can be performed within 24 hours of injury, based on the stability of the individual. If the individual is not yet medically stable, the timing of surgical debridement will be determined once respiratory and circulatory resuscitation have been achieved (Liu 2023).

Escharotomies

Eschar is a hard, leathery layer of dead tissue that results when there has been a full-thickness burn. It is dark brown to black. Tissue perfusion or quality of respiration can become compromised because of circumferential eschar constriction. An escharotomy (release of skin and subcutaneous tissue) is a surgical procedure performed to release constriction of the eschar to prevent secondary ischaemic necrosis. A longitudinal incision is made through the eschar and is extended across joints. As the eschar does not contain nerve endings the procedure is painless but is still performed under an anaesthetic. It results in open wounds, which provide a portal for infection.

Primary closure

Specialised dressings, skin closure with skin grafts or skin substitutes can all be used to achieve primary closure of a burn wound. All methods aim to achieve the same outcome of promoting healing, preventing infection and preventing scar development and contraction of scar tissue. Common methods of closure include skin grafting (split and full thickness), application of biological dressings (allografts, xenografts) or biosynthetic dressings.

Skin grafting

The ideal burn wound closure is with autograft (i.e. using the individual's own skin). It is performed as per the treatment of some deeper partial-thickness burns and in the treatment of all full-thickness burns. Skin grafting promotes healing, prevents infection and prevents the contraction of scars. It is performed as early as possible in the treatment of some partial-thickness burns and all full-thickness burns. Split-skin grafting involves the removal of thin sheets of the epidermis and some dermis (split-thickness skin graft) or all the dermis (full-thickness skin

CLINICAL INTEREST BOX 29.10 Aseptic non-touch technique (ANTT)

There are two types of ANTT: Surgical (for complex procedures) and standard (for uncomplicated procedures). The choice of Surgical-ANTT or Standard-ANTT is based on ANTT risk assessment and will also determine equipment selection and technique.

Standard aseptic non-touch technique (Standard-ANTT) in wound care is used for procedures that are technically uncomplicated, involve small Key-Parts and Key-Parts, minimal numbers of Key-Parts, and are short in duration (approximately <20 minutes). Surgical-ANTT is used for procedures that are technically complex, involve large open Key-Sites, and large or numerous numbers of Key-Parts, and last approximately >20 minutes. Correct hand hygiene (clinical handwash and '5 Moments for Hand Hygiene') and appropriate personal protective equipment must be adhered to as part of the ANTT approach.

Each procedure must be risk assessed. The ANTT technique will vary depending upon the risk assessment (i.e. size of Key-Site and number of wounds and ability to protect Key-Parts). Part of the risk assessment includes determining the length of the procedure and whether Key-Parts and Key-Sites will need to be touched during the procedure.

Gloves are single use only. Sterilised gloves are to be used for Surgical-ANTT, while non-sterile gloves are for Standard-ANTT. However, if directly touching a Key-Part is unavoidable or the person is immunocompromised, the application of sterile gloves should be used to minimise the risk of contamination.

Use of a dressing pack does not automatically make it a Surgical-ANTT procedure. Simple wound management techniques could be managed through Standard-ANTT. However, complex wounds, such as management of a wound drain, may require Surgical-ANTT.

Standard-ANTT

- Involves a small number of Key-Parts and Key-Sites
- Involves small Key-Parts and Key-Sites
- Are technically simple
- Are short in duration (e.g. <20 minutes)

Requires clinicians to

- Identify Key-Parts and Key-Sites
- Protect those Key-Parts and Key-Sites from contamination during the procedure
- Create and maintain aseptic fields
- Perform hand hygiene
- Apply non-sterile gloves
- Use a non-touch technique
- Control environmental risks

Examples of wound care:

- Removing sutures or staples
- Change simple dressing
- Manage superficial wounds

Surgical-ANTT

- Involves large number of Key-Parts
- Involves large-sized Key-Sites or Key-Parts
- Are technically complex
- Are long in duration (e.g. >20 minutes)
- Involves critical aseptic field and sterile gloves
- Avoid touching the sterile dressing surfaces that will be in contact with the wound
- Requires clinicians to:
  - Identify Key-Parts and Key-Sites
  - Protect those Key-Parts and Key-Sites from contamination during the procedure
  - Create and maintain aseptic fields
  - Perform hand hygiene
  - Apply sterile gloves
  - Use a non-touch technique whenever possible
  - Control environmental risks
- Examples of wound care:
  - Suturing of lacerations
  - Acute traumatic wounds
  - Where bone/tendon/ligament is visible
  - Surgical wounds up to 48 hours post operation if immunocompromised
  - When people are immunocompromised for both chronic and acute wounds
  - Change dressing of an invasive device (e.g. central venous catheters)

(ACSQHC 2017; The-ASAP 2019)

graft) from a donor site, often the thigh, buttocks or back, and placing the skin over the debrided burned area.

In extensive burns, the sheets of skin can be 'meshed' to give a net-like appearance and increase the body surface area to be covered. A full-thickness graft includes the epidermis and the entire dermal layer and is generally used when full-thickness skin loss has occurred.

Skin from a source other than the individual's own body may be used as a temporary cover for large, burned areas, to decrease fluid loss. The donor site is generally covered with a non-adherent dressing, a topical antimicrobial to reduce the risk of infection and graft failure, and layers of dressing material to absorb blood and serum that ooze from the wound.

To promote successful transplantation, the graft must be immobilised to prevent displacement. Immobilisation is achieved by one of several methods, such as suturing, and the graft area is covered for protection. Successful 'take' of the graft depends on many factors, including absence of infection in the area, prevention or elimination of haematomas or seromas, adequate blood circulation, nutrition and hydration, and wound management.

Skin substitutes

Common methods of temporary or permanent skin coverage are cellular and acellular skin substitutes to replace the function and form of skin. Cellular or natural skin substitutes are composed of living cells (mainly skin cells) within a matrix, which is more effective than acellular substitutes. Examples of cellular skin substitutes include TransCyte, Dermagraft, Aligraf, OrCel and Epicel. Acellular or biosynthetic skin substitutes (e.g. Biobrane, Integra, AlloDerm, Graftjacket, Omnigraft) consist of different matrices without the inclusion of cells to minimise any foreign body response. Skin substitutes provide early coverage, reduce the risk of wound contamination and infection and reduce pain and fluid loss. Different types of skin substitute can be used on various wounds—Integra and Epicel can be used for burn survivors, while Dermagroft and Apligraf can be used for VLUs, and Graftjacket and Omnigraft for treating diabetic foot ulcers (Ahangar et al 2018). (See Clinical Interest Box 29.1.)

Dressings

The initial burn dressing should be one that can remain intact for 48 hours and prevent infection. Silver dressings (e.g. Acticoat™, Mepilex® Ag) slowly release silver, which is toxic to microorganisms and use for the first 48 hours post injury has been shown to reduce infection. After 48 hours, the silver dressing is removed and an assessment of the burn injury made. Silver dressings are not routinely continued after 48 hours. Dressings that can be used after this time include hydrocolloids (e.g. Duoderm, Granuflex), which are good for low/moderate exudating burns; foams (e.g. Allevyn, Mepilex), which are suitable for highly exudating burns; alginates (e.g. Algisite, Kaltostat), which are good for moderately-to-highly exudative sloughy wounds; and hydrogels (e.g. Intrasite), which are good for dry or sloughy burns, which need some debridement (Douglas & Wood 2017). Dressing changes are performed using strict aseptic precautions and adequate pain management. For extensive burns, the individual is given an analgesic and/or anaesthesia before the dressing change or before the procedure is performed. After the dressings have been removed, the wounds are cleansed and further debridement is performed where necessary before the burns are re-dressed.

Donor site care

The donor site is generally covered with a non-adherent dressing and layers of dressing material to absorb blood and serum that ooze from the wound.

Providing adequate nutrition

In addition to the loss of erythrocytes and protein-rich serum, the hypermetabolic response of the body to a burn rapidly depletes stores of energy. The individual must be provided with adequate carbohydrates, protein, fats, minerals, vitamins and fluid. Energy and protein requirements are generally assessed using a formula, and oral dietary intake is often augmented by nasogastric feeding or parenteral therapy to meet these requirements. Accurate monitoring of tolerance to the diet enables continual assessment of nutritional requirements. Nursing responsibilities include adherence to feeding protocols, daily calorie counts, understanding the enteral formulas and regular communication with the dietitian. Micronutrients—for example, vitamins (e.g. vitamins B, C, D and E) and trace elements such as copper, zinc and selenium—are often introduced early via a parenteral route to reduce Gram-negative bacteraemia (Legrand et al 2020; NSW Agency for Clinical Innovation 2018).

Pain management

Superficial burn injury pain can be severe because nerve endings are exposed. In deeper burn injuries, the nerve endings are destroyed, and the person may say the burn does not hurt. Pain management is complex and challenging because the perception of pain has physical and psychological origins. Pain should be recognised from the individual's perspective and is the responsibility of the entire burn team. Inadequate pain management is distressing to the individual, the person's family and the burn team. Morphine is the preferred analgesia to manage pain in the acute phase of the burn injury (Trauma Victoria 2023). Ketamine is effective for burn-induced pain as part of multimodal pain management to minimise the excess use of morphine (Legrand et al 2020). Depending on the complexity of the burn and severity of the pain, intravenous analgesia provides more rapid pain relief for severe burn survivors. Nevertheless, the clinician must follow local organisational protocols on analgesia administration (Trauma Victoria 2023).

Nursing measures also include explanation and assurance to the individual to reduce fear, and careful positioning may be beneficial. The nurse has a responsibility to observe the individual continually and to be directed by the person on the level of analgesia required. (More information on pain management is provided in Chapter 33.)

Promoting mobility

Because of the nature of the injury, and its management, a person with burns may experience prolonged periods of immobility. Thus, the individual is subject to the complications of immobility, such as venous thrombosis, pneumonia, pressure injuries and contractures. (See Chapter 28 for measures to manage problems associated with immobility.) Regular and careful position changes are essential. Individuals must be positioned for comfort and repositioned frequently to prevent pressure injuries and contractures. Splints and other devices may be used to improve positioning and to prevent contractures. The individual's limbs should be correctly positioned to decrease joint flexion.

Physiotherapy is essential for a person who is immobile and involves chest physiotherapy and range-of-movement (ROM) exercises. ROM exercises may be performed actively or passively, and the degree of motion should be recorded to document progress. Ambulation is started as soon as possible and the nurse may be required to assist. However, if skin grafting has been performed, the individual is usually required to rest in bed for approximately a week unless instructed otherwise to allow the skin graft to form its own blood supply and lymphatic drainage (Black & Black 2021).

Scar and contracture management

Current management of burn scars comprises a combination of therapies from non-operative interventions to surgery for contracture release. Pressure placed directly over the healed burn tissue is commenced as soon as the new epithelium can tolerate the pressure without causing friction. Individuals with severe and extensive burns will have scarring and will normally have a tailored elastic compression garment applied. These garments are custom made to fit exactly over the burned area. Pressure garments are required to be worn between 6 months and 2 years after healing. Silicone gel sheets are also used to manage scar tissue. These can be worn under a pressure garment or on their own. Other treatments include prolonged stretching and splinting and mobilisation and massage of the scar. It is usual practice for non-operative methods to be applied before surgery is used. Surgery is required for contractures and where vital functional areas are exposed such as the eyelids (Romanelli et al 2019).

Providing psychological support

Because a burn injury can have a devastating emotional impact on the individual and their significant others, psychological support is an extremely important aspect of care. After the injury, the person will experience various emotions such as fear of death, fear of disability and fear of disfigurement. Feelings of despair, anger, frustration, depression and guilt may all be experienced at any time after the burn. (See Case Study 29.3.)

Communication between team members caring for the individual is important to achieve adequate support for both them and their significant others. The nurse can help to provide support by:

CASE STUDY 29.3

Michael, a 42-year-old, is recovering from extensive burns after an industrial accident at a manufacturing facility. He is married with two young children.

What are some of the psychosocial issues Michael may face in his recovery from his burns and the associated complications?

- Developing a therapeutic relationship and being available to listen. The nurse should encourage the person to talk through their feelings and fears.
- Providing information about all the procedures and equipment in a way that can be understood. Fear will be reduced if information is provided to the individual and significant others in a way that facilitates understanding of the injury, the treatment and the prognosis. People who are experiencing stress often have difficulty in remembering, so information should be repeated whenever necessary.
- Assisting the individual to adapt gradually to body changes, and by being supportive when the person views their injury, particularly for the first time.
- Supporting the individual's coping mechanisms for as long as necessary. The nurse should understand that any expressions of anger, aggression or intolerance are not being directed at the nurse personally. Rather, it is the person's way of reacting to the injury and its consequences.
- Involving the individual in all aspects of care as much as possible, to promote independence and self-esteem.

Complications of burns

In a severe burn, all body systems become involved as the body attempts to maintain homeostasis; complications can involve any body system.

Shock

Shock is due to loss of fluid from the circulation. The greatest loss of fluid occurs at the site of the burn, but loss also occurs throughout the body. Substances such as kinins, released by the body in response to the injury, increase capillary permeability, allowing serum to escape into the tissues. This loss of serum causes reduced blood volume (hypovolaemia), which may lead to severe shock. Hypovolaemia contributes to decreased cardiac output, a fall in blood pressure and acute renal failure and potential death.

Infection and graft failure

Infection may occur if microorganisms gain entry through areas where the skin has been damaged or destroyed. Although a burn wound is usually sterile initially, the area provides an ideal culture medium for a wide range of microorganisms. Necrotic tissue, oedema and transudate all provide a nutrient medium for bacteria. The individual's resistance to infection is reduced by factors such as shock, anaemia and electrolyte imbalance.

Septicaemia

Septicaemia occurs when there is bacterial invasion of the tissues and bloodstream and is a major cause of death in severely burned individuals. Septic shock is a form of shock that occurs in septicaemia, when endotoxins are released from bacteria in the bloodstream. The endotoxins cause decreased vascular resistance, resulting in a drastic fall in blood pressure, pyrexia, tachycardia and **multiple organ dysfunction syndrome (MODS)**, a direct poor outcome from sepsis especially in people with burns (Zhang et al 2021).

Psychological effects

A person who has been severely burned is likely to experience depression, anxiety and difficulty in adjusting to the consequences of injury. The person's significant others are likely to experience similar emotions. If a child has been burned, the parents are also likely to experience severe guilt feelings about the incident. In support of the person and relations, the nurse should not exhibit any verbal or non-verbal dislike of burn injuries or characteristics of the wound.

Contractures, hypertrophic and keloid scars

Scar formation is a normal part of wound healing and in linear wounds is minimal. In large surface area wounds, scars can create problems. Contractures, hypertrophic scarring and keloid formation frequently result after healing of a burn injury. Contractures occur over joints and functional areas. These are characterised by their interference with normal function of any joint that they cross and deformity of mobile structures. True keloid scars tend to extend beyond the margin of the original scar and continue to grow, failing to undergo scar maturation and size reduction. They can also recur after excision. Hypertrophic scars mature and reduce in size. They tend to stay within the boundaries of the original wound and after excision will tend to be a better scar than the original.

Curling's ulcer

A Curling's ulcer is a duodenal ulcer that may develop in a person with severe burns. It is thought to be the result of stress.

Preparation for discharge

Before discharge from hospital, it is important that the individual understands that the healed burned and grafted skin is very fragile and will break down more easily than normal skin. The individual must be informed that these areas are vulnerable to extremes of temperature, irritant substances and physical trauma. As part of discharge preparation, the nurse should advise the individual, or the parents of the young child, to:

- Avoid sunlight on the burned or recently healed areas due to vulnerability and sensitivity. If unavoidable, ensure adequate sun protection such as long sleeve clothing and application of low irritant sunscreen.
- Bath or shower in tepid water due to the hypersensitivity to extreme temperature.
- Use non-irritant soaps and cosmetics on the burn areas.
- Exercise care if engaging in activities such as sports in which there is the possibility that the burned areas may be bumped or damaged.
- Wear clothing made from soft fabrics that will not irritate the healed burned or grafted areas.
- Continue with prescribed management of the areas. Management may include the continual wearing of a tailored compression garment, or application of a cream to the areas. The person may also be required to follow a planned program of exercises designed to improve mobility.
- Seek appropriate help, such as psychological counselling, when there is difficulty in adapting to a changed physical appearance.

(Romanelli et al 2019; Victoria Adult Burns Service 2019)

SURGICAL WOUNDS

Care of a surgical wound is directed towards promoting healing and preventing infection. In the immediate postoperative period, assessing for haemorrhage is a major responsibility of the nurse. Both the dressing and the bed linen under the individual should be checked for signs of haemorrhage. Any increase in blood staining on the dressing or an increase of blood in a surgical drainage system must be reported immediately to the nurse in charge. Strict asepsis is necessary when caring for surgical wounds and the nurse must follow the individual healthcare facility's protocol.

Adequate oxygenation of the tissues is promoted by deep breathing and coughing exercises, and early ambulation to promote full lung expansion will enhance oxygenation of the blood. Adequate circulation of blood to the area should be promoted to transport all the substances required for healing and combating infection. Adequate blood volume can be maintained by ensuring sufficient fluid intake, and circulation can be stimulated by exercises and mobility.

Surgical wound classification

Clean wound

Clean wounds are made under aseptic conditions, such as surgery, and heal by primary intention. These wounds generally do not require drainage.

Clean contaminated wound

A clean contaminated wound is a wound made under aseptic conditions, but involving a body cavity that normally harbours microorganisms, such as the gastrointestinal, respiratory or urinary tract.

Contaminated wound

The term 'contaminated wound' applies to a wound in which microorganisms are likely to be present, and includes open, traumatic and accidental wounds, and surgical wounds in which a break in asepsis occurred.

Progress Note 29.1

05/12/2023 1230 hrs	Nursing AM: Daily skin assessment performed. Stage II pressure injury noted to left heel (intact serous fluid-filled blister size 2 × 2 × 1 cm). Area dressed with Mepilex border for protection. Skin dry and intact to all other pressure points. Patient is unable to reposition independently, pressure area care provided with assistance. Incontinence associated dermatitis (IAD) noted to right groin due to double incontinence. Area cleansed with Cavilon barrier spray and wipes. Incontinence aid changed and regular toileting offered. Moisturiser applied to all other areas. Poor nutritional intake despite encouragement and assistance. MUST score 2. Dietitian referral sent, await review. Occupational therapist referral sent and await assessment for appropriate pressure relieving device. Riskman on Stage II pressure injury to left heel completed (#267595). Patient and family notified and educated regarding pressure injury prevention and management. Medical team and RN notified re changes in skin condition. *J Smith* (SMITH), *EN*

Dirty wound

The term 'dirty wound' applies to traumatic wounds that are generally more than 4 hours old. Purulent discharge is evident. The wounds involve perforation of viscera and spillage of contents.

Infected wound

Wounds that show signs of early infection are red, swollen, hot and painful. If not treated appropriately, cellulitis develops and may lead to conditions such as lymphangitis, lymphadenitis, bacteraemia, septicaemia and possibly even death (ACSQHC 2017; IWII 2022).

Surgical wound management

To provide the conditions necessary for healing, the wound must be free of dead or infected tissue, protected against external agents that may delay healing and provided with a moist environment, which is conducive to healing.

Controversy exists about many aspects of wound care, such as the type of dressing applied, frequency of dressing changes, cleansing procedures and solutions used.

(See Clinical Skill 29.5, Clinical Skill 29.6 and Clinical Skill 29.7 for skills related to removal of sutures and staples and surgical drain tubes.)

Surgical site infection (SSI)

Surgical site infection (SSI) refers to an infection at the site of a surgery occurring within 30 days post-operation or within 1 year if it involves implant(s) (Stryja 2019). It is the most common postoperative complication and affects almost a third of those in low- and middle-income countries and approximately 160,000–300,000 SSI occur each year (Stryja 2019; WHO 2018). It is important that healthcare workers identify early signs and symptoms of possible infection and ensure they have put in place the required preventative actions outlined in the guidelines from the World Health Organization (2018):

- Achieve and maintain sterile operative environment to minimise microorganisms.
- Practise good hand hygiene.
- Aim to leave the wound intact unless instructed by the treating team.
- Use an aseptic non-touch technique (ANTT) for changing or removing dressings.

Most healthcare facilities develop their own protocols and procedures for wound management and it is the nurse's responsibility to know these procedures and be aware of the protocols and regulations relating to wound care.

The key elements of postoperative wound management include timely review of the wound, appropriate cleansing and dressing, and early recognition and intervention of wound complications (Stryja 2019).

See Clinical Skill 29.6 and Clinical Skill 29.7 on skills related to surgical drain tubes.

CRITICAL THINKING EXERCISE 29.4

What discharge education would you give an individual about their wound?

CRITICAL THINKING EXERCISE 29.5

Mr Jones, aged 85, was referred by his GP to attend the emergency department as his leg ulcer was not improving and the GP suspected that it was infected. Mr Jones was admitted for a course of intravenous (IV) antibiotics. He lives alone and his only family, an older sister, passed away 2 years ago. He is planned for discharge from hospital in the next 48 hours. When does discharge planning need to be started for Mr Jones? Explain the discharge plan for Mr Jones. Identify some additional support services that can be accessed to help Mr Jones.

CLINICAL SKILL 29.5 Removal of sutures and staples

Please adhere to the policy and procedures of the facility/organisation prior to undertaking the skill. Ensure this skill is in your scope of practice.

NMBA Decision-making Framework considerations (refer to NMBA Decision-making framework for nursing and midwifery 2020):	Equipment:
1. Am I educated? 2. Am I authorised? 3. Am I competent? If you answer 'no' to any of these, do not perform that activity. Seek guidance and support from your teacher/a nurse team leader/clinical facilitator/educator.	Sterile dressing pack Sterile dressing materials including sterile wound closure strips Sterile 0.9% sodium chloride Additional sterile gauze Sterile staple remover Sterile suture cutter Additional light source (if required) Disposable gloves Waste receptacle Sharps bin Dressing trolley Disinfectant wipes/solution

PREPARE FOR THE SKILL

(Please refer to the Standard Steps on pp. xviii–xx for related rationales.)
Mentally review the steps of the skill.
Discuss the skill with your instructor/supervisor/team leader, if required.
Confirm correct facility/organisation policy/safe operating procedures.
Validate the order in the individual's record.
Identify indication and rationale for performing the activity.
Assess for any contraindications.
Locate and gather equipment.
Perform hand hygiene.
Ensure therapeutic interaction.

Identify the individual using three individual identifiers.
Gain the individual's consent.
Assess for pain relief.
Prepare the environment.
Provide and maintain privacy.
Assist the individual to assume an appropriate position of comfort.

Skill activity	Rationale
Sutures and staples are removed once wound healing has occurred. Alternate sutures and staples may be removed with the remainder the following day.	
Assess the individual's record to determine previous appearance of wound and previous dressing.	Determines requirements for equipment and dressing requirements.

PERFORM THE SKILL

(Please refer to the Standard Steps on pp. xviii–xx for related rationales.)
Perform hand hygiene.
Apply PPE: gloves, eyewear, mask and gown as appropriate.
Ensure the individual's safety and comfort throughout skill.
Promote independence and involvement of the individual if possible and/or appropriate.
Assess the individual's tolerance to the skill throughout.
Dispose of used supplies, equipment, waste and sharps appropriately.
Remove PPE and discard or store appropriately.
Perform hand hygiene.

CLINICAL SKILL 29.5 Removal of sutures and staples—cont'd

Skill activity	Rationale
Create the aseptic field by using the sterile dressing pack and add sterile equipment including 0.9% sodium chloride to the field. Open sterile dressing pack by using corners. Open the sterile dressing products away from the aseptic field and add into the field.	Prevents contamination of sterile items and Key-Parts.
Loosen and remove the existing wound dressing for the visual wound assessment including the type and amount of exudate on the removed dressing and peri-wound condition, and count the number of sutures or staples. Dispose of wound dressing and used gloves.	Assesses the signs and symptoms of wound infection (e.g. redness, swelling, warmth, exudate amount and type). Prevents spread of microorganisms.
Rearrange and assemble the required sterile dressing and equipment in the aseptic field using ANTT without contaminating the Key-Parts.	Maintains ANTT to protect the wound from environmental contamination. Prevents contamination of the Key-Parts.
Position sterile dressing drape below or near the wound.	Protects the wound from environmental contamination.
Cleanse the wound with sterile 0.9% sodium chloride. Clean from top to bottom and from a clean area towards a less clean area, usually an outward direction.	Removes debris from the wound bed. Avoids transferring wound exudate and normal flora from the surrounding skin into the wound. Prevents wound contamination.
Reassess the suture wound for any signs of infection or dehiscence.	Assesses for any signs of infection and wound dehiscence.
Removal of sutures: • Start with the second suture, using forceps to grasp the knot and gently raise it off the skin. • Cut the suture as close to the skin as possible, away from the knot. • Pull the cut suture up and out of the skin, ensuring that the exposed portion of the suture is not pulled through the tissues. • Remove alternating sutures by using the same technique leaving the first and last sutures till last to remove.	Allows for assessment of union. Avoids risk of pulling exposed suture through the tissues, which prevents infection.
Removal of staples: • Place the staple remover's lower jaw under the centre of the staple. • Squeeze the handles of the staple remover until the jaws are completely closed. • Slightly tilt the staple remover from side to side to facilitate removal. • Gently lift the staple remover to remove the staple from the skin. • Place the staple(s) onto the extended sterile field for counting later. • Repeat the same process for alternating staples leaving first and last staple till last to remove.	The extractor reforms the shape of the staple and pulls the prongs out of the intradermal tissue. Ensures that the incision has healed before removing all staples.
Apply an appropriate sterile wound dressing using ANTT and secure.	If necessary, apply sterile wound closure strips to provide additional support in wound edge closure. Provides protection from infection and irritation if required.
Count and dispose of staples.	Ensures required number of staples were removed and disposed.

Continued

CLINICAL SKILL 29.5 Removal of sutures and staples—cont'd

AFTER THE SKILL

(Please refer to the Standard Steps on pp. xviii–xx for related rationales.)
Communicate outcome to the individual, any ongoing care and report any complications.
Restore the environment.
Report, record and document assessment findings, details of the skill performed and the individual's response.
Report, record and document any abnormalities and/or inability to perform the skill.
Reassess the individual to ensure there are no adverse effects/events from the skill.

(Adapted from ACIPC 2015; LeMone et al 2020; Berman et al 2020; Lynn 2022; The-ASAP 2019)

CLINICAL SKILL 29.6 Shortening a drain tube

Please adhere to the policy and procedures of the facility/organisation prior to undertaking the skill. Ensure this skill is in your scope of practice.

NMBA Decision-making Framework considerations (refer to NMBA Decision-making framework for nursing and midwifery 2020): 1. Am I educated? 2. Am I authorised? 3. Am I competent? If you answer 'no' to any of these, do not perform that activity. Seek guidance and support from your teacher/a nurse team leader/clinical facilitator/educator.	**Equipment:** Sterile dressing pack Sterile dressing materials Sterile gloves Disposable gloves Additional light source (if required) Sterile 0.9% sodium chloride Additional gauze Sterile scissors Sterile suture cutter Sterile safety pin Ostomy/appliance bag (if required) Protective eyewear Waste receptacle Sharps bin Dressing trolley Disinfectant wipes/solution

PREPARE FOR THE SKILL

(Please refer to the Standard Steps on pp. xviii–xx for related rationales.)
Mentally review the steps of the skill.
Discuss the skill with your instructor/supervisor/team leader, if required.
Confirm correct facility/organisation policy/safe operating procedures.
Validate the order in the individual's record.
Identify indication and rationale for performing the activity.
Assess for any contraindications.
Locate and gather equipment.
Perform hand hygiene.
Ensure therapeutic interaction.
Identify the individual using three individual identifiers.
Gain the individual's consent.
Assess for pain relief.
Prepare the environment.
Provide and maintain privacy.
Assist the individual to assume an appropriate position of comfort.

Skill activity	Rationale
Drain tubes are shortened to reduce irritation to the bottom of the wound and promote healing.	
Assess the individual's record to determine previous appearance of wound and previous dressing.	Determines requirements for equipment and dressing requirements.

CLINICAL SKILL 29.6 Shortening a drain tube—cont'd

PERFORM THE SKILL

(Please refer to the Standard Steps on pp. xviii–xx for related rationales.)
Perform hand hygiene.
Apply PPE: gloves, eyewear, mask and gown as appropriate.
Ensure the individual's safety and comfort throughout skill.
Promote independence and involvement of the individual if possible and/or appropriate.
Assess the individual's tolerance to the skill throughout.
Dispose of used supplies, equipment, waste and sharps appropriately.
Remove PPE and discard or store appropriately.
Perform hand hygiene.

Skill activity	Rationale
Create the aseptic field by using the sterile dressing pack and add sterile equipment including 0.9% sodium chloride to the field. Open sterile dressing pack by using corners. Open the sterile dressing products away from the aseptic field and add into the field.	Prevents contamination of sterile items and Key-Parts.
Loosen and remove the existing wound dressing for the visual wound assessment including the type and amount of exudate on the removed dressing and peri-wound condition. Dispose of wound dressing and used gloves.	Assesses the signs and symptoms of wound infection (e.g. redness, swelling, warmth, exudate amount and type). Prevents spread of microorganisms.
Rearrange and assemble the required sterile dressing and equipment in the aseptic field using ANTT without contaminating the Key-Parts.	Maintains ANTT to protect the wound from environmental contamination. Prevents contamination of the Key-Parts.
Position sterile dressing drape below or near the wound.	Protects the wound from environmental contamination.
Cleanse the drain tube site at the point where the tubing enters/exits with sterile 0.9% sodium chloride. Assess drain tube site. Allow to dry.	Removes debris from the wound bed. Avoids transferring wound exudate and normal flora from the surrounding skin into the wound. Observes for any signs of infection (e.g. warmth, redness, increasing amount of exudate, odour) and peri-wound condition. Prevents wound contamination.
Cut and remove the drain tube securing suture with suture cutter and remove (if present).	Enables the tube to be free for retraction and/or rotation.
Hold onto the drain tube close to the exit point. Gently rotate the drain tube before using smooth and gentle traction to withdraw/shorten the drain tube by the specified amount (cease procedure immediately if excessive force is required to withdraw drain tube).	Rotates the tube free from any adherent granulation tissue.
Place the sterile safety pin through the drain tube after shortening (open drains only). Trim excess length below the sterile safety pin.	Prevents drain tube retraction or extrusion. Prevents it pressing on the wound.
Apply an appropriate sterile wound dressing or appliance bag (e.g. ostomy bag) using ANTT and secure.	Collects exudate to facilitate moist healing environment. Covers wound and prevents spread of microorganisms.

AFTER THE SKILL

(Please refer to the Standard Steps on pp. xviii–xx for related rationales.)
Communicate outcome to the individual, any ongoing care and report any complications.
Restore the environment.
Report, record and document assessment findings, details of the skill performed and the individual's response.
Report, record and document any abnormalities and/or inability to perform the skill.
Reassess the individual to ensure there are no adverse effects/events from the skill.

(Adapted from ACIPC 2015; LeMone et al 2020; Berman et al 2020; IWII 2022; Lynn 2022; The-ASAP 2019)

CLINICAL SKILL 29.7 Removal of a drain tube

Please adhere to the policy and procedures of the facility/organisation prior to undertaking the skill. Ensure this skill is in your scope of practice.

NMBA Decision-making Framework considerations (refer to NMBA Decision-making framework for nursing and midwifery 2020):	Equipment:
1. Am I educated? 2. Am I authorised? 3. Am I competent? If you answer 'no' to any of these, do not perform that activity. Seek guidance and support from your teacher/a nurse team leader/clinical facilitator/educator.	Sterile dressing pack Sterile dressing materials Sterile gloves Disposable gloves Additional light source (if required) Sterile 0.9% sodium chloride Additional sterile gauze Sterile suture cutter Protective eyewear Waste receptacle Sharps bin Dressing trolley Disinfectant wipes/solution

PREPARE FOR THE SKILL

(Please refer to the Standard Steps on pp. xviii–xx for related rationales.)
Mentally review the steps of the skill.
Discuss the skill with your instructor/supervisor/team leader, if required.
Confirm correct facility/organisation policy/safe operating procedures.
Validate the order in the individual's record.
Identify indication and rationale for performing the activity.
Assess for any contraindications.
Locate and gather equipment.
Perform hand hygiene.
Ensure therapeutic interaction.
Identify the individual using three individual identifiers.
Gain the individual's consent.
Assess for pain relief.
Prepare the environment.
Provide and maintain privacy.
Assist the individual to assume an appropriate position of comfort.

Skill activity	Rationale
Drain tubes are removed to reduce irritation to the bottom of the wound and promote healing.	
Assess drain tube condition and output.	Inspects for signs of infection, bleeding, leakage, suction patency, the quantity and type of drain.
Dissipate suction.	Prevents trauma to tissue around the drain tube upon removal. Prevents pain associated with drain tube removal.

PERFORM THE SKILL

(Please refer to the Standard Steps on pp. xviii–xx for related rationales.)
Perform hand hygiene.
Apply PPE: gloves, eyewear, mask and gown as appropriate.
Ensure the individual's safety and comfort throughout skill.
Promote independence and involvement of the individual if possible and/or appropriate.
Assess the individual's tolerance to the skill throughout.
Dispose of used supplies, equipment, waste and sharps appropriately.
Remove PPE and discard or store appropriately.
Perform hand hygiene.

CLINICAL SKILL 29.7 Removal of a drain tube—cont'd

Skill activity	Rationale
Create the aseptic field by using the sterile dressing pack and add sterile equipment including 0.9% sodium chloride to the field. Open sterile dressing pack by using corners. Open the sterile dressing products away from the aseptic field and add into the field.	Prevents contamination of sterile items and Key-Parts.
Loosen and remove the existing wound dressing for the visual assessment of the drain tube site. Dispose of wound dressing and used gloves.	Assesses the signs and symptoms of wound infection at the drain tube site (e.g. redness, exudate amount and type). Prevents spread of microorganisms.
Rearrange and assemble the required sterile dressing and equipment in the aseptic field using ANTT without contaminating the Key-Parts.	Maintains ANTT to protect the wound from environmental contamination. Prevents contamination of the Key-Parts.
Position sterile dressing drape below or near the wound.	Protects the wound from environmental contamination.
Cleanse the drain tube site at the point where the tubing enters/exits with sterile 0.9% sodium chloride. Reassess drain tube site. Allow to dry.	Removes debris from the wound bed. Avoids transferring wound exudate and normal flora from the surrounding skin into the wound. Observes for any signs of infection (e.g. redness, exudate type and amount), and peri-wound condition. Prevents wound contamination.
Cut and remove the drain tube securing suture with suture cutter (if present).	Ensures the tube is free for retraction and/or rotation.
Hold onto the drain tube close to the exit point. Gently rotate the drain tube (if the drain tube is round), and apply smooth and gentle traction to fully remove the drain tube (avoid forceful pulling of the tube). Inspect the drain tube tip for its integrity.	Rotates the tube free from any adherent granulation tissue to facilitate removal and to minimise pain/discomfort upon drain tube removal. Gentle traction to prevent drain tube fracture from forceful pulling action. Checks for integrity of the drain tube tip and escalates concerns if tube fracture is suspected.
Apply an appropriate sterile wound dressing using ANTT and secure.	Collects exudate to facilitate moist healing environment. Covers wound and prevents spread of microorganisms.

AFTER THE SKILL

(Please refer to the Standard Steps on pp. xviii–xx for related rationales.)
Communicate outcome to the individual, any ongoing care and report any complications.
Restore the environment.
Report, record and document assessment findings, details of the skill performed and the individual's response.
Report, record and document any abnormalities and/or inability to perform the skill.
Reassess the individual to ensure there are no adverse effects/events from the skill.

(Adapted from LeMone et al 2020; Berman et al 2020; LeBlanc et al 2018; Lynn 2022; The-ASAP 2019)

Progress Note 29.2

07/12/2023 2030 hrs	Nursing: Patient sat out of bed for dinner (approx. 1 hour) and returned to bed after. Patient mobilises with four-wheelie walker under close supervision. High falls risk. Incontinent pad changed. HPU, incontinent × 1, pad changed. Pressure area care performed. Stage II pressure injury (intact serous filled blister) to left heel remains unchanged. Moisturiser applied to dry skin areas, which is improving. IAD to groin/perineum improving, continue with current regime of cleansing with Cavilon barrier spray and wipes, followed by the barrier cream. Two-hourly repositioning and heel wedge remains in situ. Encouraged oral intake and additional supplemental nutritional drinks as per dietitian's recommendation. Patient appeared comfortable and voiced same with no report of pain at time of report.
	K Jones (JONES), *EN*

DECISION-MAKING FRAMEWORK EXERCISE 29.1

A person you have been caring for has an open wound on the lower leg. You are asked to change the dressing. A dry dressing is requested in their care plan. You remove the dressing with some difficulty as it has adhered to the wound. What actions would you take as an Enrolled Nurse in this situation?

Summary

The integumentary system consists of the skin and its appendages: the hair, nails, sweat and sebaceous glands. The skin is the largest organ of the body and is composed of two layers. The epidermis is the thin outermost layer composed of epithelial cells. The dermis, or deeper layer of the skin, contains blood vessels, nerve endings, hair follicles and hairs, arrector pili muscles, sebaceous glands and sweat glands. Nails and hair protect certain areas of the body (e.g. nails protect the tips of toes and fingers, while hair protects areas such as the scalp). The major functions of the skin are protection, thermoregulation, sensory perception, excretion, immunity, synthesis of vitamin D and to act as a blood reservoir.

Wound healing and tissue repair present as a frequent priority in providing nursing care. Holistic assessment including intrinsic and extrinsic factors and knowledge of the stages of wound healing—haemostasis, inflammation, reconstruction and maturation—inform clinical practice. Important consideration is required for types of wound healing; primary, secondary, third or delayed primary intention. The links between wound bed preparation, wound care practice and dressing product selection are indispensable to promote effective wound healing.

Surgical wounds are the result of intervention by the surgeon and can range from an uncomplicated suture line to a more complex wound requiring drainage tubes or skin grafts. A surgical wound must be treated with strict aseptic technique and the nurse must be aware of the individual health organisation's protocols.

Pressure injuries result from ischaemic hypoxia of the tissues due to prolonged pressure in an area of the body, usually over a bony prominence. Both intrinsic and extrinsic predisposing factors contribute to the development of a pressure injury. Pressure injuries can be classified as stages I, II, III, IV and two temporary categories, SDTI and unstageable, depending upon degree of tissue damaged. Risk assessment and preventative strategies that are employed by the nurse play an important role in ensuring that the incidence of pressure injuries, which are largely predictable and preventable, is kept to a minimum. The nurse engages the multidisciplinary team to assist in the prevention of pressure injuries within the vulnerable individual population, such as the elderly and severely compromised.

Skin tears are a traumatic injury that can occur mainly to the frail elderly population. Implementing preventative strategies and education to improve the condition of the person's skin, the environment and safe use of equipment required for caring for this vulnerable age group are important.

Leg ulcers are a debilitating condition and the nurse is required to differentiate between the different types to employ the appropriate wound management practice. The use of compression bandaging, which can be quite effective in the management of VLUs, is contraindicated and dangerous for the management of arterial leg ulcers.

Heat, chemicals, electricity, radiation and cold injury can cause a burn. The depth of tissue injury describes a burn and the size of the burn is estimated by using either the Lund–Browder method or the rule of nines. Complications include shock, infection, scarring and contracture, and adverse psychological effects. Medical and nursing management of an individual with burn injury will vary according to the severity of the injury. The care of the individual involves fluid and electrolyte replacement,

Summary—cont'd

prevention of infection, provision of adequate nutrition, relief of pain, promotion of mobility, providing psychological support and promoting healing of the injury.

The effects that disorders of the skin have on the individual range from minor and temporary to major and life-threatening. Some serious skin disorders affect the individual to the extent that self-concept and body image are severely impaired. Disorders of the skin may have a single cause or may result from several interrelated factors, while for some disorders the cause is unknown. Tests used to diagnose skin disorders include direct examination, biopsy, microscopic examination and skin testing.

With any skin integrity deficit, the psychosocial support for the individual is of major importance. Pain management and nutritional support are also vital to achieving positive person-focused outcomes. Suitable wound care practice is essential and should include a clear understanding of the normal healing processes, wound assessment, dressing selection and management of the effect that certain pathologies have on those processes to promote healing and skin integrity.

Review Questions

1. What are the major functions of skin?
2. What are the major factors that affect skin integrity?
3. Describe the four stages of the wound-healing process.
4. What factors can affect wound healing?
5. State the benefits of moist wound healing.
6. What are the major manifestations of skin disorders?
7. Describe the four categories and two temporary categories of pressure injury.
8. What care is required to prevent and manage pressure injuries?
9. What care is required to prevent skin tears?
10. What is the difference between an arterial ulcer and a venous ulcer?

Evolve® Answer guide for the Review Questions, Critical Thinking Exercises, Decision-making Framework Exercises and Critical Thinking Questions in Case Studies is hosted on Evolve: http://evolve.elsevier.com/AU/Koutoukidis/Tabbner.

References

Ahangar, P., Woodward, M., Cowin, A.J., 2018. Advanced wound therapies. *Wound Practice & Research* 26(2), 55–68.

Ahuja, K., Lio, P., 2023. The role of trace elements in dermatology: A systematic review. *Journal of Integrative Dermatology.* Available at: <https://www.jintegrativederm.org/article/73228-the-role-of-trace-elements-in-dermatology-a-systematic-review>.

Almadani, Y.H., Vorstenbosh, J., Davison, P.G., et al. 2021. Wound healing: A comprehensive review. *Seminars in Plastic Surgery* 35(3), 141–144.

Andriessen, A., Apelqvist, J., Mosti, G., et al., 2017. Compression therapy for venous leg ulcers: Risk factors for adverse events and complications, contraindications – a review of present guidelines. *Journal of the European Academy of Dermatology and Venereology* 31(9), 1562–1568.

Artz, C.P., Moncrief, J.A., 1969. *The treatment of burns*, 2nd ed. Saunders, Philadelphia.

Atkin, L., 2019. Chronic wounds: The challenges of appropriate management. *British Journal of Community Nursing* 24(suppl 9), S26–S32.

Australian & New Zealand Burn Association (ANZBA), 2019. Care. Available at: <https://anzba.org.au>.

Australasian College for Infection Prevention and Control (ACIPC), 2015. Aseptic technique policy and practice guidelines. Available at: <https://www.acipc.org.au/aseptic-technique-resources>.

Australian Commission on Safety and Quality in Health Care (ACSQHC), 2017. Approaches to surgical site infection surveillance. Available at: <https://www.safetyandquality.gov.au/sites/default/files/2019-06/approaches-to-surgical-site-infection-surveillance.pdf>.

Australian Commission on Safety and Quality in Health Care (ACSQHC), 2018. Hospital-acquired complication – 13. Malnutrition fact sheet (long). Available at: <https://www.safetyandquality.gov.au/sites/default/files/migrated/SAQ7730_HAC_Malnutrition_LongV2.pdf>.

Australian Commission on Safety and Quality in Health Care (ACSQHC), 2020. Preventing pressure injuries and wound management. Available at: <https://www.safetyandquality.gov.au/sites/default/files/2020-10/fact_sheet_-_preventing_pressure_injuries_and_wound_management_oct_2020.pdf>.

Australian Commission on Safety and Quality in Health Care (ACSQHC), 2021. National safety and quality health service standards, 2nd ed. ACSQHC, Sydney.

Australian Commission on Safety and Quality in Health Care (ACSQHC), 2023. Antimicrobial stewardship. Available at: <https://www.safetyandquality.gov.au/our-work/antimicrobial-stewardship>.

Australian Medical Association, 2022. Solutions to the chronic wound problem in Australia. Available at: <www.ama.com.au>.

Bergstrom, N., Braden, B.J., Laguzza, A., et al., 1987. The Braden Scale for predicting pressure sore risk. *Nursing Research* 36(4), 205–210.

Berman, A., Snyder, S., Levett-Jones, T., et al., 2020. *Kozier and Erb's fundamentals of nursing*, 5th ed. Pearson, Melbourne.

Black, J., Black, J., 2021. Ten top tips: Skin grafting. *Wounds International* 12(3), 10–13.

Bishop, A., Witts, S., Martin, T., 2018. The role of nutrition in successful wound healing. *Journal of Community Nursing* 32(4), 44–50.

Bjork, R., Ehmann, S., 2019. S.T.R.I.D.E. Professional guide to compression garment selection for the lower extremity. *Journal of Wound Care* 28(6 suppl 1), 1–44.

Brown, A., 2023. Assessing and managing wound pain. *Practice Nursing* 34(1), 10–15.

Campbell, K.E., Baronoski, S., Gloeckner, M., et al., 2018. Skin tears: Prediction, prevention, assessment and management. *Nurse Prescribing* 16(12), 600–607.

Carter, M., Cole, W., Crombie, R., et al., 2023. Best practice for wound repair and regeneration use of cellular, acellular and matrix-like products (CAMPs). *Journal of Wound Care* 32(suppl 4b), S1–S31.

Carville, K., Lewin, G., Newall, N., et al., (2007). STAR: A consensus for skin tear classification. *Primary Intention* 15(1), 8–25.

Carville, K., 2023. *Wound care manual*, 8th ed. Silver Chain Nursing Association, Perth, Western Australia.

Cheng, Q., Gibb, M., Graves, N., et al., 2018. Cost-effectiveness analysis of guideline-based optimal care for venous leg ulcers in Australia. *BMC Health Services Research* 18, 421.

Clark, M., Semple, M.J., Ivins, N., et al., 2017. National audit of pressure ulcers and incontinence-associated dermatitis in hospitals across Wales: A cross-sectional study. *British Medical Journal Open* 7(8), e015616.

Cortes, R., Bennasar-Veny, M., Castro-Sanchez, E., et al., 2020. Nutrition screening tools for risk of malnutrition among hospitalized patients: A protocol for systematic review and meta analysis. *Medicine* 99(43), e22601.

Curtis, P., Duane L., 1965. Treatment of burns. *Current Problems in Surgery* 2(3), 1–40. ISSN 0011-3840. Available at: <https://doi.org/10.1016/S0011-3840(65)80012-0>.

Deans, C., Paterson, H., 2024. *Core topics in general and emergency surgery: A companion to specialist surgical practice*, 7th ed. Elsevier Ltd.

Dent, E., Chapman, I., Piantadosi, C., et al., 2017. Screening for malnutrition in hospitalised older people: Comparison of the Mini Nutritional Assessment with its short-form versions. *Australasian Journal on Ageing* 36(2), E8–E13.

Docherty, J., 2020. Understanding the elements of a holistic wound assessment. *Nursing Standard* 35(10), 69–76.

Douglas, H., Woods, F., 2017. Burns dressings. *Australian Journal for General Practitioners* 46(3), 94–97.

Dowsett, C., Pagnamenta, F., Fletcher, J., et al., 2020. Management of lower limb skin tears in adults. Available at: <https://wounds-uk.com/wp-content/uploads/sites/2/2023/02/9ec79295c0614f25f48e636b0b0ebc6e.pdf>.

Edwards, H., Finlayson, K., Parker, C., et al., 2019. Champions for skin integrity wound dressing guide. Queensland University of Technology, Brisbane. Available at: <https://research.qut.edu.au/ccm>.

Eriksson, E., Liu, P.Y., Schultz, G.S., et al., 2022. Chronic wound: Treatment consensus. *Wound Repair and Regeneration* 30(2), 156–171.

European Pressure Ulcer Advisory Panel (EPUAP), National Pressure Injury Advisory Panel (NPIAP), Pan Pacific Pressure Injury Alliance (PPPIA), Haesler, E. (ed.), 2019. *Prevention and treatment of pressure ulcers/injuries: Clinical practice guidelines*, 3rd ed. EPUAP/NPIAP/PPPIA.

Feng, H., Wu, Y., Su, C., et al., 2018. Skin injury prevalence and incidence in China: A multicentre investigation. *Journal of Wound Care* 27(suppl 10), S4–S9.

Francis, K., 2019. Damage control: Differentiating incontinence-associated dermatitis from pressure injury. *The Nurse Practitioner* 44(12), 12–17.

Fillit, H.M., 2017. *Brocklehurst's textbook of geriatric medicine and gerontology*, 8th ed. Elsevier Ltd, London.

Finch, K., Osseiran-Moisson, R., Carville, K., et al., 2018. Skin tear prevention in elderly patients using twice-daily moisturiser. *Wound Practice and Research* 26(2), 99–109.

Gawkrodger, D.J., Arden-Jones, M.R., 2021. *Dermatology: An illustrated colour text*, 7th ed. Elsevier, Edinburgh.

Gibb, M., 2023. *A to almost A of wound dressings*, 1st ed. Wound Specialist Services Pty Ltd, Samford, Queensland.

Goswami, A.G., Basu, S., Banerjee, T., et al., 2023. Biofilm and wound healing: From bench to bedside. *European Journal of Medical Research* 28, 157.

Guillamat-Prats, R., 2021. The role of MSC in wound healing, scarring and regeneration. *Cells* 10(7), 1729.

Haesler, E., 2018. Evidence summary: Prevention of pressure injuries in individuals with overweight or obesity for wound healing and management node. *Wound and Practice Research* 28(3), 158–161.

Haesler, E., Carville, K., 2023. *Australian standards for wound prevention and management*, 4th ed. Australian Health Research Alliance, Wounds Australia and WA Health Translation Network.

Hampton, S., 2018. Venous leg ulcers: Choosing the right type of compression. *Nursing & Residential Care* 20(11), 559–562.

Harding, K., Gray, D., Timmons, J., et al., 2007. Evolution or revolution? Adapting to complexity in wound management. *International Wound Journal* 4 (2), 1–12.

Healy, B., Freedman, A., 2022. Infections. In: Price, A., Grey, J.E., Patel, G.K., et al., *ABC of wound healing*, 2nd ed. John Wiley & Sons, Incorporated, Newark.

Hockenberry, M., Duffy, E., Gibbs, K., 2024. *Wong's nursing care of infants and children*, 12th ed. Elsevier Inc, St Louis.

Holman, M., 2023. Using tap water compared with normal saline for cleansing wounds in adults: A literature review of the evidence. *Journal of Wound Care* 32(8), 507–512.

Idensohn, P., Beeckman, D., Campbell, K.E., et al., 2019. Skin tears: A case-based and practical overview of prevention, assessment and management. *Journal of Community Nursing* 33(2), 32–41.

International Wound Infection Institute (IWII), 2022. Wound infection in clinical practice: Principles of best practice. Wounds International. Available at: <https://woundinfection-institute.com/wp-content/uploads/IWII-CD-2022-web-1.pdf>.

Isoherranen, K., Montero, E.C., Atkin, L., et al., 2023. Lower leg ulcer diagnosis & principles of treatment. Including recommendations for comprehensive assessment and referral pathways. *Journal of Wound Management* 24(2 suppl 1), s1–s76.

Jenkins, S., 2020. The assessment of pain in acute wounds (part 1). *Wound UK* 16(1), 26–33.

Kapp, S., Tomkins, Z., 2020. Integumentary system. In: Tomkins, Z. (eds.), *Applied anatomy & physiology: An interdisciplinary approach*. Elsevier, St Louis.

Kim, H., Shin, S., Han, D., 2022. Review of history of basic principles of burn wound management. *Medicina* 58, 400.

King, C., 2020. Changing attitudes toward maggot debridement therapy in wound treatment: A review and discussion. *Journal of Wound Care* 29(2), S28–S34.

Kirsner, R.S., Zimnitsky, D., Robinson, M., 2021. A prospective, randomized, controlled clinical study on the effectiveness of a single-use negative pressure wound therapy system, compared to traditional negative pressure wound therapy in the treatment of diabetic ulcers of the lower extremities. *Wound Repair and Regeneration* 29(6), 908–911.

LeBlanc, K., Campbell, K., Beeckman, D., et al., 2018. Best practice recommendations for prevention and management of skin tears in aged skin: An overview. *Journal of Wound, Ostomy, and Continence Nursing* 45(6), 540–542.

LeBlanc, K., Langemo, D., Woo, K., et al., 2019. Skin tears: Prevention and management. *British Journal of Community Nursing* 24(9), S12–S18.

LeBlanc, K., Baranoski, S., Holloway, S., et al., 2013. Validation of a new classification system for skin tears. *Advances in Skin and Wound Care* 26(6), 263–265.

Legrand, M., Barraud, D., Constant, I., et al., 2020. Management of severe thermal burns in the acute phase in adults and children. *Anaesthesia Critical Care & Pain Medicine* 39(2), 253–267.

LeMone, P., Bauldoff, G., Gubrud-Howe, P., et al., 2020. *Medical–surgical nursing: Critical thinking in person-centred care*, 4th ed. Pearson, Melbourne.

Liu, Y., Chinese Burn Association, 2023. Chinese expert consensus on the management of pediatric deep partial-thickness burn wounds (2023 ed). *Burns and Trauma* 11, tkad053.

Lynn, P., 2022. *Taylor's clinical nursing skills. A nursing process approach*, 6th ed. Wolters Kluwer Lippincott Williams & Wilkins, Philadelphia.

Mattox, E.A., 2017. Reducing risks associated with negative-pressure wound therapy: Strategies for clinical practice. *Critical Care Nurse* 37(5), 67–77.

McCosker, L., Tulleners, R., Cheng, Q., et al., 2019. Chronic wounds in Australia: A systematic review of key epidemiological and clinical parameters. *International Wound Journal* 16, 84–91.

Miles, S.J., Fulbrook, P., Williams, D.M., 2022. Skin tear prevalence in an Australian acute care hospital: A 10-year analysis. *International Wound Journal* 19(6), 1418–1427.

Munoz, N., Litchford, M., Cox, J., et al., 2022. Malnutrition and pressure injury risk in vulnerable populations: Application of the 2019 International Clinical Practice Guideline. *Advances in Skin & Wound Care* 35(3), 156–165.

Murphy, C., Atkin, L., Swanson, T., et al., 2020. International consensus document. Defying hard-to-heal wounds with an early antibiofilm intervention strategy: Wound hygiene. *Journal of Wound Care* 29(suppl 3b), S1–S28.

Newall, N., Lewin, G.F., Bulsara, M.K., et al., 2017. The development and testing of a skin tear risk assessment tool. *International Wound Journal* 14(1), 97–103.

NSW Agency for Clinical Innovation, 2018. *Burn patient management: Summary of evidence*, 4th ed. ACI, Chatswood.

Nursing and Midwifery Board of Australia (NMBA), 2020. Decision-making framework summary for nursing and midwifery. Available at: <https://www.nursingmidwiferyboard.gov.au/Codes-Guidelines-Statements/Frameworks.aspx>.

Nuutila, K., Eriksson, E., 2021. Moist wound healing with commonly available dressings. *Advances in Wound Care* 10(12), 685–697.

Oozageer Gunowa, N., Hutchinson, M., Brooke, J., et al., 2018. Pressure injuries in people with darker skin tones: A literature review. *Journal of Clinical Nursing* 27(17–18), 3266–3275.

Pacella, R.E., Tulleners, R., Cheng, Q., et al., 2018. Solutions to the chronic wounds problem in Australia: A call to action. *Journal of Wounds Australia* 26, 2.

Patton, K.T., Thibodeau, G.A., 2019. Skin – Anatomy and physiology. In: Patton, K.T. (eds.), *Anatomy and physiology*, adapted international ed. Elsevier, St Louis.

Paul, W., Sharma, C.P., 2021. Tissue and organ regeneration: An introduction. In: Sharma, C.P., *Regenerated organs*. Academic Press. Available at: <https://www.sciencedirect.com/science/article/pii/B9780128210857000014?via%3Dihub>.

Payne, R., Martin, M., 1993. Defining and classifying skin tears: Need for a common language. A critique and revision of the Payne-Martin classification system for skin tears. *Ostomy/Wound Management* 39, 16–20.

Peate, I., Stephens, M., 2020. *Wound care at a glance*, 2nd ed. John Wiley & Sons Incorporated, Oxford.

Potter, P.A., Perry, A.G., Stockert, P.A., et al., 2013. *Fundamentals of nursing*, 8th ed. Mosby, St Louis.

Rodgers, K., Sim, J., Clifton, R., 2021. Systematic review of pressure injury prevalence in Australian and New Zealand hospital. *Collegian* 28(3), 310–323.

Romanelli, M., Serena, T., Kimble, R., et al., 2019. Skin graft donor site management in the treatment of burns and hard-to-heal wounds. Wounds International. Available at: <https://woundsinternational.com/wp-content/uploads/sites/8/2023/02/4a138f37fac1c741cd4b5a0bc06674ec.pdf>.

Scanlon, V.C., Sanders, T., 2019. The integumentary system. In: Scanlon, V.C., Sanders, T., (eds.), *Essentials of anatomy and physiology*. F.A. Davis Company, Philadelphia.

Scheel-Sailer, A., Frotzler, A., Mueller, G., et al., 2017. Biophysical skin properties of grade 1 pressure ulcers and unaffected skin in spinal cord injured and able-bodied persons in the unloaded sacral region. *Journal of Tissue Viability* 26(2), 89–94.

Schneider, K.L., Yahia, N., 2019. Effectiveness of arginine supplementation on wound healing in older adults in acute and chronic settings: A systematic review. *Advances in Skin & Wound Care* 32(10), 457–462.

Shamsian, N., 2021. Wound bed preparation: An overview. *British Journal of Community Nursing* 26(suppl 9), S6–S11.

Sibbald, R.G., Elliot, J.A., Persaud-Jaimangal, R., et al., 2021. Wound bed preparation 2021. *Advances in Skin & Wound Care* 34(4), 183–195.

Singh, R., Kumar, A., Solanki, P., et al., 2024. *Nanotechnological aspects for next-generation wound management*. Elsevier Inc, St Louis.

Stryja, J., 2019. Ten top tips: Prevention of surgical site infections. *Wounds International* 9(2), 16–20.

Tang, S.K.Y., Marshall, W.F., 2017. Self-repairing cells: How single cells heal membrane ruptures and restore lost structures. *Science* 345(6342), 1022–1025.

The-Association for Safe Aseptic Practice (The-ASAP), 2019. Aseptic non touch technique (ANTT). The ANTT clinical practice framework V4.0. Available at: <https://www.antt.org/antt-practice-framework.html>.

Thomas, D.C., Tsu, C.I., Nain, R.A., et al., 2021. The role of debridement in wound bed preparation in chronic wound: A narrative review. *Annals of Medicine and Surgery* 71, 102876.

Torbrand, C., Anesäter, E., Borgquist, O., et al., 2018. Mechanical effects of negative pressure wound therapy on abdominal wounds – effects of different pressures and wound fillers. *International Wound Journal* 15(1), 24–28.

Trauma Victoria, 2023. Burns. Available at: <https://trauma.reach.vic.gov.au>.

Trelease, C.C., 1988. Developing standards for wound care. *Ostomy/Wound Management* 20, 46.

Victorian Adult Burns Service, 2019. Burns management guidelines. Available at: <www.vicburns.org.au>.

Vowden, P., Kerr, A., Mosti, G., 2020. Demystifying mild, moderate and high compression systems – when and how to introduce “lighter” compression. Wounds International, London. Available at: <www.woundsinternational.com>.

Wang, G., Xu, H., Zhang, H., et al., 2023. Clinical outcomes of negative pressure wound therapy with instillation vs standard negative pressure of wound therapy for wound: A meta-analysis of randomised controlled trials. *International Wound Journal* 20(5), 1739–1749.

Weir, D., Swanson, T., 2019. Back to basics: Clean it like you mean it! *International Wound Infection Institute Newsletter*, May 2019.

Wilson, L., Kapp, S., Santamaria, N., 2019. The direct cost of pressure injuries in an Australian residential aged care setting. *International Wound Journal* 16(1), 64–70.

World Health Organization (WHO), 2018. *Global guidelines for the prevention of surgical site infection*, 2nd ed. Geneva.

Wounds International, 2019. World Union of Wound Healing Societies Consensus Document: Wound exudate – Effective assessment and management. Wounds International. Available at: <https://woundsinternational.com/wp-content/uploads/sites/8/2023/02/836aed9753c3d8e3d8694bcaee336395.pdf>.

Wounds UK, 2023. Best practice statement: The use of compression therapy for peripheral oedema: Considerations in people with heart failure. Wounds UK, London. Available at: <https://wounds-uk.com/wp-content/uploads/sites/2/2023/06/ESS23_BPS_Heart-failure_WUK_web.pdf>.

Wounds UK, 2022. Best practice statement: Holistic management of venous leg ulceration, 2nd ed. Wounds UK, London. Online. Available at: <https://wounds-uk.com/wp-content/uploads/sites/2/2023/02/f45d25738c222a3361e587b6473f0665.pdf>.

Wounds UK, 2017. Best practice statement: Making day-to-day management of biofilm simple. Wounds UK, London. Available at: <https://wounds-uk.com/wp-content/uploads/sites/2/2023/02/fbf51962d868ab4ccc8eb8038963b6f8.pdf>.

Wu, S., Carter, M., Cole, W., et al, 2023. Best practice for wound repair and regeneration: Use of cellular, acellular and matrix-like products (CAMPs). *Journal of Wound Care* 32(4 suppl B), S1–S32.

Xie, T., Ye, J., Rerkasem, K., et al., 2018. The venous ulcer continues to be a clinical challenge: An update. *Burns Trauma* 6, 18.

Zerwekh, J., Garneau, A., Miller, C.J., 2017. *Digital collection of the memory notebooks of nursing*, 4th ed. Nursing Education Consultants Inc, Chandler.

Zhang, P., Zou, B., Liou, Y.C., et al., 2021. The pathogenesis and diagnosis of sepsis post burn injury. *Burns & Trauma* 9, tkaa047.

Zenith, 2018. *Medical assisting module: A textbook*. Elsevier Inc, St Louis.

Recommended Reading

Angel, D., 2019. Slough: What does it mean and how can it be managed. *Wound Practice and Research* 24(4), 164–167.

Anghel, E.L., DeFazio, M.V., Barker, J.C., et al., 2016. Current concepts in debridement: Science and strategies. *Plastic and Reconstructive Surgery* 138(3S), 82S–93S.

Australian Commission on Safety and Quality in Health Care, 2018. Hospital-acquired complication 1 pressure injury.

Australian Commission on Safety and Quality in Health Care. Available at: <https://www.safetyandquality.gov.au/wp-content/uploads/2018/06/SAQ7730_HAC_Factsheet_PressureInjury_LongV2.pdf>.

Barakat-Johnson, M., Ryan, H., Brooks, M., et al., 2023. A 'quick guide' to pressure injury management. Wounds International. Available at: <https://woundsinternational.com/wp-content/uploads/sites/8/2023/09/Mol23_SUPP_PITA_WINT-WEBv2.pdf>.

Bishop, A., 2021. Wound assessment and dressing selection: An overview. *British Journal of Nursing* 30(5), S12–S20.

Do, H.T., Edwards, H., Finlayson, K., 2016. Identifying relationships between symptom clusters and quality of life in adults with chronic mixed venous and arterial leg ulcers. *International Wound Journal* 13(5), 904–911.

Dowsett, C., von Hallern, B., 2017. The triangle of wound assessment: A holistic framework from wound assessment to management goals and treatments. *Wounds International* 8(4), 34–39.

Franks, P.J., Barker, J., 2016. Management of patients with venous leg ulcers. *Journal of Wound Care* 25(suppl 6), S1–S67.

Haesler, E., White, W., 2017. Minimising wound-related pain: A discussion of traditional wound dressings and topical agents used in low-resource communities. *Wound Practice & Research: Journal of the Australian Wound Management Association* 25(3), 138.

Haesler, E., Carville, K., 2023. *Australian standards for wound prevention and management*, 4th ed. Australian Health Research Alliance, Wounds Australia and WA Health Translation Network.

Holloway, S., Mahoney, K., 2021. Periwound skin care considerations for older adults. *Community Wound Care* 26(suppl 6), S26–S33.

Jaffe, L., Wu, S., 2017. The role of nutrition in chronic wound care management: What patients eat affects how they heal. *Podiatry Management* 36(9), 77–84.

Leaper, D.J., Schultz, G., Carville, K., et al., 2015. Extending the TIME concept: What have we learned in the past 10 years? *International Wound Journal* 9(suppl 2), 1–19.

LeBlanc, K., 2014. Skin tears best practices for care and prevention. *Nursing* 44(5), 36–46.

Murphy, C., Atkin, L., Vega de Ceniga, M., et al., 2022. International consensus document. Embedding wound hygiene into a proactive wound healing strategy. *Journal of Wound Care* 31, S1–S24.

Murphy, C., Atkin, L., Swanson, T., et al., 2020. International consensus document. Defying hard-to-heal wounds with an early antibiofilm intervention strategy: Wound hygiene. *Journal of Wound Care* 29(suppl 3b), S1–S28.

National Health and Medical Research Council (NHMRC), 2019. Australian guidelines for the prevention and control of infection in healthcare. Canberra. Available at: <https://www.nhmrc.gov.au/about-us/publications/australian-guidelines-prevention-and-control-infection-healthcare-2019>.

National Institute for Health and Care Excellence (NICE), 2020. Surgical site infections: Prevention and treatment. Available at: <https://www.nice.org.uk/guidance/ng125>.

NSW Health, 2022. NSW burn transfer guidelines—NSW Severe Burn Injury Service, 4th ed. (version 2). Available at: <https://aci.health.nsw.gov.au/__data/assets/pdf_file/0004/162634/ACI-Burn-transfer-guidelines.pdf>.

Nowak, M., Mehrholz, D., Barańska-Rybak, W., et al., 2022. Wound debridement products and techniques: Clinical examples and literature review. *Advances in Dermatology and Allergology* 39(3), 479–490.

Nursing and Midwifery Board of Australia (NMBA), 2020. Decision-making framework summary for nursing and midwifery. Available at: <https://www.nursingmidwiferyboard.gov.au/Codes-Guidelines-Statements/Frameworks.aspx>.

Percival, S.L., McCarty, S.M., Lipsky, B., 2015. Biofilms and wounds: An overview of the evidence. *Advances in Wound Care* 4(7), 373–381.

Posthauer, M.E., Banks, M., Dorner, B., et al., 2015. The role of nutrition for pressure ulcer management: National Pressure Ulcer Advisory Panel, European Pressure Ulcer Advisory Panel, and Pan Pacific Pressure Injury Alliance white paper. *Advances in Skin & Wound Care* 28(4), 175–188.

Ritchie, G., Taylor, H., 2018. Understanding compression: Part 2 – holistic assessment and clinical decision-making in leg ulcer management. *Journal of Community Nursing* 32(3), 22–29.

Sandoz, H., 2015. Negative pressure wound therapy: Clinical utility. *Chronic Wound Care Management and Research* 2, 71.

Sibbald, R.G., Goodman, L., Woo, K.Y., et al., 2012. Special considerations in wound bed preparation 2011: An update. *World Council of Enterostomal Therapists Journal* 32(2), 10–30.

Sorg, H., Tilkorn, D.J., Hager, S., et al., 2017. Skin wound healing: An update on the current knowledge and concepts. *European Surgical Research* 58, 81–94.

Stallard, Y., 2018. When and how to perform cultures on chronic wounds? *Journal of Wound, Ostomy, and Continence Nursing* 45(2), 179–186.

Wynn, M., 2021. The benefits and harms of cleansing for acute traumatic wounds: A narrative review. *Advances in Skin & Wound Care* 34, 488–492.

World Union of Wound Healing Societies (WUWHS), 2019. Consensus document. Wound exudate: Effective assessment and management. Wounds International. Available at: <https://woundsinternational.com/wp-content/uploads/sites/8/2023/02/836aed9753c3d8e3d8694bcaee336395.pdf>.

Wound Source, 2018. Types of wound dressings: Features, indications and contraindications. Available at: <https://www.woundsource.com/sites/default/files/whitepapers/types_of_wound_dressings_-_features_indications_and_contraindications.pdf>.

Online Resources

Aseptic Non-Touch Technique: <https://www.antt.org>. This website provides education, training, clinical practice, research, quality assurance and advising industry in improving standards of aseptic technique in clinical practice and supporting safe and standard practice to prevent healthcare-acquired infection (HAI).

Australasian College for Infection Prevention and Control (ACIPC): <https://www.acipc.org.au>.

Australian Commission and Safety and Quality in Health Care – Standards: <https://www.safetyandquality.gov.au/standards/nsqhs-standards>. Provide a nationally consistent statement of the level of care consumers can expect from health services organisations.

European Wound Management Association: <https://ewma.org>. EWMA website offers free access to EWMA documents and joint publications, covering different aspects of wound management as well as online courses, materials, networks and opportunities for professionals to engage in wound management education.

Hand Hygiene Australia: <https://www.hha.org.au>.

International Wound Infection Institute: <https://woundinfection-institute.com>. IWII provides up-to-date research and evidence relating to prevention, identification and management of wound infection.

JBI: <https://jbi.global>. JBI is a global organisation uses the best available evidence to promote and support evidence-based decisions that improve health and health service delivery.

National Pressure Injury Advisory Panel: <https://npiap.com>. NPIAP provides health professionals with education, public policy and research to improve patient outcomes in pressure injury prevention and management.

Nutrition Education Materials Online (NEMO) from Queensland Health: <https://www.health.qld.gov.au/nutrition>. NEMO provides access to the best nutrition education resources through the evidence-based information developed by experienced health professionals, or by providing links to the existing excellent resources.

Prevention and Treatment of Pressure Ulcers/Injuries: Clinical Practice Guidelines: <www.internationalguideline.com>. This clinical practice guideline provides the comprehensive evidence-based recommendations and good practice statements, together with implementation considerations, evidence summaries and evidence discussion.

Victorian Adult Burns Service, Alfred Health, Melbourne, Australia: <http://www.vicburns.org.au>. Victorian Adult Burns Service at The Alfred provides consistent standard of burn management for burn injuries and the direction to healthcare professionals (such as emergency department staff, general practitioners, physicians, general surgeons, nurses and paramedics) caring for adults or children with burn injuries in the primary care setting in Victoria.

Wounds Australia: <https://woundsaustralia.org/ocd.aspx>. This website provides resources on wound practice and research articles and standards and guidelines documents.

Wounds International: <https://woundsinternational.com>. This website provides resources on best practice statements and consensus documents that offer the peer-reviewed publications as well as the guiding principles in wound care.

CHAPTER 30

Nutrition

Ashleigh Djachenko

Key Terms

adipocytes
anabolism
anorexia nervosa
basal metabolic rate (BMR)
body mass index (BMI)
bulimia nervosa
carbohydrates
catabolism
disaccharides
dysphagia
enteral
essential amino acids
faltering growth
fat-soluble vitamins
malnutrition
monosaccharides
non-essential amino acids
overweight and obesity
pagophagia
polysaccharides
recommended dietary intake (RDI)
total parenteral nutrition (TPN)

Learning Outcomes

At the completion of this chapter and with further reading, learners should be able to:

- Define the key terms.
- Identify the major groups of essential nutrients.
- List the major vitamins required for health.
- List the eight major trace elements required for health.
- Identify the functions and common food sources of the essential nutrients.
- Describe the physical characteristics associated with a usual nutritional status.
- Identify factors and disorders that may affect an individual's nutritional status.
- Identify commonly used assessment techniques to measure an individual's nutritional status.
- State the components of a healthy balanced diet.
- State the principles of good nutrition throughout the lifespan.
- Recognise signs and symptoms of poor nutrition.
- Describe how the healthy balanced diet can be adapted to meet specific dietary beliefs and/or requirements.
- Apply appropriate principles to meet nutritional needs throughout the lifespan, during episodes of illness or alterations in physiological or psychological status.
- Assist in meeting an individual's nutritional needs accurately and safely in relation to assisting at mealtimes.
- Provide care for an individual requiring enteral and parenteral feeds.
- Have a clear understanding of the nurse's role in identifying malnutrition in individuals.

CHAPTER FOCUS

This chapter focuses on the nutritional needs of individuals over the lifespan and how a person's wellbeing can be affected by an alteration in the quantity and quality of absorbed nutrients. Nurses are required to assess and educate individuals to maintain nutritional health status and provide information on how to undertake care related to nutrition. Nutritional practices and requirements may vary according to age, height, sex, religion, culture, socioeconomic factors and physical and psychological status. Nurses must be able to accommodate for all these different factors when they plan care and provide health education for individuals as well as refer to the multidisciplinary team to optimise the care of the individual.

LIVED EXPERIENCE

Recently I was admitted to hospital for 10 days due to a worsening of my COPD (chronic obstructive pulmonary disease). When I was discharged, I only weighed 48 kg since I had lost 8 kg during my stay. Often meals were brought into my room, left on the table out of my reach and were made up of food that I didn't enjoy eating. When I would call the nurse, they would quickly move the tray over to me, saying they would be back later to assist with my meal. I could see they were busy and they would run out of the room before I could ask them if they would be able to help me with my meal order. Because of my shortness of breath and poor eyesight, I was unable to open a lot of the packaging and I had trouble cutting the food into smaller bites. It took me a long time to eat even a single mouthful since I often had to rest and catch my breath, and my mouth was often dry and the food hard to swallow. By the time the kitchen staff came to collect the tray, the food was cold and even more unappealing and my cup of tea was cold. After a few days my daughter spoke to the nursing unit manager and the nursing staff were asked to assist with my meals and meal order. They ensured I had my glasses on and was sitting out of bed when the meals were delivered. This meant I was better able to feed myself.

Michael, 72 years old

INTRODUCTION

Food and nutrition have long been recognised as important contributors to health. However, food and nutrition affect more than just the physical aspects of our health and wellbeing. The buying, preparing and eating of food is part of everyday life. For many cultures, including Australia, food is a focus for social interactions with family and friends. For some, it is also an economic concern (Australian Institute of Health and Welfare [AIHW] 2022a). Nutritional care in healthcare facilities requires a coordinated approach involving health professionals, support staff, the individual and their carers.

While eating has a psychosocial and cultural significance in life, the major roles of food intake are to provide nutrients necessary for the development and growth of cells and the replacement of substances required by cells to maintain efficient body function. Information about the ingestion and digestion of food and the absorption of nutrients is provided in Chapter 32. After the digested nutrients have been absorbed into the blood and lymph, they are distributed to the cells for further chemical processing, releasing the energy necessary for body function. The process of metabolism converts the nutrients into chemical forms that produce energy and rebuild body tissue. The two phases of metabolism are: **anabolism** (or constructive phase), when simple substances derived from the nutrients are converted into complex substances that can be used by the cells, and **catabolism** (or destructive phase), when these complex substances are reconverted into simpler forms to release the energy necessary for cell function (Harris et al 2019).

The term 'nutrition' is used to describe the processes by which the body uses nutrients for energy, growth, maintenance and repair (Grodner et al 2020). It is important to recognise that nutritional requirements vary in response to changes throughout the lifespan. Factors that increase the body's metabolic demand include the periods of rapid growth during infancy and adolescence, pregnancy and lactation, increased physical activity and periods of stress, disease or trauma. Metabolic requirements diminish with reduced energy demands, decreased physical activity and age (Green 2020).

Adequate nutrition is partially dependent on the ability of the body to ingest and digest food, to absorb nutrients from the intestine and to excrete waste products. Additionally, the quality and quantity of food consumed has an important influence on an individual's current and future health status. It is important that a diet contains the essential nutrients for each stage of the lifespan in order to maintain health and wellbeing.

Malnutrition is defined as a deficit, excess or imbalance of essential nutrients (DiMaria-Ghalili & McPherson 2020) and includes undernutrition (wasting, stunting or underweight), inadequate vitamins and minerals, overweight and obesity, and resulting diet-related noncommunicable diseases (WHO 2021a). Childhood and adult malnutrition can be classified into three broad groups, with the role of inflammation being a key factor. Starvation-related malnutrition refers to a clinical state in which nutritional needs are not met, causing chronic starvation without inflammation (e.g. anorexia nervosa). Chronic disease-related malnutrition occurs when tissue needs are not met due to sustained mild to moderate inflammation, even though the dietary intake would ordinarily be considered sufficient (e.g. organ failure, cancer, rheumatoid arthritis and obesity). The third category is acute disease- or injury-related malnutrition. This type of malnutrition results from a rapid increase in energy needs due to a severe inflammatory response (e.g. major infection, burns, trauma or post-surgery) (DiMaria-Ghalili & McPherson 2020).

Food is not just a source of nutrients. It is important for good social and emotional health as well as physical health. Food and eating are part of the way people live their lives. The eating patterns of individuals and families are constantly being shaped and changed by a variety of factors. Some of these include:

- availability and affordability of food
- ability to access and select culturally appropriate foods
- the amount of time available to shop for, prepare and cook food
- the dietary preferences of household members
- values, attitudes and beliefs about food and eating
- knowledge about food and nutrition (known as 'food literacy')
- conflicting messages (e.g. advertising of energy-dense but nutrient-poor foods)
- access to transport
- physical or psychological status of the individual such as allergies or an intolerance to specific foods or nutrients; difficulty in chewing or swallowing; level of independence/dependence; disorders that interfere with nutrition which may result in maldigestion, malabsorption or loss of nutrients (these, in turn, can lead to emotional states such as depression or anxiety, which may further impact on the physical or psychological status of the individual).

(AIHW 2021; 2022a)

NUTRITION ASSESSMENT

Nutrition risk screening should be inclusive of the nursing assessment on admission. It is essential to obtain information about the individual's appetite, food preferences, height, weight, food allergies, dysphagia, chronic diseases, level of activity, assistance required for eating, feeding and drinking, and social or physiological issues. Observation of an individual's general appearance provides information about their general state of health and their nutritional status. Some characteristics of altered nutritional status are presented in Table 30.1. Assessing the individual's eating pattern and their nutritional status may also identify problems or risk factors.

The Global Leadership Initiative on Malnutrition (GLIM) criteria for the diagnosis of malnutrition (Firman 2019) includes both phenotypic and etiologic criteria.

TABLE 30.1 | Clinical signs and symptoms of micronutrient deficiencies

Body region	Signs	Possible deficiencies
Skin	Petechiae	Vitamins A, C
	Purpura	Vitamins C, K
	Pigmentation	Niacin
	Oedema	Protein, vitamin B1
	Pallor	Folic acid, iron, biotin, vitamins B12, B6
	Decubitus	Protein, energy
	Seborrheic dermatitis	Vitamin B6, biotin, zinc, essential fatty acids
	Unhealed wounds	Vitamin C, protein, zinc
Nails	Pallor or white colouring Clubbing, spoon-shape, or transverse ridging /banding; excessive dryness, darkness in nails, curved nail ends	Iron, protein, vitamin B12
Head/hair	Dull/lacklustre; banding/sparse; alopecia; depigmentation of hair; scaly/flaky scalp	Protein and energy, biotin, copper, essential fatty acid

Continued

TABLE 30.1 | Clinical signs and symptoms of micronutrient deficiencies—cont'd

Body region	Signs	Possible deficiencies
Eyes	Pallor conjunctiva	Vitamin B12, folic acid, iron
	Night vision impairment	Vitamin A
	Photophobia	Zinc
Oral cavity	Glossitis	Vitamins B2, B6, B12, niacin, iron, folic acid
	Gingivitis	Vitamin C
	Fissures, stomatitis	Vitamin B2, iron, protein
	Cheilosis	Niacin, vitamins B2, B6, protein
	Pale tongue	Iron, vitamin B12
	Atrophied papillae	Vitamin B2, niacin, iron
Nervous system	Mental confusion	Vitamins B1, B2, B12, water
	Depression, lethargy	Biotin, folic acid, vitamin C
	Weakness, leg paralysis	Vitamins B1, B6, B12, pantothenic acid
	Peripheral neuropathy	Vitamins B2, B6, B12
	Ataxia	Vitamin B12
	Hyporeflexia	Vitamin B1
	Muscle cramps	Vitamin B6, calcium, magnesium
	Fatigue	Energy, biotin, magnesium, iron

(Pirlich et al 2018; Esper 2015)

A diagnosis of malnutrition requires at least one of each to be present.

Phenotypic:

- weight loss (%): >5% within past 6 months, or >10% beyond 6 months
- low body mass index: <20 if <70 years, or <22 if >70 years. Asia: <18.5 if <70 years, or <20 if >70 years
- reduced muscle mass.

Etiologic:

- reduced food intake or assimilation, or any chronic GI condition that adversely impacts food assimilation or absorption
- inflammation: acute disease/injury or chronic disease-related.

While these criteria associate malnutrition with undernutrition, it is recognised that a significant burden of malnutrition also exists in the overweight and obese population, due to inadequate micronutrient consumption and poor food quality (Freeman & Aggarwal 2020).

In addition to the physical characteristics associated with poor nutritional status, psychological symptoms may be evident. An individual with a poor nutritional status may experience irritability, lethargy, apathy or inability to concentrate. It is possible, however, that these symptoms and the physical signs presented in Table 30.1 may be related to an underlying condition and/or the person's nutritional status.

It is essential to determine the individual's nutrition risk by utilising a validated nutrition risk screening tool. The Malnutrition Screening Tool (MST) (Figure 30.1) is the most frequently reported screening tool utilised in Australian healthcare facilities. For further information on nutritional assessment see also Chapter 15. Others include the Subjective Global Assessment (SGA), the Patient Generated Subjective Global Assessment (PG-SGA) and the Mini-Nutritional Assessment (MNA) (Australian Commission on Safety and Quality in Health Care [ACSQHC] 2018). The result of nutrition risk screening must be documented in the healthcare record.

Risk factors for poor nutritional status include:

- increased age
- impaired mobility and/or frailty
- polypharmacy
- dysphagia
- chronic GIT/malabsorption conditions (e.g. Crohn's disease, cystic fibrosis)

Malnutrition Screening Tool (MST)
Please circle appropriate answer to each question.

Have you lost weight recently without trying? If No If Unsure	 0 2
If Yes, how much weight have you lost? 1–5 kg 6–10 kg 11–15 kg >15 kg Unsure	 1 2 3 4 2
Have you been eating poorly because of a decreased appetite? If No If Yes	 0 1
Total If the score is 2 or more please refer to the dietitian	
Date dietitian contacted	
Date seen by dietitian	

Figure 30.1 Malnutrition Screening Tool (MST)

(NSW Department of Health 2017)

- cognitive decline, dementia and delirium
- parkinson's disease
- pregnancy and lactating women
- eating disorders, 'fad' diets or dependencies.

(ACSQHC 2018)

Any person identified at risk of malnutrition needs prompt referral to a clinical dietitian for further nutrition assessment or to other health professionals for the management of specific issues which may affect their nutrition status. This includes swallowing, biting, chewing difficulties, impaired upper limb function affecting self-feeding, poor dentition, mental health issues or cognitive issues. To maintain or promote an appropriate intake of food and therefore a good nutritional status, individuals should be encouraged to follow the principles of a balanced healthy diet that provides the body with essential nutrients. However, it is also important when looking after individuals to take into account that while the consumption of food provides for the physiological needs of a person, it can also contribute to their social and emotional needs.

Nutritional assessment and the older person

When performing a nutritional assessment on an older person, it is important that the nurse determines the type, quantity and frequency of food eaten. Unintentional weight loss is associated with multiple poor health outcomes such as pressure injury development, depression, frailty, and decreased quality of life. In the older person, this can be attributed to a combination of protein–energy malnutrition, cachexia or physiological anorexia (a result of the ageing process on various body systems) (Mathewson et al 2021). The recent Royal Commission into Aged Care Quality and Safety (Commonwealth of Australia 2023) identified food and nutrition as one of the top four priority areas requiring immediate attention (along with dementia, restrictive practices and palliative care). Identification of poor nutrition in older persons can occur on admission to hospital, nursing homes, during follow-up outpatient appointments or at GP clinics. This can lead to improved health outcomes and better quality of life (ACSQHC 2018). Nurses should ask the older person about the following:

- any special diets (e.g. low-salt, low-carbohydrate) or self-prescribed diets
- intake of dietary fibre and prescribed or over-the-counter vitamins
- use of aperients
- weight loss and change of fit in clothing
- amount of money individuals have available to spend on food
- accessibility of food stores and suitable kitchen facilities
- variety and freshness of foods.

The ability to eat (e.g. to chew and swallow) needs to be evaluated. Poorly fitted dentures or decreased taste or smell may reduce the pleasure of eating, so individuals may eat less. Individuals with decreased vision, arthritis, immobility or tremors may have difficulty preparing meals and may injure or burn themselves when cooking. Individuals who are worried about urinary incontinence and frequency may reduce their fluid intake; as a result, they may eat less food.

While all older persons are at risk of malnutrition, individuals diagnosed with dementia are at increased risk. Throughout the assessment of the older person, it is therefore essential that cognitive function be assessed (Dementia Australia 2022).

It is important for the nurse to realise that ageing changes the interpretation of many measurements that reflect nutritional status in younger people. For example, ageing can alter height. Weight changes can reflect alterations in nutrition, fluid balance, or both. Despite these age-related changes, **body mass index (BMI)** is still useful in the older adult. If abnormalities in the nutrition history (e.g. weight loss, suspected deficiencies in essential nutrients) or BMI are identified, a thorough nutritional evaluation by the medical officer, which includes laboratory measurements, is indicated (Reber et al 2019).

CRITICAL THINKING EXERCISE 30.1

Elsa, an 86-year-old female, is admitted to the surgical ward with a fractured right neck of femur following a fall at home. On admission, you use the Malnutrition Screening Tool and she is found to be at risk of malnutrition. Discuss the importance of performing a nutritional assessment.

CRITICAL THINKING EXERCISE 30.2

Yasmin is an 18-year-old under investigation by her GP with dizziness, heat intolerance and shakiness. She has had unintentional weight loss of 8 kg over the past 5 months despite a reported healthy appetite and increased calorie intake. Other symptoms reported include intermittent palpitations, hair loss, change in menstrual cycle, sweating and irritability. The provisional diagnosis is hyperthyroidism. What care should you arrange to assist Yasmin in planning, regaining and maintaining her weight?

Healthy balanced diet

Eating a balanced diet is vital for good health and wellbeing. Food provides human bodies with the energy, protein, essential fats, vitamins and minerals to live, grow and function properly. People need a wide variety of different foods to provide the right amounts of nutrients for good health. Enjoyment of a healthy diet can also be one of the great cultural pleasures of life. The foods and dietary patterns that promote good nutrition are outlined in the Australian Dietary Guidelines (National Health and Medical Research Council [NHMRC] 2013a). There are five principal recommendations to be considered equally important in terms of public health outcomes:

1. To achieve and maintain a healthy weight, be physically active and choose amounts of nutritious food and drinks to meet your energy needs.
2. Enjoy a wide variety of nutritious foods from the five groups every day (see below).
3. Limit intake of foods containing saturated fat, added salt, added sugars and alcohol.
4. Encourage, support and promote breastfeeding.
5. Care for your food; prepare and store it safely.

(NHMRC 2013a)

The total amount of food that a person needs each day will vary depending on the person's age, sex and activity levels, and whether or not the person is pregnant or breastfeeding. The NHMRC (2017) provides **recommended dietary intake (RDI)** levels for energy and the various nutrients across various conditions, age and sex categories. The RDIs are specified in the nutrient reference values for Australia and New Zealand. RDIs or 'allowances' are the levels of intake of essential nutrients considered adequate to meet the nutritional needs of 97–98% of healthy individuals.

The Australian Guide to Healthy Eating (Figure 30.2) is Australia's current suggested food selection guide based on latest evidence and expert opinion (NHMRC 2013c). The guide aims to promote healthy eating habits throughout life to assist in reducing the risk of chronic health problems, such as heart disease, obesity and type 2 diabetes mellitus. The Australian Guide to Healthy Eating is a visual representation of the Australian Dietary Guidelines. The aim of the guide is to encourage the consumption of a variety of foods from each of the food groups every day in proportions that are consistent with the Australian Dietary Guidelines and to drink plenty of water.

The five foods groups are:

1. grain (cereal) foods—bread, cereals, rice, pasta, noodles
2. vegetables and legumes/beans
3. fruit
4. milk, yoghurt, cheese and/or alternatives
5. lean meat, fish, poultry, eggs, tofu, nuts, seeds and legumes/beans.

Furthermore, the Australian Guide to Healthy Eating highlights that fats and oils should be eaten only occasionally or in small amounts. See Figure 30.3 for information on how to understand food labels. For serve sizes, see Figure 30.4.

Nutritional needs of infants and children

Throughout all stages of development, a healthy balanced diet is necessary to provide the nutrients required for the body's needs. For information on maternal and newborn nutrition, see Chapter 45.

The WHO recommends that breastfeeding be initiated within an hour of birth and that children be exclusively breastfed for the first 6 months, meaning no other foods or liquids are provided, including water (WHO 2021b). At around 6 months of age, the child's energy requirements begin to exceed the amount provided by breast milk, so introduction of complementary or solid foods is recommended. When a child is ready to eat solids, at around 6 months of age (but not before 4 months), the parents/carers should introduce a new food every 2–3 days, starting with iron-rich foods (regardless of whether the food is thought to be highly allergenic). One new food should be introduced at a time so that reactions can be more clearly identified. If a food is tolerated, this should be continued as a part of a varied diet (ASCIA 2020).

The aim of introducing solids is to wean the infant off milk to prevent such problems as faltering growth, malnutrition and anaemia. Eating also becomes a learning process to educate the palate to different tastes and textures. Rice cereal, pureed stewed fruit and vegetables are suitable first foods. By 6–8 months of age, chewing movements begin and the infant can be introduced to more coarsely textured foods.

When the infant begins to grasp objects and put them in their mouth, they may be ready to be introduced to finger foods. An infant can take fluids from a cup at about 7–8 months of age. Giving fruit juice to a child from a bottle should be discouraged because high fructose levels may contribute to the development of jaw and tooth deformity and dental caries, and excessive volumes of fruit juice may result in diarrhoea.

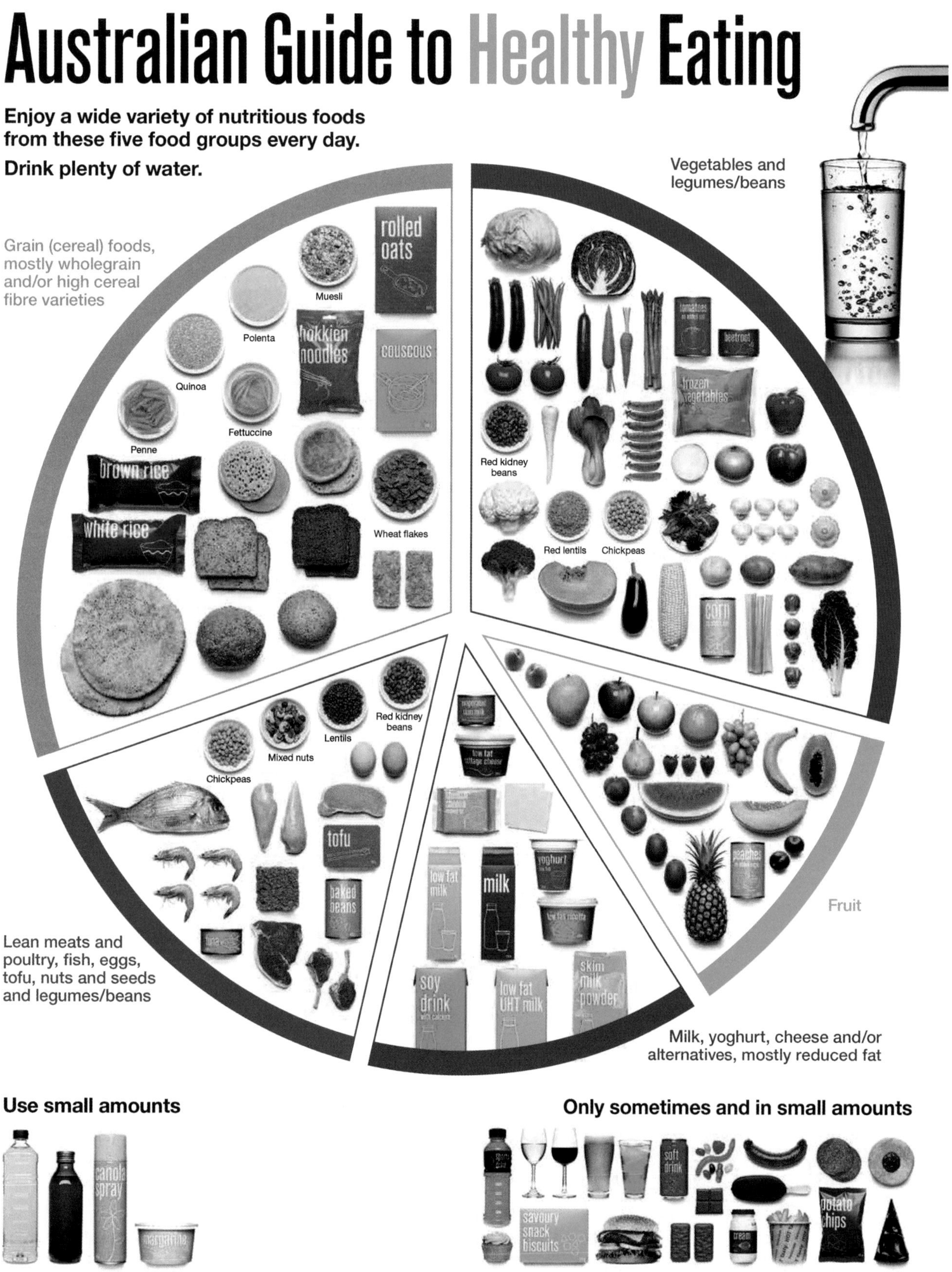
Australian Guide to Healthy Eating
Enjoy a wide variety of nutritious foods from these five food groups every day.
Drink plenty of water.
Grain (cereal) foods, mostly wholegrain and/or high cereal fibre varieties
rolled oats
Muesli
Polenta
Quinoa
hokkien noodles
couscous
Fettuccine
Penne
brown rice
white rice
Wheat flakes
Vegetables and legumes/beans
tomatoes
beetroot
frozen vegetables
Red kidney beans
Red lentils
Chickpeas
corn
Fruit
peaches
Chickpeas
Mixed nuts
Lentils
Red kidney beans
tofu
baked beans
tuna
Lean meats and poultry, fish, eggs, tofu, nuts and seeds and legumes/beans
low fat cottage cheese
yoghurt
low fat milk
milk
low fat ricotta
soy drink
low fat UHT milk
skim milk powder
Milk, yoghurt, cheese and/or alternatives, mostly reduced fat
Use small amounts
canola spray
margarine
Only sometimes and in small amounts
soft drink
savoury snack biscuits
cream
potato chips

Figure 30.2 The Australian Guide to Healthy Eating

(NHMRC 2013c)

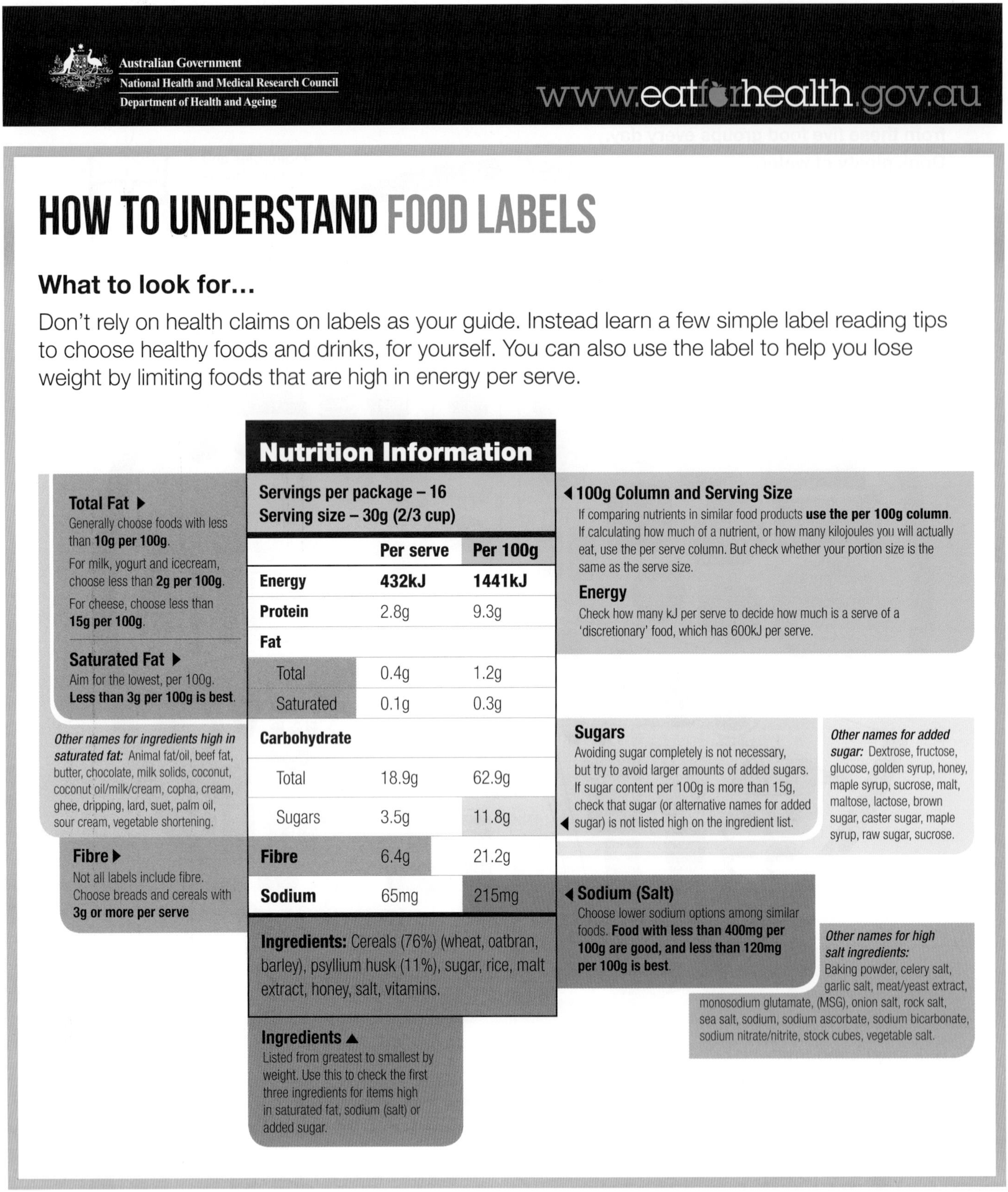
Australian Government
National Health and Medical Research Council
Department of Health and Ageing
www.eatforhealth.gov.au
HOW TO UNDERSTAND FOOD LABELS
What to look for...
Don't rely on health claims on labels as your guide. Instead learn a few simple label reading tips to choose healthy foods and drinks, for yourself. You can also use the label to help you lose weight by limiting foods that are high in energy per serve.
Nutrition Information
Servings per package – 16
Serving size – 30g (2/3 cup)
Per serve | Per 100g
Energy 432kJ 1441kJ
Protein 2.8g 9.3g
Fat
Total 0.4g 1.2g
Saturated 0.1g 0.3g
Carbohydrate
Total 18.9g 62.9g
Sugars 3.5g 11.8g
Fibre 6.4g 21.2g
Sodium 65mg 215mg
Ingredients: Cereals (76%) (wheat, oatbran, barley), psyllium husk (11%), sugar, rice, malt extract, honey, salt, vitamins.
Total Fat ▶
Generally choose foods with less than 10g per 100g.
For milk, yogurt and icecream, choose less than 2g per 100g.
For cheese, choose less than 15g per 100g.
Saturated Fat ▶
Aim for the lowest, per 100g. Less than 3g per 100g is best.
Other names for ingredients high in saturated fat: Animal fat/oil, beef fat, butter, chocolate, milk solids, coconut, coconut oil/milk/cream, copha, cream, ghee, dripping, lard, suet, palm oil, sour cream, vegetable shortening.
Fibre ▶
Not all labels include fibre. Choose breads and cereals with 3g or more per serve
◀ 100g Column and Serving Size
If comparing nutrients in similar food products use the per 100g column. If calculating how much of a nutrient, or how many kilojoules you will actually eat, use the per serve column. But check whether your portion size is the same as the serve size.
Energy
Check how many kJ per serve to decide how much is a serve of a 'discretionary' food, which has 600kJ per serve.
Sugars
Avoiding sugar completely is not necessary, but try to avoid larger amounts of added sugars. If sugar content per 100g is more than 15g, check that sugar (or alternative names for added ◀ sugar) is not listed high on the ingredient list.
Other names for added sugar: Dextrose, fructose, glucose, golden syrup, honey, maple syrup, sucrose, malt, maltose, lactose, brown sugar, caster sugar, maple syrup, raw sugar, sucrose.
◀ Sodium (Salt)
Choose lower sodium options among similar foods. Food with less than 400mg per 100g are good, and less than 120mg per 100g is best.
Other names for high salt ingredients:
Baking powder, celery salt, garlic salt, meat/yeast extract, monosodium glutamate, (MSG), onion salt, rock salt, sea salt, sodium, sodium ascorbate, sodium bicarbonate, sodium nitrate/nitrite, stock cubes, vegetable salt.
Ingredients ▲
Listed from greatest to smallest by weight. Use this to check the first three ingredients for items high in saturated fat, sodium (salt) or added sugar.

Figure 30.3 How to understand food labels

(NHMRC 2019)

SERVE SIZES

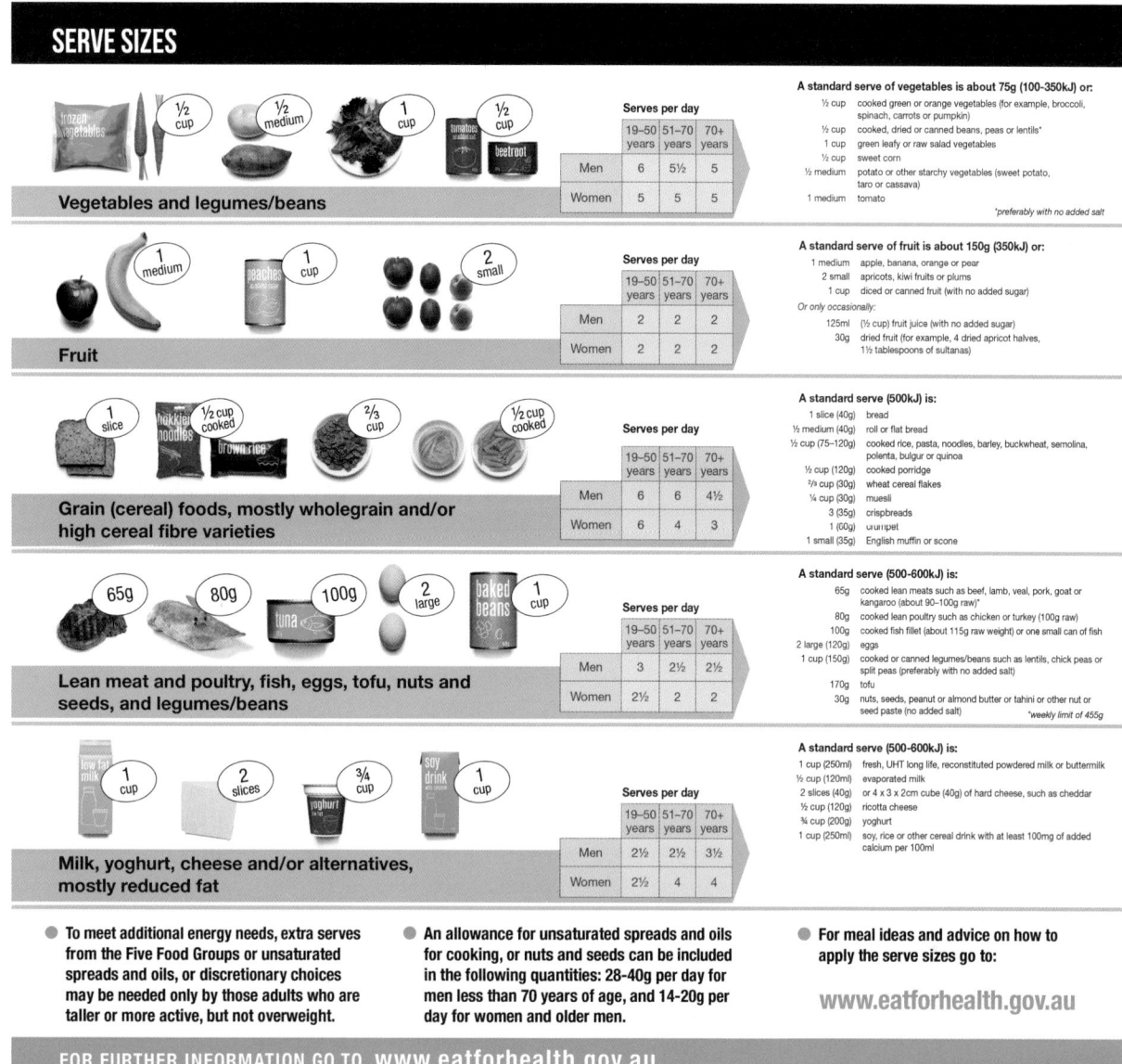

Vegetables and legumes/beans

Serves per day	19–50 years	51–70 years	70+ years
Men	6	5½	5
Women	5	5	5

A standard serve of vegetables is about 75g (100-350kJ) or:

½ cup	cooked green or orange vegetables (for example, broccoli, spinach, carrots or pumpkin)
½ cup	cooked, dried or canned beans, peas or lentils*
1 cup	green leafy or raw salad vegetables
½ cup	sweet corn
½ medium	potato or other starchy vegetables (sweet potato, taro or cassava)
1 medium	tomato

**preferably with no added salt*

Fruit

Serves per day	19–50 years	51–70 years	70+ years
Men	2	2	2
Women	2	2	2

A standard serve of fruit is about 150g (350kJ) or:

1 medium	apple, banana, orange or pear
2 small	apricots, kiwi fruits or plums
1 cup	diced or canned fruit (with no added sugar)

Or only occasionally:

125ml	(½ cup) fruit juice (with no added sugar)
30g	dried fruit (for example, 4 dried apricot halves, 1½ tablespoons of sultanas)

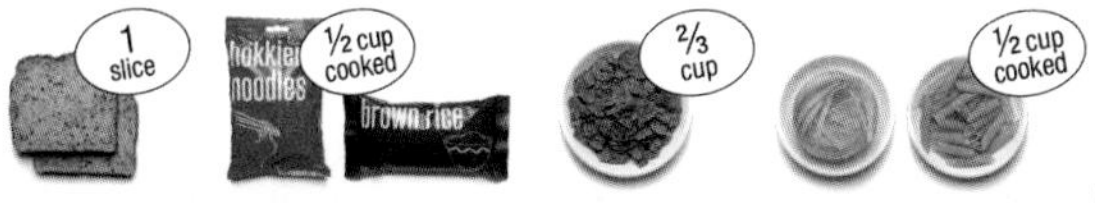

Grain (cereal) foods, mostly wholegrain and/or high cereal fibre varieties

Serves per day	19–50 years	51–70 years	70+ years
Men	6	6	4½
Women	6	4	3

A standard serve (500kJ) is:

1 slice (40g)	bread
½ medium (40g)	roll or flat bread
½ cup (75–120g)	cooked rice, pasta, noodles, barley, buckwheat, semolina, polenta, bulgur or quinoa
½ cup (120g)	cooked porridge
⅔ cup (30g)	wheat cereal flakes
¼ cup (30g)	muesli
3 (35g)	crispbreads
1 (60g)	crumpet
1 small (35g)	English muffin or scone

Lean meat and poultry, fish, eggs, tofu, nuts and seeds, and legumes/beans

Serves per day	19–50 years	51–70 years	70+ years
Men	3	2½	2½
Women	2½	2	2

A standard serve (500-600kJ) is:

65g	cooked lean meats such as beef, lamb, veal, pork, goat or kangaroo (about 90–100g raw)*
80g	cooked lean poultry such as chicken or turkey (100g raw)
100g	cooked fish fillet (about 115g raw weight) or one small can of fish
2 large (120g)	eggs
1 cup (150g)	cooked or canned legumes/beans such as lentils, chick peas or split peas (preferably with no added salt)
170g	tofu
30g	nuts, seeds, peanut or almond butter or tahini or other nut or seed paste (no added salt)

**weekly limit of 455g*

Milk, yoghurt, cheese and/or alternatives, mostly reduced fat

Serves per day	19–50 years	51–70 years	70+ years
Men	2½	2½	3½
Women	2½	4	4

A standard serve (500-600kJ) is:

1 cup (250ml)	fresh, UHT long life, reconstituted powdered milk or buttermilk
½ cup (120ml)	evaporated milk
2 slices (40g)	or 4 x 3 x 2cm cube (40g) of hard cheese, such as cheddar
½ cup (120g)	ricotta cheese
¾ cup (200g)	yoghurt
1 cup (250ml)	soy, rice or other cereal drink with at least 100mg of added calcium per 100ml

- **To meet additional energy needs, extra serves from the Five Food Groups or unsaturated spreads and oils, or discretionary choices may be needed only by those adults who are taller or more active, but not overweight.**
- **An allowance for unsaturated spreads and oils for cooking, or nuts and seeds can be included in the following quantities: 28-40g per day for men less than 70 years of age, and 14-20g per day for women and older men.**
- **For meal ideas and advice on how to apply the serve sizes go to:**

www.eatforhealth.gov.au

FOR FURTHER INFORMATION GO TO www.eatforhealth.gov.au

Figure 30.4 Serve sizes

(NHMRC 2015)

At about 12 months of age, the infant should be eating a range of basic foods. The diet should consist of bread and cereals, fruit and vegetables, meat and/or other protein foods, milk and/or milk products and small amounts of butter or margarine. Salt, sugar and fatty foods should be avoided (NHMRC 2012).

The toddler and preschool child

During this stage of development, a child's rate of growth is slower than in infancy and this is normally reflected by a decrease in appetite, although appetite is generally unpredictable during these years. Toddlers are learning to feed themselves and to eat new foods. They should eat a variety of nutritious foods from all five food groups.

CRITICAL THINKING EXERCISE 30.3

Noah, a 5-week-old infant, presents to emergency with frequent gagging and vomiting post feeds. Noah's mum, Georgia, describes the vomits as large, non-projectile undigested milk with no reports of blood visible. Georgia appears tired and describes Noah as having frequent episodes of crying, and being unable to be consoled, particularly in the late afternoon. She is concerned that Noah is not tolerating adequate amounts of breast milk and that he may become dehydrated. Noah is examined in the department and has bare weight of 4.2 kg, length 56 cm, head circumference 36.5 cm. What would you discuss with Georgia and her medical officer?

Toddlers in particular need an adequate iron and calcium intake, with low-fat diets not suitable for children less than 2 years.

Foods should be served at regular times in a calm and relaxed atmosphere. Because young children are active, snacks between meals are important. The foods offered for snacks should contribute to the nutritional needs of the child, while foods with poor nutritional value should be avoided. Small hard foods, such as nuts, raw carrots and popcorn, are potentially dangerous for the young child since these may be inhaled and obstruct airways.

The school-age child

During the first 12 months of life, the foundation is laid down for good dietary practices. By the time the child is of school age, eating patterns are usually firmly established. As the child grows and develops, their tastes can change, and foods that were previously enjoyed may be refused, while the child may acquire a taste for other foods, due in part to social interaction and their changing physiological needs and subsequent sensory changes.

Nutritional requirements are similar to those for children of preschool age, although kilojoule needs are diminished in relation to body size. However, fat and protein reserves are being laid down for the increased growth needs of the adolescent period, and the school-age child should be encouraged to consume a healthy balanced diet consisting of foods from each of the five food groups and should be discouraged from consuming foods that have poor nutritional value. If the child consumes an excessive quantity of food and/or food that is high in kilojoules, and does not exercise, they may be at risk of childhood obesity and subsequent development of conditions such as adult-onset diabetes mellitus and cardiovascular disease. The Australian Institute of Health and Welfare (AIHW) (2020) reported that in 2017–2018, about one in four (27%) children and adolescents aged 2–17 were overweight or obese and one in 12 (8.2%) were obese. Similar proportions of girls and boys were obese for children aged 2–4 and 5–17 years.

While the prevalence of childhood overweight and obesity increased in Western countries during the 1980s to the late 1990s, more recent studies have reported a significant plateau in the prevalence of both overweight and obesity since the late 1990s (AIHW 2020). Childhood obesity is associated in later life with chronic conditions such as coronary heart disease, stroke, type 2 diabetes mellitus and osteoarthritis (Weihrauch-Blüher et al 2018). Iron-deficiency anaemia is a more immediate nutritional problem in school-age children due to inadequate amounts of iron in the diet.

Adolescence

From 10 years of age, children's bodies are developing rapidly to prime the body for reproduction. A pre-puberty growth spurt occurs earlier in girls than in boys, as they store more fat, which initiates adolescence faster. (See Chapter 22.) During adolescence, the need for nutrients including energy, protein, vitamins and minerals increases. During this time there can be major changes in the selection and volume of food; however, it is important to continue choosing nutritious foods across the food groups (NHMRC 2013a). Hormones alter senses such as taste to enable the adolescent to adapt to changing nutrient requirements. Some individuals at this age may be vulnerable to self, peer and social influences that alter their perception of appearance and self-worth and drastically modify their eating habits (see the 'Eating disorders' section later in this chapter). (See Case Study 30.1.)

Older persons

The ageing process has significant impact on nutrition due to a decline in biological and physiological function. Older individuals have reduced lean body mass and basal metabolic rate as well as often reduced appetite and energy expenditure. While requirements for some nutrients are reduced, requirements for other essential nutrients (such as calcium and vitamin D) may increase (Nutrition Australia 2021).

Energy requirements

In addition to the consumption of foods from the five food groups that provide the essential nutrients, dietary requirements need to be considered in terms of energy requirements. Energy is needed for all the chemical and physical activities of the body, such as muscular activity,

CASE STUDY 30.1

Erina, an 11-year-old girl, has been brought into hospital for an adenoidectomy and tonsillectomy. While admitting her, you discover she weighs 78 kg. She is accompanied by her mother, who you notice is also overweight. As a nurse in the team looking after Erina, it is important that your care of Erina is person-centred and ensures that Erina has the best possible health outcomes both in the hospital and on discharge.

1. What are the implications Erina's weight may have on her short-term and long-term health?
2. Does Erina's weight have any implications for her preoperative and postoperative care? If yes, what are these concerns?
3. How would you as the nurse caring for Erina address her weight issue? Is it appropriate to also involve her parents in this discussion?
4. What nursing advice would you give to Erina and her family? How would you address an issue like Erina's diet, which could have health behavioural implications?

production of glandular secretions and the synthesis of substances in cells. The amount of energy required is the amount necessary to maintain physiological processes and depends on factors such as age, sex, climate, body build, height and weight, level of physical activity and usual function or dysfunction.

Energy requirements are increased during periods of rapid growth. For example, during pregnancy, infancy and adolescence and when a person engages in a high level of physical activity. Certain types of body dysfunction, such as hyperthyroidism, can also increase the amount of energy required. Energy requirements are decreased when an individual's level of physical activity is low, with certain metabolic conditions, such as hypothyroidism, and during stages of development when there is little growth, such as old age (Dains et al 2020).

The two units of measurement that specify the energy value of food are calories and joules. A calorie is defined as the amount of heat required to raise 1 g of water by 1°C. A joule, which is the standard international (SI) unit of energy and heat, is equivalent to the amount of work performed when a 1 kg mass is moved 1 m by the force of 1 newton. One calorie is equal to 4.184 joules. Since joules are very small units, it is more convenient to measure food energy in terms of kilojoules. One kilojoule (kJ) is 1000 joules.

The energy values of the three major types of nutrients are as follows:

1. 1 g protein produces about 17 kJ.
2. 1 g carbohydrate produces about 17 kJ.
3. 1 g fat produces about 38 kJ.

(NHMRC 2017)

Energy expenditure varies with the level of physical activity a person engages in and ranges from about 5 kJ/min during sleep to about 120 kJ/min during heavy physical activity. When the intake of kilojoules is increased or energy expenditure is decreased, weight gain occurs. Conversely, loss of weight occurs when the intake of kilojoules is decreased or energy expenditure is increased (Dains et al 2020). Basal metabolism is the term used to describe the minimal maintenance of all normal body functions at rest and in the absence of disease. The amount of energy required to support basal metabolism is measured when an individual is awake but at complete rest and has not eaten for at least 12 hours. The measurement is expressed as **basal metabolic rate (BMR)**, according to the number of kilojoules consumed per hour per square metre of body surface area (or per kilogram of body weight) (Harris et al 2019). The BMR is one diagnostic test commonly used to estimate nutritional needs. Variations in the BMR between individuals of the same weight and height may be due to alteration in body composition, such as muscle mass as opposed to fatty tissue, and the presence of certain disease states.

There are two types of measurement that may be used by clinicians when determining body fat and risk of chronic disease. These are the BMI and waist circumference.

The BMI is a simple index of weight-for-height that is commonly used to classify underweight, overweight and obesity in adults. It is defined as the weight in kilograms divided by the square of the height in metres (kg/m^2). For example, the BMI of a male who is 1.83 m tall and weighs 115 kg is:

$$\frac{115}{1.83^2} = \text{BMI of } 34$$

The value obtained when this formula is used should be rounded to the nearest whole number.

BMI values are age-independent and the same for both sexes. The BMI has limitations and should be used as a screening tool rather than a diagnostic standard. The BMI measurement does not account for differences based on body frame size, body fat distribution, effects of physical training, puberty or menopausal status, amputations or deformities (Grantham 2020). The health risks associated with increasing BMI are continuous and the interpretation of BMI grading in relation to risk may vary for different populations.

A BMI value below 18.5 is classified as underweight. A BMI of 18.5–24.9 is classified as within the healthy weight range. A BMI of 25–29.9 is classified as overweight, while a value of greater than 30 is classified as obese (WHO 2021c). However, BMI may not correspond to the same degree of fatness in different populations due, in part, to different body proportions. For people of Asian descent, BMI cutoff points have been adjusted downward. In these people, a BMI of 18.5–22.9 is normal, between 23–27.4 is overweight and greater than 27.5 is obese. People of Asian descent may experience delayed diagnosis of obesity and overweight if BMI values are not adjusted downward (Elsevier 2021). For graphical representation of BMI, see Figure 30.5.

The waist measurement compares closely with a person's body mass index, and is another widely utilised scale of predicting an individual's risk of developing a chronic disease and a common measure of overweight and obesity. Excessive body fat around the abdomen (central adiposity) is an indicator of internal fat deposits on the heart, kidneys, pancreas and liver. A waist measurement of greater than 94 cm for men and 80 cm for women is an indicator of increased risk of chronic disease development such as type 2 diabetes mellitus and cardiovascular disease (AIHW 2022b). An advantage of using waist circumference is that the measurement is not related to the individual's height; however, specific ethnic group waist measurements are yet to be determined (Grodner 2020).

Measuring a person's waistline is a simple check for a nurse to perform and for accurate measurement the nurse should ensure the following:

- Measurement occurs against the skin.
- The person breathes out normally.
- The tape measure is snug but does not compress the skin.

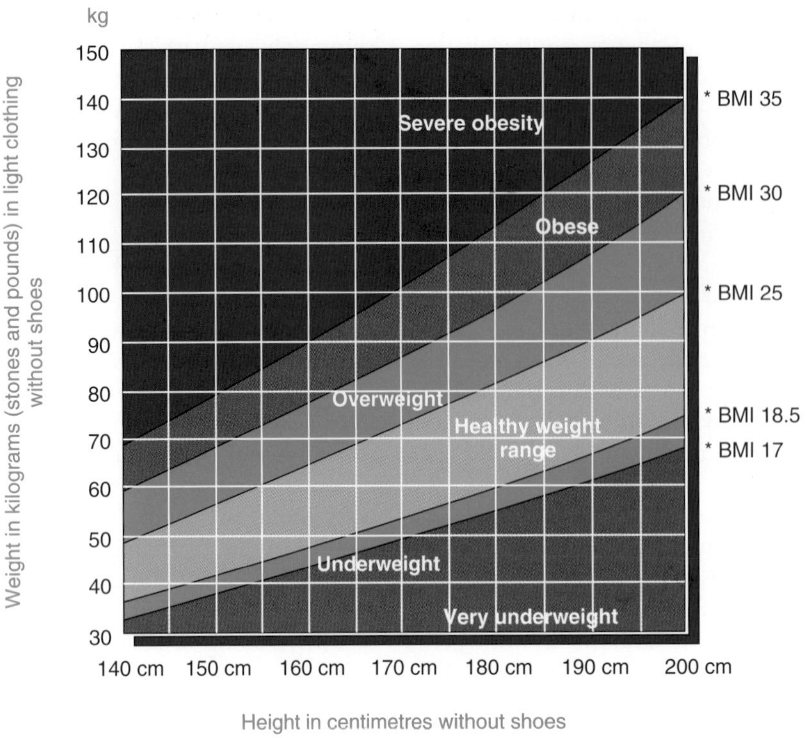

$$\text{* Body mass index (BMI)} = \frac{\text{Weight (kg)}}{\text{Height}^2\text{ (metres)}}$$

Figure 30.5 Body mass index for adults

(NHMRC 2013b)

- The correct place to measure the waist is horizontally halfway between the lowest rib and the top of the iliac crest. This is roughly in line with the individual's umbilicus (belly button).

(Kawaji & Fontanilla 2021)

Glycaemic index

Glycaemic index (GI) classifies carbohydrate foods according to how rapidly glucose is released from them and absorbed into the blood. It has traditionally been used to treat individuals with diabetes mellitus but is now being used for establishing optimal diets for the general populace. The lower the GI, the slower the rate of absorption and the slower the rate of insulin release. Complex carbohydrates such as starch provide lower GI nutrients and result in a more stable blood glucose level (Harris et al 2019).

Some simple carbohydrates, such as those found in fruits, have a lower GI value than some complex carbohydrates, such as those found in rice and potatoes. Foods with low-GI values have been used to treat hypercholesterolaemia and obesity (Vidal-Ostos et al 2022), and there is evidence to suggest that high-GI foods may contribute to overall cancer risk (Long et al 2022). Low-GI foods include multigrain breads, bran, legumes, milk, yoghurt and fruits. High-GI foods, of which there are more than 70, include rice, potatoes, wholemeal and white bread, and some cereals. Further health benefits may be gained by including foods that are high in fibre.

NUTRIENTS

Nutrients are chemical substances in food that provide energy, build and maintain cells or regulate body processes. The essential nutrients are:

- carbohydrates
- proteins
- lipids (fats)
- water
- fibre
- vitamins
- mineral salts.

Carbohydrates

Carbohydrates are a group of organic compounds that includes sugar, starch and cellulose. They are composed of one or more monosaccharide (single-sugar) units. Sugars can be classified as either simple or complex and are divided into groups according to the complexity of their molecular structure. Simple sugars, or **monosaccharides**, include glucose, fructose and galactose (Harris et al 2019).

Disaccharides, which are a combination of two sugars, include sucrose, lactose and maltose. For example, glucose and fructose combine to form sucrose. Complex sugars or **polysaccharides** are a combination of many sugars and include starch, glycogen and cellulose. Before carbohydrates can be utilised by the body cells, disaccharides and polysaccharides must be converted by chemical digestion into glucose.

Carbohydrates provide energy, assist in the metabolism of fat and act as a protein sparer (if there is insufficient carbohydrate in the diet, protein is converted to glucose and used for energy). Carbohydrate foods also supply indigestible cellulose, which adds bulk to the intestinal contents, resulting in stimulation of peristalsis. The major food sources of carbohydrates are:

- sugars, present in fruits, honey, cane sugar, milk and cereals
- starch, present in vegetables, cereals and foods made from cereals (e.g. bread and pasta)
- cellulose, present in vegetables, fruits and cereals (complex carbohydrates).

Proteins

Proteins are a group of nitrogenous compounds composed of chains of amino acid subunits. Twenty-two amino acids have been identified in humans. Eight of these, the **essential amino acids**, the body is unable to make, and they must be obtained from dietary sources. The remaining 14 **non-essential amino acids** can be synthesised by the body. Before proteins can be utilised by the cells, they must be broken down by physical and chemical digestion into their constituent amino acids. According to the number and type of amino acids present, proteins are classed as either complete (containing all essential amino acids) or incomplete (lacking one or more essential amino acids) (Harris et al 2019).

Proteins build and repair tissue and supply energy (protein that is not needed for growth and repair of tissues is converted into glucose and stored in the liver and muscles as a reserve store of energy). The major food sources of protein are meat, fish, eggs, cheese, milk, poultry and soya beans (complete [or first-class] protein), and cereals, lentils, legumes and nuts (incomplete [or second-class] protein).

Lipids (fats)

Lipids are a group of substances that are insoluble in water and are composed of fatty acids and glycerol. Fatty acids are classed as saturated or unsaturated. Saturated, or solid, fats are chiefly of animal origin, such as butter, and contain a full complement of hydrogen. Unsaturated, or soft or liquid, fats are chiefly of vegetable origin, such as margarine, and are capable of adding more hydrogen to their molecular structure.

Before fats can be utilised by the body cells, they must be broken down by chemical digestion into their constituent fatty acids and glycerol. Fat supplies energy and may be used in the tissues or stored in adipose tissue, which functions to support and protect nerves and organs from trauma, insulate the body to prevent excessive heat loss or gain and as a reserve store of fuel. Fats also supply the **fat-soluble vitamins** A, D, E and K as well as stimulating adolescence, fertility and mood, and suppressing appetite through the action of hormones such as leptin, secreted by **adipocytes** (Harris et al 2019).

The major food sources of fat are animal fats, present in meat, butter, cream, egg yolk, cheese and fish oils, and vegetable fats, present in margarine, cocoa and oils such as olive, safflower, corn and peanut.

Water

Water is a chemical compound obtained by the body from food and fluid and resulting from the metabolism of protein, fat and carbohydrate in the tissues. Water constitutes about 60% of the total body weight in an adult and is present as intracellular fluid and extracellular fluid. Water is also the basis of all body secretions and excretions.

Water is necessary for the digestion, absorption and metabolism of food, for the production of secretions and for the maintenance of body fluids. Water is also necessary for the regulation of body temperature by evaporation of sweat, and for the elimination of waste products through the kidneys, bowel, skin and lungs.

Water is present in all body fluids and as part of the cellular structure of solid foods. Foods vary in water content; fruit and vegetables contain about 80–90% water, meat contains about 70% and bread contains about 35%.

Fibre

Dietary fibre, also referred to as cellulose, consists of the non-digestible forms of carbohydrate that usually come from plant-based foods. Although fibre is not generally considered an essential nutrient, it is recognised to have a significant impact on gut flora, insulin sensitivity and overall metabolic health (Barber et al 2020). Fibre creates bulk in the stools, which enhances gut motility and defecation. Dietary fibre may prevent or minimise symptoms of certain disorders, such as haemorrhoids, diverticular disease, formation of gallstones, simple constipation and intestinal cancer (Harris et al 2019). Foods with high fibre content are fruits, vegetables and wholegrain products. Clinical Interest Box 30.1 provides discussion of the management of constipation in the older person.

Vitamins

Vitamins are a group of organic compounds that, with few exceptions, must be obtained from dietary sources. Although they have no energy value, they are essential for normal metabolic and physiological bodily function. The term 'vitamin' was first used in 1912, and letters of the alphabet were assigned to them as they were discovered. Now that more is known about their composition, the chemical name for a vitamin is frequently used.

Vitamins are classed as being either water- or fat-soluble. The water-soluble vitamins are easily destroyed during the

CLINICAL INTEREST BOX 30.1 Constipation and the older adult

Constipation can occur at any age but is common in the older adult, associated with diminished exercise, fibre and fluid intake, as well as diminished neurogenic gastrointestinal regulation. Aged-care home residents and hospital inpatients are at increased risk. Measures to avoid constipation are required to reduce the incidence of conditions such as diverticulosis, megacolon, carcinoma, stroke and heart attack. A detailed history is required including past medical and family history, medications (including any over-the-counter and laxative remedies) and symptoms. A nutritional assessment of dietary intake is required, as is examination for any underlying pathologies. Laboratory tests and abdominal imaging may be required in severe cases where the underlying cause is not identifiable. First-line treatment of constipation is to increase dietary fibre and fluid intake. Fibre is obtained mainly from grains and cereals. Synthetic bulking agents such as psyllium may be considered but an adequate fluid intake is essential, as bulking agents can worsen constipation if fluid intake is insufficient. If laxatives are deemed necessary, osmotic laxatives (such as magnesium hydroxide) are preferred to irritant laxatives (such as bisocodyl) as the latter can lead to decreased bowel motility and dependency.

(Ferri 2022)

preparation and prolonged cooking of food. If they are consumed in excess of the body's need, they are excreted in the urine. Fat-soluble vitamins are oxidised by exposure to air, light and high temperatures. Since fat-soluble vitamins are not soluble in water, any excess is stored in the body, and a condition known as hypervitaminosis may occur, which may result in organ failure (Harris et al 2019).

Excessive intake of vitamin A over long periods can result in hypervitaminosis A, a condition characterised by yellow discolouration of the skin (often mistaken as jaundice), loss of appetite and dry itchy skin. Excessive intake of vitamin B may result in allergic-type reactions. Hypervitaminosis D may occur if excessive amounts of vitamin D are taken in and is characterised by nausea, vomiting, diarrhoea, general irritability and severe impairment of kidney function. In normal circumstances, a healthy balanced diet will provide the body with sufficient quantities of all vitamins without the need for supplemental vitamin ingestion. Table 30.2 describes the functions and effects of vitamin deficiencies.

Mineral salts

Mineral salts are a group of compounds that play an important role in metabolism, maintenance of blood pressure, cardiac function, fluid and electrolyte balance, acid–base balance and the regulation of other body processes. Storage and processing of food does not alter its mineral content, although mineral salts may be lost when food is soaked or cooked in water. The elements that mineral salts contain are

TABLE 30.2 | Vitamins and health

Vitamin	Functions	Sources	Effects of deficiency
Vitamin A (retinol or carotenes)	Sustains normal vision in dim light, promotes healthy growth of epithelial tissue and bone and therefore raises resistance to infection	Cod liver oil, liver, kidney, egg yolk, milk and dairy products, yellow fruits and yellow and green vegetables	Night blindness, keratinisation of epithelial tissue (and therefore less resistance to infection), stunted growth, zinc deficiency
Thiamine (B1)	Nerve function Energy and carbohydrate metabolism	Yeast extract, wholegrain cereals, meats, leafy green vegetables	Polyneuritis, beriberi, Wernicke–Korsakoff syndrome, lack of muscular and mental development
Riboflavin (B2)	Energy and protein metabolism, cellular respiration, healthy skin and mucous membranes	Liver, yeast extract, milk and dairy products, eggs, green leafy vegetables	Fissures at the corner of mouth (cheilosis), angular stomatitis, glossitis, dermatitis, failure to thrive
Niacin (B3)	Energy utilisation; metabolism of fat, carbohydrate and protein; nervous system function	Liver, bran, meat, fish, yeast extract, legumes	Pellagra (diarrhoea, dermatitis, dementia); glossitis, anaemia
Pantothenic acid (B5)	Metabolism of carbohydrates, protein and fat; formation of haemoglobin and acetylcholine	Offal, yeast, fish, meat, egg yolk, apricots	Fatigue, sleep disturbances, headaches, personality changes, irritability

TABLE 30.2 | Vitamins and health—cont'd

Vitamin	Functions	Sources	Effects of deficiency
Pyridoxine (B6)	Protein metabolism, nervous system function, formation of red blood cells	Liver, fish, meat, wholegrain cereals, bananas, avocado, egg yolk, peanuts	Neuritis, depression, anaemia, EEG and ECG changes, cheilosis, renal stone formation
Cyanocobalamin (B12)	Formation of red cells and nucleic acids	All foods of animal origin	Pernicious anaemia, CNS atrophy, vision loss
Biotin	Synthesis of fatty acids, metabolism of carbohydrates and fat, gluconeogenesis	Liver, brewer's yeast, fish, offal, soya beans	Lethargy, dermatitis, EEG and ECG changes, hypercholesterolaemia
Folic acid (folacin, folate)	Metabolism, DNA and RNA synthesis, formation of haemoglobin	Liver, citrus fruit, offal, nuts, leafy green vegetables	Macrocytic anaemia, malabsorption
Vitamin C (ascorbic acid)	Formation of collagen, assists in wound healing, maintenance of capillaries, production of neurotransmitters, aids absorption of iron	Citrus fruits, tropical fruits, berry fruits, tomatoes, potatoes, green vegetables	Delayed healing, bleeding tendencies, scurvy, reduced nervous system and muscle function
Vitamin D (calciferol)	Calcium and phosphorus metabolism, immune function	Cod liver oil, fish, butter, margarine, egg yolk, sunlight on the skin	Rickets, osteomalacia
Vitamin E (alpha-tocopherol)	Antioxidant action protects the cell membrane, prevents heart disease and delays the ageing process (not yet confirmed)	Wheatgerm, vegetable oil, wholegrain cereals, nuts, legumes	Muscle degeneration, haemolytic anaemia in the newborn, infertility, malabsorption
Vitamin K (menadione)	Formation of clotting factors II, VII, IX and X; assists in regulating calcium metabolism	Liver, leafy green vegetables, egg yolk, synthesised by bacterial flora in the gastrointestinal tract	Bleeding tendencies

(Mann & Truswell 2017)

classed as either major or trace elements; trace elements are present in only minute quantities in the body. A mineral salt that has the property of being a conductor of electrical current is referred to as an electrolyte. The functions and effects of mineral salt deficiencies are listed in Table 30.3.

DIETS TO MEET INDIVIDUAL NEEDS

A person's normal diet depends on their age, pattern of eating and the food they choose. Dietary requirements may change during illness (e.g. an individual may avoid eating foods that cause adverse reactions such as indigestion, nausea or diarrhoea). The diet may also need to be adapted as part of their treatment during certain conditions and disease states.

While acknowledging the factors that influence a person's choice of foods and observing any restrictions to their diet in the management of disease processes, nurses should encourage the consumption of healthy balanced meals following the Australian Healthy Eating Guide principles.

Furthermore, individuals should become aware of the information in the labels of prepared and packaged foods. Notice should be taken of the expiry date and the presence of preservatives and other additives. The listing of ingredients on the packaging denotes the relative quantities of each ingredient, with the major ingredient listed first. The remainder are listed in order of decreasing quantities.

Individuals may choose, or may be prescribed, certain diets, as follows, and described further below:

- healthy balanced diet
- plant-based diet
- religious and cultural diet
- therapeutic diet
- diet for wound healing
- diet for mental health.

TABLE 30.3 | Mineral salts and health

Mineral	Functions	Sources	Effects of deficiency
Trace (macro & micro) elements found in mineral salts			
Calcium (Ca)	Formation of bones and teeth, muscle contraction, normal blood clotting, activator for enzymes and neurotransmitters	Milk, yoghurt, cheese, sardines, salmon, sesame seed paste	Osteoporosis, tetany and severe muscle spasms, osteomalacia
Copper (Cu)	Aids iron absorption; nerve function	Shellfish, nuts, wholegrain cereals	Neutropenia, hypochromic anaemia, vascular disorders
Phosphorus (P)	Formation of DNA, bones and teeth; nerve and muscle function	Milk, cheese, meat, fish, eggs	Anaemia, weight loss, abnormal growth
Sodium (Na) Potassium (K) Chloride (Cl)	Act closely together in the maintenance of osmotic pressure balance between intracellular and extracellular fluid; nerve and muscle function, maintenance of acid–base balance	Salt, fruits, vegetables, monosodium glutamate	Cell and tissue fluid abnormality, arrhythmias, muscular weakness
Magnesium (Mg)	Activator of enzymes; nerve and muscle function	Cereals, nuts, leafy green vegetables, dried beans	Anorexia, nausea
Iron (Fe)	Formation of haemoglobin, necessary for the transport of oxygen	Liver, red meats, eggs, leafy green vegetables	Iron-deficiency anaemia, pago-phagia, lethargy and exhaustion, poor tissue regeneration
Ultratrace (microminerals) elements found in mineral salts			
Cobalt (Co)	Synthesis of vitamin B12	Leafy green vegetables	Pernicious anaemia due to vitamin B12 deficiency
Iodine (I)	Formation of thyroxine	Seafoods, vegetables, iodised salt	Goitre, myxoedema and hypothyroidism, stillbirths and spontaneous abortions, mental and growth retardation, cretinism
Selenium (Se)	Antioxidant	Fish, liver, cereals	Muscular dystrophy, delayed growth, renal and cardiac degeneration
Zinc (Zn)	Metabolism, collagen formation, component of certain enzymes, healthy skin and hair	Wheatgerm, oysters, meat, cheese, wholegrain cereals	Impaired healing, poor condition of the skin, growth retardation, fatigue, hair loss, behavioural changes

(Crisp et al 2021; Patton & Thibodeau 2019)

Healthy balanced diet

A healthy balanced diet is one without dietary restrictions or modifications. An individual may select the foods they prefer within the principles of good nutrition and diets based on age, health and cultural or religious beliefs. Some individuals choose to follow a diet in which specific foods or nutrients are restricted or increased, as part of a commitment to a healthy lifestyle. Other people will follow a diet based on cultural or religious commitment.

A healthy approach to eating based on the Australian Dietary Guidelines is depicted in Figure 30.2.

Plant-based diet

Individuals may choose to follow a plant-based diet for health, personal, ecological or religious reasons. Vegetarian diets exclude all flesh foods, such as meat, fish and poultry, and have an intake high in plant foods. The lacto (milk)-ovo (egg) vegetarian diet includes milk, other dairy products and eggs, while a lacto-vegetarian diet includes milk and other dairy products but excludes eggs. The vegan diet (strict vegetarian) excludes all animal-derived products and consists of plant foods only (Nutrition Australia 2020). While it is possible to obtain sufficient nutrients on a plant-based diet, care must be taken to ensure that intake of iron, vitamin B12, calcium and omega-3 fatty acids is adequate since animal products are a major source of these nutrients.

Religious and cultural diet

Certain religious groups have particular rules concerning the choice, preparation and storage of specific items in the diet; however, individuals may vary in their adherence to religious dietary doctrines and the nurse should not assume that all people who are of a particular faith strictly follow the religious dietary restrictions. Some examples of religious dietary restrictions include the following:

- Hinduism (Hindu): People of the Hindu faith abstain from eating beef products and follow a vegetarian diet. Stimulants are forbidden.
- Buddhist: Most Buddhists are vegetarian, with consumption of alcohol considered a personal choice but not encouraged.
- Islam (Moslem, Muslim): All pork and pork products, alcohol and caffeine are forbidden. Any meat consumed must be from animals slaughtered according to strict rules (halal). Ramadan, a period of fasting, forbids eating or drinking of any substance from sunrise to sunset for one lunar month.
- Jehovah's Witness: Dietary restrictions are against any foods that are prepared with blood (e.g. some meat pies and blood sausages). Additionally, some Jehovah's Witnesses may refuse to eat meats if they are unsure if the meat presented was not properly bled. There are no specific 'rules' for correct bleeding of an animal so it is best to discuss this requirement with the individual and their family.
- Judaism (Jewish faith): Foods must be 'kosher' (prepared according to Jewish law) and only certain parts of an animal may be eaten. Fish with scales may be eaten; however, all pork, shellfish and predatory birds are prohibited. Meat and dairy products are never eaten at the same time and are required to be stored and prepared separately. Certain periods of fasting are observed, such as Yom Kippur, a 24-hour fast. Passover, lasting 8 days, prohibits the consumption of leavened (yeast-containing) bread. Cooking is not permitted on Saturdays (the Sabbath).
- Mormon (Church of Jesus Christ of Latter Day Saints): Meat, although not forbidden, is eaten infrequently. Alcohol and drinks containing caffeine (e.g. tea, coffee and cola) are not permitted. Tobacco is also forbidden.
- Roman Catholic: Ash Wednesday and Good Friday are specified days on which abstinence from meat is obligatory.
- Seventh-Day Adventist: A lacto-vegetarian diet is commonly followed and stimulants such as coffee, tea and alcohol are not permitted.

(Queensland Faith Communities Council 2023; State of Queensland 2021)

Aboriginal and Torres Strait Islander Peoples

The Australian Dietary Guidelines, while relevant to Aboriginal and Torres Strait Islander Peoples, includes specific recommendations for this population group (Australian Indigenous Health*InfoNet* 2020). The consumption of traditional bush foods, if enjoyed, should be supported as much as possible. Store-bought foods most closely resembling traditional foods are preferred, such as fresh plant foods, wholegrains, seafood and lean meats and poultry. Breastfeeding infants is recommended due to the nutritional and immunological benefits. Lactose intolerance can occur in children, so alternative sources of calcium are recommended in these cases.

Therapeutic diet

A specific diet may be prescribed to rectify a nutritional deficiency, to decrease specific nutrients or to provide modifications in the texture or consistency of food. If a therapeutic diet is prescribed, it is important that the individual understands the reasons for any restrictions or modifications. Information about various therapeutic diets is provided in Table 30.4. Nursing Care Plan 30.1 shows a sample nursing care plan for an individual on a restricted diet.

TABLE 30.4 | Therapeutic diets

Diet	Description	Indications
Clear liquid	No solids permitted and only fluids that leave no residue, are non-irritating and non-gas forming are allowed (e.g. water, black tea or coffee, clear soups and fruit drinks).	Obstruction or irritation of the gastrointestinal tract Preparation for colonoscopy Postoperatively before starting on solids
Full liquid	All fluids, plus foods that become liquid at room temperature (e.g. jelly and ice-cream) are permitted.	Progression from clear liquids Before starting on solids Inability to chew or swallow solids

Continued

TABLE 30.4 | Therapeutic diets—cont'd

Diet	Description	Indications
Soft	Semi-solid easily digested foods are permitted (e.g. soup, cooked cereal, milk pudding, mashed or pureed vegetables and fruit, eggs, soft meats and fish).	Advancing from a liquid diet Individuals with chewing or swallowing difficulties Certain gastrointestinal disorders
Low fibre	Foods that can be absorbed easily and leave no colour or residue are permitted (e.g. clear soup, tender meat, fish or chicken, eggs, refined cereal products, jelly, ice-cream).	As part of preparation for colonoscopy Colitis Before and after surgery on the lower colon
High fibre	Foods that contain residue that adds bulk to the faeces and stimulates peristalsis (e.g. fruit, vegetables, nuts, wholegrain products).	Prevention of cancer Prevention and treatment of constipation Hypercholesterolaemia
Low kilojoule	The number of kilojoules is reduced below the usual daily requirement. Foods that are low in fat or refined carbohydrate are permitted.	Weight reduction
High kilojoule	The number of kilojoules is increased above the usual daily requirements. Foods that are high in carbohydrate, protein and fat are included.	Weight gain. To replace and repair damaged tissue (e.g. after severe burns)
Low cholesterol	Foods that are high in fat and cholesterol are restricted (e.g. butter, cream, whole milk, cheese, egg yolk, meat).	Prevention or treatment of heart disease, atherosclerosis, high serum cholesterol levels
Low fat	Foods that are high in fat are restricted (e.g. butter, cream, whole milk, cheese, fatty meat).	Liver or gallbladder disorders Irritable bowel syndrome Weight reduction
Low protein	The amount of protein is restricted and fat and carbohydrate is increased.	Kidney or liver failure
High protein	The amount of protein is increased and foods high in complete protein are included (e.g. meat, fish, eggs, cheese, milk).	To replace and repair damaged tissue
High iron	Foods that are rich in iron are included (e.g. liver, red meat, green leafy vegetables).	Prevention and treatment of iron-deficiency anaemia
Controlled carbohydrate (diabetic)	The amounts of carbohydrate, kilojoules and protein are controlled to meet nutritional needs, to control blood sugar levels and to maintain an appropriate body weight.	Diabetes mellitus
Controlled sodium	Foods that are high in sodium are omitted and no salt is added to food.	Cardiovascular disease Certain kidney diseases, liver failure, fluid retention (oedema)
Gluten restricted	Foods that contain gluten are eliminated (e.g. wheat, rye, oats, malt, barley). Rice and corn are permitted.	Coeliac disease
High vitamin	A balanced healthy diet that includes foods that are high in one or more deficient vitamins.	Vitamin deficiency diseases (e.g. night blindness) Anaemia (e.g. vitamin B12, folate) Beriberi Scurvy Rickets

(Raymond & Morrow 2023)

NURSING CARE PLAN 30.1

Assessment: Marcus is a 31-year-old male, 198 cm tall and 140 kg. BMI >30, categorising him as obese. His waist circumference is 150 cm. BP 132/86 mmHg, HR 98 beats/min, fasting BGL 7.2 mmol, and reports breathlessness on minimal exertion.
Issue/s to be addressed: Nutrition altered, more than body requirements—overweight, obesity.
Goal/s: Decreased body mass index to healthy range. Decreased waist circumference to healthy range. Increased activity level to 30 minutes of exercise 5 days per week.

Care/actions	Rationale
Weekly body weight recorded.	Weight loss or gain should be recorded to determine effectiveness of care plan.
Dietitian referral.	Dietitians are a member of multidisciplinary team with a detailed understanding of nutrition to assist in weight loss.
Formulate eating plan with appropriate caloric intake and nutritional needs.	Weight loss is associated with a negative calorie input to output balance.
Educate individual to keep a daily food and fluid diary.	Quantification of intake, and a visual record may also help individual to make more appropriate food choices and serving sizes.
Facilitate water intake 2 L minimum per day.	Water assists in the excretion of byproducts of fat breakdown and helps prevent ketosis.
Discuss mindful eating and consciousness of nutritional habits.	Non-hungry eating is a commonly recognised symptom in obese individuals.
Discuss role of regular exercise.	The combination of diet and exercise promotes loss of adipose tissue.

Evaluation: Six weeks following implementation of care plan, Marcus has had a weight reduction of 8 kg and waist circumference decrease of 3 cm. He has decreased breathlessness on exertion and increased activity tolerance with walking 30 minutes 5 days per week. He has maintained a food diary of all intake during the time period. He has identified poor portion control as a trigger for his overindulgence. Marcus reports water intake of approximately 1.5 L per day with a reported effort to increase to the recommended 2 L.

Diet for wound healing

Nutrition is intricately interrelated with wound healing. It is important that appropriate nutritional support be provided to individuals as a part of their wound care plan. Malnutrition has a negative impact on wound management including delayed wound repair, decreased wound strength and increased risk of skin breakdown (Wounds Australia 2016). Alternatively, nutritional supplementation has demonstrated positive effects of accelerated wound healing (Bishop et al 2018). Large wounds cause a significant increase in an individual's metabolic rate. Bishop et al (2018) recommend a diet consisting of 20% proteins and amino acids, 40% carbohydrates and 40% fruits and vegetables to ensure optimal consumption of vitamins, iron, zinc and fats during the wound healing process. It is therefore not therapeutic for persons with chronic wounds to follow restrictive diets until wound repair has been achieved.

The National Safety and Quality Health Standards were developed to improve the quality and standardise care within Australian healthcare settings. Preventing and managing pressure injuries mandates that individuals with pressure injuries must be managed according to best practice guidelines. Improved nutrition is highlighted by the Australian Commission on Safety and Quality in Health Care (ACSQHC) as an implementation strategy to address risk reduction (ACSQHC 2018; 2021). See Chapter 29 for further information on wound healing.

Diet for mental health

Just as physical health is interrelated with nutrition, so too is mental health. Nutrient intake may influence mental health by affecting neurotransmitter levels and/or promoting vascular brain changes. Depression and anxiety, and the medications used to treat them, may negatively influence appetite and nutritional intake, leading to further mental deterioration (Harbottle 2019). Nurses should encourage people with mental illness to consume a nutrient-dense diet based on the Australian Guide to Healthy Eating (Figure 30.2), as well as promoting exercise, social interaction and adherence to medications (Harbottle 2019).

CRITICAL THINKING EXERCISE 30.4

Ada is 32 weeks pregnant with her first child. While she is usually healthy, she has been experiencing breathlessness and tiring easily throughout the day. She reports light-headedness, craving ice and leg cramps. Her GP has discussed oral iron replacement therapy; however, she is concerned regarding the side effect of constipation from this treatment. What diet and care would you recommend to Ada?

CRITICAL THINKING EXERCISE 30.5

Ian is a 77-year-old male recently diagnosed with oesophageal cancer. He presented to hospital with a history of unintentional weight loss, difficulty swallowing, loss of appetite and a persistent cough. His medical officer has recommended that Ian be discharged home with enteral feeding while he waits to commence radiotherapy and surgical treatment. What education could you provide to Ian about enteral feeding?

CRITICAL THINKING EXERCISE 30.6

Bernadette, 22 years old, who is a strict raw vegan, is hospitalised for severe abdominal pain and dysmenorrhoea. She asks you for jugs of ice to chew on, although she is allowed clear fluids. You suspect **pagophagia** (craving for ice) as a result of blood loss. She is diagnosed with uterine fibroids and iron-deficiency anaemia. What other signs or symptoms may reinforce the diagnosis of iron-deficiency anaemia and what nursing interventions could you plan and implement to improve her anaemia?

CRITICAL THINKING EXERCISE 30.7

Lucy, 35 years old, is admitted to the medical ward with mastitis. Her 4-week-old baby is rooming in so she can continue breastfeeding. What are some nutritional considerations needed?

NURSING PRACTICE AND NUTRITIONAL NEEDS

Each institution has its own system for delivering meals, and the nurse should ensure that both the individual and their immediate environment are prepared in readiness for mealtimes in accordance with local facility policy and procedure. See Chapter 18 (Clinical Interest Box 18.1) for information on bringing food for individuals into healthcare settings. The following aspects of nursing practice in meeting nutritional needs are in accordance with information taken from Australian state standards for nutrition in the healthcare setting (State of Queensland 2022; State of Victoria 2022) and the Royal Commission into Aged Care Quality and Safety (Commonwealth of Australia 2023a).

Assisting individuals at mealtimes

Key aspects related to the mealtime experience

- Mealtime should be coordinated with nursing care to minimise disruptions.
- Nursing care should be planned to ensure that there are no unpleasant sights, sounds, smells or treatments being performed during mealtimes since these could interfere with appetite.
- Individuals should be offered the use of toilet facilities, and their hygiene needs should be attended to before meals arrive in the ward.
- Individuals who require assistance/supervision during mealtimes should be identified.
- Ambulant individuals may need assistance to a table; non-ambulant individuals should be assisted into a comfortable position. Either sitting upright in bed or out of bed if appropriate.
- Eating areas should be cleared of unnecessary items to provide space for the meal tray; the tray should be placed within reaching distance for the individual.
- When the meals arrive the nurse should ensure that each individual receives the correct meal, prepared in the correct manner according to their dietary, ethnic, cultural or religious requirements and that all the necessary items meet the individual's needs. This includes the provision of adaptive aids, cutlery and drinking devices for eating and drinking.
- Medications that are required before, during or after the meal are administered (e.g. insulin).
- During mealtimes ensure allocation of appropriate staff, carers, relatives and volunteers to meet individual needs (e.g. by cutting food, opening packets, pouring fluids or help with feeding).
- Nursing staff should provide supervision and assistance with eating and drinking where there is clinical risk (e.g. suspected dysphagia, eating disorders).
- If an individual is not able to eat what has been provided, measures should be taken to obtain an alternative meal type or other form of nourishment.
- The nurse should observe the individual's intake of food and fluid, complete clinical assessment of intake and inform nursing, medical or dietitian staff if the individual's intake declines. Intake needs to subsequently be recorded in food and fluid records accurately.
- Following the meal, the nurse should ensure that the individual has the opportunity and equipment to perform normal hygiene (e.g. cleaning of hands, face and teeth or dentures).

Certain individuals may experience difficulty or be unable to feed themselves for a variety of reasons, including age, general weakness, pain due to surgery, paralysis or limitation of movement due to, for example, the presence of arm splints, intravenous lines or casts. An individual who is dependent may experience embarrassment if they require assistance at mealtimes; the nurse should therefore endeavour to make mealtimes as normal and enjoyable as possible. Clinical Skill 30.1 outlines how to assist with eating and drinking.

CLINICAL SKILL 30.1 Assisting with eating and drinking

Please adhere to the policy and procedures of the facility/organisation prior to undertaking the skill. Ensure this skill is in your scope of practice.

NMBA Decision-making Framework considerations (refer to NMBA Decision-making framework for nursing and midwifery 2020): 1. Am I educated? 2. Am I authorised? 3. Am I competent? If you answer 'no' to any of these, do not perform that activity. Seek guidance and support from your teacher/a nurse team leader/clinical facilitator/educator.	**Equipment:** Appropriate adaptive aids (e.g. plate guard) Dysphagia cup Cutlery Straw Clothes protector and/or serviette

PREPARE FOR THE SKILL

(Please refer to the Standard Steps on pp. xviii–xx for related rationales.)
Mentally review the steps of the skill.
Discuss the skill with your instructor/supervisor/team leader, if required.
Confirm correct facility/organisation policy/safe operating procedures.
Validate the order in the individual's record.
Identify indication and rationale for performing the activity.
Assess for any contraindications.
Locate and gather equipment.
Perform hand hygiene.
Ensure therapeutic interaction.
Identify the individual using three individual identifiers.
Gain the individual's consent.
Assess for pain relief.
Prepare the environment.
Provide and maintain privacy.
Assist the individual to assume an appropriate position of comfort.

Skill activity	Rationale
Critically think through the assessment data and problem-solving—level of consciousness, position of individual, dysphagia, chronic diseases that require dietary management, food allergies, appetite, assistance needed (personnel and equipment), social and psychological issues that may affect eating, appetite or food and drink choices, food texture, fluid viscosity, check if individual is wearing dentures if applicable.	Evaluate each aspect and its relationship to other data to help identify specific problems and modifications of the procedure that may be needed for the individual.
Assist the individual into the high Fowler's position or sit out of bed unless contraindicated. If contraindicated elevate head of bed >30 degrees. Individual to be centred in midline position, head flexed forwards and down.	Reduces risk of gastro-oesophageal reflux and aspiration by ensuring individual is safely positioned prior to commencement of feeding. Promotes comfort and reduces risk of choking. Sitting out of bed promotes independence of individual and increases enjoyment of meal.

PERFORM THE SKILL

(Please refer to the Standard Steps on pp. xviii–xx for related rationales.)
Perform hand hygiene.
Apply PPE: gloves, eyewear, mask and gown as appropriate.
Ensure the individual's safety and comfort throughout skill.
Promote independence and involvement of the individual if possible and/or appropriate.
Assess the individual's tolerance to the skill throughout.
Dispose of used supplies, equipment, waste and sharps appropriately.
Remove PPE and discard or store appropriately.
Perform hand hygiene.

Continued

CLINICAL SKILL 30.1 Assisting with eating and drinking—cont'd

Skill activity	Rationale
Ensure that appropriate food and fluid textures are given to individual.	Food texture checked and appropriate texture given to individual to prevent choking or aspiration. Fluid viscosity checked and appropriate viscosity given to individual to avoid aspiration.
Position a chair opposite if assistance with feeding required, so you are sitting face-to-face.	Improves communication and interaction.
Present meal in a safe manner to individual. Ensure meal tray/drink is not placed within individual's reach if it has been identified that the individual requires assistance and/or supervision for eating. Provide assistance to open packaging if required. Ensure individual is alert before commencing feeding. Ask individual for preference for food. Understand the risks associated with assisting an individual to eat and drink (e.g. suspected dysphagia, eating disorders). Assist only as necessary. Allow hot food to cool. Check food is not stuck in buccal region.	Prevents aspiration and/or injury from hot food/fluid. Assists with meal set-up. Promotes independence and involvement if possible. Prepares for potential risks and an emergency situation.
Ensure each mouthful of food is presented in a safe manner to individual. Introduce each mouthful of food verbally and visually to individual, ensuring an appropriate size. Ensure appropriate pacing is employed.	Assesses tolerance to the procedure. Alerts individual to next mouthful of food. Ensures prior mouthful is swallowed prior to next being presented.
Ensure observation is maintained throughout meal. Cease meal if there are any signs of choking, aspiration, reduced level of consciousness, food stuck in cheek, excessive spillage from mouth/drooling, food coming out of nose, not swallowing food after several attempts or regurgitation, vomiting.	Maintains individual's safety.

AFTER THE SKILL

(Please refer to the Standard Steps on pp. xviii–xx for related rationales.)
Communicate outcome to the individual, any ongoing care and to report any complications.
Restore the environment.
Report, record and document assessment findings, details of the skill performed and the individual's response.
Report, record and document any abnormalities and/or inability to perform the skill.
Reassess the individual to ensure there are no adverse effects/events from the skill.

Skill activity	Rationale
On completion of meal leave individual sitting upright, clean individual's mouth/face, remove clothes protector.	Ensures individual is treated with respect and courtesy during interactions.
Document in nutrition care plan/fluid balance chart if appropriate. Document and report dietary intake, level of assistance and any swallowing difficulties.	Ensures transfer of nutrition care and appropriate care can be planned and implemented.

(Berman et al 2020; Hall et al 2022; NSW Department of Health 2017)

Key aspects related to assisting an adult at mealtimes

- Ensure that the individual is comfortable before starting a meal.
- Elimination and hygiene needs should be attended to before a meal is started.
- The individual may require to be assisted into a comfortable position and the table adjusted to the appropriate height.
- The meal should be placed where it can be seen and smelt, to stimulate the appetite.
- Condiments (e.g. salt and pepper) should be provided and may be added to the food, provided the individual is not on a salt-restricted diet.
- The nurse should ascertain whether the individual prefers one food at a time or a combination (e.g. meat alone, or combined with a vegetable). It is also important to ensure that food or fluids are not too hot or cold.
- Suitable utensils should be selected (e.g. an individual may prefer to eat using a spoon rather than a fork). The amount of food placed on the utensil should be easily managed by the individual. The utensil should be placed gently into the front of the mouth, to avoid injury or stimulation of the gag reflex.
- The food should be presented at a rate that meets the individual's needs, giving them sufficient time to chew and swallow each mouthful and to maintain dignity.
- Sips of fluid should be offered during the meal. A flexible straw, rather than a cup or glass, may be easier for some individuals to manage.
- To maintain dignity and to promote independence, the individual should be encouraged to be as independent as possible and may be encouraged, but never forced, to eat a meal.
- Allow the individual to wipe their mouth with a serviette during the meal, or assist if necessary.
- On completion of the meal, the individual's hygiene and comfort needs should be met. The nurse should report and document the intake of food and fluid.

Key aspects related to assisting a child at mealtimes

Mealtimes in a hospital should be pleasant unhurried occasions and the environment should be one that enables the child to enjoy mealtimes. The nurse should communicate effectively with the parent/carer and child to ensure that the appropriate foods are being served. Some guidelines include the following:

- Mealtimes should be free from distractions.
- Servings need to be small to minimise the psychological reaction to a large-sized serving.
- Adequate time should be allowed for the meal to be eaten without hurrying.
- The child should be prepared for the meal. Toilet needs should be attended to, nappy changed if necessary, hands and face washed, serviette or bib provided, distractions such as toys put away and the child made comfortable in bed or seated on a chair at a table.
- The child should be discouraged from eating in front of the television or electronic devices.
- Painful or emotionally distressing procedures should not be performed immediately before or after a meal, and activities should be timed so that a child does not become too tired to eat a meal.
- Meals should be served attractively, in amounts appropriate to the age and the condition of each child.
- Children should be encouraged to feed themselves, even though they may do it in a 'messy' fashion.
- Assistance should be given if the child is unable to manage or to use distractive therapy to maintain input.
- Very young children should be supervised during mealtimes, monitoring total intake and safe consumption.

(Cole et al 2018; NSW Department of Health 2017)

Uneaten food should be removed without comment and the nurse in charge informed. If the child's illness is causing anorexia, other forms of nutrition may be offered. Refusal to eat may be an attempt by the child to gain more attention, or it may be that the foods are different in appearance, presentation, availability of condiments or timing to the meals they are used to eating. Every attempt should be made to provide nutritious foods that the child enjoys. In a clinical setting, a lot of patience may be required to assist a child to eat a healthy balanced diet, particularly if their carers are not present. The child may be apprehensive of their setting, in pain, used to different foods or their diet at home may be of a poor standard.

Children should be observed for any adverse reaction to food and the nurse in charge and/or medical officer informed if a child vomits before, during or after a meal; develops diarrhoea; or develops what may be an allergic reaction to a food, such as a rash, pruritus or breathing difficulties.

Key aspects related to the mealtime experience in aged care

Following the Royal Commission into Aged Care Quality and Safety (Commonwealth of Australia 2023a) a Food and Nutrition Expert Advisory Group was established to develop resources to promote high-quality, enjoyable dining experiences for aged-care residents (Commonwealth of Australia 2023b). Some of the recommendations include the following:

- An enjoyable dining experience should be provided regardless of what, where, how and when residents eat.
- Residents should be involved in the planning and assessment of their dining needs.
- Texture modified (blended) foods can be piped onto the plate or moulded in such a way as to resemble the original food, which makes it more appetising.
- The use of table decorations and background music can improve the overall experience.

CASE STUDY 30.2

Francis is a 73-year-old man with dementia who has recently been admitted into an aged-care home. Francis is from a remote community and his daughter and extended family are not able to visit regularly due to distance and lack of transport. You have noticed that since his admission 1 month ago Francis has become withdrawn and has lost 5 kg in weight. During his meals he eats very little and says he is not hungry.

1. What are some possible adverse effects of malnutrition on an older person?
2. What are some strategies that the nurse and the organisation can implement to improve Francis' mealtime experience?

- Providers should maximise the numbers of staff available at mealtimes.
- Mealtimes should focus on food, drink and socialising, not clinical tasks.
- Staff should be trained in the early recognition and referral of swallowing difficulties. (See Case Study 30.2.)

The general nutritional requirements of an individual with dementia are similar to those of others of the same age; however, due to cognitive decline they may require a range of interventions to support intake (Dietitians Australia 2020):

- Assistive feeding devices to promote independent provision of food and fluids.
- Finger foods may allow the person to regain the enjoyment of eating if they have experienced the loss of adequate manual dexterity to control cutlery.
- Encourage support of family and caregivers at mealtime.
- Specific diet to meet personal food taste.
- Contrasting-coloured crockery may assist the individual distinguish food/fluids.
- As oral intake diminishes artificial nutrition may be necessary. See Clinical Skill 30.1 for guidelines on assisting with eating and drinking.

Key aspects related to assisting an individual with chewing or swallowing difficulties

Some individuals who experience difficulty chewing or have dysphagia—due to, for example, glossitis, stomatitis, cerebral vascular accidents or dental conditions—are at risk of malnutrition because of limitations to the types of foods they can chew and swallow safely. Clinical Interest Box 30.2 provides an example of how gastro-oesophageal reflux can affect the nutritional status of a child. Individuals may require modifications to the consistency of food. Depending on the cause and degree of difficulty, the individual's needs may be met by:

- Referral to a speech pathologist to ascertain the cause of the problem by observing the individual's swallowing reflex and by investigations such as saliva grams, fluoroscopy or barium swallows.

CLINICAL INTEREST BOX 30.2 Gastro-oesophageal reflux and faltering growth

Faltering growth—previously called 'failure to thrive'—is a term used in paediatrics to describe an infant, toddler or child whose weight or BMI is below expected levels for their age and gender. The most common mechanism of faltering growth is inadequate energy (caloric) intake.

In infants, inadequate intake may result from gastro-oesophageal reflux (GOR), which can be due to lax cardiac sphincter muscle or changes in coordination of oesophageal peristalsis. GOR can cause oesophagitis from intermittent bathing of oesophageal tissue in stomach acid. Common symptoms may also include food refusal, diminished intake, prolonged feeding times, distractibility, sleep disorders and continued crying, which may lead some to diagnose an infant as a 'colicky baby'. Diagnosis is usually based on history, with more invasive tests such as medical imaging, biopsy and oesophageal pH monitoring less common due to their relative unreliability. Treatments may include thickening agents, postprandial prone positioning while awake, positioning up to 30 degrees from the horizontal while sleeping, peristaltic medications and gastric acid inhibitors. Changing the infant's diet is not suggested (i.e. from breast milk to formula or, if formula fed switching to an alternative formula type). In most cases symptoms resolve within 6 to 18 months.

(Ayerbe et al 2019; Tang et al 2021)

- Providing meals comprised of soft foods or thickened fluids.
- Initiating the swallowing reflex by gentle pressure on the tongue with the feeding utensil.
- Offering all food and fluid carefully and monitoring to avoid or detect aspiration.
- Placing the food into the unaffected side of the mouth in individuals with a facial paralysis (e.g. Bell's palsy) or after a cerebrovascular accident. The nurse should ensure that food does not accumulate in the cheek of the affected side.

(Department of Communities, Disability Services and Seniors 2019)

Key aspects related to assisting an individual with vision impairment at mealtimes

- It is important to encourage independence; the nurse should therefore consult the individual about the type of assistance that would be most beneficial. For example, individuals may find it helpful if the nurse describes the meal by referring to the plate as a clock face. The nurse should state where each food on the plate may be located (e.g. the meat at 2 o'clock, the potatoes at 4 o'clock and the beans at 6 o'clock).

- To avoid injury the individual should be made aware of the proximity and location of hot articles (e.g. cups of tea or coffee) and the nurse should ask if assistance to pour the fluids is required.
- If the individual is unable to feed themself, they should be asked to indicate when they are ready for the next mouthful.
- Self-feeding should be encouraged at all ages to promote independence and dignity. When an individual is being fed, the nurse should perform the procedure in a relaxed and confident manner, with due regard for maintaining their dignity. A variety of self-help devices are available to assist individuals in feeding themselves (Figure 30.6).

(Vision Australia 2023)

Assistive feeding devices

Self-help feeding devices (Figure 30.6) may be helpful for an individual who has poor vision, limited arm mobility, limited grasp or reduced coordination and include the following:

- Plate guards, which attach to one side of the plate and are used to assist an individual to place food on the eating utensils.
- Angled or swivelling utensils (e.g. forks and spoons that are angled to assist individuals with a limited range of arm or hand movement).
- Weighted utensils for individuals with limited hand control (e.g. Parkinson's disease).
- Utensils with built-up handles. The thicker handles are beneficial for individuals with diminished grasp or who experience joint pain or discomfort (e.g. arthritis).

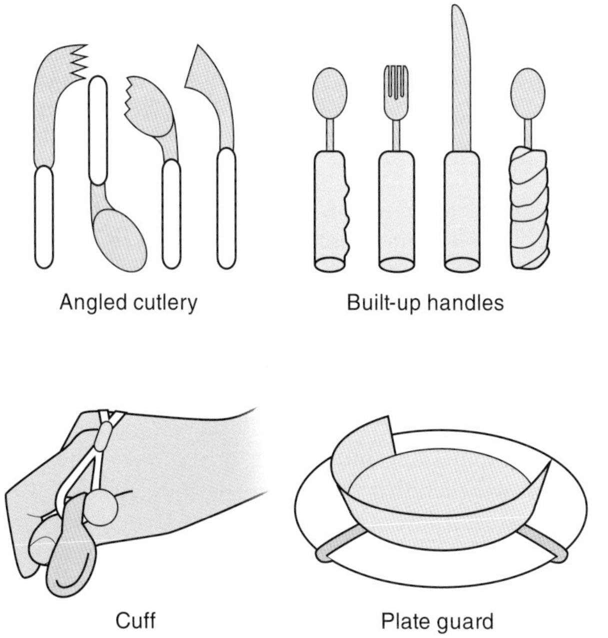

Figure 30.6 Assistive feeding devices

(Djachenko, A.)

- Cuffs, which are placed over an individual's hand, with a spoon or fork inserted into the slot in the cuff. A cuff may be beneficial for an individual with diminished grasp or movement.

COMMON DISORDERS ASSOCIATED WITH NUTRITION

Although many disorders are related to a specific nutrient deficiency, the common disorders of nutrition may be classified as malnutrition, obesity, eating disorders and nutrient loss as a result of vomiting or diarrhoea.

Malnutrition

Malnutrition occurs as a consequence of continued poor nutrition status and may be described as the condition in which nutrients are being used or lost by the body in excess of the intake and absorption or utilisation of nutrients. Identifying factors that put an individual at risk is an important step in ensuring that all individuals have their individual nutritional needs met. People who are at risk of malnutrition include those who:

- are experiencing increased metabolic demands or protracted loss of nutrients (e.g. due to burns, surgery, inflammatory conditions or infections, vomiting, diarrhoea, physical or psychological trauma, hormonal imbalance or prolonged pyrexia)
- are not consuming oral food or fluid for more than a few days
- have a BMI value below 20 or who have recently experienced a loss of more than 10% of their normal body weight
- are alcohol- or drug-dependent
- are receiving medications or treatments that have an anti-nutrient or have catabolic properties (e.g. immunosuppressants or anti-tumour agents)
- have a disorder that results in defective digestion, utilisation or absorption of nutrients (e.g. gastrectomy, diabetes mellitus, Crohn's disease).

Malnutrition in hospitals is frequently undetected and/or unreported. An estimated 20–50% of adults experience malnutrition on admission, with many experiencing further deterioration during the course of their stay (Cass & Charlton 2022). Information on the rate of hospital-acquired malnutrition in Australian hospitals was collected in 2015–2016 and found to be 12 per 10,000 hospitalisations (AIHW 2017a). In 2018, the Australian Commission on Safety and Quality in Health Care provided selected best practices and suggestions for improvement for clinicians and health system managers to address hospital-acquired malnutrition (ACSQHC 2018).

Early identification of individuals at risk of malnutrition enables early nutrition intervention to be initiated. If the risk of becoming malnourished, or malnutrition, is identified and addressed in a timely manner, there are positive outcomes for the individual and the health system.

For the individual

- Improved wound healing
- Reduced risk of falls and pressure injuries
- Reduced muscle wasting and weakness
- Reduced prevalence of adverse drug reactions and drug interactions
- Reduced infection rates
- Improved hydration
- Reduced diarrhoea and constipation
- Improved metabolic profiles
- Reduced apathy and depression

For the health system

- Reduced length of stay
- Reduced antibiotic use
- Reduced clinical complications
- Reduced staff time per patient
- Reduced rates of readmission
- Reduced healthcare costs

(Agency for Clinical Innovation 2021)

Treatment includes identifying the cause and providing adequate nutrients. See Clinical Interest Box 30.3 on high rates of malnutrition in older adults.

CLINICAL INTEREST BOX 30.3 High rates of malnutrition in hospitalised individuals

Agarwal et al (2010) conducted a ground-breaking Australian study involving 56 hospitals across Australia and New Zealand. The 3122 participants were involved in an audit of nutritional status and dietary intake of adult hospitalised individuals using the Malnutrition Screening Tool. This study revealed alarming levels of malnutrition. In hospitalised persons, based on the International Classification of Diseases (Australian modification), participants were deemed malnourished if their body mass index was $<18.5\,kg/m^2$. Malnutrition prevalence was recorded as 32% with a further 41% of the participants deemed 'at risk' of malnutrition. Fifty-five per cent of malnourished participants consumed ≤50% of the food offered, with 'Not hungry' the most common reason for poor food consumption. A more recent audit of five Australian hospitals showed that hospital-acquired malnutrition was significantly associated with increased length of stay, pressure injury, falls and developing a cognitive impairment. With the burden of increased morbidity and mortality surrounding malnutrition as well as the associated financial burden on the healthcare system, it is essential nursing staff implement early nutrition interventions and referral to members of multidisciplinary teams.

(Agarwal et al 2010; Woodward et al 2020)

Overweight and obesity

Overweight and obesity are defined as abnormal or excessive fat accumulation that may impair health (WHO 2020a). They generally arise from a sustained energy imbalance when energy intake through eating and drinking is more than energy expended through physical activity (AIHW 2022a). Obesity is determined by calculating the individual's BMI or waist measurement. Genetic and environmental factors play a role (AIHW 2017c). Obesity may result from excessive kilojoule intake, metabolic disturbances, side effects of drugs such as steroids, an inadequate expenditure of energy or from a combination of factors. Overweight and obesity among adults increases the likelihood of developing many chronic conditions, including some cancers, cardiovascular disease, asthma, back pain and problems, chronic kidney disease, dementia, diabetes mellitus, gallbladder disease, gout and osteoarthritis (AIHW 2017b). Obese people may also demonstrate undernourishment in essential vitamins and minerals, even though excess food is consumed (Berman et al 2020).

Principles of treatment include reducing dietary intake and any causative drugs or hormones, while planning exercise, dietary and behaviour modification. The NSW Healthy Eating and Active Living Strategy 2022–2032 provides a whole-of-government framework to promote and support healthy eating and active living in NSW to address overweight and obesity and to reduce the impact of lifestyle-related chronic diseases (NSW Ministry of Health [MoH] 2022). The administration of medications such as appetite suppressants, hormonal therapy or oral substances containing, for example, cellulose, may be required. Surgical interventions are sometimes indicated in instances of morbid obesity. A variety of surgical procedures is available and most are aimed at reducing the capacity of the stomach (Morgan 2019). See Nursing Care Plan 30.1 for an example of the nursing care required for obese individuals.

Eating disorders

Eating disorders are serious and potentially life-threatening mental illnesses characterised by disturbances in behaviours, thoughts and attitudes towards food, eating, body weight and shape (National Eating Disorders Collaboration nd). The two most recognised disorders are anorexia nervosa and bulimia nervosa. **Anorexia nervosa** is characterised by self-imposed starvation, weight phobia and consequent emaciation. Body image, with a consequential loss of weight, becomes the individual's prime focus and is the result of a belief that their body is too fat, even when extreme emaciation is evident with BMI <18.5 (Daven 2022). **Bulimia nervosa** is characterised by episodes of 'bingeing' on large quantities of food, followed by purging with laxatives or self-induced vomiting.

The causes of both disorders are difficult to determine, but most experts agree that they result from an interaction of biological, psychological and sociocultural factors. Treatment, which is difficult and varied, includes behaviour modification, psychotherapy and, in some cases, hospitalisation until the desired weight is achieved (National Eating Disorders Collaboration 2021).

Nutrient loss as a result of vomiting

Vomiting, if prolonged, may result in significant nutrient deficiency, dehydration and electrolyte disturbance. To correct the imbalance, oral, enteral, intravenous therapy or total parenteral nutrition (TPN) may be indicated. Vomiting is not a disease itself but is a symptom of disease and may occur as a result of:

- diseases of the stomach, intestines, liver, biliary system, pancreas or peritoneum
- hypersensitivity to certain foods
- ingestion or presence of irritants
- acidosis, either metabolic or respiratory
- pain
- adverse reaction to, or a side effect of, certain medications
- hormonal changes during early pregnancy
- disturbances of equilibrium (e.g. travel sickness, vertigo)
- disorders of the central nervous system (e.g. concussion, cerebral oedema, brain tumours)
- psychological factors (e.g. apprehension, unpleasant sights or smells).

Vomiting (emesis) is the expulsion of the contents of the stomach or small intestine and is a reflex action caused by stimulation of the emesis centre in the medulla oblongata. When this centre is stimulated the glottis and nasopharynx close, the cardiac sphincter of the stomach relaxes and contractions of the diaphragm and abdominal muscles occur. As a result of the increased intra-abdominal pressure, the stomach or intestinal contents are forced upwards and are expelled through the mouth. Vomiting may be preceded by a feeling of sickness (nausea) and accompanied by salivation, sweating and pallor. In conditions such as intestinal or sphincter obstruction, 'projectile' vomiting may occur, in which the vomited material is ejected with great force (Harris et al 2019).

Vomiting should be assessed in terms of the nature of vomiting (effortless or projectile) and the characteristics of the material vomited (vomitus). Observations made of the vomitus may assist in determining the cause of vomiting and include observations of the:

- Consistency: The vomitus may consist of fluid, partially digested or undigested food.
- Colour: Vomitus may vary in colour from clear to yellow, to brown or green. The presence of bile tends to colour vomitus yellow or green and may indicate propulsion of the contents of the small intestine into the stomach.
- Presence of blood: Blood may be present as bright red streaks or clots, or may have a 'coffee grounds' appearance. The latter occurs when blood has been partially digested by gastric acid secretions. Vomiting of blood is called haematemesis. Forceful vomiting may induce blood-stained vomit (e.g. Weismann's tear).
- Odour: Vomitus is usually sour smelling, but a 'faecal' odour indicates reflux of bowel contents due to an intestinal obstruction (e.g. paralytic ileus).
- Quantity: If possible, vomitus should be measured in millilitres to assess the amount of fluid being lost, particularly if haematemesis is present.

Key aspects related to care of an individual who is vomiting

- If the individual is sitting, place an emesis bowl under the chin and position a towel to protect clothes and bedding.
- If the individual is lying down, lift and turn the head to one side to reduce the risk of aspiration.
- Ensure privacy, as individuals will feel distressed and embarrassed by the incident.
- Ensure dentures do not become dislodged.
- The nurse should stay with the individual to provide comfort and support, to ensure aspiration is recognised or prevented and to splint an abdominal wound or area of pain to reduce further pain or dehiscence of wounds, if present.
- The vomitus should be removed as soon as the episode is over to reduce the risk of a recurrence caused by the sight, smell or thought of the vomitus.
- Soiled linen or clothing should be changed and removed immediately from the room.
- Hands and face should be washed to refresh the individual and to remove any vomitus.
- Oral hygiene should be attended to by cleaning teeth, plates or dentures and providing a suitable mouth rinse to eliminate any unpleasant aftertaste.
- The individual should be assisted into a position of comfort and permitted to rest quietly.
- If antiemetics are ordered they should be administered by appropriate nursing staff.
- Assess hydration status including urine output, mucous membranes, thirst, skin turgor and capillary refill.
- Take measurement of individual's blood glucose level to recognise/treat hypoglycaemia.
- The nurse should report and document (in healthcare record, fluid balance chart) the incident so that appropriate nursing or medical actions may be implemented. An antiemetic medication may be prescribed by a medical officer and administered to reduce nausea and to prevent further vomiting.

(Emergency Care Institute 2023)

Alternative methods to meet nutritional needs

An alternative method of meeting nutritional needs may be indicated when an individual is unable to consume food or fluid orally. Alternative methods include total parenteral nutrition (TPN), intravenous therapy and tube feeding via orogastric, nasogastric, nasoduodenal, nasojejunal, gastrostomy, gastroduodenal or gastrojejunal tubes.

Total parenteral nutrition

Total parenteral nutrition (TPN) is sometimes referred to as hyperalimentation and involves the parenteral administration of a complete nutritional preparation that contains high concentrations of essential nutrients and which may include intralipid solutions, containing fats (Harris et al 2019). This method of feeding may be indicated when it is not possible for the individual's nutritional needs to be met via the digestive tract.

Hypertonic solutions are administered through a catheter that has been inserted into a large vein, such as the subclavian vein. The solution containing nutrients enters directly into the bloodstream. TPN solutions administered by this route provide a medium for rapid bacterial growth and, because the tubing provides access for the entry of microorganisms, contamination and septicaemia must be prevented. The catheter is inserted by a medical officer using sterile equipment and technique. Care of the equipment throughout the course of treatment requires strict asepsis.

Management of an individual who is receiving TPN is the responsibility of the RN, and the individual must be monitored continually to prevent or detect possible complications. Complications that may result from TPN include:

- hyperglycaemia or hypoglycaemia
- fluid and electrolyte imbalance
- catheter-related septicaemia
- infection of the catheter site
- extravasation of blood from the vein due to catheter trauma
- air emboli
- liver failure
- diarrhoea or constipation.

The Enrolled Nurse may be required to assist with the care of an individual receiving TPN and must be aware of the scope of their role in promoting safety and comfort. ENs should refer to the Nursing and Midwifery Board of Australia's (NMBA) Decision-Making Framework to guide clinical decision-making, particularly in regards to scope of practice and delegated tasks (NMBA 2020).

Intravenous therapy

Intravenous therapy involves the introduction of a solution or solutions into a peripheral or central vein. Information about intravenous therapy is provided in Chapter 26.

Enteral tube feeding

Naso-enteric tubes are orogastric, nasogastric, nasoduodenal or nasojejunal tubes used to administer a range of nutritional feeds to an individual for a variety of reasons, including:

- malabsorption (e.g. inflammatory bowel disorders)
- surgery (e.g. oral or throat surgery)
- central nervous system disorders (e.g. paraplegia, unconsciousness, pharyngeal paralysis)
- metabolic disorders (e.g. hyperinsulinaemia, hypoglycaemia)
- food refusal or **dysphagia**, when the individual is too ill or weak to eat normally.

Selecting the most appropriate device for an individual is multifactorial. The device selection should always include the individual and include consideration of anticipated feeding duration and the individual's clinical condition and social circumstances (Bloom & Seckel 2021).

The nurse should be aware of the policies and regulations regarding their role and responsibilities in both insertion and management of **enteral** tubes.

Nasogastric tubes

Feeds given by a nasogastric tube inserted via the nares into the stomach (Figure 30.7) are normally administered to individuals who experience short-term difficulties in nutrition, or when surgically placed tubes such as gastrostomy tubes (see below) may be contraindicated by the individual's physical condition. For information on insertion of a nasogastric tube, see Clinical Skill 30.2. Following insertion, it is essential nursing progress notes are

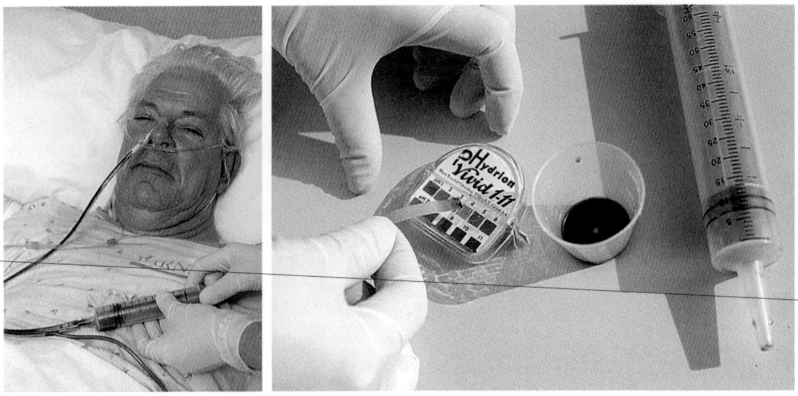

A

Figure 30.7 Administering enteral feeds via nasogastric tubes

A: Confirm placement,

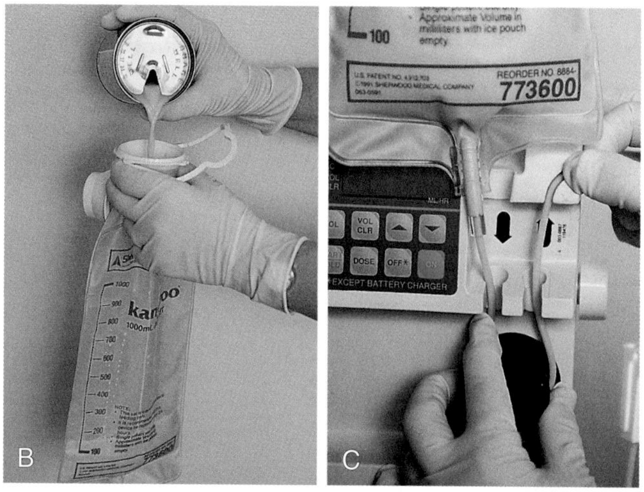

Figure 30.7—Cont'd.

B: Pour formula into feeding container, **C:** Connect tubing through infusion pump.

(Crisp et al 2021)

CLINICAL SKILL 30.2 Inserting a nasogastric tube

Please adhere to the policy and procedures of the facility/organisation prior to undertaking the skill. Ensure this skill is in your scope of practice.

NMBA Decision-making Framework considerations (refer to NMBA Decision-making framework for nursing and midwifery 2020): 1. Am I educated? 2. Am I authorised? 3. Am I competent? If you answer 'no' to any of these, do not perform that activity. Seek guidance and support from your teacher/a nurse team leader/clinical facilitator/educator.	**Equipment:** Appropriate-sized nasogastric tube (large or fine bore tube) Nasofix or hypoallergenic tape (approx. 7 cm × 2.5 cm split in half for 5 cm of its length to look 'Y-shaped' Lubricant (KY gel) if tube not self-lubricating 10 mL and 20 mL syringes Water or moist cotton buds (if permitted) Kidney dish Disposable gloves Protective eyewear Yankauer sucker and suction Emesis bag/bowl Tissues Protective sheet Plastic bag Equipment for observations (O_2 saturation) Safety pin Spigot or drainage bag if required pH indicator paper/strip

Continued

CLINICAL SKILL 30.2 Inserting a nasogastric tube—cont'd

PREPARE FOR THE SKILL

(Please refer to the Standard Steps on pp. xviii–xx for related rationales.)
Mentally review the steps of the skill.
Discuss the skill with your instructor/supervisor/team leader, if required.
Confirm correct facility/organisation policy/safe operating procedures.
Validate the order in the individual's record.
Identify indication and rationale for performing the activity.
Assess for any contraindications.
Locate and gather equipment.
Perform hand hygiene.
Ensure therapeutic interaction.
Identify the individual using three individual identifiers.
Gain the individual's consent.
Assess for pain relief.
Prepare the environment.
Provide and maintain privacy.
Assist the individual to assume an appropriate position of comfort.

Skill activity	Rationale
Critically think through the assessment data and problem-solving—special precautions for nasogastric tube insertion.	Evaluate each aspect and its relationship to other data to help identify specific problems and modifications of the procedure that may be needed for the individual.
Assist the individual into the high Fowler's position with neck flexed unless contraindicated. Spinal and neurological individuals must be positioned as per medical orders.	Facilitates tube insertion and reduces risk of gastro-oesophageal reflux and aspiration. Avoids neck extension as it closes oesophagus, opens trachea and promotes aspiration.

PERFORM THE SKILL

(Please refer to the Standard Steps on pp. xviii–xx for related rationales.)
Perform hand hygiene.
Apply PPE: gloves, eyewear, mask and gown as appropriate.
Ensure the individual's safety and comfort throughout skill.
Promote independence and involvement of the individual if possible and/or appropriate.
Assess the individual's tolerance to the skill throughout.
Dispose of used supplies, equipment, waste and sharps appropriately.
Remove PPE and discard or store appropriately.
Perform hand hygiene.

Skill activity	Rationale
Clean nares if necessary and examine nostrils for deformity/obstruction and nasal surgery to determine best side for insertion. If nasogastric tube is being reinserted the other nostril should be used.	Asking the individual to breathe through one nostril while occluding the other will help ascertain if one nostril has an occlusion. Minimises risk of irritation and pressure necrosis around the nose.
Measure the portion of tube to be inserted by extending it from the tip of the individual's nose to the earlobe and from the earlobe to the xiphoid process. Note length and mark this measurement on the tube.	Determines the insertion length of the tube to ensure the tube is inserted an adequate distance so that the distal tip rests in the stomach.
Flush fine bore nasogastric tube with 10 mL of water to activate the Hydromer coating.	Ensures easy removal of stylet after insertion and confirms correct positioning.
Lubricate the first 5–10 cm of the tube with water-soluble lubricant. **Note:** Some small-bore tubes self-lubricate when dipped in water.	The use of lubricant will ease insertion by decreasing friction.

CLINICAL SKILL 30.2 Inserting a nasogastric tube—cont'd	
Grasp the tube with your hand and gently insert it into the nostril guiding it posteriorly and inferiorly straight back along the floor of the nose. Ask the individual to sniff to ease the passage of the tube from nose to oropharynx. Have an emesis basin and tissues in the individual's lap. Pause a moment if the individual is coughing or gagging.	Insertion of the nasogastric tube can stimulate the gag reflex.
Instruct the individual to tilt the head slightly forwards.	Flexing the head forwards allows the tube to follow the posterior wall of the nasopharynx and enter the oesophagus rather than the trachea.
Instruct the individual to swallow while you gently but steadily advance the tube. Coincide advancement of the tube with the individual swallowing. Sips of water may be given to assist swallowing if safe and not contraindicated.	The muscular movement of swallowing helps advance the tube. Minimises risk of aspiration.
If resistance is met, withdraw the tube 1–2 cm and rotate the tube slowly with downward advancement towards the closest ear. Do not force the nasogastric tube. Abort procedure and attempt other nostril. Withdraw the tube immediately if the individual exhibits signs of distress or a change in respiratory status, if individual begins to cough or change colour or if the tube coils in the individual's mouth. Should two failed attempts occur, cease the procedure and escalate to a more experienced staff member.	Prevents adverse individual outcome such as pneumothorax, aspiration, trauma to surrounding tissues, incorrect tube placement into lungs or cranium.
Advance tube until the pre-measured mark is reached. When the pre-measured mark has been reached secure the tube to the individual's nose using Nasofix or hypoallergenic tape ensuring the tube does not cause pressure on the naris. If inserting a fine-bore nasogastric tube, do not remove stylet until correct placement has been confirmed by X-ray and documented in individual's health record. To prevent tension on the tube, place a piece of tape onto the nasogastric tube (distal end) and attach it to individual's clothing.	Ensures the tube does not move out of the stomach.
Perform and document observations and compare to pre-procedure observations.	Ensures individual has not been compromised by insertion of nasogastric tube.
Ensure correct position of the nasogastric tube. Aspirate 5 to 10 mL of gastrointestinal fluid. Observe amount and colour and test pH using pH indicator paper/strip. Obtain post-insertion chest/upper abdominal X-ray. The medical officer must document correct placement in the individual's file prior to the administration of any medications, fluids or formula.	Ensures the tube is in the correct location and not in the trachea. Gastric fluid pH is usually 1.0–4.0, indicating the tube is in correct position. pH of pleural fluid is usually >6, indicating incorrect position. Radiological confirmation should be obtained if pH is greater than 5.
Once correct placement has been confirmed and documented, reactivate the Hydromer coating with another 10 mL of water before removing the stylet. The stylet must not be reinserted. If using a large-bore tube for aspiration, attach a spigot or drainage bag to the main lumen of the nasogastric tube.	

Continued

CLINICAL SKILL 30.2 Inserting a nasogastric tube—cont'd

AFTER THE SKILL

(Please refer to the Standard Steps on pp. xviii–xx for related rationales.)
Communicate outcome to the individual, any ongoing care and to report any complications.
Restore the environment.
Report, record and document assessment findings, details of the skill performed and the individual's response.
Report, record and document any abnormalities and/or inability to perform the skill.
Reassess the individual to ensure there are no adverse effects/events from the skill.

Skill activity	Rationale
Document reason for nasogastric tube insertion, nostril used, type and size of tube, insertion distance and the external length of the tube (from nostril to tip).	Ensures transfer of information.

(Berman et al 2020; Crisp et al 2021; Hall et al 2022; LeMone et al 2020; NSW Department of Health 2023; Rebeiro et al 2021)

completed abiding to institution documentation policies. (See Progress Note 30.1.)

Nasoduodenal and nasojejunal tubes

Tubes placed into the duodenum or jejunum are used for individuals with gastric disorders that contraindicate gastric placement, such as severe reflux, partial or total gastrectomy and malabsorption.

Gastrostomy tubes

Feeding via a gastrostomy tube may be indicated if there has been recent surgery or an obstruction in the upper part of the digestive tract, or as a long-term treatment for feeding difficulties. A gastrostomy tube is a hollow tube, often composed of silicone, inserted through the abdomen into the stomach by a surgeon either through an external approach via an incision through the abdominal wall or endoscopically via the mouth through the stomach and through the abdominal wall. The opening around the tube may be sutured to prevent leakage or accidental removal (Figure 30.8) or held in place with an inflatable balloon and a flange or similar device that applies pressure to hold the tube against the inside wall of the stomach.

Gastrostomy (percutaneous endoscopic gastrostomy [PEG]) and jejunostomy (percutaneous endoscopic jejunostomy [PEJ]) devices are used for long-term nutritional support, generally more than 6–8 weeks (Berman et al 2020). Fluid enteral feeds are normally introduced 24 hours later through the tube, into the lumen of the stomach, duodenum or jejunum. Some tubes may require replacement to prevent or treat occlusion or disintegration; long-term silastic tubes may be left in situ indefinitely. In the event of accidental tube removal, the individual should have a Foley or Malecot catheter available, to enable a medical officer to ensure the stoma's patency and continuity of feed.

Prepared enteral feeds are administered by either:

- Intermittent or bolus feeds, in which a solution is administered at regular intervals (e.g. every 4 hours). Administered to individuals who can tolerate volumes at a rate they could normally drink orally. A syringe or giving set is attached to the end of the nasogastric tube and filled with the feed or fluid, which is allowed to flow in slowly by gravity or by the use of an enteral feeding pump. The rate of administration can be adjusted (e.g. by the height at which the syringe or set is held at, or by adjusting the enteral pumping rate).
- Continuous feeds, in which a gravity infusion set or a controlled enteral feeding pump is used that can deliver the fluid at a regulated rate over a predetermined time. Continuous feeds are administered to individuals who have difficulty tolerating bolus doses, or for individuals with malabsorption, reactive hyperinsulinaemia, diarrhoea or other metabolic problems.

Depending on the institution and the nutrition required, the enteral feed may come pre-packaged (e.g. in cans) and will not require refrigeration, while other solutions stored in containers such as waxed cardboard or made in-house do require refrigeration.

The nurse should be aware of the policies and regulations in their healthcare setting regarding their role and responsibilities in checking the location of the tip of the nasogastric tube. (See Clinical Skill 30.3.)

Care specific to gastrostomy type tubes

For individuals who may be discharged home or to encourage independence with enteral tubes in situ, the individual may be taught how to test, administer and perform the care required independently. Part of the education involves discussing some of the complications and how to deal with them, as described below.

Care and cleaning of gastrostomy tube and equipment

Abdominal distension. Determine tube position by testing the aspirate with pH-sensitive paper. Before administering an enteral feed or fluid, gas may be vented (released) from the stomach to avoid distension. Venting is achieved by removing a spigot, unscrewing a cap and/or releasing an

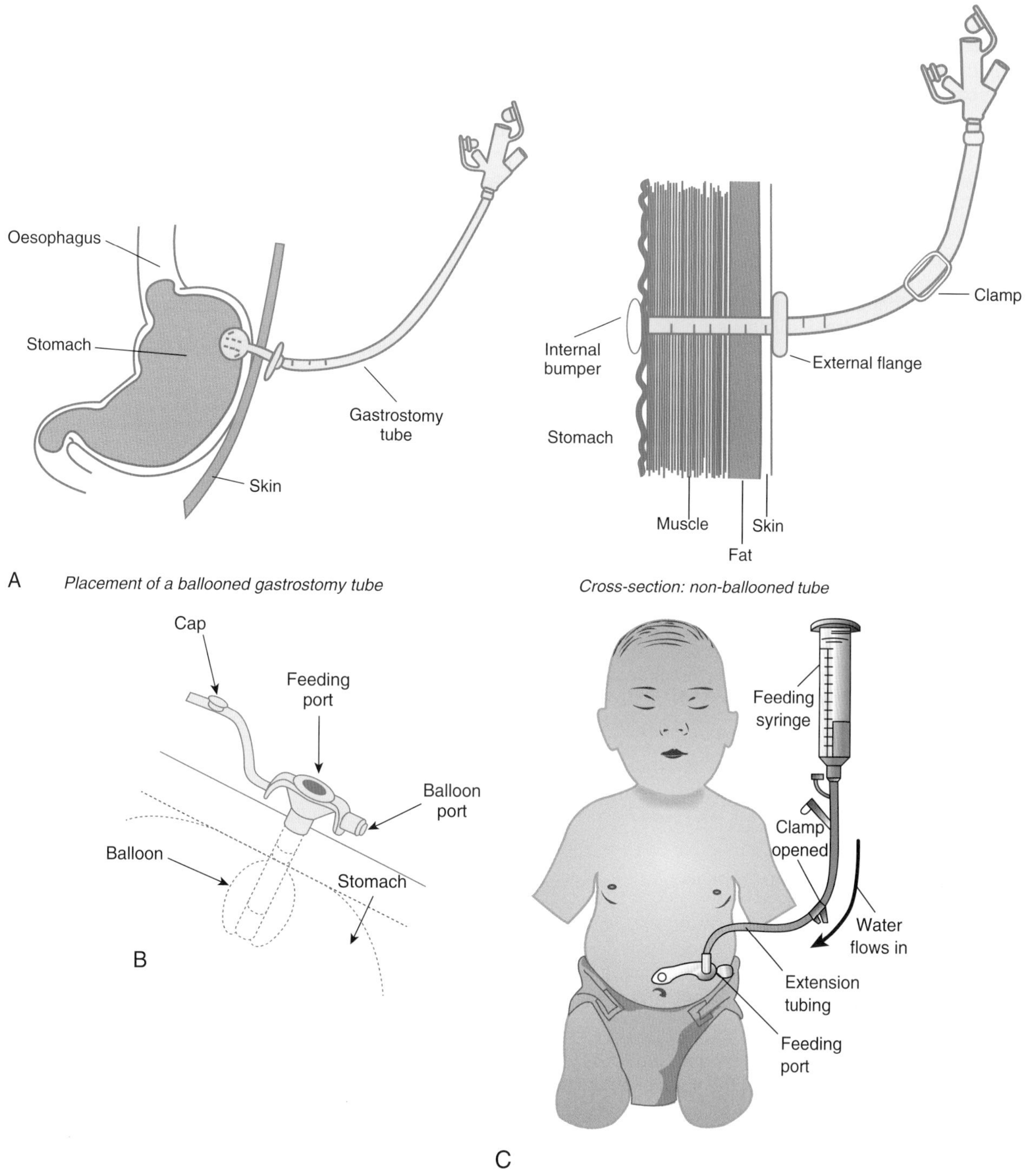

Figure 30.8 Gastrostomy feeding

A: Gastrostomy placement, **B:** When not in use the end of the tube is capped, **C:** Administration of bolus feed.

obstructive clamp, or by inserting a catheter and raising the tube to a vertical position.

Hanging times. In a warm environment, feeds can be contaminated by pathogens. For maximum hanging times local policies and procedures should be abided by. Times may vary depending on the individual's condition (e.g. immunocompromised), the type of feed and environment (e.g. hospital setting or person's home).

Home cleaning. Feeding equipment, syringes, etc. can be washed with warm soapy water and left to air-dry and can be used for 3 days. The equipment should be washed again in warm soapy water immediately before each use.

Flushing. Flush tube pre and post feeding. Flush tube pre and post medications. If the individual is on continuous feeding, the gastrostomy tube should be flushed every 4 hours.

CLINICAL SKILL 30.3 Enteral feed

Please adhere to the policy and procedures of the facility/organisation prior to undertaking the skill. Ensure this skill is in your scope of practice.

NMBA Decision-making Framework considerations (refer to NMBA Decision-making framework for nursing and midwifery 2020):	**Equipment:**
1. Am I educated? 2. Am I authorised? 3. Am I competent? If you answer 'no' to any of these, do not perform that activity. Seek guidance and support from your teacher/a nurse team leader/clinical facilitator/educator.	Enteral feeding pump Enteral feeding set Prescribed enteral feed or ready-to-hang formula IV pole Disposable gloves 20 mL oral/enteral syringe pH indicator paper/strip Stethoscope Glucometer to obtain blood glucose by finger-stick

PREPARE FOR THE SKILL

(Please refer to the Standard Steps on pp. xviii–xx for related rationales.)
Mentally review the steps of the skill.
Discuss the skill with your instructor/supervisor/team leader, if required.
Confirm correct facility/organisation policy/safe operating procedures.
Validate the order in the individual's record.
Identify indication and rationale for performing the activity.
Assess for any contraindications.
Locate and gather equipment.
Perform hand hygiene.
Ensure therapeutic interaction.
Identify the individual using three individual identifiers.
Gain the individual's consent.
Assess for pain relief.
Prepare the environment.
Provide and maintain privacy.
Assist the individual to assume an appropriate position of comfort.

Skill activity	Rationale
Critically think through assessment data and problem-solving—correct position of nasogastric tube, documentation of order, individual's baseline weight and laboratory values, electrolyte and metabolic abnormalities such as hyperglycaemia and fluid volume excess or deficit and auscultate for bowel sounds.	Evaluate each aspect and its relationship to other data to help identify specific problems and modifications of the procedure that may be needed for the individual. Baseline objective data is used to measure the effectiveness of the feeds. Absent bowel sounds may indicate decreased ability of GI tract to digest or absorb nutrients.
Confirm documentation of enteral feeding regimen (type, route, volume and flow rate) by medical officer and dietitian. Ensure correct position of nasogastric tube has been confirmed by a post-insertion chest/upper abdominal X-ray and documented by medical officer in individual's health records prior to administration of medications or fluids.	Ensures correct feeding regimen. Ensures correct position of nasogastric tube prior to administration of medication or fluids.

PERFORM THE SKILL

(Please refer to the Standard Steps on pp. xviii–xx for related rationales.)
Perform hand hygiene.
Apply PPE: gloves, eyewear, mask and gown as appropriate.
Ensure the individual's safety and comfort throughout skill.
Promote independence and involvement of the individual if possible and/or appropriate.
Assess the individual's tolerance to the skill throughout.
Dispose of used supplies, equipment, waste and sharps appropriately.
Remove PPE and discard or store appropriately.
Perform hand hygiene.

CLINICAL SKILL 30.3 Enteral feed—cont'd

Skill activity	Rationale
Check the tube length measurement at the nostril is unchanged compared to the documented correct tube length confirmed by the medical officer by post-insertion X-ray.	Checks correct tube placement prior to commencement of the formula.
Placement on chest/upper abdominal X-ray must be confirmed and documented by a medical officer where there is suspicion of tube displacement or if the individual has been retching, vomiting or violent coughing. With a torch, examine the back of the individual's mouth to ensure tube has not curled up in the back of the throat. Aspirate gastric contents to check for gastric residual. Return aspirated contents to stomach unless the volume exceeds 150 mL. Measure pH of aspirated gastrointestinal contents. Test pH by using pH indicator paper/strips. Gastric aspirate has a pH <5. Observe the aspirate appearance.	Presence of gastric secretions indicates that the distal end of the tube is in the stomach. Residual volume of greater than 150 mL may indicate gastric emptying is delayed. The pH of fluid aspirated from tube of fasting individuals is helpful in differentiating between gastric and respiratory placement and gastric and small bowel placement. Gastric fluid is usually cloudy and grassy green or tan to off-white in colour.
Individual should be positioned in high Fowler's position or elevate head of bed >30 degrees. Where this is contraindicated, the individual should be positioned laterally (left side) to protect the airway during and for at least 60 minutes post cessation of enteral feeding.	Reduces risk of gastro-oesophageal reflux and aspiration by ensuring individual is safely positioned prior to commencement of feeding.
A closed enteral feeding system ready to hang is generally used; it has a maximum 24-hour hang time post connection with a giving set. Giving set must be changed at time of a closed enteral feeding system being hung. Decanted formula should not be hung for more than 8 hours. Ensure non-touch technique when preparing and handling formula and nasogastric tube. Enteral feeding delivery set must be replaced at least every 24 hours. Time and date should be specified on giving set label.	Ensures correct enteral feed and hang time. Prevents contamination of formula and nasogastric tube. Tubing and formula must be free of contamination to prevent bacterial growth.
Ensure formula is at room temperature. Shake formula container well. Close roller clamp at lower end of spike giving set to prevent air entering the tube. Connect tubing to container or prepare ready-to-hang container and fill container and tubing with formula. Connect distal end of tubing to the proximal end of the feeding tube. Hang pack on IV pole and adjust height. Connect tubing through enteral feed pump, prime line as per manufacturer's instruction. Set flow rate as ordered.	Ensures correct administration of formula. Cold formula may cause gastric cramping and discomfort.

AFTER THE SKILL

(Please refer to the Standard Steps on pp. xviii–xx for related rationales.)
Communicate outcome to the individual, any ongoing care and to report any complications.
Restore the environment.
Report, record and document assessment findings, details of the skill performed and the individual's response.
Report, record and document any abnormalities and/or inability to perform the skill.
Reassess the individual to ensure there are no adverse effects/events from the skill.

Continued

CLINICAL SKILL 30.3 Enteral feed—cont'd

Skill activity	Rationale
Assess individual while feeding is in progress for signs of intolerance to enteral feeding (e.g. vomiting, reflux, nausea, diarrhoea, distension, large residual aspirate volumes).	Ensures formula is tolerated by individual.
During continual enteral feeding, the nasogastric tube should be flushed with 30 mL of tap water three times a day unless clinical indication prevents this volume of fluid. Chart the amount of water used to flush on fluid balance chart. Consult with RN if the feeding tube is blocked. Measure amount of residual aspirate every 4 hours. When tube feedings are not being administered, cap or clamp the proximal end of the feeding tube after flushing the tube with 30 mL water.	Continuous feeding delivers a prescribed hourly rate of feeding which reduces risk of abdominal discomfort. Flushing the tube with water reduces the risk of sediment forming and blocking the tubing. Individuals receiving continuous feeding should have tube placement confirmed and residual aspirate checked every 4 hours. Prevents air entering the stomach between feeds.
Monitor the cleanliness and effectiveness of the tape securing the nasogastric tube to the nose. Tape should be replaced daily. During tape change observe for signs of pressure necrosis around the nose.	Ensures the correct tube placement and absence of pressure areas.
Monitor blood glucose level (BGL) as per facility/organisation policy. Document intake on fluid balance chart. Monitor intake and output every 24 hours. Weigh individual daily until administration rate is reached for 24 hours then three times per week. Observe return of normal laboratory values. Record and report amount and type of feed, individual's tolerance of feed, adverse effects and patency and placement of tube.	Monitors individual's tolerance of glucose. Ensures accurate intake is recorded. Intake and output are indications of fluid balance or fluid volume excess or deficit. Weight gain is an indicator of improved nutritional status. Sudden gain of more than 900 g in 24 hours may indicate fluid retention. Improving laboratory values indicate improved nutritional status.

(Berman et al 2020; Crisp et al 2021; Hall et al 2022; LeMone et al 2020; NSW Department of Health 2023; Rebeiro et al 2021)

Skin care

The area around the gastrostomy site requires daily cleaning with warm soapy water to remove build-up of secretions from the stoma site and to prevent infection. Creams and dressings are not recommended if there is no redness or inflammation. The tube and the surrounding pressure device should be rotated in the stoma daily to prevent adhesion or ulceration of the surrounding skin. The skin around the site should be inspected for redness, oozing, swelling or bleeding (Boeykens et al 2022).

Common problems associated with enteral feeding

Aspiration

This is a potentially life-threatening complication and occurs when gastric contents, saliva, food or nasopharyngeal secretions have been inhaled into the respiratory tract. Signs and symptoms of aspiration include tachypnoea, increased work of breathing, wheeze, crackles, hypoxaemia, fever, cyanosis and cough (Guenter & Lyman 2021). Feed should be immediately ceased and not recommenced until reviewed by medical officer.

Tube occlusion

Occasionally, tubes can become occluded because of inadequate flushing, feeds being too thick, the tube too long and/or too narrow, or the administration of certain crushed medications (Guenter & Lyman 2021). To unblock the tube, a volume of 20–30 mL (adults) of lukewarm water can be administered into the tube with pulsatile ('back and forth') pressure for about 5 minutes. Carbonated acidic soft drinks can be tried although their effect is not superior to water (Boeykens et al 2022).

Tube migration/obstruction

Verify placement and discontinue feeding until medical review.

Accidental removal

Rinse tube and replace it as soon as possible—do not recommence feeds until tube position has been verified.

Balloon burst

Check balloon volume by withdrawing water into syringe and change tube.

Bleeding

Bleeding may indicate the presence of an infection or trauma to the tube. Bleeding is stopped by localised pressure or 'stomahesive' dressing, and the incident documented and reported.

Redness

Localised redness with or without swelling may indicate inflammation from acidic gastric contents due to, for example, the tube being too small for the stoma, the flange being too loose on the skin or perishing or bursting of the balloon in the stomach. Any ooze can be checked for acidity using pH-sensitive paper. If acid is detected, a waterproof cream can be applied to prevent further irritation of the skin by acid (O'Flynn 2019). The use of dressings to soak up the fluid or topical antacids may cause further skin breakdown. The size of the tube and the flange's location need to be checked daily to prevent migration. An indelible pen can be used to mark the lower limit of the tube, and the measurement is recorded on the care plan. In some cases, an individual may require a tube to be replaced with a larger-diameter one.

Complications with tubes or flanges are reported to a medical officer or a stomal therapist. In some situations, particularly after surgery, primary and/or secondary peritonitis may be caused by inadequate pressure from the flange and balloon, and subsequent poor sealing of underlying tissues.

Diarrhoea

If the feeds are administered too rapidly or the individual is intolerant to the feed, diarrhoea may develop. This may be minimised by slowing the rate of the feed or changing the feed type. If symptoms persist a medical officer should be contacted.

Granulation of gastrostomy site

Granulation of the surrounding tissue occurs as a healing response but can interfere with the comfort of the tube. To prevent granulation, the site should be kept as dry as possible and properly secured to minimise friction (Boeykens et al 2022). Treatments for hypergranulation include silver nitrate cauterisation (Rackham 2022), topical low-dose steroid application, topical antimicrobials and foam dressings (Mitchell & Llumigusin 2021).

Hypoglycaemia

Individuals who have bolus feeds administered too rapidly, in excessive quantities or who may have a lax pyloric sphincter are at risk of the feeds entering the duodenum too rapidly and causing hyperinsulinaemia and consequential hypoglycaemia. See Clinical Interest Box 30.4 for other electrolyte disturbances that may result.

CLINICAL INTEREST BOX 30.4 COVID-19 and nutrition

The respiratory disease known as COVID-19 was declared a global pandemic in March 2020. The COVID-19 pandemic is an ongoing challenge that imposes a significant burden on public health resources.

Research into the impact of COVID-19 on nutrition is continually emerging but it is known that people with existing conditions including malnutrition might be more vulnerable to COVID-19 and similar infections. COVID-19 negatively impacts on nutrition status since the affected person will have increased nutritional requirements and simultaneously a lower food intake. Impacts of COVID-19 on dietary intake include:

- respiratory issues such as coughing, sneezing and shortness of breath
- loss of taste and smell
- fever, which increases inflammatory responses and nutritional requirements
- fatigue and malaise, which impacts on a person's ability to undertake normal ADLs such as shopping or cooking
- severe illness requiring mechanical ventilation
- quarantine/isolation, which may reduce carer support and limit social interactions that would normally accompany eating.

Nutritional screening and intervention should be considered an integral part of COVID-19 treatment. Foods likely to be of benefit are anti-inflammatory foods such as omega-3 rich foods, vitamin D supplementation and foods that are known to prevent/reduce obesity. Prescription of oral nutritional supplements should be considered in persons with inadequate dietary intake.

(Garofolo et al 2020; Holdoway 2020; WHO 2023; Tsagari & Kyriazis 2021)

Progress Note 30.1

12/05/2024 0810 hrs	Nursing: NG inserted by RN D Nelson as per Dr Smith orders above. NG size 16F inserted left naris to 30 cm without difficulty. Placement confirmed with universal paper pH 4. pH witnessed by both RN D Nelson and myself. NG Gastrolyte commenced as per fluid order. Dr Smith aware of same. *H Joy* (JOY), *EN*

DECISION-MAKING FRAMEWORK EXERCISE 30.1

You are working on a gastrointestinal ward and caring for Dimitri, a 52-year-old male, day 4 post bowel resection for chronic diverticulitis. This morning he has been vomiting and complaining of severe cramping abdominal pain. On taking his vital signs, you find he is tachycardic and diaphoretic. His abdomen is distended and on auscultation has decreased bowel sounds. In response, you call the medical emergency team to review Dimitri. The medical officer requests you insert a nasogastric tube (NGT) immediately to alleviate a paralytic ileus. During your course you had NGT insertion demonstrated and had practised in the nursing lab. Since starting on the ward, you have assisted with multiple insertions and have almost completed the local hospital accreditation course.

Using the nursing practice decision-making framework:

1. What would your response be to the medical officer's request?
2. What would be the appropriate nursing action to ensure Dimitri receives the requested treatment?

Summary

Nutrition is necessary for the development and growth of cells and for the replacement of substances required by the cells to maintain efficient body function. A diet that contains the essential nutrients is important throughout each stage of the lifespan, and people should be encouraged to follow the principles of good nutrition and to eat a balanced healthy diet. Food provides energy that is necessary for the chemical and physical activities of the body. Energy requirements vary according to age, sex, body composition and presence of ailments or conditions. Each nutrient performs a specific function, and a nutrient deficiency may result in body dysfunction.

Many factors influence an individual's eating pattern, and choice of foods and illness may necessitate certain changes in dietary intake. Modification of the consistency of food may be indicated, or a specific diet may be prescribed for therapeutic purposes. The nurse should assist individuals to meet their nutritional needs and the nurse may need to assist or feed an individual who is unable to feed themself. If an individual is unable to consume food or fluid orally, an alternative method of meeting their nutritional needs may be necessary.

Problems associated with nutrition should be identified so that appropriate medical, nursing and dietitian care can be planned and implemented to meet the individual's nutritional needs.

Review Questions

1. What information should be included in the nutrition assessment of an individual?
2. What are the national healthy eating guidelines?
3. Should individuals be recommended a low or high GI diet? Why?
4. List the essential nutrients.
5. What are the common disorders associated with nutrition?
6. What are principles of good nutrition suggested by the NHMRC?
7. What other diets are there to meet individual needs?
8. What are potential alternative methods to meet nutritional needs and when should these be considered?
9. What are the common problems associated with gastrostomy tubes?
10. Define the term 'TPN' and explain potential indications and nursing care for individuals receiving TPN.
11. What are some of the positive outcomes for the individual and health system if malnutrition is identified and addressed in a timely manner?

Evolve® Answer guide for the Review Questions, Critical Thinking Exercises, Decision-making Framework Exercises and Critical Thinking Questions in Case Studies is hosted on Evolve: http://evolve.elsevier.com/AU/Koutoukidis/Tabbner.

References

Agarwal, E., Ferguson, M., Banks, M., et al., 2010. Nutritional status and dietary intake of acute care patients: Results from the Australasian day survey. *Clinical Nutrition* 31(1), 41–47.

Agency for Clinical Intervention, 2021. South Eastern Sydney Local Health District – I AM: Identifying and addressing malnutrition. Available at: <https://aci.health.nsw.gov.au/ie/projects/i-am>.

Australasian Society of Clinical Immunologists and Allergists (ASCIA), 2020. ASCIA guidelines—infant feeding and allergy prevention. Available at: <https://www.allergy.org.au/images/pcc/ASCIA_Guidelines_Infant_Feeding_and_Allergy_Prevention_2020.pdf>.

Australian Commission on Safety and Quality in Health Care (ACSQHC), 2018. Hospital-acquired complication 13 malnutrition. Available at: <https://www.safetyandquality.gov.au/publications-and-resources/resource-library/hospital-acquired-complication-13-malnutrition-fact-sheet>.

Australian Commission on Safety and Quality in Health Care (ACSQHC), 2021. National safety and quality health service standards, 2nd ed. ACSQHC, Sydney.

Australian Indigenous Health*InfoNet*, 2020. Summary of nutrition among Aboriginal and Torres Strait Islander people. Available at <https://healthinfonet.ecu.edu.au/healthinfonet/getContent.php?linkid=642619&title=Summary+of+nutrition+among+Aboriginal+and+Torres+Strait+Islander+people&contentid=40271_1>.

Australian Institute of Health and Welfare (AIHW), 2017a. Admitted patient care 2015–16: Australian hospital statistics. Health services series no. 75. Cat. no. HSE 185. AIHW, Canberra. Available at: <https://www.aihw.gov.au/getmedia/3e1d7d7e-26d9-44fb-8549-aa30ccff100a/20742.pdf.aspx?inline=true>.

Australian Institute of Health and Welfare (AIHW), 2017b. Impact of overweight and obesity as a risk factor for chronic conditions: Australian burden of disease study. Australian burden of disease study series no. 11. Cat. no. BOD 12. AIHW, Canberra.

Australian Institute of Health and Welfare (AIHW), 2017c. Risk factors to health. Available at: <https://www.aihw.gov.au/reports/risk-factors/risk-factors-to-health/contents/overweight-and-obesity/causes-of-overweight-and-obesity>.

Australian Institute of Health and Welfare (AIHW), 2020. Overweight and obesity among Australian children and adolescents. Available at: <https://www.aihw.gov.au/reports/overweight-obesity/overweight-obesity-australian-children-adolescents/summary>.

Australian Institute of Health and Welfare (AIHW), 2021. Australia's youth: Nutrition. Available at: <https://www.aihw.gov.au/reports/children-youth/nutrition>.

Australian Institute of Health and Welfare (AIHW), 2022a. Australia's health: Topic summaries. Available at: <https://www.aihw.gov.au/australias-health/summaries>.

Australian Institute of Health and Welfare (AIHW), 2022b. Food and nutrition. Available at: <https://www.aihw.gov.au/reports-data/behaviours-risk-factors/food-nutrition/overview>.

Ayerbe, J., Hauser, B., Salvatore, S., Vandenplas, V., 2019. Diagnosis and management of gastroesophageal reflux disease in infants and children: From guidelines to clinical practice. *Pediatric Gastroenterology, Hepatology & Nutrition* 22(2), 107–121. Available at: <https://doi.org/10.5223/pghn.2019.22.2.107>.

Barber, T., Kabisch, S., Pfeiffer, A., Weickert, M., 2020. The health benefits of dietary fibre. *Nutrients* 12(10), 3209. Available at: <https://doi.org/10.3390/nu12103209>.

Berman, A., Snyder, S., Levett-Jones, T., et al., 2020. *Kozier and Erb's fundamentals of nursing*, 5th ed. Pearson, Frenchs Forest.

Bishop, A., Witts, S., Martin, T., 2018. The role of nutrition in successful wound healing. *Journal of Community Nursing* 32(4), 44–50.

Bloom, L., Seckel, M., 2021. Placement of nasogastric feeding tube and postinsertion care review. *AACN Advanced Critical Care* 33(1), 68–84.

Boeykens, K., Duysburgh, I., Verlinden, W., 2022. Prevention and management of minor complications in percutaneous endoscopic gastrostomy. *BMJ Open Gastroenterology* 9, e000975. doi: 10.1136/bmjgast-2022-000975.

Cass, A., Charlton, K., 2022. Prevalence of hospital-acquired malnutrition and modifiable determinants of nutritional deterioration during inpatient admissions: A systematic review of the evidence. *Journal of Human Nutrition and Dietetics* 35(6), 1043–1058. Available at: <https://doi.org/10.1111/jhn.13009>.

Cole, N., Musaad, S., Lee, S-Y., Donovan, S., STRONG Kids Team, 2018. Home feeding environment and picky eating behavior in preschool-aged children: A prospective analysis. *Eating Behaviors* 30, 76–82. doi: 10.1016/j.eatbeh.2018.06.003.

Commonwealth of Australia, 2023a. Royal Commission into Aged Care Quality and Safety. Available at: <https://agedcare.royalcommission.gov.au>.

Commonwealth of Australia, 2023b. Food, dining and nutrition resources (providers). Available at: <https://www.agedcarequality.gov.au/providers/quality-care-resources/food-dining-and-nutrition-resources-providers>.

Crisp, J., Douglas, S., Rebeiro, G., et al. (eds.), 2021. *Potter and Perry's fundamentals of nursing*, 6th ed. Elsevier, Sydney.

Dains, J., Baumann, L,. Scheibel, P., 2020. Unintentional weight loss or gain. In: *Advanced health assessment & clinical diagnosis in primary care*, 6th ed. Elsevier, Sydney.

Daven, J., Hellzen, O., Haggstrom, M., 2022. Encountering patients with anorexia nervosa – An emotional roller coaster. Nurses' lived experiences of encounters in psychiatric inpatient care. *International Journal of Qualitative Studies on Health and Well-being* 17. Available at: <https://doi.org/10.1080/17482631.2022.2069651>.

Dementia Australia, 2022. Nutrition. Available at: <https://www.dementia.org.au/support-and-services/families-and-friends/personal-care/nutrition>.

Department of Communities, Disability Services and Seniors, 2019. Mealtime support resources. Centre of Excellence for Clinical Innovation and Behaviour Support, Queensland

Government. Available at: <https://publications.qld.gov.au/dataset/mealtime-support-resources>.

Dietitians Australia, 2020. Mealtimes and dining experience in aged care. Available at: <https://dietitiansaustralia.org.au/advocacy-andpolicy/position-statements/mealtimes-and-diningexperience-aged-care-position-statement>.

DiMaria-Ghalili, R., McPherson, B., 2020. Nursing management: Nutritional problems. In: Brown, D., *Lewis's medical-surgical nursing*, 5th ed. Elsevier, Sydney.

Elsevier ClinicalKey, 2021. Clinical overview: Obesity in adults. Available at: <https://elsevier.health/en-US/preview/clinical-overview-obesity-in-adults>.

Emergency Care Institute, 2023. Vomiting and diarrhoea. Nurse management guidelines. Available at: <https://www.aci.health.nsw.gov.au/networks/eci/clinical/ndec/vomiting-and-diarrhoea-nmg>.

Esper, D.H., 2015. Utilization of nutrition-focused physical assessment in identifying micronutrient deficiencies. *Nutrition in Clinical Practice* 30, 194–202. doi: 10.1177/0884533615573054.

Ferri, F., 2022. Clinical overview: Constipation in older adults. Available at: <https://clinicalkey.com.au>.

Firman, G., 2019. GLIM criteria for the diagnosis of malnutrition. Available at: <https://medicalcriteria.com/web/glim-malnutrition>.

Flood, C., Parker, E., Kaul, N., et al., 2021. A benchmarking study of home enteral nutrition services. *Clinical Nutrition ESPEN* 44, 387–396. Available at: <https://doi.org/10.1016/j.clnesp.2021.05.007>.

Freeman, A., Aggarwal, M., 2020. Malnutrition in the obese: Commonly overlooked but with serious consequences. *Journal of the American College of Cardiology* 76(7), 841–843.

Garofolo, A., Qiao, L., dos Santos Maia-Lemos, P., 2020. Approach to nutrition in cancer patients in the context of the coronavirus disease 2019 (COVID-19) pandemic: Perspectives. *Nutrition and Cancer* 73(8), 1293–1301. Available at: <https://doi.org/10.1080/01635581.2020.1797126>.

Guenter, P., Lyman, B., 2021. Evidence-based strategies to prevent enteral nutrition complications. *American Nurse Journal* 16(6), 18–21.

Grantham, S., 2020. Obesity and weight management. In: *Primary care*, 6th ed. Elsevier, Missouri.

Green, S., 2020. Nutrition and health. In: Peate, I., *Alexander's nursing practice: Hospital and home*, 5th ed. Elsevier, Edinburgh.

Grodner, M., Escott-Stump, S., Dorner, S., 2020. *Nutritional foundations and clinical applications*, 7th ed. Elsevier, Sydney.

Harbottle, L., 2019. The effect of nutrition on older people's mental health. *British Journal of Community Nursing* 24(7), S12–16.

Harris, P., Nagy, S., Vardaxis, N. (eds.), 2019. *Mosby's dictionary of medicine, nursing & health professions*, 3rd ed. Elsevier, Sydney.

Hall, H., Glew, P., Rhodes, J., 2022. *Fundamentals of nursing and midwifery: A person-centred approach to care*, 4th ed. Australian and New Zealand ed. Lippincott, Williams and Wilkins Australia, Sydney.

Holdoway, A., 2020. Nutritional management of patients during and after COVID-19 illness. *British Journal of Community Nursing* 25(8), S6–S10. doi: 10.12968/bjcn.2020.25.Sup8.S6.

Kawaji, L., Fontanilla, J., 2021. Accuracy of waist circumference measurement using the WHO versus NIH protocol in predicting visceral adiposity using bioelectrical impedance analysis among overweight and obese adult Filipinos in a tertiary hospital. *Journal of the ASEAN Federation of Endocrine Societies* 36(2), 180–188. doi: 10.15605/jafes.036.02.13.

Koletzko, B., Fishbein, M., Lee, W., et al., 2020. Prevention of childhood obesity: A position paper of the Global Federation of International Societies of Paediatric Gastroenterology, Hepatology and Nutrition (FISPGHAN). *Journal of Pediatric Gastroenterology and Nutrition* 70(5), 702–710. doi: 10.1097/MPG.0000000000002708.

LeMone, P., Burke, K., Bauldoff, G., et al., 2020. *Medical–surgical nursing: Critical thinking for person-centred care*, 4th ed. Pearson, Melbourne.

Long, T., Liu, K., Long, J., Li, J., Cheng, L., 2022. Dietary glycemic index, glycemic load and cancer risk: A meta-analysis of prospective cohort studies. *European Journal of Nutrition* 61, 2115–2127. Available at: <https://doi.org/10.1007/s00394-022-02797-z>.

Mann, J., Truswell, A.S., 2017. *Essentials of human nutrition*, 5th ed. Oxford University Press, New York.

Mathewson, S., Azevedo, P., Gordon, A., et al., 2021. Overcoming protein-energy malnutrition in older adults in the residential care setting: A narrative review of causes and interventions. *Ageing Research Reviews* 70, 101401. doi: 10.1016/j.arr.2021.101401.

Mitchell, A., Llumigusin, D., 2021. The assessment and management of hypergranulation. *British Journal of Nursing* 30(5).

Morgan, Y., 2019. Obesity, metabolic and surgery outcomes. *The Dissector* 47(2), 18–22.

National Eating Disorders Collaboration, nd. What is an eating disorder? Available at: <https://nedc.com.au/eating-disorders/eating-disorders-explained/the-facts/whats-an-eating-disorder>.

National Eating Disorders Collaboration, 2021. Eating disorders in Australia. Available at: <https://www.nedc.com.au/assets/Fact-Sheets/Eating-Disorders-in-Australia-ENG.pdf>.

National Health and Medical Research Council (NHMRC), 2012. Eat for health. Infant feeding guidelines: Information for health workers. Available at: <https://nhmrc.gov.au/about-us/publications/infant-feeding-guidelines-information-health-workers>.

National Health and Medical Research Council (NHMRC), 2013a. Eat for health. Australian dietary guidelines: Providing the scientific evidence for healthier Australian diets. NHMRC, Canberra.

National Health and Medical Research Council (NHMRC), 2013b. Clinical practice guidelines for the management of overweight and obesity in adults, adolescents and children in Australia. NHMRC, Canberra.

National Health and Medical Research Council (NHMRC), 2013c. The Australian guide to healthy eating. Guidelines for healthy foods and drinks supplied in school canteens. Available at: <https://www1.health.gov.au/internet/publications/publishing.nsf/Content/nhsc-guidelines[aus-guide-healthy-eating>.

National Health and Medical Research Council (NHMRC), 2015. Serve sizes. Available at: <https://www.eatforhealth.gov.au/food-essentials/how-much-do-we-need-each-day/serve-sizes>.

National Health and Medical Research Council (NHMRC), 2017. Nutrient reference values for Australia and New Zealand including recommended dietary intake. NHMRC, Canberra.

National Health and Medical Research Council (NHMRC), 2019. How to understand food labels. Available at: <https://www.eatforhealth.gov.au/eating-well/how-understand-food-labels>.

NSW Department of Health, 2023. Guideline: Insertion and management of nasogastric and orogastric tubes in adults. Available at: <https://www1.health.nsw.gov.au/pds/ActivePDSDocuments/GL2023_001.pdf>.

NSW Department of Health, 2017. Policy directive: Nutrition care. Pd2017_041. NSW Health, Sydney. Available at: <https://www1.health.nsw.gov.au/pds/ActivePDSDocuments/PD2017_041.pdf>.

NSW Ministry of Health (MoH), 2022. The NSW Healthy Eating and Active Living Strategy 2022–2032. Available at: <https://www.health.nsw.gov.au/heal/publications/nsw-healthy-eating-strategy.pdf>.

Nursing and Midwifery Board of Australia (NMBA), 2020. Decision-making framework summary for nursing and midwifery. Available at: <https://www.nursingmidwiferyboard.gov.au/Codes-Guidelines-Statements/Frameworks.aspx>.

Nutrition Australia, 2020. Plant-based diets: What's the fuss? Available at: <https://nutritionaustralia.org/division/nsw/plant-based-diets-whats-the-fuss>.

Nutrition Australia, 2021. Nutrition and older adults. Available at: <https://nutritionaustralia.org/app/uploads/2022/03/Nutrition-and-older-adults.pdf>.

O'Flynn, S., 2019. Peristomal skin damage: Assessment, prevention and treatment. *The British Journal of Nursing* 28(5), S6–S12. doi: 10.12968/bjon.2019.28.5.S6.

Patton, K.T., Thibodeau, G.A., 2019. *Anatomy and physiology*, 10th ed. Mosby Elsevier, St Louis.

Pirlich, M., Norman, K., 2018. Bestimmung des Ernährungszustands (inkl. Bestimmung der Körperzusammensetzung und ernährungsmedizinisches Screening) in Biesalski, rnährungsmedizin. Georg Thieme Verlag KG; Stuttgart, Germany.

Rackham, F., 2022. 'Being savvy with silver': Clinical indications, cautions and constituents of silver nitrate in stomal therapy. *Journal of Stomal Therapy Australia* 42(2), 20–22.

Raymond, J., Morrow, K., 2023. *Krause and Mahan's food and the nutrition care process*, 16th ed. Elsevier, St Louis.

Rebeiro, G., Wilson, D., Fuller, S., 2021. *Fundamentals of nursing: Clinical skills workbook*, 4th ed. Elsevier, Chatswood.

Reber, E., Gomes, F., Vasiloglou, M., et al., 2019. Nutritional risk screening and assessment. *Journal of Clinical Medicine* 8(7), 1065. doi: 10.3390/jcm8071065.

State of Queensland, 2021. Multicultural nutrition resources. Available at: <https://metrosouth.health.qld.gov.au/multicultural-nutrition-resources>.

State of Queensland, 2022. Queensland Health nutrition standards for meals and menus revised 2022. Available at: <https://www.health.qld.gov.au/__data/assets/pdf_file/0030/156288/qh-nutrition-standards.pdf>.

State of Victoria, 2022. Nutrition and quality food standards for adults in Victorian public hospitals and residential aged care services. Available at: <https://www.health.vic.gov.au/quality-safety-service/nutrition-and-food-quality-standards-for-health-services>.

Tang, M., Adolphe, S., Rogers, S. Frank, D., 2021. Failure to thrive or growth faltering: Medical, developmental/behavioural, nutritional, and social dimensions. *Pediatrics in Review* 42(11), 590–603.

Tsagari, A., Kyriazis, I., 2021. Nutritional care of the COVID-19 patient. *International Journal of Caring Sciences* 14(1), 794–799.

Vidal-Ostos, F., Ramos-Lopez, O., Jebb, S., et al., 2022. Dietary protein and the glycemic index handle insulin resistance within a nutritional program for avoiding weight regain after energy-restricted induced weight loss. *Nutrition & Metabolism* 19(71), 1–15. Available at: <https://doi.org/10.1186/s12986-022-00707-y>.

Vision Australia, 2023. Helpful resources. Available at: <https://www.visionaustralia.org/services/helpful-resources/carers>.

Weihrauch-Blüher, S., Wiegand, S., 2018. Risk factors and implications of childhood obesity. *Current Obesity Reports* 7, 254–259. Available at: <https://doi.org/10.1007/s13679-018-0320-0>.

Woodward, T., Josephson, C., Ross, L. et al., 2020. A retrospective study of the incidence and characteristics of long-stay adult inpatients with hospital-acquired malnutrition across five Australian public hospitals. *European Journal of Clinical Nutrition* 74, 1668–1676. Available at: <https://doi.org/10.1038/s41430-020-0648-x>.

Wounds Australia, 2016. *Standards for wound prevention and management*, 3rd ed.

World Health Organization (WHO), 2020a. Fact sheets. Obesity and overweight. WHO, Geneva. Available at: <https://www.who.int/news-room/fact-sheets/detail/obesity-and-overweight>.

World Health Organization (WHO), 2021a. Fact sheets. Malnutrition. Available at: <https://www.who.int/news-room/fact-sheets/detail/malnutrition>.

World Health Organization (WHO), 2021b. Infant and young child feeding. Available at: <https://www.who.int/news-room/fact-sheets/detail/infant-and-young-child-feeding>.

World Health Organization (WHO), 2021c. Obesity and overweight. Available at: <https://www.who.int/news-room/fact-sheets/detail/obesity-and-overweight>.

World Health Organization (WHO), 2023. Timeline: WHO's COVID-19 response. Available at: <https://www.who.int/emergencies/diseases/novel-coronavirus-2019/interactive-timeline#!>.

Recommended Reading

Australian Government Department of Health, 2022. Get up and grow: Healthy eating and physical activity for early childhood resources. Available at: <https://www.health.gov.au/resources/collections/get-up-grow-resource-collection>.

Brown, J., 2020. *Nutrition through the life cycle*, 7th ed. Cengage Learning, Stamford.

Butte, N., Stuebe, A., 2020. Patient education: Maternal health and nutrition during breastfeeding (beyond the basics). Available at: <https://www.uptodate.com/contents/maternal-health-and-nutrition-during-breastfeeding-beyond-the-basics>.

Dudek, S.G., 2021. *Nutritional essentials for nursing practice*, 9th ed. Wolters Kluwer, Philadelphia.

Koletzko, B., Fishbein, M., Lee, W., et al., 2020. Prevention of childhood obesity: A position paper of the Global Federation of International Societies of Paediatric Gastroenterology, Hepatology and Nutrition (FISPGHAN). *Journal of Pediatric Gastroenterology and Nutrition* 70(5), 702–710. doi: 10.1097/MPG.0000000000002708.

Neiman, D.C., 2019. *Nutritional assessment*, 7th ed. McGraw Hill, New York.

Nix, S., 2017. *Williams basic nutrition & diet therapy*, 5th ed. Elsevier Mosby, St Louis. Available from ProQuest database.

Oostenbach, L.H., Slits, E., Robinson, E., et al., 2019. Systematic review of the impact of nutrition claims related to fat, sugar and energy content on food choices and energy intake. *BMC Public Health* 19, 1296. Available at: <https://doi.org/10.1186/s12889-019-7622>.

Whitney, E., Rolfes, S.R., Crowe, T., et al., 2019. *Understanding nutrition*, Australian and New Zealand ed, 4th ed. Cengage Learning, Melbourne.

Zhang, C., Hu, L., Qiang, Y., et al., 2022. Home enteral nutrition for patients with esophageal cancer undergoing esophagectomy: A systematic review and meta-analysis. *Frontier Nutrition* 9. Available at: <https://doi.org/10.3389/fnut.2022.895422>.

Online Resources

Dietitians Australia: <https://dietitiansaustralia.org.au>.

Food Standards Australia and New Zealand: <https://www.foodstandards.gov.au>.

National Health and Medical Research Council. Nutrition: <https://www.nhmrc.gov.au/health-advice/public-health/nutrition>.

Nutrition Australia: <https://nutritionaustralia.org>.

World Health Organization: Nutrition: <https://www.who.int/health-topics/nutrition#tab=tab_1>.

CHAPTER

31

Urinary health

Marie V Long

Key Terms

anuria
bladder
chronic kidney disease (CKD)
cystitis
diuresis
dysuria
enuresis
haematuria
incontinence-associated dermatitis (IAD)
kidney
micturition
oliguria
polyuria
postoperative urinary retention (POUR)
pyelonephritis
ureter
urethra
urethritis
urinalysis
urinary calculi
urinary incontinence (UI)
urinary retention
voiding

Learning Outcomes

At the completion of this chapter and with further reading, learners should be able to:

- Define the key terms.
- Describe the transport mechanisms in the body related to the urinary system.
- Explain homeostasis as related to the urinary system.
- Identify the principal components of the urinary system and describe the structure and function of each part.
- Identify the common factors that affect urinary elimination throughout the lifespan.
- Describe the common disorders of the urinary system.
- Describe the types of urinary incontinence and possible causes.
- Outline the major components of a nursing assessment of urinary tract function.
- Describe the common diagnostic tests used to assess urinary system function.
- Describe the nursing interventions to promote normal voiding patterns and promote continence and identify how these can be incorporated into day-to-day practice.
- Assist in planning and implementing nursing care for the person with dysfunction of the urinary system.

CHAPTER FOCUS

The urinary system can be divided into two sections: the upper urinary tract and the lower urinary tract. The upper urinary system consists of two kidneys and two ureters, while the lower urinary system consists of the urinary bladder and the urethra. Urine is formed in the kidneys, descends through the ureters where it is then stored in the bladder before being eliminated from the body through the ureter. The urinary system plays an important role in the homeostatic balance of the body and interacts with other body systems to maintain that balance.

Many factors can affect the formation of urine and the subsequent excretion of urine, including normal ageing. Urinary elimination problems can have a significant impact on a person's quality of life and wellbeing. Recognising the impacts on the person and maintaining the person's dignity is a major focus of care planning.

LIVED EXPERIENCE

The following quotes from a qualitative study by Javanmardifard et al (2022) gives some insight into the lived experience of older women with urinary incontinence:

'I often try to not go out of the house. Even if I have to go shopping, I try to go back home before anything happens. I do not wait. I come back home immediately.' (p. 6)

Another participant also expressed: *'My condition depends on the amount of fluid I drink. I drink less tea: half a glass in the morning and half a glass in the evening, not more. I don't even drink this amount of tea if I need to go out.' (p. 14)*

INTRODUCTION

The urinary system (Figure 31.1) filters waste products from the blood and excretes them in the form of urine. The kidneys account for 20–25% of cardiac output and approximately 1200 mL/min of blood flows to the kidneys (Turnball 2023). The urinary system is also instrumental in regulating the rates of elimination of water and electrolytes from the body. By regulating the volume of the body fluid, the urinary system helps maintain blood pressure and the electrolyte content and pH of the blood. The urinary system consists of the **kidneys**, which filter blood; the **ureters**, which transport urine to the bladder; and the **bladder**, which stores the urine until it is excreted via the **urethra**.

The kidneys

The adult kidney weighs approximately 120–175 g, is 10–13 cm in length, 5–6 cm wide and 3–4 cm thick. The kidneys are protected and supported by renal fascia and by layers of perirenal fat. They are positioned at approximately vertebral level of T12–L3. The right kidney is usually slightly lower than the left due to its location inferior to the liver. An adrenal gland lies on top of each kidney (Turnbull 2023).

Each kidney contains at least 1 million nephrons, together with their collecting tubules or ducts. The nephron (Figure 31.2) is the functional unit of the kidney. Each nephron is composed of a vascular and tubular system that allows for the formation of urine. Each nephron is composed of the glomerulus, the Bowman's capsule and a tubular system. The blood enters via the afferent vessel from the renal artery to the glomerulus where filtration begins. It then passes through the Bowman's capsule into the proximal convoluted tubule, down the loop of Henle and through the distal convoluted tubule before exiting the nephron via the efferent vessel (Turnbull 2023). (See Figure 31.2.) The nephrons are located in the renal tissue, with most (approximately 85%) in the cortex (the outer layer of the kidney) and some extending deep into the medulla (inner layer) of the kidney.

Homeostasis is the process that controls the body's internal environment. The urinary system maintains homeostasis by filtering the blood to:

- Regulate water and electrolyte balance.
- Regulate acid–base balance in the blood.
- Eliminate wastes from the blood and reabsorb required substances back in the blood.
- Regulate blood pressure.

(Kirov & Needham 2023)

The kidneys produce erythropoietin, prostaglandins, renin, and activated vitamin D, which are important to the production of red blood cells, blood pressure regulation and bone mineralisation:

- Erythropoietin functions within the bone marrow to stimulate red blood cell production and maturation. This protein is secreted in response to hypoxia and decreased renal blood flow.
- Prostaglandins produced specifically in the kidney help regulate glomerular filtration, kidney vascular resistance, and renin production. They also increase sodium and water excretion.
- Renin activates the renin-aldosterone pathway, causing aldosterone to be released from the adrenal cortex.

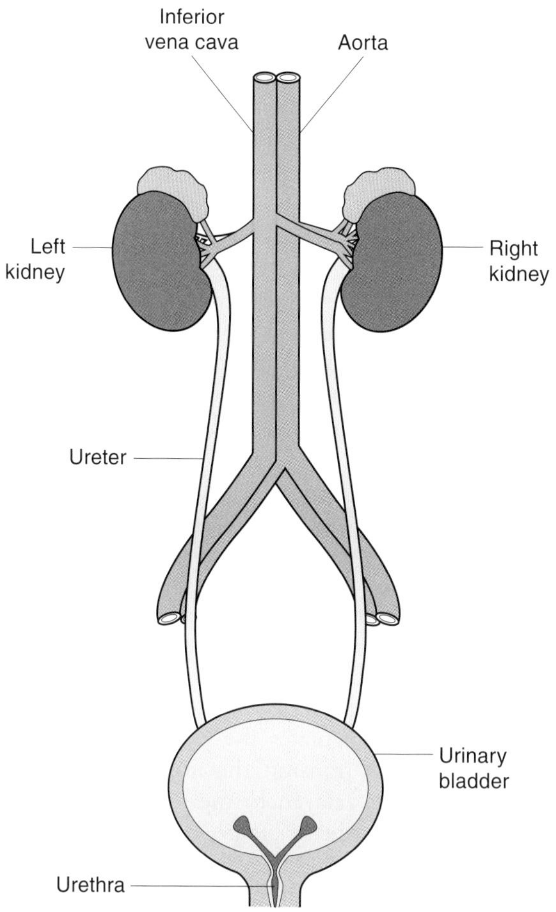

Figure 31.1 The urinary system

Aldosterone causes retention of sodium and water, thus increasing blood volume, raising blood pressure and renal blood flow.

- Vitamin D is converted into calcitriol, which regulates calcium homeostasis.

(McCance & Huther 2023; Turnball 2023)

Composition of urine

Urine is composed of water and dissolved substances that are in excess of the body's needs, and includes by-products of metabolism, such as urea. Normally, urine is a clear, light amber-coloured, slightly acidic fluid with a non-offensive odour and is composed of 95% water and 5% electrolytes and waste substances (Turnball 2023; Hryciw 2023). The kidneys excrete approximately 1500–2000 mL in 24 hours, but this amount varies with intake, physical activity and general health.

The ureters

The ureters are two narrow, thick-walled muscular tubes, 25–30 cm long and approximately 3–4 mm in diameter, which originate in the renal pelvis of each kidney (Kirov & Needham 2023; Hryciw 2023). They pass down the posterior abdominal wall and into the pelvic cavity to enter the posterior base of the bladder. The ureters enter the bladder at an oblique angle, forming a valve mechanism so that, as the bladder fills and contracts, urine is not forced back towards the kidneys. The walls of the ureters consist of an outer fibrous coat that is continuous with the renal capsule, a middle coat of involuntary muscle, and a lining of transitional epithelium. The function of the ureters is to carry

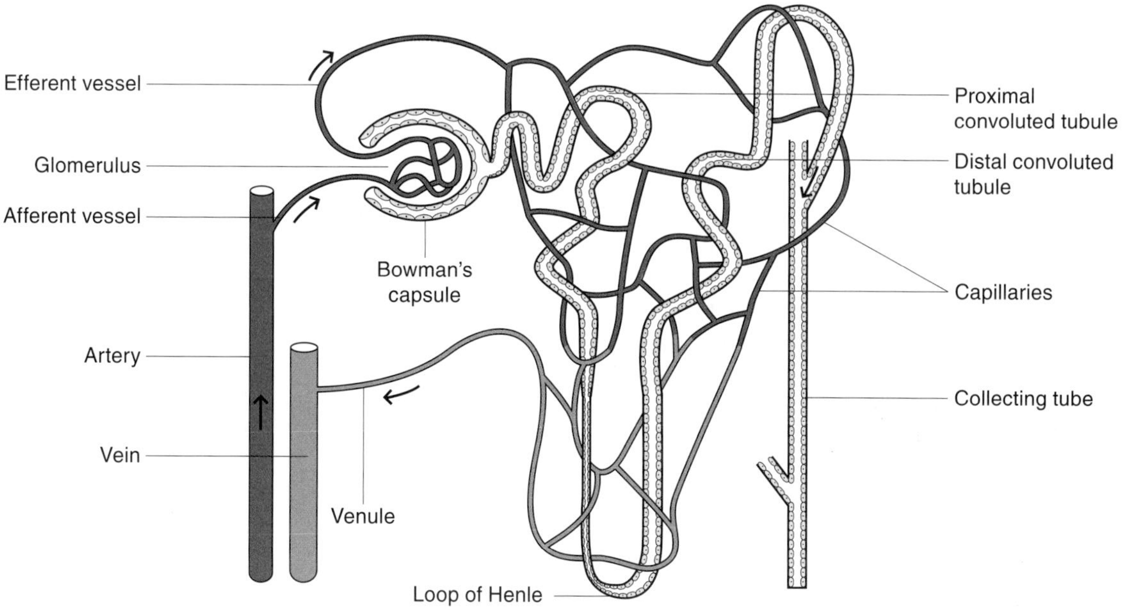

Figure 31.2 The nephron

urine from the kidneys to the bladder by means of peristaltic action (Turnball 2023). The involuntary muscle layer in the walls of the ureters contract one to five times per minute to force urine into the bladder (Kirov & Needham 2023).

The urinary bladder

The urinary bladder is a muscular organ (detrusor muscle) that acts as a reservoir for urine. The detrusor muscle is a layer of the urinary bladder wall made of smooth muscle fibres arranged in spiral, longitudinal and circular bundles; its competency is vital to maintaining continence. In women, the bladder is anterior to the vagina. In men, it is anterior to the rectum. The peritoneum covers the upper portion (the fundus) of the bladder. The walls of the bladder consist of four layers:

- an outer serous coating
- a layer of involuntary muscle
- a submucous layer of connective tissue
- a layer comprised of mucous membranes that are formed into folds (rugae), which increase the surface areas of the bladder, enabling the bladder to expand when full and contract when empty.

(Kirov & Needham 2023)

The trigone of the bladder is a smooth triangular area formed by the two ureteric orifices, where the ureters enter the bladder, and the urethral orifice at the bladder neck. This area contains a large number of sensory nerve fibres, which respond to stretch as the bladder fills with urine (Kirov & Needham 2023).

The urethra

The urethra (Figure 31.3) is a muscular tube extending from the neck of the bladder to the urethral meatus. The function of the urethra is to provide a passage for urine from the bladder, out of the body. In the male, it also forms a passage for semen (Kirov & Needham 2023).

In women, the urethra is about 3.5–5.5 cm long, with the urethral meatus located anterior to the vaginal opening and posterior to the clitoris. The external urethral sphincter enables voluntary flow of urine. In the male, the urethra is approximately 18–23 cm long, terminating at the tip of the penis. The male urethra has three sections: the prostatic urethra; the membranous urethra, which passes through the muscles of the pelvic floor; and the spongy or penile urethra (Turnball 2023). There is an internal sphincter within the prostatic urethra and the membranous urethra. The prostate gland encircles the urethra at the base of the bladder.

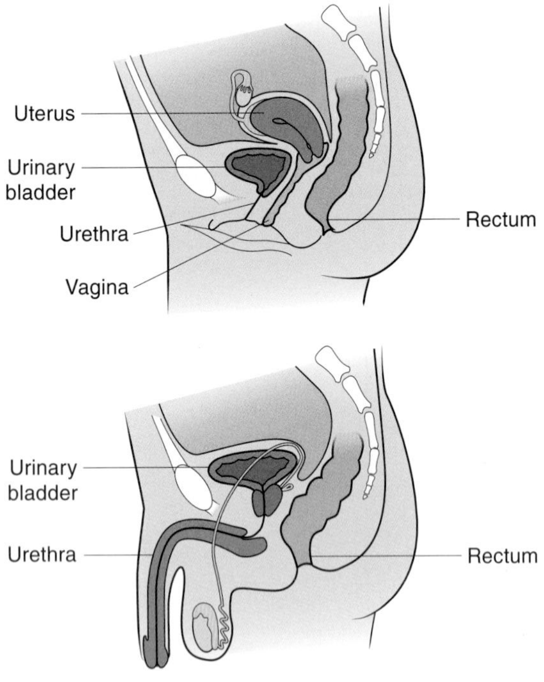

Figure 31.3 Position of the female and male urethra

Micturition

Micturition (or **voiding**) is the act of passing urine. While the normal capacity of the adult urinary bladder is about 300–400 mL, the bladder is capable of expanding to hold larger amounts. The bladder fills gradually over a period of time and, when it holds about 200–300 mL, a desire to empty the bladder is experienced (Turnball 2023). A reflex initiated by impulses from stretch receptors in the bladder wall regulates the process of micturition. The sensory neurons transmit the impulses to the spinal cord, where they are relayed to the brain, which in turn stimulates parasympathetic neurons that innervate the bladder wall (Turnball 2023). When a person is ready to void, these impulses cause the bladder muscles to contract, the internal urethral sphincter relaxes and the desire to urinate is activated. The person is then able to voluntarily relax the external sphincter and void at an appropriate time and place. Normal urinary output is calculated at 1–2 mL/kg/hr (Hryciw 2023).

FACTORS THAT AFFECT URINARY SYSTEM FUNCTIONING

In the previous section, we discussed that the kidneys regulate the rates of elimination of water, electrolytes, waste and toxic substances, and contribute to the maintenance of a constant blood pH and blood pressure. Therefore, any dysfunction in the formation or excretion of urine can have major adverse effects on homeostasis and impact on a person's quality of life.

Changes with ageing

Development of daytime urinary continence occurs within the first 2–3 years of life when the child becomes aware of bladder filling and begins to be able to inhibit voiding. In addition, the child needs to be able to store urine for long periods, have the motor skills needed for toileting and bladder emptying, and the understanding to complete toileting in a socially acceptable manner (Hryciw 2023). Many children experience nocturnal **enuresis** (bedwetting) into the early school years.

There are changes that occur with normal ageing that predispose the older person to problems related to their kidneys or bladder function. As a person ages, there is a progressive decrease in renal blood flow and tubular function, thus reducing the filtration rate of the kidney (Hryciw 2023). Older people may experience an increase in the need to void at night (nocturia) and an increase in urinary frequency due to changes in the muscle tone and capacity of the bladder (Cooper & Gosnell 2023). This can also affect the ability of the bladder to contract, resulting in incomplete emptying of the bladder after voiding (residual urine) (Cardozo et al 2023).

For women, changes that occur during pregnancy and menopause can alter urinary function. For example, during pregnancy the growing foetus and uterus place pressure on the bladder (and bowel) and can lead to urinary frequency. Changes to the pelvic floor muscles and nerves during childbirth can result in reduced pelvic floor muscle tone and predispose the woman to urinary incontinence (Hryciw 2023). Hormone changes that occur in menopause can change the urethral mucosa and tissues that support the urethra, resulting in an increased risk of infection and urinary urgency (McCance & Huther 2023).

As the individual ages, a number of chronic health conditions impact urinary continence. These include chronic heart failure, dementia, arthritis, diabetes mellitus, Parkinson's disease, stroke and mental health (Continence Foundation of Australia 2023a). As the individual ages, the detrusor muscle can become impaired. It may become overactive and contract while the bladder is still filling, which leads to urinary urgency or it may not contract fully during urination, resulting in residual urine in the bladder (Patton 2021). Older individuals may experience **incontinence-associated dermatitis (IAD)**, which is a type of skin irritation or damage due to prolonged contact with urine or faeces (Department of Health and Aged Care 2022).

Fluid balance

Water accounts for half or more of young adult body weight. It may be intracellular (within the cell) or extracellular (outside the cell). Extracellular fluid consists of blood plasma and interstitial fluid. Small changes in the electrolyte concentration in each of the fluid compartments will cause water to move from one compartment to another. Normally, the intake of fluids and food balances with the output of water in urine, faeces and insensible losses in perspiration and breathing. However, if the kidneys are unable to concentrate the urine by regulating reabsorption, the loss of a large amount of dilute urine may result in fluid imbalance. If the kidneys fail to excrete sufficient water, the increase in total circulating fluid volume may impede cardiovascular function. Changes in renal function may also result in abnormal retention or loss of electrolytes such as sodium, potassium, calcium or phosphorus. Drinks that contain caffeine (e.g. coffee, tea and cola drinks) promote increased urine formation (Burchum & Rosenthal 2022). Alcohol inhibits the release of antidiuretic hormone, causing an increase in water loss in the urine (**diuresis**).

Changes to renal function

The structure and function of the kidneys can be affected by disease processes that impact renal function. These can be acute or chronic:

- prerenal causes—a decrease in renal blood flow or perfusion (e.g. dehydration, haemorrhage, shock)
- renal causes—anything that causes injury to structure or function (e.g. diabetes mellitus, renal tumours, glomerulonephritis)
- post-renal causes—resulting from obstruction to flow of urine in the renal pelvis, the ureter, the bladder or urethra, usually causing an increase in pressure within the kidney and/or ureter (e.g. an enlarged prostate, urinary calculi, tumours or strictures).

(Lough 2022)

Changes to bladder function

In addition to changes to normal bladder function that can occur with ageing, several systemic diseases can affect bladder function. For example, diabetes, multiple sclerosis or spinal cord injury cause changes to peripheral nerves related to bladder function that can result in loss of bladder tone, diminished sensation of bladder filling and difficulty in controlling voiding (Jarvis & Eckhardt 2021).

Illness and frailty

Any health condition that reduces the person's mobility, ability to care for themselves or perceive the need for toileting can affect urinary elimination. For example, the person may not be able to recognise the need to void or place to void because of cognitive dysfunction such as dementia. A person who has impaired mobility or a disability may not be able to toilet independently or reach the toilet in a timely manner (Gulanick & Myers 2022). Any inflammation in the urinary tract can cause pain and a reluctance to void or may irritate the lining of the bladder and urethra, resulting in a sense of urgency to void. A change in medication may also directly affect the function of the kidneys and bladder.

Environment

People who have cognitive changes are particularly affected by changes in environment (Patton 2021). A person who has dementia may experience increased confusion when hospitalised, putting them at risk of injury from falls, and which may also increase the likelihood of urinary (and/or faecal) incontinence (Cardozo et al 2023).

Being a patient in hospital is a confronting experience. The usual privacy that we have in our own home is not available in hospital, with many individuals needing to share toilet facilities with others. They may also be required to rest in bed and need assistance with toileting and use of a urinal or bedpan.

COMMON DISORDERS OF THE URINARY SYSTEM

The most common health issues related to the urinary system involve disturbances that impair bladder or kidney function, obstruct the flow of urine or affect the ability to voluntarily control micturition. The following section will outline common disorders of the urinary system, including urinary tract infection, urinary incontinence, benign prostatic hypertrophy, prostate cancer, urinary calculi and chronic kidney disease. For more detailed information refer to a medical–surgical nursing textbook or specialist urology textbook.

Urinary tract infection

Infection may occur in any part of the urinary tract because urine provides an ideal medium for the growth of microorganisms. Urinary tract infections (UTIs) are common, particularly in women and older people (Brandt 2022). UTIs can affect the bladder only (lower urinary tract infection) or the kidneys (upper urinary tract infection), which is known as **pyelonephritis**. The most common bacteria to cause infection in the urine (bacteriuria) is *Escherichia coli* (Jones & Steggal 2020). Microorganisms usually enter the urinary tract via the urethra to the mucosal lining of the bladder. Here, they can multiply and cause infection. The risk factors for developing a UTI include being a woman (shortness of the urethra), sexual activity in women, pregnancy and the presence of an underlying congenital or acquired structural anomaly (e.g. vesicoureteral reflux, obstruction anywhere in the urinary tract, urinary calculi, history of recurrent UTI) or being an older person or a person with generalised ill-health (Jarvis & Eckhardt 2021).

Symptoms in children and adults include painful urination (**dysuria**), frequent voiding, difficulty starting a stream of urine (hesitancy), feeling the need to void urgently (urgency), difficulty emptying the bladder, urinary incontinence and bladder pain (suprapubic tenderness). The presentation may be atypical in older people, particularly frail older people, who may present with functional and cognitive decline, falls and dehydration (Jarvis & Eckhardt 2021). A person with acute pyelonephritis may experience severe pain or a continual dull ache in the kidney region, as well as pyrexia, nausea and vomiting, and fatigue. Rigours may be present, and urination may be frequent and painful. Table 31.1 summarises the age-related symptoms of UTI.

Initial screening for UTI is done with dipstick urinalysis of a freshly collected urine sample to detect the presence of protein, blood, leucocytes and nitrites. The presence of bacteria and white blood cells in the urine contributes to an unpleasant odour, often concentrated appearance and cloudiness of the urine (Brandt 2022). The inflammation caused by the infection in the bladder can cause the presence of macroscopic or microscopic blood in the urine (**haematuria**).

Urinary incontinence

Urinary incontinence (UI) is the complaint of any involuntary loss of urine (Cardozo et al 2023) and may occur across the entire lifespan. Urinary incontinence is common: 38% of Australians have experienced incontinence and, of these, 80% are women (Continence Foundation of Australia 2023a). UI can seriously impact on the person's quality of life. People who have incontinence report reduced general wellbeing and a negative impact on their daily activities, sexuality, self-image and self-esteem (Patton 2021). Caring for someone with a continence problem has also been found to have a negative impact on the quality of life of carers (Bradway 2018; Collis et al 2019). This is a significant point to note when caring for older people who have a continence problem; supporting the carer should also be a priority on the plan of care.

UI can be transient or ongoing and is defined according to the person's symptoms: urge, stress, mixed, functional,

TABLE 31.1 | Age-related symptoms of urinary tract infection (UTI)

Younger persons (symptoms tend to be specific)	Older persons (symptoms tend to be less specific)
Frequency/urge	May/may not be present
Usually continent	May have episodes of incontinence
Pyrexia/chills	Not always present
Dysuria	Seldom present
Suprapubic pain	Suprapubic pain
Lethargy	Lethargy
Loss of appetite/nausea	Loss of appetite
Mentally alert	Altered mental state, usually an acute change—confusion, delirium may be present

(Adapted from Jarvis & Eckhardt 2021; Brandt 2022)

TABLE 31.2 | Types of urinary incontinence (UI)

Description	Symptoms
Urge urinary incontinence Involuntary leakage of urine after a strong sense of urgency to void	Significant urinary urgency—inability to defer voiding once the urge has occurred, often with frequency (more often than every 2 hours).
Stress urinary incontinence Involuntary leakage of urine on exertion or effort, or on sneezing or coughing	Loss of urine with increased intra-abdominal pressure. Usually small amounts of urine lost.
Mixed urinary incontinence Involuntary leakage of urine associated with urgency and also with exertion or effort, or on sneezing or coughing	Loss of urine with increased intra-abdominal pressure, urinary urgency and frequency. Can be a small or large amount of urine lost.
Functional urinary incontinence Involuntary urine loss that occurs because of impaired functional status—impaired cognitive status, impaired mobility and dexterity and/or environmental barriers that block toilet access	Inability to get to the toilet in time, inability to undress, re-dress or manage personal hygiene. The person with cognitive changes may have forgotten what to do or not recognise the place to void.
Nocturnal enuresis Involuntary loss of urine occurring during sleep	Urine loss while asleep.
Overactive bladder Symptoms of urgency with or without urge incontinence, usually with frequency and nocturia	Diagnosed with urodynamic testing. Bothersome urgency usually associated with frequency and nocturia.
Post-micturition dribble Feeling of involuntary urine loss immediately after finishing voiding	Men will complain of urine loss immediately after voiding; women will complain of urine loss on rising from the toilet.

(Adapted from Cardozo et al 2023)

nocturnal enuresis, overactive bladder or post-micturition dribble (Cardozo et al 2023). Table 31.2 outlines the definitions and typical symptoms of each type of UI. The aetiology of UI is wide-ranging and includes weakened pelvic floor muscles; decreased bladder capacity; UTI; frailty or disability; neurological disorders (e.g. stroke, Parkinson's disease, spinal cord injury); endocrine disorders (e.g. diabetes mellitus, menopause); pregnancy; sensory, cognitive or mobility deficits; post prostatectomy in men; and the side effects of some medications (Cardozo et al 2023; Gulanick & Myers 2022).

Benign prostatic hypertrophy

Benign prostatic hypertrophy (BPH) is an enlargement of the prostate gland surrounding the male urethra, which may cause obstruction to the passage of urine out of the bladder. About 80% of males will have prostatic enlargement before age 80 years and there is a 25–30% lifetime chance of needing prostatectomy for benign prostatic hyperplasia once a man reaches 50 years of age (Hogwarth & Smith 2023). The main function of the prostate gland is to supply the proteins and electrolytes that form the main constituents of seminal fluid (Grodesky 2022). The cause of hypertrophy of the prostate gland is not fully understood but is probably related to hormonal changes that occur with ageing.

Typically, men with BPH present with lower urinary tract symptoms (LUTS) that have developed over a long period of time, such as weak urinary stream, hesitancy, intermittent flow, urgency, daytime frequency and nocturia (Robertson 2023). See Table 31.3 for a description of common alterations in urinary elimination patterns. Diagnosis is made by a careful assessment of the symptoms and the severity of the symptoms on a male's quality of life. A physical examination would include a digital rectal examination to examine the size and consistency of the prostate gland (Hogwarth & Smith 2023). In some men, the obstruction to the urethra causes urinary retention, which can be acute or chronic (see below). Treatment options depend on the severity of the symptoms and include ongoing assessment of the symptoms, medical management (medications that aim to relax the smooth muscles at the bladder neck or to reduce the size of the prostate gland) and surgical management (e.g. transurethral resection of the prostate [TURP]) (Robertson 2023; Gulanick & Myers 2022). (See Case Study 31.1.)

Prostate cancer

Prostate cancer is the most common cancer in Australian men (Australian Institute of Health & Welfare [AIHW] 2021).

TABLE 31.3 | Common alterations in urinary elimination patterns

Term	Definition
Changes in urine output	
Anuria	A urinary output <100 mL/24 hours
Oliguria	An abnormally low urinary output of between 100 mL and 400 mL/24 hours
Polyuria	The excretion of an abnormally large volume of urine (usually >3 L/24 hours)
Lower urinary tract symptoms	
Dysuria	Pain and burning on micturition—usually associated with bladder infection (cystitis), trauma or inflammation of the urethra (urethritis)
Hesitancy	Difficulty initiating urination and delay in onset of voiding—usually associated with prostate enlargement, anxiety, urethral oedema
Feeling of incomplete bladder emptying	Complaint that the bladder does not feel empty after voiding has ceased—usually associated with abnormal bladder sensations, bladder outlet obstruction, neurological diseases, pelvic organ prolapse
Frequency (daytime)	Voiding more frequently than normal during the day—usually more than eight times per day (but this varies)—associated with high fluid intake, bladder inflammation (usually from infection), increased pressure on bladder (pregnancy, psychological stress), overactive bladder
Nocturia	Waking from sleep to void more than once per night (or more than twice/night if aged >65)—associated with excessive fluid intake before bed (especially coffee or alcohol), renal disease, ageing process, prostate enlargement, heart failure, use of sedatives and hypnotics
Urgency	Strong and immediate need to void immediately that is not easily deferred—associated with bladder irritation or inflammation from infection, incompetent urethral sphincter, psychological stress
Retention of urine (can be acute or chronic)	The accumulation of urine in the bladder as a result of being unable to empty the bladder completely
Residual urine	The volume of urine remaining after voiding

(Adapted from Kirov & Needham 2023)

CASE STUDY 31.1

Exploring one of the disorders of the urinary system

Mr Ivan Kowalski, a 69-year-old, has been to see his general practitioner (GP) for a routine check-up. He reports good health and is active. He has been retired for 4 years from his career as a police officer. He has no significant medical history and is taking no medications. He says he is very busy with his family, playing golf three times per week and volunteering. However, he discloses that he has been experiencing urinary frequency, hesitancy and slow urinary stream for several months. He is also needing to go to the toilet at least three times overnight. His GP recommends, in addition to a general health check, a digital rectal examination to check the size and consistency of his prostate. The general physical examination was normal. The examination of the prostate revealed a smooth, symmetrical, enlarged prostate gland.

1. What do the symptoms Mr Kowalski described and the findings of the digital rectal examination suggest?
2. What are the treatment options for Mr Kowalski?

The risk of developing prostate cancer to age 75 years is 1 in 23 and to age 85 is one in nine for Australian men (AIHW 2021). The majority of men diagnosed with prostate cancer are over 60 years of age. The cause of prostate cancer is unclear, although contributing factors are obesity, and metabolic syndrome in middle age. Men who have a family history of prostate cancer are at highest risk of developing the disease (Prostate Cancer Foundation of Australia [PCFA] and Cancer Council Australia [CCA] 2019). Most men do not have any symptoms until the late stage of the disease. Diagnosis is made through health assessment, a prostatic-specific antigen (PSA) blood test, digital rectal examination, multiparametric magnetic resonance imaging (MRI) and prostate biopsy (PCFA & CCA 2019). Treatment options include continuing to observe and assess (active surveillance), surgery (radical prostatectomy), androgen deprivation therapy, radiation therapy, chemotherapy and immunotherapy. Most treatment options can severely impact on the man's bladder function, including incontinence from surgery or bladder irritation from radiation therapy, or sexual function (erectile dysfunction).

Chronic kidney disease

Chronic kidney disease (CKD) is the gradual loss of renal function that is evidenced by a reduced eGFR (estimated glomerular filtration rate) blood test result lasting more than 3 months (AIHW 2022). Approximately 1 in 10 Australians have some biochemical evidence of CKD and Aboriginal and Torres Strait Islander Peoples have more than double the risk than non-Aboriginal and Torres Strait Islander Peoples (AIHW 2022).

A major risk factor for CKD is diabetes mellitus. Other risk factors include cigarette smoking, hypertension, obesity, a family history of CKD and being over 50 years of age (AIHW 2023). CKD produces major changes in all body systems and a significant decrease in quality of life. When kidney function decreases to a point where the person can no longer maintain homeostasis, they will experience fluid and electrolyte disturbances and symptoms such as nausea, vomiting, headache and, finally, coma and convulsions (Childress 2022).

In the early stages of CKD, the treatment options include dietary and fluid restrictions. If the kidney failure progresses (end-stage kidney disease), renal replacement therapies such as dialysis and renal transplant need to be commenced. There are two main types of dialysis: haemodialysis and peritoneal dialysis. Haemodialysis involves the use of a machine that has a filter membrane (artificial kidney) that removes waste products from the blood via a vascular access device (Childress 2022). Peritoneal dialysis uses the peritoneum as the filter membrane. Dialysis fluid is infused into the abdomen via a special catheter that is surgically inserted. The fluid is left in the abdomen for a period of time to allow time for waste products to be diffused or osmosed, then drained (Childress 2022). Renal transplantation is another option in end-stage kidney disease. A renal transplant involves the surgical implantation of a healthy kidney from a living or deceased donor that is of a compatible blood and tissue type. The person will require ongoing immunosuppressive treatment to prevent rejection of the transplanted organ. Unlike dialysis, transplantation has the potential for the person to return to normal kidney function for the life of the transplanted kidney (Williams-Taylor 2022).

Urinary retention

Urinary retention is the inability to void or inability to empty the bladder despite persistent effort (International Continence Society [ICS] 2023). Urinary retention can be acute or chronic. In acute retention, there is a rapid onset of bladder distension, usually suprapubic pain, and an inability to void over several hours. The bladder may hold as much as 2000–3000 mL (or more) of urine and it is treated as a medical emergency (Cooper & Gosnell 2023). Acute retention is most common in men due to obstruction of the urethra from BPH. It can also occur in people in the postoperative period, particularly following a long surgical procedure, in people who have had an epidural anaesthetic or infusion, following removal of an indwelling catheter, in people who have poorly controlled pain and after vaginal birth (Gersch 2021). **Postoperative urinary retention (POUR)** affects up to 70% of individuals following anaesthesia. The inability to void is usually temporary, but may be prolonged in some individuals (Potter et al 2023). Common risk factors are:

- person-specific: older age, male gender, history of POUR, neurological disease, or prior pelvic surgery
- procedure-specific: anorectal surgery, joint arthroplasty, hernia repair, or incontinence surgery
- anaesthesia-specific: excessive intraoperative fluid administration, medication-related (e.g. use of opioids, anticholinergic agents, sympathomimetics), prolonged anaesthesia, or type of anaesthesia.

(Potter et al 2023)

Bladder scanning is a non-invasive way to confirm an overdistended bladder and is used when the individual has risk factors for POUR or is unable to void 4 hours postoperatively. If >600 mL of urine is measured on bladder scan, a single-time catheterisation is recommended.

Chronic retention results from incomplete bladder emptying over a period of time despite being able to pass some urine (ICS 2023). It is caused by either a partial obstruction of the urethra (e.g. enlarged prostate, chronic constipation) and/or from reduced ability of the detrusor (bladder) muscle to contract during voiding (e.g. spinal cord injury or nerve damage from diabetes mellitus) (Cooper & Gosnell 2023). The person may have an urge to void but is only able to void small amounts, or they may also have intermittent episodes of incontinence or constant dribbling of urine. Depending on the cause of the chronic retention, the person may or may not be aware of the incomplete bladder emptying. Chronic retention can result in increased pressures within the urinary tract, causing damage to the kidneys, and can predispose the person to UTIs (Gersch 2021).

Urinary calculi

Urinary calculi are stones that form in any part of the urinary tract. Most stones form in the kidneys and pass down into the ureters or bladder. The calculi can vary in size from microscopic to several centimetres in diameter. Approximately 4–8% of Australian adults experience urinary calculi at some stage in their lives (Kidney Health Australia 2020). Urinary stones are classified according to their composition and one or more substances may form them. They are usually composed of calcium salts or uric acid. Multiple small calculi may remain in the renal pelvis or pass down the ureter, while a staghorn calculus remains in the kidneys.

The major symptom of urinary calculi is pain, felt as a dull ache if the stone remains in the kidney. If the stone moves within the urinary tract, the person will experience severe pain, usually of sudden onset, and may have microscopic or macroscopic haematuria, nausea and vomiting (Gersch 2021). The person may find it difficult to void because of pain or obstruction.

Treatment options for urinary calculi can be classified as either non-invasive (watchful waiting or extracorporeal shockwave lithotripsy) or invasive (percutaneous or open surgical removal). Initial acute management may include intravenous fluids, treatment of nausea and vomiting and pain relief (Gersch 2021).

NURSING ASSESSMENT OF URINARY SYSTEM FUNCTION

Because health problems related to the urinary system are common, assessment related to urinary system function should be included on each admission nursing assessment. Many people who are hospitalised have a pre-existing urinary tract health issue or may develop a problem as the result of medical or surgical intervention and general ill-health. However, some will be reluctant to discuss urinary tract problems, especially urinary incontinence, because of embarrassment, so the nurse needs to approach the assessment with tact and empathy. Urinary tract health may also affect or be affected by other areas such as skin, bowel function, activity and exercise, cognition and nutrition.

Subjective data (nursing history)

The following areas form the basis of a nursing history related to urinary tract function:

- Presenting concern with urinary tract function. Does the person perceive they have a problem? How long has this been happening? How has this affected their usual daily living?
- Usual urinary pattern—pattern of voiding day and overnight. Because people are usually unable to detail urinary output or pattern accurately, data from a fluid balance chart or voiding diary may be needed to establish the usual voiding pattern.
- Characteristics of the urine—the person's description of the colour, odour and clarity of the urine.
- Fluid intake—type and amount over a 24-hour period; data may be collected on a fluid balance chart (see about objective data below).
- History of change or disturbance to urinary tract function. Ask the person to detail the changes, how long this has been happening and what they have been doing about it.
- Pain—location, character, onset, duration, severity, pattern, associated factors. Pain is more common in acute rather than chronic disorders of the kidneys and urinary tract. Pain that originates from the kidneys is generally experienced as a dull ache in the flank and may radiate to the lower abdominal area. Pain associated with renal colic is sudden and severe. It is felt in the flank and may radiate to the groin area. If the pain is severe, there may be nausea and vomiting. Suprapubic or lower abdominal pain may result from spasms or over-distension of the bladder, as happens in acute retention of urine. An infection of the lower urinary tract, such as **cystitis** or **urethritis** (inflammation of the urethra), may cause pain and burning during and/or after voiding (dysuria).
- Lower urinary tract symptoms—daytime voiding frequency, urgency, nocturia, urinary incontinence, reduced urinary stream, straining, post-micturition symptoms (dribble, feeling of incomplete emptying), difficulty voiding, lack of sensation of the need to void. (See Table 31.3.)
- Other symptoms—fever, nausea and vomiting, weight gain/loss, peripheral oedema, fatigue, constipation, erectile dysfunction, itchy skin, headache.
- Past history—of urinary tract health problems, diabetes, neurological disorders, mental health problems. For men—history of BPH or prostate cancer. For women—obstetric history, obesity, surgical history (e.g. gynaecological, spinal, bowel).
- Health and lifestyle management—activity and exercise, smoking, use of continence aids and appliances, medications, prostate screening for men over 50 years.
- Environmental issues related to bladder function—mobility and dexterity, home and work environment.

(Watt 2021)

Objective data (physical examination and specimen screening)

While the focus of objective data collection will be primarily related to urinary tract function, the nurse may also need to assess the skin (especially if the person has urinary incontinence), abdomen, mobility and dexterity, bowel function and mental status (Watt 2021). Start with vital signs:

- Vital signs—temperature, pulse, blood pressure. Check for fever, which may be related to infection. Hypertension is associated with chronic kidney disease.
- Inspection of urine—collect a fresh clean specimen of urine in a urinal, jug or bedpan. Measure the volume of urine. Inspect the urine for colour and clarity, assess the odour. Normally, urine would be clear, pale yellow in colour, and have a non-offensive odour.

- Specimen screening (dipstick or routine **urinalysis**)—collect a fresh clean specimen of urine in a urinal, jug or bedpan. Measure the volume of urine (the same specimen as collected for inspection of the urine can be used). The urine should not be contaminated by faeces or menstrual blood since an inaccurate finding may result. Dipstick (reagent urine testing strips) are used to screen urine samples. This test can give useful information about the person's general health status, as well as bladder and kidney function. Check each container of reagent strips is within the use-by date, that the strips are dry, and that the container has an efficient closure. Each manufacturer may vary slightly in application of the test and the sequence and type of reagent pads, so check information as to how to read the strip and the time needed for a result before commencing the test (Figure 31.4). See Table 31.4 for interpretation of

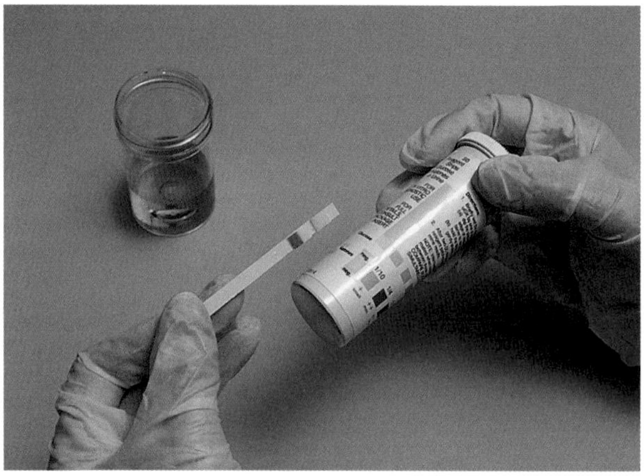

Figure 31.4 Checking urine test result of a chemical reagent strip (dipstick)

(Crisp et al 2021)

TABLE 31.4 | Interpretation of urinalysis findings

Test	Normal values	Interpretation
Glucose	Nil	Individuals with diabetes have glucose in urine as a result of inability of tubules to reabsorb high glucose concentrations. Ingestion of high concentrations of glucose may cause some glucose to appear in urine of healthy people. Not a reliable test for gestational diabetes.
Bilirubin	Nil–trace	Positive in obstructive jaundice and hepatitis.
Ketones	Nil	Individuals whose diabetes mellitus is poorly controlled experience breakdown of fatty acids. End products of fat metabolism are ketones. Individuals with dehydration or starvation also may have ketonuria.
Specific gravity (SG)	1.003–1.030	Specific gravity measures concentration of particles in urine. High specific gravity reflects concentrated urine, and low specific gravity reflects diluted urine. Dehydration, reduced renal blood flow and increased antidiuretic hormone (ADH) secretion elevate specific gravity. Overhydration, early renal disease and inadequate ADH secretion reduce specific gravity. Dipstick evaluations may be falsely high when the urine pH is <6 and falsely low when the pH is >7.
Blood	Nil	Damage to glomeruli or tubules may allow red blood cells (RBCs) to enter the urine. Trauma, disease or surgery of the lower urinary tract also may cause blood to be present. In women, blood in a routine urine specimen may be contaminated with menstrual fluid.
pH	4.5–8.0; average 5.0–6.0	pH helps indicate acid–base balance. Urine that stands for several hours becomes alkaline. An acid pH helps protect against bacterial growth, Illness, diet, fluids and medications can affect urinary pH.
Protein	Nil	Protein is not normally present in urine. It is seen in renal disease because damage to glomeruli or tubules allows protein to enter urine.
Urobilinogen	0.1–1.0	Positive in cirrhosis, chronic hepatic failure, hepatitis, hyperthyroidism but not a reliable guide to liver disease.
Nitrite	Nil	Nitrites are produced by bacteria. It will be positive in UTI; however, a negative test does not rule out infection because some organisms do not produce nitrites.
Leucocytes	Nil	Detects significant numbers of white blood cells (WBCs) which are suggestive of urinary tract infection. When combined with the nitrite test, it has a predictive value of 74% for UTI if both tests are positive.

(Adapted from The Royal College of Pathologists of Australasia 2019; Watt 2021)

urinalysis findings. Routine urinalysis is described in Clinical Skill 31.1. (See Case Study 31.2.)

- Fluid balance chart/voiding diary—a fluid balance chart is often used for hospitalised people. The data is recorded on a fluid balance chart, and intake and output are compared over a 24-hour period (see example in Figure 31.5). Urine output should be close to fluid intake over a 24-hour period. In an average-sized adult, the rate of urine production is approximately 30–40 mL per hour.
- The information in a voiding diary (which is different from a fluid balance chart) will also help determine the amount and types of fluid that the person usually consumes, volume voided, lower urinary

CLINICAL SKILL 31.1 Routine urinalysis

Please adhere to the policy and procedures of the facility/organisation prior to undertaking the skill. Ensure this skill is in your scope of practice.

NMBA Decision-making Framework considerations (refer to NMBA Decision-making framework for nursing and midwifery 2020):	Equipment:
1. Am I educated? 2. Am I authorised? 3. Am I competent? If you answer 'no' to any of these, do not perform that activity. Seek guidance and support from your teacher/a nurse team leader/clinical facilitator/educator.	Urinalysis reagent testing strip (dipstick)—check use-by date Paper towel Urine collection container Disposable gloves Watch or timer to measure time required for reaction to occur on the test strip (from immediate to 60 seconds)

PREPARE FOR THE SKILL

(Please refer to the Standard Steps on pp. xviii–xx for related rationales.)
Mentally review the steps of the skill.
Discuss the skill with your instructor/supervisor/team leader, if required.
Confirm correct facility/organisation policy/safe operating procedures.
Validate the order in the individual's record.
Identify indication and rationale for performing the activity.
Assess for any contraindications.
Locate and gather equipment.
Perform hand hygiene.
Ensure therapeutic interaction.
Identify the individual using three individual identifiers.
Gain the individual's consent.
Assess for pain relief.
Prepare the environment.
Provide and maintain privacy.
Assist the individual to assume an appropriate position of comfort.

Skill activity	Rationale
Collect a fresh urine specimen from the person in appropriate container (may be a bedpan or urinal) and taken to the pan room for testing.	A fresh specimen is more likely to yield accurate results.

PERFORM THE SKILL

(Please refer to the Standard Steps on pp. xviii–xx for related rationales.)
Perform hand hygiene.
Apply PPE: gloves, eyewear, mask and gown as appropriate.
Ensure the individual's safety and comfort throughout use of the skill.
Promote independence and involvement of the individual if possible and/or appropriate.
Assess the individual's tolerance to the skill throughout.
Dispose of used supplies, equipment, waste and sharps appropriately.
Remove PPE and discard or store appropriately.
Perform hand hygiene.

CLINICAL SKILL 31.1 Routine urinalysis—cont'd

Skill activity	Rationale
Inspect urine for colour, amount, odour and clarity.	Abnormalities in the appearance of the urine may indicate abnormalities.
Prepare testing area by placing absorbent paper towel onto benchtop.	Paper towel will absorb any urine spilt.
Check test strips are within the use-by date.	Out-of-date test strips or inaccurate timing may not give an accurate result.
Uncap bottle and remove reagent strip from bottle. Recap bottle.	Prevents contamination of remaining strips in bottle.
Note the time the reagent strip is inserted into the urine.	Not all tests are read at the same time.
Dip reagent strip into the collected urine, making sure to cover all testing areas on the strip.	Ensures the chemical reaction will occur on each test patch area of the strip.
Lift the test strip out of the urine and blot the side of the stick on the paper towel.	Reduces the risk of urine dripping on the test strip container when reading the results.
Holding the reagent strip container on its side, without touching the test strip against the bottle, match the test areas of the reagent strip against the chart on the container. Wait the required time from dipping the strip in the urine to reading the result (from immediate to 60 seconds). Each individual test has a required time for the reaction to complete. Note the results on the chart as the time elapses.	Test results are noted against colour matching on the reagent test strip container chart. Touching the strip against the bottle will lead to cross-contamination. Timing of the reaction for each test ensures accuracy of the results.
Dispose of urine sample, test strip and absorbent towel into correct receptacles.	Correct disposal prevents cross-contamination and spread of infection.

AFTER THE SKILL

(Please refer to the Standard Steps on pp. xviii–xx for related rationales.)
Communicate outcome to the individual, any ongoing care and to report any complications.
Restore the environment.
Report, record and document assessment findings, details of the skill performed and the individual's response.
Report, record and document any abnormalities and/or inability to perform the skill.
Reassess the individual to ensure there are no adverse effects/events from the skill.

(Patton et al 2024; Watt 2021)

CASE STUDY 31.2

Mrs Jane Smith is an 85-year-old who resides in an aged-care home. She is in good health and has always been very friendly and talkative with the staff. During handover, you are informed that Mrs Smith has been experiencing urge frequency and incontinence. You have commenced your shift and, upon entering the room, you notice that Mrs Smith is unusually quiet and will not make eye contact with you. She has been incontinent of urine and you notice that her urine smells malodourous. Her observations are BP 145/90 mmHg, RR 22 breaths/min, temp 38.5°, HR 115 beats/min. Mrs Smith is diaphoretic, and she starts to become agitated.

1. What clinical assessments could indicate that Mrs Smith has a delirium?
2. What clinical assessment intervention/skill should be undertaken to determine if Mrs Smith has a UTI?
3. What are your responsibilities as an EN in this situation?

Bladder diary

Fill in this diary for three or more days in a row.

Name:

Day and time		Drinks/fluid intake		Urine (wee)				Pads or clothing	What happened at the time of the leak?	Bowel movement
Day	Time	Type of drink or fluid	Amount of drink/ fluid (ml)	Amount of urine passed (ml)	How urgent was your need to pass urine (wee)? 1 = no urge to 3 = normal urge to 5 = strong urge	Did you leak or wet yourself? (Yes or No)	How much did you leak? (Spot, small, medium, large)	Did you change your pad or clothing? (Yes or No)	Where you were and what you were doing at the time you leaked urine	Did you pass a bowel motion (poo)?
Examples: Monday 3 March	*7.00am*			*250ml*	*5*	*Yes*	*Medium*	*Yes - my underwear and pyjama pants*	*I woke up and got out of bed.*	*No*
Monday 3 March	*8.00am*	*Coffee*	*200ml*							

Figure 31.5 Bladder diary

(Continence Foundation of Australia 2021)

tract symptoms including incontinence, precipitating factors (such as coughing) and use of continence pads. For a continence assessment, this data is usually collected for three consecutive, 24-hour days.

Other areas for assessment—these may vary, depending on where the nurse is practising, local hospital policy and skill level:

- *Abdominal examination*—inspection and light palpation to determine bladder distension. The bladder is not normally felt above the symphysis pubis after voiding.
- *Post-void residual urine volume (PVR)*—assessed by use of a portable ultrasound bladder scanner. The person is asked to void normally and then the scan is performed to detect the volume of any residual urine left in the bladder. Normally, no more than 50 mL PVR would be expected. If there is more than 200 mL, this is considered to be inadequate emptying (Crisp et al 2021) and the person should be referred for further assessment by an RN or medical practitioner.

CRITICAL THINKING EXERCISE 31.1

You have accepted care from the morning shift of a person with an IDC in situ post an abdominal hysterectomy. You note at 1400 hrs that there is no urine in the catheter bag. IV fluids are running at 100 mL/hr. The last documented urine output was at 0600 hrs and the bag was emptied of 40 mL at that time. The person you are caring for is confused, febrile, hypertensive, has shortness of breath, is nauseous and is complaining of left flank and chest pain.

1. What is your first response?
2. What is the medical terminology for this volume of urine output?
3. What could the observations and symptoms indicate?

Common diagnostic tests

Mid-stream urine specimen

When urinary tract infection is suspected, a mid-stream urine specimen may be required. This type of specimen is needed to culture urine to determine the presence of bacteriuria and to check for antibiotic sensitivity (microculture and sensitivity or MCS test). The test is conducted by microbiologists. To obtain a urine sample that is relatively free of the microorganisms growing in the lower urethra, the person will need to be instructed about the method for obtaining a mid-stream urine specimen. If the person is unable to manage the required perineal or penile cleansing and collection of the specimen or unable to follow instructions, the nurse needs to perform the specimen collection. It generally takes 24 hours to culture the bacteria and 48 hours to identify sensitivity to antimicrobial agents. The procedure for collecting a mid-stream urine specimen is outlined in Clinical Skill 31.2.

Urine collection over a period of time

Several tests of renal function and urine composition (e.g. creatinine clearance or hormone studies) require collection of urine over a specified period of time, most commonly 24 hours. The urine is collected in a clean container each time the person voids and immediately emptied into a specially labelled large container over the prescribed period of time. The timed collection period begins after the person urinates. For example, for a 24-hour collection the person first voids at 0900. This sample is discarded, and the 24-hour time period begins. All urine from this time onwards is saved until 0900 the next day. The person voids as close as possible to 0900 at the end of the collection period. This urine is added to the collection container and the time period is completed. It is important to make sure that the person understands that all urine in the time period needs to be collected. Any missed specimens will make the results inaccurate.

Catheter urine specimen

Urinalysis (see Case Study 31.2) using dipsticks and collection of a urine specimen for laboratory analysis can be done on a person who has a urinary catheter; however, the following points should be noted:

- The specimen should *not* be collected from the drainage bag. Bacteria grow rapidly in the drainage bag and could cause an inaccurate result.
- The aim is to obtain a fresh urine sample while maintaining the closed system between the catheter and the urine drainage bag.
- The sample needs to be drawn from the needleless sampling port in the drainage bag tubing. The catheter should not be disconnected from the drainage bag tubing, nor a needle inserted into the catheter or the drainage bag tubing. Breaking the closed system (catheter and drainage bag tubing) should be avoided since this increases the risk of catheter-associated urinary tract infection (CAUTI).
- Place the urine drainage bag tubing so that a loop near the drainage port is lying flat on the individual's bed or chair (so that urine will collect in the tubing).
- After performing hand hygiene, put on non-sterile gloves. A sterile 10 mL syringe will also be required.
- If the specimen is for microbiological analysis, a sterile pathology specimen will be needed (do not touch the inside of the container or the lid). Make sure that the container is labelled with the person's details, date and time of the specimen collection, and that the urine was obtained from an individual with an indwelling catheter.
- Wipe the needleless port on the drainage bag tubing with an alcohol swab. When this has dried, carefully insert the hub of the syringe through the needleless port into the drainage bag tubing lumen. Aspirate 5–10 mL of urine and remove the syringe from the sampling port. Transfer the urine into the sterile container using an aseptic technique.

CLINICAL SKILL 31.2 Mid-stream urine collection

Please adhere to the policy and procedures of the facility/organisation prior to undertaking the skill. Ensure this skill is in your scope of practice.

NMBA Decision-making Framework considerations (refer to NMBA Decision-making framework for nursing and midwifery 2020):	Equipment:
1. Am I educated? 2. Am I authorised? 3. Am I competent? If you answer 'no' to any of these, do not perform that activity. Seek guidance and support from your teacher/a nurse team leader/clinical facilitator/educator.	Sterile specimen container with wide opening and lid Commercially produced water wipe or mild soap and water to wash genital area Laboratory request form (signed by a medical practitioner or Nurse Practitioner—may be an electronic document) Disposable gloves Biohazard specimen transport bag

PREPARE FOR THE SKILL

(Please refer to the Standard Steps on pp. xviii–xx for related rationales.)
Mentally review the steps of the skill.
Discuss the skill with your instructor/supervisor/team leader, if required.
Confirm correct facility/organisation policy/safe operating procedures.
Validate the order in the individual's record.
Identify indication and rationale for performing the activity.
Assess for any contraindications.
Locate and gather equipment.
Perform hand hygiene.
Ensure therapeutic interaction.
Identify the individual using three individual identifiers.
Gain the individual's consent.
Assess for pain relief.
Prepare the environment.
Provide and maintain privacy.
Assist the individual to assume an appropriate position of comfort.

Skill activity	Rationale
Mid-stream urine (MSU) specimen obtains a urine specimen that is not contaminated by microorganisms from the hands or urethra. Accurate urine collection for an MSU can only be achieved if the individual is able to follow instructions. If the person is unable to follow instructions, the nurse will need to assist to obtain the specimen.	
Explain to the person how to obtain a specimen that is free of toilet paper and stool.	To promote collection of an uncontaminated specimen.

PERFORM THE SKILL

(Please refer to the Standard Steps on pp. xviii–xx for related rationales.)
Perform hand hygiene.
Apply PPE: gloves, eyewear, mask and gown as appropriate.
Ensure the individual's safety and comfort throughout use of the skill.
Promote independence and involvement of the individual if possible and/or appropriate.
Assess the individual's tolerance to the skill throughout.
Dispose of used supplies, equipment, waste and sharps appropriately.
Remove PPE and discard or store appropriately.
Perform hand hygiene.

CLINICAL SKILL 31.2 Mid-stream urine collection—cont'd

Skill activity	Rationale
Explain to the person how to: • Perform hand hygiene. • Wash genital area. • Female: hold labia open. Male: draw back foreskin if uncircumcised. • Void a small amount of urine into the toilet (keeping the labia held open with one hand). • While not interrupting the flow of urine, with the other hand, place the specimen container in a position to catch the urine, taking care not to touch the inside of the container or touch the container onto the skin of the genital area. Fill approximately half the container. • Remove the container, replace the lid securely without touching the inside surface and place on a secure surface. • Pass the remaining urine into the toilet, wipe as needed, re-dress and wash hands. For a man—make sure the foreskin is replaced to its normal position covering the glans penis. *Note:* If the person is unable to collect the specimen themselves, the nurse will need to assist (with disposable gloves on). Follow the same procedure as above. It may be easier to collect the urine in a larger sterile container and, when collected, pour the specimen into the smaller sterile container for transport to the laboratory. All other steps are the same.	Promotes cooperation and individual's participation. Where appropriate, the individual can collect a clean-voided specimen independently. All actions are an attempt to collect the most uncontaminated specimen possible.
Specimen container may need wiping with an absorbent paper towel. Label the specimen container with the person's name, date of birth, hospital or patient number and the date and time of the specimen collection.	Ensures that the correct specimen is sent for testing and that it is for the correct person.
Specimen container is placed in the zip lock section of the plastic biohazard bag.	Standard infection control precaution.
Pathology request form is checked for the person's details. The pathology request form is placed in the other section of the bag. Indicate on laboratory slip if individual is menstruating.	Ensures correct form and specimen are sent to pathology department and correct test will be undertaken in the pathology department.

AFTER THE SKILL

(Please refer to the Standard Steps on pp. xviii–xx for related rationales.)
Communicate outcome to the individual, any ongoing care and to report any complications.
Restore the environment.
Report, record and document assessment findings, details of the skill performed and the individual's response.
Report, record and document any abnormalities and/or inability to perform the skill.
Reassess the individual to ensure there are no adverse effects/events from the skill.

Skill activity	Rationale
The specimen should be transported to the laboratory as soon as possible, or stored in a refrigerator until transport can be arranged.	Decomposition and cell growth occur if urine is left standing, and may provide an inaccurate result.

(Patton et al 2024; Rebeiro et al 2021; Watt 2021)

- Return the drainage bag tubing to the usual position so that urine will flow freely into the drainage bag.
- Remove the gloves and properly dispose of equipment. Perform hand hygiene.
- The specimen is transferred to the laboratory in a sealed biohazard plastic bag with the request slip for testing.

Other diagnostic tests

Tests that may be performed to assist or confirm the diagnosis of urinary system disorders include the following. Only the most common tests are discussed.

Blood tests

Renal function is assessed via the eGFR, which is based on the detection of waste products in the blood in conjunction with a urine test for the protein albumin. Other blood tests may include:

- serum electrolytes (the kidneys regulate electrolyte levels)
- urea and creatinine (urea and creatinine are waste products of protein breakdown and muscle metabolism)
- full blood count (FBC) (the kidneys produce erythropoietin, which controls red blood cell production).

(The Royal College of Pathologists of Australasia 2019)

Ultrasound and other imaging diagnostic studies

Ultrasound is a non-invasive diagnostic tool in the assessment of urinary disorders. Ultrasound makes use of high-frequency inaudible soundwaves that reflect from tissue structures (Cooper & Gosnell 2023). Ultrasound is often used to identify gross renal structures and structural abnormalities of the kidneys or lower urinary tract, and to assist with biopsy procedures. An intravenous pyelogram (IVP) is an X-ray examination of the urinary tract in which an injection of dye is given into a vein so that the function of the kidneys is shown by passage of the dye through the kidneys and down the ureters that drain them to the bladder (Cooper & Gosnell 2023). A retrograde pyelogram involves the insertion of catheters into the ureters through a cystoscope. Contrast medium is introduced through the ureteric catheters into the pelvis or the kidneys, and X-ray films are taken (Cooper & Gosnell 2023).

A renal scan allows indirect viewing of urinary tract structures after an intravenous injection of radioactive isotopes, which circulates through the kidneys and is excreted. No precautions against radioactive exposure are needed except for the use of disposable gloves if the individual uses a bedpan or urinal to void after the procedure (Cooper & Gosnell 2023). The scan enables assessment of renal blood flow, anatomy and function.

A computed tomography (CT) scan is a computerised X-ray procedure used to obtain detailed images of structures within a selected plane of the body. With this procedure it is possible to see abnormal pathological conditions such as tumours, obstructions, retroperitoneal masses and lymph node enlargement (Cooper & Gosnell 2023). Some CT procedures require oral or intravenous contrast material and/or bowel preparation prior to the procedure.

Magnetic resonance imaging (MRI) uses radiowaves to alter magnetic fields produced by the body. The detail of the MRI scan can be enhanced with the use of an intravenous injection of a contrast media (Cooper & Gosnell 2023).

Cystoscopy

A cystoscope is an endoscopic instrument that is passed into the bladder through the urethra in order to inspect the interior of the bladder and urethra, and collect urine and tissue specimens (Phillips & Hornacky 2021). The procedure is carried out either under a general anaesthetic with a rigid instrument or under local anaesthesia (anaesthetic gel inserted into the urethra) with a flexible cystoscope. The person should be observed after the procedure to make sure they are voiding normally (they have no urinary retention) and the colour and characteristics of the urine should be recorded (Cooper & Gosnell 2023).

NURSING INTERVENTIONS

There are many factors that can affect a person's normal voiding pattern (Crisp et al 2021), especially in those hospitalised. These include:

- anxiety, stress, nervousness or embarrassment associated with the need to use toilet aids or to void in the presence of others
- the need to remain in a supine position when using a bedpan or, for males, and not being able to stand to void
- the effects of medications, anaesthesia or the acute stress of surgery
- pain following surgery or a dysuria which can lead to reluctance to void
- altered cognitive state, such as dementia or delirium
- constipation
- being in an unfamiliar environment.

Promoting normal voiding patterns

Nursing interventions that may be implemented to promote normal voiding patterns include the following:

- Ensuring adequate privacy and sufficient time for the person to void. If possible, the person should be left alone to use the toilet aids (e.g. commode, bedpan or urinal) since they may be self-conscious about the need to void in the presence of others. Ensure that bedside curtains are drawn, room doors are closed if appropriate and that the call bell is accessible. Allow adequate time to void.
- Explaining the need for the person to press the call bell to get assistance with voiding.
- Assessing for cultural differences in toileting habits.
- Making sure that the person's need to void is responded to promptly. If they feel no-one is coming to assist them, they are likely to become anxious, it may increase the risk of incontinence and the person's safety may be at risk if they try to get to the toilet unassisted.

- Relieving pain. If a person is experiencing pain, the cause should be identified and treated. Nursing interventions to relieve pain include assessing the type, location and nature of the pain; ensuring that the person is positioned comfortably; and making sure that the person gets pain relief if required.
- Assisting the person to assume a natural voiding position. Whenever possible the person should be permitted to use the toilet but, if this is contraindicated, an upright position on a bedpan may assist (see Figure 31.6). Males may find it easier to pass urine if assisted to stand, even if they are semi-sitting and leaning on the side of the bed (Patton 2021). (Refer to Clinical Skill 31.3.) Make sure that the person is safe and comfortable, and that toilet paper and the call bell are easy to reach. If the person requires assistance at the bedside or cannot go to the toilet, make sure that they have assistance with wiping after voiding if needed. The person should be offered a warm bowl of water, hand soap and a towel to wash their hands after toileting.
- Using clear signage and lighting to indicate the location of toilet facilities.

(Rebeiro et al 2021)

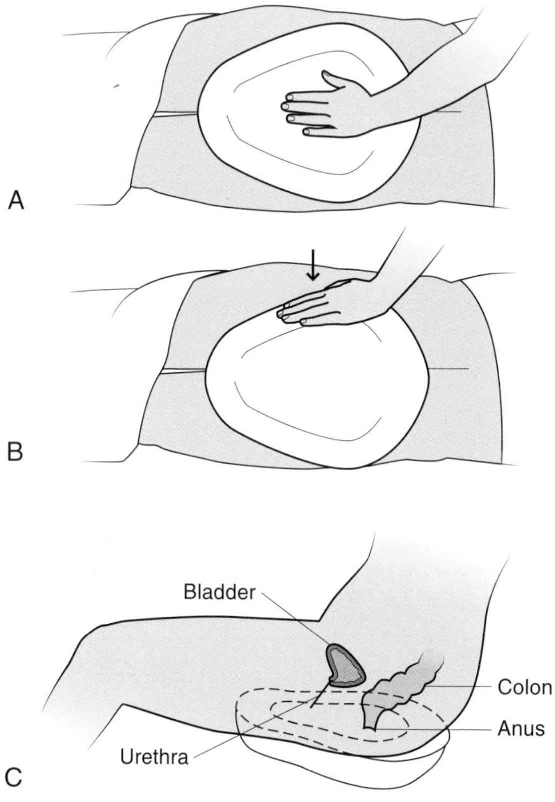

Figure 31.6 Positioning a bedpan

(A) Another method of placing a bedpan is used when the person is unable to help. The person lies on one side and the bedpan is placed firmly against the buttocks, **(B)** The nurse pushes down on the bedpan and towards the person, **(C)** The person is positioned on the bedpan so that the urethra and anus are directly over the opening.

Stimulating the micturition reflex

To be able to void, the person needs to be able to recognise the urge to void, be able to control when they are ready to void and be able to relax during voiding. As mentioned previously, privacy and positioning are important; however, assisting the person to relax is of equal importance. Unless contraindicated, a warm shower or bath, or the pouring of warm water over the genitalia of a female, may stimulate micturition. Another stimulation technique is the sound of running water (e.g. turning on a nearby tap) (Patton 2021).

Promoting adequate fluid intake

Encourage the person to drink adequate amounts of fluids, unless this is contraindicated (e.g. renal impairment, heart failure). The recommended fluid intake for adults is 1500–2000 mL per day, preferably water (Continence Foundation of Australia 2023b). An adequate fluid intake will keep the urine dilute, reducing the risk of UTI. If the person is on fluid restriction, make sure to plan out their intake so they can access fluids throughout the day.

Promoting normal bowel function

Prevention of constipation should be a priority of care for all individuals who are hospitalised. Many people will have a history of constipation; however, illness or surgery, the need for pain medication, change of diet and environment are all likely to make the individual at risk of constipation. (See Chapter 32 for details.) Constipation can impact on urinary function and, if severe enough, can contribute to incomplete bladder emptying and urinary retention (Chiba et al 2022). Persistent straining to defecate can weaken the pelvic floor muscles and the external anal sphincter (Chiba et al 2022).

Promoting continence

All of the interventions mentioned above contribute to promotion of continence. While many people nurses care for will have risk factors for incontinence, in many cases, incontinence can be prevented by simple measures that are easy to incorporate into a nursing care plan and everyday life. These interventions should be part of every individual's care plan, not just those who have established urinary or bowel incontinence.

Healthy bowel and bladder habits

The Continence Foundation of Australia (2023b) recommends five important steps aimed at promoting good bowel and bladder habits that should form part of health promotion activities. These include:

- Drinking well—maintaining a fluid intake of at least 1.5–2 L per day. People should be encouraged to drink water and limit their intake of caffeine and alcohol as these are irritants to the bladder (and also avoid cola-based drinks, which are high in caffeine).
- Eating a healthy diet—high fibre with plenty of fresh fruit and vegetables.
- Leading a positive lifestyle—maintaining a healthy weight, not smoking. An obese person may require a

CLINICAL SKILL 31.3 Assisting with toileting: bedpan, urinal, commode

Please adhere to the policy and procedures of the facility/organisation prior to undertaking the skill. Ensure this skill is in your scope of practice.

NMBA Decision-making Framework considerations (refer to NMBA Decision-making framework for nursing and midwifery 2020): 1. Am I educated? 2. Am I authorised? 3. Am I competent? If you answer 'no' to any of these, do not perform that activity. Seek guidance and support from your teacher/a nurse team leader/clinical facilitator/educator.	**Equipment:** Bedpan traditional or slipper type/urinal/commode chair Pan/urinal cover Waterproof sheet/'bluey'/absorbent pad (if using a bedpan) Disposable gloves Toilet paper Hand hygiene available for the person—water, face washer, towel, disposable wipes If the person can assist with moving themselves onto the bedpan, they will need an overhead trapeze bar. If the person is unable to assist in lifting themselves, another person will be needed to assist with rolling them onto the pan or a lifting machine.

PREPARE FOR THE SKILL

(Please refer to the Standard Steps on pp. xviii–xx for related rationales.)
Mentally review the steps of the skill.
Discuss the skill with your instructor/supervisor/team leader, if required.
Confirm correct facility/organisation policy/safe operating procedures.
Validate the order in the individual's record.
Identify indication and rationale for performing the activity.
Assess for any contraindications.
Locate and gather equipment.
Perform hand hygiene.
Ensure therapeutic interaction.
Identify the individual using three individual identifiers.
Gain the individual's consent.
Assess for pain relief.
Prepare the environment.
Provide and maintain privacy.
Assist the individual to assume an appropriate position of comfort.

Skill activity	Rationale
Assist with toileting using bedpan/urinal	
A bedpan or urinal is used to assist an individual with toileting when they are unable to move from the bed to the toilet or a commode chair beside the bed.	
Assist the person to a sitting or semi-Fowler's position if the person's health condition allows.	Provides ease of access to insert bedpan. Enables the person to assist by lifting themselves by the overhead trapeze.

PERFORM THE SKILL

(Please refer to the Standard Steps on pp. xviii–xx for related rationales)
Perform hand hygiene.
Apply PPE: gloves, eyewear, mask and gown as appropriate.
Ensure the individual's safety and comfort throughout use of the skill.
Promote independence and involvement of the individual if possible and/or appropriate.
Assess the individual's tolerance to the skill throughout.
Dispose of used supplies, equipment, waste and sharps appropriately.
Remove PPE and discard or store appropriately.

Skill activity	Rationale
Place waterproof sheet/'bluey'/absorbent pad under the person's buttock area.	Absorbent pad will collect any spilt urine and prevent bed from becoming wet.

CLINICAL SKILL 31.3 Assisting with toileting: bedpan, urinal, commode—cont'd

Place bedpan under the person's buttocks, on top of the waterproof pad. A urinal is placed between a man's thighs (the handle upwards). The penis is placed into the neck of the urinal.	Ensures that urine or faeces will go into the bedpan/urinal and not soil the bedding.
Assist the person with use of toilet paper.	To remove urine and faecal matter from the perineal area.
Remove bedpan/urinal and place the paper cover.	Prevents contents from being viewed during transportation to pan room/flusher.
Provide for hand hygiene (bowl of warm water, hand wash, towel etc.).	Prevents the spread of infection. Provides hygiene requirements for the person.
Volume measurement, urinalysis, use Bristol Stool Chart for documenting faeces.	Measurement required for maintaining fluid balance.
Place the bedpan/urinal in the pan flusher for cleaning/sterilising.	Standard infection control measure.
Assist with toileting using commode	
A commode chair is used to assist an individual with toileting when they are unable to move from the bed to the toilet but are able to sit out of bed with assistance. Use of a commode chair provides a more normal position for toileting than use of a bedpan. However, where possible, the person should be assisted to the toilet.	
Commode is placed close to the bed or chair with brakes applied.	Provides ease of access. Brakes prevent chair from moving.
Pan placed into commode chair.	Collects urine or faeces.
Individual is assisted onto the commode (may need more than one person to assist).	Prevents individual from falling.
Provide call bell for individual and allow for privacy.	Dignity and privacy are maintained.
Assist individual with use of toilet paper.	To remove urine and faecal matter from the perineal area.
Assist individual into the bed or chair.	To maintain safety.
Provide for hand hygiene (such as a bowl of warm water, hand wash, towel).	Prevents the spread of infection. Provides hygiene requirements for the person.
Remove commode and transport to the pan room.	Remove from vicinity of individual's bedside. Contents are disposed of in the correct manner.
Volume measurement, urinalysis, use Bristol Stool Chart for documenting faeces.	Measurement required for maintaining fluid balance.

AFTER THE SKILL

(Please refer to the Standard Steps on pp. xviii–xx for related rationales.)
Communicate outcome to the individual, any ongoing care and to report any complications.
Restore the environment.
Report, record and document assessment findings, details of the skill performed and the individual's response.
Report, record and document any abnormalities and/or inability to perform the skill.
Reassess the individual to ensure there are no adverse effects/events from the skill.

(Patton et al 2024; Potter et al 2023; Watt 2021)

program of weight reduction; a 5% weight reduction is associated with a significant improvement in urinary incontinence (Cardozo et al 2023).
- Being active.
- Practising good toilet habits—it is normal for people to void between four and eight times per day and no more than once at night. Good toileting habits include not going to the toilet 'just in case' because this may result in a smaller functional bladder capacity over time. People should be encouraged to go to the toilet only when their bladder is full and they have the need to void (except before going to bed at night, which most people do routinely). People should also be encouraged to take their time when voiding so that their bladder has the opportunity to empty completely (Patton 2021). Incomplete emptying can result in UTI, particularly in women.

Pelvic floor muscle exercises

All women should be doing regular pelvic floor exercises (PFEs) as part of their general fitness program. PFEs are designed to improve the strength of pelvic floor muscles. They consist of repetitive contractions of specific muscle groups (Touhy 2022). For pregnant women, pelvic floor exercises help the body to cope with the increasing weight of the baby and aid in recovery after birth. Pelvic floor exercises are also prescribed for men, especially following surgery for BPH or prostate cancer (Gulanick & Myers 2022). A health education program should include information about the location of the muscles and therefore which muscles need to be contracted, the pattern of contractions and how often they need to be contracted. Because PFEs involve the identification and conscious recruitment of the pelvic floor muscles, the person must be able to follow instructions and repeat a series of exercises without supervision over a long period of time. (See Clinical Interest Box 31.1 for details.) The Continence Foundation of Australia has excellent brochures, posters and teaching materials related to PFEs.

CLINICAL INTEREST BOX 31.1
Pelvic floor muscle exercises

It is important for the person to understand the anatomy and function of the pelvic floor muscles and factors that can contribute to weakness of the muscles.

Provide the person with written information with instructions and anatomical diagrams that can be obtained online or in hard copy from the Continence Foundation of Australia.

It is important that the right muscles are being contracted. If the person is unsure, refer to a nurse continence specialist or continence physiotherapist to confirm that the correct muscles are being contracted.

Finding the right muscles

Have the person lie on their back and tighten the muscles around the anus by imagining that they are trying to stop passing wind. When on the toilet, attempt to stop the flow of urine. Pull the muscles up into the body and get the sense of squeezing and lifting the pelvic floor muscles without squeezing the buttocks or abdominal muscles. Then relax and finish passing urine. This action should not be continued once the person is familiar with contracting the correct muscles.

Exercising

Have the person squeeze the muscle identified and hold for a count of 8 (or the best they can do). Relax for a count of 8 seconds. Repeat the squeeze and lift 8–12 times, then relax and repeat three times.

Advise the person to repeat these exercises three times per day (8–12 squeeze and lifts), then relax and repeat three times per day. Try to do the exercises in various positions (e.g. lying, sitting, standing).

It may take time to work up to 10-second squeezes; reassure the person that it will improve over time.

(Adapted from Continence Foundation of Australia 2023c)

Seeking help when symptoms persist

All healthcare professionals have an obligation to provide information for people so they can make informed choices about the healthcare that will best suit their needs. This means that the healthcare professional has to be informed about the services that are available. All people with a continence problem need to be encouraged to talk to their GP or practice nurse about their concerns. They can also call the National Continence Helpline (free call—1800 33 00 66), where they can talk with a nurse continence specialist, get information and find out where their local continence service is located. There is no need for a medical referral to a continence service; the person can refer themselves (or the nurse can refer on their behalf).

Interventions for urinary incontinence

One of the biggest barriers to effective and excellent continence care is community attitudes and, in particular, the attitudes of healthcare staff. Some staff members will believe that nothing can be done to improve continence, that it is part of ageing or that 2-hourly toileting and pads are the only solution (Cardozo et al 2023). All nurses have a role in continence promotion and management and need to be informed about appropriate evidence-based interventions. The continence promotion strategies listed previously should be part of the care plan for all individuals.

Before interventions can be selected that address the person's health goals, a comprehensive continence assessment needs to be conducted so that the specific continence issue/s can be identified. For many people, this will mean they need referral to a nurse continence specialist, continence physiotherapist and/or a medical practitioner who specialises in continence care. Enrolled Nurses will also frequently be involved in the implementation of a continence care plan. (See Nursing Care Plan 31.1.)

NURSING CARE PLAN 31.1 Caring for a person with urinary incontinence

Mrs Mary O'Connor (82 years old) was admitted to the acute medical ward the previous evening following a fall after tripping on a wet floor at the supermarket. This morning the nurse noticed that the sheets were damp and Mrs O'Connor was very distressed about it. On further questioning, Mrs O'Connor acknowledged she has had several episodes of losing small amounts of urine and is deeply traumatised by the event. She repeatedly asked the nurse not to tell anyone and said that she managed well at home. The nurse reassures Mrs O'Connor and says that she would like to ask her a few more questions and test her urine so that a plan of care can be developed to meet her health needs.

Further assessment

- The incontinence has only been an issue for about 6 months. More likely to occur when she is lifting groceries, carrying the washing basket to the line, when she laughs or sneezes. No urine loss overnight. Happens once or twice a day. Sometimes needs to change her underwear, which she finds distressing and annoying. She has not mentioned this to family members or her GP.
- Bowels normally opened once per day. Bristol 4 score.
- Has never used continence pads.
- Has three children, all born vaginally, forceps used for the first delivery.
- Is keen to do something about the incontinence.
- Current medications: Panadol Osteo PRN for osteoarthritic pain in knees and hips, vitamin D3—1000 IU per day. No other regular medications.
- Urinalysis: urine clear, non-offensive odour, pH 6, SG 1010, no abnormalities detected.
- No evidence of skin excoriation on thighs or perineum.

Reporting

The Enrolled Nurse reported to the Registered Nurse the situation with Mrs O'Connor and the further assessment that had already been undertaken. Following discussion of the findings, the following collaborative plan was developed with Mrs O'Connor.

Issue/s to be addressed

Type of urinary incontinence needs to be identified through further assessment.
Plan to discuss the continence problem with her attending medical officer when they review her later in the day.
Reassure Mrs O'Connor and keep her informed of the plan.

Goal/s

Mrs O'Connor will report a decrease in incidence of urinary incontinence episodes (which may take several months).
During the assessment process Mrs O'Connor will be able to maintain social continence.
Mrs O'Connor will be able to discuss good bowel and bladder habits within 2 days.
Mrs O'Connor will gain confidence in ability to self-manage her continence problem.
Mrs O'Connor will have a referral and appointment to attend the local continence service before discharge from hospital.

Care/actions	Rationale
Maintain standard precautions. Maintain bladder diary for at least 72 hours. Review person's fluid intake and types of fluid consumed. Discuss the normal anatomy and physiology of the bladder and bowel. Discuss good bowel and bladder habits (including pelvic floor muscle exercises). Provide written resources (e.g. from the Continence Foundation of Australia). Discuss use of a low-volume continence pad to manage the small leakages until she sees the nurse continence specialist at an outpatient's appointment. Provide reassurance to Mrs O'Connor that her incontinence is likely to be improved and probably is curable.	To reduce the transmission of infection. To establish continence pattern, acts as a baseline to measure improvement with interventions. To check if the person is taking any fluids which might irritate the bladder (e.g. drinks containing caffeine) as this can irritate the bladder in some people. Dilute urine reduces bladder irritation. Information so that individual understands bodily processes. Promotes continence and normal bowel and bladder function. Provides individual with information she can refer to later. The Continence Foundation is a good source of further information and support. The person can contact the helpline herself for further assistance. Will give Mrs O'Connor social continence and is likely to reduce her distress over concern about urinary leakage. Will give her encouragement to engage in the treatment plan.

Evaluation

Mrs O'Connor is able to describe normal bladder and bowel function.
Mrs O'Connor is able to describe good bowel and bladder habits.
Mrs O'Connor reports feeling dry and comfortable.
Mrs O'Connor's fluid intake is at least 1.5–2 L per day.
Mrs O'Connor is able to state where she can get further assistance when discharged from hospital.
Mrs O'Connor is able to outline the plan following discharge from hospital (referral to continence service).

Voiding programs

The aim of a bladder training program is to increase the person's functional bladder capacity and to try to reduce the frequency of voiding. People with incontinence often have tried to manage the problem themselves, decreasing their fluid intake and going to the toilet more frequently in order to reduce incontinence episodes. A voiding program is then developed based on the person's current voiding pattern and aims to increase the interval between voids to a normal 3–4-hour period. The program starts with education about how the bladder works and how continence is maintained (Cooper & Gosnell 2023). These programs may take some time to achieve the goal of a normal voiding pattern, especially if the person is having significant urge symptoms. The person will need ongoing encouragement and support to defer voiding since they are likely to fear incontinent episodes. Many people with significant urge symptoms will need an appropriate continence pad to make them feel secure during the early stages of a program.

Habit training, timed voiding and prompted voiding are methods of bladder re-education aimed at re-establishing a normal voiding pattern. These programs are used for people with stress, urge and mixed incontinence and are often used with frail or cognitively impaired people to reduce incontinence episodes (Cooper & Gosnell 2023). Habit training involves identification of the person's usual voiding pattern and pre-empting incontinence episodes by decreasing voiding intervals, while keeping these intervals as long as possible. Timed voiding is a program of voiding according to a schedule that is determined from a voiding diary (not just every 2 hours). Prompted voiding is a program in which the nurse checks the person at regular intervals to see if they are wet or dry, provides feedback to the person about their own perception of being wet or dry, and offers assistance with toileting. Positive responses are praised, and incontinent episodes are managed without comment. This type of voiding program is most suited to people with mild to moderate cognitive impairment or with functional incontinence due to immobility (Cardozo et al 2023).

Continence aids and appliances

Continence aids and appliances are the key to achieving social continence. Social continence refers to the capacity of a person to engage socially with confidence that there will be containment of involuntary loss of urine or faeces. Continence aids and appliances are an important part of active treatment plans for many people because they give the person the confidence they need to engage in normal daily activities and social interactions. They include body-worn absorbent products (continence pads), bed and chair pads, external collection devices (urinary sheath/condom) and aids to toileting. These are described briefly below. Urinary catheters can also be considered to be a continence aid; however, these are discussed separately.

Assessing the needs of the person

There are a number of criteria that need to be considered when selecting appropriate continence aids and appliances. These include:

- The volume of urine that is being lost—continence pads have different absorbency levels according to the degree of incontinence. The amount of urine that the person is losing can be estimated based on the results of a voiding diary.
- Rate of urine loss—if urine is lost quickly (e.g. in people with significant urge incontinence), the absorbency of the pad will need to be higher to accommodate the rate.
- Gender—some continence aids and appliances are made specifically for women, and some specifically for men.
- Size of the person—affects the choice of many products (e.g. size of a urinary catheter, size of a urinary sheath, some pads need to be sized to the person's waist circumference). There are bariatric-sized continence pads available for obese people.
- Short- or long-term use—may influence choice of aid or appliance.
- Whether the person also has faecal incontinence—in this case, containment becomes more important than absorption.
- The person's mobility, manual dexterity and cognitive function—these become important considerations in choice. There is no point choosing an aid or appliance that the person is unable to use.
- The cost and the person's personal preference—cost will be a significant factor for many people. People should always be given several options to try so they can work out which suits them the best.
- Disposal facilities—this becomes an issue for people who are working or spend a lot of time away from home.

(Watt 2021)

Continence pads

Continence pads come in a variety of sizes, shapes and absorbency. The absorbency varies from quite small (panty liners) to large pant-like products that are designed to accommodate large volumes over extended periods of time (e.g. overnight), with a capacity of approximately 3000 mL or more. While most continence pads are disposable, washable pads are available. Each type has its own benefits.

Getting the right pad for the person requires significant assessment and knowledge. It is definitely not the case that 'one size fits all'. This is a problem in many long-term care facilities where only one or two pads may be available for all residents. Often, when the pad is not effective, it is the person that is blamed, rather than recognising that the pad was not right for the person's individual situation.

A nurse continence specialist will have knowledge of the range of possible products. Many suppliers and manufacturers of continence pads will provide free samples; some may have guides to assist selection. The National Continence Helpline staff (free call—1800 33 00 66) will also be able to advise on selection of continence products. Nurses and other healthcare workers can call the helpline for professional advice. A useful resource for those working in aged-care services is the Continence Support Now website (see Online Resources). This is an initiative of the Continence Foundation of Australia and provides a pocket guide to in-home and aged-care and disability workers providing bladder and bowel support. This site has excellent information, including videos on a range of continence-related topics including care of a person who uses continence pads.

Sheath (condom) drainage

Condom (sometimes known as 'sheaths' or external catheters) drainage may be suitable for some men with urinary incontinence. It has the advantage of keeping the groin area dry and can be used for both ambulant and non-ambulant men, but does require some assessment and regular management with daily fitting and cleaning, and effectively removes the capacity to use the toilet for voiding (Perry et al 2022). Condom drainage can be used 24 hours/day, daytime only, night time only or for special occasions. It is not suitable for men with urinary obstruction.

Most continence condoms are 'one piece'; they have built-in adhesive to secure them to the penis. Less common are 'two piece', which have an adhesive strip, generally hydrocolloid and which adheres to the penile skin on one side and the condom on the other. Selection of the continence condom should be based on prior sizing, with inspection for penile shaft length and use of a sizing guide, as the condoms are available in a variety of lengths and diameters (Perry et al 2022).

The condom is attached to an overnight bag (usually 1500–2000 mL) or bottle (usually 2000–4000 mL), or a leg bag (commonly 500 mL, but may be 350–900 mL). Leg bags are secured with leg bag straps or a 'sleeve' with a pocket for the bag. The tubing between the condom and the bag or bottle should be secured with a fixation device.

The penis should be observed for oedema or discolouration (the condoms are usually clear or translucent). If detected, the appliance is removed immediately and the sizing reassessed since they can potentially cause significant skin damage (Perry et al 2022; Watt 2021). At least every 24 hours, remove the condom, and ensure the penis is cleaned and dried before reapplication. Use of such appliances should be discontinued at least temporarily if there are signs of skin excoriation, persistent oedema of the penis or UTI (Perry et al 2022). (See Clinical Skill 31.4.)

CLINICAL SKILL 31.4 Applying a sheath/condom drainage device

Please adhere to the policy and procedures of the facility/organisation prior to undertaking the skill. Ensure this skill is in your scope of practice.

NMBA Decision-making Framework considerations (refer to NMBA Decision-making framework for nursing and midwifery 2020): 1. Am I educated? 2. Am I authorised? 3. Am I competent? If you answer 'no' to any of these, do not perform that activity. Seek guidance and support from your teacher/a nurse team leader/clinical facilitator/educator.	**Equipment:** Silicone sheath/condom catheters in a variety of sizes and sizing guide Disposable razor or personal hair clippers (individual supplied) Urine drainage bag or leg bag and straps Disposable gloves Basin with warm water, soap, washcloth, towel

PREPARE FOR THE SKILL

(Please refer to the Standard Steps on pp. xviii–xx for related rationales.)

Mentally review the steps of the skill.
Discuss the skill with your instructor/supervisor/team leader, if required.
Confirm correct facility/organisation policy/safe operating procedures.
Validate the order in the individual's record.
Identify indication and rationale for performing the activity.
Assess for any contraindications.
Locate and gather equipment.
Perform hand hygiene.
Ensure therapeutic interaction.
Identify the individual using three individual identifiers.
Gain the individual's consent.
Assess for pain relief.
Prepare the environment.
Provide and maintain privacy.
Assist the individual to assume an appropriate position of comfort.

Continued

CLINICAL SKILL 31.4 Applying a sheath/condom drainage device—cont'd

Skill activity	Rationale
A sheath/condom catheter is used for a male who is incontinent but can void on his own and who prefers this method rather than continence pads. It should not be used when the person has any skin disease or irritation on the penis or if they have allergies to adhesives, or in men who have a very short retracted penis (the sheath will not stay in place).	
Assess the condition of the skin on the penis. Use a disposable sizing guide to measure the circumference of penis—assess for shaft length. Select an appropriately sized sheath.	Urinary incontinence increases the risk of skin breakdown or irritation. Enables the correct size to be used and reduces the risk of leakage of urine.

PERFORM THE SKILL

(Please refer to the Standard Steps on pp. xviii–xx for related rationales.)
Perform hand hygiene.
Apply PPE: gloves, eyewear, mask and gown as appropriate.
Ensure the individual's safety and comfort throughout use of the skill.
Promote independence and involvement of the individual if possible and/or appropriate.
Assess the individual's tolerance to the skill throughout.
Dispose of used supplies, equipment, waste and sharps appropriately.
Remove PPE and discard or store appropriately.
Perform hand hygiene.

Skill activity	Rationale
Ask the man to wash and dry the penis and surrounding skin, including the penile glans (in an uncircumcised man). Hand hygiene provided for individual (such as a bowl of warm water, soap, washcloth, towel). If the man cannot assist, the nurse can do this for him. Make sure that the foreskin is replaced back to its normal position. If needed, clip as much hair as possible from the base of the penis.	Cleanses the skin before application of the condom device. Moisture will reduce the adhesion. Prevents the spread of infection. Provides hygiene requirements for the person. The foreskin must be replaced to its normal position or it can swell and form a constriction ring, which will be painful and can impact on the penile circulation. Assists in the adherence of the sheath.
Prepare the urinary drainage bag for easy attachment to the sheath.	Prepares the system for use.
Grasp the penis along the shaft. The foreskin should be in its natural position (or very slightly extended so that when the condom is fitted, as the foreskin resumes its normal location, the condom is drawn closer to the body). Place the sheath at the tip of the penis and smoothly roll the sheath onto the penis, leaving a small amount of space between the tip of the penis and the drainage tube of the condom sheath. When applied, gently grip the condom around the penile shaft and squeeze for a few seconds to assist adhesion.	Positions the condom catheter on the penis. Inspects the applied condom to ensure it is the right size. It should appear neither too tight nor too loose. Reduces irritation and discomfort. The adhesive is on the inside of the silicone sheath.
Connect the sheath to the urine drainage bag tubing and check for kinks. Apply fixation device to upper thigh. Fit the drainage bag to a hanger for attachment to, for example, a bed rail, or to a stand on the floor.	Allows urine to flow into the collection bag. Secures tubing and limits tension on the condom.

CLINICAL SKILL 31.4 Applying a sheath/condom drainage device—cont'd

AFTER THE SKILL

(Please refer to the Standard Steps on pp. xviii–xx for related rationales.)
Communicate outcome to the individual, any ongoing care and to report any complications.
Restore the environment.
Report, record and document assessment findings, details of the skill performed and the individual's response.
Report, record and document any abnormalities and/or inability to perform the skill.
Reassess the individual to ensure there are no adverse effects/events from the skill.

Skill activity	Rationale
Explain how the sheath works, how the male can manage it himself and what to be aware of (pain, irritation, change in urine etc.). Provide written information on care of sheath drainage.	Health education is empowering and encourages independence.
Document the date, reason for the procedure, condition of the genital area, size and type of sheath applied, type of drainage bag attached to the sheath and if there were any difficulties applying the sheath.	Medicolegal requirement. Allows for the planning and implementation of care.
Check the penis after 30 minutes to ensure that the system is comfortable, not restricting penile blood flow and not leaking.	Assessment reduces risk of complications.

(Patton et al 2024; Rebeiro et al 2021; Watt 2021)

Environment and personal factors

An important part of a care plan for a person with incontinence is assessment of the environment and personal factors that can impact on the ability of the person to get to and use the toilet, particularly in hospitals and residential care facilities. For example:

- Provide easy access for people to get to the toilet and have suitable rails and/or equipment to assist them to void comfortably.
- People with perceptual problems (impaired eyesight or impaired cognition) may benefit from assistive signage and attention to lighting to identify the location of the toilet.
- People confined to bed should be provided with toileting aids (such as bedpans, urinals) appropriate to their individual needs. Any request for use of the toilet should be responded to promptly.
- If the person does have an incontinence episode, the wet clothing or bedclothes should be changed immediately. The person should be provided, or assisted with, personal hygiene to ensure that no urine or faeces is left on the skin (see also 'Maintaining skin integrity' below). They should be provided with clean, dry clothing and appropriate continence aids.
- Planning for outings may assist in preventing episodes of incontinence. For example, consider recommending or assisting with voiding before an outing, and before coming home. The National Public Toilet Map may assist in locating toilets when away from home.

(Gulanick & Myers 2022; Cardozo et al 2023)

Maintaining skin integrity

The skin of any person with incontinence is at risk of breakdown; however, frail older people are most at risk. Selecting the right aids and appliances is crucial to the maintenance of healthy skin as they are specifically designed to draw urine away from the skin. Incontinence-associated dermatitis (IAD) is the term used to describe the erythema and oedema of the surface of the skin in people who have incontinence (Sim et al 2020; Department of Health and Aged Care 2022). (See Clinical Interest Box 31.2.) It arises from the chemical irritation of urine (or faeces) on the skin and the physical irritation on the skin from prolonged exposure to moisture (Potter et al 2023; Department of Health and Aged Care 2022).

Skin care should be a priority in the care of anyone with incontinence. The following interventions for the prevention and treatment of IAD are recommended:

- Frequent checking of the individual and prompt changing of wet or soiled continence pads.
- Implementing a structured skin-care program for people with incontinence, which consists of washing, cleansing, moisturising and protecting the skin.
- Using skin cleansers (pH balanced, non-perfumed liquids or wipes) rather than soap and water, especially when skin cleansing is required frequently.
- Gentle but thorough cleaning is essential, taking care with skin folds and crevices.
- Effective drying of the skin after cleansing.
- Routine application of a pH balanced, non-perfumed moisturising cream or gel and a moisture barrier product (these may be combined in one product).

CLINICAL INTEREST BOX 31.2 Quality indicator reporting of incontinence-associated dermatitis (IAD) in residential aged care

Incontinence-associated dermatitis (IAD) is common in residential aged care. The risk factors associated with this include incontinence of urine and/or faeces, pre-existing skin conditions, poor mobility and the individual's inability to attend to their own personal hygiene. For the purposes of the National Aged Care Mandatory Quality Indicator Program, approved providers of residential aged care must collect and report on the percentage of care recipients who experienced incontinence-associated dermatitis quarterly. Incontinence-associated dermatitis is assessed using the Ghent Global IAD Categorisation Tool, and includes the following categories:

1A Persistent redness without clinical signs of infection
1B Persistent redness with clinical signs of infection
2A Skin loss without clinical signs of infection
2B Skin loss with clinical signs of infection

(Department of Health and Aged Care 2022)

- Ongoing assessment and reporting of skin integrity (at least daily). Report to a more senior staff member if the individual's skin condition is not improving or is deteriorating.

(Clinical Excellence Commission 2021; Potter et al 2023; Sim et al 2020)

CRITICAL THINKING EXERCISE 31.2

Consider your own values and beliefs about incontinence and how you feel about caring for a person who is incontinent.

1. Write down your thoughts and feelings.
2. Reflect on how these thoughts and feelings may impact on how you care for people who have a continence problem.

URINARY CATHETERISATION

A catheter is a tube that is inserted into the bladder to drain urine. There are several ways to achieve drainage of urine from the bladder:

- Indwelling urethral catheterisation—an indwelling catheter is inserted aseptically into the bladder via the urethra. A self-retaining catheter (Foley catheter) is used for this purpose. It has a small inflatable balloon that sits at the neck of the bladder to prevent the catheter falling out (Cooper & Gosnell 2023). The catheter balloon is filled with sterile water after the catheter is inserted. The catheter will have two or three lumens: one for drainage of urine, one for inflation of the balloon and possibly one for the installation of fluids or medication into the bladder (see Figure 31.7). This type of catheterisation can be used short term or long term. Long-term catheters need to be changed periodically, depending on the needs of the individuals.
- Suprapubic catheterisation—a catheter is surgically inserted into the bladder by a puncture wound on the lower abdomen. This type of catheterisation is used in people who have chronic retention of urine, neurological disorders (such as spinal cord injury), prior to pelvic surgery, urethral trauma and who need long-term bladder drainage (Cooper & Gosnell 2023). Suprapubic catheters are also self-retaining. They need to be changed periodically; the timeframe varies from person to person. An RN who has specific knowledge and skill is able to change this type of catheter.
- Intermittent catheterisation—a non-retaining catheter is inserted into the bladder and then removed when the bladder has been emptied. Intermittent catheterisation can be repeated as often as needed throughout the day. Where possible, people who need ongoing intermittent catheterisation are taught to do it themselves (intermittent self-catheterisation).

Reasons for urinary catheterisation

There are many reasons for a catheter to be used. The most common reason is short-term use following surgery or serious ill-health where accurate and frequent measurement of urinary output is required. Urinary catheterisation should only be used as a treatment option for incontinence when all other measures have failed.

Selection of an appropriate catheter

Catheters are made of a variety of materials and sizes. The best catheter will be one that causes the least trauma and discomfort and is the smallest lumen to effectively drain the bladder. Points to consider when selecting an appropriate catheter are described in Clinical Interest Box 31.3.

Catheter bags—the closed drainage system

After catheter insertion, the catheter is attached to a sterile single-use urine drainage bag. This forms a closed system to reduce the risk of UTI. Urinary drainage bags are made of a soft plastic material which can hold about 1000–1500 mL of urine. The bag has drainage tubing, which connects directly with the end of the catheter and a sealable emptying port at

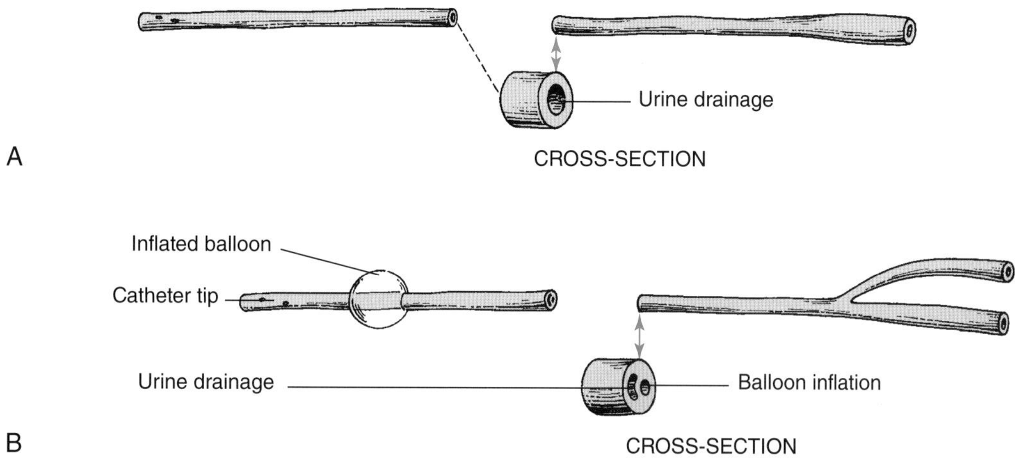

Figure 31.7 Types of urinary catheters

CLINICAL INTEREST BOX 31.3 Selecting an appropriate urinary catheter

Size

- The French system (French gauge; FG) is used; the larger the gauge number, the larger the catheter size. One FG ⅓ of a millimetre.
- Usually, women require a 12–14 FG and men require a 14–16 FG.
- To prevent trauma, the smallest effective catheter size should be selected.

Material selection (main types)

- The expected time required for the catheterisation and presence of latex allergy will determine the catheter material selection.
- Hydrogel-coated catheters are recommended for use up to 3 months; they increase the individual's comfort since they produce a slippery outside surface (in the urethra), which reduces friction and protects the urethra. These are latex covered with hydrogel, so check for a history of latex allergy.
- Silicone-coated latex catheters are recommended for use up to 1 month. They provide minimal urethral irritation and smooth insertion. Latex hypersensitivity can occur since the coating dissolves over time.
- Pure silicone catheters are best suited for long-term use (2–3 months) because they cause less encrustation at the urethral meatus. They have a large lumen because they are not coated and are more rigid.
- PVC catheters are suitable only for intermittent use due to their rigidity.

Balloon size

- Balloon size is important in selecting an indwelling catheter. Use the smallest balloon size possible since the larger the balloon, the more irritation at the bladder neck is likely to occur. In adults, the 10 mL is the most common. A 30 mL size is used after some prostate surgery to provide haemostasis of the prostatic bed.
- Only sterile water should be used to inflate the balloon.

(Adapted from Cooper & Gosnell 2023)

the bottom of the bag. At the catheter end of the drainage bag tubing, there will be a sampling port for collection of urine samples. The closed drainage system should not be broken to take urine samples (Cooper & Gosnell 2023). If it is necessary to disconnect any part of the system, an aseptic technique must be used.

Where frequent measurement (usually hourly) of urine output is required, choose a drainage bag that has a measuring burette, a rigid plastic container that is part of the drainage system that is calibrated to measure small volumes. When the hourly reading is performed, the urine is drained into the larger drainage bag.

For the person who will go home from hospital with an indwelling urinary catheter, a smaller leg bag is aseptically connected to the catheter so that they can carry on their usual daily activities without having to carry a large urine bag. Because the leg bag only holds approximately 500 mL of urine, it will need to be emptied frequently throughout the day, into a toilet or plastic jug (see Figure 31.8). A larger overnight bag is connected to the outlet of the leg bag

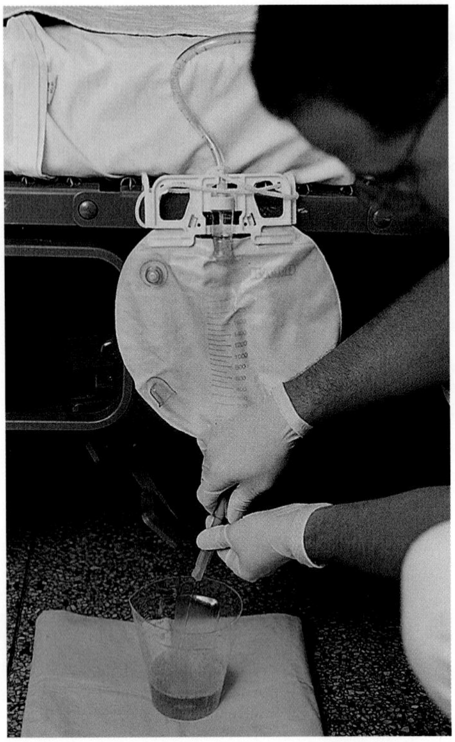

Figure 31.8 Emptying a urine drainage bag

(Crisp et al 2021)

before the person goes to bed, so that their sleep is not interrupted by the need to empty the smaller leg bag. The key steps related to emptying urine collection bags are outlined in Clinical Skill 31.5.

Routine catheter care

Urinary catheters are not without complications. There are significant risks associated with indwelling catheterisation, including discomfort and pain, bladder spasm, symptomatic UTI, generalised sepsis, urethral trauma, bladder calculi, encrustation and blockage, urethral stricture and stenosis (Cooper & Gosnell 2023). Urinary catheterisation also has significant impact on a person's body image, sexuality and general wellbeing (Markiewicz et al 2020; Cooper & Gosnell 2023). Catheter-associated urinary tract infection (CAUTI) is said to be one of the most common healthcare-associated infections worldwide, with greater than 90% of individuals developing bacteriuria within 30 days of indwelling catheter insertion (Cooper & Gosnell 2023). Prevention of hospital-acquired infection, such as catheter-associated urinary tract infections, is one of the priority areas identified in the National Safety and Quality Health Service (NSQHS) Standards (Australian Commission on Safety and Quality in Health Care 2021).

CLINICAL SKILL 31.5 Emptying a urine drainage bag

Please adhere to the policy and procedures of the facility/organisation prior to undertaking the skill. Ensure this skill is in your scope of practice.

NMBA Decision-making Framework considerations (refer to NMBA Decision-making framework for nursing and midwifery 2020):	Equipment:
1. Am I educated? 2. Am I authorised? 3. Am I competent? If you answer 'no' to any of these, do not perform that activity. Seek guidance and support from your teacher/a nurse team leader/clinical facilitator/educator.	Disposable gloves Alcohol wipe Urine jug Protective eyewear Paper towel × 2 (to prevent spillage of urine on the floor; to cover urine jug while taking it to the pan room or bathroom)

PREPARE FOR THE SKILL

(Please refer to the Standard Steps on pp. xviii–xx for related rationales.)

Mentally review the steps of the skill.
Discuss the skill with your instructor/supervisor/team leader, if required.
Confirm correct facility/organisation policy/safe operating procedures.
Validate the order in the individual's record.
Identify indication and rationale for performing the activity.
Assess for any contraindications.
Locate and gather equipment.
Perform hand hygiene.
Ensure therapeutic interaction.
Identify the individual using three individual identifiers.
Gain the individual's consent.
Assess for pain relief.
Prepare the environment.
Provide and maintain privacy.
Assist the individual to assume an appropriate position of comfort.

CLINICAL SKILL 31.5 Emptying a urine drainage bag—cont'd

Skill activity	Rationale

Drainage bags need to be emptied at regular intervals (often once per 8 hours) from the drainage port at the base of the drainage bag. The closed system (drainage bag tubing connected to the urethral catheter) should not be broken to reduce the risk of catheter-associated urinary tract infection (CAUTI).

PERFORM THE SKILL

(Please refer to the Standard Steps on pp. xviii–xx for related rationales.)
Perform hand hygiene.
Apply PPE: gloves, eyewear, mask and gown as appropriate.
Ensure the individual's safety and comfort throughout use of the skill.
Promote independence and involvement of the individual if possible and/or appropriate.
Assess the individual's tolerance to the skill throughout.
Dispose of used supplies, equipment, waste and sharps appropriately.
Remove PPE and discard or store appropriately.
Perform hand hygiene.

Skill activity	Rationale
Cleanse the end of the valve at the base of the drainage bag with the alcohol wipe and allow to dry. Place the jug below the valve and open valve, avoid splashing and prevent contact of the drainage valve with the urine jug.	Allows urine to drain from the bag into the jug. Reduces the risk of bacterial contamination of the urine drainage bag.
When the bag is empty, close the valve.	Prevents subsequent drainage of urine out of the bag.
Remove the jug, cover with a piece of paper towel. Remove the paper towel on the floor and dispose of appropriately. Take the urine to the pan room.	Safe transport of a bodily fluid.
Inspect the urine for colour, clarity and odour. Measure the volume.	The person is at risk of CAUTI. Maintain fluid balance chart.
Empty urine from jug into pan flusher or toilet, rinse the jug, place the jug in the pan washer.	Prevents cross-contamination.

AFTER THE SKILL

(Please refer to the Standard Steps on pp. xviii–xx for related rationales.)
Communicate outcome to the individual, any ongoing care and to report any complications.
Restore the environment.
Report, record and document assessment findings, details of the skill performed and the individual's response.
Report, record and document any abnormalities and/or inability to perform the skill.
Reassess the individual to ensure there are no adverse effects/events from the skill.

(ACSQHC 2021; Patton et al 2024; Watt 2021)

Nursing care of a person with an indwelling catheter is similar for both males and females and is planned and implemented to promote comfort, maintain the flow of urine and minimise the possibility of a CAUTI (Cooper & Gosnell 2023):

- Make sure the person is fully informed about the purpose of their catheter, possible complications and when to seek help.
- The catheter must be securely fixed to the thigh or lower abdomen (for men) to reduce movement of the tube in the urethra to minimise the risk of infection and discomfort. A range of catheter fixation devices exist, including belts and adhesive devices.
- The bag should hang on the bed frame or wheelchair without touching the floor (Figure 31.9). The urine bag should be kept below the person's waist level to promote free drainage. However, most drainage bags contain an anti-reflux valve to prevent urine in the bag from re-entering the drainage tubing and contaminating the person's bladder.

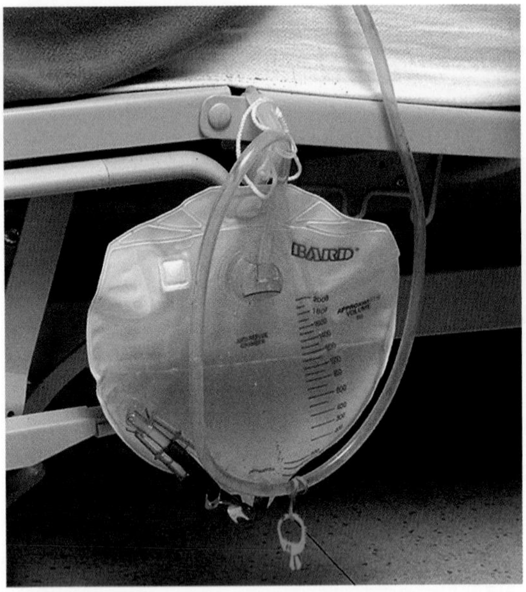

Figure 31.9 Closed urinary drainage system

(Fairchild et al 2022)

- Nursing assessment—assess the patency of the system at least once per shift (every 8 hours) or more frequently if there have been problems with the catheter. Assess the person's comfort/pain level, fluid intake and the colour, characteristics and amount of urine. Also check for kinks in the tubing and that the catheter is securely strapped to the person's thigh or lower abdomen. If there is any leakage of urine around the catheter, the person has the feeling they need to void or they have pain, report your findings to the RN or medical officer for further investigation. This may be caused by bladder spasm, blockage of the catheter or tubing or insertion of a catheter of incorrect size (usually too large). Document your assessment in the progress notes. (See Clinical Interest Box 31.4.)
- The collection bag is emptied at specified intervals or when it is almost full, using standard infection control precautions.
- Encourage the person to drink at least 2000 mL daily, unless this is contraindicated. This will help flush urine through the bladder and reduce the risk of sediment forming in the system.
- For most people, usual genital hygiene during a daily shower will be sufficient. In people who have faecal incontinence, it may be necessary to cleanse the perineum and genital area, especially in women. Use skin cleansers (pH balanced, non-perfumed liquids or wipes) rather than soap and water, especially when skin cleansing is required frequently. For an uncircumcised male, the foreskin should be retracted before cleansing, and replaced to its normal position after cleansing. Where possible, the person should be assisted to clean themselves.
- Prevent constipation—a hard faecal mass in the rectum can obstruct the catheter. (See Chapter 32.)

Insertion and removal of a urinary catheter

Urinary catheterisation usually requires a written request from a medical practitioner, Nurse Practitioner, nurse continence specialist or urology nurse specialist. The procedure of catheter insertion is called catheterisation and is performed using sterile equipment and aseptic technique. (See Clinical Skill 31.6 and Clinical Skill 31.7.)

Removal of a urinary catheter also requires a written request. The aim is to remove the catheter with minimal trauma to the bladder neck or urethra. Removing a catheter requires aseptic technique. (Refer to Clinical Skill 31.8.) After catheter removal, the person should be encouraged to drink plenty of fluids. The person's urine output, including volume of each void, should be assessed and recorded until a normal voiding pattern is established. In addition, assess for and report any difficulty with voiding, voiding small amounts, incontinence, dribbling, urgency, dysuria or frequency (Cooper & Gosnell 2023). Some people will have ongoing difficulty with voiding and may need the catheter to be reinserted.

CLINICAL INTEREST BOX 31.4
Tubing positioning

If an individual with an indwelling catheter reports that they have a feeling to void, ensure that you investigate this. The problem could be caused by the catheter being kinked, twisted or blocked.

CRITICAL THINKING EXERCISE 31.3

You are asked by the nurse manager to develop a presentation that will be given to the nursing staff on the ward as a quality improvement activity. The topic you need to address is continence promotion for the individuals on an acute medical ward.

1. What information would you include in the presentation?
2. Where would you access quality, evidence-based information and resources?
3. Make a list of the resources you would recommend for the ward to assist nursing staff to promote continence in their day-to-day clinical practice.

CLINICAL SKILL 31.6 Urinary catheterisation (female)

Please adhere to the policy and procedures of the facility/organisation prior to undertaking the skill. Ensure this skill is in your scope of practice.

NMBA Decision-making Framework considerations (refer to NMBA Decision-making framework for nursing and midwifery 2020):	Equipment:
1. Am I educated? 2. Am I authorised? 3. Am I competent? If you answer 'no' to any of these, do not perform that activity. Seek guidance and support from your teacher/a nurse team leader/clinical facilitator/educator.	Procedure trolley/suitable clean surface if in community setting Catheter pack (basic) containing: • Gloves (extra pair optional) • Drapes, one fenestrated • Lubricant (usually water-based or xylocaine gel [2%] in a pre-filled syringe) • Antiseptic cleaning solution (aqueous chlorhexidine), normal saline or sterile water • Gauze swabs • Forceps • Syringe with sterile water to inflate the balloon of indwelling catheter • Receptacle or basin (usually bottom of disposable catheterisation tray) Catheter of correct size and type for procedure (i.e. intermittent or indwelling) Sterile urine drainage bag Catheter strap or other catheter fixation device Urine drainage bag bedside hanger Protective eyewear Blanket/large towel to cover individual Disposable waterproof pad Procedure light/torch

PREPARE FOR THE SKILL

(Please refer to the Standard Steps on pp. xviii–xx for related rationales.)
Mentally review the steps of the skill.
Discuss the skill with your instructor/supervisor/team leader, if required.
Confirm correct facility/organisation policy/safe operating procedures.
Validate the order in the individual's record.
Identify indication and rationale for performing the activity.
Assess for any contraindications.
Locate and gather equipment.
Perform hand hygiene.
Ensure therapeutic interaction.
Identify the individual using three individual identifiers.
Gain the individual's consent.
Assess for pain relief.
Prepare the environment.
Provide and maintain privacy.
Assist the individual to assume an appropriate position of comfort.

Skill activity	Rationale
Make an assessment of the need for another nurse to assist (e.g. if the person is confused or uncooperative, or unable to position their legs during the procedure).	Reduces anxiety. Provides assistance.
Assist the person to a semi-Fowler's position. Assist them to remove underwear, place a disposable waterproof pad under the buttocks and drape with a blanket or towel. Position extra lighting if needed.	Promotes comfort and facilitates performance of the procedure. Assists visualisation.

Continued

CLINICAL SKILL 31.6 Urinary catheterisation (female)—cont'd

PERFORM THE SKILL

(Please refer to the Standard Steps on pp. xviii–xx for related rationales.)
Perform hand hygiene.
Apply PPE: gloves, eyewear, mask and gown as appropriate.
Ensure the individual's safety and comfort throughout use of the skill.
Promote independence and involvement of the individual if possible and/or appropriate.
Assess the individual's tolerance to the skill throughout.
Dispose of used supplies, equipment, waste and sharps appropriately.
Remove PPE and discard or store appropriately.
Perform hand hygiene.

Skill activity	Rationale
Open the outer cover of the catheterisation pack, ensuring aseptic technique is maintained, and slide the pack onto the top shelf of the trolley.	Maintains the sterile field. Reduces risk of transmission of infection.
Using a non-touch technique, open each side of the sterile cover of the catheter pack. Carefully open and place other sterile equipment onto the sterile field, ensuring aseptic technique is maintained (depending on what equipment is in the catheter pack): • Sterile, self-retaining urinary catheter • Urinary drainage bag	Prepares equipment. Maintains the sterile field and therefore reduces the risk of CAUTI.
Organise catheter pack contents and other equipment on sterile field, ensuring aseptic technique is maintained—for example, draw up sterile water into syringe (amount usually 10 mL—check on the catheter balloon port), open lubricant and squeeze out near the edge of one of the plastic trays, open cleansing solution and moisten gauze swabs on the other tray, ready for cleansing the urethral meatus. Remove the top part of the plastic covering the catheter. Place a small amount of lubricating gel on the tip of the catheter and leave on one of the sterile plastic trays.	Maintains an asepsis, which will reduce the risk of CAUTI.
Ask the person (or another nurse) to position the knees so they are flexed and separated, and feet slightly apart on the bed.	Provides a clear view of the urethral meatus.
Carefully pick up the sterile plastic tray with cleansing solution and moistened gauze and place close to the individual (either on/near the thigh or between open legs).	Makes it easier to perform cleansing procedure.
With the non-dominant hand, separate the labia minora so that the urethral meatus is visualised. Cleanse both the labia and around the urethral orifice with sterile cleansing solution, using single downward strokes. Keep the labia open with non-dominant hand (or leave a sterile piece of gauze in the labia).	Reduces risk of introducing microorganisms from the genital/anal area into the urinary tract. Provides better access to the urethral orifice and helps to prevent labial contamination of the catheter.
Remove used tray and drop into waste bag/bin without contaminating the gloved hand.	Prevents cross-contamination and decreases risk of contaminating the field.
Apply fenestrated drape to genital area.	Creates and extends protective field.
Place sterile paper drape across the person's thighs.	Reduces risk of equipment becoming contaminated during the procedure and extends sterile area.

CLINICAL SKILL 31.6 Urinary catheterisation (female)—cont'd

Place the second sterile tray with the catheter in it onto the sterile drape between the person's legs. Pick up the lubricated catheter with dominant hand and insert in the urethral meatus. Gently advance the catheter along the urethra until urine flows out into the tray. Insert the catheter approximately 2 cm further.	Gives a good view of the meatus and minimises the risk of contamination of the urethra. Inadvertent inflation of the balloon in the urethra causes pain and urethral trauma. Length of catheter inserted must be in relation to the anatomical structure of the urethra.
Connect the syringe with the correct amount of sterile water (usually 10 mL) to the balloon port of the catheter, ensure syringe is firmly in place and inflate the balloon slowly with a gentle constant force.	The inflated balloon keeps the catheter in the bladder. Inadvertent inflation with the balloon in the urethra causes trauma and pain. Use of less or more than recommended volume can result in an asymmetrically inflated balloon, the catheter falling out or bursting of the balloon.
Connect the sterile drainage bag tubing and ensure it is securely connected.	Ensures the closed system is maintained, reducing the risk of CAUTI.
Make sure the person's genital area is dry. Remove fenestrated drape and equipment from bed. The person's legs may be straightened.	Ensures comfort.
Attach the drainage bag to a bedside hanger and frequently check for kinks in the tubing. Ensure bag is not touching the floor. Ensure the drainage bag is kept lower than the catheter and the person's bladder.	Failure to keep drainage bag below the level of the bladder, or looped or kinked tubing, can slow the flow of urine, causing discomfort and backflow within the system.
Secure the catheter to the individual's inner thigh using a catheter strap device. The securement should be placed where the catheter is stiffest, typically just below the bifurcation. Ensure that the catheter does not become pulled when person is moving.	Stabilising urethral catheters can reduce adverse events such as dislodgement, tissue trauma, inflammation and UTI. Movement-induced trauma (urethral erosion) can lead to UTIs and tissue necrosis.
Depending on the reason for catheterisation, measurement of the amount of urine drained shortly after catheterisation may be required.	In cases of urinary retention.

AFTER THE SKILL

(Please refer to the Standard Steps on pp. xviii–xx for related rationales.)
Communicate outcome to the individual, any ongoing care and to report any complications.
Restore the environment.
Report, record and document assessment findings, details of the skill performed and the individual's response.
Report, record and document any abnormalities and/or inability to perform the skill.
Reassess the individual to ensure there are no adverse effects/events from the skill.

Skill activity	Rationale
Document reason for catheterisation or changing catheter, catheter type and size, balloon size and amount of sterile water in the balloon, batch number/lot number (on the outside label of the catheter packaging), expiry date, date and time of insertion. Description of urine, colour and volume drained.	To provide a point of reference or comparison in the event of later queries. It may be helpful to keep the product identification section from the catheter packaging.
If the person is to go home with the catheter, commence a health education program including troubleshooting and signs and symptoms that indicate they need to seek professional advice. Provide written information about catheter care and management of the urine bag.	The person is likely to have more confidence. Encourages the person to report any problems that may occur while catheter in situ.

(ACSQHC 2021; Cooper & Gosnell 2023; Rebeiro et al 2021; Watt 2021)

CLINICAL SKILL 31.7 Urinary catheterisation (male)

Please adhere to the policy and procedures of the facility/organisation prior to undertaking the skill. Ensure this skill is in your scope of practice.

NMBA Decision-making Framework considerations (refer to NMBA Decision-making framework for nursing and midwifery 2020):

1. Am I educated?
2. Am I authorised?
3. Am I competent?

If you answer 'no' to any of these, do not perform that activity. Seek guidance and support from your teacher/a nurse team leader/clinical facilitator/educator.

Equipment:

Procedure trolley/suitable clean surface if in community setting
Catheter pack (basic) containing:

- Gloves (extra pair optional)
- Drapes, one fenestrated
- Lubricant (usually water-based or xylocaine gel [2%] in a pre-filled syringe)
- Antiseptic cleaning solution (aqueous chlorhexidine), normal saline or sterile water
- Gauze swabs
- Forceps
- Syringe with sterile water to inflate the balloon of indwelling catheter
- Receptacle or basin (usually bottom of disposable catheterisation tray)

Catheter of correct size and type for procedure (i.e. intermittent or indwelling)
Sterile urine drainage bag
Catheter strap or other catheter fixation device
Urine drainage bag bedside hanger
Protective eyewear
Blanket/large towel to cover individual
Disposable waterproof pad
Procedure light/torch

PREPARE FOR THE SKILL

(Please refer to the Standard Steps on pp. xviii–xx for related rationales.)
Mentally review the steps of the skill.
Discuss the skill with your instructor/supervisor/team leader, if required.
Confirm correct facility/organisation policy/safe operating procedures.
Validate the order in the individual's record.
Identify indication and rationale for performing the activity.
Assess for any contraindications.
Locate and gather equipment.
Perform hand hygiene.
Ensure therapeutic interaction.
Identify the individual using three individual identifiers.
Gain the individual's consent.
Assess for pain relief.
Prepare the environment.
Provide and maintain privacy.
Assist the individual to assume an appropriate position of comfort.

Skill activity	Rationale
Make an assessment of the need for another nurse to assist (e.g. if the person is confused or uncooperative, or unable to position their legs during the procedure).	Reduces anxiety. Provides assistance.
Assist the person to a supine position with legs extended and flat on bed. Assist them to remove underwear, place a disposable waterproof pad under the buttocks and drape with a blanket or towel. Position extra lighting if needed.	Promotes comfort and facilitates performance of the procedure. Assists visualisation.

CLINICAL SKILL 31.7 Urinary catheterisation (male)—cont'd

PERFORM THE SKILL

(Please refer to the Standard Steps on pp. xviii–xx for related rationales.)
Perform hand hygiene.
Apply PPE: gloves, eyewear, mask and gown as appropriate.
Ensure the individual's safety and comfort throughout use of the skill.
Promote independence and involvement of the individual if possible and/or appropriate.
Assess the individual's tolerance to the skill throughout.
Dispose of used supplies, equipment, waste and sharps appropriately.
Remove PPE and discard or store appropriately.
Perform hand hygiene.

Skill activity	Rationale
Open the outer cover of the catheterisation pack, ensuring aseptic technique is maintained, and slide the pack onto the top shelf of the trolley.	Maintains the sterile field. Reduces risk of transmission of infection.
Using a non-touch technique, open each side of the sterile cover of the catheter pack. Carefully open and place other sterile equipment onto the sterile field, ensuring aseptic technique is maintained (depending on what equipment is in the catheter pack): • Sterile, self-retaining urinary catheter • Urinary drainage bag	Prepares equipment. Maintains the sterile field and therefore reduces the risk of CAUTI.
Organise catheter pack contents and other equipment on sterile field, ensuring aseptic technique is maintained; for example, draw up sterile water into syringe (amount usually 10 mL—check on the catheter balloon port), open lubricant and squeeze out near the edge of one of the plastic trays, open cleansing solution and moisten gauze swabs on the other tray, ready for cleansing the urethral meatus. Remove the top part of the plastic covering the catheter. Place a small amount of lubricating gel on the tip of the catheter and leave on one of the sterile plastic trays.	Maintains an asepsis, which will reduce the risk of CAUTI.
Carefully pick up the sterile plastic tray with cleansing solution and moistened gauze and place close to the individual (either on/near the thigh or between open legs).	Makes it easier to perform cleansing procedure.
With the non-dominant hand, grasp the penis just below the glans and hold upright. If the individual is uncircumcised, retract the foreskin. With the dominant hand, clean the glans around the urethral orifice with sterile cleansing solution in a circular motion. Keep the penis in non-dominant hand.	Reduces risk of introducing microorganisms into the urinary tract. The urethra has two curves in it as it passes through the penis and can be straightened out by lifting the penis in an upright position. Provides better access to the urethral orifice and helps to prevent contamination of the catheter.
Remove used tray and drop into waste bag/bin without contaminating the gloved hand.	Prevents cross-contamination and decreases risk of contaminating the field.
Apply fenestrated drape to genital area.	Creates and extends protective field.
Place sterile paper drape across the person's thighs.	Reduces risk of equipment becoming contaminated during the procedure and extends sterile area.

Continued

CLINICAL SKILL 31.7 Urinary catheterisation (male)—cont'd

Place the second sterile tray with the catheter in it onto the sterile drape between the person's legs. With the non-dominant hand gently straighten and stretch the penis to an angle of 60 to 90 degrees. A pre-filled syringe of lidocaine (uro-jet) can be used to anaesthetise the urinary canal. Pick up the lubricated catheter with dominant hand and insert in the urethral meatus. Gently advance the catheter along the urethra until urine flows out into the tray (to the Y section of the catheter). Replace foreskin if uncircumcised.	Gives a good view of the meatus and minimises the risk of contamination of the urethra. Local anaesthetic to minimise discomfort. Inadvertent inflation of the balloon in the urethra causes pain and urethral trauma. Length of catheter inserted must be in relation to the anatomical structure of the urethra.
Connect the syringe with the correct amount of sterile water (usually 10 mL) to the balloon port of the catheter, ensure syringe is firmly in place, inflate the balloon slowly with a gentle constant force.	The inflated balloon keeps the catheter in the bladder. Inadvertent inflation with the balloon in the urethra causes trauma and pain. Use of less or more than recommended volume can result in an asymmetrically inflated balloon, the catheter falling out or bursting of the balloon.
Connect the sterile drainage bag tubing and ensure it is securely connected.	Ensures the closed system is maintained, reducing the risk of CAUTI.
Make sure the person's genital area is dry. Remove fenestrated drape and equipment from bed.	Ensures comfort.
Attach the drainage bag to a bedside hanger and frequently check for kinks in the tubing. Ensure bag is not touching the floor. Ensure the drainage bag is kept lower than the catheter and the person's bladder.	Failure to keep drainage bag below the level of the bladder, or looped or kinked tubing, can slow the flow of urine, causing discomfort and backflow within the system.
Secure the catheter to the individual's inner thigh using a catheter strap device. The securement should be placed where the catheter is stiffest, typically just below the bifurcation. Ensure that the catheter does not become pulled when person is moving.	Stabilising urethral catheters can reduce adverse events such as dislodgement, tissue trauma, inflammation and UTI. Movement-induced trauma (urethral erosion) can lead to UTIs and tissue necrosis.

AFTER THE SKILL

(Please refer to the Standard Steps on pp. xviii–xx for related rationales.)
Communicate outcome to the individual, any ongoing care and to report any complications.
Restore the environment.
Report, record and document assessment findings, details of the skill performed and the individual's response.
Report, record and document any abnormalities and/or inability to perform the skill.
Reassess the individual to ensure there are no adverse effects/events from the skill.

Skill activity	Rationale
Document reason for catheterisation or changing catheter, catheter type and size, balloon size and amount of sterile water in the balloon, batch number/ lot number (on the outside label of the catheter packaging), expiry date, date and time of insertion. Description of urine, colour and volume drained.	To provide a point of reference or comparison in the event of later queries. It may be helpful to keep the product identification section from the catheter packaging.
If the person is to go home with the catheter, commence a health education program including troubleshooting and signs and symptoms that indicate they need to seek professional advice. Provide written information about catheter care and management of the urine bag.	The person is likely to have more confidence. Encourages the person to report any problems that may occur while catheter in situ.

(ACSQHC 2021; Cooper & Gosnell 2023; Rebeiro et al 2021; Watt 2021)

CLINICAL SKILL 31.8 Removal of indwelling urinary catheter

Please adhere to the policy and procedures of the facility/organisation prior to undertaking the skill. Ensure this skill is in your scope of practice.

NMBA Decision-making Framework considerations (refer to NMBA Decision-making framework for nursing and midwifery 2020): 1. Am I educated? 2. Am I authorised? 3. Am I competent? If you answer 'no' to any of these, do not perform that activity. Seek guidance and support from your teacher/a nurse team leader/clinical facilitator/educator.	**Equipment:** Disposable gloves Protective eyewear Sterile syringe for deflating balloon Disposable bed protector pad Waste bin or bag

PREPARE FOR THE SKILL

(Please refer to the Standard Steps on pp. xviii–xx for related rationales.)
Mentally review the steps of the skill.
Discuss the skill with your instructor/supervisor/team leader, if required.
Confirm correct facility/organisation policy/safe operating procedures.
Validate the order in the individual's record.
Identify indication and rationale for performing the activity.
Assess for any contraindications.
Locate and gather equipment.
Perform hand hygiene.
Ensure therapeutic interaction.
Identify the individual using three individual identifiers.
Gain the individual's consent.
Assess for pain relief.
Prepare the environment.
Provide and maintain privacy.
Assist the individual to assume an appropriate position of comfort.

Skill activity	Rationale
Self-retaining urinary catheters need to have the balloon deflated before removal. It is important to make sure that the full amount of water is removed so that the removal does not cause trauma to the urethra or pain. Make sure that the drainage bag is emptied before you start the procedure.	
Check volume of water that was inflated into the balloon (this will be written in nursing progress note from insertion and is also located on the port for balloon inflation/deflation).	To confirm how much water is in the balloon. To ensure balloon is completely deflated before removing catheter.

PERFORM THE SKILL

(Please refer to the Standard Steps on pp. xviii–xx for related rationales.)
Perform hand hygiene.
Apply PPE: gloves, eyewear, mask and gown as appropriate.
Ensure the individual's safety and comfort throughout use of the skill.
Promote independence and involvement of the individual if possible and/or appropriate.
Assess the individual's tolerance to the skill throughout.
Dispose of used supplies, equipment, waste and sharps appropriately.
Remove PPE and discard or store appropriately.
Perform hand hygiene.

Skill activity	Rationale
Place bed protector pad under the person's buttocks. Remove the catheter securing device from the person's thigh.	Comfort of the person.

Continued

CLINICAL SKILL 31.8 Removal of indwelling urinary catheter—cont'd

Open syringe and insert the tip into the balloon port. Allow the pressure within the port to force the plunger back and fill the syringe with water. Do not use suction on the syringe but allow the sterile water to come back spontaneously (or if needed only use minimal suction to get the flow started).	Reduces the likelihood of damaging the balloon port or tubing.
Check amount of fluid in syringe corresponds to the amount used at insertion. Remove syringe.	Ensures balloon is completely deflated before removing catheter.
Ask individual to breathe in and then out: as individual exhales, gently remove the catheter. Inspect the catheter to make sure that it is intact and place it on the waterproof sheet for wrapping and disposal. *Note:* If catheter does not easily come out, stop the procedure, reassure the individual and inform the RN. **Do not** place a needle in the tubing or cut the tubing.	Distracts the person while the tubing is being removed. Failure of balloon to deflate. Ruins the integrity of the catheter.

AFTER THE SKILL

(Please refer to the Standard Steps on pp. xviii–xx for related rationales.)
Communicate outcome to the individual, any ongoing care and to report any complications.
Restore the environment.
Report, record and document assessment findings, details of the skill performed and the individual's response.
Report, record and document any abnormalities and/or inability to perform the skill.
Reassess the individual to ensure there are no adverse effects/events from the skill.

Skill activity	Rationale
Ask the person to notify a nurse when they feel the desire to void and that they must void into a container for measurement. Encourage them to increase their fluid intake (approx. 250 mL per hour until normal voiding pattern is established unless contraindicated). If the person is voiding small amounts of urine, has symptoms of UTI or voiding frequently, report to the RN.	Assesses whether the person has returned to a normal voiding frequency and volume.
Document time of removal, description of urine, colour and volume drained, time of first void post removal and frequency of voiding.	Accurate recording of individual's progress. Assists with the planning and implementation of care.

(Patton et al 2024; Watt 2021)

DECISION-MAKING FRAMEWORK EXERCISE 31.1

You are the Enrolled Nurse who is caring for Ms Jane Stewart (52 years of age) 4 hours post laparoscopic hysterectomy. Jane reports that she cannot pass urine and has abdominal pain with a scale of 8/10. The Registered Nurse (RN) you are working with performed an abdominal assessment, which revealed a distended bladder on light palpation, and a bladder scan that demonstrated an 800 mL urine volume. Pain relief was administered and Ms Stewart was assisted to the toilet. She was unable to pass urine and was becoming more distressed. The medical officer was informed and requested that an indwelling catheter was to be inserted, left in overnight and then removed in the morning. The RN asks you to insert the catheter. You have only inserted a catheter once as a student and you do not feel confident in making decisions about the catheter type and size or the procedure of catheter insertion. (Review Progress Note 31.1 as a sample of how this case information should be documented.)

1. Why did the RN perform an abdominal assessment and bladder scan?
2. Given your lack of confidence with knowledge and skill related to catheter insertion, what would you do in this situation and why?
3. What would be an appropriate catheter type and size for this situation?

Progress Note 31.1

24/06/24 1430 hrs	Nursing: Ms Jane Stewart at 1230 hrs reported that she was not able to pass urine and had an abdominal pain score of 8/10. Chris Blake RN was informed—abdominal examination revealed a distended bladder. Bladder scan—800 mL bladder volume (refer to print-out). She was given pain relief (with good effect, see chart) and assisted to the toilet, but was unable to pass urine. Dr Williams was informed and requested an indwelling catheter to be inserted. A hydrogel-coated self-retaining catheter, size 12 FG, with 10 mL balloon was inserted aseptically by Chris Blake RN at 1330 hrs. Catheter drained 750 mL of clear urine. The catheter is to be left in overnight on free drainage, then removed in the morning—for trial of void. A catheter strap was applied to her upper thigh. Ms Stewart stated she felt more comfortable post catheter insertion. The function of the catheter, the removal procedure and trial of void process was explained to her. She was encouraged to increase her fluid intake.
	E Lewis (LEWIS), *Enrolled Nurse*

Summary

The urinary system is essential for homeostasis. It is the means by which the body rids itself of a variety of metabolic wastes and maintains fluid and electrolyte balance. The urinary system consists of the kidneys, the ureters, the urinary bladder and the urethra. The kidneys filter the blood to maintain its normal composition, volume and pH. In carrying out this function, the kidneys secrete urine.

Common disorders of the urinary system include urinary tract infection, urinary incontinence, benign prostatic hypertrophy, prostate cancer, chronic kidney disease, urinary retention and urinary calculi. All people admitted to hospital, residential or home care should be screened for urinary tract disorders.

Nursing assessment includes subjective data collection to gather information about the person's usual urinary pattern, the characteristics of the urine, changes in urinary tract function, the presence of pain and lower urinary tract symptoms, fluid intake, past medical history, health and lifestyle management, presence of other symptoms and environmental factors related to urinary function. Objective data collection includes vital signs, inspection of the urine, dipstick urinalysis and analysis of the fluid balance chart or voiding diary.

Common diagnostic tests that are used to assess urinary system function include mid-stream urine collection for microbiological culture and sensitivity, urine collection over a time period, blood tests, ultrasound and other imaging diagnostic studies, and cystoscopy.

There are many factors that can affect the person's normal voiding pattern, especially when hospitalised (e.g. lack of privacy, pain, voiding position and lack of familiarity with the environment). These factors need to be considered when developing a plan of care for a hospitalised person. Nursing interventions that promote normal voiding include stimulating the micturition reflex and promoting adequate fluid intake, normal bowel function and continence. Nursing interventions to treat urinary incontinence include voiding programs, use of continence aids and appliances, attention to environmental and personal factors and maintaining skin integrity.

Urinary tract dysfunction can have a significant impact on a person's quality of life. Some conditions are life-changing and in many cases the person may delay seeking assessment and treatment because of embarrassment. The attitude and approach of the nurse and other healthcare workers is important in helping people ask for and accept help. There is a need to approach care of the person with a urinary system dysfunction with compassion and sensitivity in order to maintain and promote the person's dignity and self-esteem.

Review Questions

1. Interpret the following results from a dipstick urinalysis:
   a. Urine sample clear and dark yellow, 300 mL voided
   b. pH 6.5, specific gravity 1025
   c. Glucose, bilirubin, ketones, protein, urobilinogen negative
   d. Blood—trace, leucocytes—small, nitrite—positive
2. Describe the likely signs and symptoms of a urinary tract infection in a 90-year-old man.
3. Identify nursing interventions that could promote normal voiding patterns in an individual who is hospitalised.
4. A 55-year-old woman complains of involuntary loss of urine when she sneezes, coughs and laughs. What is the most likely type of urinary incontinence she is experiencing?
   a. Urge urinary incontinence
   b. Mixed urinary incontinence
   c. Stress urinary incontinence
   d. Functional urinary incontinence

5. What are the important factors to take into account when choosing a continence aid or appliance?
6. Describe the nursing care for a person with an indwelling urinary catheter.
7. What education needs to be given to an individual to collect a mid-stream specimen of urine (MSU)?

Evolve® Answer guide for the Review Questions, Critical Thinking Exercises, Decision-making Framework Exercises and Critical Thinking Questions in Case Studies is hosted on Evolve: http://evolve.elsevier.com/AU/Koutoukidis/Tabbner.

References

Australian Commission on Safety and Quality in Health Care (ACSQHC), 2021. *National Safety and Quality Health Service Standards*, 2nd ed. ACSQHC, Sydney.

Australian Institute of Health and Welfare (AIHW), 2021. Cancer in Australia—web report. Cat. No: CAN 144. AIH W, Canberra. Available at: <https://www.aihw.gov.au/reports/cancer/cancer-in-australia-2021/summary>.

Australian Institute of Health and Welfare (AIHW), 2022. Australia's health 2022. Australia's health series no.18. AUS 240. AIHW, Canberra. Available at: <https://www.aihw.gov.au/reports/australias-health/australias-health-2022-data-insights/about>.

Australian Institute of Health and Welfare (AIHW), 2023. Chronic kidney disease: Australian facts. AIHW, Canberra. Available at: <https://www.aihw.gov.au/getmedia/c7a13869-0c7c-429e-bbda-70d4da6e2eed/Chronic-kidney-disease-Australian-facts.pdf.aspx?inline=true>.

Bradway, C., 2018. Caring for men with lower urinary tract symptoms and Parkinson's disease: Coping experiences of female spouses. *Urologic Nursing* 38(3), 113–120.

Brandt, C.L., 2022. Disorders of the lower urinary tract – pathophysiology. In Banasik, J., *Pathophysiology*, 7th ed, pp. 620–635. Elsevier, Missouri.

Burchum, J.R., Rosenthal, L.D., 2022. *Lehne's pharmacology for nursing care*, 11th ed. Elsevier, Missouri.

Cardozo, L., Rovner, E., Wein, A., Abrams, P. (eds.), 2023. *Incontinence*, 7th ed. ICI-ICS, International Continence Society, Bristol.

Chiba, T., Kikuchi, S., Omori, S., Seino, K., 2022. Chronic constipation and acute urinary retention. *European Journal of Gastroenterology & Hepatology* 34(1), e1–e3.

Childress, K., 2022. Acute kidney injury in chronic kidney disease. In: Banasik, J., *Pathophysiology*, 7th ed, pp. 603–619. Elsevier, Missouri.

Clinical Excellence Commission, 2021. Incontinence Associated Dermatitis (IAD) best practice principles. Available at: <https://www.cec.health.nsw.gov.au/__data/assets/pdf_file/0015/424401/Incontinence-Associated-Dermatitis-IAD-Best-Practice-Principles.pdf>.

Collis, D., Kennedy Behr, A., Kearney, L., 2019. The impact of bowel and bladder problems on children's quality of life and their parents: A scoping review. *Child: Care, Health and Development* 45(1), 1–14.

Continence Foundation of Australia, 2021. Bladder Diary with instructions. Continence Foundation of Australia. Available at: <https://www.continence.org.au/resource/bladder-diary-instructions?v=8452>.

Continence Foundation of Australia, 2023a. Continence in Australia: A snapshot. Continence Foundation of Australia, Melbourne. Available at: <https://continence.org.au/data/files/Reports/Continence_in_Australia_Snapshot.pdf>.

Continence Foundation of Australia, 2023b. Prevention. Available at: <https://www.continence.org.au/pages/prevention.html>.

Continence Foundation of Australia, 2023c. Pelvic floor. Available at: <www.continence.org.au/pages/pelvic-floor-women.html>.

Cooper, K., Gosnell, K., 2023. *Adult health nursing*, 9th ed. Elsevier, Missouri.

Crisp, J., Douglas, C., Rebeiro, G., et al. (eds.), 2021. *Potter and Perry's fundamentals of nursing*, 6th ed. Elsevier, Sydney.

Department of Health and Aged Care, 2022. National aged care mandatory quality indicator program (QI) program manual 3.0 – Part A. Commonwealth of Australia.

Fairchild, S.L., O'Shea, R.K., Washington, R.D., 2022. *Pierson and Fairchild's principles and techniques of patient care*, 7th ed. Elsevier, St Louis.

Gersch, C., 2021. Concepts of care for patients with urinary problems. In: Ignatavicius, D., Workman, L., Rebar, C., et al., *Medical-surgical nursing: Concepts for interprofessional collaborative care*, pp. 1325–1354. Elsevier, Missouri.

Grodesky, M., 2022. Male genital and reproductive function. In: Banasik, J., *Pathophysiology*, 7th ed, pp. 636–650. Elsevier, Missouri.

Gulanick, M., Myers, J.L., 2022. *Nursing care plans*, 10th ed. Elsevier, Missouri.

International Continence Society (ICS), 2023. ICS glossary. Available at: <https://www.ics.org/glossary>.

Hryciw, D., 2023. The structure and function of the urinary system. In: Craft, J.A., Gordon, C.J., Huether, S.E., et al., *Understanding pathophysiology* Australia and New Zealand edition, pp. 862–885. Elsevier, Chatswood.

Hogwarth, K., Smith, K., 2023. Alterations of the reproduction systems across the lifestyle. In: Craft, J.A., Gordon, C.J., Huether, S.E., et al., *Understanding pathophysiology* Australia and New Zealand edition, pp. 986–1032. Elsevier, Chatswood.

Javanmardifard, S., Gheibizadeah, M., Shirazi, F., et al., 2022. Experiences of urinary incontinence management in older women. A qualitative study. *Frontiers in Public Health* 9: 738202.

Jarvis, C., Eckhardt, A., 2021. *Jarvis's health assessment and physical examination*, 8th ed. Elsevier, Chatswood.

Jones, K., Steggal, M., 2020. Nursing patients with urinary disorders. In: Peate, I., *Alexander's nursing practice: Hospital and home*, pp 225–280. Elsevier.

Kidney Health Australia, 2020. Kidney stones. Available at: <https://kidney.org.au/your-kidneys/what-is-kidney-disease/types-of-kidney-disease/kidney-stones#:,:text=The%20development%20of%20kidney%20stones%20is%20one%20of,history%20of%20kidney%20stones%2C%20or%20if%20you%E2%80%99re%20elderly>.

Kirov. E., Needham, A., 2023. *Foundations of anatomy and physiology*. Elsevier, Chatswood.

Lough, M., 2022. Kidney disorders and therapeutic management – critical care nursing. In: Urden, L.D., Stacy, K.M., Lough, M., *Critical care nursing*, pp. 641–651. Elsevier, Missouri.

Markiewicz, A., Goldstine, J., Nichols, T., 2020. Emotional attributes, social connectivity and quality of life associated with intermittent catherisation. *International Journal of Urological Nursing* 14(10), 27–35.

McCance, K.L., Huether, S.E., 2023. *Pathophysiology: The biologic basis for disease in adults and children*, 9th ed. Elsevier, St Louis.

Nursing and Midwifery Board of Australia (NMBA), 2020. Decision-making framework for nursing and midwifery. Available at: <https://www.nursingmidwiferyboard.gov.au/Codes-Guidelines-Statements/Frameworks.aspx>.

Patton, V.E., 2021. Elimination – gerontological nursing. In: Vafeas, C., Slater, S., *Gerontological nursing*, pp. 137–154. Elsevier, Chatswood.

Patton, K.T., Bell, F., Thompson, T., Williamson, P., 2024. *The human body in health and disease*, 8th ed. Elsevier, Missouri.

Perry, A.G., Potter, P.A., Ostendorf, W., Laplaten, N., 2022. *Clinical nursing skills and techniques*. Elsevier, Missouri.

Potter, P., Perry, A.G., Stockert, P.A., et al., 2023. *Fundamentals of nursing*, 11th ed. Elsevier, Missouri.

Phillips, N., Hornacky, A. 2021. *Berry's & Kohn's operating technique*, 14th ed, pp. 712–741. Elsevier, Missouri.

Prostate Cancer Foundation of Australia (PCFA) and Cancer Council Australia (CCA), 2019. PSA Testing Guidelines Expert Advisory Panel. Clinical practice guidelines PSA Testing and Early Management of Test-Detected Prostate Cancer. Cancer Council Australia, Sydney. Available at: <https://wiki.cancer.org.au/australia/Guidelines:PSA_Testing>.

Rebeiro, G., Wilson, D., Fuller, S., 2021. *Potter & Perry's fundamentals of nursing workbook*, 4th ed. Elsevier, Chatswood.

Robertson, J., 2023. Men's reproductive health. In: McCuistion, L.K., DiMaggio, K.V., Windon, M.B., Yeager, J.J. *Pharmacology: A patient-centred nursing process approach*, 11th ed, pp. 713–721. Elsevier, Missouri.

Sim, J., Campbell, J., 2020. Skin integrity issues – wound care. In: Coleman, K. (ed.), *Wound care*, pp. 113–134. Elsevier, Australia.

The Royal College of Pathologists of Australasia, 2019. Manual. Available at: <https://www.rcpa.edu.au/Manuals/RCPA-Manual/Pathology-Tests/U/Urinalysis>.

Touhy, T.A., 2022. *Ebersole and Hess' gerontological nursing and healthy aging*, 6th ed. Elsevier, Missouri.

Turnball, T., Assessment: Urinary system. In: Harding, M., Kwong, J., Hagler, D., 2023, *Lewis's medical–surgical nursing*, 12th ed, pp. 1177–1194. Elsevier, Missouri. Available at: <https://doi.org/10.12968/bjcn.2019.24.1.32>.

Watt, E., 2021. Maintaining continence. In: Crisp, J., Douglas, C., Rebeiro, G., et al. (eds.), 2021. *Potter and Perry's fundamentals of nursing*, 6th ed, pp. 1043–1089. Elsevier, Sydney.

Williams-Taylor, S.P., 2022. Organ donation and transplantation. In: Urden, L.D., Stacy, K.M., Lough, M., *Critical care nursing*, pp. 889–932. Elsevier, Missouri.

Recommended Reading

Collins, L., 2019. Diagnosis and management of a urinary tract infection. *British Journal of Nursing* 28(2), 84–88.

Crisp, J., Douglas, C., Rebeiro, G., et al. (eds.), 2021. *Potter and Perry's fundamentals of nursing*, 6th ed. Elsevier, Sydney.

Harding, M., Kwong, J., Hagler, D., 2023, *Lewis's medical–surgical nursing*, 12th ed. Elsevier, Missouri.

Marieb, E., Keller, S., 2021. *Essentials of human anatomy & physiology*, 13th ed. Pearson Global, New York.

McCuistion, L.K., DiMaggio, K.V., Windon, M.B., Yeager, J.J., 2023. *Pharmacology: A patient-centred nursing process approach*, 11th ed. Elsevier, Missouri.

Newman, D.K., 2019. Prompted voiding for individuals with urinary incontinence. *Journal of Gerontological Nursing* 45(2), 14–26.

Serlin, D.C., Heidelbaugh, J.J., Stoffel, J.T., 2018. Urinary retention in adults: Evaluation and initial management. *American Family Physician* 98(8), 496–503.

Slade, S.C., Hay-Smith, J., Mastwyk, S., et al., 2018. Barriers and enablers to implementation of pelvic floor muscle training interventions for urinary incontinence. *Australian and New Zealand Continence Journal* 24(4), 11.

van Wissen, K., Blanchard, D., 2019. Preventing and treating incontinence-associated dermatitis in adults. *British Journal of Community Nursing* 24(1), 32–33. Available at: <https://doi.org/10.12968/bjcn.2019.24.1.32>.

Yates, A., 2019. Understanding incontinence in the older person in community settings. *British Journal of Community Nursing* 24(2), 72–76.

Online Resources

Continence Foundation of Australia.:<www.continence.org.au>.

Continence New Zealand: <www.continence.org.nz>.

Continence Support Now: <https://www.continencesupportnow.com>.

Healthy Male (Andrology Australia): <www.healthymale.org.au>.

Kidney Health Australia: <https://kidney.org.au>.

CHAPTER 32

Bowel health

Heather Wakefield

Key Terms

anal fissures
appendicitis
bowel obstruction
cholecystitis
coeliac disease
colon
colostomy
constipation
defecation
diarrhoea
diverticulitis
endoscopy
enema
enzyme
faeces
flatulence
gastritis
gastroenteritis
gastro-oesophageal reflux disease (GORD)
haemorrhoids
hepatitis
hernia
ileostomy
impaction
incontinence
inflammatory bowel disease (IBD)
irritable bowel syndrome (IBS)
parotitis
peristalsis
peritoneum
peritonitis
pilonidal sinus
polyp
prolapse
saliva
stoma
stomatitis
suppository
xerostomia

LEARNING OUTCOMES

At the completion of this chapter and with further reading, learners should be able to:

- Define the key terms relating to the digestive system.
- Describe the anatomical position and structure of the digestive system and accessory organs.
- Describe the physiological functions of the digestive system and accessory organs.
- Describe normal faeces and the defecation process.
- Identify the factors that affect bowel elimination.
- Identify appropriate nursing actions to assist the individual to meet their bowel elimination needs.
- Perform procedures described in this chapter accurately and safely, including the observation, collection and testing of faeces, assisting individuals with bowel elimination and changing ostomy devices.
- Briefly describe the pathophysiology, clinical manifestations and management of the specific disorders of the digestive system.
- Describe the diagnostic tests that may be performed to assess digestive system function.
- Outline nursing assessments specific to the digestive system.
- Employ critical thinking to provide care for individuals with alterations in bowel elimination.

CHAPTER FOCUS

Ingestion, digestion, absorption and elimination are the primary functions of the digestive system. Consumed food and fluids are broken down into nutrients and electrolytes that can be absorbed by the body for cell energy and function. Various factors that influence normal bowel elimination are explored in this chapter. Assessment of the individual's ability to eliminate faeces, together with observation of the faeces, provides the nurse with information about the individual's bowel elimination status. As a result, nursing care may be planned and implemented in conjunction with the individual and other healthcare providers, to meet bowel elimination needs in a dignified and appropriate manner.

LIVED EXPERIENCE

Besides trying to manage bouts of pain and diarrhoea, some days I cannot find the energy to get out of bed. My doctor said that fatigue is linked to my chronic inflammatory bowel disease. The doctor prescribed me a high energy diet, encouraged exercise as well as rest, and I'm starting to feel a little better.

Joanne, 70 years old, Retiree

INTRODUCTION

The digestive process enables consumed food and fluids to be broken down into nutrients and electrolytes that can be absorbed by the body for cell energy and function. This process is achieved through four basic activities: ingestion, digestion, absorption and elimination (Harding et al 2023). Any condition that causes a change in these activities can have a detrimental impact on a person's health and quality of life. Healthy bowel function is maintained by routine elimination habits, a nutritional diet with the recommended amount of fibre and fluid intake, and daily mild exercise to stimulate colonic motility. The various factors that can affect normal digestion and bowel elimination are explored in this chapter. Observation of the individual's ability to eliminate faeces, together with observation of the faeces, provides the nurse with an objective assessment of the individual's bowel elimination status.

The digestive process

The digestive system comprises the gastrointestinal (GI) or alimentary tract, the organs of the gastrointestinal tract, and the accessory organs of digestion that include salivary glands, the liver, pancreas and gallbladder (Berman et al 2021; Harding et al 2023). The GI tract is a muscular tube about 9–10 metres in length, which extends from the mouth to the anus (Figure 32.1). The structure of the GI tract is similar for most of its length and consists of four layers—an outer serosa covering, middle layers of involuntary muscle and connective tissue (submucosa), and an inner mucous membrane lining or mucosa (Harding et al 2023) (See Figure 32.2.)

The inner mucous membrane lining, which can be found in the mouth and the oesophagus, protects against wear and tear caused by food travelling through the oesophagus. This layer also secretes mucus into the digestive tract to lubricate the walls of the GI tract and protect against digestive enzyme damage (Waugh & Grant 2023).

The submucosa is composed of connective tissue, which contains many large blood and lymph vessels, and collagen and elastic fibres. It binds the mucosa to the muscle layer. The involuntary muscle layer pushes the contents of the GI

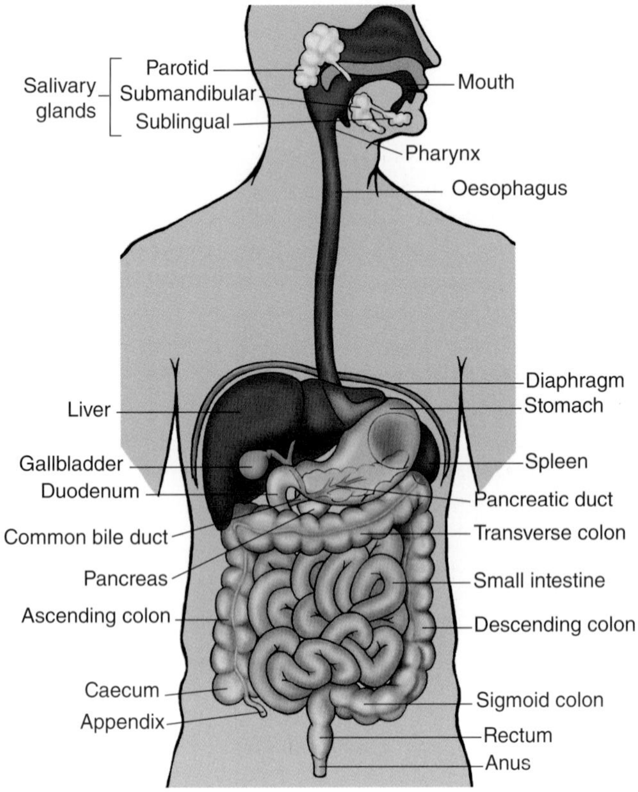

Figure 32.1 The gastrointestinal system

(Monahan & Neighbors 1998)

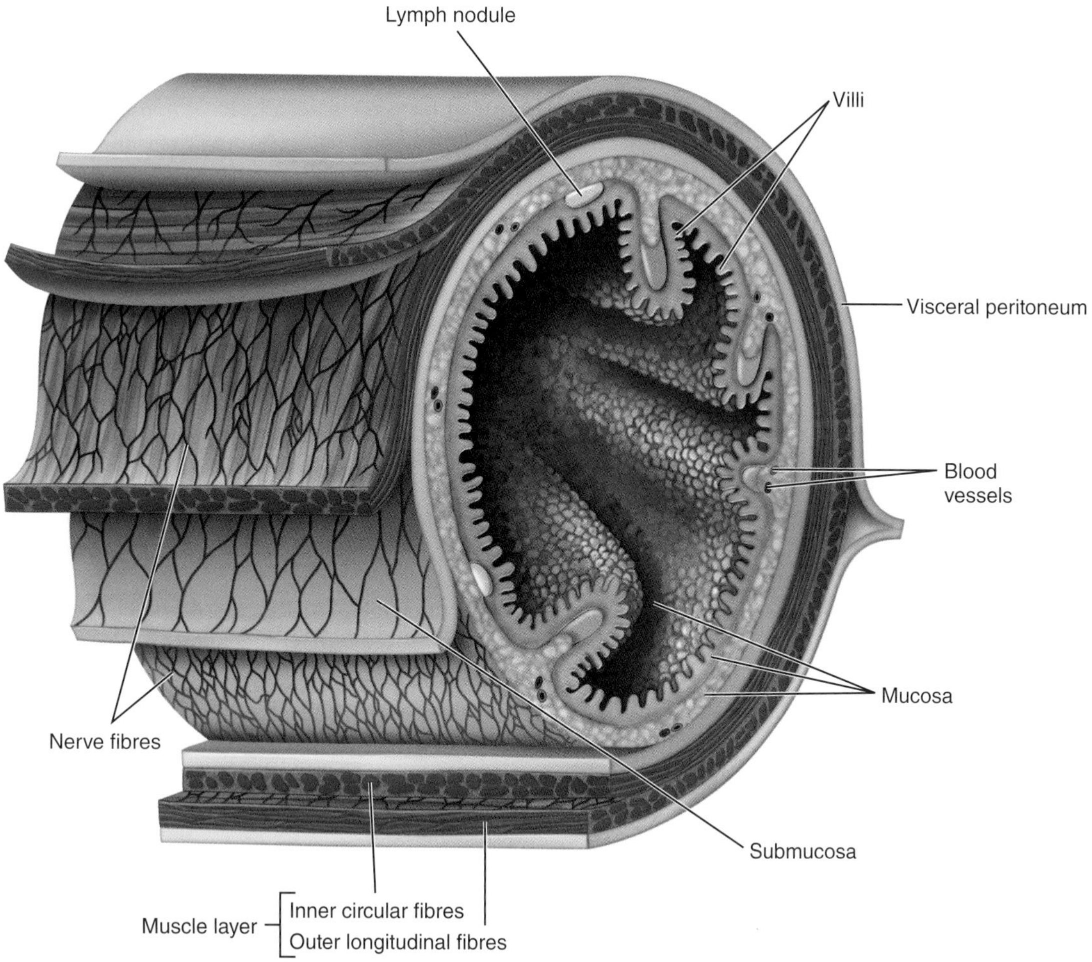

Figure 32.2 Cross-section through the wall of the GI tract

(Solomon 2016)

tract onwards by peristalsis, and helps mix food with digestive juices (Waugh & Grant 2023).

The outer covering of the GI tract consists of fibrous tissue (the serosa) or, in the abdomen, the peritoneum. The **peritoneum** is a double-layer serous membrane that secretes serous fluid to prevent friction between the layers. The parietal peritoneum lines the abdominal wall, and the visceral peritoneum covers the organs and abdominal and pelvic cavities. The mesentery, which is formed by the peritoneum, covers the intestines and attaches them to the posterior abdominal wall (Waugh & Grant 2023).

The organs that make up the GI tract are the mouth, the oropharynx, the oesophagus, the stomach, the small intestine and the large intestine.

The mouth

The process of ingestion usually begins in the mouth. Ingestion is the intake of food and is directed by appetite (Harding et al 2023). The mouth, or oral cavity, has boundaries of muscle and bone and is lined by mucous membrane. The lips surround the opening of the mouth, keep food in the mouth and contribute to speech (Harding et al 2023). The cheeks form the lateral walls, the hard palate forms its anterior roof and the soft palate forms its posterior roof. The mouth also contains the uvula, a curved fold of mucous-membrane-covered muscle, hanging down from the midline border of the soft palate (Waugh & Grant 2023).

Components of the mouth

The mouth contains the tongue, the teeth and the salivary glands. Once food is placed in the mouth, the teeth break down the food into smaller particles through chewing. The teeth are embedded in the maxillae and the mandible. All teeth have the same basic structural organisation but differ in shape and size. Each tooth is made up of an ivory-like substance called dentine; a central pulp cavity containing blood and lymphatic vessels, nerves and connective tissue; and a thin layer of enamel covering the crown. In children, there are 20 deciduous (milk) teeth, consisting of 10 in each jaw; in adults, there are 16 permanent teeth in each jaw. In each jaw, there are four incisors, used for biting; two canines, used for tearing; four premolars, used for crushing;

and six molars, used for grinding. A wisdom tooth is the third molar tooth and it is the last tooth to erupt. Wisdom teeth usually erupt from ages 18 to 25 years.

The salivary glands (an accessory digestive organ), of which there are three pairs, pour secretions into the mouth. **Saliva** is a watery fluid containing ions, mucin and the digestive enzyme salivary amylase. Salivation is largely initiated by sensory stimulation, including the presence of food in the mouth, and by taste and smell. Saliva has the following functions:

- moistens and softens food
- contains mucin, which acts as a lubricant to aid swallowing
- moistens the mouth
- has an antibacterial activity
- enables molecules to dissolve on the surface of the tongue and stimulate the tastebuds
- contains the enzyme salivary beta-amylase, which begins the chemical digestion of starch.

The salivary glands produce approximately 1 L of saliva per day (Patton et al 2022).

The tongue consists of a mass of voluntary muscle and is covered by squamous epithelium on its superior surface. On the upper surface of the tongue, there are many small projections called papillae, which contain tastebuds, the sensory endings of the nerve that perceives taste. The tastebuds also stimulate secretions from the stomach, pancreas and gallbladder in preparation for the digestion of food. The tongue is a very mobile organ, important in the chewing (mastication) of food, the formation of a bolus and swallowing the formed bolus of food, and is also essential for speech (Waugh & Grant 2023).

The pharynx

The next phase of digestion involves the movement of food. From the mouth, the food is moved into the pharynx. The pharynx is a muscular tube lined with mucous membrane that begins behind the nose and ends at the top of the oesophagus and trachea. The pharynx is divided into three sections: the oropharynx, the laryngopharynx and the nasopharynx (Waugh & Grant 2023).

The oropharynx is the muscular canal forming the passage between the oral cavity and the oesophagus. Food or liquid in the oropharynx stimulates receptors to initiate the swallow reflex. The laryngopharynx is a common passageway for both respiratory and digestive systems. The epiglottis prevents food from entering the respiratory tract and this ensures that food progresses through to the oesophagus (Harding et al 2023).

The oesophagus

The function of the oesophagus is to carry food to the stomach by means of peristaltic action.

Food continues its movement through the digestive system by moving from the pharynx to the oesophagus. The oesophagus is a muscular tube about 20–25 cm long and 2 cm in diameter, extending from the pharynx above to join the stomach below. It lies behind the trachea, is midline through the neck and thorax, and passes through the diaphragm to join the stomach. The oesophagus has an outer layer of fibrous tissue, a layer of involuntary muscle, a layer of connective tissue (submucosa) and an inner mucosa (Waugh & Grant 2023).

Peristalsis is a wave-like progression of alternate contraction and relaxation of the muscle fibres of the oesophagus or intestines, by which contents are propelled along the GI tract. The mucosa of the oesophagus secretes mucus, which acts as a lubricant and assists in the movement of food (Waugh & Grant 2023). At rest, the oesophagus is collapsed and the opening between the oesophagus and pharynx (upper oesophageal sphincter) is closed. Swallowing causes the upper oesophageal sphincter to relax and a peristaltic wave pushes the bolus of food to pass down into the oesophagus. A wave of contraction in the circular muscle layer then propels the bolus downwards to the stomach (Harding et al 2023). As the peristaltic wave approaches the lower oesophageal sphincter, the muscle relaxes and allows food to enter the stomach. The sphincter then closes again and prevents regurgitation of gastric contents back into the oesophagus. It remains closed except during swallowing, burping or vomiting, preventing reflux of gastric acid (Harding et al 2023).

The stomach

The stomach (Figure 32.3) is where the process of digestion begins. It is located in the upper left quadrant of the abdomen and is commonly described as being 'J-shaped'. The stomach is divided into three regions: the body, the fundus and the pylorus. The body of the stomach includes the lower oesophageal sphincter or entrance to the stomach. The fundus is the upper portion of the stomach, and the

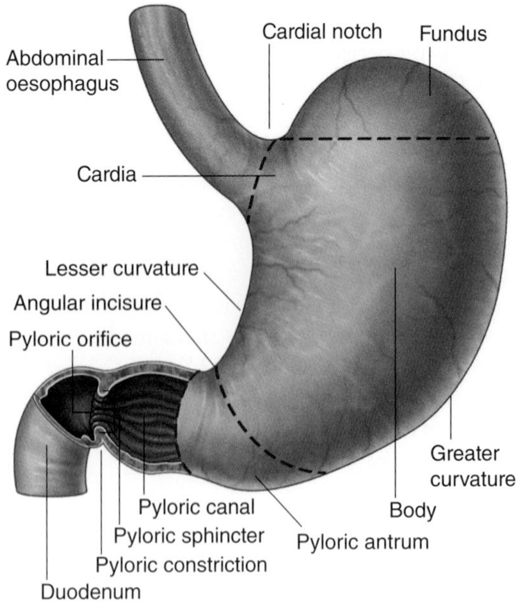

Figure 32.3 Anatomy of the stomach

(Odom-Forren 2024)

pylorus contains the pyloric sphincter, or exit of the stomach (Waugh & Grant 2023).

Stomach size varies according to the volume of food it contains. Food accumulates and remains in the stomach for some time after eating. Approximately 1 hour after a meal, gastric juice is secreted into the stomach. Contraction of the stomach muscles mixes the food with gastric juices and assists in breaking down the ingested food. The body produces an estimated 2 L of gastric secretions a day (Waugh & Grant 2023), which include:

- hydrochloric acid, which is released in response to the hormone gastrin, and activates pepsins, providing an optimal pH for pepsin activity, and destroys bacteria
- intrinsic factor, which is vital for the absorption of vitamin B12 from the diet, which is needed for the development of erythrocytes
- mucus, which is secreted by the surface cells of the stomach mucosa and forms a lining that protects the mucosal cells from the gastric contents
- gastric enzymes (pepsinogens), which are inactive until exposed to hydrochloric acid, when the active pepsins are released. Pepsins act as a catalyst in the chemical breakdown of protein, forming polypeptides and free amino acids.

Functions of the stomach include:

- temporary storage of the food bolus
- chemical digestion of protein
- mechanical churning and breakdown of the food into chyme (partially digested food)
- limited absorption of water, alcohol and some drugs
- non-specific antimicrobial defence
- mineral and vitamin preparation and absorption
- regulation of movement of gastric contents into the duodenum.

The rate at which the stomach empties depends on the type of food eaten. A carbohydrate meal is the quickest to leave the stomach, while a fatty meal is the slowest (Waugh & Grant 2023).

The small intestine

The process of digestion and absorption continues in the small intestine. The small intestine is a coiled muscular tube about 7 m in length, extending from the pyloric end of the stomach to the large intestine (Harding et al 2023). The small intestine is divided into the duodenum, the jejunum and the ileum. The ileocaecal valve is at the end of the small intestine and prevents reflux of the large intestine's contents back into the small intestine (Harding et al 2023). The surface area of the small intestine is greatly increased by circular folds of mucous membrane, which is covered by villi and microvilli. Nutrients, vitamins, mineral salts and water are absorbed from the small intestine into the blood capillaries surrounding the villi (Waugh & Grant 2023).

Functions of the small intestine are to:

- Move chyme onwards by peristalsis.
- Secrete intestinal juice to mix with pancreatic juice from the pancreas and bile from the liver.
- Complete chemical digestion of proteins, fats and carbohydrates.
- Protect against infection by lymph follicles.
- Secrete hormones.
- Absorb nutrients.

(Waugh & Grant 2023)

The large intestine

The large intestine, or **colon**, is a muscular tube about 1.5 m in length and 6 cm in diameter, which extends from the end of the ileum to the anus (Figure 32.4). It commences at the

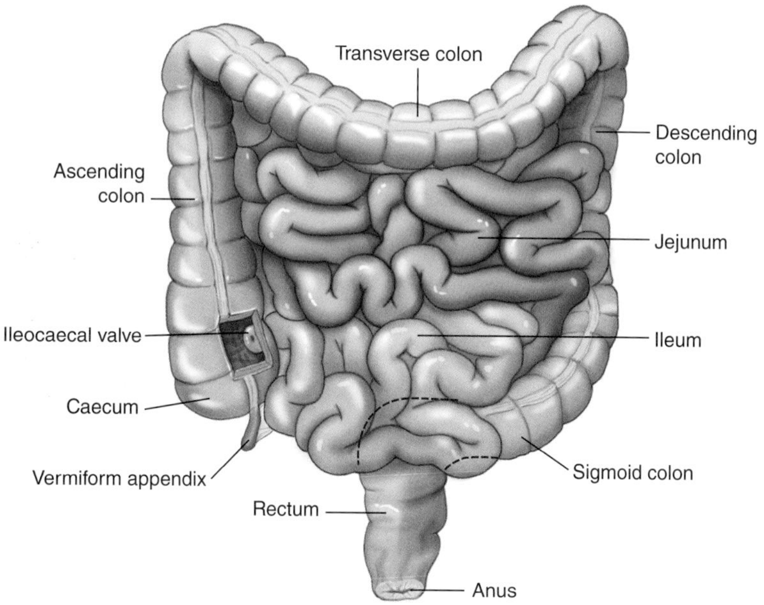

Figure 32.4 Small and large intestines

(Shiland 2022)

caecum and ends at the anus. It is divided into the caecum, ascending colon, transverse colon, descending colon, sigmoid colon and anus:

- The caecum contains the ileocaecal valve and appendix, and is approximately 8–9 cm long.
- The ascending colon passes up the right side of the abdominal cavity from the caecum to the liver.
- The transverse colon crosses the upper abdomen from right to left, to near the spleen.
- The descending colon passes down the left side of the abdominal cavity towards the midline.
- The sigmoid colon is 'S'-shaped and continues downward to become the rectum.
- The rectum joins the sigmoid colon and anal canal.
- The anal canal opens up to the exterior anus. Two sphincters, the involuntary internal and voluntary external, control the expulsion of faeces.

(Waugh & Grant 2023)

Functions of the large intestine include absorption of water (by osmosis), mineral salts, vitamins and some drugs into the capillaries. Another function is synthesis of vitamin K and folic acid by bacteria that exist in the colon. The colon produces flatus, moves faecal matter along its length by mass movement (gastrocolic reflex) and defecates the faecal matter through the anus. **Faeces** is made up of water, indigestible fibre, dead and live bacteria, shed epithelial cells, fatty acids and mucus secreted by the epithelial lining of the colon (Waugh & Grant 2023).

The accessory digestive organs

The accessory digestive organs are vital in the digestive process. Although food does not pass through these organs, digestion could not occur without them. The accessory organs secrete enzymes that are actively involved in the process of digestion into the GI tract. An **enzyme** is a substance, usually protein in nature, that initiates and accelerates a chemical reaction. The accessory organs are the salivary glands, pancreas, liver and biliary tract.

Salivary glands

Three main pairs of salivary glands release approximately 1000–1500 mL/day of saliva into the mouth when stimulated by the presence of food in the mouth, or even by the sight, smell or thought of food (Waugh & Grant 2023). Saliva lubricates the mouth, facilitates swallowing and begins a small amount of chemical digestion of food in the mouth (Urden et al 2021).

The pancreas

The pancreas is a long, slender gland lying across the abdominal cavity behind the stomach. It is divided into a head, which fits into the curve of the duodenum, and a body and a tail, which extend out to the spleen. The pancreatic duct extends along the length of the pancreas and joins the common bile duct from the liver to enter the duodenum (Figure 32.5) (Harding et al 2023).

The pancreas has both endocrine and exocrine functions. The exocrine function of the pancreas is to secrete enzymes crucial to protein, fat and carbohydrate digestion. Approximately 700 mL of pancreatic juice is secreted each day (Harding et al 2023).

The primary endocrine function of the pancreas is to secrete insulin and glucagon. Scattered among the exocrine tissue are groups of hormone-secreting cells, the islets of Langerhans, which contain four distinct cells, of which the beta cells are crucial to the production of insulin (Harding et al 2023).

The liver

The liver is the largest internal organ in the body; it is situated in the right upper quadrant of the abdominal cavity, immediately beneath the diaphragm (Patton et al 2022). Although the greater part of the liver lies in the right upper abdomen, the organ extends across to the left upper abdomen (Figure 32.5). The liver has four lobes: the anterior right and left lobes and, posteriorly, the caudate and quadrate lobes.

The liver has many functions but those involved in the digestive process include:

- Synthesis and secretion of bile. Approximately 500–1000 mL of bile is secreted by the liver daily. Bile emulsifies fats in the small intestine, aiding digestion. Bile salts make fatty acids and cholesterol more water soluble and aid fat-soluble vitamins to be absorbed.
- Carbohydrate metabolism and storage of glucose as glycogen.
- Protein metabolism for excretion in urine.
- Production of plasma proteins and clotting factors.
- Breakdown of red blood cells.
- Microbial defence.
- Inactivation of drugs and hormones.
- Production of heat.

(Harding et al 2023)

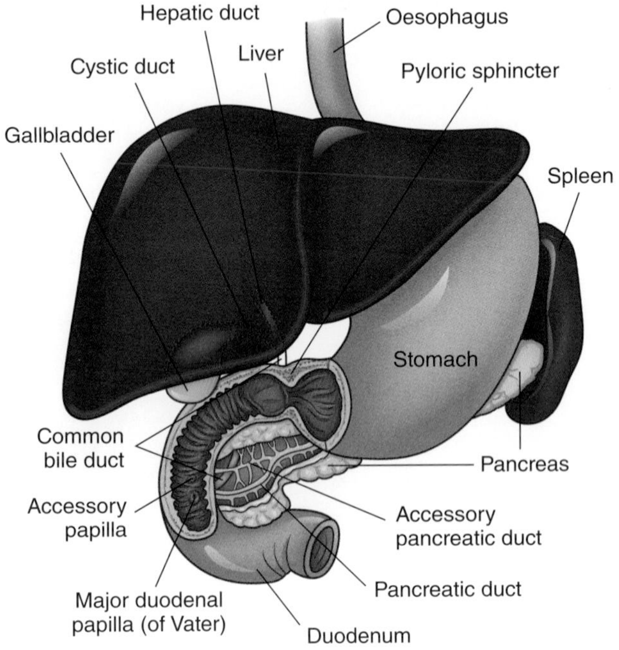

Figure 32.5 Gross structure of the liver, gallbladder, pancreas and duct system

(Rogers 2023)

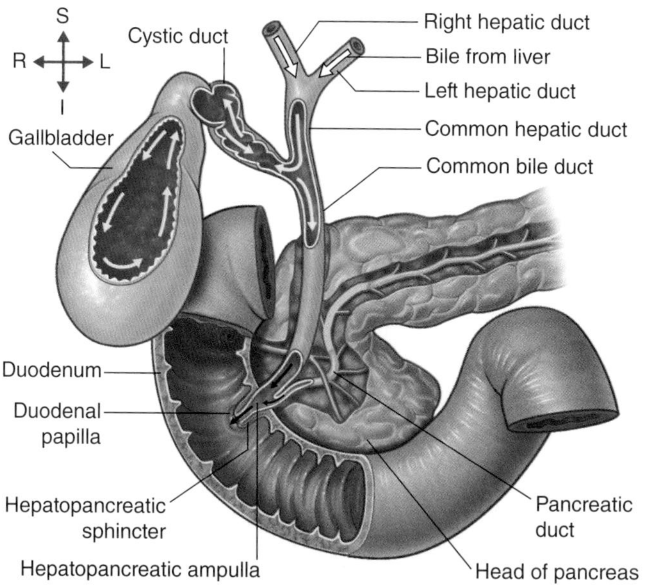

Figure 32.6 Direction of the flow of bile from the liver to the duodenum

(Waugh & Grant 2023)

The biliary tract connects the liver, gallbladder and duodenum, and consists of the left and right hepatic ducts, the common hepatic duct, the cystic duct, the gallbladder and the common bile duct (Figure 32.6) (Harding et al 2023).

The gallbladder

The gallbladder is a small, pear-shaped, muscular sac that is attached to the posterior of the liver. The main function of the gallbladder is to store and concentrate bile until it is needed for digestion. The presence of fat and acid in the duodenum stimulates contraction of the gallbladder and release of bile into the bile duct and duodenum (Waugh & Grant 2023).

Faecal matter and defecation

Frequency of defecation is individual to the person and depends on diet habits, fluid intake, activity level, drugs, disability, age and privacy. An individual may defecate two to three times a day, or two to three times a week. Normal stools are brown and semi-soft (Sorrentino & Remmert 2021).

Faeces collect in the sigmoid colon before entering the rectum. Most of the time the rectum is empty of faeces until a mass movement forces faeces into the rectum. As the faecal mass enters the rectum, the defecation reflex and the desire to defecate are initiated. If it is not convenient, **defecation** can be delayed temporarily, as within a few seconds the reflex contractions cease and the rectal walls relax (Berman et al 2021; Marieb & Keller 2022). An individual with healthy bowel function is able to voluntarily relax their external anal sphincter when the desire to defecate is felt and evacuate their rectum completely (Harding et al 2023). Optimal bowel function for adults means that the individual should be able to:

- Hold on for a short period of time, after feeling the first urge to defecate, so they can access a toilet and remove clothing without incident.
- Pass a stool within 60 seconds of sitting down on the toilet.
- Pass a stool without straining or pain.
- Completely empty the rectum when a stool is passed.

(Continence Foundation of Australia 2021)

Meeting elimination needs

A focused nursing assessment can establish an individual's elimination status. In addition to a systematic physical assessment, the following information regarding bowel elimination should be ascertained:

- Presenting signs and symptoms, especially if the individual perceives that their bowel function is abnormal (pain, blood, changes in frequency).
- Usual bowel elimination pattern including frequency, usual time of day and description of the stool.
- Usual diet since certain foods may change stool characteristics and frequency of elimination.
- Daily fluid intake. Recommended daily fluid intake is approximately 1.5–2 L/day. Inadequate fluid intake can cause hardening of the stool.
- Medication history. Some medications such as iron supplements, analgesics and diuretics may alter stool characteristics and defecation patterns. Excessive use of aperients may lead to an atonic bowel (sluggish or lacking in muscular tone).
- Activity and exercise patterns. Physical activity stimulates peristalsis, and lack of exercise is linked to constipation.
- Mobility and dexterity. Relates to the ability to access a toilet, undress, re-dress and perform hand hygiene. This also includes the ability to assume an optimal position for defecation (knees at or above hip height).
- Routines of bowel elimination including time of day, and triggers such as a hot drink, laxative or specific meal.
- Age. Infants have rapid peristalsis and lack of neuromuscular control. Older individuals' bowel function may be influenced by chronic disease, immobility and medication.
- Pain. Chronic diseases, haemorrhoids, anal fissures and surgical interventions may result in discomfort, and therefore the individual may ignore the 'call to stool' urge to avoid pain.
- Privacy or lack thereof due to shared bathroom facilities, limited mobility requiring the use of a bedpan or commode, or even the need to be assisted or supervised by nursing staff impact on privacy during defecation. This may lead to individuals ignoring the urge to defecate to avoid embarrassment.
- Pregnancy. Peristalsis slows in the third trimester.
- Psychological state. Emotional stress accelerates peristalsis, which may lead to diarrhoea and abdominal distension.

- Nosocomial infections. Can present as abdominal pain and diarrhoea.
- Surgery. Can lead to a period of reduced peristalsis.
- Anaesthetic agents may cause temporary stoppage of peristalsis.

(Crisp et al 2021)

Promoting a healthy bowel elimination program

A program to promote bowel elimination is an important part of the nursing care plan for an individual. The goal of a bowel management program is to establish regular bowel elimination, promote behaviour that maintains normal bowel function and avoid the use of aperients. This can be achieved by promoting privacy and increasing physical activity and high-fibre foods (12 g/day) and an adequate fluid intake of 1500–2000 mL/day. Care staff should also encourage toileting when the individual's urge to defecate is the strongest, and educate the individual to assume an optimal position to defecate, preferably on the toilet (Williams 2022). (See Clinical Interest Box 32.1.)

Diet

The role of diet is pivotal for a functioning digestive system and the individual's overall health. Dietary fibre and fluids enhance normal defecation; therefore, it is important that the individual includes adequate dietary fibre in their diet. Fibre adds bulk to the stool, softens it and stimulates bowel actions. While a high-fibre diet is indicated with constipation, a low-fibre diet is required in the presence of diarrhoea. Fluid liquefies intestinal contents, promoting ease of passage through the large intestine. Fluid intake of at least 2 L/day is recommended, but consider additional fluid during hot summer months and also take into consideration individuals with disease that may contraindicate fluid intake (Williams 2022).

CLINICAL INTEREST BOX 32.1 Nursing assessment relating to bowel problems

- Past history
- Vital signs, weight, height and BMI
- Assessment of stool, habits and frequency
- Hydration and nutrition status
- Mobility
- Hygiene
- Medications
- Coexisting medical conditions
- Psychosocial (including cultural influences) and environmental factors
- Cognitive function
- Continence status
- Skin integrity assessment

(Crisp et al 2021)

Individuals who are lactose intolerant are unable to digest lactose (dairy products) and present with signs and symptoms of diarrhoea, abdominal cramping and abdominal distension (Crisp et al 2021). If an individual requires modification of diet due to an allergy or intolerance, special effort must be made to ensure regular, healthy bowel function is maintained.

Monitoring elimination

Daily bowel charts recording bowel movements within a 24-hour period and analysis of a pattern over seven complete consecutive days, or one complete month, will demonstrate any changes. Bowel charts record the following: frequency of defecation per day, stool consistency as per the Bristol Stool Chart, volume passed, presence of incontinence, medications used to promote defecation, pain on defecation and urgency. Additional information to be collected includes food and fluid intake, physical activity levels, medications and any recent changes to lifestyle (Yates 2018). (See Clinical Interest Box 32.2.)

Examining faeces

To detect and identify abnormalities, faeces are examined by observation (see Table 32.1 and the Bristol Stool Chart in Figure 32.7), by chemical testing in the workplace or by analysis in the laboratory. Laboratory analysis of faeces provides information about the condition and functioning of the digestive system. Faeces is analysed for presence of leukocytes, erythrocytes, ova, parasites, bile and fat. Specimens for laboratory analysis need to be collected in a clean, dry container, uncontaminated by urine and delivered to the lab immediately (Linton & Matteson 2023).

Environment and positioning

Bowel evacuation is for most adults an intensely private function, preferably done away from people listening. Squatting is the optimal, normal position during defecation. Modern toilets are designed to replicate this position, allowing the individual to position their knees higher than their hips, lean forward, apply intraabdominal pressure and contract thigh muscles (Crisp et al 2021).

CLINICAL INTEREST BOX 32.2 Clinical consideration when assessing bowel patterns

Some individuals may be embarrassed when nurses ask them about their bowel functioning. Therefore, it is important to ensure that questioning is conducted in an appropriate way, place and time. Nurses should adapt their use of terminology to the individual they are dealing with. For example, the nurse may ask a child, 'Have you had a poo today?' instead of 'Have you used your bowels today?'

(Williams 2021)

TABLE 32.1 | Common characteristics of altered presentation of faeces

Colour	Odour	Presentation	What it may mean
Grey, 'clay-coloured'	Strong	Within normal range	Flow of bile blocked.
Dark/black	Strong	'Tarry', 'sticky'	Intestinal bleeding.
Dark/black	Slight	'Tarry'	Taking iron pills or other drugs.
Pale yellow	Strong	'Greasy'	Pancreatic malfunction.
Pale yellow	Slight to strong		Use of 'diet pills'.
Fresh blood	Slight	Within normal range	Haemorrhoids.
Red	Slight	Within normal range	Ingestion of foods (e.g. beetroot).
Green	Strong	Within normal range or loose	Rapid transit through the intestines.
Meconium	None	Viscous and sticky	Only evident in newborn babies; disappears in the first few days of life.
Mucus			Inconsistent or increasing amounts may indicate underlying disease (e.g. Crohn's disease, ulcerative colitis).
Undigested food			If occurs infrequently and with no other symptoms (e.g. diarrhoea), unlikely to be of concern.

(Berman et al 2021)

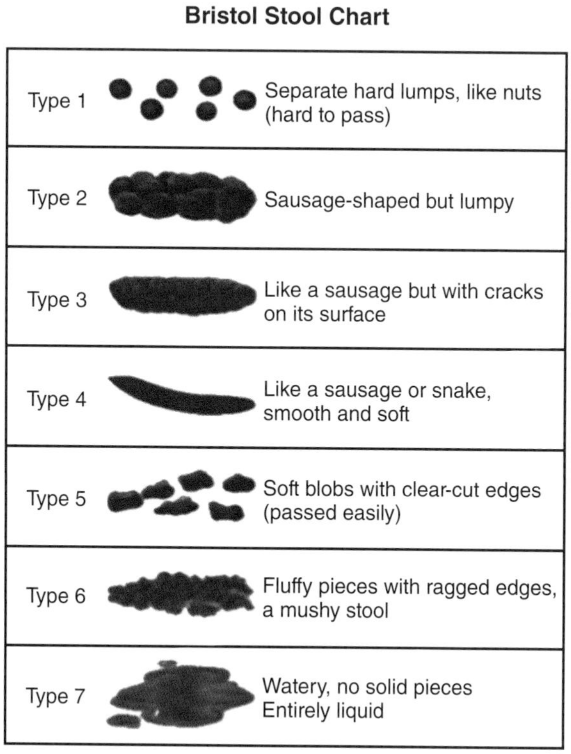
Bristol Stool Chart
Type 1
Separate hard lumps, like nuts (hard to pass)
Type 2
Sausage-shaped but lumpy
Type 3
Like a sausage but with cracks on its surface
Type 4
Like a sausage or snake, smooth and soft
Type 5
Soft blobs with clear-cut edges (passed easily)
Type 6
Fluffy pieces with ragged edges, a mushy stool
Type 7
Watery, no solid pieces Entirely liquid

Figure 32.7 Bristol Stool Chart

(Meiner & Yeager 2019)

The individual's sitting position on the toilet may need investigation to optimise a relaxed and natural posture to aid elimination. Privacy and time are also important to allow the individual to relax and empty their bowels completely.

Common problems associated with elimination of faeces

Constipation

Constipation is the infrequent passage of dry, hard stools, accompanied by straining and prolonged evacuation time, bloating and abdominal discomfort. Constipation affects women two to three times more than men, and is suggested to be experienced by 40% of adults older than 65 years (Touhy & Jett 2019).

The Rome III criteria for determining chronic functional constipation in adults states that an individual must have experienced two or more of the following for at least 12 weeks in the past year:

- straining with defecation 25% of the time
- lumpy or hard stools 25% of the time
- manual manoeuvres to promote emptying in greater than 25% of defecation efforts
- less than three bowel movements per week.

(Touhy & Jett 2019)

Primary constipation is intrinsically related to colonic (transit) or anorectal (outlet) dysfunction. Secondary constipation reflects chronic illness, poor toileting habits, diet and fluid intake, medications, physical inactivity and voluntary suppression of defecation (Crisp et al 2021).

Natural measures to prevent constipation include:

- Sufficient dietary fibre: Foods such as wholegrains, fruit and vegetables, and lean meats, which trap water in the stool and provide bulk. This in turn stimulates the normal defecation reflex.
- Adequate fluid input: At least 1500 mL/day is necessary to prevent excessive fluid reabsorption from the stool making it harder, drier and more difficult to pass.
- Acknowledging and responding to the urge to defecate as soon as possible.
- Maintaining a regular time for bowel movement; establishing a routine.
- Maintaining daily exercise to stimulate peristalsis.
- Assuming an upright, seated or squatting position for defecation.
- Avoiding undue anxiety about bowel habits and accepting the 'normal' pattern for defecation. Privacy reduces embarrassment.

(Williams 2022)

Other measures to assist elimination from the bowel may be necessary, including:

- Laxatives: Substances taken orally that promote evacuation of the bowel by increasing bulk, increasing moisture content of the stool, retaining water in the colon, and stimulating peristalsis (see Table 32.2).
- Suppositories: Small, cone-shaped, solid medications inserted into the rectum to promote the evacuation of faeces.
- Enemas: The introduction of fluid through the anus into the rectum to promote the evacuation of faeces and relieve constipation, faecal impaction and flatulence, or cleanse the bowel of faeces before diagnostic procedures or certain surgeries.

(Scott et al 2018).

Consequences of constipation include adverse health effects such as haemorrhoids and faecal impaction, impaired quality of life, distress, pain and increased healthcare costs (Touhy & Jett 2019). (See Case Study 32.1.)

Suppositories

Suppositories may be ordered and inserted into the rectum to promote the evacuation of faeces or to facilitate rectal administration of a drug. (See Chapter 20.)

TABLE 32.2 | Laxatives in common use

Category	Example	Action	Route	Time frame
Bulking agents	Psyllium (e.g. Metamucil) Ispaghula (e.g. Fybogel)	Increase weight and water-absorbent properties of the faeces, which stimulate peristalsis.	Oral	12–24 hours
Stimulant laxatives	Bisacodyl (e.g. Dulcolax)	Increases water and electrolyte content in colon, causing increased peristalsis.	Oral	6–12 hours
	Glycerol suppositories	Increase water and electrolyte content in colon, causing increased peristalsis.	Rectal	15–30 minutes
Faecal softeners	Liquid paraffin (e.g. Agarol) Docusate sodium (e.g. Coloxyl) Sodium picosulfate (e.g. Picolax)	Oil softens the faeces by decreasing surface tension.	Oral	24–72 hours
Osmotic agents	Colon electrolyte lavage (e.g. ColonLYTELY)	Induces diarrhoea.	Oral	3–4 hours
	Magnesium salts (e.g. Epsom salts)	Increase the water content of faeces, increasing bulk and stimulating peristalsis.	Oral	1–2 hours
	Lactulose (e.g. Duphalac)	A bulk forming and irritant laxative.	Oral	4–72 hours
	Microlax enema	Inserted rectally to draw water into the rectum to increase stool bulk and stimulate peristalsis.	Rectal	30 mins

(Tiziani 2021)

CASE STUDY 32.1

Margot, 83 years old, is admitted with abdominal pain associated with severe constipation. While you are interviewing Margot, she states that she has managed her constipation in the past with laxatives and that because of stress incontinence she restricts her fluid intake. Additionally, Margot is awaiting a hip replacement and has not been as physically active recently.

1. What do you think may be contributing to Margot's constipation?
2. What key changes can you suggest to Margot to maintain a regular bowel elimination program?

Suppositories prescribed to promote a bowel action are composed of various substances, such as glycerine. Evacuant suppositories act by softening and lubricating the faeces to facilitate easy passage and excretion, or by increasing peristalsis through the irritation of intestinal sensory nerve endings. The nurse must be aware of the different types of suppositories available and work within the scope of practice regarding the checking and administration of drugs. Types of medications that may be administered rectally by suppository include those used to relieve constipation, and medications used for the treatment of nausea and pain. (See Figure 32.8.)

Enemas

To give an **enema** is to introduce a solution into the rectum and sigmoid colon (see Clinical Skill 20.3 in Chapter 20). Most commonly, it is ordered and administered to promote the evacuation of faeces and alleviate constipation, to prepare a bowel for diagnostic procedures or surgery or to begin a bowel training program.

Impaction

Impaction is the prolonged retention and build-up of hardened faeces in the rectum, which prevents the individual from defecating. Signs and symptoms of faecal impaction include abdominal discomfort, nausea, rectal pain, poor appetite and confusion (in older individuals). Liquid faeces may pass around the faecal mass in the rectum and overflow from the anus (Scott et al 2018). Debilitated, confused older individual, unconscious individual, or individual with intellectual disabilities are most at risk of faecal impaction (Crisp et al 2021).

Treating impacted faeces

When the condition occurs, it is a result of prolonged constipation, poor bowel habits, inactivity, dehydration, use of constipation-inducing drugs or incomplete bowel cleansing after a barium swallow or enema. If measures to promote a bowel action, such as a suppository or enema, are ineffectual, surgical removal of the mass may be prescribed. If medically approved, encourage fluids and exercise once evacuation is complete and the individual is rested (Berman et al 2021; Crisp et al 2021).

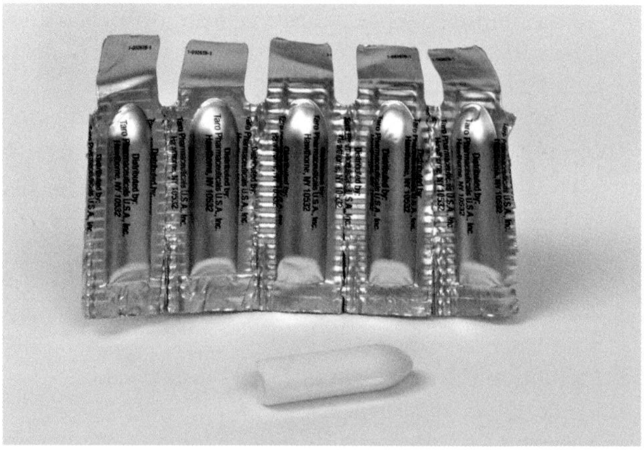

Figure 32.8 Examples of suppositories

(Davis & Guerra 2022)

Flatulence

Excessive formation of gas in the intestines is called **flatulence**. If the gas is not expelled, the intestines become distended and the person may experience abdominal fullness, pain and cramping. Flatus is the term used for gas in the intestine that is expelled through the anus. Flatulence may result from swallowed air, the consumption of gas-forming food or liquid, bacterial action within the intestines, irritable bowel syndrome, anxiety disorders and food poisoning (Crisp et al 2021; Ferri 2023).

Diarrhoea

Diarrhoea is defined as greater than three loose, watery stools per day. Diarrhoea may be accompanied by bloating, flatulence and abdominal pain, and may be classified as acute or chronic. Diarrhoea is a symptom of various conditions, including:

- irritation or inflammation of the gastrointestinal tract (e.g. due to pathogenic infection, highly spiced foods or medications that increase intestinal motility)
- intestinal malabsorption disorders
- disorders that increase secretion and function of bile or pancreatic juice, such as in obstructive jaundice
- increased intestinal motility associated with inflammatory bowel disease
- side effects of medications such as antibiotics
- radiation therapy
- enteral feeds
- emotional states such as anxiety or stress.

(Gulanick & Myers 2022)

Diarrhoea should be assessed in terms of the frequency of defecation and the characteristics of the faeces. The cause of diarrhoea must be investigated and treated. Key aspects related to the care of an individual with diarrhoea include:

- Stool culture to test for infectious cause.
- Reducing intestinal peristalsis: Dietary management of an adult individual involves the withholding of food until the diarrhoea diminishes, then the gradual reintroduction of bland (low-fibre) foods.

- Administering any prescribed medications such as antidiarrhoeal medications, antispasmodic preparations to reduce abdominal cramps and pains, and antimicrobial therapy if infectious causes are diagnosed (Gulanick & Myers 2022).
- Oral rehydration therapy to replace lost fluids and to prevent dehydration; 1500–2000 mL per day plus 200 mL per loose stool in adults is recommended unless contraindicated. Input and output should be observed and documented as part of the individual's fluid balance assessment.
- Probiotics to re-establish intestinal flora balance (Anderson et al 2023).
- Ensuring that the individual has adequate privacy whenever toilet facilities are being used, and that used toilet utensils are removed from the room immediately.
- Ensuring that the individual's hygiene needs are met. After each bowel action the anal area and buttocks should be cleansed with a mild soap and thoroughly dried. A protective barrier cream may be applied to reduce discomfort, and the area should be observed for signs of excoriation.
- Hand hygiene of the individual and carer must be implemented to prevent cross-infection.
- When using a bedpan or commode chair, the individual may be embarrassed by the odours associated with diarrhoea, so measures to eliminate odours should be taken. Any soiled linen should be changed and removed from the room immediately. The room should be well ventilated, and room deodorants may be used with discretion.
- A private room and isolation precautions should be considered until diagnosis of the cause (e.g. pathogenic infection) to prevent cross-infection (Gulanick & Myers 2022). (See Nursing Care Plan 32.1.)

CRITICAL THINKING EXERCISE 32.1

Jason, aged 22, is admitted to your unit with dehydration and diarrhoea after returning from a backpacking holiday around Indonesia. Jason says the diarrhoea started 2 weeks prior. What are the nursing implications of this? Describe appropriate nursing interventions for Jason.

CRITICAL THINKING EXERCISE 32.2

It is the middle of a hot summer. Ernest, an older adult who lives alone, is admitted with a history of 3 days of diarrhoea. What are the possible causes of diarrhoea? What is your primary concern for this individual? What key information should be charted regarding the bowel actions?

Faecal incontinence

Faecal **incontinence** is the inability to control the excretion of faeces and flatus through the anus (Sorrentino & Remmert 2021). Risk factors for faecal incontinence include increasing age, poor physical or mental health, some medications, anorectal procedures, diarrhoea and faecal impaction. Other contributing factors are chronic illness, nervous system disorders and injuries, intestinal disease, decreased mobility, difficulty removing clothing, finding a bathroom in time and vaginal childbirth. Management includes continence products, bowel training, toileting regimens and assistance, skin care, pelvic floor training and drug therapy. Specific interventions are to increase fluid intake to 3 L/day unless contraindicated, and to encourage ingestion of food that is naturally stool bulking, such as bananas and rice (Gulanick & Myers 2022).

NURSING CARE PLAN 32.1

Assessment: Individual experiencing diarrhoea.
Issue/s to be addressed: Risk of perineal skin excoriation.
Goal/s: Perineal skin will show no signs of redness or excoriation.

Care/actions	Rationale
Ensure skin is cleaned and patted dry after each episode of diarrhoea. Use barrier cream on sacral area. Stay hydrated (at least 2 L fluid per day unless contraindicated). Modify diet to bland foods. Skin should be checked regularly for signs of irritation and excoriation.	Reduces risk of skin irritation and excoriation. Acts as a protective barrier for skin. Reduces risk of dehydration related to additional fluid loss in watery stools. Bland foods are less likely to irritate gastric mucosa/stimulate diarrhoea episodes.

Evaluation: Skin integrity intact, nil signs excoriation.

Artificial openings into the intestine

An intestinal **stoma** is when the small or large intestine is surgically opened and brought through, and secured to the surface of the abdomen. Instead of faeces discharging from the anus, faecal elimination occurs through the stoma, which may be created as a temporary or a permanent measure. Indications for bowel diversion surgery include to divert faecal matter away from an obstruction or surgical anastomosis, or to provide an outlet for faeces in the absence of a functioning rectum (Gulanick & Myers 2022).

There are two different types of stomas that can be created: a colostomy and an ileostomy. A **colostomy** is created when a loop or end of the large bowel or colon is diverted through a surgical incision made in the abdominal wall. The faecal matter produced from this type of stoma is soft but formed and the colostomy may function approximately one to three times a day. An **ileostomy** is fashioned from a loop or end of part of the ileum, that is redirected through the abdominal wall. An ileostomy produces a more liquid stool and may produce 800–1000 mL of output per day (Thomas et al 2021).

Care of individual with a stoma

A stoma may be created in order to be used permanently or temporarily. A temporary stoma may be created to divert faecal contents to allow the bowel to rest (e.g. as part of the treatment regimen in an inflammatory bowel disease). A permanent stoma is indicated principally when a partial or total colectomy has been performed. The site is selected according to which part of the bowel is affected and with consideration to the individual's physique, belt line, manual dexterity and any other factors that may influence the individual's ability to successfully manage the care of the stoma (Harding et al 2023).

In many healthcare institutions, a stoma therapist liaises with the individual and surgeon to select the most appropriate site and commence education about the procedure and care afterwards. The type of the stoma—ileostomy or colostomy (Figure 32.9)—will determine the consistency of the faecal matter excreted through it. The closer the stoma is to the small intestine, the more liquid the faeces will be. Figure 32.10 illustrates the types of colostomy that may be created. An ileostomy will produce approximately

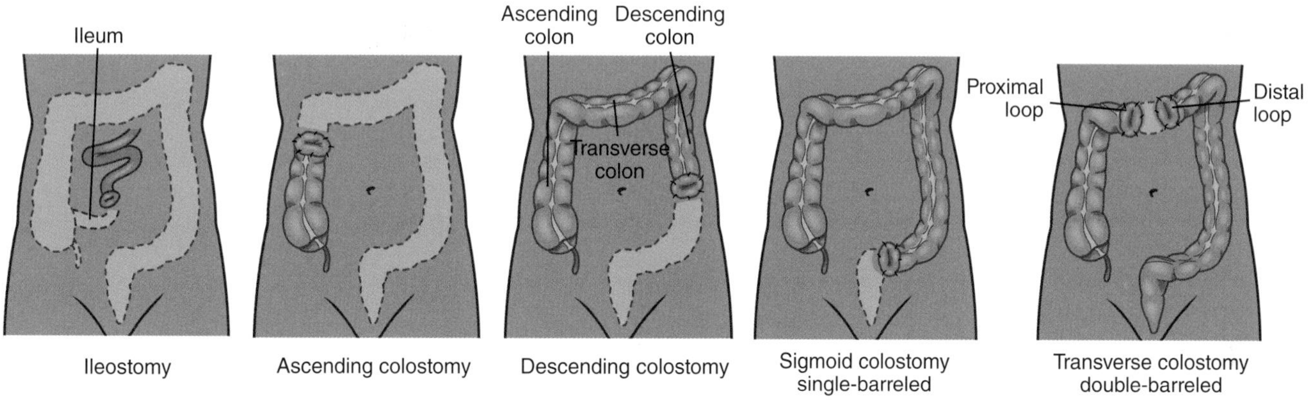

Figure 32.9 Types of ostomies

(Harding et al 2023)

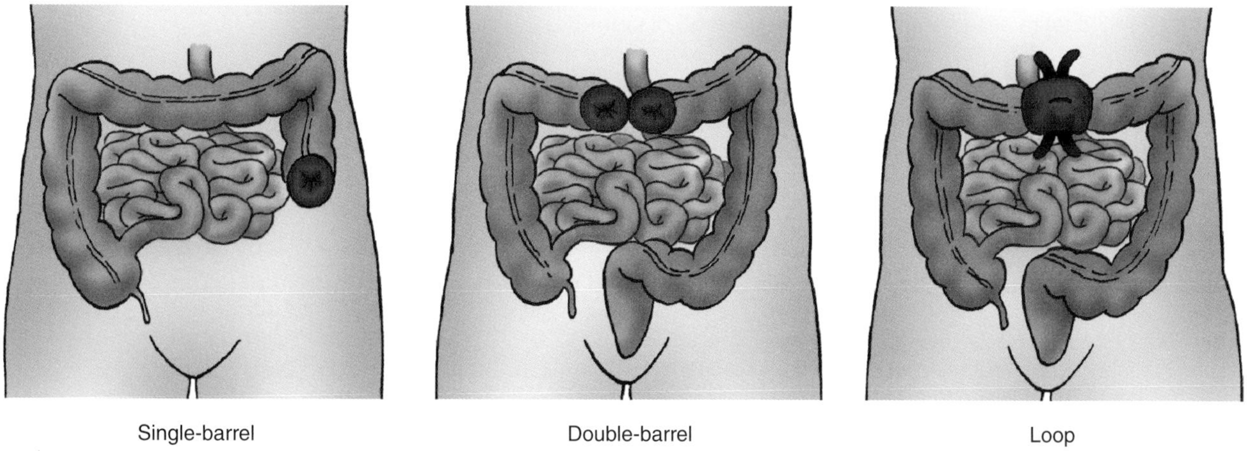

Figure 32.10 Types of colostomies

(Linton & Matteson 2023)

800–1000 mL of faecal matter daily, requiring the stoma appliance to be emptied three to four times a day. The colostomy should be active daily with multiple episodes of flatus being noted (Thomas et al 2021). The stoma appliance will require changing depending on the type used and frequency and volume of bowel actions. (See Clinical Skill 32.1.)

Care of the individual with a stoma includes the selection and management of appliances (Figure 32.11), care of the stoma and surrounding skin, meeting nutritional needs, discussing foods to avoid or take care with, and providing psychological support. A stomal therapist may be available to assist in the preparation of the individual and

CLINICAL SKILL 32.1 Changing an ostomy appliance

Please adhere to the policy and procedures of the facility/organisation prior to undertaking the skill. Ensure this skill is in your scope of practice.

NMBA Decision-making Framework considerations (refer to NMBA Decision-making framework for nursing and midwifery 2020):	**Equipment:**
1. Am I educated? 2. Am I authorised? 3. Am I competent? If you answer ‘no’ to any of these, do not perform that activity. Seek guidance and support from your teacher/a nurse team leader/clinical facilitator/educator.	One piece, adhesive, clear drainable colostomy/ileostomy appliance in correct size Pouch closure device Adhesive remover Disposable gloves Deodorant if indicated Gauze pads or washcloth Towel or disposable waterproof pad Basin with warm water Scissors Skin barrier paste Skin barrier wipes

PREPARE FOR THE SKILL

(Please refer to the Standard Steps on pp. xviii–xx for related rationales.)
Mentally review the steps of the skill.
Discuss the skill with your instructor/supervisor/team leader, if required.
Confirm correct facility/organisation policy/safe operating procedures.
Validate the order in the individual’s record.
Identify indication and rationale for performing the activity.
Assess for any contraindications.
Locate and gather equipment.
Perform hand hygiene.
Ensure therapeutic interaction.
Identify the individual using three individual identifiers.
Gain the individual’s consent.
Assess for pain relief.
Prepare the environment.
Provide and maintain privacy.
Assist the individual to assume an appropriate position of comfort.

Skill activity	**Rationale**
Review care plan and current treatment orders to determine type, size of device and length of time in place.	Provides information about individual’s treatment, equipment/supplies needed. To minimise skin irritation, avoid unnecessary changing of entire system.

PERFORM THE SKILL

(Please refer to the Standard Steps on pp. xviii–xx for related rationales.)
Perform hand hygiene.
Apply PPE: gloves, eyewear, mask and gown as appropriate.
Ensure the individual’s safety and comfort throughout skill.
Promote independence and involvement of the individual if possible and/or appropriate.
Assess the individual’s tolerance to the skill throughout.
Dispose of used supplies, equipment, waste and sharps appropriately.

CLINICAL SKILL 32.1 Changing an ostomy appliance—cont'd

Remove PPE and discard or store appropriately.
Perform hand hygiene.

Skill activity	Rationale
Place towel or disposable waterproof pad under the person. Remove the old appliance gently and place it in a plastic bag.	Promotes comfort. Avoids damage to surrounding skin surface.
Wipe the stoma and surrounding skin, using gauze pads or washcloth and warm water. Pat dry.	Cleanses the skin of mucus and faecal drainage.
Inspect the stoma and surrounding skin. The stoma should be pink or red, and free from excoriation.	Deviations from normal must be reported immediately so that appropriate action can be planned.
Apply the skin barrier wipe to the surrounding skin.	Protects the skin from excoriation when applying and removing appliance.
Remove the adhesive backing and place the new appliance over the stoma. Ensure that it is secured firmly in position with no gaps exposing the skin around the base of the stoma, and that the stoma is not being 'choked'.	Prevents leakage of faeces.
Ensure opening of the appliance is distal to the stoma.	To facilitate drainage.

AFTER THE SKILL

(Please refer to the Standard Steps on pp. xviii–xx for related rationales.)
Communicate outcome to the individual, any ongoing care and to report any complications.
Restore the environment.
Report, record and document assessment findings, details of the skill performed and the individual's response.
Report, record and document any abnormalities and/or inability to perform the skill.
Reassess the individual to ensure there are no adverse effects/events from the skill.

(Australian Council of Stoma Associations Inc. 2021; Rebeiro et al 2021; Tollefson et al 2022)

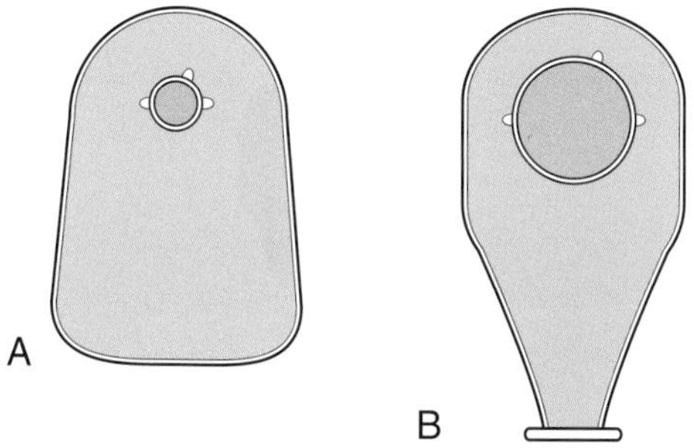

Figure 32.11 Ostomy appliances

A: Non-drainable stoma bag, **B:** Drainable stoma bag

their significant others before the operation and also plays a major role in providing support and education after the operation. Dietary changes may be necessary and are made in partnership with the individual, stomal therapy nurse and dietitian. If an individual has a colostomy, 1500–2000 mL of fluid and a high-fibre diet is recommended to promote regular bowel movements. To reduce the frequency and volume of bowel movements in the individual with an ileostomy, it is recommended that refined cereals are consumed, and fibre-rich food reintroduced slowly. Again, fluid intake must be encouraged to avoid dehydration from water loss in the liquid stools (Altomare & Rotelli 2019).

An individual's response to their stoma may be positive or negative. The formation of a stoma may affect an individual's social, professional, family and emotional life, self-esteem and identity. Education and support are key to empowering the individual to learn and care for themselves; however, they may not be capable of this in the short or long term due to a variety of reasons such as feelings of disgust, denial or disability. The stomal therapist may need to refer the individual, their caregiver or intimate partner to professional help to overcome changes associated with interpersonal or intimate relationships.

As part of the discharge process, the stomal therapist needs to refer the individual to a local ostomy association for not only stoma supplies, but support groups and stomal care specialists. Additionally, the stomal therapist needs to consider if the individual requires home-care services (Lataillade & Chabal 2021).

For the latest information and research findings on this subject, see the Australian Council of Stoma Associations website (www.australianstoma.com.au).

CASE STUDY 32.2

Michael Kramer, a 71-year-old gentleman, has been admitted to your ward for revision of his Parkinson's medication. Michael has a colostomy that was formed 2 years ago. Michael is quite self-caring of the colostomy; however, when you observe him change the appliance, you notice that the surrounding skin is very excoriated and in fact the appliance was not sticking to the skin in places. When questioned, Michael admits that it has been like that for a while.

1. What factors may contribute to excoriated peristomal skin?
2. Outline nursing interventions that may promote skin healing.
3. Discuss any education you will give Michael regarding his stoma and care.

See Progress Note 32.1 for documenting the changing of a colostomy appliance. (See Case Study 32.2.)

DISORDERS OF THE DIGESTIVE SYSTEM

Specific disorders

Any changes to the nutritional status of the individual will impact on their elimination process and may be ongoing, depending on the nature of the disease process. There are many and varied disorders of the alimentary tract but the following are some of the disorders commonly encountered in practice.

Stomatitis

Stomatitis is inflammation of the oral mucosa, including the cheek, lips, tongue, gingiva, palate and floor of the mouth (Hockenberry et al 2022). It may be a primary condition or a symptom of another disease. Stomatitis is characterised by pain, bleeding, swelling, ulceration and halitosis. It may be infectious or non-infectious and caused by local factors, such as biting the cheek, or systemic factors, such as herpes simplex virus. Management of stomatitis includes pain relief, mouth care, maintaining adequate hydration and modifying diet and fluids to bland while the mouth is painful (Hockenberry et al 2022).

Parotitis

Parotitis is inflammation of the parotid gland, presenting as localised pain, oedema, fever, chills, anorexia and malaise. Parotitis may be caused by decreased salivary flow associated with medication use, chronic illness, immunocompromised host, poor oral hygiene, salivary duct obstruction, recent surgery, radiotherapy and hypovolaemia. Infectious parotitis (mumps) is an acute viral disease, but bacteria, fungi or mycobacterial invasion may also cause parotitis (Buttaro et al 2020).

Management of parotitis may include antibiotic therapy, fluid and electrolyte replacement, oral hygiene, analgesia and medication to stimulate saliva flow (Buttaro et al 2020).

Xerostomia

Xerostomia (dry mouth) is a result of salivary gland hypofunction. Primary causes of xerostomia are due to a direct effect on salivary glands and include autoimmune conditions, viral infections and endocrine disorders such as diabetes mellitus. Secondary 'indirect' causes of xerostomia include radiotherapy, chemotherapy, medications, alcohol and tobacco abuse. Xerostomia can present as mouth pain; gum, tongue and mucosal irritations and lesions; mouth infections; taste changes; bad breath; and dental cavities (Buttaro et al 2020). Treatment of xerostomia begins with correcting the cause, if possible, frequent water consumption, oral lubricants, saliva substitutes, salivary stimulants and oral hygiene (Saxena et al 2019).

Gastro-oesophageal reflux disease

Gastro-oesophageal reflux disease (GORD) is a disorder of regurgitation of gastric contents back into the oesophagus, with or without mucosal damage. GORD may be caused by oesophagogastric motility defects, lower oesophageal sphincter impairment, delayed gastric emptying or a hiatal hernia (Buttaro et al 2020). (See Figure 32.12.) Symptoms include persistent heartburn and acid regurgitation, hypersalivation, nausea and vomiting, chronic cough, a hoarse voice and chest pain (Cooper & Urso 2018). Changes to diet and lifestyle, such as decreased alcohol consumption,

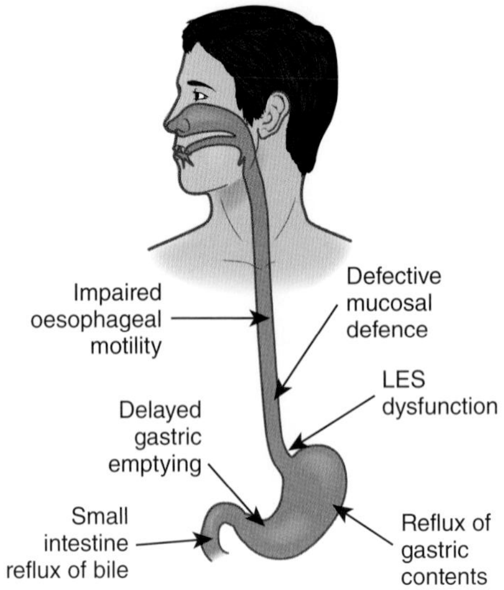

Figure 32.12 Factors involved in the pathogenesis of gastrointestinal reflux disease

Lower oesophageal sphincter

(Harding et al 2023)

decreased dietary fat, decreased meal size and weight loss, may aid the individual. Certain prescription medications, including antacids and proton pump inhibitors, can reduce gastric acid secretion and, in some cases, surgical intervention may also be required (Buttaro et al 2020; Tiziani 2021).

Gastritis

Gastritis is inflammation of the gastric mucosa and may be acute or chronic (Rogers 2023). Acute gastritis is caused by injury to the gastric mucosa by drugs, chemicals, *Helicobacter pylori*, smoking, stress, some foods, alcohol and caffeine. Manifestations of acute gastritis include fever, epigastric pain, headache, nausea and vomiting, and loss of appetite (Cooper & Gosnell 2023). Chronic gastritis involves chronic inflammation and gastric mucosal changes. It is commonly associated with an underlying disorder such as rheumatoid arthritis or type 1 diabetes mellitus, alcohol, tobacco and non-steroidal anti-inflammatory drugs. Many people with chronic gastritis have no symptoms, while others experience anorexia, a feeling of fullness, nausea and vomiting, eructation (burping) and vague epigastric pain. There is an increased risk of gastric ulcer formation and bleeding (Rogers 2023). Haemorrhage may occur, presenting as haematemesis (vomited blood) and/or occult blood in the faeces, or melaena.

Gastritis management, whether acute or chronic, focuses on relieving nausea and vomiting, fluid replacement, drug therapy to decrease acid secretion and antibiotic therapy to eradicate *H. pylori* (Harding et al 2023).

Gastroenteritis

Gastroenteritis is inflammation of the stomach and intestines. It is an acute disorder characterised by diarrhoea, nausea, vomiting and abdominal cramps. Gastroenteritis has many causes, including the ingestion of bacteria, amoebae, parasites, viruses, toxins or food allergens, and drug reactions (Gulanick & Myers 2022). Viral gastroenteritis is extremely contagious; therefore, hand hygiene, general hygiene and disposal of faecally contaminated items is crucial. Infants, older adults and individuals who are debilitated are more vulnerable to the rapid loss of fluid and electrolytes that occurs with the condition. Fluid replacement is vital for management of gastroenteritis (Gulanick & Myers 2022).

Haemorrhage

Gastrointestinal haemorrhage can occur anywhere from the mouth to the anus and may be a result of a variety of disorders. Common causes of bleeding from the upper digestive tract are peptic ulcer disease, oesophageal varices, malignancy and erosive gastritis, and oesophagitis (Buttaro et al 2020). Upper gastrointestinal haemorrhage may be accompanied by haematemesis or melaena. Causes of bleeding from the lower digestive tract include haemorrhoids, fissures, inflammatory bowel disease, polyps, diverticular disease and malignancy. Haemorrhage from the lower intestinal tract may present as bright-red blood excreted through the anus, or as occult blood present in the faeces. In addition, the individual may display signs and symptoms of dyspnoea, angina, postural hypotension and shock. Management requires stabilisation of the individual and identification of the cause of bleeding, usually by endoscopy (Buttaro et al 2020). (See Figure 32.13.)

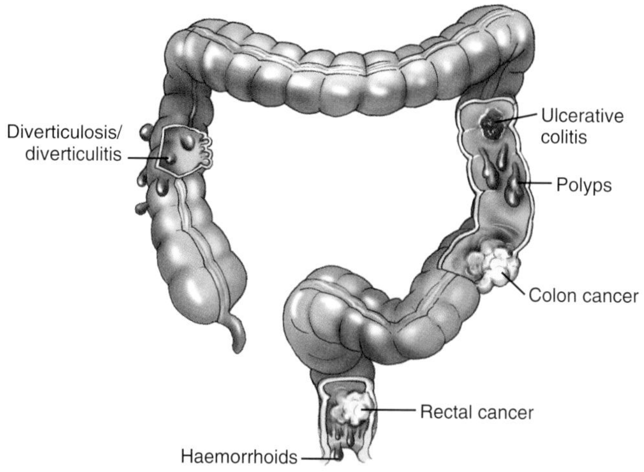

Figure 32.13 Common causes of lower gastrointestinal bleeding
(Leonard 2022)

Peptic ulcer

A peptic ulcer is a localised area of erosion and ulceration occurring in the mucosa of the stomach or duodenum. Common causes of peptic ulcers are hyperacidity, non-steroidal anti-inflammatory drug use, stress, altered gastric emptying or presence of *H. pylori* bacteria (Gulanick & Myers 2022).

Sometimes asymptomatic, primary signs and symptoms of peptic ulcers are dyspepsia and epigastric pain, post-eating belching, a feeling of fullness, intolerance of fatty food, and nausea and vomiting. Treatment aims to decrease gastric acid secretion and includes antibiotic therapy in the presence of *H. pylori* (Buttaro et al 2020).

Cholecystitis

Cholecystitis is inflammation of the gallbladder. Cholecystitis may be acute or chronic. Cholecystitis is most commonly associated with obstruction caused by gallstones or biliary sludge. Obstruction of the duct causes the gallbladder wall to become congested and oedematous followed by haemorrhage and necrosis, suppuration and infection (Gallaher & Charles 2022; Harding et al 2023).

Risk factors for cholecystitis include increasing age, female gender, obesity or rapid weight loss, certain ethnic groups and pregnancy. Symptoms include right upper quadrant pain that may radiate to the right shoulder or back, nausea, vomiting and loss of appetite. Pain exacerbated by inspiration effort (Murphy's sign) is usually present. Murphy's sign is defined as increased tenderness and stoppage of inspired breathing when the right upper quadrant is palpated (Elisha et al 2022; Ferri 2023). Choledocholithiasis is the presence of gallstones in the common bile duct (Ferri 2023). Major manifestations of choledocholithiasis are similar to those of cholecystitis. If a stone obstructs the common bile duct, right upper quadrant pain and jaundice may be evident. Gallstones may be formed by cholesterol that is supersaturated in fat, instigated by stasis of bile from immobility, pregnancy and lesions in the biliary system (Harding et al 2023).

CRITICAL THINKING EXERCISE 32.3

Peter has arrived in the emergency department reporting a sharp pain in his abdomen and right shoulder. He states he feels nauseous, especially when eating and that his appetite is reduced. His ECG is normal. What other assessments should you make and why?

Hepatitis

Hepatitis, which is inflammation of the liver, may be viral or non-viral in origin. Viral hepatitis is classified as infection with hepatitis A virus (HAV), hepatitis B (HBV), hepatitis C (HCV), hepatitis D (HDV) or hepatitis E (HEV).

Hepatitis B, C and D usually occur as a result of parenteral contact with infected body fluids. Hepatitis A and E are typically caused by ingestion of contaminated food or water (World Health Organization [WHO] 2022a). The individual may have few symptoms or may experience headaches, fatigue, anorexia, pyrexia, dark urine, pale faeces, liver enlargement, jaundice and pruritus. Healthcare workers are at risk of contracting hepatitis B and C through body fluids and, therefore, standard precautions must be scrupulously adhered to at all times.

Hepatitis A is a viral infection of the liver generally spread via the faecal–oral route when food or water contaminated by faeces of an infected person is ingested. The course of the infection is usually short term, but can cause acute liver failure. A vaccination against hepatitis A is available (WHO 2022a).

Hepatitis B (serum hepatitis) is generally transmitted parentally by contact with infected blood. The virus may also be spread via contact with body secretions such as saliva, vaginal secretions, menstrual blood and semen, and from an infected mother to her baby during passage through the birth canal or via breast milk (WHO 2022b). The incidence of hepatitis B is higher in people who receive blood or blood products, use or share contaminated needles or razors, or engage in unprotected sexual practices (WHO 2022b). The infection may be asymptomatic in the acute phase, but some individuals experience symptoms of jaundice, fatigue, nausea and vomiting and abdominal pain. The WHO (2022b) reports that there are 257 million people worldwide who are chronically infected with hepatitis B and death is due to acute liver failure. Adult vaccination against hepatitis B involves three doses given over 6 months, and is 95% effective in preventing infection.

Hepatitis C is a virus that presents as jaundice, abnormal liver function tests, flu-like symptoms and right upper quadrant pain. It is spread through blood-to-blood contact, such as blood transfusions, infected needles and IV drug use, and can lead to cirrhosis and end-stage liver disease. There is no vaccination currently available for hepatitis C and treatment is with antiviral drugs. For individuals with severe liver disease secondary to the hepatitis C infection, a liver transplant may be indicated (Dawson & Meader 2018).

Hepatitis D is an inflammation of the liver caused by the hepatitis D virus (HDV), which requires HBV for its replication. Hepatitis D infection cannot occur in the absence of hepatitis B virus and is most commonly seen in developing countries. Vaccination against hepatitis B can also protect individuals from the D strain of the virus (Hepatitis Victoria nd). Hepatitis E is a viral disease more common in developing countries. The highest rates of hepatitis E infection occur in regions where there is poor sanitation and sewage management that promotes the transmission of the virus, such as Central and South-east Asia, North and West Africa and Mexico. In most cases, hepatitis E infection will resolve by itself (WHO 2022c).

Non-viral hepatitis generally results from exposure to certain toxins and medications and excessive use of alcohol. Manifestations of the disorder are similar to those of viral hepatitis.

Diverticular disease

Diverticula are outpouchings of mucosa in the colon, and diverticulosis is the presence of multiple non-inflamed diverticula. **Diverticulitis** is inflammation of one or more of the diverticula, which may have trapped faeces. Diverticulitis causes mild to severe lower abdominal pain, bloating, a change in bowel habits, intestinal perforation, abscesses, fistula, colitis and peritonitis. Risk factors for diverticular disease are age, a diet high in refined foods, obesity, smoking, a sedentary lifestyle and alcohol (Harding et al 2023). (See Figure 32.13.)

Polyps

Polyps are projections of the mucosal surface of an organ and may develop in the stomach or intestine, and have the potential to be malignant. They may be attached flush to the mucosal wall or by a 'stalk'. Polyps may be asymptomatic or they may cause diarrhoea or haemorrhage, or they may be the manifestations of intestinal obstruction. Familial colonic polyposis is a hereditary disorder characterised by hundreds, or potentially thousands, of polyps, and has a high association with colonic malignancy (Hagler et al 2022). (See Figure 32.13.)

Irritable bowel syndrome

Irritable bowel syndrome (IBS) is a gastrointestinal disorder characterised by alteration of bowel pattern and symptoms of constipation and diarrhoea. The condition is thought to result from food intolerance and psychological stressors. It is familial, affects 50% more women than men and is more prevalent in Western countries. Treatment may involve the use of antispasmodics, antidepressants, antidiarrhoeals, anticonstipation medications, lifestyle coaching, dietary modification and an increased intake of probiotics (Buttaro et al 2020).

CRITICAL THINKING EXERCISE 32.4

Jack, 31 years old, has been diagnosed with IBS. What are the classic symptoms associated with IBS? What individual education points related to diet and lifestyle can you suggest to help Jack manage his IBS?

Coeliac disease

Coeliac disease is an abnormal response to wheat, barley and rye by the immune system, causing damage to the mucosa of the small bowel. Symptoms include diarrhoea, steatorrhoea, flatulence, abdominal distension and malabsorption. Atypical signs and symptoms include weight loss, iron deficiency anaemia and peripheral neuropathy. Treatment requires a continuing gluten-free diet to resolve the symptoms (LeMone et al 2020).

Hernia

A **hernia** is the protrusion of an organ or the fascia of an organ through an abnormal opening in the wall of a cavity. Various types of hernias are named according to their location: umbilical (abdomen), inguinal (groin), femoral (groin), hiatal (diaphragm) and incisional, the last occurring at the site of an abdominal incision. If the protrusion can be pushed back into the cavity, the hernia is said to be reducible. The major complication of an intestinal hernia is strangulation, when the blood flow to the protruding loop of bowel may be obstructed, resulting in necrosis. Signs and symptoms of this include severe pain, vomiting, cramping, distension and symptoms of a bowel obstruction. Repair of the hernia involves surgery to place mesh over the hernia orifice, thus preventing the protrusion of the organ (Hagler et al 2022; Harding et al 2023).

Bowel obstruction

Bowel obstruction (intestinal obstruction) is a mechanical or functional obstruction of the intestines, preventing the normal progression of bowel contents. Mechanical or simple obstructions are often caused by fibrous adhesions of the small intestine. Functional obstruction is triggered by such things as abdominal surgery, intestinal infection and acute pancreatitis and is a failure of normal intestinal motility. Chronic obstructions are associated with inflammatory disorders and tumours. Acute obstructions usually have mechanical causes such as hernias and adhesions. Signs and symptoms of large bowel obstruction include pain, abdominal distension and vomiting late in the process. Small bowel obstruction presents with abdominal distension, pain, nausea and vomiting, sweating and tachycardia. Further manifestations of bowel obstruction may include fluid and electrolyte imbalance because of progressive dehydration, fever related to ischaemia and subsequent infection of the affected bowel. Complications of intestinal obstruction include peritonitis, ischaemia and necrosis of the bowel. Management of a bowel obstruction focuses on identifying and eradicating the cause of obstruction, treating the fluid and electrolyte imbalance, and resting the bowel. Treatment also includes pain relief and gastrointestinal decompression via nasogastric tube (Rogers 2023).

Haemorrhoids

Haemorrhoids are distended veins in the anal area, and they can be internal or external. Internal haemorrhoids commonly present with prolapse or painless rectal bleeding. External haemorrhoids cause bleeding and can cause acute pain if thrombosed. Haemorrhoids commonly result from increased pressure in the anal area related to constipation, straining to defecate, obesity, pregnancy and prolonged sitting or standing. The individual commonly experiences pain in, and bleeding from, the anus, particularly during defecation. Management includes increasing oral fluids, increasing exercise, avoiding straining, topical creams, rubber band ligation and surgery (Hagler et al 2022; Harding et al 2023).

Anal fissure

An **anal fissure** is a linear tear in the mucosa of the anal canal and is associated with increased pressure in the anal area from trauma such as large bowel movements, frequent diarrhoea or local trauma during labour and childbirth. Sudden occurrence is characterised by a tearing or burning pain during or immediately after defecation, and bleeding. An anal fissure may heal spontaneously or it may partially heal and recur. A chronic fissure (lasting 6 weeks or longer) produces scar tissue, which may impede normal defecation (LeMone et al 2020). Basic treatment strategies include increasing fluid and fibre intake to soften the stool, sitz (salt) baths to promote hygiene, and topical analgesia and medications to improve blood flow to the area and therefore healing. Second line treatments include botulinum toxin injections and surgery (Yu 2022).

Rectal prolapse

Rectal **prolapse** is the protrusion of one or more layers of the wall of the rectum through the anal canal. Prolapse may be partial (anal or rectal mucosa only) or complete—with displacement of the anal sphincter and rectum (Ferri 2023). Risk factors for this condition include increasing age (especially women), massive diarrhoea, chronic constipation and straining on defecation, and childbirth. When a rectal prolapse occurs, protrusion of tissue from the rectum is evident, and the individual may experience a sensation of rectal fullness, bleeding and rectal and abdominal pain, as well as associated symptoms of constipation, faecal incontinence, urinary incontinence, and protrusion of pelvic organs such as the uterus and bladder (Lee 2022a).

Inflammatory and infectious disorders

Inflammatory and/or infectious disorders of the digestive system may be related to internal or external irritation or to the proliferation of pathogenic microorganisms.

Appendicitis

Appendicitis is the acute inflammation of the vermiform appendix that leads to appendix distension and ischaemia, and possibly necrosis, perforation and peritonitis. The individual typically presents with acute abdominal pain starting in the mid-abdomen, later localising to the right lower quadrant. Symptoms may include fever, anorexia, nausea, vomiting and elevation of the neutrophil count. The condition commonly results from an obstruction of the lumen of the appendix (e.g. by a faecal mass, lymphoid tissue, tumour, parasite or foreign body). Analgesia, fluid resuscitation, antibiotic therapy and a surgical assessment are required to treat appendicitis (Garzon et al 2020).

Peritonitis

Peritonitis is inflammation of the peritoneum. Primarily, peritonitis is caused by infective organisms entering the abdominal cavity. Secondary peritonitis occurs when the peritoneum is contaminated by gastrointestinal or urinary tract contents, due to perforation or rupture of these organs (Ross et al 2018). Causes of peritonitis include end-stage liver disease, ruptured appendix, ruptured diverticula, peritoneal dialysis, and abdominal trauma. The onset of peritonitis may be acute, or slow and progressive. The inflammatory process causes accumulation of fluid in the abdominal cavity, formation of adhesions, decreased motility and obstruction, leading to abdominal distension and rigidity, severe pain, nausea and vomiting. As a result of loss of fluid and electrolytes into the abdominal cavity, the individual displays signs of hypovolaemic shock. Other potential complications include septic shock, acute renal failure, liver failure and gastrointestinal bleeding (Cooper & Gosnell 2023). Treatment commonly includes antibiotics, analgesics, antiemetics, surgery and supportive care such as supplemental oxygen, blood transfusions and fluid and electrolyte replacement (Harding et al 2023).

Pilonidal sinus

A **pilonidal sinus** occurs when a hair tunnels inwards, causing a tract under the skin, between the buttocks at the base of the spine. Sinuses occur primarily in men between the ages of 15 and 40 years. Symptoms of a pilonidal sinus range from a painful, tender abscess forming from acute inflammation to a chronic, painful sinus tract with purulent exudate. Management of a pilonidal sinus may initially be with antibiotics to improve inflammation; however, the majority of cases require a surgical incision and drainage (Lee 2022b). Nursing care includes analgesia, wound care, promotion of hygiene (sitz baths) and education (LeMone et al 2020).

Inflammatory bowel disease

Inflammatory bowel disease (IBD) describes a chronic inflammation of the gastrointestinal tract characterised by active and remission periods (Harding et al 2023). The two main conditions associated with IBD are Crohn's disease and ulcerative colitis (Figure 32.14). Although the precise cause of IBD is unknown, factors that have been implicated include genetics, infection, autoimmune reactions to intestinal flora, dietary choices, age and tobacco. The effect of the disease causes altered mobility and fatigue, as well as changes to perception of body image and alteration in quality of life (Harding et al 2023).

Ulcerative colitis primarily affects the mucosal and submucosal layers of the colon. The inflammation associated with the disorder causes ulceration, bleeding, increased production of mucus and necrosis. Symptoms include abdominal pain and bloody diarrhoea. The faeces are generally watery and may contain blood and mucus (Harding et al 2023).

Crohn's disease can affect any part of the digestive tract from the mouth to the anus, but it most commonly affects the small intestine and/or colon (Crohn's and Colitis Australia [CCA] 2023a). There may be healthy sections of the intestine between the diseased sections. Crohn's disease can affect all layers of the intestinal wall and can lead to complications such as strictures, abscesses, fistulae and fissures (CCA 2023a). Symptoms vary according to the site and

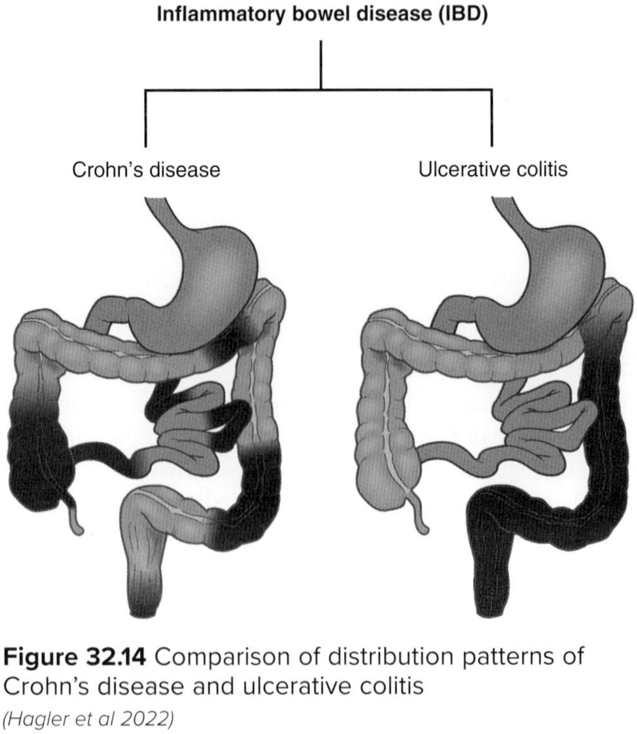

Figure 32.14 Comparison of distribution patterns of Crohn's disease and ulcerative colitis
(Hagler et al 2022)

extent of the lesions and, in acute episodes, the individual experiences abdominal pain and cramps, flatulence, diarrhoea, pyrexia and nausea and vomiting. The faeces may contain large quantities of blood and mucus. Chronic or prolonged episodes of IBD lead to nutritional imbalances, marked weight loss and an increased risk of colon cancer (CCA 2023b).

Complications of IBD are both local and systemic, and include haemorrhage, fistulas, toxic megacolon and colorectal cancer. Medications used to manage IBD include anti-inflammatories, antimicrobials and immunosuppressants. Surgery is often indicated to resect diseased bowel. Nursing care aims to control pain, fluid and electrolyte replacement, and nutritional support (Harding et al 2023).

Neoplastic disorders

Gastrointestinal system malignancies include cancers of the mouth, oesophagus, stomach, intestines, rectum, liver or pancreas. The manifestations and prognosis of cancer of the digestive system vary according to the site (Swearingen & Wright 2018).

Colorectal cancer is the most common cancer of the digestive system and is the third most commonly diagnosed cancer worldwide (World Cancer Research Fund 2023). It can develop with few, if any, early warning symptoms. Symptoms of bowel cancer include:

- bleeding from the anus or any sign of blood after a bowel motion
- a recent and persistent change in bowel habit (e.g. looser bowel motions, severe constipation and/or needing to go to the toilet more than usual)
- unexplained fatigue (a symptom of anaemia) and weight loss, anorexia, shortness of breath or angina
- abdominal pain, especially after meals.

Risk factors for developing colorectal cancer include age, familial history, ethnicity, history of IBD and a diet low in fibre, fruits and vegetables and high in fat and red meat (Simonson 2018).

Screening tests for occult blood assist in early diagnosis of colorectal cancers, improving treatment options and chances of survival. Bowel cancer can be treated successfully in 90% of cases of early identification. Care of the individual with colorectal cancer requires gastroenterological, oncological and surgical management (Buttaro et al 2020).

Traumatic disorders

Trauma to parts of the digestive system may be related to injury or to irritation, such as the ingestion of a corrosive substance. Abdominal trauma may be localised or it may involve more than one abdominal structure. When a part of the digestive system is damaged, the processes of digestion, absorption and elimination may be impaired. As a consequence, alterations in nutritional, electrolyte and fluid status occur. Depending on the type and extent of injury, the manifestations include external bruising, abdominal distension, pain, altered bowel sounds and haemorrhage, either internal and concealed, or presenting as haematemesis and/or melaena. Complications of trauma to the digestive system include haemorrhage, shock, infection, peritonitis and obstruction (Berman et al 2021; Crisp et al 2021).

End-of-life care

Nausea and vomiting from the bowel disease process, treatment and medications contribute to a decreased appetite and decrease in oral intake. Narcotics and decreased mobility may result in decreased peristalsis, whilst decreased fibre intake and reduced fluid intake contribute to constipation. Diarrhoea may result from the disease process, treatment and medications, which, in turn, may cause incontinence. If possible, the cause of the problem should be diagnosed so appropriate interventions can be put into place. Antiemetics, stool softeners and incontinence aids promote dignity, comfort and potential relief (Crisp et al 2021).

CRITICAL THINKING EXERCISE 32.5

Lorraine has end-stage dementia and is under a palliative care plan. What aspects of her bowel elimination care need considering?

Diagnostic tests

Certain tests may be performed to assist or confirm the diagnosis of digestive system disorders.

Digital rectal examination

A digital examination is done with a gloved finger inserted through the anus into the rectum to identify anal abnormalities, sphincter tone, pain, impaction, rectal prolapse and haemorrhoids. This is an invasive and uncomfortable procedure and the individual needs privacy and reassurance (Buttaro et al 2022).

Screening

Screening is recognised as one method in the early detection of bowel cancer (Bowel Cancer Australia 2020). Individuals are now able to screen for unseen blood in their stool, which may be an indicator of a disease process. The faecal occult blood test (FOBT) involves placing small samples of stool on special cards (faecal immunochemical test [FIT]) and sending them to a pathology laboratory for analysis. The results are then sent back to the individual and their designated medical officer (Bowel Cancer Australia 2020).

Laboratory tests

Specimens that may be obtained from the individual for laboratory analysis include blood, faeces, gastric or peritoneal fluid, urine and samples of tissue. Laboratory tests include:

- Histology, microbiology and cytology of stools.
- The blood may be tested to determine haemoglobin level, haematocrit, leucocyte count, serum electrolytes,

bilirubin levels, glucose levels or pancreatic enzyme levels.
- The faeces may be tested to identify bleeding disorders, biliary obstruction, infections and disorders of digestion or absorption.
- Gastric fluid analysis involves examination of gastric secretions, and may be performed by examining a specimen of vomitus or by testing a sample of the gastric contents aspirated via a nasogastric tube.
- Peritoneal fluid analysis assesses a sample of peritoneal fluid obtained by abdominal paracentesis. The test may be performed when bleeding or infection is suspected by a medical officer. Abdominal paracentesis involves the insertion of a trocar and cannula through the abdominal wall to aspirate a quantity of peritoneal fluid.
- The urine may be tested to detect the presence of any abnormal substance (e.g. bilirubin) that may be excreted in the urine as a result of a digestive system disorder.
- Biopsy: Specimens of tissue may be obtained during endoscopic examinations or surgery. The specimens are examined microscopically for changes in cellular structure, to confirm diagnosis or to determine the cause of a disease (e.g. malignancy).

(Berman et al 2021; CCA 2023b; Crisp et al 2021)

Radiological examination

Several different types of radiological investigation may be performed to assist or confirm the diagnosis of digestive system disorders:
- Plain X-rays may be taken to aid in the diagnosis of abdominal masses, bowel obstruction, trauma to abdominal organs and ascites.
- Computerised tomography (CT) scanning involves the direction of a narrow X-ray beam at parts of the body, from various angles. Contrast medium is often administered intravenously to enhance visualisation. A computer reconstructs the information as a three-dimensional image on a screen.
- Ultrasound involves the use of soundwaves to visualise body structures. A transducer is passed over the area, such as the abdomen, and receives echoes, which are bounced off body structures. The echoes are converted into electrical impulses, which may be viewed on a screen or photographed.
- Fluoroscopy (visualisation with motion) involves use of a contrast agent (e.g. barium sulfate), which can be visualised as it passes through and outlines structures in the digestive tract. Fluoroscopic examination of the digestive tract includes barium swallow, barium meal and barium enema.
- Defecating proctogram is an X-ray of the rectal region during defecation. A simulated stool is an oral contrast agent, composed of barium and a liquid, starchy substance and the individual is required to pass this agent.
- **Endoscopy** is the visual examination of part of the digestive tract using a flexible fibreoptic endoscope. The endoscope also provides a channel for the introduction of instruments for the purpose of obtaining a sample of tissue for microscopic examination. The various forms of endoscopy derive their names from the part of the body being examined:
  - oesophagoscopy (the oesophagus)
  - gastroscopy (the stomach)
  - duodenoscopy (the duodenum)
  - proctoscopy (the anus and rectum)
  - sigmoidoscopy (the sigmoid colon)
  - colonoscopy (the colon).

(Crisp et al 2021; Berman et al 2021)

CRITICAL THINKING EXERCISE 32.6

Bill, 50 years old, is admitted for a colonoscopy because he has seen blood in his bowel actions and has a family history of diverticulitis. What education can you provide Bill with about this procedure?

Care of the individual with a digestive system disorder

Although specific nursing actions and medical management may vary depending on the disorder, the main aims of care are to:
- Maintain standard precautions.
- Monitor and maintain accurate bowel frequency and stool form scale (see Clinical Skill 32.2).
- Ensure accurate documentation and assessment to aid all health professionals in treatment.
- Ensure hygiene needs are met (e.g. that handwash or sanitisers are available following bowel action).
- Maintain skin integrity and appropriate personal hygiene.
- Ensure environment is clean, fresh and appropriate to age and ability of the individual.
- Encourage appropriate fluids and diet, monitor intake and output.
- Identify foods that may trigger discomfort or alterations in bowel elimination.
- Provide education about medications.
- Encourage ambulation.
- Ensure the individual is in partnership with the health team in care planning and support individual in accessing further information.
- Investigate culturally sensitive issues specific to the lifestyle of the individual.
- Maintain individual dignity and support self-image deficits through exploration of potential for altered relationships (both physical and emotional) with significant others.
- Consider emotional, psychosocial and spiritual needs.

(Ringos Beach et al 2018)

CLINICAL SKILL 32.2 Stool assessment/collection

Please adhere to the policy and procedures of the facility/organisation prior to undertaking the skill. Ensure this skill is in your scope of practice.

NMBA Decision-making Framework considerations	Equipment:
NMBA Decision-making Framework considerations (refer to NMBA Decision-making framework for nursing and midwifery 2020): 1. Am I educated? 2. Am I authorised? 3. Am I competent? If you answer 'no' to any of these, do not perform that activity. Seek guidance and support from your teacher/a nurse team leader/clinical facilitator/educator.	**Equipment:** Faecal specimen container Laboratory request form (signed by a medical practitioner or Nurse Practitioner—may be an electronic document) Biohazard specimen transport bag Bedpan/collection pan Disposable gloves

PREPARE FOR THE SKILL

(Please refer to the Standard Steps on pp. xviii–xx for related rationales.)
Mentally review the steps of the skill.
Discuss the skill with your instructor/supervisor/team leader, if required.
Confirm correct facility/organisation policy/safe operating procedures.
Validate the order in the individual's record.
Identify indication and rationale for performing the activity.
Assess for any contraindications.
Locate and gather equipment.
Perform hand hygiene.
Ensure therapeutic interaction.
Identify the individual using three individual identifiers.
Gain the individual's consent.
Assess for pain relief.
Prepare the environment.
Provide and maintain privacy.
Assist the individual to assume an appropriate position of comfort.

Skill activity	Rationale
Provide the individual with a bedpan/collection pan. Explain to the person how to obtain a specimen that is free of toilet paper and urine: encourage the individual to void prior to providing the stool sample.	Ideally, the stool sample should be uncontaminated by urine, although this might not always be possible.

PERFORM THE SKILL

(Please refer to the Standard Steps on pp. xviii–xx for related rationales.)
Perform hand hygiene.
Apply PPE: gloves, eyewear, mask and gown as appropriate.
Ensure the individual's safety and comfort throughout skill.
Promote independence and involvement of the individual if possible and/or appropriate.
Assess the individual's tolerance to the skill throughout.
Dispose of used supplies, equipment, waste and sharps appropriately.
Remove PPE and discard or store appropriately.
Perform hand hygiene.

Skill activity	Rationale
Visually assess the stool sample. The size, shape, colour and consistency of the stool should be observed.	Changes in the size, shape, colour and consistency of the stool can be a sign of an underlying medical condition.
Specimen container may need wiping with an absorbent paper towel. Label the specimen container with the person's name, date of birth, hospital or patient number and the date and time of the specimen collection.	Ensures that the correct specimen is sent for testing and that it is for the correct person.

Continued

CLINICAL SKILL 32.2 Stool assessment/collection—cont'd

Using the scooped lid of the faecal specimen container, place a portion of the stool into the container. Place the lid on the container.	All stool samples must be placed into the faecal specimen container.
Specimen container is placed in the ziplock section of the plastic biohazard bag.	Standard infection control precaution.
Pathology request form is checked for the person's details. The pathology request form is placed in the other section of the bag.	Ensures correct form and specimen are sent to pathology department and correct test will be undertaken in the pathology department.

AFTER THE SKILL

(Please refer to the Standard Steps on pp. xviii–xx for related rationales.)
Communicate outcome to the individual, any ongoing care and report any complications.
Restore the environment.
Report, record and document assessment findings, details of the skill performed and the individual's response.
Report, record and document any abnormalities and/or inability to perform the skill.
Reassess the individual to ensure there are no adverse effects/events from the skill.

Skill activity	Rationale
The specimen should be transported to the laboratory as soon as possible, or stored in a refrigerator until transport can be arranged.	Decomposition and cell growth occur if faeces is left standing, and may provide an inaccurate result.

(Linton & Matteson 2023)

It is vital that infection control principles are adhered to when handling any stool sample. The Australian Commission on Safety and Quality in Health Care (ACSQHC) has recognised the importance of infection control and made the reduction of harm through healthcare-associated infections one of the national safety and quality health service standards. Nurses have a central role to play in this by using effective, evidence-based hand hygiene practices and educating individuals to do the same (ACSQHC 2021).

Specific nursing activities include implementing measures to assist elimination from the bowel, observing and collecting excreta, and care of an individual with a stoma.

Progress Note 32.1

12/02/2024 1430	Nursing: Individual assisted with changing of the ileostomy appliance. Skin surrounding stoma is intact, nil signs of excoriation. Stoma is pink, warm and moist. Flatus and 400 mL semi-formed, brown stool passed this shift. One piece, drainable appliance applied. *JJ Grey* (GREY), *EN*

DECISION-MAKING FRAMEWORK EXERCISE 32.1

Patrick Brown, who has a partial spinal cord injury, has been admitted for a surgical procedure. During his admission he reports to you that he has not had a bowel action for 4 days. Patrick states he usually gives himself a warm water enema to help him open his bowels and asks whether you would do this for him. You have never performed this procedure before and do not feel confident in doing so. Patrick reassures you that it is easy and he will talk you through the process.

How should you respond to this situation in accordance with legal and ethical aspects of nursing, and the decision-making framework for nurses?

Refer to the Decision-making framework summary: Nursing (NMBA 2020) for steps to guide actions in this situation.
The steps are:

1. Identify potential risks/hazards associated with mobilising this patient.
2. Reflect on whether the nurse has the necessary educational preparation, experience, capacity, confidence and competence to safely perform the activity.
3. Decide whether there is a justifiable, evidence-based reason to perform the activity.
4. Identify strategies to meet the patient's needs without compromising their safety.

Summary

The functions of the digestive system are to ingest and digest foods so that nutrients can be absorbed into the bloodstream, and to eliminate waste products of digestion from the body. Normal functioning may be impaired as a result of disorders in swallowing, digestion, secretory function, gastric motility, absorption or elimination. Disorders of the digestive system can be classified as those occurring from inflammation or infection, as a result of neoplasms, obstruction or as a result of injury. Diagnostic tests used to assess digestive system function include laboratory analysis of body fluids, excretions or tissues; radiological examinations; and endoscopy.

Care of the individual with a digestive system disorder includes preventing and managing altered elimination patterns and processes, promoting comfort, maintaining skin and mucous membrane integrity, and maintaining nutritional and fluid status. These tasks need to be balanced by supporting the individual through often undignified and embarrassing procedures. Maintaining an individual's self-esteem and encouraging a team approach from all healthcare providers to ensure an optimum lifestyle for the individual is crucial for satisfactory person-centred outcomes.

Review Questions

1. Outline the role of the accessory organs of the digestive system.
2. Describe the difference between an ileostomy and a colostomy.
3. What factors may impact an individual's ability to ingest food?
4. Describe the digestion process in the large intestine.
5. Consider the psychosocial impact of bowel disease on the individual and their family.
6. Describe the different types of hepatitis.
7. Identify the factors that affect bowel elimination.
8. Outline five causes for the onset of diarrhoea in an individual.
9. Explain how diet can influence bowel elimination.

Evolve® Answer guide for the Review Questions, Critical Thinking Exercises, Decision-making Framework Exercises and Critical Thinking Questions in Case Studies is hosted on Evolve: http://evolve.elsevier.com/AU/Koutoukidis/Tabbner.

References

Altomare, D.F., Rotelli, M.T., 2019. *Nutritional support after gastrointestinal surgery*, 1st ed. 2019. [Online]. Cham: Springer International Publishing.

Anderson, C., Shilkofski, N., Kapoor, S., et al., 2023. *The Harriet Lane handbook*, 23rd ed. Elsevier, Philadelphia.

Australian Council of Stoma Associations Inc., 2021. Colostomy hints and tips. Available at: <https://australianstoma.com.au/wp-content/uploads/HInts-and-Tips-for-Colostomy.pdf>.

Australian Commission on Safety and Quality in Health Care (ACSQHC), 2021. National safety and quality health service standards, 2nd ed. ACSQHC, Sydney. Available at: <https://www.safetyandquality.gov.au/publications-and-resources/resource-library/national-safety-and-quality-health-service-standards-second-edition>.

Berman, A., Frandsen, G., Snyder, S.J., et al., 2021. *Kozier and Erb's fundamentals of nursing*, 5th ed. Pearson Australia, Melbourne.

Bowel Cancer Australia, 2020. Bowel cancer screening. Available at: <https://www.bowelcanceraustralia.org/national-bowel-cancer-screening-program>.

Garzon, D.L., Starr, N., Brady, M., et al. 2020. *Burn's pediatric primary care*, 7th ed. Elsevier, St Louis.

Buttaro, T.M., Trybulski, J., Polgar-Bailey, P., et al., 2020. *Primary care*, 6th ed. Elsevier, St Louis.

Continence Foundation of Australia, 2021. Bristol stool chart. Available at: <https://www.continence.org.au/pages/bristol-stool-chart.html>.

Cooper, C.A., Urso, P.P., 2018. Gastroesophageal reflux in the intensive care unit patient. *Critical Care Nursing Clinics of North America* 30(1), 123–135.

Cooper, K., Gosnell, K., 2023. *Adult health nursing*, 9th ed. Mosby Elsevier, St Louis.

Crisp, J., Douglas, C., Rebeiro, G., Waters, D., 2021. *Potter & Perry's fundamentals of nursing*, 6th ed. Elsevier, Sydney.

Crohn's and Colitis Australia (CCA), 2023a. About Crohn's disease. Available at: <https://crohnsandcolitis.org.au/about-crohns-colitis/crohns-disease/about-crohns-disease>.

Crohn's and Colitis Australia (CCA), 2023b. About Crohn's and colitis. Available at: <https://www.crohnsandcolitis.com.au/about-crohns-colitis/>.

Davis, K., Guerra, A., 2022. *Mosby's pharmacy technician: Principles and practice*, 6th ed. Elsevier, St Louis.

Dawson, S., Meader, E., 2018. Hepatitis C. *InnovAiT* 11(2), 101–108.

Elisha, S., Heiner, J.S., Nagelhout, J.J., 2022. *Nurse anaesthesia*, 7th ed. Elsevier, St Louis.

Ferri, F.F., 2023. *Ferri's clinical advisor 2023*. Elsevier, Philadelphia.

Gallaher, J.R., Charles, A., 2022. Acute cholecystitis: A review. *JAMA* 327(10), 965–975.

Gulanick, M., Myers, J.L., 2022. *Nursing care plans: Diagnoses, interventions, and outcomes*, 10th ed. Elsevier Mosby, St Louis.

Hagler, D., Harding, M., Kwong, J., et al., 2022. *Clinical companion to medical-surgical nursing*, 12th ed. Elsevier, St Louis.

Hepatitis Victoria, n.d. An overview of hepatitis A, B, C, D, and E. Available at: <https://liverwell.org.au/wp-content/uploads/2020/11/A-B-C-D-E-OVERVIEW.pdf>.

Hockenberry, M.J., Wilson, D., Rodgers, C.C., 2022. *Wong's essentials of paediatric nursing*, 11th ed. Elsevier, St Louis.

Lataillade, L., Chabal, L., 2021.Therapeutic patient education: A multifaceted approach to ostomy care. *Advances in Skin & Wound Care* 34(1), 36–42.

Lee, G., 2022a. Rectal prolapse. In: Steele, S.R., Hull, T.L., Hyman, N., et al., 2022. *The ASCRS textbook of colon and rectal surgery*, 4th ed, pp. 95–103. Springer International Publishing, Cham.

Lee, E.L., 2022b. Pilonidal disease. In: Steele, S.R., Hull, T.L., Hyman, N., et al., 2022. *The ASCRS textbook of colon and rectal surgery*, 4th ed, pp. 124–128. Springer International Publishing, Cham.

LeMone, P., Bauldoff, G., Gubrud-Howe, P., et al., 2020. *Medical–surgical nursing: Critical thinking in person-centred care*, 4th ed. Pearson, Melbourne.

Leonard, P., 2022. *Building a medical vocabulary: With Spanish translations*, 11th ed. Elsevier, St Louis.

Linton, A.D., Matteson, M.A., 2023. *Medical–surgical nursing*, 8th ed. Elsevier Saunders, St Louis.

Marieb, K.N., Keller, S.M., 2022. *Essentials of human anatomy and physiology*, 13th ed. Pearson, San Francisco.

Meiner, S.E., Yeager, J.J., 2019. *Gerontologic nursing*, 6th ed. Elsevier, St Louis.

Monahan, F.D., Neighbors, M., 1998. *Medical-surgical nursing*, 2nd ed. Saunders, Philadelphia.

Nursing and Midwifery Board of Australia (NMBA), 2020. Decision-making framework for nursing and midwifery. Available at: <https://www.nursingmidwiferyboard.gov.au/codes-guidelines-statements/frameworks.aspx>.

Odom-Forren, J., 2024. *Drain's peri anaesthesia nursing*, 8th ed. Elsevier, St Louis.

Patton, K., Bell, F., Thompson, T., Williamson, P., 2022. *Anatomy & physiology*, 11th ed. Elsevier/Mosby, St Louis.

Rebeiro, G., Wilson, D., Fuller, S., 2021. *Potter and Perry's fundamentals of nursing workbook*, 4th ed. Elsevier, Chatswood.

Ringos Beach, P., Hussey, L., De Ranieri, J.T., 2018. Caring for the hospitalized adult patient with ulcerative colitis. Elsevier Clinical Update. Available at: <https://www.clinicalkey.com.au/nursing/#!/content/clinical_updates/54-s2.0-195965>.

Rogers, J.L. 2023. *McCance & Huether's pathophysiology*, 9th ed. Elsevier, St Louis.

Ross, J.T., Matthay, M.A., Harris, H.W., 2018. Secondary peritonitis: Principles of diagnosis and intervention. *British Medical Journal* 361, k1407.

Saxena, A., Ongole, R., Ahmed, J., 2019. Medical management of xerostomia: An update for general dental practitioners. *New York State Dental Journal* 85(4), 32–38.

Scott, K., Webb, M., Kostelnick, C., 2018. *Long-term caring*, 4th ed. Elsevier, Chatswood.

Shiland, B.J., 2022. *Mastering healthcare terminology*, 7th ed. Elsevier, St Louis.

Simonson, C., 2018. Colorectal cancer—an update for primary care nurse practitioners. *Journal for Nurse Practitioners* 14(4), 344–350.

Solomon, E.P., 2016. *Introduction to human anatomy and physiology*, 4th ed. Saunders Elsevier, St Louis.

Sorrentino, S.A., Remmert, L.N., 2021. *Mosby's textbook for nursing assistants*, 10th ed. Elsevier, St Louis.

Swearingen, P.L., Wright, J., 2018. *All-in-one nursing care planning resource*, 5th ed. Elsevier, St Louis.

Thomas, M., MacLean, A., McDermott, B., Epstein, J., 2021. Stomas. *InnovAiT* 14(10), 623–628.

Tiziani, A., 2021. *Havard's nursing guide to drugs*, 11th ed. Elsevier, Chatswood.

Tollefson, J., Watson, G., Jelly, E., Tambree, K., 2022. *Essential clinical skills: Enrolled nurses*, 5th ed. Cengage, South Melbourne.

Touhy, T.A., Jett, K., 2019. *Ebersole & Hess' toward healthy aging*, 10th ed. Elsevier, St Louis.

Urden, L.D., Stacy, K.M., Lough, M.E., 2021. *Critical care nursing*, 9th ed. Elsevier, Maryland Heights.

Waugh, A., Grant, A., 2023. *Ross and Wilson anatomy and physiology in health and illness*, 14th ed. Elsevier, Edinburgh.

Williams, P., 2022. *Basic geriatric nursing*, 8th ed. Elsevier, St Louis.

Williams, P., 2021. *Fundamental concepts and skills for nursing*, 6th ed. Elsevier, St Louis.

World Cancer Research Fund, 2023. Cancer trends. Available at: <https://www.wcrf.org/cancer-trends/colorectal-cancer-statistics>.

World Health Organization (WHO), 2022a. Hepatitis A fact sheet. Available at: <https://www.who.int/news-room/fact-sheets/detail/hepatitis-a>.

World Health Organization (WHO), 2022b. Hepatitis B fact sheet. Available at: <https://www.who.int/news-room/fact-sheets/detail/hepatitis-b>.

World Health Organization (WHO), 2022c. Hepatitis E fact sheet. Available at: <https://www.who.int/news-room/fact-sheets/detail/hepatitis-e>.

Yates, A., 2018. How to perform a comprehensive baseline continence assessment. *Nursing Times* 114(5), 26–29. Available at: <https://search-proquest-com.ezproxy.lib.swin.edu.au/docview/2061036521/DF20BAE5F37F4F97PQ/11?accountid=14205>.

Yu, S. 2022. Anal fissure. In: Steele, S.R., Hull, T.L., Hyman, N., et al., 2022. *The ASCRS textbook of colon and rectal surgery*, 4th ed, pp. 46–54. Springer International Publishing, Cham.

Recommended Reading

Bladder and Bowel Health Australia, 2019. Available at: <https://www.health.gov.au/topics/bladder-and-bowel/about-bladder-and-bowel-health>.

CareSearch, 2021. Constipation. Available at: <https://caresearch.com.au/tabid/6222/Default.aspx>.

Kirkland-Kyhn, H., Martin, S., Zaartkiewicz, S., et al., 2018. Ostomy care at home. *American Journal of Nursing* 118 (4), 63–68.

Queensland Health, 2020. Managing Irritable Bowel Syndrome (IBS). Available at: <https://www.health.qld.gov.au/__data/assets/pdf_file/0034/674386/gastro_ibs.pdf>.

Online Resources

Australian Council of Stoma Associations Inc. (ACSA): <www.australianstoma.com.au>.

Bowel Cancer Australia: <www.bowelcanceraustralia.org>.

Coeliac Australia: <https://www.coeliac.org.au>.

Continence Foundation of Australia: <www.continence.org.au>.

Crohn's and Colitis Australia: <www.crohnsandcolitis.com.au>.

Hepatitis Australia: <www.hepatitisaustralia.com>.

IBIS Irritable Bowel Information & Support Association of Australia Inc.: <www.ibis-australia.org>.

CHAPTER 33

Pain

Andrea Zivin and Jasmin Rigby-Day

Key Terms

acute pain
analgesic
chronic pain
co-analgesic
endorphins
epidural analgesia
gate control theory
pain
pain assessment tool
pain management
patient-controlled analgesia (PCA)
threshold

Learning Outcomes

At the completion of this chapter and with further reading, learners should be able to:

- Define the key terms.
- Describe the physiological basis of pain perception.
- Describe the factors influencing an individual's experience of pain.
- Describe the differences in approach to pain assessment across the lifespan.
- Describe various methods of pain management, including both non-pharmacological and pharmacological approaches.
- Apply appropriate principles in planning and implementing nursing actions to prevent and to alleviate an individual's pain.

CHAPTER FOCUS

Pain is generally the primary reason for individuals seeking medical care. Pain can be described as a biopsychosocial phenomenon caused by actual or potential physiological damage, which manifests in emotions and behavioural responses often modulated by socioenvironmental and cultural factors. Pain is complex because the stimuli for pain can be perceived as pleasurable in other contexts. Pain is a subjective experience and individuals without diagnosable pathophysiology may report experiences of severe pain. This is captured in a seminal statement by Margo McCaffery in 1968, who identified that 'pain is what the person says it is and exists when he [sic] says it does' (McCaffery & Pasero 1999). The absence of the verbal expression of pain or physical display of pain does not mean an individual is not experiencing pain, especially when working with young children or people with an intellectual disability. Therefore, nurses should be adequately equipped with cross-cultural, interdisciplinary, and age-appropriate skills to assess and manage pain effectively, as they spend the most amount of time with individuals in clinical settings. This chapter focuses on the pathophysiology, assessment and management of pain.

LIVED EXPERIENCE

I've always been an active and vibrant person. I used to enjoy hiking, dancing and spending time with my friends and family. However, life for me took an unexpected turn when I hurt my back and ruptured discs 3 years ago while doing deadlifts at the gym. Since then, I've had four epidural steroidal injections for the pain associated with the ruptured discs. I recently went to my local GP clinic because I just didn't know how I could go on like this. The pain used to be tolerable until 2 days ago. I'm hurting so bad, and am struggling to do basic things like go to the toilet. I'm at the point of tears, and can't help but pace around since it's excruciating pain to sit down.

Emily, 27, with chronic pain syndrome

INTRODUCTION

Pain is defined by the International Association for the Study of Pain (IASP) (2021), as 'an unpleasant sensory and emotional experience associated with, or resembling that associated with, actual or potential tissue damage'. Pain is a protective factor of actual or impending tissue damage, but can exist in the absence of tissue damage. For example, burning oneself on a hot oven, the sensation of pain, is what pulls the person away from further damage. Each episode of pain is unique and subjective and is influenced by a variety of factors such as age, culture, beliefs and previous experience. Consequently, it is important for the nurse to appreciate that pain is what the person says it is.

Melzack and Casey (1968) outlined a conceptual model that described pain in terms of three hierarchical components: sensory-discriminant (location, intensity and quality), motivational-affective (depression and anxiety) and cognitive evaluative (thoughts on pain's cause and significance). Recognising psychological influences, this model acknowledged pain may not always relate to tissue damage, impacting mental wellbeing. Pain's sensory-discriminative role is evolutionary, signalling potential harm. Avoidance of pain is instinctive, seen throughout the lifespan, such as the recoiling response to pain in the newborn age. Controlling and managing pain requires understanding its occurrence and pathophysiological regulation (Craft et al 2023).

Although the mechanism of the physiology and psychology of pain is not fully understood, several theories of pain process have been put forward. The leading theory is the gate control theory developed by Melzack and Wall in 1965. The **gate control theory** of pain suggests that neural mechanisms in the dorsal horns of the spinal cord can act like 'gates', which control transmission of pain impulses to the brain and, ultimately, the perception of pain. The activity of large diameter nerve fibres can close the gate and block pain impulses, resulting in a decrease or elimination of pain sensation. According to this theory, it is possible to block pain impulses travelling to the brain by stimulating the large 'A' nerve fibres that 'close the gate'. This theory may help to explain why rubbing on an injury can relieve pain, exploring that the stimulation of non-painful nerve fibres can 'confuse' messages and suppress pain signals (Crisp et al 2021).

Pain can be inhibited along the course of transmission of the signals to the brain. To achieve this, peripheral tissues connect to the cerebral cortex through a three-neuronal pain pathway (Figure 33.1 and Figure 33.2). The first-order neuron carries information from the periphery to the spinal cord, synapsing with the second-order neuron. The second-order neuron transmits information to various brain sites, including the thalamus. Autonomic nervous system responses are triggered, but conscious perception of tissue damage occurs via the third-order neuron, relaying information to the cerebral cortex. This ensures widespread connectivity to the cerebral cortex, where conscious awareness of pain occurs (Craft et al 2023).

In addition to neural pathways, various substances can influence pain pathways collectively known as neuromodulators.

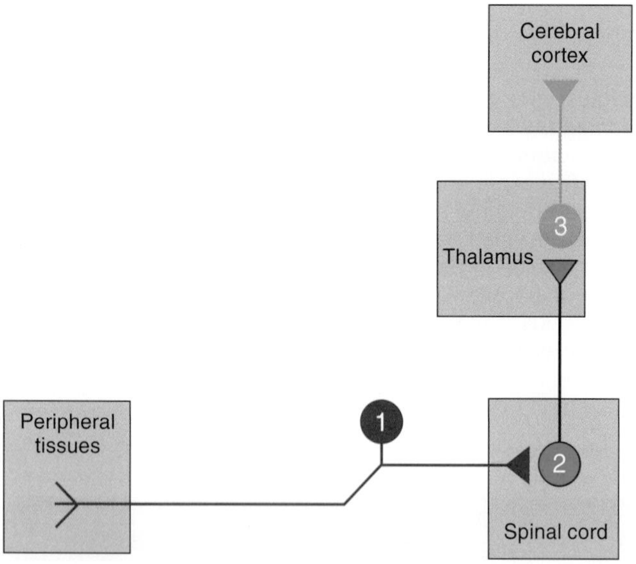

Figure 33.1 The transmission of pain
(Craft et al 2023)

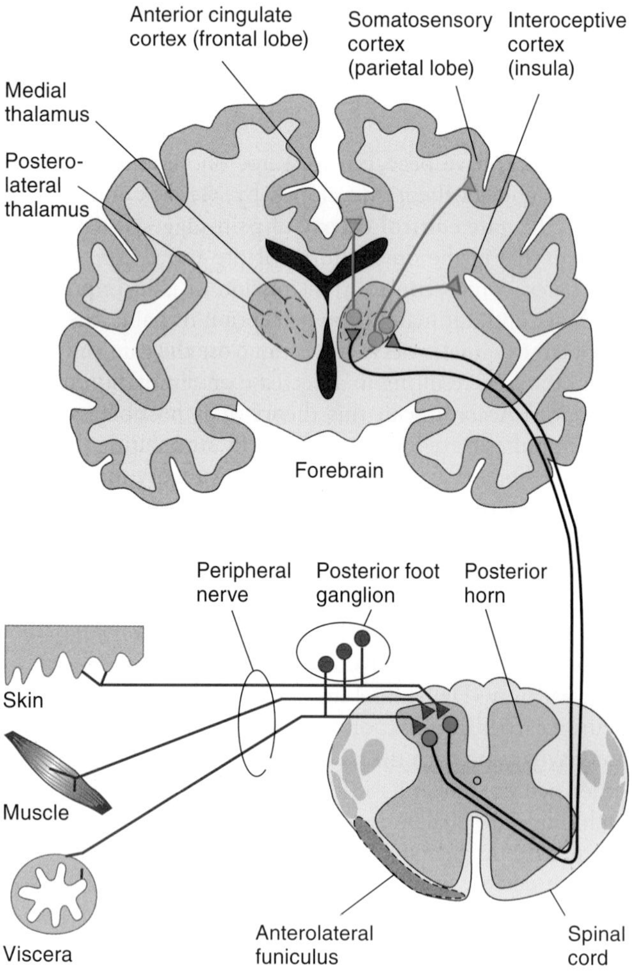

Figure 33.2 The transmission of pain
(Craft et al 2023)

These substances, distinct from neurotransmitters, are released by neurons and alter the activities of other neurons in the pathways that convey information about painful stimuli throughout the nervous system. An example of a neuromodulator is endorphins (Craft et al 2023). **Endorphins** inhibit pain in the spinal cord and brain, by binding to opioid receptors which combine with the same receptors as morphine and other opioids to produce the analgesic effect (Knights et al 2023). They act as neurotransmitters that mediate the transmission of pain information between nerve fibres. As a result of pain or stress, an impulse from the brain may trigger the release of endorphins from pain-inhibiting neurons in the dorsal horn, which block transmission of the pain impulse before it reaches the brain (Figure 33.3).

> **CRITICAL THINKING EXERCISE 33.1**
>
> Explain the pathophysiology of why some individuals may not experience pain, for example a person with diabetic peripheral neuropathy, and what this may mean for their perception of actual or potential tissue damage.

Classification of pain

There are two major classifications of pain: acute pain and chronic pain. This is based upon the duration of the pain's presence. There are also a variety of types and subtypes of pain categorised based on their pathology and generation: nociceptive, neuropathic and nociplastic pain (see Table 33.1). These types include both classifications of acute and chronic pain.

Acute pain is the sudden, time-limited pain of varying intensity. It is often perceived as severe, with precise location and description. It may arise from injury, infection or surgery and includes conditions like postoperative pain, burns and trauma. Mild cases may require no intervention, while more severe pain can be successfully managed.

Chronic pain is defined as persistent pain lasting 3 months or more. It is often resistant to natural resolution or intervention, and no longer signals imminent danger or tissue damage. Chronic pain includes both pain associated with cancer and non-cancer pain, such as migraine or phantom pain (Crisp et al 2021). Chronic pain can be difficult to manage, as it may include an overlap of nociceptive, neuropathic and/or nociplastic pain.

Before assessing pain, it is important the nurse addresses their own biases and misconceptions about the experience of pain (Clinical Interest Box 33.1). Two people with the same pathophysiology may have very different experiences of pain, due to differences with how pain is expressed culturally, socially and across the lifespan. (See Table 33.2.)

Nurses, having continuous proximity to individuals around the clock, play a pivotal role in the diagnosis and treatment of pain. Given the subjective nature of pain,

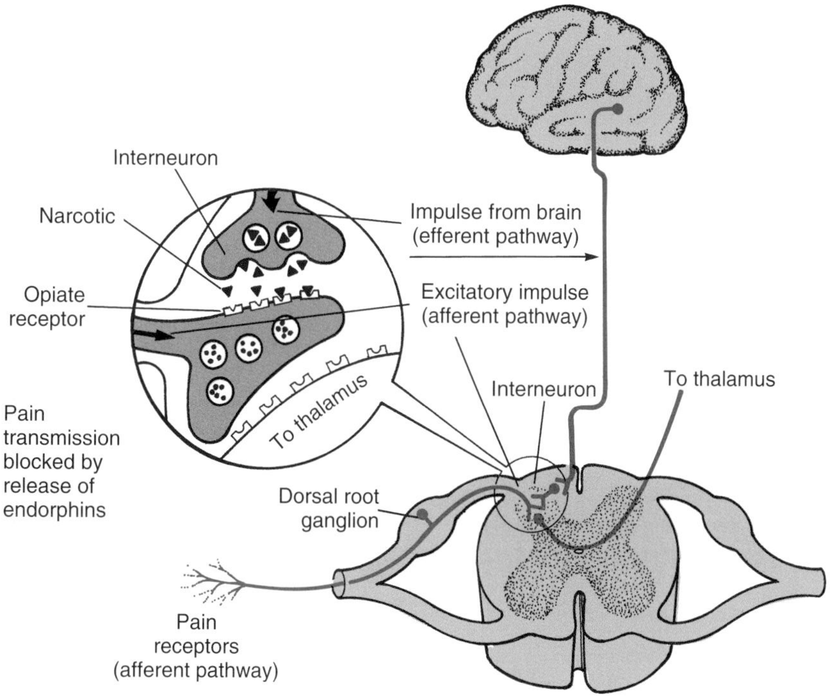

Figure 33.3 Modulation of pain by endorphins
(Craft et al 2023)

TABLE 33.1 | Classification of pain based on pathophysiology

Type of pain	Pathophysiology
Nociceptive	*Nociceptive (physiological) pain* is sustained by activation of the sensory systems that process noxious stimuli. It is the result of actual or potential damage to somatic or visceral tissues sufficient to activate the pain transmission process. Examples include pain associated with trauma, surgery, burns and tumour growth. Pain impulses, whether fast or slow, reach the dorsal root ganglia, synapsing with neurons in the grey matter's posterior horns. These sensations then travel to the brain via the thalamus, where they are perceived and interpreted. (See Figure 33.2.) *Somatic pain* occurs when pain receptors in tissues (including the skin, muscles, skeleton, joints and connective tissues) are activated. Typically, stimuli such as force, temperature, vibration or swelling activate these receptors. This type of pain is often described as sharp or gnawing. *Visceral pain* describes pain emanating from the internal thoracic, pelvic or abdominal organs. Unlike somatic pain, visceral pain is generally vague, poorly localised, and characterised by hypersensitivity to a stimulus such as organ distension. This type of pain is often described as dull or aching. *Referred pain* is typically pain felt in a part of the body other than its actual source, due to nerve root distribution, such as the shoulder pain associated with cardiac conditions. (See Figure 33.4.)
Neuropathic	*Neuropathic (pathophysiological) pain* is sustained by a lesion or disease of the central or peripheral nervous system. Neuropathic pain is caused by abnormal processing of stimuli. Neuropathic pain problems are common in diseases affecting the nervous system, such as diabetes mellitus, herpes zoster and multiple sclerosis. It may also result from surgery and/or trauma to nervous tissue. Individuals may present with symptoms of neuropathic pain without an objective cause. The pain may be difficult for the individual to describe, but common symptoms are qualities such as shooting or burning, numbness, pain in response to light touch and increased sensitivity to pain. *Neuralgic pain* is pain in the distribution of a nerve or nerves. Typically described as shooting, stabbing or burning sensations. *Migraine pain* is often characterised by a throbbing or pounding feeling. Although they are frequently one-sided, they may occur anywhere on the head, neck and face—or all over. At their worst, they are typically associated with sensitivity to light, noise and/or smells. Sometimes can be preceded with warning signs (aura).

Continued

TABLE 33.1 | Classification of pain based on pathophysiology—cont'd

Type of pain	Pathophysiology
	Neuropathy is a disturbance of function or pathological change in a nerve, which may be associated with pain and/or numbness. *Phantom pain* is a pain sensation resulting from body parts that have been surgically removed.
Nociplastic	*Nociplastic pain* emerges from modified nociception without clear evidence of actual or threatened tissue damage activating peripheral nociceptors or a somatosensory or central/peripheral nervous system disease or lesion causing the pain. The individual may experience a combination of nociceptive, neuropathic and nociplastic pain simultaneously. This is very common after major surgery and with cancer pain.

(Berman et al 2020; Crisp et al 2021; IASP 2021)

CLINICAL INTEREST BOX 33.1 Common biases and misconceptions about pain

The following statements are false:

- Substance abusers and alcoholics overreact to discomforts.
- Individuals with minor illnesses have less pain than those with severe physical alteration.
- Administering analgesics regularly will lead to drug addiction.
- The amount of tissue damage in an injury can accurately indicate pain intensity.
- Healthcare personnel are the best authorities on the nature of an individual's pain.
- Nociplastic pain is not real.
- Chronic pain is psychological.
- Individuals should expect to have pain in hospital.
- Individuals who cannot speak do not feel pain.

(Crisp et al 2021)

TABLE 33.2 | Factors influencing the experience of pain

Factor	Rationale
Age	Infants and young children may not have their pain recognised due to a lack of verbal expression ability. Misconceptions, like the belief that infants do not feel pain, persist. Behavioural cues, such as facial activity and crying, indicate pain. Children may hide pain due to societal expectations, while older individuals might associate pain with the impact on their activities and goals, leading to increased anxiety. Tolerance for pain generally increases with age, influenced by societal expectations of 'adult' behaviour. Misconceptions also surround pain in older adults, particularly those with cognitive impairment, resulting in underestimation and under-management of pain, as seen in individuals with a diagnosis of dementia. Clinical Interest Box 33.2 provides more information about pain management in individuals with cognitive impairment.
Gender	Societal norms may have stereotypes regarding gender and pain. This is changing over time; however, it may still be seen. It is vital for the nurse to be aware of this and able to ask appropriate questions to enable comprehensive understanding of the individual's experience of pain.
Culture	Cultural values shape individuals' expression of pain. While in some cultures it is normal to adopt a stoic approach and conceal suffering, others openly express pain, seeking immediate relief. It is essential for the nurse to recognise that the nurse's own cultural norms regarding pain expression may be different to the individual's cultural norms and that this should not impact pain assessment and management.

TABLE 33.2 | Factors influencing the experience of pain—cont'd

Factor	Rationale
Emotional state	A person who is emotionally or physically exhausted often has a reduced capacity to tolerate pain. Individual resistance to, and control over, reactions to pain may be severely decreased. This is often a cyclical phenomenon; continual pain may lead to anxiety and fear, which exacerbates pain. Positive emotions usually decrease experienced pain. Attention, expectancy and appraisal can either increase or decrease pain experiences depending on their specific focus and content; this is why distraction techniques may assist in pain management.
Social support	The support of family, friends and caregivers significantly shapes pain experiences. Individuals in pain commonly rely on family or close friends for support, assistance or protection. While the pain may persist, the presence of a loved one can reduce feelings of loneliness and fear. This is especially important for individuals who may not be able to express their pain experiences, such as those with cognitive impairment or young children. Conversely, the absence of family or friends can intensify the stress associated with the pain experience. For children in pain, the presence of parents is particularly crucial since parents can contribute to pain assessment and treatment. Partners and caregivers, while eager to help manage their loved one's pain, may be unsure of their role and it is important for the nurse to guide caregivers. Insufficient support increases vulnerability and predisposes the individual to heightened stress and pain.
Time of the day	Night, with accompanying darkness and reduced sensory input (resulting in lack of distractions), often increases a person's sensation of pain. Fear and anxiety may be increased and, as a result, so too is the sensation of pain. The effects of pain-relieving medication may also be reduced overnight, depending on dosage and duration of efficacy.
Previous experience	Previous episodes of severe pain often cause great apprehension, and pain may be increased if individuals anticipate the recurrence of a previous experience of severe pain. Previous pain experience may at times be useful as a form of comparison when assessing a subsequent pain episode.

(Adapted from Crisp et al 2021)

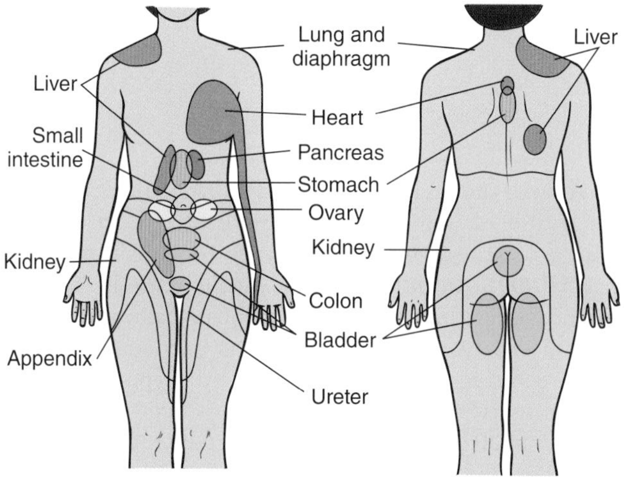

Figure 33.4 Referred pain sites: Cutaneous areas to which pain from certain viscera is referred
(Craft et al 2023)

CLINICAL INTEREST BOX 33.2 Pain management in individuals with cognitive impairment

Individuals with cognitive impairment experience pain equally to those without. Individuals with dementia and progressive deficits of cognition, particularly those in long-term care facilities, suffer significant unrelieved pain and discomfort, often due to poor assessment and management by caregivers.

Assessing pain in these individuals may require a different approach, such as the use of the faces pain scale (Figure 33.5) or Abbey Pain Scale (Figure 33.6) for those with a diagnosis of dementia.

(Crisp et al 2021)

nurses must be aware that it is a lived experience shaped by internal and external stimuli and the whole individual (Brown et al 2020). Nurses bear the responsibility of observing visible signs of pain, attentively listening to the individual's descriptions, and implementing preventative or treatment measures. They also monitor and report the effectiveness of prescribed pain management.

Assessing pain

Pain is the fifth vital sign, alongside classic vital signs such a blood pressure, pulse, respiration and temperature (Crisp et al 2021). Incomplete assessment of individuals leads to

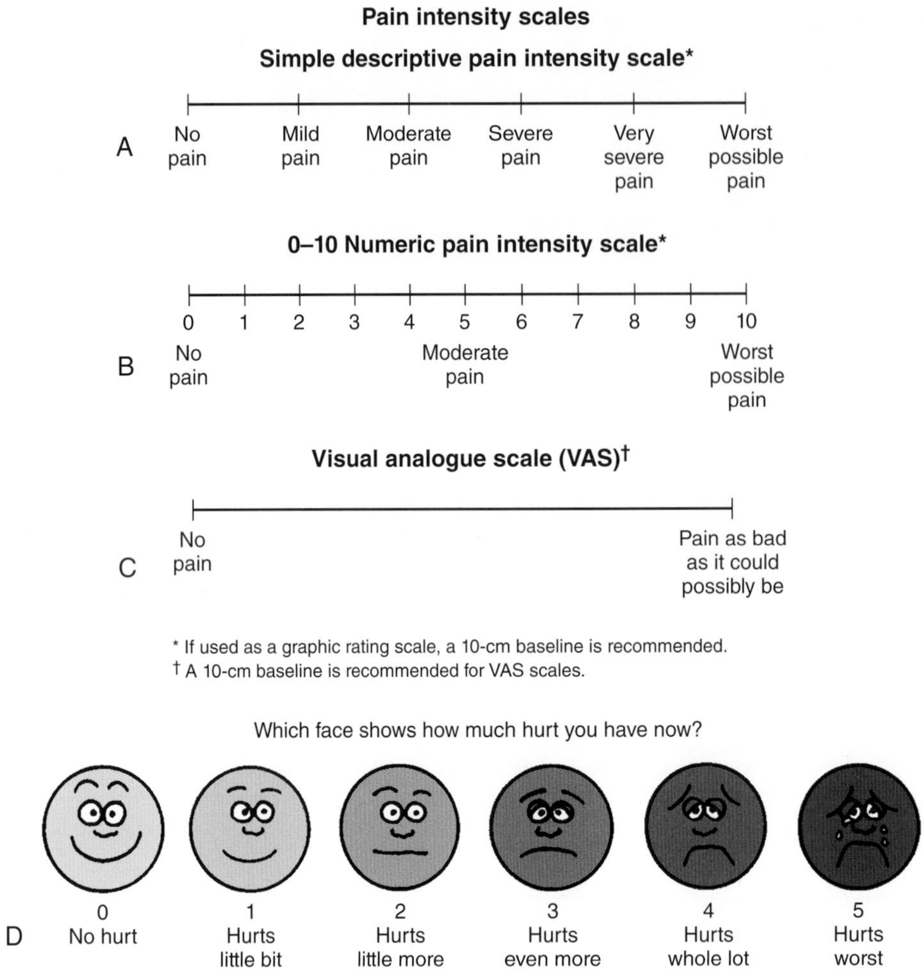

Figure 33.5 Scales for rating the intensity of pain

(Acute Pain Management Guideline Panel 1992)

inadequate pain management, which in turn interferes with the healing process.

The assessment process involves obtaining both subjective and objective data (Table 33.3 and Table 33.4). The data must be comprehensive, covering both the physiological and the behavioural manifestations of pain (Clinical Interest Box 33.3) (Crisp et al 2021). Assessment begins with a comprehensive pain history and use of the PQRST or PQRSTU mnemonic (Table 33.3) is recommended (Chang & Johnson 2022; Crisp et al 2021). This includes provoking/palliative factors, quality, region, and radiation, severity and temporal pattern (onset, duration and pattern). The questions must be designed to enable the individual to describe the pain in their own words. In circumstances when individuals cannot describe their pain, appropriate assessment questions and tools should be used. These circumstances could be younger children, language or cultural barriers and individuals with cognitive impairment (refer to Clinical Interest Box 33.2 and Clinical Interest Box 33.3).

A nurse should never ignore an individual's statement of pain and should remember that 'pain is what the person says it is', as described by McCaffery in 1968 (McCaffery & Pasero 1999). An individual can usually sense if the nurse does not believe that they are experiencing pain, and this can increase anxiety. Therefore, the person may compensate by under-reporting pain or by anxiously over-reporting. Either reaction aggravates the cycle of mistrust–anxiety–more pain (Crisp et al 2021). When assessing an individual's pain, the nurse should obtain sufficient and appropriate information through observation, questioning and conducting a physical examination. (See Case Study 33.1, Nursing Care Plan 33.1 and Progress Note 33.1.) (See also Clinical Skill 33.1.)

CRITICAL THINKING EXERCISE 33.2

Discuss the rationale for ensuring that pain assessment is undertaken in a non-judgmental manner.

Place identification label here

Name: ....
DOB: ....
Room No: ....

ABBEY PAIN SCALE

For measurement of pain in people with dementia who cannot verbalise

How to use scale: While observing the resident, score questions 1 to 6.

Name of person completing the scale:..
Date: .... Time: .... Designation:....................................
Latest pain relief given was .... at .... hrs.

Q1 Vocalisation **Q1** ☐
(e.g. whimpering, groaning, crying)
Absent 0 Mild 1 Moderate 2 Severe 3

Q2 Facial expression **Q2** ☐
(e.g. looking tense, frowning, grimacing, looking frightened)
Absent 0 Mild 1 Moderate 2 Severe 3

Q3 Change in body language **Q3** ☐
(e.g. fidgeting, rocking, guarding part of body, withdrawn)
Absent 0 Mild 1 Moderate 2 Severe 3

Q4 Behavioural change **Q4** ☐
(e.g. increased confusion, refusing to eat, alteration in usual patterns)
Absent 0 Mild 1 Moderate 2 Severe 3

Q5 Physiological change **Q5** ☐
(e.g. temperature, pulse or blood pressure outside normal limits, perspiring, flushing or pallor)
Absent 0 Mild 1 Moderate 2 Severe 3

Q6 Physical changes **Q6** ☐
(e.g. skin tears, pressure areas, arthritis, contractures, previous injuries)
Absent 0 Mild 1 Moderate 2 Severe 3

Add scores for 1–6 and record here **Total Pain Score** ☐

Now tick the box that matches the Total Pain Score

0–2 No pain	3–7 Mild	8–13 Moderate	14+ Severe

Finally tick the box which matches the type of pain

Chronic	Acute	Acute on Chronic

Abbey, J; Do Bellis, A; Piller, N; Esterman, A; Giles, I; Parker, D and Lowcay, B.
Funded by the JH & JD Gunn M Medical Research Foundation 1998–2002
(This document may be reproduced with this acknowledgement retained)
Taken from: www.health.gov.au/acc/reports/download/

Figure 33.6 The Abbey Pain Scale
(Abbey et al 2004)

Pain assessment tools

There are a variety of **pain assessment tools** used for individuals across the lifespan (Figures 33.5, 33.6 and 33.7). The aim of these tools is to standardise and objectify assessment. These tools include:

- pain intensity scale (Figure 33.5A)
- pain distress scale (Figure 33.5B)
- facial pain scale for children (Figure 33.5C)
- facial pain scale for adults (Figure 33.5D)
- Abbey Pain Scale (Figure 33.6)
- FLACC (Faces, Legs, Activity, Cry & Consolability) (see Figure 33.7).

To manage pain effectively, an understanding of the classification of pain is important. The taxonomy of pain and pain syndromes has continued to increase and evolve over recent decades (IASP 2021).

TABLE 33.3 | Assessing pain—subjective data

SUBJECTIVE DATA

Domain	Assessment questions	Rationale
Pain history	PQRSTU	PQRSTU is a simple mnemonic to remember when obtaining a pain history. PQRSTU identifies the nature, source and aggravating factors of pain and what is beneficial to the person in reducing this discomfort.
	P—Provoking/Palliative *What were you doing when the pain started?* *What makes the pain worse?* *Is there something that helps relieve the pain?* *What caused it?*	It is imperative to understand the person's perspective on their pain. It is important the nurse understands what the cause or aggravating factors are and what helps to reduce this discomfort.
	Q—Quality *What does the pain feel like? Try to describe it in your own words.*	It is important the nurse understands from the individual's own words what it feels like. Some words that may be used by the individual include gripping, knife-like, burning, prickling, tingling, dull, ache, cramping, throbbing, stabbing, shooting etc ...
	R—Region/Radiation *Where is the pain located?* *Does the pain travel anywhere else?* *Do you feel it is related to any other pain? If so, tell me more.*	The nurse is required to understand exactly where the pain of the individual is located. It may be demonstrated through words or pointing to oneself. Does the pain travel to anywhere else in the body?
	S—Severity *How severe is the pain?* *Can you rate the pain from 0–10 (use a numerical scale or faces scale or any other tool that is appropriate for the individual)* Use the assessment scales here (e.g. NRS, VAS, Abbey Pain Scale etc.) (Refer to Figure 33.6 and Figure 33.7.)	Understanding the level of pain directly from the person enables the nurse to plan management and implement appropriate interventions. Body language and facial expressions can also be a good indicator.
	T—Time (onset, duration and pattern) *When did the pain start?* *How long has the pain been present?* *Is the pain consistent or intermittent?*	This is important for the nurse to understand further detail about whether the pain is an acute or chronic concern for the individual.
	U—Understanding *How does the pain affect you?* *What treatments have been tried?* *What is the goal of treatment?*	The nurse needs to assess what the individual understands about their own attitudes and beliefs towards pain, treatment options and overarching goals of management of pain. This provides important information to enable relevant, realistic and appropriate education.
Medication history	*What medication have you currently taken to treat the pain? Has it been effective?* *What medications are you currently taking? Any over-the-counter vitamins or supplements?* *Have you been prescribed medications in the past to treat this pain? Is it different to the current medication? Is it helpful?*	Asking these questions provides invaluable information about what has previously and currently worked/not worked for the person. The information obtained can shape the treatment and management plan.

TABLE 33.3 | Assessing pain—subjective data—cont'd

Cognitive dimensions	*Is the individual cognitively impaired?* *What are the beliefs of the individual related to pain?* *Does the person have any reason preventing them from treating their pain?* *What is the meaning of the pain for the person?*	A person's self-perception can influence a reaction to pain. For example, gender stereotypes, cognitive impairments and personal beliefs may distort their perception of pain and influence their ability to verbalise this to the nurse.
Psychological status	*How is the individual coping with the pain? Is there any functional impairment from the pain?* *What are your expectations of the pain and treatment plan? Is this realistic and achievable?*	It is important for the nurse to understand the current and previous coping mechanisms to pain. Also understand the expectations of the individual's pain and consequently their goal of pain management. For example, post-surgery, a person may expect to have severe pain, but an expectation of zero pain after analgesia may be unrealistic. Therefore, it is vital for nurses to assist the person to set realistic expectations.
Social and family history	*What are the social pressures?* *How is the pain affecting the social role of the individual?* *Does the individual have any support from the family?* *How is the family coping?*	Assessment should include whether the pain interferes with lifestyle or the performance of any activities of daily living (e.g. does it affect the ability to eat, move freely or sleep?). Are roles and relationships being affected in a significant way by the pain being experienced?
Cultural and spiritual aspects	*What is the cultural background?* *What gives meaning to the individual?* *How does this help during the painful experience?*	Cultural values, attitudes and feelings contribute to the way people react to pain. Some people have a matter-of-fact attitude to pain, with little outward expression of their suffering, while others are more expressive and seek immediate pain relief. Various cultures have differences in their expression and management of pain.

(Adapted from Brown et al 2020; Crisp et al 2021)

TABLE 33.4 | Assessing pain—objective data

OBJECTIVE DATA

Domain	Rationale
Vital signs	The individual's temperature, pulse, respirations, oxygen saturations and blood pressure should be measured when pain is experienced and regularly reviewed. Any abnormal finding should be reported to the appropriate healthcare professional. When acute pain occurs, the autonomic response is activated—every individual responds differently—but this could potentially cause: • Heart rate increase • Blood pressure rise • Breathing becoming rapid and shallow.
Physical examination	A head-to-toe assessment using inspection, auscultation, palpation and percussion is warranted to assess the location and type of the pain. This provides an overall picture of the pain status of the person. It can also be used to determine if other interventions are an issue. • Muscles tense. • Blood flow to the hands and feet is constricted, and they become cold. • The skin becomes pale and sweaty. • Nausea and vomiting may occur.
Investigations	The medical practitioner may order further investigations to help diagnose the source of pain. This may include pathology or medical imaging.

(Adapted from Brown et al 2020; Crisp et al 2021)

CLINICAL INTEREST BOX 33.3 Behavioural indicators of effects of pain

Vocalisations

- Sighing, groaning, moaning
- Grunting, screaming, calling out
- Aggressive/offensive speech
- Noisy breathing
- Asking for assistance

Facial expressions

- Frowning, sad or frightened face
- Grimacing, wincing, eye tightening
- Distorted facial expressions—brow raising/lowering, cheek raising, nose wrinkling, lip corner pulling
- Rapid blinking

Body movement

- Tense posture, guarded, rigid
- Fidgeting
- Pacing, rocking or repetitive movements
- Reduced or restricted movement
- Altered gait

Social interaction

- Aggressive or disruptive behaviour
- Socially inappropriate behaviour
- Decreased social interactions
- Withdrawn

Changes in activities

- Appetite change, refusing food
- Increase in rest periods
- Sleep or rest pattern changes
- Increased wandering

(Schofield 2018)

PAIN MANAGEMENT ACROSS THE LIFESPAN

Pain management encompasses the application of non-pharmacological or pharmacological nursing interventions to holistically address discomfort and enhance the quality of life for individuals. It requires vigilant monitoring through a multidisciplinary approach, emphasising that it goes beyond the simple administration of prescribed analgesics (Brown et al 2020). The primary objective is to minimise pain, thereby enhancing overall quality of life and functional wellbeing. In palliative care (see Chapter 38), pain management is critical and allows individuals to experience a good quality of life while living with a terminal diagnosis and to die with dignity as their condition progresses.

Pain management involves addressing the underlying disease, managing symptoms, and utilising both non-pharmacological and pharmacological therapies. The nurse

CASE STUDY 33.1

Mrs Corowa, 86 years old, is an Aboriginal and Torres Strait Islander woman. Two months ago, her family decided to move her into an aged-care home since they could no longer care for her in the home. The facility is called ACES and is dedicated to Aboriginal and Torres Strait Islander cultured individuals. Mrs Corowa has a medical history of dementia, uncontrolled type 2 diabetes mellitus, osteoarthritis and rheumatic heart disease. Chronic pain is a major ongoing issue for her, and she is not inclined to take medication.

Describe the assessment and management of Mrs Corowa's pain.

NURSING CARE PLAN 33.1

Assessment: Mrs Corowa is 86 and is an Aboriginal and Torres Strait Islander woman. She recently moved into the aged-care home. She is very close to her family and is experiencing sadness and loneliness. She has a medical history of dementia (severely progressed), uncontrolled type 2 diabetes mellitus, osteoarthritis, and rheumatic heart disease. Chronic pain is a major issue for her.

Issue/s to be addressed:

- Chronic pain, related to joint inflammation, from osteoarthritis.
- Impaired functionality, ADL's and mobility related to dementia and osteoarthritis.
- Activity intolerance, related to the chronic pain, osteoarthritis and dementia.
- Glucose management, due to type 2 diabetes mellitus.

Goal/s:

- Effective pain management.
- Minimise joint stress with ADLs.
- Increase glucose control.

Continued

NURSING CARE PLAN 33.1—cont'd

Care/actions	Rationale
Assess (physical and psychosocial) client including vital signs, pain, and BGL reading, and pathology testing (including liver function test and renal function test).	Obtain baseline and understanding for the health concerns. Enables an appropriate management plan to be determined.
Assess the level of pain using the Abbey Pain Scale regularly throughout the day.	Due to the diagnosis of dementia, age, and minimal English, the Abbey Pain Scale enables the nurse to assess pain level and then treat appropriately.
Schedule paracetamol osteo at equal intervals (TDS) throughout the day.	Aids to provide underlying analgesia. Helping pain management.
Plan for PRN analgesia.	In case pain intensifies, need to have additional and stronger analgesic to be given as required.
Regularly revise positioning.	Repositioning is important to prevent pressure ulcers/sores, which further pain. Also used to minimise acute episodes of pain.
Performing gentle range of motion (ROM) exercises in shower or bathtub.	Reduces joint stiffness by allowing heat to relax the muscles and joints.
Apply local heat; use cold packs as needed.	Reduces pain and increases joint mobility.
Provide information about the Arthritis Foundation of Australia to the family.	Family is key to Aboriginal and Torres Strait Islander culture, and their involvement aids communication with the person as well as treatment decision-making.
Provide information about the disease process and its manifestations, prescribed medications with desired and adverse effects, and the importance of balancing rest and activity.	Empowers the individual and the family.

Evaluation: Verbalises effective pain management strategies.
Uses assistive devices to minimise joint stress with ADLs.
Verbalises a plan to reduce responsibilities for home maintenance.
Expresses a willingness to plan rest breaks during the day.
Demonstrates understanding of the prescribed therapeutic regimen and its importance for both short- and long-term benefit.

should also evaluate lifespan issues when managing pain. Older adults may experience many painful conditions such as neoplasms, injuries and other external causes, and diseases of the musculoskeletal and connective tissues systems. Older adults often have decreased renal function with a reduced creatinine clearance rate, resulting in a longer elimination half-life of analgesic medications. Some older adults believe that pain is a normal process of ageing and is something they must learn to accept as normal. Treatment of pain in pregnant women requires consultation with the clinical pharmacist to consider both the mother and baby (Sole et al 2021). Preparing the child/young person is an important part of undertaking a painful procedure. Play therapists can help prepare children/young people for procedures and support the healthcare team (Glasper et al 2021).

Nursing interventions include minimising stimuli causing or contributing to pain, providing supportive care and assisting individuals in self-managing pain. Importantly, even the simple act of providing information and explanations can significantly empower individuals in feeling more in control of their pain management situation (Craft et al 2023).

Barriers to effective pain management

There are multiple barriers to adequate pain management—these place individuals at risk of under-treatment. Individuals recognised to be at risk are those in the extremes of age (i.e. children and the elderly), individuals with psychiatric disorders, people with a cognitive impairment, individuals with a history of past or current substance use/misuse and those with a diagnosis of chronic pain. The perception of pain is individual and is different for each person. Table 33.2 outlines the factors that can influence the experience of pain.

CLINICAL SKILL 33.1 Focused pain assessment

Please adhere to the policy and procedures of the facility/organisation prior to undertaking the skill. Ensure this skill is in your scope of practice.

NMBA Decision-making Framework considerations (refer to NMBA Decision-making framework for nursing and midwifery 2020):

1. Am I educated?
2. Am I authorised?
3. Am I competent?

If you answer 'no' to any of these, do not perform that activity. Seek guidance and support from your teacher/a nurse team leader/clinical facilitator/educator.

Equipment:

Appropriate pain assessment scale such as:
- Pain intensity scale
- Pain distress scale
- Visual analogue scale (VAS)
- Facial pain scale
- FLACC
- Abbey Pain Scale

Vital sign equipment:
- Sphygmomanometer
- Pulse oximeter
- Thermometer probe

PREPARE FOR THE SKILL

(Please refer to the Standard Steps on pp. xviii–xx for related rationales.)
Mentally review the steps of the skill.
Discuss the skill with your instructor/supervisor/team leader, if required.
Confirm correct facility/organisation policy/safe operating procedures.
Validate the order in the individual's record.
Identify indication and rationale for performing the activity.
Assess for any contraindications.
Locate and gather equipment.
Perform hand hygiene.
Ensure therapeutic interaction.
Identify the individual using three individual identifiers.
Gain the individual's consent.
Assess for pain relief.
Prepare the environment.
Provide and maintain privacy.
Assist the individual to assume an appropriate position of comfort.

Skill activity	Rationale
Collate known history from healthcare record (including paper based and/or electronic records) including: • Pain history & correlated BP, HR, RR, SaO_2 and temperature • Recent invasive procedures (e.g. blood tests, surgery) • Current medical conditions and comorbidities (including cognitive capabilities) • Person's previous response to analgesia (both pharmaceutical and non-pharmaceutical).	Subjective and objective data identify key information to focus your pain assessment and enable safe guidance with effective dosing of pain medication and implementation of non-pharmacological pain-management interventions. It can provide baseline information and the bigger picture of the person's health status.
Verify the indication for the pain assessment including selecting the most appropriate pain tool. This may take into consideration person's age, culture and language/cognition.	It is important that the nurse understands why the individual is receiving this assessment and uses the most appropriate tool to achieve the most accurate data.

PERFORM THE SKILL

(Please refer to the Standard Steps on pp. xviii–xx for related rationales.)
Perform hand hygiene.
Apply PPE: gloves, eyewear, mask and gown as appropriate.
Ensure the individual's safety and comfort throughout skill.
Promote independence and involvement of the individual if possible and/or appropriate.

CLINICAL SKILL 33.1 Focused pain assessment—cont'd

Assess the individual's tolerance to the skill throughout.
Dispose of used supplies, equipment, waste and sharps appropriately.
Remove PPE and discard or store appropriately.
Perform hand hygiene.

Skill activity	Rationale
Assess person, family and caregiver knowledge of health including: • Prior experience with pain • Prior experience with pain management • Understanding and feelings about completing this assessment.	Ensures that the person, family and/or caregiver have the capacity to gather, communicate, process and understand health information. Reveals any clarification, instructions and/or supports required.
Conduct a pain history, assessing each of the following characteristics of the pain using the PQRSTU mnemonic: **P—Provoking/Palliative** *What were you doing when the pain started?* *What makes the pain worse?* *Is there something that helps relieve the pain?* *What caused it?*	This is a simple mnemonic to remember when obtaining a pain history. PQRSTU identifies the nature, source and aggravating factors of pain and what is beneficial to the person in reducing this discomfort. It is important to understand the person's perspective on their pain.
Q—Quality *What does the pain feel like? Try to describe in own words.*	This information is helpful in understanding the underlying pain mechanism (e.g. neuropathic or nociceptive) and may assist in the type of pain treatment chosen. Some words that may be used by the individual include gripping, knife-like, burning, prickling, tingling, dull, ache, cramping, throbbing, stabbing, shooting etc.
R—Region/Radiation *Where is the pain located?* *Does the pain travel anywhere else?* *Do you feel it is related to any other pain? If so, tell me more.*	The location(s) and distribution of the pain are helpful in determining the pain mechanism. It may be demonstrated through words or pointing to oneself.
S—Severity *How severe is the pain?* *Can you rate the pain from 0–10? (Use a numerical scale or faces scale or any other tool that is appropriate for the individual.)* Use the assessment scales here (e.g. NRS, VAS, Abbey Pain Scale etc.).	Understanding the level of pain directly from the person enables the nurse to plan management and implement appropriate interventions. Body language and facial expressions can also be a good indicator.
T—Time (onset, duration, and pattern) *When did the pain start?* *How long has the pain been present?* *Is the pain consistent or intermittent?*	May provide further detail about whether the pain is acute or chronic and the pathophysiological background of the pain.
U—Understanding *How does the pain affect you?* *What treatments have been tried?* *What is the goal of treatment?*	Assesses what the individual understands about their own attitudes and beliefs towards: pain, treatment options and overarching goals of management of pain. Determines the success of other pain interventions. Provides important information to enable relevant, realistic and appropriate education.
When pain is self-reported, assess physical, behavioural and emotional signs and symptoms, including non-verbal indicators of pain: • moaning, crying, whimpering, groaning, vocalisations • decreased activity	Signs and symptoms may reveal source and nature of pain. Non-verbal responses to pain are useful in assessing pain in individuals who are cognitively impaired or unable to self-report.

Continued

CLINICAL SKILL 33.1 Focused pain assessment—cont'd

• facial expressions (e.g. grimace, clenched teeth) • change in usual behaviour (e.g. less active, irritable) • abnormal gait (e.g. shuffling) and posture (e.g. bent, leaning) • guarding a body part; functional impairment such as decreased range of motion (ROM) • diaphoresis • depression, hopelessness, anger, fear, social withdrawal • assess for decreased gastrointestinal (GI) motility, constipation, nausea and vomiting • assess for insomnia, anorexia and fatigue.	Experiencing pain may decrease opportunities to engage in activities, experiences or relationships, causing a negative affect that contributes to feelings of depression, hopelessness, anger, fear and social withdrawal. Constipation can occur with most pain medications; however, it is most common with opioid therapy. Co-occurrence of pain and insomnia or fatigue is common and is strongly associated with reduced functional ability.
Examine site of pain or discomfort when possible: inspect for discoloration, swelling or drainage; palpate for change in temperature, area of altered sensation, painful area or areas that trigger pain; assess range of motion of involved joints.	Reveals nature of pain and directs towards appropriate interventions.
Assess vital signs (objective data): • blood pressure • heart rate • respiratory rate • oxygen saturation • temperature.	Can indicate (while not always sensitive) the presence of pain and provide further insight to any other potential concerns underlying in the person. Also provides continuity to observe for trends over time.
Analyse and interpret the findings from the above assessment. Is intervention required? If so, discuss with the individual. Make an appropriate decision in conjunction with the person on what would be most beneficial for them: • pharmacological intervention • non-pharmacological intervention.	Based on the PQRSTU findings, and in conjunction with the person, decide the best course of management. Take into consideration allergens, previous responses to interventions and the severity/location of the pain.

AFTER THE SKILL

(Please refer to the Standard Steps on pp. xviii–xx for related rationales.)
Communicate outcome to the individual, any ongoing care and to report any complications.
Restore the environment.
Report, record and document assessment findings, details of the skill performed and the individual's response.
Report, record and document any abnormalities and/or inability to perform the skill.
Reassess the individual to ensure there are no adverse effects/events from the skill.

Skill activity	Rationale
Plan for next assessment of effectiveness of intervention, and pain assessment. For example, reassess pain level 30–60 mins post intervention. Provide education as needed.	It is important to continually reassess pain, to keep the person as comfortable as possible and determine if the chosen intervention is effective. Keeps individual informed and creates an opportunity to initiate education.

(Brown et al 2020; Crisp et al 2021; Rebeiro et al 2021)

Category	Score		
	0	**1**	**2**
Face	No particular expression or smile	Occasional grimace or frown, withdrawn, disinterested	Frequent-to-constant quivering chin, clenched jaw
Legs	Normal position or relaxed	Uneasy, restless, tense	Kicking, or legs drawn up
Activity	Lying quietly, normal position, moves easily	Squirming, shifting back and forth, tense	Arched, rigid, or jerking
Cry	No cry (awake or asleep)	Moans or whimpers, occasional complaint	Crying steadily, screams or sobs, or frequent complaints
Consolability	Content, relaxed	Reassured by occasional touching, hugging, or being talked to, distractible	Difficult to console or comfort

Each of the five categories–(F) Face, (L) Legs, (A) Activity, (C) Cry, (C) Consolability–is scored from 0–2, which results in a total score between 0 and 10.

Figure 33.7 FLACC scale for pain assessment used for paediatrics or cognitively impaired persons
(Workman & LaCharity 2024)

As the experience of pain is individual, some will express pain much earlier than others. All individuals have a similar sensation **threshold** to pain, but the ways in which different people react to pain may vary tremendously and many factors may be involved (Knights et al 2023; Rogers 2023). (See Figure 33.8.) The pain threshold is the point at which a stimulus, such as pressure, activates pain receptors and produces a sensation of pain (Brown et al 2020).

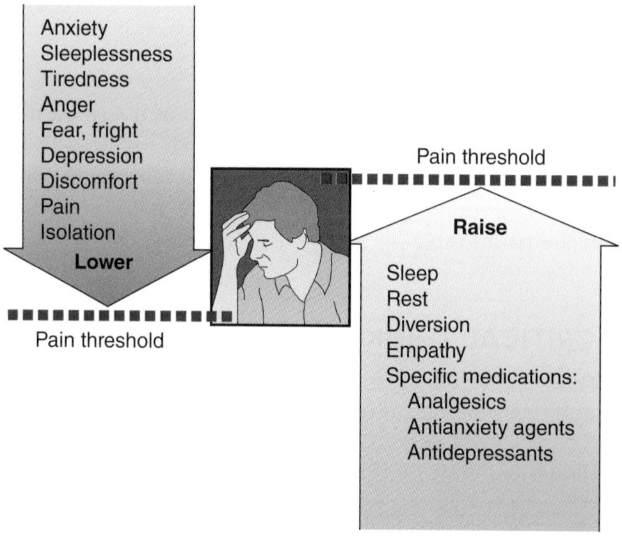

Figure 33.8 Factors that alter the pain threshold
(McKenry et al 2006)

NURSING INTERVENTIONS FOR AN INDIVIDUAL EXPERIENCING PAIN

The nurse has a responsibility to try to eliminate or minimise the stimulus (if present) that is causing pain. The nurse should also observe the individual who is experiencing pain, report and document their observations and implement nursing measures accordingly to alleviate pain. Continued assessment and monitoring of the individual is necessary to evaluate the effectiveness of any prescribed therapy (Brown et al 2020). Particular attention must be paid to individuals who cannot clearly articulate their needs or feelings, such as infants and small children and those with cognitive or communicative impairment (Crisp et al 2021). Pain management, both of a non-pharmacological and pharmacological nature, must be implemented and responses evaluated. The nurse also plays a role in supporting the individual's significant others who are usually distressed by the pain experience of their loved one, particularly when the pain is chronic or is a result of terminal illness.

The importance of clear and effective communication between the nurse and the individual and significant others cannot be overemphasised. A positive relationship facilitates effective communication, which can affect the individual's response to pain and pain relief. The individual should be encouraged to express feelings openly, in an atmosphere of trust. The nurse should learn to listen actively to the individual, so that not only the verbal interactions are heard but any non-verbal cues are also detected and acted on. For example, individuals may deny pain, or state that they are not experiencing much pain, but the body language and tone of voice may indicate otherwise. To promote peace of mind and to reduce anxiety, individuals should be provided with information about their illness, including expected pain and its management.

TABLE 33.5 | Nursing considerations for an individual receiving analgesics

Medication	Nursing considerations
Paracetamol	Nurses should make sure the dosage limits are maintained as paracetamol can cause liver toxicity. Nurses need to be mindful when dispensing and administering paracetamol since other medication may contain paracetamol within it (e.g. cold and flu tablets). Paracetamol is safe to use in pregnancy.
NSAIDs Salicylates (aspirin) Propionic acid derivatives (ibuprofen and naproxen) Acetic acid derivatives (indomethacin)	Medications must be given with food since they can cause gastrointestinal discomfort and ulcers. Care needs to be taken when used with gastrointestinal tract disorders and renal damage. Since these medications may reduce coagulation, nurses should monitor for signs of bleeding, especially with individuals who have a diagnosis of a bleeding disorder.
Opioid products (such as codeine, morphine, oxycodone)	Monitor vital signs regularly as these medications can cause respiratory depression, hypotension, bradycardia and changes to cognition such as drowsiness or euphoria. Nurses should also monitor bowels and encourage fluids and fibre since these medications typically cause constipation. Long-term use of these medications can be addictive and withdrawal symptoms can occur if they are suddenly stopped.

(Adapted from Knights et al 2023; Tiziani 2022)

Individuals have a right to pain relief and that various pain-relieving measures are available. It is important to prevent or reduce the cycle of pain–stress–anxiety–pain. A variety of nursing measures may help to minimise or alleviate pain (Table 33.5).

CRITICAL THINKING EXERCISE 33.3

Older individuals who live in supported care, such as aged-care homes, are among the most under-treated for pain. Why do you think this may occur? What can the nurse do to improve this situation?

Non-pharmacological therapy

Pain management may be achieved by a variety of non-pharmacological interventions, such as the use of heat or cold, massage and psychological methods.

Application of heat or cold

Typically, application of heat is for chronic pain, while application of cold is for acute injuries. Heat applied to the skin causes dilation of the local blood vessels and, as a result, may improve the blood supply to an area, relax muscles and relieve spasm, promote healing and relieve pain. Cold applications may also be used to relieve swelling and pain. Cold has a numbing effect by reducing blood flow (and histamines) to the area, which help to reduce pain. The use of heat and cold depends on the individual's preferences and hospital policy and, if used, should include education on potential risks and safe use (Brown et al 2020). Heat packs have been associated with burns, especially in individuals with altered sensation, such as peripheral neuropathy. The Therapeutic Goods Administration (TGA) advises consumers to follow manufacturer instructions and to use heat packs listed on the Australian Register of Therapeutic Goods (ARTG).

Change of position

At times pain can result from, or be increased by, an uncomfortable posture. The individual should be assisted into a more comfortable position, with appropriate pillows arranged for support. It is important to ensure that the individual's body is in alignment (where possible), and the placement of a pillow under a painful limb may further enhance comfort. Correct positioning should ensure that there is no stress on incisions, and no pressure is applied to any tubing or medical devices present (e.g. surgical drain tube, splints or urinary catheter). (See Chapter 28.)

Massage

Massage involves the manipulation of soft tissue to increase circulation, reduce muscle tension, relax the individual and relieve pain. Sensory stimulation may act to alter the individual's conscious awareness of pain, such as when an individual wriggles their toes when receiving a vaccination. Aromatherapy and massage using essential oils may also be of benefit in some situations. Soothing touch and gentle rocking motion to promote contact, warmth and closeness may help to soothe an infant in pain.

Psychological methods

Various techniques may be used to promote general relaxation and a state of calm with the individual. It is vital for the nurse to have knowledge on these techniques and educate the person with pain of its benefit and use. The most common of these techniques the nurse encourages is deep breathing exercises. This aids in slowing breathing down in a controlled rhythmic way. Distraction techniques such as music, television, prayer, puzzles and mindful colouring can lessen the focus on the pain, which in turn can reduce the severity.

Acupuncture

Acupuncture, which is a form of traditional Chinese medicine, involves the insertion of fine needles into the skin at selected points on the body. It may be used to manage both acute and chronic pain, and there are several theories about how it relieves pain. Acupuncture may provide analgesia by stimulating the release of endorphins or by stimulating the large diameter nerve fibres that effectively close the gate and block pain impulses (Amir et al 1980; Bowen et al 1987; Brown et al 2020; Knights et al 2023).

Transcutaneous electrical nerve stimulation

A specific technique of peripheral nerve stimulation, transcutaneous electrical nerve stimulation (TENS), involves the application of electrodes to trigger points on the skin. The electrodes are activated by a battery-powered device to produce a tingling or vibrating sensation in the painful area. The impulses block the transmission of pain impulses to the brain (Brown et al 2020; Knights et al 2023). TENS is regularly used in childbirth. It should not be used for individuals with cardiac pacemakers since it can interfere with pacemaker function.

CRITICAL THINKING EXERCISE 33.4

Discuss the rationale/benefits for use of non-pharmacological pain management strategies for:

1. a young child
2. an adolescent
3. an older adult.

Biofeedback

Biofeedback is a method that assists a person to become aware of, and subsequently to control, certain autonomic physiological responses, such as blood pressure, muscle tension and heart rate. Through concentration the individual can learn to control and modify these processes, which are normally involuntary. The technique of biofeedback is more effective when accompanied by other relaxation techniques, and words to reduce the person's experience of pain.

Placebo therapy

Placebo therapy involves the administration of inactive substances (such as lactose pills or sterile water) and may be effective for certain people in certain situations. It is thought that placebos relieve pain or other symptoms by causing the body to release endorphins, combined with an expectation that the treatment will be effective (McCaffery & Arnstein 2006). The use of placebos involves a degree of recipient deception and poses many ethical and moral problems (McCaffery & Arnstein 2006). Its use in mainstream pain management is limited and sometimes restricted to clinical trials and chronic pain management.

Pain clinics

People who experience chronic pain may be helped by attending a multidisciplinary pain clinic. Pain clinics tailor the use of pain medication for the individual and help individuals resume normal activities and restore a positive self-image. Management includes a thorough physical and psychological examination before a program is designed for the individual. The pain regimens are reviewed, side effects managed and potential new drugs trialled. It is a holistic approach to managing chronic pain. The individual may be taught alternative ways of carrying out ADLs so that associated pain is minimised.

Pharmacological therapy

Medications prescribed by a medical practitioner to relieve pain may be either local or systemic (e.g. anaesthetic), analgesic (e.g. morphine) or co-analgesic (e.g. corticosteroids). The use of medical cannabis for pain management is a recent development in most countries (see Clinical Interest Box 33.4). The nurse's role in relation to medication administration involves assessment and monitoring of individual responses to therapeutic treatments ordered. When medications have been prescribed, it may be within the nurse's scope of practice to administer them. Figure 33.9 is a flowchart for a standardised approach to pharmacological management of pain.

Nerve block

Peripheral nerve transmission of pain can be interrupted temporarily by the injection of a local anaesthetic (e.g. lignocaine), or permanently by injecting a sclerosing agent into the nerve root area. As the latter method can result in destruction of tissue adjacent to the injected area, other pain-relieving methods are usually preferred, with this being an option in cases when other pain-relieving methods have been unsuccessful.

Counter-irritants

Counter-irritants, such as mentholated ointments and heat rubs, applied locally to the skin, can produce a topical inflammatory response, thereby relieving inflammation in underlying tissues.

Radiotherapy and/or chemotherapy

The pain associated with malignant disease may be relieved by radiation, which shrinks a tumour that is actively causing compression in an area. Chemotherapy (also considered as pharmacological therapy) may sometimes control pain if the tumour is sensitive to the medications

CLINICAL INTEREST BOX 33.4 The use of medicinal cannabis (cannabinoid/CBD)

The use of medical cannabis for pain management is a recent development in most countries. In Australia, it was approved in 2016 and New Zealand 2017. Marijuana (the plant) has not been approved as a medicine and remains an illegal substance in many jurisdictions. However, the chemical cannaboids (derived from marijuana) have been approved for use in Australia (Crisp et al 2021). Prescribers need to be registered and approval for the use of cannabis needs to come from the Therapeutic Goods Administration (TGA). Each state's and territory's laws manage the prescribing, administration and storage of medicinal cannaboids. Nurses should ensure they are familiar with the requirements where they practise.

Medical cannabis has been found to be a beneficial option for chronic pain, neuropathic pain and cancer pain. A challenge with medicinal cannabis involves finding the appropriate dosage for analgesia. Therefore, it is recommended to commence at a low dose and titrate upward. Adverse effects of too high a dose include disorientation, vertigo and loss of coordination (Brown 2020; Knights et al 2023).

Cannabis may be directed for individuals where other medications are ineffective. It is medically indicated for use in chronic pain syndromes, migraine, opioid withdrawal and neurological diseases with painful spasticity such as stroke and multiple sclerosis. Individuals who require the use of cannabis typically commence treatment on low doses (Brown 2020).

Despite these medications being available through legal measures, there is evidence that many people continue to use illegal measures to access such medications. Reasons for this include the high financial cost and difficulties associated with discussing medicinal cannabis with health professionals (Crisp et al 2021). For this reason, a comprehensive history-taking by the nurse on admission, including asking the individual about the use of both prescribed and non-prescribed substances, is needed.

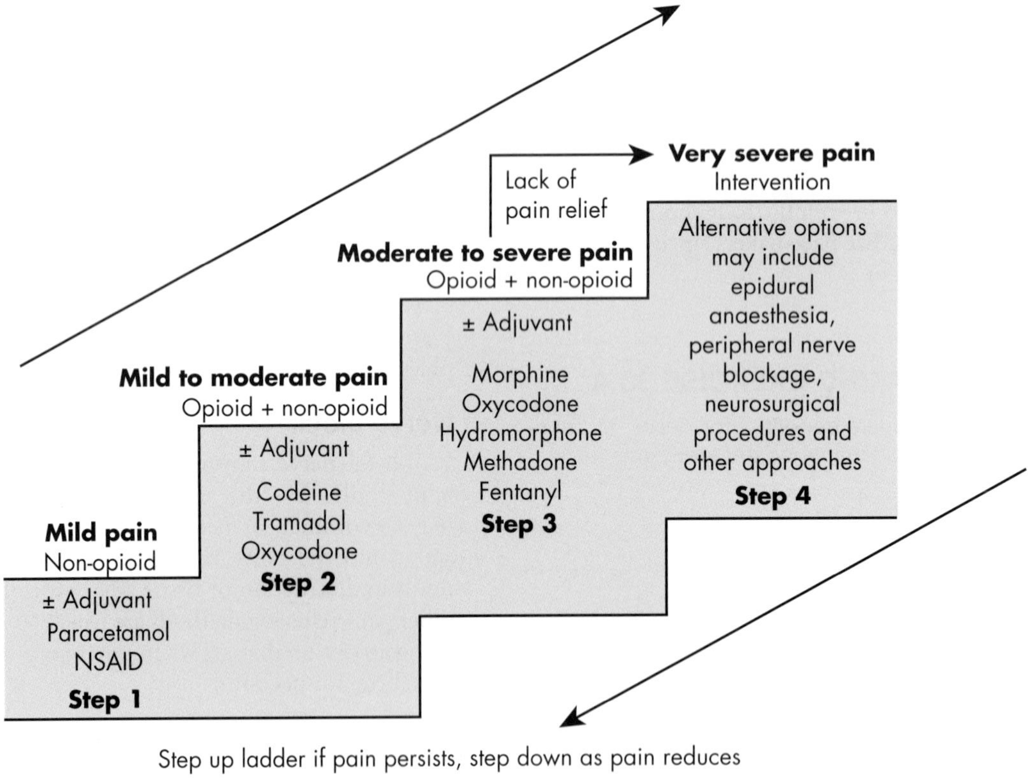

Figure 33.9 Flowchart for pharmacological management of pain
(Craft et al 2023)

used. Both radiation and chemotherapy may cause pain as a side effect of treatment (e.g. radiotherapy burns and mucositis). Because of these side effects, the use of these treatments requires a sensitive and person-tailored approach, and they may not be appropriate for all people or in all circumstances. Assessment and management of pain related to these treatments may be undertaken by the nurse, subject to their scope of practice.

Analgesic

Analgesic or pain-relieving medications may be mild (e.g. non-opioids such as acetylsalicylic acid [aspirin] or paracetamol) or strong (e.g. opioids such as morphine or oxycodone). Analgesics may be administered via several routes, including orally, by injection or infusion (intramuscularly, subcutaneously, intravenously or into the epidural space), or in some instances they may be applied topically (via creams or patches onto the skin) (see Chapter 20). The type, dosage and route of analgesic medications given will be prescribed by the medical practitioner according to the individual's needs. Good pain control, especially in postoperative and acute pain situations, is usually achieved by administering effective and appropriate medication at regular intervals, thus avoiding the experience of peaks and troughs of pain. In some cases, analgesia is ordered on a 'PRN' (as required) basis, which may be used for intermittent episodes of pain. Clinical Interest Box 33.5 provides a caution related to pain management in the older adult.

Analgesics are frequently given intravenously for severe pain, either as a bolus dose (a concentrated dose given in a short period of time) or as an infusion, which has the advantage of avoiding repeated injections and establishes a constant blood level of analgesic medication, thus avoiding considerable pain between doses. This can be done using an intravenous (IV) pump controlled by the individual (patient-controlled analgesia, or PCA) or a programmable pump with a catheter placed in the epidural space.

Patient-controlled analgesia (PCA) uses IV opioids and a programmable pump. A dose of medication is delivered each time the individual pushes a button, within limitations set by the medical practitioner. This allows the individual to choose how often and when to receive the medication, and often enables them to establish a greater sense of control over pain management.

Epidural analgesia is an alternative method of pain control that uses a fine catheter inserted into the epidural space of the spine, again connected to a programmable pump. This method of pain relief is effective in controlling pain while allowing the individual to remain alert. It is frequently used in obstetrics, postoperatively and, sometimes, in individuals with cancer. The primary responsibility of caring for individuals with either opioid or epidural infusions remains with the Registered Nurse (RN). Nonetheless, response to medications and evaluation of pain control measures are within the scope of practice of all nurses.

Co-analgesic medications, while not true analgesics in the pharmacological sense, act to augment pain relief, either alone or in combination with analgesics. Examples of medications that may be used as co-analgesics are corticosteroids and non-steroidal anti-inflammatory drugs (NSAIDs), both of which may act to decrease inflammation and oedema (Knights et al 2023). The use of anti-anxiety and anti-spasmodic medication may also be incorporated into a treatment plan. Sometimes a dose of co-analgesic medication together with an analgesic can produce greater pain relief than a higher dose of an analgesic alone. Table 33.5 outlines the nursing considerations for an individual receiving specific analgesics and Table 33.6 presents the actions of analgesics.

CLINICAL INTEREST BOX 33.5 Pain and the older adult

Pain is prevalent in older people and has significant debilitating outcomes. It is associated with decreased mobility, social isolation, frequent falls, insomnia and depression, among other manifestations. This is exacerbated by the existence of multiple comorbidities and polypharmacy. Therefore, nursing older people requires an understanding of the pharmacokinetics and pharmacodynamics of analgesics in older people and the careful monitoring of side effects. Older people are susceptible to confusion if given higher doses of opioids, for example.

(Knights et al 2023)

TABLE 33.6 | Action of analgesics

Drug category	Example	Site of action	Mechanism
Antipyretic	Paracetamol	Damaged cells	Decrease production of prostaglandins thereby reducing inflammation.
Non-steroidal anti-inflammatory drugs (NSAIDs)	Aspirin Ibuprofen Indomethacin Piroxicam Ketorolac Celecoxib	Damaged cells	Decrease production of prostaglandins thereby reducing inflammation.
Opioids	Codeine Pethidine Tramadol Oxycodone Morphine Fentanyl	Brain	Bind to natural endorphin stimulant receptor in the brain. This depresses pain perception.

Continued

TABLE 33.6 | Action of analgesics—cont'd

	Adjuvents		
Anaesthetics	Lignocaine Ketamine	Brain and peripheral nerve fibres	Block perception and transmission of pain.
Antidepressants	Amitriptyline Venlafaxine Fluoxetine	Brain	May reduce pain perception in some individuals.
Anticonvulsants	Carbamazepine Gabapentin Pregabalin	Brain	Block/modulate transmission of pain.
Antiemetics	Metoclopramide Ondansetron	Mainly brain but metoclo-pramide is also a prokinetic (promotes movement—e.g. GI tract)	Acute pain is associated with nausea and opioids can also cause nausea and vomiting.
Corticosteroid	Betamethasone Budesonide Dexamethasone Hydrocortisone	Depends on administration (systemic versus targeted)	Reduces inflammation.
Cannaboids (see Clinical Interest Box 33.4)	CBD oil (oral mucosa spray)	CNS	Acts on the endogenous cannaboidal system regulating GABA receptors.

(Adapted from Knights et al 2023; Tiziani 2022)

Progress Note 33.1

20/04/2024 1020 hrs

Nursing: Mrs Corowa is 86 and is an Aboriginal and Torres Strait Islander woman. She recently moved into the aged-care home. She is very close to her family and is experiencing sadness and loneliness. She is isolated and not engaged with other residents. This AM, she has presented as moderately confused and disoriented. Her BP is 160/87 mmHg, HR 88 beats/minute, RR 18 breaths/minute, SpO_2 95% on RA, Temp 36.5°C and BGL 11.5 (pre-breakfast). GCS 14/15, PEARL and pain assessed using Abbey Pain Scale equated to moderate level (13). Regular paracetamol osteo and PRN tramadol given as per medication chart. Heat packs were also applied, but due to her confused and disoriented status, was unable to keep in use. She uses a 4WF on exertion requiring assistance with ADLs. Her pathology results were within normal limits. Her children are planning to visit this PM. Nil other concerns identified.

S Stewart (STEWART), *EN*

DECISION-MAKING FRAMEWORK EXERCISE 33.1

You are an Enrolled Nurse who has just commenced working in the Greenslopes Hospice. You have been asked to assist Craig with his breakfast. You notice that Craig has medications sitting on his tray in a cup. Craig tells you they are his pain-relief tablets, and he likes to take them with his breakfast. He cannot take them on his own and asks you to assist him in taking them.

What action should you take? Use the decision-making framework to assist your decision, utilising the following headings:

1. Identify individual need/benefit.
2. Reflect on scope of practice and nursing practice standards.
3. Consider context of practice/organisational support.
4. Select appropriate, competent person to perform the activity.

Summary

Pain, which is often a protective signal of actual or impending tissue damage, can be both an unpleasant physical sensation and an emotional experience. Each episode of pain is unique and subjective, and it is important for the nurse to appreciate that 'pain is what the individual says it is'. Pain may be mild or severe, acute, or it may be chronic, physical or psychological.

Pain receptors transmit impulses along nerve fibres to the brain, where the impulses are received and interpreted. The body has some internal mechanisms that may be activated to help manage pain and its reaction, such as the gate control mechanism and the endorphin system.

The experience of pain varies with the individual; therefore, some people will experience pain much sooner and more intensely than others. Many factors influence an individual's reaction to pain, including age, gender, culture and emotional state, history of pain, the time of day and social support. Although everyone's behavioural reaction to pain is different, the physiological responses to acute pain are the same.

The nurse has a responsibility to assess an individual's pain in terms of site, time it occurs, duration, precipitating factors, type, intensity, associated signs and symptoms, body posture, vital signs and emotional state.

The management of pain includes non-pharmacological and pharmacological therapy and depends on the individual's needs. The nurse has a responsibility to minimise painful stimuli by planning, analysing and implementing supportive nursing measures.

Review Questions

1. What is pain?
2. What are the different types of pain?
3. Explain why individuals can feel pain in limbs that have been removed.
4. List potential nursing issues that could affect someone with chronic pain.
5. What are the nursing considerations for someone receiving an opioid medication?
6. What is the difference between paracetamol and aspirin? Explain the side effects of NSAIDs.
7. Why do we feel pain?
8. Explain why rubbing/massage can relieve pain.
9. If individuals experience nociplastic pain, should we dismiss it as attention seeking?
10. What would be the general psychosocial impact of chronic pain on a middle-aged individual?
11. How do age, gender and culture or background affect the individual's perception of pain?
12. What is the pain threshold?
13. How different would the perception of pain be in an individual who already suffers from chronic pain?
14. What is the appropriate assessment tool that could be used to assess:
    a. Children in pain?
    b. Adult individuals who do not speak English?
    c. An individual with dementia?

Evolve® Answer guide for the Review Questions, Critical Thinking Exercises, Decision-making Framework Exercises and Critical Thinking Questions in Case Studies is hosted on Evolve: http://evolve.elsevier.com/AU/Koutoukidis/Tabbner.

References

Abbey, J., Piller, N., DeBellis, A., et al., 2004. The Abbey Pain Scale. A 1-minute numerical indicator for people with late-stage dementia. *International Journal of Palliative Nursing* 10(1), 6–13.

Acute Pain Management Guideline Panel, 1992. Acute pain management in adults: Operative procedures: Quick reference guide for clinicians, AHCPR Pub No. 92-0019. Agency for Health Care Policy and Research, Rockville, MD.

Amir, S., Brown, Z.W., Amit, Z., 1980. The role of endorphins in stress: Evidence and speculations. *Neuroscience and Biobehavioral Reviews* 4, 77–86.

Berman, A., Snyder, S., Levett-Jones, T., et al., 2020. *Kozier and Erb's fundamentals of nursing*, 5th ed. Pearson Australia, Frenchs Forest.

Bowen, W.D., Hellewell, S.B., Kelemen, M., et al., 1987. Affinity labelling of delta-opiate receptors using (D-Ala2, Leu5, Cys6) enkephalin. Covalent attachment via thiol-disulfide exchange. *Journal of Biology Chemistry* 262, 13,434–13,439.

Brown, D., Edwards, H., Buckley, T., et al., 2020. *Lewis's medical-surgical nursing*, 5th ed. Elsevier, Sydney.

Chang, E., Johnson, A., 2022. *Living with chronic illness & disability: Principles for nursing practice*, 4th ed. Elsevier, Sydney.

Craft, J., Gordon, C., Heuther, S., et al., 2023. *Understanding pathophysiology*, 4th ed. Elsevier, Sydney.

Crisp, J., Douglas, C., Rebeiro, G., et al., 2021. *Potter and Perry's fundamentals of nursing*, 6th ed. Elsevier, Sydney.

Glasper, E., Richardson, J., Randall, D., 2021. *A textbook of children's and young people's nursing*, 3rd ed. Elsevier Limited.

International Association for the Study of Pain (IASP), 2021. IASP terminology—pain terms. Available at: <https://www.iasp-pain.org/Education/Content.aspx?ItemNumber=1698>.

Knights, K., Darroch, S., Rowland, A., et al., 2023. *Pharmacology for health professionals*, 6th ed. Elsevier, Sydney.

McCaffery, M., Arnstein, P., 2006. The debate over placebos in pain management. The ASPMN disagrees with a recent placebo position statement. *American Journal of Nursing* 106(2), 62–65.

McCaffery, M., Pasero, C., 1999. *Pain clinical manual*, 2nd ed. Mosby, St Louis.

McKenry, L., Tessier, E., Hogan, M., 2006. *Mosby's pharmacology in nursing*, 22nd ed. Mosby, St. Louis.

Melzack, R., Casey, K.L., 1968. Sensory, motivational, and central control determinants of pain: A new conceptual model. In: Kenshalo, D. (ed.), *The skin senses*. Charles C Thomas, Springfield, pp. 423–429.

Melzack, R., Wall, P., 1965. Pain mechanisms: A new theory. *Science* 150, 171–179.

Nursing and Midwifery Board of Australia (NMBA), 2020. Decision-making framework for nursing and midwifery. Available at: <https://www.nursingmidwiferyboard.gov.au/Codes-Guidelines-Statements/Frameworks.aspx>.

Rebeiro, G., Wilson, D., Fuller, S., 2021. *Fundamentals of nursing: Clinical skills workbook*, 4th ed. Elsevier, Chatswood.

Rogers, P., 2023. *McCance and Huether's pathophysiology*, 9th ed. Elsevier, St Louis.

Schofield, P., 2018. The assessment of pain in older people: UK national guidelines. *Age and Ageing* 47(1), i1–i22. doi: 10.1093/ageing/afx192.

Sole, M., Klein, D., Moseley, M., et al., 2021. *Introduction to critical care nursing*, 8th ed. Elsevier Inc.

Tiziani, A., 2022. *Havard's nursing guide to drugs*, 11th ed. Elsevier, Sydney.

Workman, M., LaCharity, L., 2024. *Understanding pharmacology: Essentials for medication safety*, 3rd ed. Elsevier Inc.

Recommended Reading

Australian Commission on Safety and Quality in Health Care (ACSQHC), 2022. Opioid analgesic stewardship in acute pain clinical care standard. Available at: <https://www.safetyandquality.gov.au/publications-and-resources/resource-library/opioid-analgesic-stewardship-acute-pain-clinical-care-standard-2022>.

Belvisi, M.G., Hele, D.J., 2009. Cough sensors. III. Opioid and cannabinoid receptors on vagal sensory nerves. *Handbook of Experimental Pharmacology* 187, 63–76.

Department of Health, 2019. National strategic action plan for pain management. Available at: <https://www.painaustralia.org.au/static/uploads/files/national-action-plan-11-06-2019-wfflaefbxbdy.pdf>.

Ford, C., 2019. Adult pain assessment and management. *British Journal of Nursing* 28(7). Available at: <https://www.britishjournalofnursing.com/content/clinical/adult-pain-assessment-and-management>.

Karch, M., 2017. *Focus on nursing pharmacology*, 7th ed. Lippincott Williams & Wilkins, Philadelphia.

Lynch, M., 2001. Pain: The fifth vital sign. Comprehensive assessment leads to proper treatment. *Advance Nurse Practitioner* 9(11), 28–36.

Marieb, E., 2019. *Human anatomy and physiology*, 11th ed. Benjamin Cummings, San Francisco.

Royal Children's Hospital, 2022. Pain assessment and management guidelines. Available at: <https://www.rch.org.au/rchcpg/hospital_clinical_guideline_index/Pain_assessment_and_measurement/#Pain%20Assessment%20Tool>.

Schug, S.A., Scott, D.A., Mott, J.F., et al., 2020. APM:SE Working Group of the Australian and New Zealand College of Anaesthetists and Faculty of Pain Medicine, Acute Pain Management: Scientific Evidence (5th ed), ANZCA & FPM, Melbourne.

Williams, P., 2021. *Fundamental concepts and skills for nursing*, 6th ed. WB Saunders, St Louis.

World Health Organization (WHO), 2019. WHO revision of pain management guidelines. Available at: <https://www.who.int/news/item/27-08-2019-who-revision-of-pain-management-guidelines>.

Online Resources

Australian Pain Management Association: <www.painmanagement.org.au>.

Australian Pain Society: <www.apsoc.org.au>.

Chronic Pain Australia: <www.chronicpainaustralia.org.au>.

International Association for the Study of Pain: <https://www.iasp-pain.org>.

Pain assessment tools: <https://www.caresearch.com.au/tabid/7464/Default.aspx>.

Pain Australia: <https://www.painaustralia.org.au>.

CHAPTER 34

Sensory health

Megan Christophers

Key Terms

ageusia
anosmia
cacogeusia
chemoreceptors
convergence
diplopia
dysgeusia
hyperopia
hypogeusia
hyposmia
myopia
nystagmus
otalgia
parosmia
presbycusis
presbyopia
proprioception
refraction
tinnitus

Learning Outcomes

At the completion of this chapter and with further reading, learners should be able to:

- Define the key terms.
- Describe the position and structure of each sense organ.
- Describe the physiology of taste, smell, sight and hearing.
- Describe the factors affecting sensory functions in the sense organs.
- Describe the major manifestations of disorders of the eye and ear.
- Describe diagnostic tests that may be used to assess eye and ear function.
- Plan and implement nursing care for the person with altered sensory function.

CHAPTER FOCUS

The sensory abilities of taste, smell, touch, sight and hearing enable the person to 'sense' changes in their external and internal environments. This is an essential requirement for maintaining homeostasis, so we can interact with the world around us (Patton & Thibodeau 2018). Perception of stimuli has its origin in the five special sense organs, which are adapted to receive specific stimuli: tongue (taste); nose (smell); skin (touch); eyes (sight); and ears (hearing and maintenance of balance). Receptors in the sensory organs pick up stimuli from the environment, which is known as sensory input. The information is transmitted to the brain via pathways in the nervous system. In the brain, the information is processed and interpreted in a process known as integration (Marieb & Keller 2021).

A person's senses are essential for growth, development and survival. A person can initiate protective reflexes only if they can see or sense a change or danger. Sensory stimuli give meaning to events in the environment. Alterations in sensory function may lead to dysfunctions of sight, hearing, smell, taste, balance or coordination.

Since the eyes and ears are the two major structures by which an individual receives information about the external environment, this chapter focuses on the care of these two organs. The eye is the means by which light is reflected from objects and travels to the retina so that an image is formed. Nerve endings in the retina transmit electrical impulses along the optic nerve to the brain for interpretation. The ear is the means by which soundwaves are collected and amplified. Nerve endings in the inner ear transmit electrical impulses along the auditory pathways to the brain for interpretation. The auditory system is also responsible for maintenance of balance (Patton & Thibodeau 2018).

LIVED EXPERIENCE

Around 18 years old, I started to have random bouts of double vision. It took years of seeking out support and visiting countless doctors and optometrists before I was diagnosed with esotropia. By the age of 23 years, I was considered legally blind. I wasn't allowed to drive, I had trouble seeing things at night and on a few occasions was almost hit by a car when trying to cross the road.

I often felt like a burden to friends and family and my mental health suffered, but I found ways to adjust. Asking people to stand on my left side, linking arms when crossing roads or in crowds and making sure to communicate with the people around me when I was struggling to see.

I was eventually able to undergo surgery at the age of 24 years. I had a significant improvement in my vision, though I still experienced periods of double vision even 3 years later. I will likely need more surgery in the years to come, but I will ensure that I stay connected with my health team and communicate my experience with the people around me.

Jackleen, 27 years old

INTRODUCTION

Sense organs can be classified as special and general sense organs. Special sense organs, such as the eye and the ear, are characterised as being large and complex organs or having localised groups of special receptors for specific and specialised detection of stimuli. The general sense organs are for detecting stimuli such as pain and touch. They have microscopic receptors and are distributed throughout the entire body (see Table 34.1). An example of a general sense organ is the skin (Patton & Thibodeau 2018). Receptors in general sense organs are scattered over almost the entire body. The skin over different parts of the body will respond differently because of the differing numbers of touch receptors. Touch receptors are distributed closely together over the fingertips and far apart across the back and torso. Stimulation of some receptors will lead to the sensation of vibration, while others give the sensation of pressure, pain (pain receptors) or temperature (thermoreceptors).

Many general receptors are present in deep tissue; there are stretch receptors in the stomach that signal when it is full. There are important chemoreceptors in the aorta that detect changes in blood pH and carbon dioxide levels (Patton & Thibodeau 2018).

ALTERED SENSES

People become accustomed to certain sensory stimuli and, when these change, the individual may experience discomfort. Factors that contribute to alterations in behaviour include sensory deprivation, sensory overload and sensory deficits.

Sensory deprivation

Sensory deprivation is thought of as a decrease or lack of meaningful stimuli. Because of reduced stimulation, a person becomes more acutely aware of the remaining stimuli and often perceives these in a distorted manner. The individual often experiences alterations in perception, cognition and emotion.

TABLE 34.1 | General sense organs

Type		Main locations	General senses
Free nerve endings			
(Naked nerve ending; several types exist)	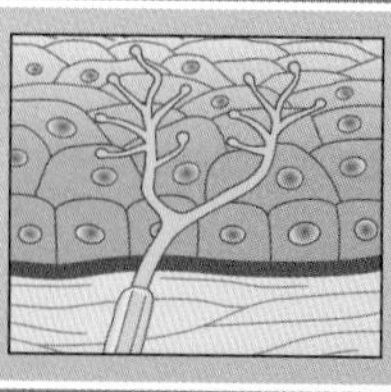	Skin and mucosa (epithelial layers)	Pain, discriminative touch, tickle and temperature
Encapsulated nerve endings			
Bulboid (Krause) corpuscle	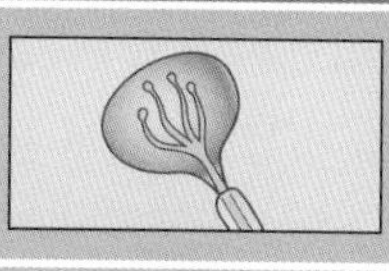	Skin (dermal layer), subcutaneous tissue, mucosa of lips and eyelids, and external genitals	Touch and possibly cold
Lamellar (Pacini) corpuscle	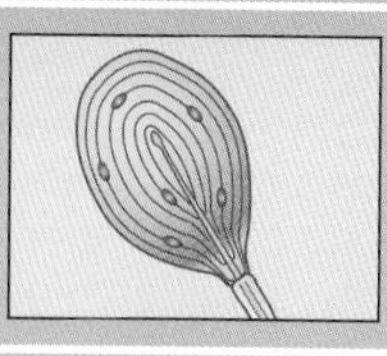	Subcutaneous, submucous and subserous tissues; around joints; in mammary glands; and external genitals of both sexes	Pressure and high-frequency vibration
Tactile (Meissner) corpuscle	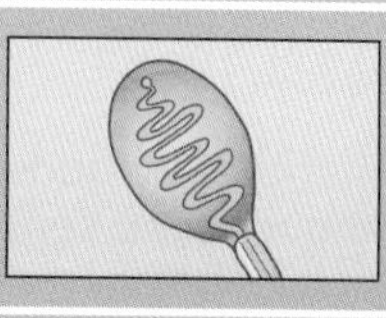	Skin (in papillae of dermis) and fingertips and lips (numerous)	Fine touch and low-frequency vibration
Bulbous (Ruffini) corpuscle	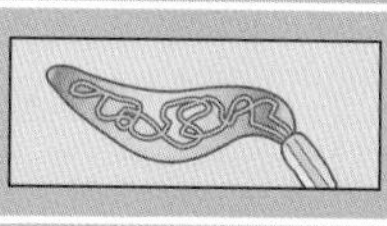	Skin (dermal layer) and subcutaneous tissue of fingers	Touch and pressure
Golgi tendon receptor	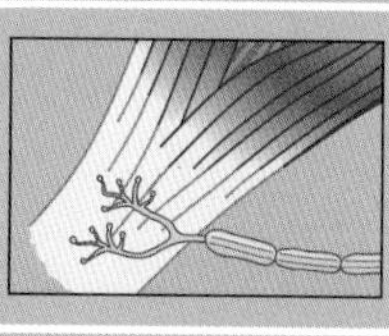	Near junction of tendons and muscles	**Proprioception** (sense of muscle tension)
Muscle spindle	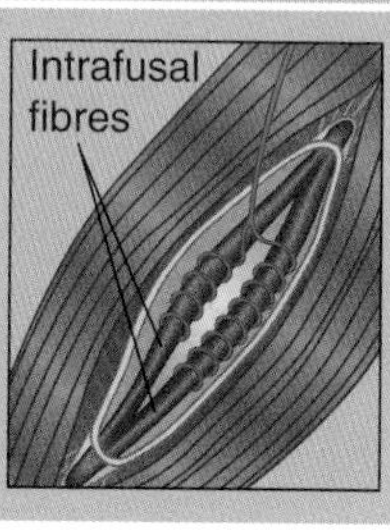	Skeletal muscles	Proprioception (sense of muscle length)

(Patton & Thibodeau 2018)

Sensory overload

Sensory overload generally occurs when a person is unable to process or manage the amount or intensity of sensory stimuli. Factors that can contribute to sensory overload are:

- pain, dyspnoea, and anxiety
- a noisy healthcare setting, intrusive diagnostic studies, contact with many strangers
- nervous system disturbances, certain medication.

Sensory overload can prevent the brain from ignoring or responding to specific stimuli. Some signs of sensory overload can include feelings of fatigue, irritability, anxiety, disorientation, reduced cognitive function and inability to concentrate (Patton & Thibodeau 2018).

Sensory deficits

A sensory deficit is impaired reception, perception, or both, of one or more of the senses. Impaired hearing and sight are sensory deficits. When only one sense is affected, other senses may become more acute to compensate for the loss. However, sudden loss of one of our senses can lead to confusion, disorientation and emotional distress. When there is a gradual loss of sensory function, people often develop behaviours to compensate for the loss. For example, a person with gradual hearing loss in the right ear may unconsciously turn the left ear towards the speaker. Persons with sensory deficits are at risk of both sensory deprivation and sensory overload (Berman et al 2021).

FACTORS AFFECTING SENSORY FUNCTION

A range of factors affect the amount and quality of sensory stimulation, including a person's developmental stage, culture, level of stress, medications, illness and lifestyle. These are outlined in Clinical Interest Box 34.1 and Clinical Interest Box 34.2.

CLINICAL INTEREST BOX 34.1 Factors that influence sensory function

Age

- Infants are unable to discriminate sensory stimuli. Nerve pathways are immature.
- Visual changes during adulthood include presbyopia (inability to focus on near objects) and the need for glasses for reading (usually occurring from age 40–50).
- Hearing changes, which begin at age 30, include decreased hearing acuity, speech intelligibility, pitch discrimination and hearing threshold. Tinnitus often accompanies a hearing loss as a side effect of drugs. Older adults hear low-pitched sounds the best but have difficulty hearing conversation over background noise.
- Older adults have reduced visual fields, increased glare sensitivity, impaired night vision and reduced accommodation, depth perception and colour discrimination.
- Older adults have difficulty discriminating the consonants (*f, s, th, ch*). Speech sounds are garbled and there is a delayed reception and reaction to speech.
- Gustatory and olfactory changes include a decrease in the number of taste buds in later years and reduction of olfactory nerve fibres by age 50. Reduced taste discrimination and reduced sensitivity to odours are common.
- Proprioceptive changes after age 60 include increased difficulty with balance, spatial orientation and coordination.
- Older adults experience tactile changes, including declining sensitivity to pain, pressure and temperature.

Medications

- Some antibiotics (e.g. streptomycin, gentamicin) are ototoxic and can permanently damage the auditory nerve; chloramphenicol can irritate the optic nerve. Narcotic analgesics, sedatives and antidepressant medications can alter the perception of stimuli.

Environment

- Excessive environmental stimuli (e.g. equipment noise and staff conversation in an intensive care unit) can result in sensory overload, marked by confusion, disorientation and the inability to make decisions. Restricted environmental stimulation (e.g. with protective isolation) can lead to sensory deprivation. Poor-quality environmental stimuli (e.g. reduced lighting, narrow walkways, background noise) can worsen sensory impairment.

Comfort level

- Pain and fatigue alter the way a person perceives and reacts to stimuli.

Pre-existing illness

- Peripheral vascular disease can cause reduced sensation in the extremities and impaired cognition. Chronic diabetes mellitus can lead to reduced vision, blindness or peripheral neuropathy. Strokes often produce loss of speech. Some neurological disorders impair motor function and sensory reception.

Smoking

- Chronic tobacco use can cause the taste buds to atrophy, lessening the perception of flavours.

Noise levels

- Constant exposure to high noise levels (e.g. on a construction job site) can cause hearing loss.

Endotracheal intubation

- Temporary loss of speech results from insertion of an endotracheal tube through the mouth or nose into the trachea.

(Crisp et al 2021; Brown et al 2020)

CLINICAL INTEREST BOX 34.2 Cultural considerations affecting sensory function

An individual's culture often determines the amount of stimulation that a person considers normal. The normal amount of stimulation associated with ethnic origin, religious affiliation and income level also affects the amount of stimulation an individual desires and believes to be meaningful.

It is important for nurses to be sensitive to what stimulation is culturally acceptable to everyone (e.g. in some cultures, touching is comforting, whereas in others it is offensive).

(Crisp et al 2021; Brown et al 2020)

ASSESSING SENSORY FUNCTION

Nursing assessment of sensory perceptual functioning includes:

- nursing history: a guide to assessing a person's sensory perceptual functioning
- mental status, including level of consciousness, orientation, memory and attention span
- physical examination: the person's specific visual and hearing abilities; perception of heat, cold, light touch, and pain in the limbs; and awareness of the position of body parts
- the person's environment: assess for quantity, quality, and type of stimuli
- social support network: the degree of isolation a person feels is significantly influenced by the quality and quantity of support from family and friends.

Clinical Interest Box 34.3 provides further detail.

SPECIAL SENSE ORGANS

The taste receptors

The chemical receptors (**chemoreceptors**) that generate the nervous impulses that result in the sense of taste are called the taste buds. Taste buds are scattered in the oral cavity, with most concentrated over the surface of the tongue and a few found on the soft palate and the inner surface of the cheeks. These chemoreceptors respond to substances present in food and generate nerve impulses that are transmitted to the brain for interpretation. The upper surface of the tongue is covered with small projections (papillae), some of which contain a taste bud. Each taste bud consists of sensory and supporting cells situated in the epithelium and opening into the surface through a small gustatory pore.

Between the cells of the taste bud lie the endings of afferent nerve fibres derived from several cranial nerves. Taste buds on the anterior two-thirds of the tongue connect with fibres of the facial (seventh cranial) nerve. Taste buds on the

CLINICAL INTEREST BOX 34.3 Interview to assess a person's sensory perceptual functioning

Visual

- How would you rate your vision (excellent, good, fair or poor)?
- Do you wear glasses or contact lenses?
- Describe any recent changes in your vision.
- Do you have any difficulty seeing near or far objects?
- Do you have any difficulty seeing at night?
- Have you ever experienced blurred vision, double vision, spots moving in front of your eyes, blind spots, light sensitivity, flashing lights or halos around objects?
- When did you last visit an eye doctor?

Auditory

- How would you rate your hearing (excellent, good, fair or poor)?
- Do you wear a hearing aid or cochlear implant?
- Describe any recent changes in your hearing.
- Can you locate the direction of sounds and distinguish various voices?
- Do you experience any dizziness or vertigo?
- Do you experience any ringing, buzzing, humming or crackling noises or fullness in the ears?

Gustatory

- Have you experienced any changes in taste (e.g. difficulty in differentiating sweet, sour, salty and bitter tastes)?
- Do you enjoy the taste of foods as you did previously?

Olfactory

- Have you experienced any changes in your sense of smell?
- Do things (foods, flowers, perfumes etc) smell the same as previously?
- Can you distinguish foods by their odours and tell when something is burning?
- Have you experienced any changes in appetite? (Changes in appetite may be related to an impaired sense of smell.)

Tactile

- Are you experiencing any pain or discomfort?
- Have you experienced any decrease in your ability to perceive heat, cold or pain in your limbs?
- Do you have any numbness or tingling in your extremities?

Kinaesthetic

- Have you noticed any difficulty in perceiving the position of parts of your body?

(Berman et al 2021)

posterior one-third of the tongue are associated with the fibres of the glossopharyngeal (ninth cranial) nerve, while pharyngeal taste buds send impulses to the brain via the vagus (tenth cranial) nerve (Marieb & Keller 2021).

These taste buds can differentiate sweet, salty, sour and bitter stimuli. The tip of the tongue is the most sensitive to sweet and salty substances; the edges of the tongue are most sensitive to bitter substances. Substances must be in solution (saliva) so that they can reach every opening in a taste bud and stimulate the nerve ending. Molecules pass into solution on the surface of the tongue and combine with the surface membranes of the receptor cells. Transmitter substances are released, which evoke action potentials on the sensory nerve fibres. Fibres from the seventh, ninth and tenth cranial nerves carry the taste impulses via the brainstem to an area of the cerebral cortex where the taste is experienced (Patton & Thibodeau 2018).

The sense of taste is intricately linked with the sense of smell, and the sense of taste depends on stimulation of the olfactory receptors (see Figure 34.1). The ability of a person to taste and smell starts to diminish by their mid-40s, due to a gradual decrease in the presents of these receptor cells. Virtually half of people over the age of 80 will lose their sense of smell, which will reduce their sense of taste. This may explain why older adults prefer their food to be highly seasoned or they may lose their appetite completely (Marieb & Keller 2021).

Both senses have a protective function. For example, in detecting substances that may be harmful or poisonous—an example being that humans will often have an aversion to bitter tastes since this is a common taste in poisons and spoilt food. Interruption of the transmission of taste stimuli to the brain may cause taste abnormalities. Taste abnormalities may result from trauma, infection, vitamin or mineral deficiencies, neurological or oral disorders and the effects of drugs. Because tastes are most accurately perceived in a fluid medium, mouth dryness may interfere with taste. Alterations in taste may include **ageusia** (a complete loss of taste), **hypogeusia** (a partial loss of taste), **dysgeusia** (a distorted sense of taste) and **cacogeusia** (an unpleasant taste).

The smell receptors

The chemoreceptors responsible for the sense of smell are located in a small area of epithelial tissue in the upper part of the nasal cavity (Figure 34.2). These chemoreceptors are known as the olfactory receptors. They respond to airborne chemicals and generate impulses that are transmitted to the brain for interpretation. These receptors adapt quickly when exposed to an unchanging stimulus, which means that the person can become accustomed to an odour when constantly exposed to it.

Permanent alterations in the sense usually result when the olfactory neuroepithelium or part of the olfactory nerve is destroyed. Permanent or temporary loss can occur from inhaling irritants such as acid fumes that paralyse nasal cilia. Conditions such as ageing, COVID-19, Parkinson's disease, and Alzheimer's disease have been shown to alter the sense of smell. Alterations in smell include **anosmia** (a total loss of sense of smell), **hyposmia** (an impaired sense of smell)

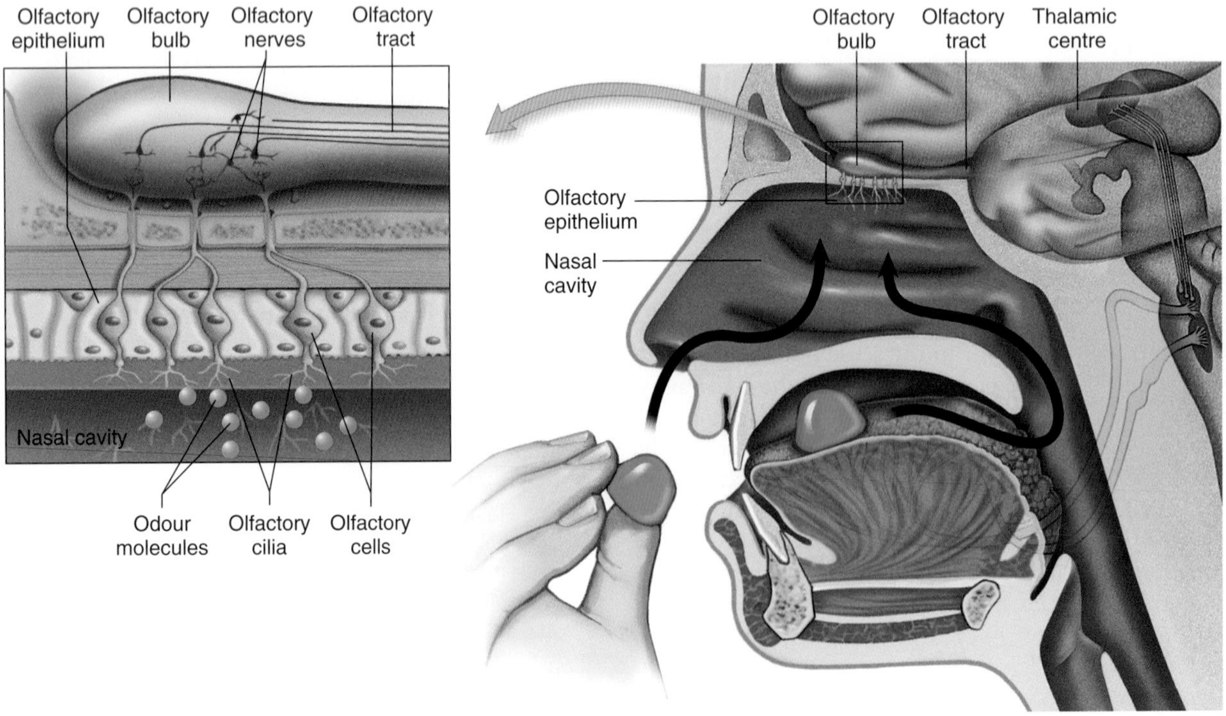

Figure 34.1 Olfactory structures

(Patton & Thibodeau 2024)

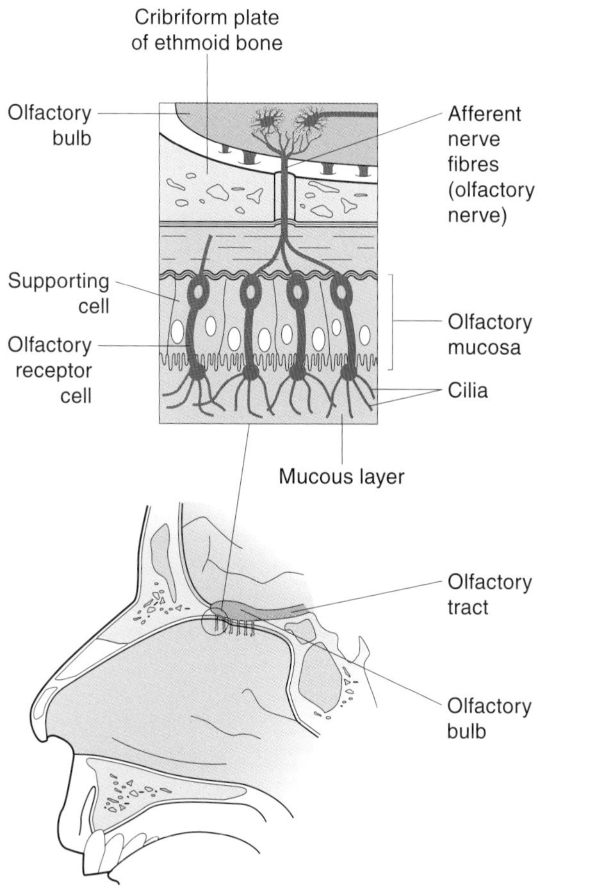

Figure 34.2 The location and structure of the olfactory receptors in the nose

and **parosmia** (an abnormal sense of smell) (Patton & Thibodeau 2018).

There is a close relationship between the sense of smell and the sense of taste, and therefore it can be difficult to distinguish between the two. The sensations of smell and taste play an important part in stimulating the secretions of digestive juices (Berman et al 2021).

The nurse plays an important role in promoting the sense of taste and stimulating the sense of smell when caring for a person with altered sensory function. Health education regarding good oral hygiene practices will enhance taste perception. Discuss with the person which foods are the most taste appealing. If taste perception is improved, we will typically see food intake and appetite improve. Taste perception is increased when food is seasoned. The person's sense of smell can be stimulated by pleasant aromas such as flowers, perfumes and food.

THE EYE

Structure of the eye

The eye is a spherical structure (Figure 34.3) about 2.5 cm in diameter, consisting of three principal layers (Patton & Thibodeau 2018).

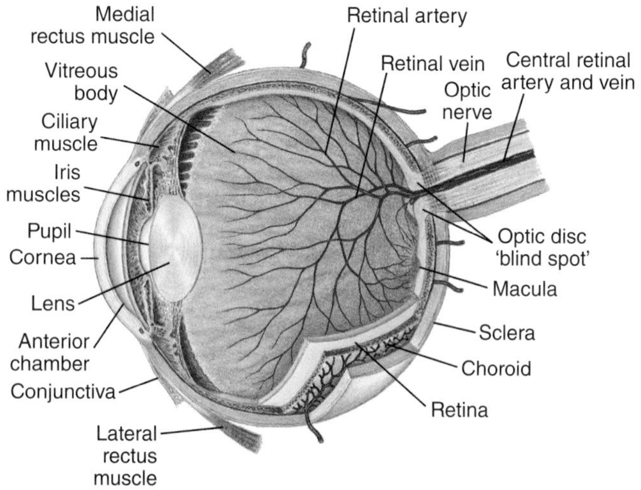

Figure 34.3 The eye cut in horizontal section

(Ball et al 2023)

The outer layer

The outer layer of the eye is also known as the fibrous layer. It consists of the sclera 'the white of the eye' and the cornea, known as the 'window', which is a transparent structure continuous with the sclera. About five-sixths of the outer surface is made up of a tough white opaque fibrous layer (sclera), while the cornea comprises the anterior one-sixth. Both the sclera and the cornea consist of layers of collagen fibres. In the cornea, the fibres are regular in size and arrangement, which accounts for its transparency. It holds a large concentration of nerve endings, which supports in the protective mechanisms of the eye, such as tear production and blinking.

The middle layer

The middle pigmented vascular layer of the eye is composed of three structures: the choroid, the iris and the ciliary body. The choroid is a layer of tissue that lies between the sclera and the retina. It is composed largely of blood vessels and contains highly pigmented cells that absorb light and prevent it from being reflected within the eyeball.

The iris is a pigmented circular membrane between the cornea and the lens and gives the eye its colour. Sphincter and dilator muscles within the iris regulate the central aperture (the pupil). By either dilation or constriction of the pupil, the amount of light entering the eye is regulated. The pupil appears black because light rays entering the eye are absorbed by the choroid and are not reflected.

The ciliary body is a thickened area of the choroid, lying anterior to the choroid, extending to the root of the iris. A circular array of fibres stretches from the ciliary body to the lens to hold it in place. The ciliary body controls focusing of the lens and contains glands that secrete aqueous humour (Marieb & Keller 2021).

The innermost layer

The innermost layer of the eye is a thin structure called the retina. The retina lines the inner wall of the posterior portion of the eyeball and comprises several layers. The two main layers are the pigmented layer (the outermost layer of the retina, lying next to the choroid, and whose cells contain melanin) and the rod and cone layer, which lies next to the pigmented layer and is highly sensitive to light.

Rods and cones (specialised nerve endings) are distributed as a tightly packed mass throughout the retina, except at a point where the ganglionic fibres converge to form the optic nerve. This area, which is about 1.5 mm in diameter, is termed the optic disc. Since it possesses no photosensitive cells, it is also known as the 'blind spot'. The prime function of rods and cones is to absorb light. Rods can be stimulated by dim light and allow perception of shapes and movement in dim light. Rods also provide far peripheral vision. Cones are specialised for fine visual discrimination of colour perception. There are three types of cones: one type responds mostly to blue light, another to red light and the third to green light (Patton & Thibodeau 2018).

In the centre of the retina is an oval yellowish area, the macula lutea, and in the centre of the macula lutea is a small depression, the fovea centralis. The photosensitive cells in the centre of the retina are more exposed to light than the rest of the retina; therefore, visual acuity is at its highest here (Marieb & Keller 2021).

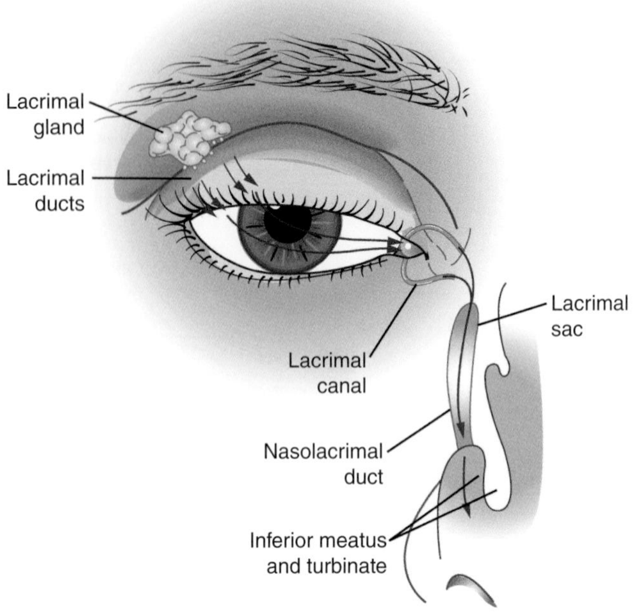

Figure 34.4 The lacrimal apparatus of the eye

(Applegate, 2011)

Extraocular structure—accessory structures

Extraocular, or accessory, structures of the eye are portions of the eye outside the eyeball. These structures consist of the eyebrows, eyelids, eyelashes and lacrimal apparatus. The eyeball is anchored into position by several structures, including the extraocular muscles, the conjunctiva and the eyelids. The eyeball is surrounded and protected by a bony orbit, the eyebrow ridge and some fatty tissue. The eyeball is lubricated by the lacrimal glands.

The extraocular muscles bring about rotational movements of the eyeball. The muscles arise from the orbit and consist of four rectus muscles, which are attached to the sclera, and two oblique muscles. The oblique muscles are arranged so that for part of their length they lie around the circumference of the eyeball. The eyebrows and eyelashes are short coarse hairs that shade the eyes and protect the eyes from dust and sweat. The eyelids consist of connective tissue covered by skin and lined with mucous membrane. The lining is reflected over the eyeballs and is called the conjunctiva. The eyelids protect the eye from foreign bodies and excessive light, as well as distributing tears by blinking (Patton & Thibodeau 2018).

The lacrimal apparatus consists of the lacrimal gland, which is situated over the eye at the upper outer corner and secretes tears, which constantly wash over the conjunctiva (Figure 34.4). Tears leave the gland via several small ducts and pass over the front of the eye, eventually draining into the lacrimal sac, which is the expanded end of the nasolacrimal duct. Tears are secreted on to the anterior surface of the eyeball and are spread over it by the blinking movements of the eyelids. Antimicrobial substances, such as water, protein, glucose, sodium, potassium, chloride, urea and lysozyme (bacterial enzyme), in tears protect the eyes against microorganisms. Excess tears drain down the nasal cavity. The lacrimal glands are stimulated in response to chemical and mechanical irritants, thus producing tears to wash away irritants. Tears may also be produced as a result of emotion such as sadness or happiness (Rothrock 2023).

The refractive media

The refractive media are the transparent parts of the eye and have the ability to bend light rays at the surfaces of two transparent media. The refractive media are the cornea, the lens, the aqueous humour and the vitreous humour. The cornea functions as a refracting and protective layer through which light rays pass en route to the brain (Patton & Thibodeau 2018).

The lens is a transparent, biconvex encapsulated structure suspended from the ciliary body posterior to the iris. The lens is an elastic structure, and this allows its shape to change when the eye is focused. The function of the lens is to refract (bend) light rays and to focus them on the retina.

Aqueous humour is a clear watery fluid that fills the cavities around the lens. These cavities are called the anterior and posterior chambers. Aqueous humour is derived from the plasma in the capillaries of the ciliary body and passes into the posterior chamber. It then passes forwards through the pupil to the anterior chamber, where it is absorbed into the ciliary veins. The rate of secretion and reabsorption is balanced so that intraocular pressure is regulated. Aqueous humour serves as a refractory medium and provides nutrients to the lens and cornea (Marieb & Keller 2021).

Vitreous humour is a clear jelly-like substance that fills the intraocular space from the posterior lens to the retina. Because it does not regenerate, any significant loss of vitreous humour—for example, as a result of injury to the eye—may distort other ocular structures. Vitreous humour helps to maintain the shape of the eyeball, helps keep the retina in position and helps with the refraction of light rays (Marieb & Keller 2021).

The physiology of sight

Light travels from its source to various objects, where it undergoes reflection. This reflected light can then travel towards the eye, where it passes through the cornea, the aqueous humour, the lens and the vitreous humour, before forming an image on the retina. Nerve endings in the retina transmit electrical impulses along the optic nerve to the brain. A coordinated process of refraction, accommodation, regulation of pupil size and convergence makes normal binocular vision possible (Patton & Thibodeau 2018).

Refraction

Refraction, or bending of light rays, occurs as the light waves pass through the cornea, aqueous humour, lens and vitreous humour. At the lens, the light is bent so that it converges at a single point on the retina (Stromberg 2023).

Accommodation

Accommodation is the process whereby the curvature of the lens is altered so that the eye can focus light from objects at close distances (approximately objects six metres away or closer). As an object moves closer to the eye, the curvature of the lens increases so that the image remains in focus on the retina (Marieb & Keller 2021).

Regulation of pupil size

The diameter of the pupil influences image formation, and the muscles of the iris respond to changes in light intensity. An increase in light intensity initiates constriction of the pupil, whereas a decrease in light intensity causes dilation of the pupil. Adjustment of pupil size therefore regulates the amount of light entering the eyes. Too much light may damage the retina, and too little fails to stimulate it (Patton & Thibodeau 2018).

Convergence

Convergence is the medial movements of the two eyeballs so that they are both directed towards the object being viewed. Convergence allows light rays to fall and stimulate two identical spots on the retinas, resulting in the perception of a single image.

After an image has been formed on the retina by the processes of refraction, accommodation, regulation of pupil size and convergence, light impulses are converted into nerve impulses by the rods and cones. The light breaks down the photosensitive chemical in either rods or cones, which stimulates electrical impulses to the brain for interpretation.

Nerve impulses travel from the retina along the optic nerve. The optic nerve emerges from the back of the eyeball and passes to the optic chiasma, an area at the base of the brain.

The fibres then form the left and right optic tracts, which continue to the visual areas of the brain in the occipital lobes. Here, further processing occurs so that the image is given meaning (Stromberg 2023).

DISORDERS OF THE EYE

Healthy vision requires three processes:

1. formation of an image on the retina (refraction)
2. stimulation of rods and cones
3. conduction of nerve impulses to the brain.

Normal eye function can be altered by a malfunction of any of these processes. Some of the pathophysiological causes of disruption of eye function can be congenital, degenerative, infectious, neoplastic or traumatic. The effects may be mild and temporary, severe or permanent. Disorders of vision include alterations in visual acuity, ocular movement, accommodation, refraction and colour vision (Berman et al 2021; Marieb & Keller 2020).

Refraction disorders

Focusing a clear image on the retina is essential for good vision. In the normal eye, light rays enter the eye and are focused into a clear, upside-down image on the retina. The brain rights the image in our conscious perception but cannot correct an image that is not sharply focused. If the eyeballs are elongated, the image focuses in front of the retina, giving the retina a fuzzy image; this is known as **myopia** or near-sightedness. This can be corrected by refractive eye surgery or by using contact lenses or glasses. If our eyeballs are shorter than normal, the image focuses behind the retina, also producing a fuzzy image; this condition is known as hypermetropia, **hyperopia** or farsightedness (see Figure 34.5). This can also be corrected by eye surgery or glasses (Brown et al 2020).

As people age, they can develop an inability to focus the lens properly; this is known as **presbyopia** and is the reason most people, once they pass through middle age, require reading glasses. The lens becomes firm and loses its elasticity; the ageing lens loses its ability to focus light rays and near objects appear blurred. People may also state that they are experiencing 'halos', which are coloured rings encircling bright lights, caused by alteration in the ocular media. Small moving spots or flecks seen before the eyes are commonly called floaters and may be due to the ageing process as the vitreous material degenerates. Floaters may also be caused by retinal laceration, diabetic neuropathy or hypertension. Visual changes also include double vision, or **diplopia**. Photophobia may be caused by inflammation of the cornea or the iris and ciliary bodies. An irregular, uneven curvature of the cornea or lens—astigmatism—can also be corrected by glasses (Patton & Thibodeau 2018).

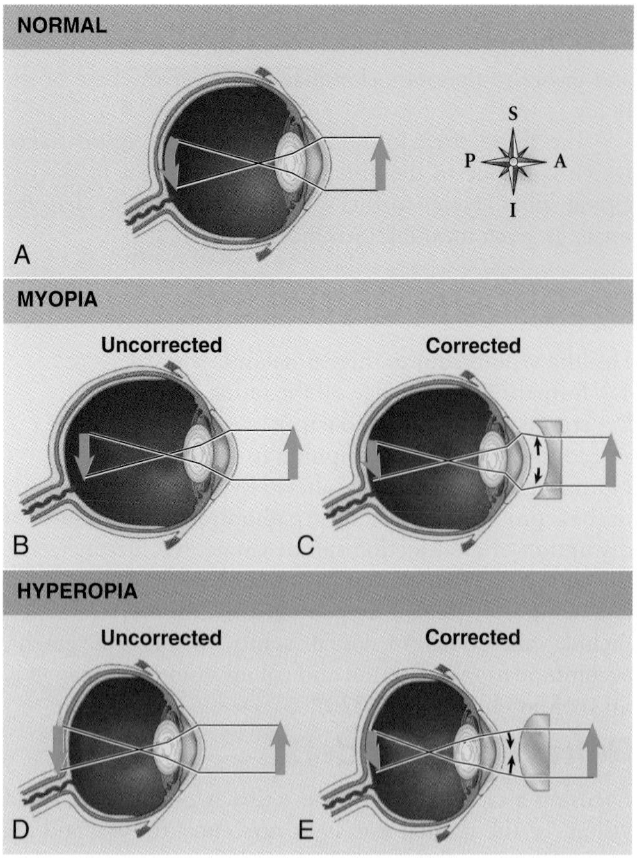

Figure 34.5 Structure and function of the body of the eye

(Patton & Thibodeau 2024)

Cataracts

There are three classifications of cataracts: congenital, traumatic and age-related. By definition, a cataract is a clouding of the lens in the eye. Cataracts generally develop bilaterally, with each progressing independently, except for congenital and traumatic cataracts. Causes include the ageing process, inflammation, malignancy, metabolic factors, toxins, heredity and trauma. Manifestations generally begin with a decrease in visual acuity. The person complains of not being able to see clearly. They may also complain of blurred vision, glare and a decrease in colour perception. As the cataract progresses, the pupil appears milky white. Surgical removal of the cataract from the lens is indicated when activities of daily living are affected (Brown et al 2020).

See Nursing Care Plan 34.1 and associated Progress Note 34.1 for an individual admitted for cataract surgery.

Infectious disorders

Infections of the eye and its associated structures also have the potential to impair vision, sometimes permanently.

Stye

A hordeolum (stye) is a localised staphylococcal infection of a sebaceous gland of the eyelid. This gland is the base of a hair follicle or eyelash. It can be an internal stye that forms on the inside of the eyelid or an external stye that forms on the outside of the eyelid. Manifestations include localised inflammation, swelling and pain (Brown et al 2020).

Blepharitis

Blepharitis is inflammation of the eyelid margins. It may be caused by bacterial infection or an allergic reaction to smoke, dust or chemicals. Seborrhoea, a disorder of the sebaceous gland, may also cause blepharitis. Manifestations include itching, burning, redness of the eyelid margins, chronic conjunctivitis and yellow purulent discharge crusts on the lashes (Stromberg 2023).

Conjunctivitis

Conjunctivitis is the inflammation of the conjunctiva and may be caused by excessive exposure to wind, sun, heat, cold, allergens or chemicals, or by bacterial, viral or fungal infection. Manifestations include itching, burning, excessive tearing and pain. Allergic conjunctivitis may cause considerable swelling (Stromberg 2023).

Trachoma

Trachoma is a chronic form of keratoconjunctivitis that causes permanent damage to the cornea which, if untreated, can result in blindness. The condition results from infection by *Chlamydia trachomatis* and is associated with poor personal and community hygiene and lack of available clean water. There is a high incidence of trachoma in Aboriginal and Torres Strait Islander Peoples. Manifestations, which may not become apparent for years, are like those for severe conjunctivitis. There is corneal inflammation and scarring, due to the eyelids turning inwards, which causes the lashes to rub against the cornea. Severe corneal scarring may result in blindness (Brown et al 2020).

Keratitis

Keratitis is inflammation of the cornea and is frequently caused by trauma or infection. It usually affects only one eye, and frequently presents as a secondary infection to an upper respiratory tract infection involving cold sores (herpes simplex infection). Manifestations include opacity of the cornea, irritation, excessive tearing, blurred vision, redness and photophobia (Brown et al 2020).

Orbital cellulitis

Orbital cellulitis is an acute infection of the orbital tissues and eyelids that does not involve the eyeball. The condition is generally secondary to infection of nearby structures and requires an immediate medical response. If orbital cellulitis is not treated, the infection may spread to the sinuses and meninges. Manifestations include unilateral eyelid oedema, inflammation of the orbital tissues and eyelids, pain, impaired eye movement and purulent discharge from indurated areas (Jarvis & Eckhardt 2021).

NURSING CARE PLAN 34.1

Assessment: Mrs Biel has been admitted for cataract extraction and intraocular lens replacement.
Issue/s to be addressed: Health education regarding the upcoming procedure.
Poor vision.
Discharge planning.
Goal/s: Mrs Biel verbalises understanding of upcoming surgery and expected outcomes.
Mrs Biel has daily needs assisted as required.
Mrs Biel is given appropriate postoperative care.
Mrs Biel understands the importance of going home to a supportive environment; family/support persons are informed.

Care/actions	Rationale
Provide preoperative health education to ensure the individual understands the procedure. Ensure this is culturally appropriate and offer verbal and written instructions in language of choice. If required, obtain assistance from interpreter service. Offer Mrs Biel assistance with daily activities including hygiene and nutrition. Ensure layout of room is explained, ensure call bell is accessible and any excess furniture or belongings are removed. Provide any nutritional aids or support such as explaining what food is where on the plate and bright-coloured utensils. Postoperative observations as per surgeon's instructions. Perform eye care as per surgeon's instructions. Mobilise as soon as able. Provide Mrs Biel and her carers with culturally appropriate information on what to expect post discharge. Have transport arranged for her on discharge and ensure she has support at home for the initial postoperative period.	Mrs Biel will feel less anxious and more prepared for surgery if all aspects of the surgery are explained in the best mode for her. Due to cataracts, Mrs Biel has poor vision and being in an unfamiliar environment will require some assistance with activities of daily living. Keeping environment clutter free and explaining the layout will minimise the risk of injury. Maintaining nutrition while in hospital will aid in recovery. Post-anaesthetic observations and mobilisation are required to ensure there are no adverse side effects. Being prepared for discharge prevents risks of readmission as Mrs Biel understands what to expect once she is at home. Ensuring transport will ensure Mrs Biel's safety and to expedite discharge.

Evaluation: Mrs Biel and her family/carers verbalise a thorough understanding of the procedure, and she appears and purports to be relaxed and comfortable.
Mrs Biel is able to perform all her required daily activities while in hospital and expresses her satisfaction.
Mrs Biel recovers from surgery as per expected outcome without any complications.
Mrs Biel and her family verbalise their understanding of what to expect on discharge and provide details of transport mode home.

Disorders of the retina

Damage to the retina impairs vision because even a well-focused image cannot be perceived if some or all of the light receptors do not function properly (e.g., in retinal detachment when part of the retina falls away from the tissue supporting it). The condition can result from normal ageing, eye tumours or a sudden blow to the head. Common warning signs are:

- sudden appearance of floating spots
- odd 'flashes of light' that appear when the eye moves.

If left untreated, the retina may detach completely and can cause total blindness (Patton & Thibodeau 2018).

Diabetic retinopathy

Diabetes mellitus may cause a condition known as diabetic retinopathy, which causes small haemorrhages in retinal blood vessels to disrupt the oxygen supply to the photoreceptors. The eye responds by building new, but abnormal, vessels that block vision and which may cause detachment of the retina (Jarvis & Eckhardt 2021). See Clinical Interest Box 34.4 for more information on diabetic retinopathy.

Glaucoma

Another common condition that can damage the retina is glaucoma. This is excessive intraocular pressure caused by abnormal accumulation of aqueous humour. As fluid pressure (intraocular pressure) against the retina increases, blood flow to the retina slows. The reduced blood flow causes degeneration of the retina and thus a loss of vision. There are various forms of glaucoma: primary open-angle, primary closed-angle, secondary, congenital and absolute.

Glaucoma progresses slowly and may or may not be symptomatic. According to Glaucoma Australia (2023), 'about 1 in 10,000 babies are born with glaucoma, and by the age of 40, about 1 in 200 have glaucoma, rising to 1 in

CLINICAL INTEREST BOX 34.4 Diabetic retinopathy

Diabetes is becoming more common throughout the world, particularly in the developing world, where lifestyle and diet are rapidly changing. According to Diabetes Australia (2022), 1,487,300 people with diabetes are registered with the National Diabetes Service Scheme (NDSS). Over the past 12 months, 116,864 people with diabetes registered. This figure is equivalent to 320 new registrants every day.

As diabetes becomes more prevalent around the world, the number of people with diabetic retinopathy is also becoming more common and has the potential to become a leading cause of blindness.

What is diabetic retinopathy?

Diabetic retinopathy is a condition in which the retina is damaged by sustained and poor control of high blood sugar levels due to diabetes. It can cause reduced vision and blindness, particularly in its later stages.

What causes diabetic retinopathy?

Diabetic retinopathy is damage to the tiniest blood vessels of the retina and the capillaries by the high and abnormally varying levels of blood sugar associated with diabetes. The site of damage is mainly the lining or endothelial cells of these vessels. These cells are necessary for the normal functioning of the capillaries including actual blood flow.

This damage causes three basic problems:

1. Leakage from the capillaries. The accumulation of fluid, protein, fat and whole blood from leaking, damaged capillaries in the retina disturbs the retina's delicate organisation and complex functions. This leakage is prone to occur at the macula, the part of the retina that is most critical for sharp vision.
2. Poor blood circulation. Because of damage to endothelial cells, the capillaries can fail to deliver oxygen and nutrients to the retina and fail to remove toxic waste products. This causes reduced function or failure of parts of the retina, affecting vision.
3. Growth of abnormal new vessels in the retina. The lack of oxygen and perhaps some other metabolic features of diabetic retinopathy can stimulate new blood vessels to grow on or out from the surface of the retina. These often cause serious problems because they can bleed, sometimes massively, and they promote the formation of scar tissue that can stretch or distort the retina. In advanced cases, this process can pull the retina off the internal surface of the eye (traction retinal detachment). If this occurs, the affected eye will almost always lose all useful vision.

Most people who have diabetic retinopathy start with mild signs as described above but may progress to the more severe stages.

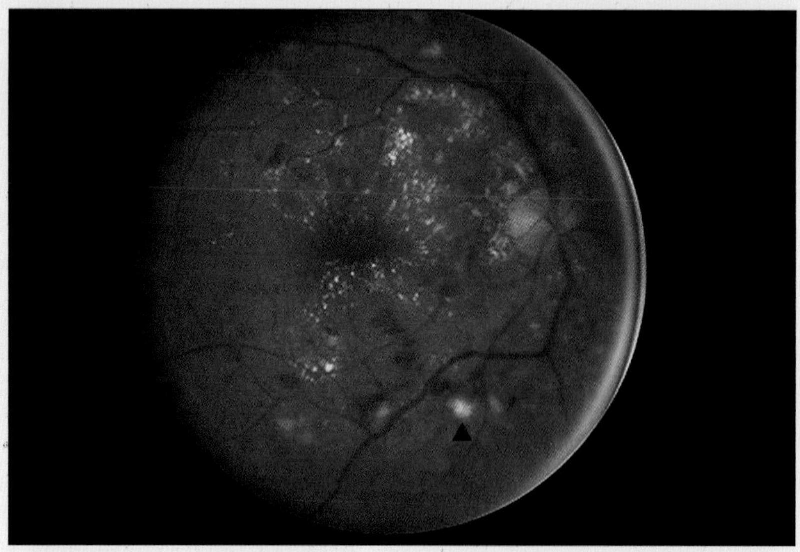

(McCance & Huether's pathophysiology, 9th ed. Copyright © 2023, 2019, 2014, 2010, 2006, 2002, 1998, 1994, 1990 Elsevier, Missouri)

Symptoms of diabetic retinopathy

Often in mild diabetic retinopathy, a person will have no symptoms. Once the disease becomes more advanced, they may experience:

- blurred vision
- floaters
- sudden catastrophic loss of vision in one or both eyes.

CLINICAL INTEREST BOX 34.4 Diabetic retinopathy—cont'd

Contributing factors

Length of disease

The longer the person has diabetes, the more likely it is that they will develop diabetic retinopathy. Once it is present it tends to worsen as time passes. It is rare to see much diabetic retinopathy in people who have had diabetes for less than 5 years, but it does happen at times. Diabetes can remain undiagnosed for a period; therefore, people can have diabetes longer than they realise and it is possible for diabetic retinopathy to be present at the time of diagnosis of diabetes.

Blood glucose levels

The poorer the control of blood sugar levels, the more likely it is that diabetic retinopathy will develop and the more likely it is that it will worsen.

Other vascular risk factors

Control of blood lipids (e.g. cholesterol) and blood pressure are also very important in the delay of onset of diabetic retinopathy. Lifestyle choices play a big part in the control of these factors. Healthy eating, weight control and exercise should be encouraged, along with quitting smoking and reducing or ceasing alcohol intake.

Prevention and slowing progression

Diabetics should have regular eye examinations from time of diagnosis. This is the single most important measure in the prevention of blindness from diabetes.

Treatment

Treatment of diabetic retinopathy should begin as soon as possible, before significant symptoms are evident and before the disease has progressed too far. This represents one of the great challenges in the care of diabetic retinopathy in both developed and developing countries.

Laser treatment

The current treatment for most people is laser. Laser treatment is usually applied through a special contact lens in an outpatient setting and the individual can go home after having it. The treatment is not usually painful. The affected areas of the retina are treated with tiny laser burns, particularly where there is significant leakage of fluid, especially at or near the macula, or where there are areas of ischaemia.

The aim of treatment is to help prevent further leakage, to promote reabsorption of fluid from the retina and reduce the stimulus to new vessel growth. Where there is severe ischaemia or when new blood vessels are already present, treatment aims to cause the new vessels to regress and prevent any further vessels from developing.

Often treatment is required to be repeated several times. In advanced diabetic retinopathy, laser treatments may fail to improve sight significantly and disease progression may continue, often leading to blindness in both eyes.

Surgical interventions

Surgical interventions may be indicated in very advanced cases of diabetic retinopathy where there has been severe bleeding in the eye, scar formation or retinal detachment. However, this intervention is usually only undertaken when all other treatments have failed to stop progression of the disease.

Other treatment

There are new and emerging forms of treatment including injecting drugs into the eye to reduce swelling in the retina and suppress new vessel growth. These are similar drugs to those used in the treatment of some forms of macular degeneration but, at present, they are too costly for routine use in some countries.

(Crisp et al 2021; Brown et al 2020)

8 at age 80. Overall, the incidence in Australia is about 2.3% of the population'. The condition may be caused by over-production of aqueous humour or obstruction to the outflow of aqueous humour, both of which result in accumulation of fluid and a rise in intraocular pressure. Manifestations of primary open-angle glaucoma are gradual and progressive; the person is unable to perceive changes in colour and experiences blurred vision and persistent aching eyes. Manifestations of primary closed-angle glaucoma occur suddenly. The person experiences intense pain, loss of vision, nausea and vomiting. The affected eye appears red, and the pupil is fixed, dilated and unresponsive (Glaucoma Australia 2023; Jarvis & Eckhardt 2021).

The manifestations of secondary glaucoma are like those of the primary form, depending on the cause. Congenital glaucoma is a rare disorder generally associated with other abnormalities, and manifests as a large-diameter cornea. Absolute glaucoma is the end result of any uncontrolled glaucoma resulting in blindness (Jarvis & Eckhardt 2021; Vision Australia 2023).

CLINICAL INTEREST BOX 34.5 Glaucoma prevention and preservation of sight

Routine eye screenings are recommended for early detection of glaucoma. Although it cannot at this time be predicted, prevented or cured, in most cases glaucoma can be controlled, and vision preserved by early diagnosis. The person needs to be aware that certain prescription and over-the-counter medications can cause increased intraocular pressure and should not be taken without consulting their doctor. The person who has experienced an episode of acute angle-closure glaucoma is taught about the risks, warning signs and management of future attacks. Persons need to understand the importance of lifetime therapy and periodic eye examinations with intraocular measurement in controlling the disease and preventing blindness. The nurse should assess the person's compliance with routine health screening.

(Glaucoma Australia 2023)

Clinical Interest Box 34.5 provides information on glaucoma prevention and preservation of sight.

Degenerative diseases of the retina

Macular degeneration (MD), also known as age-related macular degeneration (AMD), is the most common cause of untreatable blindness in developed countries. There are two types of MD: the most common form is *non-neovascular*, or *atrophic* (dry), and the most severe form is *neovascular* (wet). MD is becoming more common throughout the world as the average age of the population increases. It is caused by degenerative changes in the central part of the retina. The exact cause of the degeneration is unknown, but the risk of developing this condition increases with age after reaching 50 years. Other risk factors are cigarette smoking and a family history of the disorder.

Manifestations include loss of central vision, and activities that require fine detailed vision becoming impossible. The disease usually develops slowly and painlessly, and both eyes are generally affected. Vision may be improved in some cases by laser surgery. In extreme cases, it can cause legal blindness; however, most people usually retain good peripheral vision (Jarvis & Eckhardt 2021).

Degeneration of the retina can cause difficulty in seeing at night or in dim light. This condition, nyctalopia, or night blindness, can be caused by a deficiency in vitamin A. Vitamin A is needed to make photo pigment in rod cells. Photo pigment is a light-sensitive chemical that triggers stimulation of the visual nerve pathway. A lack of vitamin A may result in a lack of photo pigment in rods, a condition that impairs dim-light vision (Patton & Thibodeau 2018).

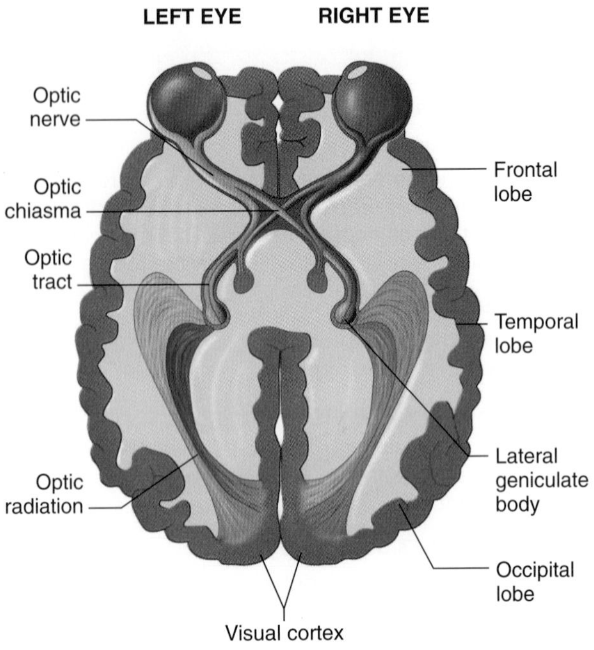

Figure 34.6 The optic (visual) pathway

(Patton & Thibodeau 2024)

Disorders of the visual pathway

Damage or degeneration in the optic nerve, the brain or any part of the visual pathway can impair vision (see Figure 34.6). This can include damage from stroke, multiple sclerosis or trauma, among others. Damage to the visual pathway does not always result in total loss of vision; depending on where the damage has occurred, only part of the visual field may be affected (Patton & Thibodeau 2018).

OTHER DISORDERS OF THE EYE

Congenital disorders

Strabismus

Strabismus is a condition of eye deviation in which the eyes fail to look in the same direction at the same time. The eyes may have uncoordinated appearance and the person may experience diplopia. Congenital strabismus is an anomaly in which there is a defect in the position and fusion ability of the two eyes. The condition is usually easily observed and, in addition to crossed eyes, the person may squint, tilt the head or close one eye to improve vision. Occasionally, the brain compensates for an error in the visual field. Though, in severe cases of strabismus, the brain may not be able to bring the two images into a single picture (Patton & Thibodeau 2018).

Ptosis

Ptosis, drooping of the upper eyelid, may be unilateral or bilateral. Congenital ptosis is a rare condition resulting from the failure of the levator muscle in the upper eyelid to develop. It is present from birth or occurs within the first year of life.

Manifestations are usually obvious; the lid appears smooth and flat, and the person may tilt the head back to compensate if the lid droops over the pupil. Ptosis can cause functional, cosmetic or psychological issues for children and adults; therefore, close monitoring of the person's visual function is necessary to preserve their sight. Depending on the severity of ptosis, surgical treatment may be necessary (Rothrock 2023).

Neoplastic disorders

Benign or malignant tumours may arise in the tissues surrounding the eye and can be a disorder found in both children and adults. Depending on the type of tumour, it may cause proptosis, pain, diplopia and vision loss. If a neoplastic disorder is suspected, a full examination and neuroimaging (e.g. CT, MRI) is taken; however, for confirmation a biopsy is required (Harding et al 2023).

Choroidal melanoma

A choroidal melanoma is a tumour that develops in the layer of tissue called the choroid (known as the uvea). This ocular malignant tumour can develop in adults around the age of 65, without predisposing risk factors such as genetic or environmental factors. Many people with choroidal melanoma are asymptomatic, while others may develop blurred vision. They tend to be slow growing tumours that are mainly identified on a routine examination (Waugh & Grant 2023).

Retinoblastoma

Retinoblastoma is a congenital hereditary neoplasm that develops from retinal germ cells. Manifestations include diminished vision, strabismus, retinal detachment, and an abnormal papillary reflex. It represents the most common childhood intraocular malignancy and accounts for 10–15% of cancers occurring within the first year of life. The tumour grows rapidly and may invade the brain and metastasise to distant sites (Waugh & Grant 2023).

Traumatic disorders

Abrasions

Abrasions are superficial scratches on the eyelid, conjunctiva or cornea. Corneal abrasions may be caused by foreign bodies or over-wearing of contact lenses. Manifestations include excessive tearing, pain, photophobia and a sensation of something in the eye.

Lacerations

Lacerations may involve the eyelids or the eyeball. Lacerations of the eyeball may lead to intraocular infection, cataract formation or loss of vision. Manifestations of a lacerated eyeball include severe pain and shock.

Contusions

Contusions of the eyeball involve a bruising injury in which intraocular damage occurs. The injury may result in bleeding into the anterior chamber (hyphema) or into the vitreous of surrounding tissues. Contusions generally result from a severe blow to the eye, such as from a fist, golf or squash ball. Manifestations include impaired vision, pain, bruising of the tissues surrounding the eye and blood in the anterior chamber.

Foreign bodies

Foreign bodies may enter the conjunctiva or cornea, or they may penetrate and perforate the eyeball. Examples of foreign bodies that gain entry include eyelashes, dirt and small particles of metal, dust and glass. Manifestations include irritation, pain, excessive tearing and photophobia.

Burns

Burns to the eye may result from exposure to a chemical, radiant energy or high temperatures. The extent of damage to the eye depends on the duration of exposure and the causative agent. Manifestations include extreme pain, excessive tearing, photophobia, inflammation or destruction of tissue and vision impairment (Cooper & Gosnell 2023).

Health promotion and education

The nurse is in a key position to educate individuals and their families about the ways by which eyesight can be protected and preserved in children. For adults, screening of visual function is imperative to detect problems early. Regular eye examinations are important, especially for persons with a family history of eye disorders and for persons who are more vulnerable to ocular complications such as diabetes mellitus. Recommended screening guidelines are structured based on age. People under 40 years of age should have periodic eye checks as required. Those aged 40–64 should have a complete eye examination every 2 years, and those aged 65 years and over should have a complete eye examination every year. Examination of the eyes is also recommended if a person experiences any disturbances of vision, pain, sudden appearance of floaters, photophobia, purulent discharge, trauma to the eye or pupil irregularities.

Prevention of the spread of infection is a principal objective for nursing care of an eye infection. Hand hygiene and the use of personal protective equipment (PPE) is crucial before touching infectious or inflamed eyes.

Avoid the use of eye make-up during this time since it can cause further irritation. Replacement of eye make-up is highly recommended after an infection has occurred, since there is a possibility for make-up to harbour bacteria, and replacement is recommended every 3–6 months thereafter. Each person should avoid sharing any eye make-up, eye drops or ointment since they should be only used by the one individual to stop any chance of the spread of infection (Cooper & Gosnell 2023; Crisp et al 2021).

Education is particularly important for persons involved in high-risk occupations and activities. Education should focus on strategies for prevention and first aid measures. Teach people what immediate care to give to prevent permanent loss of sight, such as immediately flushing the eye with copious amounts of water if a chemical splash occurs. Prevention of injury includes wearing eye protection when working with chemicals or when the eyes may be exposed to dust, wood, metal or glass fragments. Protective eyewear should also be worn during recreational or sporting activities in which sticks or balls may contact the eye, such as squash. Excessive exposure to strong sunlight or sunlamps should be avoided, as these may damage the eyes. A common form of cataract, which can result from frequent exposure to intense sunlight, can largely be prevented if sun hats and good quality sunglasses are worn.

Prevention of eye fatigue includes using adequate illumination when reading or writing, resting the eyes often during prolonged use and reducing screen glare when using a visual display unit such as a computer screen. The nurse should inform the person and family of the importance of follow-up treatment and stress the importance of complying with prescribed activity restriction to prevent further eye damage, and of safe and careful application and correct storage of prescribed eye drops or ointments (Vision Australia 2023).

See Clinical Interest Box 34.6 for information on childhood screening.

CRITICAL THINKING EXERCISE 34.1

Maria Russo is a 73-year-old woman who presented to the GP and Nurse Practitioner with progressive central blurred vision. She has a medical history of obesity and is a current smoker.

1. What health education would you provide to her within the clinic appointment?
2. Provide an explanation of the cause of her symptoms.

Diagnostic tests

Tests used to diagnose eye disorders may be classified as subjective, objective or special procedures. Subjective tests require oral responses from the person that must be interpreted by the examiner. Objective tests are those in which the examiner obtains precise measurements or directly visualises the interior of the eyes.

Subjective eye tests

A visual acuity test evaluates the person's ability to distinguish the form and detail of an object. Visual acuity is measured using a Snellen chart. The person is required to read letters on this chart from a distance of 6 metres. Generally, the smaller the symbol the person can identify, the sharper their visual acuity.

Colour vision tests evaluate the person's ability to recognise differences in colour. The most common colour vision tests use plates made up of patterns of dots of primary colours, superimposed on backgrounds of randomly mixed colours. A person with typical colour vision can identify the patterns (Marieb & Keller 2021).

CLINICAL INTEREST BOX 34.6
Childhood preventative screening

The most common visual problem during childhood is refractive error, such as near-sightedness. In early childhood, parents may be alerted to a vision problem by reduced eye contact from their infant or the infant's failure to react to light. Recommended screening guidelines are usually structured based on age, and preventative screening occurs in pre-school-age children (ages 4–5 years), where the nurse's role is one of detection and referral.

At school entry (age around 5 years):

- Examine eyes and observe for fixation, following, nystagmus, strabismus.
- Test visual acuity.
- Test hearing; perform otoscopy on children failing audiometry to determine appropriate action.
- Address parental concerns regarding vision and hearing.

For more information visit Department of Education and Early Childhood Development: <racgp.org.au/clinical-resources/clinical-guidelines/key-racgp-guidelines/view-all-racgp-guidelines/guidelines-for-preventive-activities-in-general-pr/preventive-activities-in-children-and-young-people>

Accommodation tests evaluate the ability of the eyes to adjust to the curvature of the lenses. The examiner may perform this test by questioning the person concerning their visual acuity, while placing trial lenses before their eyes. Alternatively, the test can be performed using an ophthalmoscope.

Visual field tests evaluate the functions of the retina, optic nerve and optic pathways. The person's peripheral and central visual fields are assessed when the examiner moves an object from outside the field into the field, on a radial line, until the person states that they can see the object. Tangent screen examinations detect visual field loss. In this examination, a screen is used and test objects from 1–50 mm in size are placed on the screen. Each eye is individually tested for visualisation of the objects (Berman et al 2021; Cooper & Gosnell 2023).

Objective eye tests

Intraocular pressure is assessed using a tonometer. A topical anaesthetic is instilled, and the examiner places the tonometer on the apex of the cornea to determine pressure in the eye. An alternative method involves the use of an 'air-puff' tonometer that does not contact the eye. Tonometry serves as a valuable screening test for early detection of glaucoma.

Ophthalmoscopic examination involves the use of an ophthalmoscope to view the interior structures of the eye. The ophthalmoscope examines the fundus, or interior aspect, of the eye, allowing magnified examination of the optic disc, retinal vessels, macula and retina.

Slit-lamp examination allows the examiner to visualise in detail the anterior segment of the eye. Before the examination, dilating eye drops (mydriatics) may be instilled. The person sits with their chin on a rest and their forehead against a bar attached to the lamp. Slit-lamp examination helps determine corneal abrasions, dermatitis and cataracts.

Fluorescein staining is a technique in which staining the eye's surface with dye provides a better view of the anterior portion of the eye. The test is generally performed when conjunctival or corneal abrasions are suspected. Surface defects absorb more dye than normal areas (Berman et al 2021).

Special procedures for assessing the eye

Fluorescein angiography involves rapid-sequence photographs of the fundus after intravenous injection of a contrast medium. Fluorescein angiography records the appearance of blood vessels inside the eye.

A culture to determine the microorganism causing ocular infection may be obtained by passing a sterile swab over the conjunctival surface.

Computerised tomography (CT) of the orbit may be used to detect abnormalities such as intraocular foreign bodies or retinoblastoma. Contrast dye is injected, and the eyeball scanned.

Ocular ultrasonography involves the transmission of high-frequency soundwaves through the eye, and measurement of their reflection forms the ocular structures.

Ultrasonography can identify abnormalities that are undetectable through ophthalmoscopy and may be used to locate intraocular foreign bodies.

Care of the person with an eye disorder

While the general care of the person with a disorder of the eye is directed towards helping them to meet their needs, the three main aspects of care are:

1. maintaining a safe environment
2. education
3. providing local eye care.

Maintaining a safe environment

Blindness or loss of vision can mean that the individual is susceptible to injury; therefore, the nurse has a responsibility to protect them from environmental hazards. These hazards may include such things as low levels of lighting, poor colour contrast or badly positioned furniture or clutter. When possible, the nurse should communicate with the client to identify any preferences with their environment and the management of such. To support the person, the nurse should describe the layout of the room to the individual. If the individual is ambulant, the nurse can guide them to locate various pieces of furniture so that they become familiar with their position in the room. Leave furniture and personal belongings in the same position and make sure that any clutter, rubbish or trip hazards are removed. Ensure that any doors are either fully closed or open since a person who is blind or has low vision can easily be injured if a door is left ajar.

Nurses can foster independence in the hospitalised blind or low-vision person by encouraging self-sufficiency in completing activities of daily living and improving self-esteem as the person attempts and masters activities (Vision Australia 2023).

Education

Education involves assisting the individual to adjust to their blindness or loss of vision. The nurse should initially describe to the individual with the alteration to visual function what has occurred. The person who is experiencing vision loss that is either temporary or permanent needs assistance to adjust to the physical and psychosocial implications. Care of the person includes encouraging them to express reactions and feelings to their vision loss. The person experiencing vision loss may lose the ability to observe body language and the reading and writing components of communication. It is important for the individual to be able to interact with people they encounter. Communication methods may also be taught to family members and significant others. Ensuring person-centred care and autonomy means that, when possible, the consultation with the individual should be utilised to determine their preferences and needs from social supports.

Key aspects related to assisting the vision-impaired person

- Encourage as much self-care as possible. The person who is experiencing recent loss of vision may need assistance until they adjust to their condition. A person who has been blind or low vision for some time will probably have developed considerable self-reliance. The nurse should always consult the person when uncertain whether assistance is required.
- Address the person by name and identify yourself, visitors or others in the room. This avoids frightening the person and assists them in knowing who is in the room. It is also important to knock before entering and to inform them when you are about to leave the room.
- Speak to the person in the same manner as you would a fully sighted person. The nurse must suppress the urge to speak more loudly than usual, which people often do when conversing with a person who is blind or low vision. There is no need to exclude words such as 'look' and 'see' from normal conversation.
- Any vision aids that the person uses should be kept in close proximity (Table 34.2). The person should have easy accessibility to the call bell if required.
- Encourage the person to maintain an interest in the outside environment through listening to the radio or television and discussing newspaper items.
- Provide full descriptions of people, places and things.
- Provide items that can compensate for diminished vision, such as bright non-glare lighting, large-print books,

TABLE 34.2 | Aids for people who are blind or low-vision

Aid	Description
Magnifiers	Hand-held or standing magnifiers can be used to enlarge print, or for fine detail.
Enlarged print	Large-print books, magazines and newspapers may be borrowed from the local library.
Audiobooks	Books are often available in audio form through various websites and smartphone applications. Tapes of books may be available on loan from agencies for the blind or from public libraries.
Telephone aids	Accessibility features on smartphones are often easy to set up and can support people with text-to-audio features, contrasting colours and larger text. Special dials are available for land line telephones in both large print and braille.
Braille	The braille system of writing and printing uses tangible points or dots, which the individual feels and 'reads' with the fingertips.
Optical-to-tactile/ audio converters	Consist of devices that convert vision into tactile sensation, by reproducing the outline of a letter on a tactile screen. Similar programs can convert written text to audio/spoken word.
Canes	Various types of canes are available (e.g. a white or collapsible cane), which help the individual to locate obstacles in the environment. Laser canes also locate objects and can identify changes in the region from as far away as 6 metres.
Guide dogs	Trained guide dogs allow greater mobility and independence for the vision-impaired person. The individual holds a U-shaped handle, which is attached to a harness on the dog. Communication between the two takes place through the movements of the harness. When a guide dog is working (i.e. when it is in harness), other people should not approach or pat the dog without the handler's permission because the dog may become distracted.

(Vision Australia 2023)

talking books, telephones with enlarged buttons and a clock with numbers and hands that can be felt.

- At mealtimes, it may be necessary for the nurse to describe the position of foods on the plate (such as, peas are at 9 o'clock, potatoes at 12 o'clock, pumpkin at 3 o'clock and chicken at 6 o'clock).
- It is of particular importance to thoroughly explain any procedure or treatment before it is started. Whenever possible, if it will not affect sterility, the person should be allowed to feel any items used during a procedure.
- Provide contrasting colours (e.g. non-white crockery and brightly coloured telephones, handles, borders or edges allow familiar objects to become more visible). Coloured tape, paint or nail polish can be used to colour-code appliance dials.
- Painting the edge of stairs with bright paint can help the person distinguish the edge of the step more clearly.
- Inform the person when they are approaching stairs or steps, remembering to let them know whether they are up or down.
- When walking with the person, the nurse should walk slightly ahead and let the person take their elbow. This technique ensures that the person senses the direction they are walking towards. The nurse should encourage the use of handrails while ambulating and warn the person of any hazards as they are approached.
- Cultural aspects of care should always be considered when caring for a person who has vision loss.
- On discharge, review specific hazards in the home with the person and family. It is possible the person will need an assessment by an occupational therapist prior or soon after discharge. Assessment must be made of both indoor and outdoor living arrangements. The person's living quarters should not be altered after they have become familiar with placement of furniture.
- Inform the person and family that progress will be slow and that they will need to seek support from outside agencies. Encourage families to explore community resources available to persons with partial or total loss of vision, and the rehabilitation programs available to them. This may include a referral to allied health to support in accessing National Disability Insurance Scheme if applicable. Some of the current community services available include Association for the Blind; state and territory guide dog associations and Seeing Eye Dogs Australia; Australian Braille Authority; Vision Australia; Blind Welfare Australia; and Blind Citizens Australia. All can provide services and resources for people who are blind or low-vision.

Local eye care

Various nursing procedures involving the eye should be performed in accordance with the policies of the healthcare institution. General principles that should be followed in all ophthalmic procedures include the following:

- Explain what you are going to do.
- Ensure that the person is sitting or lying with their head well supported.
- Ensure that there is adequate lighting; lights should never be allowed to shine directly into the person's eyes.
- Wash hands thoroughly before and after the procedure and wear disposable gloves to prevent cross-infection.
- Use gentle unhurried movements and refrain from exerting any pressure on the eye.
- Avoid all sudden movements.
- Avoid touching the cornea with the fingers or equipment, to prevent corneal damage.
- Use aseptic technique. When only one eye is infected or inflamed, the unaffected eye must receive attention first to prevent cross-infection.
- Ensure that if an eye pad is to be applied, the eyelid is closed firmly to avoid corneal abrasion.

(See Clinical Skill 34.1.)

CLINICAL SKILL 34.1 Application of eye pad

Please adhere to the policy and procedures of the facility/organisation prior to undertaking the skill. Ensure this skill is in your scope of practice.

NMBA Decision-making Framework considerations (refer to NMBA Decision-making framework for nursing and midwifery 2020): 1. Am I educated? 2. Am I authorised? 3. Am I competent? If you answer 'no' to any of these, do not perform that activity. Seek guidance and support from your teacher/a nurse team leader/clinical facilitator/educator.	**Equipment:** Sterile eye pad Disposable gloves Tape

PREPARE FOR THE SKILL

(Please refer to the Standard Steps on pp. xviii–xx for related rationales.)
Mentally review the steps of the skill.
Discuss the skill with your instructor/supervisor/team leader, if required.
Confirm correct facility/organisation policy/safe operating procedures.
Validate the order in the individual's record.
Identify indication and rationale for performing the activity.
Assess for any contraindications.
Locate and gather equipment.
Perform hand hygiene.
Ensure therapeutic interaction.
Identify the individual using three individual identifiers.
Gain the individual's consent.
Assess for pain relief.
Prepare the environment.
Provide and maintain privacy.
Assist the individual to assume an appropriate position of comfort.

Ensure that the person is sitting or lying with their head well supported and there is adequate lighting.	Ensures the person is relaxed and comfortable and therefore less likely to move during procedure and cause corneal damage.

PERFORM THE SKILL

(Please refer to the Standard Steps on pp. xviii–xx for related rationales.)
Perform hand hygiene.
Apply PPE: gloves, eyewear, mask and gown as appropriate.
Ensure the individual's safety and comfort throughout skill.
Promote independence and involvement of the individual if possible and/or appropriate.
Assess the individual's tolerance to the skill throughout.
Dispose of used supplies, equipment, waste and sharps appropriately.
Remove PPE and discard or store appropriately.
Perform hand hygiene.

Continued

CLINICAL SKILL 34.1 Application of eye pad—cont'd

Skill activity	Rationale
Before the eye pad is applied, the person is asked to close their eyelid firmly.	Ensures the eye is not directly in contact with the eye pad and prevents corneal damage.
Use gentle unhurried movements and avoid all sudden movements.	Prevents person from moving or flinching to prevent corneal damage.
The pad should be applied so that the eyelid cannot be opened. Check medical orders since sometimes double padding is required.	Ensures the eye is not directly in contact with the eye pad and prevents corneal damage.
Pressure should not be applied, unless prescribed by a medical officer.	Pressure can damage the eye.
The eye pad is secured into position using hypoallergenic tape. Place the tape diagonally from forehead to cheek.	Prevents exposure of the eye. Placing tape at an angle reduces the risk of pressure on the eye.
Ask the individual to report any complications during and post procedure if able. Explain that their range of vision and depth perception may be altered.	Provides anticipatory guidance so that the individual takes more care when ambulating or feeding themselves.

AFTER THE SKILL

(Please refer to the Standard Steps on pp. xviii–xx for related rationales.)
Communicate outcome to the individual, any ongoing care and to report any complications.
Restore the environment.
Report, record and document assessment findings, details of the skill performed and the individual's response.
Report, record and document any abnormalities and/or inability to perform the skill.
Reassess the individual to ensure there are no adverse effects/events from the skill.

(Australian Commission on Safety and Quality in Health Care [ACSQHC] 2021; Berman et al 2021; Tollefson et al 2022)

Application of eye pads

A light eye pad may be applied to prevent further injury after trauma to the eye or to avoid eye damage after administration of a local anaesthetic. Before the eye pad is applied the individual is asked to close their eyelid firmly. The pad should be applied so that the eyelid cannot be opened. Pressure should not be applied unless a medical officer has prescribed it. The eye pad is secured into position using hypoallergenic tape, placing the tape diagonally from forehead to cheek.

Eye irrigation

Irrigation is a technique performed to flush secretions, chemicals or foreign bodies from the conjunctival sac. Chemical injuries to the eye require flushing of the conjunctival sac with copious amounts of solution. It may be necessary to cleanse the eyelids before irrigation (e.g. if there is excessive discharge or crusting). A suggested technique for eye irrigation is outlined in Clinical Skill 34.2.

Eye prostheses

Two types of eye prosthesis are contact lenses and artificial eyes.

Contact lenses: A contact lens is a small plastic disc that is positioned on the cornea and held in place by surface tension. A person who has a refractive error (e.g. astigmatism) may wear contact lenses in place of glasses. A variety of lenses are available including hard, soft, gas permeable, extended wear, daily wear, coloured and disposable. It is important to know that all lenses require care and must be removed periodically to prevent corneal damage and eye infection. Education is required regarding proper lens care (e.g. daily wear lenses should be removed overnight for cleaning and disinfection). Only the recommended solutions should be used for cleaning, soaking and storing lenses. Wetting lenses with contact lens solution before insertion minimises discomfort. Keeping fingernails short and clean and washing and drying hands before inserting or removing lenses will help with infection control (Cooper & Gosnell 2023; Crisp et al 2021).

Artificial eyes: An artificial eye may be inserted after surgical removal of an eye. Persons with artificial eyes have had enucleation of an entire eyeball. An artificial eye may be removed from the socket, cleaned, and replaced. Alternatively, the prosthesis may remain in the socket permanently. Most persons prefer to care for their own eyes but there may be times when assistance from the nurse is required. When a

CLINICAL SKILL 34.2 Eye irrigation

Please adhere to the policy and procedures of the facility/organisation prior to undertaking the skill. Ensure this skill is in your scope of practice.

NMBA Decision-making Framework considerations	Equipment:
NMBA Decision-making Framework considerations (refer to NMBA Decision-making framework for nursing and midwifery 2020): 1. Am I educated? 2. Am I authorised? 3. Am I competent? If you answer 'no' to any of these, do not perform that activity. Seek guidance and support from your teacher/a nurse team leader/clinical facilitator/educator.	**Equipment:** Dressing pack or sterile gauze and kidney dish or another receptacle Sterile eye irrigating solution Gloves Towel or absorbent mat

PREPARE FOR THE SKILL

(Please refer to the Standard Steps on pp. xviii–xx for related rationales.)
Mentally review the steps of the skill.
Discuss the skill with your instructor/supervisor/team leader, if required.
Confirm correct facility/organisation policy/safe operating procedures.
Validate the order in the individual's record.
Identify indication and rationale for performing the activity.
Assess for any contraindications.
Locate and gather equipment.
Perform hand hygiene.
Ensure therapeutic interaction.
Identify the individual using three individual identifiers.
Gain the individual's consent.
Assess for pain relief.
Prepare the environment.
Provide and maintain privacy.
Assist the individual to assume an appropriate position of comfort.

Assist the person into a recumbent position, with the head tilted towards the affected side.	Prevents the solution running either over the cheek into the other eye or out of the affected eye and down the side of the nose.

PERFORM THE SKILL

(Please refer to the Standard Steps on pp. xviii–xx for related rationales.)
Perform hand hygiene.
Apply PPE: gloves, eyewear, mask and gown as appropriate.
Ensure the individual's safety and comfort throughout skill.
Promote independence and involvement of the individual if possible and/or appropriate.
Assess the individual's tolerance to the skill throughout.
Dispose of used supplies, equipment, waste and sharps appropriately.
Remove PPE and discard or store appropriately.
Perform hand hygiene.

Skill activity	Rationale
Place a towel under the head on the affected side and across the neck. Place a kidney dish against the person's cheek and ask the individual to hold it in position.	Prevents solution from flowing down the neck.
Pour irrigating solution into the sterile receptacle or open the container of eye wash. Gently hold the eyelid open with one hand.	A person will instinctively try to close the eye.
Hold the fluid container 2.5 cm away from the eye.	If the fluid container is held too high, fluid will flow at increased pressure, causing discomfort and possible damage to the eye.

Continued

CLINICAL SKILL 34.2 Eye irrigation—cont'd

Pour a little solution over the cheek first.	Accustoms the person to the feel of the solution and prevents person moving during procedure.
Direct the flow of solution from the nasal corner outwards.	Because the head is tilted, the stream of irrigating solution will flow over the eyeball and prevent contamination of the other eye.
Avoid directing the stream forcefully onto the eyeball, and avoid touching the eye's structures.	Prevents discomfort and damage to the eye.
Ask the person to look up and down and to either side while irrigating.	Ensures that the whole area is washed.
When the eye has been thoroughly irrigated, ask the person to close the eyes, and use a new gauze swab to dry the lids.	Promotes comfort.

AFTER THE SKILL

(Please refer to the Standard Steps on pp. xviii–xx for related rationales.)
Communicate outcome to the individual, any ongoing care and to report any complications.
Restore the environment.
Report, record and document assessment findings, details of the skill performed and the individual's response.
Report, record and document any abnormalities and/or inability to perform the skill.
Reassess the individual to ensure there are no adverse effects/events from the skill.

(ACSQHC 2021; Berman et al 2021; Stromberg 2023; Tollefson et al 2022)

prosthesis is removed from the socket, it is placed in warm normal saline for cleansing (Crisp et al 2021).

Eye surgery

Laser eye surgery is commonly performed to correct refractive errors such as myopia, hyperopia and astigmatism. A laser is used to permanently change the shape of the cornea and, in most cases, the need to use corrective lenses is reduced or eliminated. Several surgical procedures are now available:

- laser in situ keratomileusis (LASIK)
- photorefractive keratectomy (PRK)
- laser epithelial keratomileusis (LASEK)
- laser thermokeratoplasty (LTK)

These procedures reshape the cornea using laser technology to remove a thin layer of epithelial cells or to shrink and reshape the cornea. Candidates for laser vision correction should be in good health and must have adequate corneal thickness to ensure that the risk of perforation does not occur.

Following surgery, persons may experience a temporary loss of contrast sharpness (where images do not appear crisp as with corrective lenses), over-correction or under-correction of visual acuity, dry eyes or temporarily decreased night vision with halos, glare and starbursts.

Corneal transplant, known as 'keratoplasty', is when corneal tissue from one human eye is grafted to another in order to improve vision, as once the cornea has become scarred and opaque, no treatment can restore clarity. The first successful corneal transplant was performed in 1906. Corneas are harvested from cadavers of uninfected adults who were under the age of 65 and who die as a result of acute trauma or illness. Corneal transplantation is usually an elective procedure, although emergency transplantation may be required in the case of perforation of the cornea (Stromberg 2023).

THE EAR

The ear is specially adapted as the organ of hearing, but it is also concerned with the sense of position, balance and equilibrium. Hearing is a special sense that allows individuals to experience the world in which we live by providing a pathway for sounds to reach the brain. Hearing is a complex mechanism in which the ears receive soundwaves and convert them into nerve impulses. The nerve impulses are transmitted by the acoustic nerve to the brain, where they are interpreted. The externally visible portion of each ear is located on the lateral surface of the head on each side. The remaining parts of each ear are embedded in the bone of the skull (Marieb & Keller 2021).

Structure of the ears

Each ear can be divided into three areas: the external, the middle and the inner ear (Figure 34.7).

The external ear

The external ear consists of the auricle (pinna) and the external auditory canal. The auricle consists of a piece

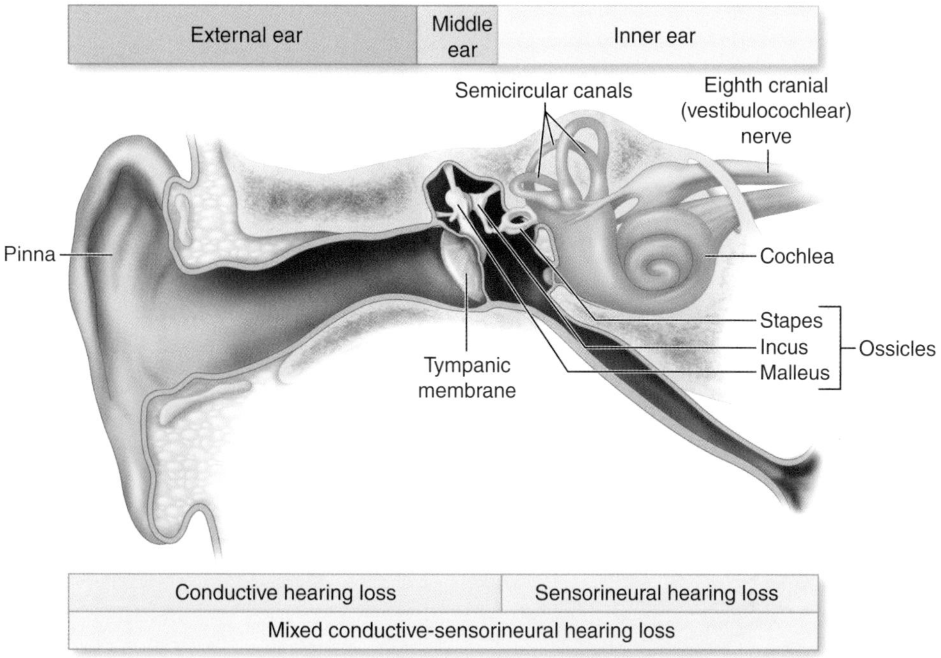

Figure 34.7 Anatomy of the middle and inner ear

(Silvestri & Silvestri 2023)

of elastic cartilage with several associated ligaments and muscles and has a small amount of adipose tissue in the earlobe. The skin of the auricle is covered with fine hairs and is continuous with the skin lining the external auditory canal. The external auditory canal is an S-shaped canal about 2.5 cm long. It extends from the auricle to the tympanic membrane (eardrum). The skin lining the canal contains glands that produce cerumen (wax) that protects the lining from damage and keeps dust particles away from the eardrum. The tympanic membrane lies between the external ear and the middle ear. It is a semi-transparent sheet consisting of three layers. The outermost layer consists of hairless skin, the middle layer is connective tissue, and the innermost layer is continuous with the mucous membrane lining of the ear (Patton & Thibodeau 2018).

The middle ear

The middle ear, or tympanic cavity, is a small chamber within the temporal bone. Three small bones, or ossicles, lying in the middle ear, transmit sound from the tympanic membrane to the oval window. Because of their shapes, the bones are named the malleus (the mallet), the incus (the anvil) and the stapes (the stirrup). The malleus is attached to the tympanic membrane; the stapes is attached to the oval window; and the incus articulates with the other two ossicles. The three ossicles are attached to the wall of the middle ear by ligaments. The auditory tube (or eustachian tube) connects the middle ear with air from the nasopharynx. It is about 3–6 cm long and is lined with mucous membrane. Normally, the tube is flattened and closed at the pharyngeal orifice but swallowing or yawning opens it briefly (Patton & Thibodeau 2018).

The inner ear

The inner ear (Figure 34.8) consists of a bony cavity within the temporal bone known as the osseous labyrinth. It is lined with periosteum and filled with a fluid called perilymph. The three divisions of the osseous labyrinth are the cochlea, the vestibule and the semi-circular canals. The cochlea is a spiralling bony cavity that resembles the shell of a snail. It houses the organ of Corti, the receptor organ of hearing. The vestibule lies between the cochlea and the semi-circular canals. It contains structures responsible for maintaining equilibrium during movement of the head. The semi-circular canals consist of three canals (in each ear), arranged at right angles to each other. They are filled with endolymph (the fluid inside the membranous labyrinth at the ear) and contain specialised nerve endings that are stimulated by the movement of the endolymph. The semi-circular canals assist the body to adjust to changes of direction. The movement of fluid in this area can cause the person to experience a feeling of dizziness.

The membranous labyrinth is a membrane consisting of three layers and lies within the osseous labyrinth. In the areas where it is not attached to the osseous labyrinth, it is surrounded by perilymph. The fluid contained within the membranous labyrinth is known as endolymph. Part of the membranous labyrinth is concerned with hearing and part is concerned with the position of the head in space (Marieb & Keller 2021).

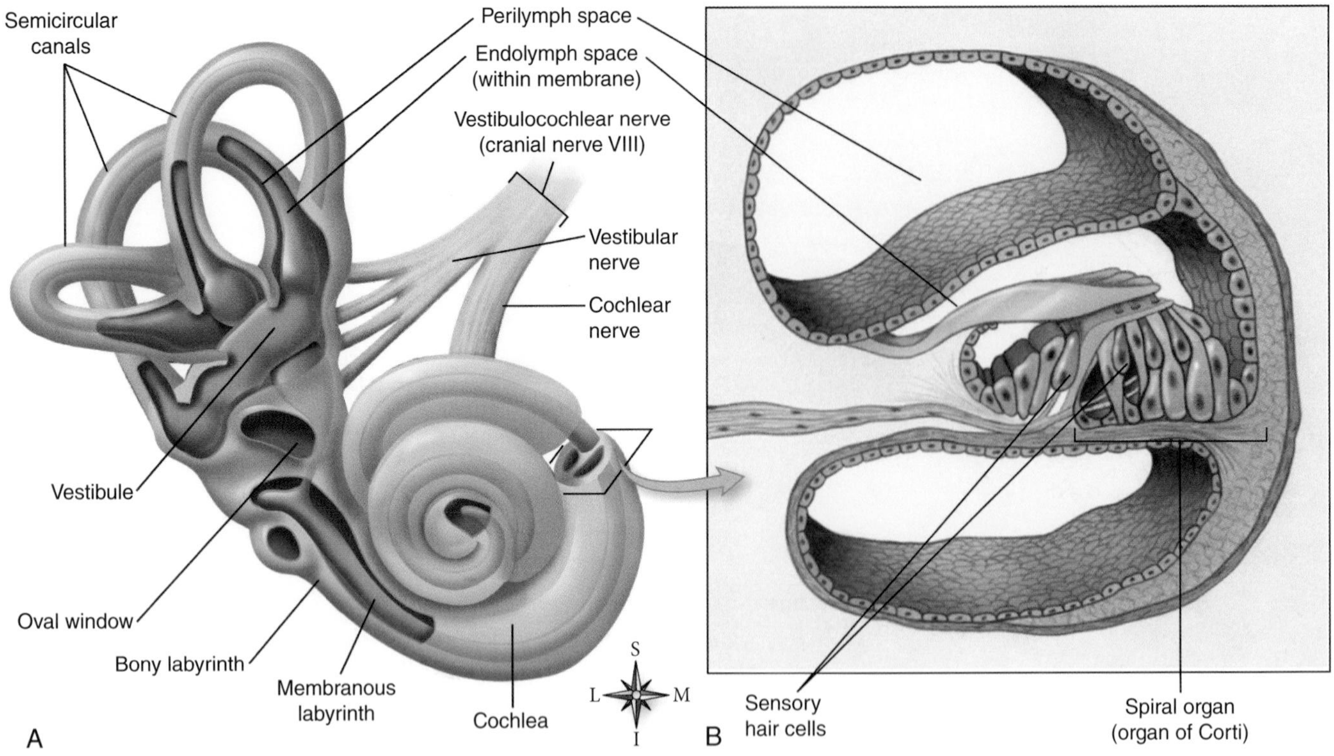

Figure 34.8 A section of membranous cochlea showing the organ of Corti

(Patton & Thibodeau 2024)

The physiology of hearing

Hearing is a sense that enables sound to be perceived. Soundwaves are collected and directed by the auricle into the external auditory canal, where they pass through and cause the tympanic membrane to vibrate. They then pass through the middle ear by vibration of the ossicles, and into the internal ear. From the internal ear, soundwaves are transmitted to the brain, via the acoustic nerve, for interpretation. Perception of sound involves interpretation of pitch and intensity. The entire process of hearing involves the following steps:

- Movement of air molecules causes a soundwave to form.
- The soundwave travels through the air to the auricle, which directs it into the external auditory canal.
- The soundwave enters the auditory canal and comes in contact with the tympanic membrane, causing it to vibrate.
- The vibrations are transferred to the ossicles, which begin to vibrate, and the soundwave is transmitted across the middle-ear cavity to the oval window and into the fluid-filled internal ear.
- The soundwaves set the cochlear fluids into motion. The receptor cells are stimulated, and the soundwaves are transmitted along the acoustic nerve to the temporal lobe of the brain for interpretation.

(Patton & Thibodeau 2018)

Two qualities of sound—pitch and intensity—are important in the interpretation of sound. Pitch is related to the frequency of the soundwave. A high-frequency sound stimulates the neurons supplying the cells near the base of the cochlea. Low-frequency sounds stimulate neurons nearer the apex of the cochlea. Intensity is related to the loudness of sound and is measured in decibels (dB). A loud sound causes the nerve endings to be stimulated at a greater rate than does a softer sound. The intensity of normal conversational speech is about 60 dB, and a decibel level of 160 can cause bursting of the tympanic membrane.

Maintenance of equilibrium (balance)

Two structures within the internal ear, the semi-circular canals and the vestibule, work together to help the individual maintain balance and equilibrium. Components of the semicircular canals alert the brain to rotational movement, and components of the vestibule alert the brain to gravitational movement. Movement of fluid in the canals gives a constant flow of information about body position and the speed and direction of any body movement. This information is used to coordinate movements and to maintain balance (Marieb & Keller 2021).

Pathophysiology of the ear

Normal function of the ear can be altered by a variety of pathophysiological factors including those that are congenital, degenerative, infectious, obstructive, neoplastic or traumatic (Marieb & Keller 2021).

Congenital factors

Congenital alterations, which may be either hereditary or acquired, include structural malformations that can lead to hearing loss or deafness, disorders resulting from maternal infection during pregnancy or trauma incurred during pregnancy or delivery, or before maturity. Congenital disorders may be caused by a genetic defect or may result from prenatal trauma or toxicity. Some disorders affect the cosmetic appearance only, while others result in varying degrees of hearing loss. Congenital disorders include partial or total absence of the external ear (auricle), protruding ears, fused or absent ossicles and malformation of the cochlea (Patton & Thibodeau 2018).

Cochlear implants are surgically implanted electronic devices that consist of two parts: one external and one internal. The inner ear implant picks up signals from the sound processor, which then stimulates the nerve fibres in the inner ear. Nerve signals then travel to the brain, to be interpreted as sound. These implants can be inserted into a baby as young as 6 months old (Healthdirect 2022). In Australia, around 12 in every 10,000 babies born will have moderate or above hearing loss in both ears, and a further 23 children will require a hearing device by the age of 17. When hearing loss is not responded to appropriately, there can be a significant impact on receptive and expressive language development and communication. Impacts on learning can result in increased likelihood of lifelong disability (Rothrock 2023).

Degenerative factors

Degenerative changes in the bones and joints of the ossicles can result in conductive hearing loss, while narrowing of blood vessels to the inner ear can result in tinnitus, vertigo or hearing loss. Gradual sensorineural hearing loss can result from a decrease in the number of hair cells and nerve fibres in the auditory system because of the ageing process. **Presbycusis** is a slowly progressive bilateral hearing loss resulting from physiological changes of ageing. It results from a loss of hair cells in the organ of Corti and causes sensorineural hearing loss, usually of high-frequency tones. Manifestations include gradual progressive hearing loss, which may be accompanied by tinnitus and dizziness, depression or irritability. Bone conductive hearing devices or aids (known as BAHA) are effective in helping people with conduction deafness to hear, as they use skull bones to conduct sound vibrations within the inner ear (Marieb & Keller 2021).

Infectious factors

Microorganisms can cause external, middle or inner ear infections, all of which result in pain and varying degrees of conductive hearing loss. Otitis externa, which may be acute or chronic, is inflammation of the external ear canal and auricle; the most common causative organism is *Streptococcus pyogenes*, although *Proteus vulgaris*, *Staphylococcus aureus*, *Candida albicans* and *Aspergillus niger* may be responsible for infection. Predisposing factors include swimming in contaminated water, abrasion of the ear canal from inserting sharp or small objects to clean the ear, exposure to irritants and constant use of earphones or earplugs. Manifestations include otalgia, which is exacerbated on chewing or opening the mouth, lymphadenopathy, pyrexia, regional cellulitis, offensive smelling discharge, pruritus and partial hearing loss.

Otitis media, also known as 'swimmer's ear' or 'tropical ear', which may be acute (over 95% of cases) or chronic, is inflammation of the middle ear. Causative organisms include *Haemophilus influenzae*, pneumococci and beta-haemolytic streptococci. Predisposing factors include the wider, shorter and more horizontal pharyngotympanic tube in infants and children, anatomical abnormalities such as cleft palate and respiratory tract infection. Manifestations include severe otalgia, pyrexia, hearing loss, dizziness, nausea and vomiting. If the tympanic membrane ruptures, there is often purulent discharge from the ear canal.

Obstructive factors

Obstruction of the auditory system, which may result in conductive or sensorineural hearing loss, includes impacted cerumen, foreign bodies, oedema and neoplasms. An obstruction can impede the passage of soundwaves, causing an imbalance of pressure on either side of the tympanic membrane, or it may disrupt the transmission of sound to the inner ear.

Neoplastic factors

Neoplasms, which may be benign or malignant, can affect the external middle or inner ear. The effects of a neoplasm include pain, discharge, vertigo, tinnitus and hearing loss. An acoustic neuroma is a benign tumour arising from the eighth cranial nerve and occurring within the internal auditory canal. As the tumour grows, the cochlear branch of the eighth cranial nerve becomes involved. Manifestations include tinnitus followed by an increasing high-frequency hearing loss. As the tumour increases in size, symptoms of other cranial nerve involvement occur, such as trigeminal pain and loss of taste in part of the tongue. Nystagmus and ataxia may occur (Stromberg 2023).

Traumatic factors

Trauma to the external ear includes bruising, lacerations and frostbite. Trauma to the head can result in fractures of the temporal bone, dislocation of the ossicles, rupture of the tympanic membrane and damage to the auditory nerve. Trauma can lead to vertigo, tinnitus, nystagmus, pain, bleeding and hearing loss. Hearing loss can also result from sudden exposure to a loud explosive sound or from continued exposure to loud noise.

Abrasion: Because of its vulnerable position, the external ear may sustain abrasion of the canal, burns or contusions of the pinna. Foreign bodies may be inserted into the canal and become lodged, or insects may fly into the ear, causing irritation.

Perforated eardrum: A perforated tympanic membrane may be caused by a variety of factors, such as the introduction of a sharp object to clean the canal, unskilled irrigation of the auditory canal, middle-ear infection, trauma to the head or sudden exposure to loud noise. Most traumatic perforations heal spontaneously, but a perforated tympanic membrane results in scarring and renders the person susceptible to chronic ear infections and hearing loss. Manifestations include sudden severe pain inside the ear, loss of hearing, tinnitus and bleeding.

Barotrauma: Barotrauma is injury caused by changes of air pressure to the wall of the pharyngotympanic tube and mucous membrane of the middle ear. It is caused by failure of the pharyngotympanic tube to open sufficiently, resulting in unequal pressure between the middle ear and the atmospheric pressure. It may occur during take-off or landing in planes, or during deep-sea diving. Manifestations include severe pain, decreased hearing, tinnitus and vertigo.

Noise-induced hearing loss: This condition develops gradually as a result of continued exposure to environmental or industrial noise. Acoustic trauma is sudden hearing loss from brief exposure to a high-intensity sound at close range, such as gunshots. Manifestations of noise trauma include hearing loss, tinnitus, and a feeling of fullness within the ear.

Ototoxicity: Ototoxicity is a toxic reaction to medications or chemicals that can damage the auditory and/or vestibular system. Auditory damage may be permanent, whereas vestibular damage may be reversed after the drug therapy is discontinued. A variety of substances may result in ototoxic reactions, including diuretics, alcohol, lead, carbon monoxide, aspirin and antibiotics. Manifestations include bilateral hearing loss, tinnitus, vertigo and ataxia (Berman et al 2021; Jarvis & Eckhardt 2021).

Major symptoms of ear disorders

The major manifestations of ear disorders are pain, discharge, tinnitus, vertigo, nystagmus and hearing loss. Table 34.3 is a representation of these manifestations.

TABLE 34.3 | Major manifestations of ear disorders

Pain	Earache (**otalgia**) is a common manifestation of many ear disorders. Middle-ear pain associated with otitis media is often described as deep seated and throbbing, whereas the pain associated with otitis externa is often described as tenderness of the pinna only. Ear pain can also result from referred pain via various cranial or cervical nerves as occurs with tonsillitis.
Discharge	Discharge from the ear, also known as otorrhoea, is generally associated with infections of the middle ear (otitis media). Purulent or haemopurulent discharge may drain from the middle ear through a perforation in the tympanic membrane. Otitis externa can sometimes produce a prolific discharge but is less likely than with otitis media.
Hearing loss	Hearing loss is a common manifestation in ear disorders. There are two types of hearing loss: *Conductive* hearing loss is caused by blockage or damage in the outer ear, middle ear, or both. Some of the causes of conductive hearing loss include ear infections, otosclerosis, otitis media, barotrauma, damage to tympanic membrane or blockage of the ear canal by wax or foreign objects. *Sensorineural* hearing loss (perceptive or nerve) is caused by damage to, or a malfunction of, the cochlea (the sensory part) or the nerve (the neural part). It can be hereditary or genetic; it can also be caused by the ageing process, excessive noise exposure, diseases such as meningitis or Ménière's disease and viruses such as mumps or measles. Some hearing loss is caused by a mixture of both above types, known as mixed hearing loss.
Tinnitus	The term '**tinnitus**' is used to describe a noise in the inner ear when there is no actual external noise. The word 'tinnitus' means 'tinkling or ringing like a bell' and is of Latin origin; it is usually pronounced tinn-i-tus, the 'i' as in 'sit'. It can be constant or intermittent, and may be described as ringing, buzzing, hissing or roaring noises. There are many possible causes of tinnitus, including trauma, obstruction, inflammation and malignancies. However, little research has been conducted in this area and there is no known cure.
Vertigo	Vertigo is a sensation of spinning. People describe it as feeling as though their head is spinning or the room is going around. Causes can include trauma, malignancies, Ménière's disease and obstruction.
Nystagmus	**Nystagmus** is the involuntary, rhythmic movement of the eyes. Movement may be horizontal, vertical, rotary or mixed. Nystagmus can be a sign of disorders of the inner ear but can also be present in some neurological disorders. Nystagmus can also be induced by introducing cold or warm water into the external auditory canal.

(Brown et al 2020; Crisp et al 2021)

CRITICAL THINKING EXERCISE 34.2

Parents Marc and Alex have presented to the clinic with their 18-month-old child Aisha. The doctor has just informed Marc and Alex that Aisha may have severe hearing loss involving both ears and has referred Aisha to an audiologist. What type of behaviour do you think Aisha has displayed for her parents to bring her to the clinic? What allied health members and community services do you think will be introduced into Aisha's life?

Disorders of multiple causes

Otosclerosis is a disorder in which the spongy temporal bone becomes a dense sclerotic mass, eventually immobilising the stapedial footplate and causing a conductive hearing loss. Although no definite cause has been identified, heredity is a significant factor. Females have a higher incidence of the disorder than males. Manifestations are slowly progressive and include bilateral conductive hearing loss and mild tinnitus (Patton & Thibodeau 2018).

Ménière's disease is a disorder of the inner ear that results from over-production or decreased absorption of endolymph. The resulting dilation of the membranous labyrinth can progress to herniation and rupture. Manifestations are exacerbation and remissions of three symptoms: vertigo, tinnitus and sensorineural hearing loss. During an acute episode, the person may experience nausea and vomiting, sweating, giddiness, nystagmus and ataxia (Marieb & Keller 2021).

CRITICAL THINKING EXERCISE 34.3

Peter is a 48-year-old man with Ménière's disease. He is experiencing frequent episodes of nausea when he tries to stand up and expresses to his partner that 'the room keeps spinning'. Peter has been unable to leave the house and go to work for the past week.

1. What is this 'spinning feeling' that Peter is experiencing?
2. What could be the cause of Peter's condition?
3. How can Peter manage his condition at home?

Health promotion

Health promotion focuses on identifying persons with potential ear disorders (see Case Study 34.1). Persistent episodes of dizziness, ringing in the ears, balance problems or loss of hearing should be reported to a healthcare provider. The nurse is in a key position to educate persons about the ways in which hearing can be protected and preserved:

- Regular hearing examinations are important for the early detection of hearing problems, especially for children, whose ability to learn can be compromised by hearing loss and consequential social and environmental barriers.

CASE STUDY 34.1

Henry Goldfield is a 48-year-old man working as a car salesman. Over the past 2 months Henry progressively had trouble hearing clients talking on the telephone. Henry also complained to his boss that he is feeling dizzy and suggested he should not take clients for a test drive until the dizziness stops. This week Henry was admitted to the hospital with left-sided facial pain, discharge from the left ear and a reduced sense of taste.

1. What do you think is happening to Henry?
2. What are some of the nursing care considerations you need to take into account when caring for Henry?

- Regular screening is also important for the person over age 65 because the ageing process is commonly accompanied by degenerative ear changes. Recommended preventative screening should be carried out for all ages as required.
- Prevention of trauma to the ears includes education, such as the importance of never putting small or sharp objects into ears.
- Excessive cleaning of the ear canal is contraindicated since it removes the cerumen, which has a protective function.
- Protection of the ears from contamination by water when swimming or diving is particularly important if the person has experienced ear infections.
- Infections that could involve the ear (e.g. upper respiratory tract infections) require adequate treatment.
- Protection of the ears from damage by noise: prolonged exposure to noise levels greater than 85–90 dB causes cochlear damage. People working in areas of high noise levels are required to wear protective devices such as earplugs or earmuffs. Exposure to loud volume from live music, audio equipment and headphones should be avoided.
- Nurse assessment of the person's understanding of the importance and necessity of routine health screening.
- Monitoring for vertigo, nystagmus, nausea, vomiting and hearing loss.
- Instructing the person not to get up without assistance during episodes of vertigo due to increased falls risk.
- Education to avoid sudden head movements or position changes.
- Discussion of the effect of unilateral hearing loss on the ability to identify the direction of sounds.

(Berman et al 2021; Crisp et al 2021)

Diagnostic tests

Tests used to assist in the diagnosis of ear disorders assess auditory and vestibular function.

Auditory tests

Otoscopic examination is the direct visualisation of the external auditory canal and the tympanic membrane through an otoscope (auroscope). Otoscopy is performed to detect foreign bodies or cerumen in the external canal, or to detect external and middle-ear pathology. Tuning forks detect hearing loss and provide information as to the type of loss. Some auditory tests include the following:

- The Weber test determines whether the individual lateralises the tone of the tuning fork to one ear.
- The Rinne's test evaluates air and bone conduction in both ears.

(Ball 2023)

Audiometry: Pure tone audiometry is the testing of each ear separately for air conduction via earphones, and for bone conduction via a vibrating tuning fork placed on the mastoid bone. The faintest point at which the individual hears the tone is called the hearing threshold level. Comparison of air and bone thresholds can suggest a conductive, sensorineural or mixed-type hearing loss.

Speech audiometry tests the person's ability to understand and discriminate sounds. Two-syllable words are presented through earphones to measure how loud speech must be before it is heard.

Speech discrimination testing measures the person's ability to distinguish phonetic elements of speech and thus understand what is heard. The examiner presents one-syllable words through the earphones.

Impedance audiometry evaluates middle-ear function by measuring the flow of sound energy into the ear, and the resistance to that flow. The objective is to determine the resistance (impedance) of flexibility (compliance) of the tympanic membrane (Patton & Thibodeau 2018).

Vestibular tests

Electronystagmography (ENG) evaluates vestibular function by measuring the effect of the semi-circular canals on the ocular muscles. Electrodes are positioned at precise points on the face and eye, with movements in response to specific stimuli recorded on a graph.

Caloric tests compare the nystagmus produced by warm and cold stimulation in each ear. Each ear is irrigated with water to stimulate mild vertigo and nystagmus. No response indicates that the labyrinth is non-functional.

Other tests used to diagnose ear disorders include cultures of secretions to detect the source of an infection, and radiological examination of the temporal bone (Cooper & Gosnell 2023).

Care of a person with an ear disorder

While the general care of the person with a disorder of the ear is directed towards helping them to meet their needs, three main aspects of care should be implemented:

- maintaining a safe environment
- education
- providing any prescribed local ear care.

Maintaining a safe environment

Impact from loss of hearing or issue with the inner ear can render the person susceptible to accidents and injury. Any environment can heighten or reduce sensory stimulation. The nurse must assess the person's environment in the healthcare setting as well as assisting the person and the family to identify hazards in the person's regular environment and recommend appropriate adaptations and referrals. Persons with vestibular disorders are at risk of losing their balance and falling. If identified as a risk, it is important to ensure that bathrooms have a non-skid surface in the shower and bath, grab bars are installed and that the nurse provides the person and their family with education regarding supervision of the person when ambulant, to minimise the risk of falls (Crisp et al 2021).

Education

The person who is experiencing hearing loss that is either temporary or permanent needs assistance to adjust to the physical and psychosocial implications. Communication is a key component of assisting the person who is deaf or hard of hearing. Initially, the person may withdraw by avoiding communication or socialisation with others to cope with the hearing loss. This can lead to social isolation and low self-esteem. The nurse should encourage the person to discuss feelings of fear and frustration with their family members and social supports relevant to them (Cooper & Gosnell 2023).

Australian Sign Language (Auslan) and the use of interpreters

Australian Sign Language (more commonly referred to as Auslan) is the language of the Australian deaf community. In the Australian deaf community Auslan is used as the primary mode of communication and because of this the community will often class themselves as a cultural and linguistic group. In recent census data, it was found that more than 16,000 people use Auslan in Australia (Deaf Connect 2022).

It is common that deaf people who use Auslan or other sign languages will have little or no concern regarding their hearing loss and will instead show a sense of pride linked to their language, community and resilience in overcoming social barriers. When working with deaf people who use sign languages, it may be that they have no interest in improving their level of hearing and will already be independent in their daily life.

According to Deaf Australia (2021), deaf people commonly report ongoing barriers to the provision of appropriate healthcare and because of this will avoid accessing services, experience higher rates of health trauma and often report poorer outcomes.

When working with deaf people who use Auslan, it is critical that qualified interpreters are used similar to when working with other patients who do not speak English. By supporting accessible healthcare, we can see improvements in the access to services, health literacy and outcomes for our patients.

CLINICAL INTEREST BOX 34.7 Hearing aid care

A hearing aid helps to capture, amplify and funnel soundwaves to the auditory nerve in a person with sensorineural hearing loss. Hearing aids are delicate and must be protected from heat, moisture and breakage. The manufacturer's guidelines for instructions specific to the person's hearing aid should be read by the person and/or family members. The aid is turned on to be certain it is working, then the ear mould is gently inserted into the ear canal. Once the mould has been inserted, the individual adjusts the volume. The tube, if fitted, is placed over the ear and attached to the battery device. Key aspects related to care of aids include:

- Ensuring that the ear mould and tubing are not blocked by wax or moisture. The hearing aid may be wiped with a soft tissue to remove any oils or waxes.
- Keeping the aid dry and away from high temperatures (e.g. direct sunlight).
- Removing the aid before the person showers or washes their hair.
- Switching off the aid when it is not in use.
- Checking the battery and replacing it when necessary. Ensure that the battery is inserted correctly.
- Checking that the hearing aid is switched on when in use and that the volume is adjusted.
- Investigating the cause of any 'whistling', which can result in embarrassment and annoyance. Causes of whistling include a poorly fitting ear mould, ear mould incorrectly positioned, cracked or broken tubing and the volume turned up too high.
- Notifying the audiologist or hearing-aid specialist if the aid is malfunctioning.

Research has resulted in the development of an implantable device to improve hearing—the cochlear implant. A cochlear implant is an electronic device that is surgically implanted. The device picks up environmental sounds and converts them to electrical impulses, which are relayed to an implant receiver. Direct electrical stimulation to the nerve fibres of cranial nerve VIII sometimes enables profoundly deaf persons to hear some sounds.

(Perry et al 2020)

Clinical Interest Box 34.7 provides an overview of hearing aid care and education.

Key aspects related to assisting a person who is deaf or hard of hearing

- Reduce background noise; attract the person's attention before speaking by moving into their line of sight or by using vibrations through the floor or furniture such as tables.
- Stand directly in front of the person or, if in a group setting, arrange semi-circular seating. This enables the person to see facial expressions, body gestures and lip patterns. Vision becomes a primary sense for the person who is deaf and hard of hearing. The nurse should avoid covering the mouth while speaking and shift items that may be blocking the line of sight.
- If the person uses Auslan as their preferred language, a qualified interpreter should be booked and whenever possible, critical conversations should be held off until the interpreter is present.
- Communication can be improved by employing non-verbal cues to help convey the meaning of your conversation (e.g. written communication, facial expression, visual cues and gestures).
- Allow the person time to insert, or adjust, any hearing aid or cochlear implant before you speak.
- Speak clearly and more slowly than usual but avoid exaggerated movements or shouting. Shouting distorts sound and is painful to the wearer of a hearing aid.
- Rephrase your words if the person has not understood. It may be helpful to write out the message if you remain uncertain whether the person has understood.
- If the person who is deaf or hard of hearing uses speech and you do not understand their communication, do not pretend to have done so. The person should be encouraged to repeat the sentence or to use other words or gestures to get the message across.
- Organisations such as the Word of Mouth Technology and Queensland Health have resources and packaged kits for healthcare institutions, designed to assist deaf and hard of hearing persons and staff. The kit generally includes visual pain guides, alerts for staff when entering the room of a deaf or hard hearing person and information sheets.
- Other assistive devices may be required, such as smartphones and watches and telephones and alarm clocks with enhanced noise or flashing lights.
- Cultural aspects of care should always be taken into account when caring for the person who is deaf or hard of hearing. This includes persons who may identify as culturally deaf rather than through the commonly understood medical model of deafness.

On discharge, the nurse should encourage the person and their family to explore community resources available to people with partial or total loss of hearing, and support programs that aid in performing the activities of daily living and language (signed and/or spoken) (Cooper & Gosnell 2023; Crisp et al 2021).

Table 34.4 provides examples of aids for deaf and hard of hearing persons.

Local ear care

Various nursing procedures involving the ear should be performed in accordance with the policies of the healthcare facility. The general principles should include:

- Explain the procedure to the person.
- Ensure the person is sitting or lying with their head well supported.

TABLE 34.4 | Aids available to people who are deaf or hard of hearing

Aid	Description
Hearing aid	Hearing aids are devices that receive speech and environmental sounds through a microphone and amplify these sounds. Various styles include those worn in the ear canal, behind the ear or on the arm of spectacles. Some styles may be used with an induction coil or transmitter for use with television, telephone and when working or listening to an individual speaker (such as a teacher or work colleague).
Modified telephone	This is a telephone fitted with volume control and induction coil.
Radio and television	Devices used in conjunction with headphones, induction coils, infrared and FM transmitters. Settings for captioning are also often available for television.
National Relay Service	A service delivered by the federal government where people can make calls via a relay officer through text message or online website. The officer will read the text written by the deaf or hard of hearing person and relay it to the receiver of the phone call. Anything spoken will be relayed back to the deaf or hard of hearing person in written form.
Flashing doorbells, fire alarms and alarm clocks	Devices that can be set up around the home and can often interact with a smart device though not always necessary for set-up. When triggered, the device can flash, vibrate loudly and/or send a notification to a person's smart device.
Interpreters	Qualified interpreters can be used when a deaf person has or is developing an understanding of Auslan. They can be used in various situations such as education, social settings or healthcare. Spoken English will be interpreted into a visual or tactile language and when the deaf or hard of hearing person signs, this will be voiced into English by the interpreter.

(Soundfair 2023)

- Ensure adequate lighting.
- Wash hands thoroughly before and after the procedure to prevent cross-infection.
- Warm solutions and eardrops to body temperature since hot or cold temperatures stimulate the inner ear, causing vertigo and sometimes nausea and vomiting.

(Berman et al 2021)

Instillation of eardrops

Eardrops that may be prescribed include those that combat infection and those that soften wax. Eardrops are instilled only when they have been prescribed by a medical officer, and the nurse must follow the regulations and policies regarding the administration of medications. Key aspects regarding the use of otic medications are the same as those for using ophthalmic medications (see Chapter 20).

Progress Note 34.1

02/12/2020 0700 hrs	Nursing: Mrs Biel has been admitted for removal of cataracts and insertion of intraocular lens. She currently has low/poor vision. She requires assistance with her daily activities and meals. She has been seen by the surgeon—refer to notes. She has expressed some nervousness about her operation and was supported with reassurance and education. A thorough explanation of the procedure has been provided to her and her family. To assist in her adjustment, staff need to spend time explaining their activities to Mrs Biel before they are carried out. *R Thompson-Lee* (THOMPSON-LEE), *EN*

DECISION-MAKING FRAMEWORK EXERCISE 34.1

Imogen is an Enrolled Nurse working alone within the community setting undertaking home visits. Upon arriving at the home of an individual she discovers that the person is charted for medicated eardrops daily. Imogen is unsure if it is within her scope of practice to administer the medicated eardrops.

What steps must she work through to decide if she can administer the medicated eardrops?

Summary

The sensory organs are those that contain receptors that pick up a stimulus from the environment and transmit impulses to the brain for interpretation. These unique organs are the tongue, eye, ear, nose and skin. With these organs taste, smell, touch, sight and sound are experienced.

The tongue contains taste buds that allow individuals to differentiate from sweet, salty and bitter tastes when substances are in solution. The information is transmitted to the brain via nerve impulses to be interpreted. The sensations of taste, sight and smell are closely related, and play an important part in stimulating appetite and the secretion of gastric juices.

One of the functions of the skin is the perception of touch, making it an organ of sensation. The sensation of touch allows individuals to be aware of pressure, heat, cold and pain—necessary to protect individuals from harm as well as to feel pleasure. The impulses that travel to the brain for interpretation enable individuals to distinguish if the intensity of the sensation is harmful.

Sight is the result of light rays reaching the retina in the eyes and the image being transmitted to the brain for interpretation of that image. This process requires several components that allow the right amount of light into the eye, the retina to be exposed to the light rays and the inner workings of the eye to be able to ensure the image is in focus and true to colour.

The ears enable individuals to hear sounds and interpret them into meaningful communication. The sense of hearing is closely linked with our ability to speak.

Soundwaves enter the outer ear and travel to the tympanic membrane where nerve endings carry the resulting vibrations to the brain for interpretation. With the complex mechanisms required for hearing, individuals can interpret intensity of sound and pitch. Structures within the ear help to maintain balance.

The sense organs enable the individual to react and respond to their environment. Caring for a person with impaired sensory function requires the nurse to maintain a safe environment for the person to interact in and to be sensitive to the sensory loss being experienced.

Review Questions

1. What are some of the traumatic disorders of the eye?
2. What are the three structures of the middle layer of the eye?
3. What nursing considerations should be made if a person has an infectious disorder of the eye?
4. What are the three classifications of cataracts?
5. What is glaucoma?
6. What is the connection between diabetes mellitus and disorders of the eye?
7. What is the most common cause of blindness in developed countries?
8. What is macular degeneration? Are there different types?
9. What are common symptoms of an ear disorder?
10. What is vertigo?

Evolve® Answer guide for the Review Questions, Critical Thinking Exercises, Decision-making Framework Exercises and Critical Thinking Questions in Case Studies is hosted on Evolve: http://evolve.elsevier.com/AU/Koutoukidis/Tabbner.

References

Australian Commission on Safety and Quality in Health Care (ACSQHC), 2021. National safety and quality health service standards, 2nd ed updated. ACSQHC, Sydney.

Applegate, E., 2011. *The anatomy and physiology learning system*, 4th ed. St Louis, Saunders.

Ball, J., Dains, J., Flynn, J., et al., 2023. *Seidel's guide to physical examination*, 10th ed. Elsevier, St Louis.

Berman, A., Frandsen, G., Snyder, S., et al., 2021 *Kozier and Erb's fundamentals of nursing*, 5th ed. Pearson Education Australia, Melbourne.

Brown, D., Edwards, H., Buckley, T., et al., 2020. *Lewis's medical-surgical nursing*, 5th ed. Elsevier, Sydney.

Cooper, K., Gosnell, K., 2023. *Adult health nursing: Care of the patient with a sensory disorder*. Elsevier, St Louis, Ch. 13, pp. 608–655.

Crisp, J., Douglas, C., Rebeiro, G., et al., 2021. *Potter and Perry's fundamentals of nursing*, 6th ed. Elsevier, Sydney.

Deaf Australia, 2021. Accessible services for deaf people who use Auslan in hospitals and health services. Available at: <https://deafaustralia.org.au/wp-content/uploads/2022/09/Accessible-Services-for-Deaf-People-who-use-Auslan-in-the-Hospitals-and-Health-Services.pdf>

Deaf Connect, 2022. Auslan User Statistics 2021 Census. Available at: <www.deafconnect.com>.

Diabetes Australia, 2022. National diabetes service scheme (NDSS), Data Snapshot: December 2022. Available at: <https://www.ndss.com.au/wp-content/uploads/ndss-data-snapshot-202212-all-types-diabetes.pdf>.

Glaucoma Australia, 2023. What is glaucoma? Available at: <http://www.glaucoma.org.au>.

Harding, M., Kwong, J., Hagler, D., et al., 2023. *Lewis's medical-surgical nursing*, 12th ed. Elsevier Inc, St Louis.

Healthdirect, 2022. Cochlear implant. Available at: <https://www.healthdirect.gov.au/cochlear-implant>.

Ignatavicius, D., et al., 2021. *Medical-surgical nursing*, 10th ed. Elsevier, St Louis.

Jarvis, C., Eckhardt, A., 2021. *Jarvis's health assessment and physical examination: Eye function*, 3rd ed. Elsevier, St Louis.

Marieb, E., Keller, S., 2021. *Essentials of human anatomy and physiology*, 13th ed. Pearson Education Limited, United Kingdom.

Rothrock, J., 2023. *Alexander's care of the patient in surgery*, 17th ed. Elsevier, St Louis.

Nursing and Midwifery Board of Australia (NMBA), 2020. Decision-making framework for nursing and midwifery. Available at: <https://www.nursingmidwiferyboard.gov.au/Codes-Guidelines-Statements/Frameworks.aspx>.

Patton, K., Thibodeau, G.A., 2018. *The human body in health and disease*, 7th ed. Elsevier, St Louis.

Patton, K., Thibodeau, G.A., 2024. *The human body in health and disease*, 8th ed. Elsevier, St Louis.

Perry, A., Potter, P., Ostendorf, W., 2020. *Nursing interventions and nursing clinical skills: Care of the eye and ear*, 7th ed. Elsevier, St Louis, Ch. 12, pp. 283–298.

Silvestri, L.A., Silvestri, A., 2023. *Saunders comprehensive review for the NCLEX-RN® examination*, 9th ed. St. Louis, Saunders.

Stromberg, H., 2023. *Medical-surgical nursing: Concepts and practice*, 5th ed. Elsevier Inc, St Louis.

Tullefson, J., Watson, G., Jelly, E., et al., 2022. *Essential clinical skills of enrolled nurses*, 5th ed. South Melbourne, Melbourne.

Vision Australia, 2023. Available at: <www.visionaustralia.org.au>.

Waugh, A., Grant, A., 2023. *Ross and Wilson anatomy and physiology in health and illness: The special senses*, 14th ed. Elsevier, Edinburgh.

Online Resources

Australian Commission on Safety and Quality in Health Care: <www.safetyandquality.gov.au>.

Australian Health Practitioner Regulation Agency (Ahpra): <www.ahpra.gov.au>.

Australian Nursing and Midwifery Federation: <www.anmf.org.au>.

Australian Nursing and Midwifery Accreditation Council: <www.anmac.org.au>.

Better Hearing Australia: <https://www.betterhearingaustralia.online>.

Deaf Australia: <https://deafaustralia.org.au>.

Department of Education and Early Childhood Development: <http://www.vic.gov.au/education>.

JBI: <https://jbi.global>.

Soundfair Australia: <www.soundfair.org.au>.

The Fred Hollows Foundation: <www.hollows.org/au/home>.

Vision Australia Foundation: <www.visionaustralia.org.au>.

CHAPTER 35

Neurological health

Anne MacLeod

Key Terms

aneurysm
aphasia
apraxia
ataxia
autonomic nervous system
brainstem
central nervous system (CNS)
cephalalgia
cerebrovascular accident (stroke)
cerebrospinal fluid (CSF)
cerebrum
chorea
cranial nerves
decerebrate
decorticate
diencephalon
dysphasia
frontal lobe
haematoma
hemiparesis
hemiplegia
hydrocephalus
medulla oblongata
meninges
midbrain
neuralgia
neuritis
neurons
neurotransmitter
occipital lobe
paraplegia
parasympathetic nervous system
parietal lobe
peripheral nervous system
pons
quadriplegia
spinal cord
spinal nerves
sympathetic nervous system
synapse
temporal lobe
transient ischaemic attack (TIA)

Learning Outcomes

At the completion of this chapter and with further reading, learners should be able to:

- Define the key terms.
- Describe the function and structure of the nervous system.
- Describe the location of each part of the nervous system.
- Describe the functions of the nervous system.
- State the pathophysiological influences and effects associated with disorders of the nervous system.
- Describe the major manifestations of nervous system disorders.
- Briefly describe the specific disorders of the nervous system outlined in this chapter.
- Apply principles of neurological assessment.
- Apply principles of neurovascular assessment.
- Demonstrate accurate documentation of a neurological assessment.
- Discuss the nursing management of an individual with a nervous system disorder.
- Discuss the nursing management of an individual with a spinal cord injury.
- State the diagnostic tests that may be used to assess nervous system function.
- Assist in planning and implementing nursing care for the individual with a nervous system disorder.

CHAPTER FOCUS

The nervous system is responsible for the coordination of all other systems. It provides a network for communication within the body, and between the body and its environment. The brain is informed of events occurring both intrinsically and extrinsically to the body by nerve impulses that originate at sensory receptors. The receptors, which may be nerve endings, single specialised cells or a group of cells forming a sense organ, convert the energy of a stimulus into impulses that pass to specific areas of the brain. An understanding of this complex and dynamic system underpins many aspects of individual care since almost all medical conditions can affect the human nervous system in some way.

The workings of the human brain, and indeed the entire nervous system, have both fascinated and mystified scientists for centuries. The knowledge that has been uncovered has enabled healthcare professionals to make more accurate assessments of individuals, allowing implementation of safer and more effective treatments. While application of this knowledge has significantly improved the expected outcomes for many individuals affected by disorders of the nervous system, there is still much research to be carried out to fully explain the workings of this intricate system.

This chapter focuses on the function and structure of the neurological system, pathophysiological influences, and effects of disorders of the nervous system, neurological assessment and the care of an individual with a nervous system disorder.

LIVED EXPERIENCE

My life changed the day I had a fall. I'm an 83-year-old male who, up until I fell, had remained physically active. I played lawn bowls twice a week, gardened and had a close group of friends who I saw regularly.

I remember tripping over the garden edge and getting to my feet thinking that it was fortunate that I hadn't broken anything. A slight bump to my head after hitting a pot plant and a small skin tear to my forearm was the only injury I thought I'd sustained. I remember walking into my house to get a band aid for the skin tear and that is the last thing I can recall prior to waking up in intensive care.

The bump to my head was more significant than I first realised. I'd sustained an extradural haemorrhage. An extradural haemorrhage is a traumatic brain injury that occurs when bleeding develops between the inner and outer layer of the skull. I've been told it was the result of a blood vessel tearing when I fell, not uncommon in someone my age due to shrinking of the brain. While I thought I was alright following the fall, I was bleeding and this was causing pressure on my brain. My wife found me confused and I was unsteady on my feet. She called an ambulance.

I was fortunate. I've had the haemorrhage drained and after 4 weeks in rehabilitation to regain my mobility and improve my independence, I have returned home. I still attend day rehab where I see an occupational therapist and physiotherapist. I've had to make some lifestyle modifications since the haemorrhage. I'm still unable to drive, and I'm not as confident on my feet as I used to be and while I don't think I am confused my wife tells me that I am at times. The neurosurgeon has indicated that I may still improve, for which I'm very thankful. In the meantime, I'm just grateful to still be alive.

Alan

INTRODUCTION

Nervous tissue

Neurons

Neurons, 'nerve cells' (Figure 35.1a & b), are the primary components of the nervous system. Functioning alone, or as units, neurons detect internal and external changes and initiate body responses needed to maintain homeostasis. Each neuron is composed of a cell body, with projections forming dendrites, and one long axon. The dendrites are short-branched fibres, which receive impulses and conduct them towards the cell body of a neuron. The axon, which may vary in length from miniscule to over a metre, conducts impulses away from the cell body of a neuron. A single neuron may have many dendrites. Each axon has a covering called a neurilemma, and most have a fatty sheath, the myelin sheath. The myelin sheath protects and insulates the axon and increases the transmission rate of nervous impulses. Neurons are supported by many types of cells that support, insulate and protect, called neuroglia or 'nerve glue' (Marieb & Keller 2021).

Neuroglia

The neuroglia include many types of cells that support and protect the neurons. They play a role in regulating neuronal activity, and in providing neurons with nutrients.

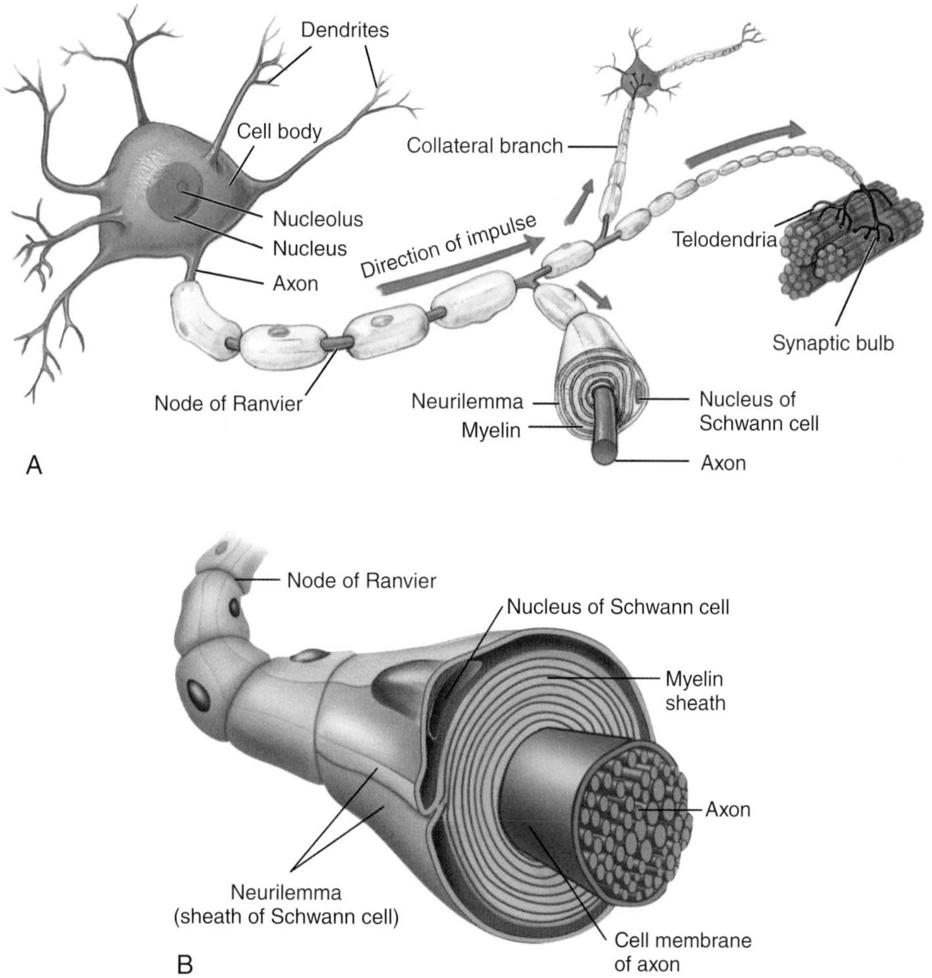

Figure 35.1 Structure of a neuron

A: Diagram of a typical neuron showing dendrites, a cell body and an axon, **B:** Segment of a myelinated axon cut to show detail of the concentric layers of the Schwann cell filled with myelin.

*(**A:** Patton et al 2024; **B:** Applegate 2011)*

Neuroglia differ from neurons in that they are not capable of transmitting nerve impulses and never lose their ability to divide. The neuroglia in the central nervous system comprise five types of cells: *astrocytes*—cells with small cell bodies and processes like dendrites and which protect the neurons from harmful substances that may be in the blood by forming a living barrier between the capillary blood supply and the neurons; *oligodendrocytes* in the central nervous system, which have few processes and produce the myelin sheath around the processes of the neurons; *microglia*, which are phagocytes that dispose of debris; *ependymal cells*, which line the cavities of the brain and spinal cord; and *Schwann and satellite cells* within the peripheral nervous system. The Schwann cells protect, nourish and form myelin and the satellite cells protect and cushion (Marieb & Keller 2021).

Functions of neurons

Neurons have two major functional properties: irritability and conductivity. Irritability is the ability to respond to a stimulus and convert it into a nerve impulse. Conductivity is the ability to transmit the impulse to other neurons, muscles or glands. An impulse is a complex electrical and chemical signal transmitted along a nerve pathway in response to a stimulus. The speed of transmission varies with the size of the nerve fibre and may be as much as 120 metres per second.

A **synapse** is the space between the terminal axon of one neuron and the dendrites of another. By means of a chemical substance (**neurotransmitter**) released by the axons, impulses are transmitted through this space from one neuron to another. Examples of neurotransmitters are acetylcholine and noradrenaline. Many different types of stimuli (electrical, mechanical or chemical) can excite neurons so that they become active and generate an impulse. Most neurons are excited by the neurotransmitters released by other neurons, but other stimuli can excite neurons. For example, sound excites some of the neuronal receptors of the ear, and pressure excites some cutaneous receptors of the skin. Receptors, or sensory nerve terminals, act as transducers, converting the energy of a stimulus into impulses that pass to the brain.

The nervous system can be divided into two primary divisions: the central nervous system, consisting of the brain and spinal cord; and the peripheral nervous system, consisting of nerves that connect the central nervous system with the body tissues (Marieb & Keller 2021; Patton et al 2019; Patton & Thibodeau 2019).

The central nervous system (CNS)

The **central nervous system (CNS)** is composed of nervous tissue, which is commonly described as grey and white matter. Examination of a section of the brain reveals that it is grey on the outside and white on the inside. Microscopic examination reveals that the grey matter is composed of neuron cell bodies responsible for processing information, and white matter, which is made up of myelinated fibres, which allows communication to and from grey matter areas, and between the grey matter and the other parts of the body (Marieb & Keller 2021).

The brain

The brain is a large organ weighing approximately1.4 kg in adults, held in position within the skull by membranes called the meninges. In most parts of the brain, the outer portion, or cortex, consists of grey matter, while white matter forms the inner portion. The grey matter is convoluted to provide a greater surface area. The brain is divided into the:

- cerebrum, comprising the left and right cerebral hemispheres
- **diencephalon**, comprising the left and right thalamus and hypothalamus
- **brainstem**, comprising the midbrain, pons and medulla oblongata—the stalk-like section that connects the brain to the spinal cord
- cerebellum.

(Patton & Thibodeau 2019)

The cerebrum

The **cerebrum** (Figure 35.2) is the largest part of the brain, filling the vault of the cranium from front to back. It is divided by fissures into the left and right hemispheres, and each hemisphere is further divided by fissures into four main lobes and the insula lobe. The insula lobe lies medial to the lateral sulcus and is thought to be involved in sensory and motor visceral functions as well as taste perception. The four main lobes are:

1. the **frontal lobe**, responsible for voluntary motor function, motivation, aggression, personality, sense of smell and mood
2. the parietal lobe, which receives and evaluates sensory information
3. the **temporal lobe**, which receives input for smell and hearing and has an important role in memory
4. the **occipital lobe**, responsible for reception and integration of visual input.

The left hemisphere of the brain controls the right side of the body, and the right hemisphere controls the left side of the body. The hemispheres are connected by the corpus callosum which allows the cerebral hemispheres to communicate with each other.

The cerebrum is divided into several areas, some of which are sensory and some of which are motor areas. The sensory areas of each hemisphere receive and interpret sensations from the opposite side of the body, including touch, temperature, pain, pressure and an awareness of the position of the body in its environment. The motor areas of each hemisphere control all voluntary movement on the opposite side of the body. The centres of special sense are located in the various lobes, including the centres for hearing, speech, smell, taste and sight (Figure 35.3).

The functions of the cerebrum are therefore to receive and interpret impulses from the sensory organs, to initiate and control the movements of skeletal muscles and to perform the higher levels of mental activity such as thinking, reasoning, intelligence, learning and memory (Marieb & Keller 2021; Patton & Thibodeau 2019).

The diencephalon

The diencephalon consists of three major structures: the thalamus, the hypothalamus and the pineal gland. It is located between the midbrain and cerebrum. The thalami are two oval masses of grey matter that form the lateral walls of the third ventricle. Each thalamus is subdivided into a number of nuclei. Most sensory pathways (except smell) synapse here, serving as the major relay station for sensory impulses. The thalamus plays an important role in the control of somatic motor activity and influences mood and strong emotions.

The hypothalamus lies beneath the thalamus and the pituitary gland is closely connected to it. The hypothalamus controls all the activities of the autonomic nervous system, which is described later in this chapter. The hypothalamus is important in controlling the endocrine system since it regulates pituitary gland function.

The pineal gland is located posterior to the thalamus, receives sensory information about the strength of light seen by the eyes and varies the secretion of the hormone melatonin (Marieb & Keller 2021; Patton & Thibodeau 2019).

The brainstem

The **midbrain** is a short narrow segment connecting the cerebrum with the pons. It is composed primarily of ascending and descending fibre tracts. Its functions are to provide a pathway for impulses passing between the cerebrum and spinal cord, and to receive stimuli that initiate eye and postural movements.

The **pons** lies just above the medulla oblongata. It contains two respiratory centres: the pneumotaxic centre and the apneustic centre. Its functions are to act as a relay station from the cerebrum to the cerebellum, and to modify the activity of the medullary respiratory centres through the pneumotaxic and apneustic centres.

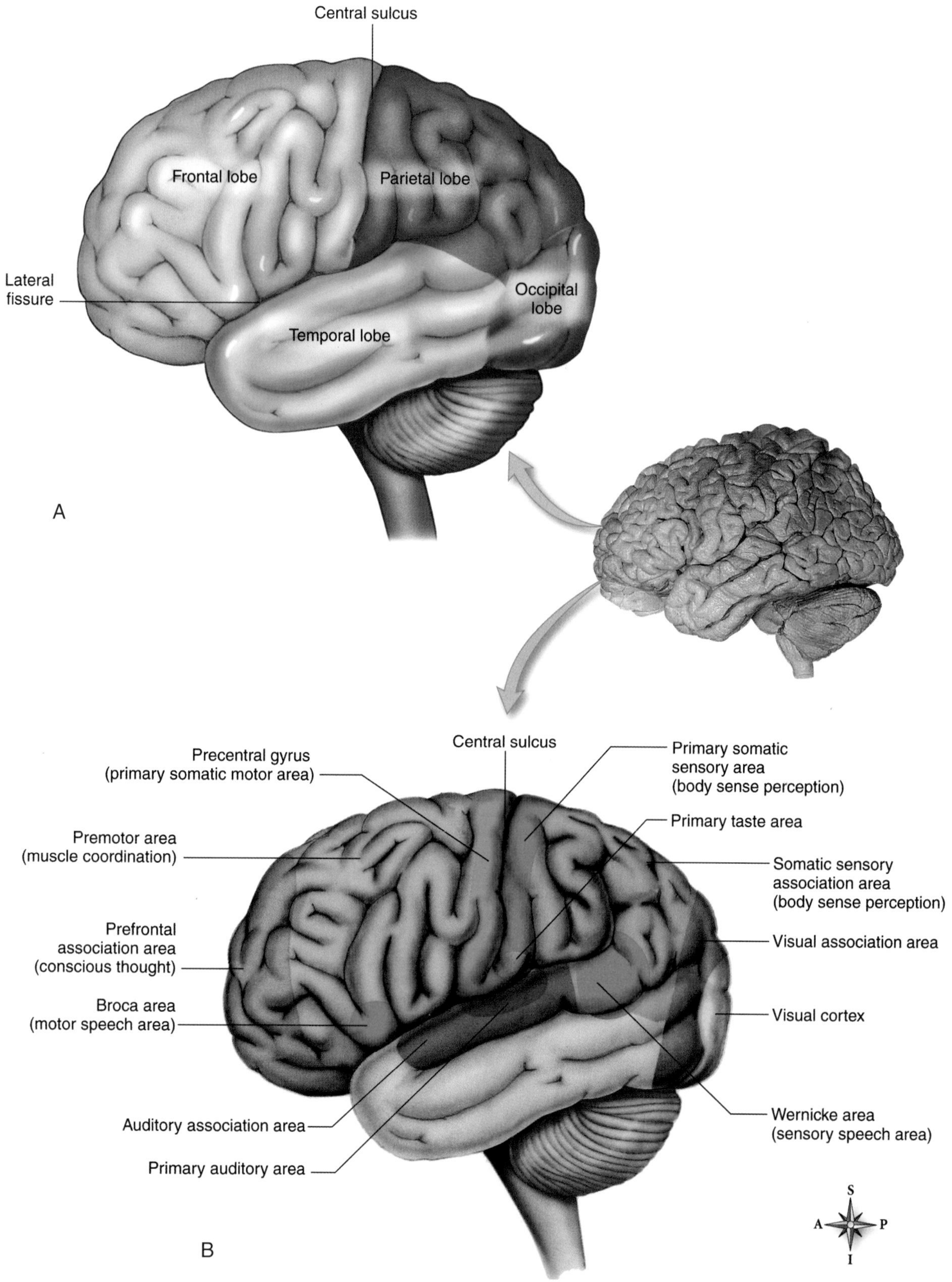

Figure 35.2 Cerebrum

A: The lobes of the cerebrum. The insula lobe is hidden from view, as it folds behind the lateral fissure, **B:** Functional regions of the cerebral cortex. Association areas are so named because they put together (associate) information from many different parts of the brain.

(Patton et al 2024)

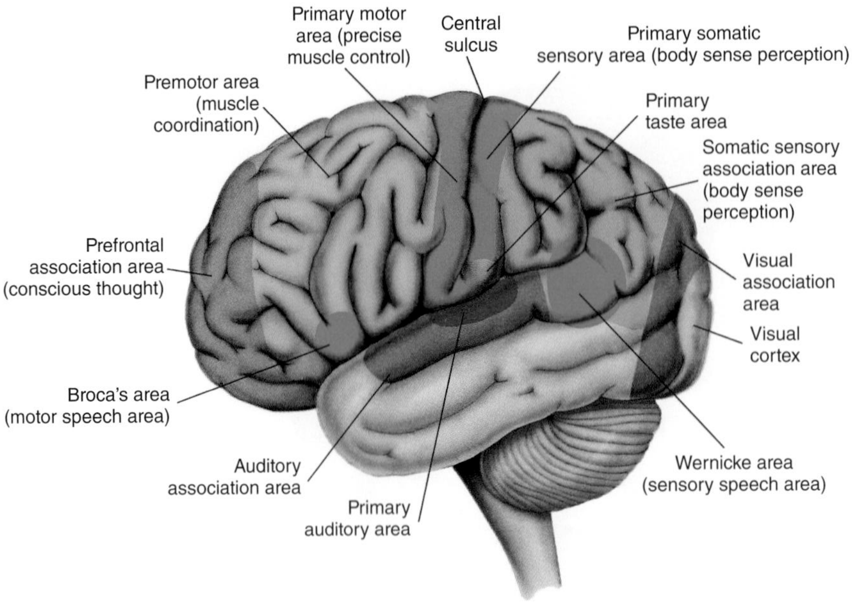

Figure 35.3 Functional regions of the cerebral cortex

(Patton & Thibodeau 2018)

The **medulla oblongata** lies between the pons and the spinal cord. It provides the link between the brain and the spinal cord and contains the cardiac, respiratory, vasomotor and reflex centres. Its functions are:

- to provide a pathway where nerve fibres to and from the brain cross over to the opposite side
- to control heartbeat (through the cardiac centre)
- to control ventilation (through the respiratory centre)
- to control constriction and dilation of blood vessels (through the vasomotor centre).
- to initiate the reflex actions of swallowing, vomiting, coughing and sneezing (through the reflex centres).

(Marieb & Keller 2021)

The cerebellum

The cerebellum lies behind the pons and medulla and below the occipital lobes of the cerebrum. Like the cerebrum, the cerebellum is divided into two hemispheres that have shallow convolutions in their surface of grey matter. Its functions are coordination of muscular activity and regulation of muscle tone, and maintenance of balance and posture (Marieb & Keller 2021).

Blood supply to the brain

The carotid and the vertebral arteries supply blood to the brain. These arteries branch and join up again, forming a circle of arteries at the base of the brain called the circle of Willis. From here, smaller cerebral arteries branch off to supply each region of the brain. Blood returns from the brain via the jugular veins to the superior vena cava.

The blood–brain barrier is a barrier that prevents or delays the entry of certain substances into brain tissue. The relatively low permeability of the capillaries supplying the brain means that some substances are either completely or partially prevented from gaining access to brain tissue. The blood–brain barrier thus acts as a protective mechanism, preventing substances such as bilirubin, which could disrupt brain function, from crossing the barrier. Water, oxygen, carbon dioxide and glucose cross the blood–brain barrier easily (Marieb & Keller 2021).

The spinal cord

The **spinal cord** is a cylindrical structure that lies within a canal inside the vertebral column. It extends from an opening on the underside of the skull (the foramen magnum) to the level of the first or second lumbar vertebra. Below this level, the vertebral canal is occupied by nerves from the lumbar and sacral segments of the cord and the conus medullaris, the most distal bulbous part of the spinal cord, which continues as the filum terminale: these constitute the cauda equina ('horse's tail'). The spinal cord, which is about 46 cm in length, consists of nervous tissue, with the white matter on the outside and the grey matter arranged roughly in an 'H' formation in the centre (Figure 35.4). The two anterior projections of grey matter are called the anterior horns, and the posterior projections are called the posterior horns. Sensory nerve fibres enter the posterior horns, and motor nerve fibres leave the anterior horns.

Leaving the spinal cord at intervals throughout its length are 31 pairs of spinal nerves. The functions of the spinal cord are:

- to receive sensory impulses from the tissues and convey them to the sensory areas of the brain via ascending (afferent) pathways
- to convey motor impulses from the brain to various parts of the body via descending (efferent) pathways
- to provide a pathway through which reflex actions take place.

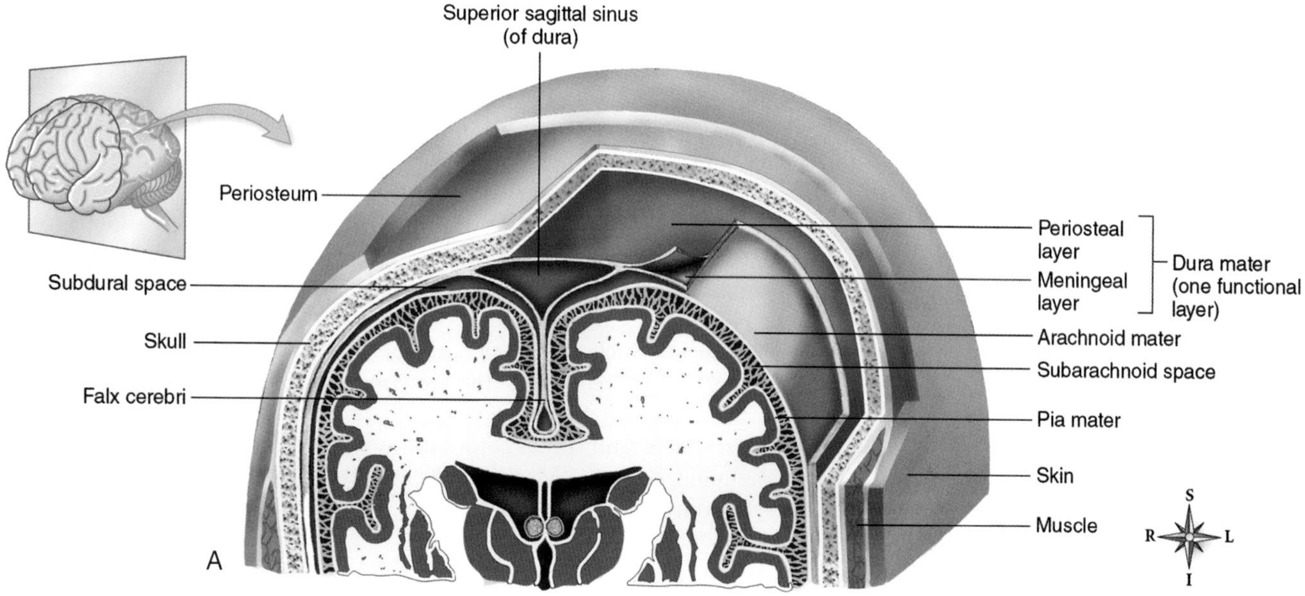

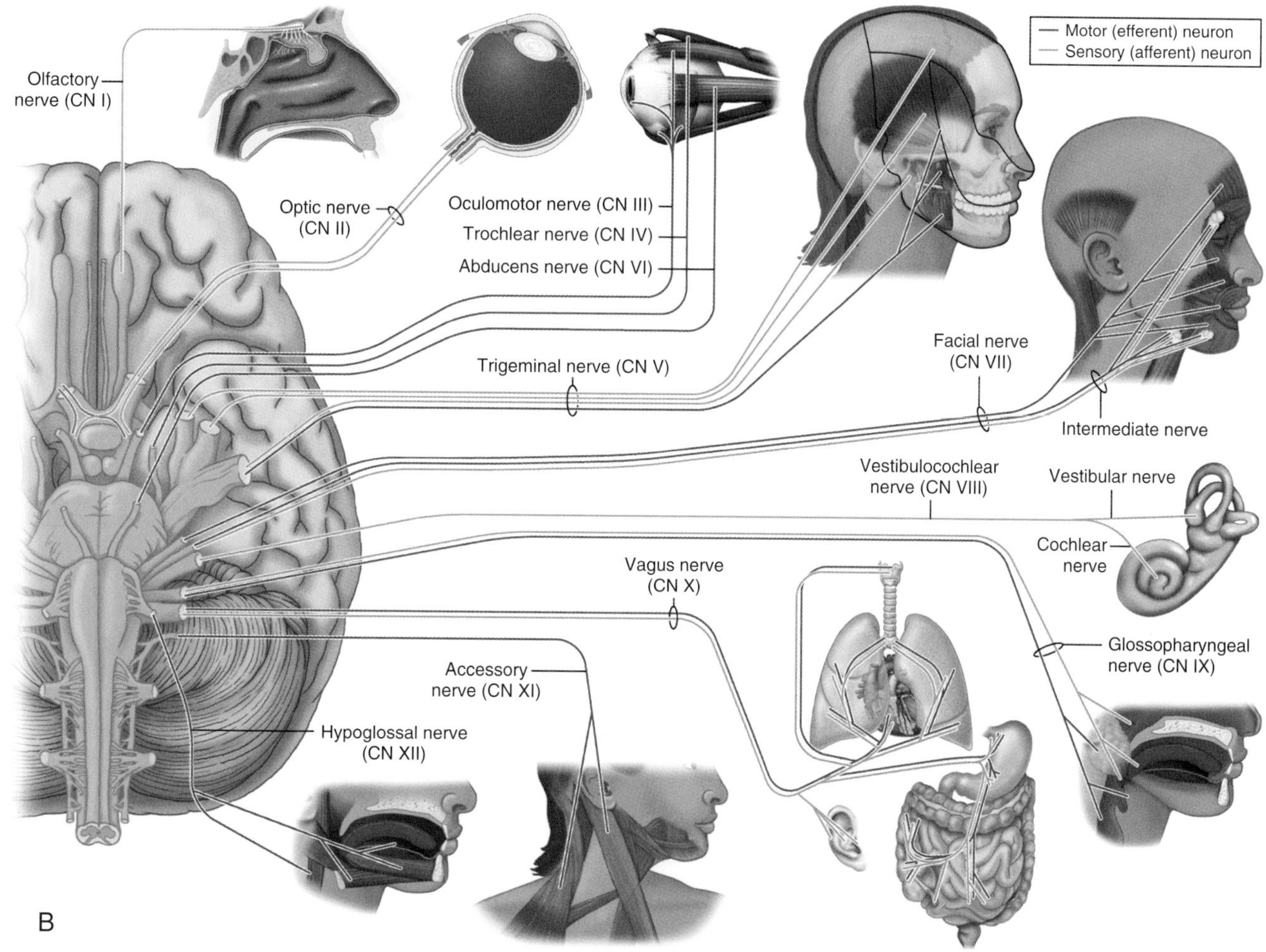

Figure 35.4 A: Coverings of the brain, **B:** Coverings of the spinal cord

*(**A:** Patton et al 2022; **B:** Banasik & Copstead 2019)*

A reflex action, or arc, is an automatic motor response to a sensory stimulus without conscious involvement (Figure 35.5). Most reflex actions are protective in nature and take place more quickly than voluntary actions. The structures involved in a reflex action are:

- a sensory organ (e.g. the skin) to receive the stimulus
- a sensory (afferent) nerve fibre to carry the impulse to the posterior horn of the spinal cord
- an association neuron in the spinal cord to receive the impulse and transmit it directly to the anterior horn
- a motor (efferent) neuron in the anterior horn to receive the impulse and transmit it to the motor organ
- a motor organ (e.g. a muscle) to receive and respond to the stimulus.

An example of a reflex action is when the hand comes into contact with a very hot object. The skin on the hand receives the stimulus of heat, and an impulse travels from the sensory nerve endings in the skin to the posterior horn of the spinal cord. From there, the impulse is transmitted to the anterior horn, then passed along the motor nerves to the muscles of the shoulder, arm and hand. As a result, the hand is pulled rapidly away from the source of heat before the brain has even processed the information (Marieb & Keller 2021; Patton et al 2019; Patton & Thibodeau 2019).

The meninges

The **meninges** are the three membranes that cover the brain and the spinal cord. The individual membranes are:

1. The dura mater (meaning 'hard mother') is the tough outermost layer. It consists of two layers of fibrous connective tissue, with one layer forming the periosteum covering the inner surface of the skull bones, and the other layer covering the brain and spinal cord.
2. The arachnoid mater (meaning 'mother like a spider's web') is the middle layer. The name refers to the fact that it is so thin that, when viewed under a microscope, it resembles a spider's web.
3. The pia mater (meaning 'gentle mother') is the delicate innermost layer. It adheres closely to the surface of the brain and spinal cord, dipping down into the convolutions and fissures. The pia mater is richly supplied with blood vessels that carry blood to the brain and spinal cord.

The subarachnoid space is the space between the arachnoid mater and pia mater, filled with cerebrospinal fluid in circulation. The functions of the meninges are to form a protective covering against physical injury around the brain and spinal cord, and to help secure the brain to the cranial vault (Marieb & Keller 2021; Patton et al 2019; Patton & Thibodeau 2019).

Cerebrospinal fluid

Cerebrospinal fluid (CSF) is a clear watery fluid with a composition similar to plasma. It contains substances including water, glucose, sodium, chloride, potassium, protein and waste products such as urea. The CSF is formed from the blood and is produced by a combination of filtration and active secretory processes by the choroid plexus in the ventricles of the brain. CSF circulates in the subarachnoid space surrounding the brain and spinal cord (Figure 35.6) (Wilson & Giddens 2020). The total volume of the CSF is about 140 mL. The fluid is formed continuously in the ventricles at a rate of about 500 mL/day and is reabsorbed into the blood at about the same rate. The functions of CSF are to:

- Form a protective cushion around the brain and spinal cord.

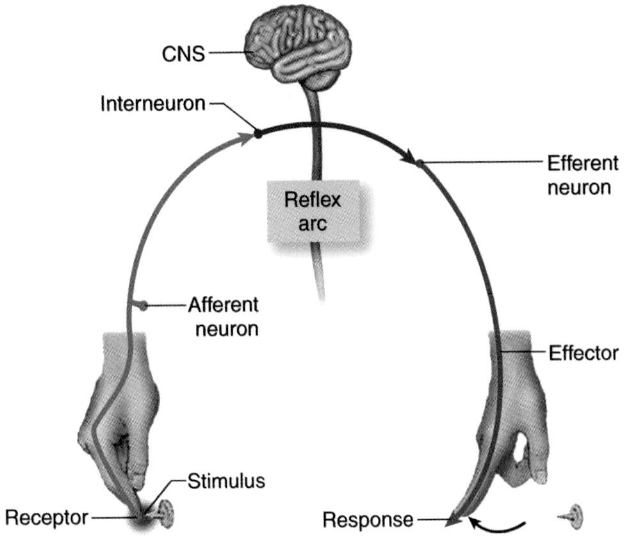

Figure 35.5 The reflex arc
(Patton et al 2022)

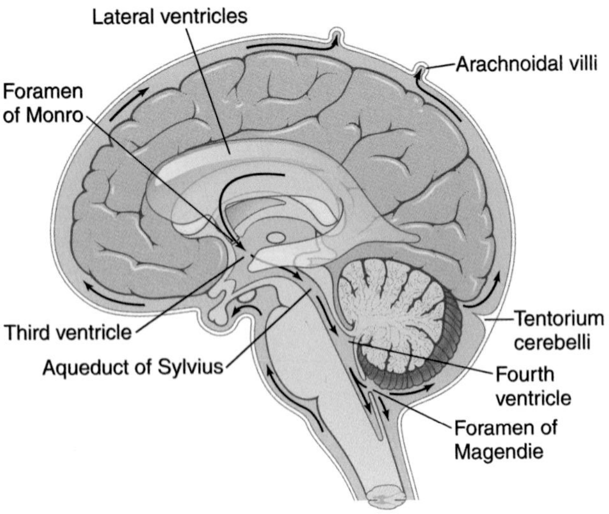

Figure 35.6 The arrows show the pathway of cerebrospinal fluid flow from the choroid plexuses in the lateral ventricles to the arachnoidal villi protruding into the dural sinuses
(Hall & Hall 2021)

- Maintain normal pressure around the brain and spinal cord.
- Provide a medium for the exchange of nutrients and waste products between the bloodstream and the nervous tissue.

(Marieb & Keller 2021; Patton et al 2019)

The peripheral nervous system (PNS)

The peripheral nervous system (PNS) consists of the 12 pairs of cranial nerves, and 31 pairs of spinal nerves that leave the spinal cord. The peripheral nerves may be sensory, motor or mixed. Sensory (afferent) nerves carry impulses to the brain and spinal cord. Motor (efferent) nerves carry impulses from the brain and spinal cord to the muscles, organs and tissues. Mixed nerves are composed of both sensory and motor fibres and transmit impulses in both directions. The motor PNS has two functional divisions:

1. The somatic nervous system, which allows us to consciously, or voluntarily, control our skeletal muscles. This division is often called the voluntary motor system, but it also includes involuntary reflexes.
2. The autonomic nervous system, which regulates events that are automatic, or involuntary, such as the activity of smooth and cardiac muscle and glands. The autonomic nervous system itself has two parts: the sympathetic nervous system and parasympathetic nervous system (described further below).

(Marieb & Keller 2021; Patton et al 2019)

The cranial nerves

Twelve pairs of **cranial nerves** leave the brainstem. The numbers (Roman numerals are the convention), names and functions of the cranial nerves are:

I. olfactory nerve: sensory—the nerve of smell
II. optic nerve: sensory—the nerve of sight
III. oculomotor nerve: motor—supplies the muscle of the eye
IV. trochlear nerve: motor—supplies one of the eye muscles
V. trigeminal nerve: mixed—sensory fibres receive stimuli from most of the skin of the head and face, the membranes of the nose and mouth, the orbits, the upper and lower jaws, and teeth; motor fibres supply the muscles of mastication
VI. abducent nerve: motor—supplies one of the eye muscles
VII. facial nerve: mixed—sensory fibres convey the sensation of taste from the anterior portion of the tongue; motor fibres supply the muscles of facial expressions
VIII. auditory nerve: sensory—the nerve of hearing and balance
IX. glossopharyngeal nerve: mixed—sensory fibres convey taste sensations from the posterior part of the tongue; motor fibres supply the pharynx
X. vagus nerve: mixed—controls secretion and movement of the internal organs (e.g. oesophagus, larynx, trachea, heart, stomach, intestines, pancreas, spleen, kidneys and blood vessels)
XI. accessory nerve: motor—supplies the muscles of the neck, and the pharynx and larynx
XII. hypoglossal nerve: motor—supplies the tongue muscles.

(Marieb & Keller 2021; Patton et al 2019)

The spinal nerves

The **spinal nerves** project out of the vertebral canal, one pair emerging below each vertebra, and one pair emerging between the cranium and the first cervical vertebra. The spinal nerves are mixed nerves, containing both sensory and motor fibres. They allow for sensation and movement in peripheral parts of the body not supplied by the cranial nerves, such as skin, muscles, bones and joints of the trunk and limbs. The spinal nerves are arranged in groups according to their region of origin in the cord. There are:

- eight pairs of cervical nerves (C1–C8)
- twelve pairs of thoracic nerves (T1–T12)
- five pairs of lumbar nerves (L1–L5)
- five pairs of sacral nerves (S1–S5)
- one pair of coccygeal nerves.

In some regions, the nerves divide immediately after leaving the cord. These then branch and unite with each other to form what is called a plexus (meaning braid). The major plexuses are:

- the cervical plexus, which supplies the muscles of the neck and shoulders, and gives rise to the phrenic nerves that supply the diaphragm
- the brachial plexus, which gives rise to the radial, median and ulna nerves, which supply the arm
- the lumbar plexus, which gives rise to the femoral nerve, which supplies the thigh muscles
- the sacral plexus, from which the sciatic nerve arises.

The sciatic nerve is the largest nerve in the body, running over the hip posteriorly down the back of the thigh to the knee where it divides into the peroneal nerve and tibial nerve (Marieb & Keller 2021; Patton et al 2019).

The autonomic nervous system

The **autonomic nervous system** is the division of the PNS concerned with involuntary activity of the body. It supplies nerves to all the structures in the body that are not under conscious control. The autonomic nervous system consists of two divisions: the sympathetic and the parasympathetic nervous systems (Marieb & Keller 2021).

The sympathetic nervous system

The **sympathetic nervous system** arises from grey matter in the spinal cord from T1 through to L2. Sympathetic nerves then synapse in a chain of ganglia that lies on either side of the vertebral column, before reaching organs or tissues. A ganglion (plural ganglia) is a knot-like mass of cell bodies. Plexuses are formed by fibres from these ganglia.

For example, the solar plexus lying behind the stomach and supplying the abdominal organs, and the cardiac plexus supplying the heart and lungs (Marieb & Keller 2021).

The parasympathetic nervous system

The **parasympathetic nervous system** consists of cranial nerves III, VII, IX and X and nerves that emerge from the sacral region of the spinal cord. The vagus nerve (cranial nerve X) is the largest autonomic nerve (Marieb & Keller 2021).

Vasovagal syncope

When the vagus nerve is overstimulated the body's blood vessels dilate causing the heart rate to slow and lowering the BP, which may cause sweating and a loss of consciousness. There are many causes for vasovagal syncope, including nausea, gastrointestinal cramping, straining during a bowel movement, the sight of blood, standing for too long or emotional or physical stressors that over-stimulate the vagus nerve (Mayo Clinic 2023).

Functions of the autonomic nervous system

The functions of the autonomic nervous system are to control the movements of internal organs and the secretions of glands. The system provides dual control: the activity of an organ is stimulated by one set of nerves and inhibited by the other set of nerves. This dual control achieves smooth rhythmic action of involuntary muscles and internal organs, maintaining a balance between activity and rest.

The sympathetic nerves are called adrenergic nerve fibres and release the neurotransmitter noradrenaline. These nerves can be affected by strong emotions such as anger, fear or excitement, and have a stimulating effect on most organs. The effect resembles that produced by adrenaline: a hormone secreted by the adrenal glands. This effect is called the 'fright, fight or flight' effect, in which the body responds to a fright either by preparing to fight or by running away. The response of the body includes:

- dilation of the pupils of the eyes
- increased force and rate of heartbeat, increasing circulation
- increased blood pressure and constriction of arterioles in the skin and abdominal organs to divert blood to all skeletal muscles, heart, lungs and brain
- dilation of the bronchi to allow more oxygen to enter
- slowing of digestion so that the digestive organs can receive a reduced blood supply, enabling blood to be diverted to vital structures
- increased production of sweat by sweat glands
- a rise in blood sugar level, as the liver is stimulated to release more glucose for increased energy needs.

The parasympathetic nerves are called cholinergic fibres and release the neurotransmitter acetylcholine. These nerves tend to slow down body processes, so that the end result of the antagonistic action of each division of the autonomic nervous system is a balance between acceleration and retardation. After the 'fright' or stressful situation is over, the parasympathetic nervous system returns things to normal. The digestive organs receive more blood, the glands increase their secretions, the heartbeat is decreased and blood pressure falls. The effects of sympathetic and parasympathetic stimulation on various body organs are compared in Table 35.1 (LeMone et al 2020; Marieb & Keller 2021; Patton et al 2019).

TABLE 35.1 | Effects of sympathetic and parasympathetic stimulation

Organ	Sympathetic stimulation	Parasympathetic stimulation
Heart	Increases rate/strength of heartbeat Dilates coronary arteries to increase blood supply to the heart muscle.	Decreases rate/strength of heartbeat. Constricts coronary arteries to decrease supply of blood to the heart muscle.
Bronchi	Dilates bronchi, allowing more air to enter the lungs.	Constricts bronchi, limiting air intake.
Digestive system	Decreases activity of the system and constricts digestive system sphincters. Inhibits production of saliva.	Increases peristalsis and relaxes sphincters. Stimulates production of saliva.
Urinary bladder	Relaxes bladder wall. Contracts internal sphincter muscle.	Contracts bladder wall. Relaxes internal sphincter muscle.
Eye	Dilates the pupil. Retracts the eyelids.	Constricts the pupil. Closes the eyelids.
Skin	Stimulates perspiration. Stimulates smooth muscles attached to hair follicles, producing 'goosebumps'.	No effect on sweat glands. No effect on muscles/hair follicles.

(Marieb & Keller 2021; Patton & Thibodeau 2019)

PATHOPHYSIOLOGICAL INFLUENCES AND EFFECTS OF DISORDERS OF THE NERVOUS SYSTEM

The pathophysiological changes that can disrupt normal function of part or all of the nervous system can be due to congenital or developmental disorders, infectious or inflammatory conditions, trauma, neoplasia, degenerative conditions and metabolic or endocrine disorders. Any pathophysiological change is capable of causing various types and degrees of dysfunction.

Aetiology of nervous system disorders

Congenital disorders

The CNS of the developing foetus is very vulnerable to damage. Factors that may cause nervous system damage include the passage of microorganisms and drugs across the placental barrier into the foetal circulation. Other factors that may cause nervous system defects and result in physical and intellectual deterioration include chromosomal abnormalities, metabolic disorders, cranial malformations and structural abnormalities. The CNS may also be damaged during the birth process (e.g. by cerebral anoxia or cerebral haemorrhage) (National Institute of Neurological Disorders and Stroke 2023).

Inflammatory and infectious conditions

Bacterial or viral infective processes affecting the CNS may result in the destruction of nervous tissue through the action of toxins released by the living microorganisms and from the material released from dead microorganisms, which stimulates the inflammatory process. Infection and inflammation of nervous tissue may result in altered behaviour, altered consciousness and sensory or motor deficits. Brain and spinal cord infections can cause dangerous inflammation with a wide range of symptoms, including raised temperature, headache, seizures, change in individual behaviour or confusion, brain damage, stroke or even death. Infection of the meninges is called meningitis and inflammation of the brain is called encephalitis. Myelitis refers to inflammation of the spinal cord. When both the brain and the spinal cord are involved, the condition is called encephalomyelitis (National Institute of Neurological Disorders and Stroke 2023d).

Trauma

Trauma to the nervous system may result from elements within the system or from external forces. Trauma occurring from elements within the nervous system includes bleeding from an **aneurysm**, a local dilation of a blood vessel, usually an artery or ruptured intracranial vessel; transient interruption of the cerebral blood flow, causing ischaemia; and occlusion of a cerebral blood vessel by a thrombus or embolus. The most common causative factors in these conditions are hypertension and atherosclerosis.

Trauma from external forces may be caused by a direct or an indirect injury. A direct acceleration brain injury occurs when the head is struck by a moving object, and a direct deceleration injury occurs when the head in motion strikes a stationary object. In an indirect brain injury, the traumatic force is transmitted to the head through an impact to another part of the body, such as the neck or buttocks.

In open head trauma, a penetrating injury damages the integrity of the skull and/or meninges and brain. Infection may occur, as the injury allows the entry of microorganisms. A closed head injury is non-penetrating, with generally no disruption to the integrity of the cerebral meninges. Closed head injuries can result in jarring, bruising or tearing of brain tissue, which can cause haemorrhage, cranial nerve damage and cerebral oedema. An important event in closed head injury is known as coup and contrecoup. The coup injury is cerebral bruising resulting from impact to the skull, and contrecoup refers to the rebound effect of the injury—the movement of the brain opposite to the site of impact.

The nervous system response to trauma, which may cause more damage than the actual injury, results in oedema, bleeding and increased ICP. These factors destroy nervous tissue by compression or restriction of the circulation.

The spinal cord may be damaged because of a crushing or penetrating injury, dislocation of the spinal column, prolapsed intravertebral discs or neoplasia. In addition to tearing of, and pressure on, the spinal cord tissues, damage may be caused by haemorrhage, oedema or disruption of the blood supply to the spinal cord.

Damage to the peripheral nerves may result in loss of sensory and/or motor function (LeMone et al 2020).

CRITICAL THINKING EXERCISE 35.1

What is the significance of discolouration over the mastoid process and clear drainage coming from the nose? What is the clear drainage and what two places may the drainage come from? What is the leakage called that comes from both places?

Neoplasia

Tumours of the nervous system, which may be either benign or malignant, cause symptoms related to pressure, destruction of nervous tissue, oedema and disruption of the blood supply. The neurological manifestations of a tumour affecting the nervous system depend on the location of the tumour and on its rate of growth. Examples of neoplasia include astrocytomas, which arise from astrocytes and gliomas, which arise from glial cells (LeMone et al 2020).

Degenerative conditions

The causes of degenerative disorders of the nervous system are varied and involve atrophy of neurons and nerve fibres.

The course of a degenerative disorder is generally gradual and progressive over many years. The effects of degenerative disorders include progressive muscular atrophy; impaired speech, chewing, swallowing and breathing; deterioration of intellectual capacity; impaired motor function; and dementia. Examples of degenerative conditions include Parkinson's disease, motor neurone disease and Alzheimer's disease.

Metabolic and endocrine disorders

Nervous system dysfunction may result from the effects of certain metabolic and endocrine disorders. Some nutritional deficiencies may affect nerve cells, resulting in their damage or death. For example, degeneration of the posterior and lateral columns of the spinal cord may occur from the vitamin B12 deficiency of pernicious anaemia. Disorders of cortical function, leading to confusion or coma, may result from a deficiency of thiamine (vitamin B1).

Specific endocrine disorders such as hypothyroidism result in decreased metabolic rate, and hypothermia can develop. If the body temperature falls below 30°C, unconsciousness will result. Myxoedema coma (hypothyroid state) is characterised by exaggeration of the signs and symptoms of hypothyroidism, with neurological impairment leading to loss of consciousness (LeMone et al 2020).

Major manifestations of nervous system disorders

The manifestations of a nervous system disorder will vary depending on the type and severity of the disorder.

Headaches (cephalalgia)

Headaches, or **cephalalgia**, are common in a variety of disorders and situations ranging from functional disturbances of blood vessels to tension and stress. In neurological disorders, headaches are one of the most common symptoms. Headaches can result from compression, traction, displacement or inflammation of the cranial periosteum, the dura mater, cerebral arteries or branches of the cranial nerves. Headaches may also occur as a result of tension within extracranial structures such as muscles, air sinuses and blood vessels. Headaches are commonly classified as vascular, tension or traction-inflammatory.

Vascular headaches include migraine, cluster headaches, hypertension headaches and headaches resulting from temporal arteritis. Although the mechanisms of migraine are not completely understood, migraine appears to result from an inherited predisposition and seems to be precipitated by trigger factors such as stress, abrupt falls in oestrogen levels, low blood glucose levels and dietary intake. One theory is that migraine results from spasm of intracranial blood vessels and dilation of extracranial blood vessels. The classic characteristics of migraine headache include throbbing and a tendency for the attacks to be unilateral. Some attacks are preceded by a variety of visual disturbances, such as loss of half of the visual field or flashing lights across the visual fields. Some individuals experience vertigo, nausea and vomiting.

Cluster headaches are a rapid succession of attacks over several days, followed by remission. Previously thought to be caused by histamine sensitisation, cluster headaches are now considered to have a vascular cause. Headaches associated with severe hypertension may be intense and similar to those caused by intracranial lesions. Temporal arteritis causes severe, throbbing headaches in the region of the temporal artery and is sometimes accompanied by visual loss.

Tension headaches are caused by prolonged contraction (tension) of the neck, head or facial muscles. Tension headaches are frequently associated with psychological factors such as anxiety or depression. The pain tends to be bilateral and, unlike vascular headaches, is not throbbing in character.

Traction–inflammatory headaches are related to increased intracranial pressure, which causes irritation of, and traction on, blood vessels and the dura mater within the skull. Inflammation of the meninges (meningitis) can also result in severe headache. Headaches of intracranial origin related to increased intracranial pressure vary from mild to excruciating depending on the location and cause, such as a tumour, lesion, or cerebral oedema (Brown et al 2020; LeMone et al 2020; National Institute of Neurological Disorders and Stroke 2023c).

Sensory changes

Sensory changes, which can result from disorders of the brain, spinal cord, or peripheral nerves, include alterations in the sense of touch, pain, temperature sensitivity and the loss of a sense of position. The loss of these sensations may be partial or complete. Common sensory disturbances include neuritis, inflammation of a nerve with pain, tenderness and loss of function and **neuralgia**, sharp stabbing pain usually along the course of a nerve. **Neuritis**, characterised by pain and tenderness along the path of a nerve, can progress to complete loss of sensory and motor function. Neuralgia is characterised by severe stabbing pain and can be caused by a variety of disorders affecting the nervous system. Other sensory changes that may accompany nervous system disorders include a loss of taste or smell, visual changes and hearing loss (LeMone et al 2020).

Motor changes

Alterations in motor function include localised or generalised weakness, with difficulty in moving normally. Muscle tone may be abnormally increased or decreased. A pronounced increase in tone is referred to as rigidity. Spasticity of muscles is an increased resistance to passive stretch, with rapid flexion of a joint. Abnormal movements include:

- twitching: localised spasmodic contraction of a single muscle group
- tremor: rhythmic quivering movements resulting from involuntary alternating contraction and relaxation of opposing groups of muscles
- myoclonus: spasm of a muscle or a group of muscles
- dystonia: intense irregular muscle spasms

- athetosis: slow, writhing involuntary movements of the extremities
- **chorea**: involuntary, purposeless, rapid jerky movements
- dyskinesia: involuntary twitching of the limbs or facial muscles.

Ataxia, a condition characterised by impaired ability to coordinate movement, may be caused by a lesion in the spinal cord or cerebellum. Symptoms of ataxia are failure of muscle coordination resulting in jerky movements, unsteadiness in standing and walking. Dizziness or vertigo, when the individual is unable to maintain normal balance in a standing or seated position, may also be related to a disorder of the nervous system. Unusual gait or stance may result from motor or sensory deficits caused by a disorder of the nervous system, such as Parkinson's disease. Paralysis, a symptom of motor disturbances, can occur in varying degrees with many nervous system disorders. Upper motor neuron lesions, in which the reflex area remains intact, generally cause spastic paralysis. Flaccid paralysis generally occurs in lower motor neuron lesions, which disrupt the reflex area (LeMone et al 2020).

Reflex changes

Reflex changes can provide evidence of damage to the nervous system. The absences of normal reflexes, or the presence of abnormal reflexes, generally indicate nervous system dysfunction. Reflexes are classed as either superficial (cutaneous) or deep tendon (muscle stretch). Superficial reflexes are elicited when a stimulus is applied to the skin surface or to mucous membrane. Deep tendon reflexes are elicited when a stimulus is applied to a tendon, bone or joint (LeMone et al 2020; Patton et al 2020).

Altered awareness, personality or level of consciousness

A neurological disorder that results in altered brain structure may cause impairment of a person's cognitive functions. They may experience difficulty in being able to think, remember, reason or understand. The person may also be confused in that orientation to time, place and person is impaired. Signs of reduced alertness or responsiveness may also be shown. Brain damage (e.g. as a result of a head injury) can cause a confused state characterised by fluctuating disorientation and incoherence.

Cerebral impairment may also cause mood changes and/or inappropriate emotional responses. Diffuse brain damage such as that caused by a large cerebral infarction may result in emotional instability or lability (a tendency to show alternating states of happiness and sadness that seem to be inappropriate). The person may also show signs of emotional flatness or apathy, demonstrated by a reactive absence of emotions. Alternatively, the individual may become euphoric.

Damage to the brain can also result in altered states of consciousness, ranging from drowsiness and difficulty in being aroused by normal stimuli, to coma. More information on assessment of level of consciousness is provided later in this chapter (Brown et al 2020; LeMone et al 2020).

Seizures

Seizures, which are paroxysmal events associated with sudden abnormal discharges of electrical energy in the neurons of the brain, may be secondary to CNS disease. Seizure disorders are described later in this chapter.

ASSESSING NEUROLOGICAL STATUS

Assessment is of prime importance in the care of an individual with a neurological disorder. The nurse must recognise the signs that indicate a change in condition since these changes can occur rapidly and dramatically or develop over a period of days or weeks.

Intracranial pressure

Intracranial pressure (ICP) is the pressure exerted by the CSF within the ventricles of the brain. However, it is more accurate to think in terms of intracranial 'pressures' rather than a single pressure, as the rigid skull is filled with brain tissue, intravascular blood and CSF. If any one of these three components increases in volume without a reciprocal change in volume of the other two, ICP will rise. Increased ICP affects the cerebral perfusion pressure, causing hypoxia, ischaemia, irreversible neurological damage and even death. Unless increased ICP is treated, the outcome will be herniation of a portion of the cerebrum through the tentorium, with pressure being exerted on the brainstem. The brainstem will then herniate through the foramen magnum, the only opening in the closed cranial vault.

Common causes of increased ICP include space-occupying masses such as tumours, haematomas, abscesses or cerebral oedema; conditions that increase cerebral blood volume; and conditions that increase CSF. It is important to identify early signs of increased ICP so that actions can be implemented to prevent or minimise irreversible brain damage. The manifestations of increased ICP include:

- early signs and symptoms: deterioration in the level of consciousness (confusion, restlessness, lethargy), pupillary dysfunction, motor weakness such as **hemiparesis**, paralysis of one side of the body and possible headaches
- later signs and symptoms: continued deterioration in the level of consciousness (coma), possible vomiting, hemiplegia, paralysis of one side of the body usually due to cerebral disease or injury, decortication, decerebration, increasing systolic blood pressure, bradycardia and decreasing or irregular ventilations.

(Crisp et al 2021; LeMone et al 2020)

Neurological assessment

Neurological assessment includes checking the level of consciousness, the pupils, motor function, sensory function and the vital signs. The frequency with which assessment is performed and documented depends on the individual's condition and on the healthcare institution's policy (see Clinical Skill 35.1).

CLINICAL SKILL 35.1 Performing a neurological assessment

Please adhere to the policy and procedures of the facility/organisation prior to undertaking the skill. Ensure this skill is in your scope of practice.

NMBA Decision-making Framework considerations (refer to NMBA Decision-making framework for nursing and midwifery 2020):	Equipment:
1. Am I educated? 2. Am I authorised? 3. Am I competent? If you answer 'no' to any of these, do not perform that activity. Seek guidance and support from your teacher/a nurse team leader/clinical facilitator/educator.	Sphygmomanometer BP cuff Stethoscope Thermometer Watch (with a second hand) Penlight and pupil gauge Neurological observations chart (must include Glasgow Coma Scale [GCS])

PREPARE FOR THE SKILL

(Please refer to the Standard Steps on pp. xviii–xx for related rationales.)
Mentally review the steps of the skill.
Discuss the skill with your instructor/supervisor/team leader, if required.
Confirm correct facility/organisation policy/safe operating procedures.
Validate the order in the individual's record.
Identify indication and rationale for performing the activity.
Assess for any contraindications.
Locate and gather equipment.
Perform hand hygiene.
Ensure therapeutic interaction.
Identify the individual using three individual identifiers.
Gain the individual's consent.
Assess for pain relief.
Prepare the environment.
Provide and maintain privacy.
Assist the individual to assume an appropriate position of comfort.

Skill activity	Rationale
Determine the need for neurological assessment and validate the medical orders in the individual's record.	Ensures correct procedure is about to take place. Physical signs and symptoms such as confusion, decreased level of consciousness and limb weakness may indicate alterations in neurological function.

PERFORM THE SKILL

(Please refer to the Standard Steps on pp. xviii–xx for related rationales.)
Perform hand hygiene.
Apply PPE: gloves, eyewear, mask and gown as appropriate.
Ensure the individual's safety and comfort throughout skill.
Promote independence and involvement of the individual if possible and/or appropriate.
Assess the individual's tolerance to the skill throughout.
Dispose of used supplies, equipment, waste and sharps appropriately.
Remove PPE and discard or store appropriately.
Perform hand hygiene.

CLINICAL SKILL 35.1 Performing a neurological assessment—cont'd

Skill activity	Rationale
Eyes opening (E)	
Assess arousal or wakefulness: • Assess for eye opening by observing the individual as you approach him/her—if he/she opens eyes spontaneously (spontaneous, score 4). • If the individual's eyes remain closed, speak in a clear strong voice by calling the individual by name to elicit a response. If eyes open (to speech, score 3). • If there is no response to speech, exert a painful stimulus (e.g. trapezium squeeze/supra-orbital pressure or sternal rub—used as a last measure). • If eyes open (to pain, score 2).	Altered level of consciousness is a key indicator to brain function. The GCS assesses the individual's level of consciousness. A fully conscious individual responds to questions spontaneously. As level of consciousness decreases individual may show irritability, a shortened attention span or an unwillingness to cooperate. Watch the individual for any response. If no response is gained, the individual is spoken to at first quietly then more loudly. Response is opening the eyes.
• If there is no eye opening following the application of painful stimulus (none, score 1). • Record (C) if the eye is closed due to trauma or swelling. **Note:** Record the best response only in this chart section.	If there is no auditory response, gentle touch is used, then use a central painful stimulus. If the individual has periorbital oedema due to trauma or surgery, a 'c' for closed can be documented next to 'None' (1) column.
Assess best motor response (M)	
Assess overall awareness and ability to respond to external stimuli by recording best arm response: • Ask the individual to perform a simple motor task (e.g. 'raise your arm' or 'squeeze and let go of my hands'). If the individual follows the command even weakly (obeys commands, score 6). • If the individual does not respond to verbal commands, apply a central painful stimulus (e.g. trapezium squeeze/supra-orbital pressure or sternal rub—used as a last measure) to determine the best arm response. • If the individual demonstrates purposeful movement to locate and remove the source of painful stimulus by bringing the hand up to at least nipple line, it is recorded as localising (localise to pain, score 5). • If the individual's hand or body moves away from the source of pain, it is recorded as withdraws (withdraws, score 4). • The individual may respond by flexing an arm demonstrating abnormal posturing (decorticate) (flexion to pain, score 3). • The individual may respond by extending an elbow and internally rotating wrist (decerebrate posturing). This response is recorded as abnormal extension (extension to pain, score 2). • If there is no response to the painful stimulus (none, score 1). **Note:** Record the best response only in this chart section.	When spoken to, a fully conscious individual should reply with an appropriate verbal response. A person with a decreased level of consciousness may respond in a puzzled way or may not respond at all, showing no response even when someone speaks directly into their ear. The individual who is able to respond is asked a series of simple questions (e.g. identify themself, what month, season or year it is). Impaired hearing may affect response. If the individual is not oriented to person, place or time, ascertain their best verbal response. Scores on the GCS are confused, inappropriate words, incomprehensible sounds and no response.
GCS is out of 15 and recorded on neurological observation chart. Overall score or change in score determines need to report to Registered Nurse (RN) and medical officer. Refer to facility/organisation policy regarding clinical review/rapid response criteria.	The GCS allows the evaluation of an individual's neurological status. The higher the score, the more normal the level of neurological functioning.

Continued

<table>
<tr><th colspan="2">CLINICAL SKILL 35.1 Performing a neurological assessment—cont'd</th></tr>
<tr><td>Assess pupillary activity:
• Note the size (mm), shape and equality of both the pupils in normal lighting.
• Shine a penlight torch, moving from the outer aspect of the eye to the pupil. Observe the reaction of the pupil.
• Test each eye separately and record reaction:
> yes '+'
> no '−'
> closed 'C'
> sluggish 'SL'.
• Pupillary response should be brisk constriction to light.
• Pupils are assessed for equality (are both pupils the same size?).
• Report to RN and medical officer if pupils become unequal or if one becomes more sluggish than the other.</td><td>Evaluating the pupils provides vital information about the brain and raised intracranial pressure.
Pupil size (1–8 mm) is determined using the pupil gauge before the light reflex is used.
Pupil shape is determined as round, oval or drawn to indicate abnormality.
Pupil reactivity to light is assessed by bringing the penlight from the lateral side of the individual's head towards the nose. Observe for pupil constriction (direct response) and repeat with the other eye.
Document a lack of consensual reaction (opposite pupil fails to constrict when light is shone in eye) in healthcare record.
Do not confuse a prosthetic eye with a fixed pupil. There will be no response from a blind eye.
If pupils are not the same size, 'unequal' differences are noted between the right and left sections of the chart.</td></tr>
<tr><td colspan="2">Assess limb strength</td></tr>
<tr><td>Testing limb strength gives an indication of the part of the brain that is affected as opposed to testing level of consciousness.
Bilateral upper limb muscle strength:
• Instruct individual to move arms, lift limb against gravity, move limb against your resistance.
• Ask the individual to squeeze both the assessor's hands followed by asking the individual to:
> Pull your hands towards them against resistance.
> Push your hands away against resistance (normal power).
• Active movement of body part against gravity with some resistance (mild weakness).
• Active movement of body part against gravity (severe weakness).
• Active movement of body part when effect of gravity is removed (spastic flexion).
• Only a trace or flicker of movement is seen or felt in the muscle (extension).
• No detectable muscle contraction (no response).
Bilateral lower limb muscle strength:
• Instruct individual to move legs laterally on bed; lift limb against gravity; move limb against your resistance.
Note: Record the response for each limb separately in this section of the chart as per upper limb muscle assessment:
• (normal power)
• (mild weakness)
• (severe weakness)
• (extension)
• (no response).</td><td>Assessment of limb strength usually focuses on the arms and legs, and the identification of significant changes are important for denoting improvement, stabilisation or deterioration in the individual's condition. The techniques used to evaluate limb strength depend on the individual's level of consciousness.
Each extremity is assessed unless contraindicated.
The individual is given clear commands such as 'squeeze my hands' or 'push against my hands'. Compare both sides. Record right (R) and left (L) separately if there is a difference between the two sides.
Response is recorded as normal, mild weakness, severe weakness, flexion, extension or no response.</td></tr>
</table>

CLINICAL SKILL 35.1 Performing a neurological assessment—cont'd

Assess vital signs	
Initially, vital signs are monitored every 15 minutes until stable then hourly or as per organisational/facility guidelines.	Vital sign changes are late changes in brain deterioration. A drop in level of consciousness is the earliest sign of neurological deterioration. Change in vital signs can indicate a worsening neurological condition, and therefore vital signs are always recorded at the same time as other neurological observations. Change in vital signs may also provide clues as to other medical problems in an unconscious individual who cannot tell staff what symptoms they are experiencing. Vital sign changes associated with raised intracranial pressure: • bradycardia • tachycardia (very late sign) • hypertension (typically, an elevated systolic blood pressure combined with a widening pulse pressure) • irregular respirations.

AFTER THE SKILL

(Please refer to the Standard Steps on pp. xviii–xx for related rationales.)
Communicate outcome to the individual, any ongoing care and to report any complications.
Restore the environment.
Report, record and document assessment findings, details of the skill performed and the individual's response.
Report, record and document any abnormalities and/or inability to perform the skill.
Reassess the individual to ensure there are no adverse effects/events from the skill.

(ACSQHC 2021a; Berman et al 2021; Crisp et al 2021; Hall et al 2022; LeMone et al 2020; Rebeiro et al 2021)

Level of consciousness

The level of consciousness is a most important factor in neurological assessment, providing valid information about changes in neurological status. Change can occur slowly over the course of many days, or it can occur rapidly in a few minutes or hours. The rapidity of change is an indicator of the severity of the neurological problem. The individual's level of consciousness is evaluated by providing stimuli and observing the response. Sound and pain are the major stimuli used. Speaking to the individual is the most common method of applying an auditory stimulus, while painful stimuli are reserved for the individual with obviously decreased levels of consciousness. When spoken to, a fully conscious individual should reply with an appropriate verbal response. A person with a decreased level of consciousness may respond in a puzzled way or may not respond at all, showing no response even when someone speaks directly into their ear (Agency for Clinical Innovation 2013; Crisp et al 2021; Hall et al 2022; LeMone et al 2020; Rebeiro et al 2021).

Painful tactile stimuli

Painful tactile stimuli may be necessary to arouse the semi comatose individual. Painful stimuli can be provided by exerting firm digital pressure on the nail beds, the Achilles tendon, or the gastrocnemius muscle. Response to painful stimuli can be classified into:

- purposeful, when the individual winces, pushes the assessor away or withdraws the affected body part
- non-purposeful, when the individual moves the stimulated body part only slightly, or when the application of painful stimuli causes an extensor response (a contraction of muscles) only
- unresponsive, when the individual shows no sign of reacting to painful stimuli.

The Glasgow Coma Scale (GCS) (Table 35.2) was originally designed to assess the level of consciousness in people with head injuries, but it is now used in a variety of settings. It has gained increasing acceptance as an accurate and effective means of evaluating levels of consciousness. Using the GCS, a score of 15 reflects a fully alert, well-oriented person, while a score of 8 or less is considered to indicate coma. The lowest possible score of 3 is indicative of brain death. The GCS is standardised worldwide (Agency for Clinical Innovation 2013; Hall et al 2022; Rebeiro et al 2021).

Evaluation of the pupils

Evaluating the pupils provides vital information about the brain and raised ICP. The findings in one pupil are compared with the findings in the other, and the differences

TABLE 35.2 | Levels of consciousness: Glasgow Coma Scale

Faculty measured	Response	Score
Eye opening	Spontaneous	4
	To verbal command	3
	To pain	2
	No response	1
Motor response	To verbal command	6
	To localised pain	5
	Flexes and withdraws	4
	Flexes abnormally	3
	Extends abnormally	2
	No response	1
Verbal response	Oriented, converses	5
	Disoriented, converses	4
	Uses inappropriate words	3
	Makes incomprehensible sounds	2
	No response	1

(Jain & Iverson 2023)

between the two pupils are documented. The pupils are assessed for size, shape and reaction to light. Normally the pupils are equal in size (average diameter of 3.5 mm), round and they constrict briskly when light is shone into the eye. A pupil gauge may be used to estimate the size of each pupil. Abnormal responses of a pupil to light may be described as sluggish, non-reactive or fixed. Generally, any change in a pupil's size, shape or reaction is indicative of an intracranial change.

Assessment of motor function

Assessment of motor function usually focuses on the arms and legs, and the identification of significant changes is important for denoting improvement, stabilisation or deterioration in the individual's condition. The techniques used to evaluate motor function depend on the individual's level of consciousness. In the conscious individual, the assessment can be made by observing motor responses to directions (e.g. by asking the individual to squeeze the assessor's hands). If the individual is unconscious or is unable to provide accurate responses, the assessor must rely on observational skills to evaluate motor function.

Assessment of sensory function

Assessment of sensory function is described earlier in this chapter.

Assessment of the vital signs

Assessing the vital signs (see also Chapter 16) provides data concerning vital functions of the body. The individual's temperature, pulse, ventilations and blood pressure are monitored and documented at a frequency that depends on their condition. Data from neurological assessments are documented according to the healthcare institution's policy. Many institutions use a special neurological assessment chart. If clinical deterioration is recognised, the response to be implemented is in accordance with the health service organisation policy and procedures (ACSQHC 2021b; Hall et al 2022; LeMone et al 2020).

DIAGNOSTIC TESTS

Specific tests may be performed for diagnostic purposes or to aid in evaluation of an individual's condition.

The neurological examination

The purpose of the neurological examination is to determine the presence or absence of disease in the nervous system by assessing cerebral, cranial nerve, motor, sensory and reflex function. Evaluation of cerebral function is performed by assessing the individual's general behaviour and cognitive functions, such as orientation to time and place, concentration, memory, vocabulary and abstract reasoning. Evaluation of the cranial nerves involves assessing:

- The olfactory nerve: The sense of smell is tested by obstructing one nostril while testing the other. A variety of substances is placed near the unobstructed nostril and the individual is asked to identify the odour of each.
- The optic nerve: Each eye is tested to assess visual acuity and visual fields. The fundus of each eye is assessed by ophthalmoscopic examination.
- The oculomotor, trochlear and abducens nerves: These three nerves are generally tested together because they supply the various muscles that rotate the eyeball. The ophthalmoscope is used during the assessment; the pupils are observed for size, shape and equality, and movement of the eyes is evaluated by requesting the individual to follow a finger through the six cardinal areas of vision.
- The trigeminal nerve: The sensory component of this nerve is tested with the individual's eyes closed. Test tubes of warm and cold water are brought into contact with the skin of the face to check temperature perception. Touching the face with a wisp of cotton checks perception of light touch. Pain perception is evaluated either by applying pressure or by touching areas of the face with the point of a pin. The motor component of the trigeminal nerve is evaluated by asking the individual to clench and unclench the

teeth, and by observing their ability to open the mouth against resistance. The corneal reflex is assessed by lightly stroking the cornea with a wisp of cotton. If the corneal reflex is intact, the individual will automatically blink.
- The facial nerve: The sensory component of this nerve is assessed by placing sweet, salty, sour and bitter substances on various areas of the tongue and asking the individual to identify each taste. The motor component of the facial nerve is assessed by requesting the individual to perform specific facial movements such as smiling, closing the eyes, pursing the lips and wrinkling the forehead.
- The acoustic nerve: Generally, unless the individual has a history of vertigo, only the hearing branch of this nerve is assessed. A series of hearing tests is performed, and hearing in both ears is compared. For a more precise assessment of hearing acuity, a tuning fork is used.
- The glossopharyngeal and vagus nerves: These nerves are usually tested together, as they are closely related both anatomically and functionally. A series of tests is performed to assess the gag and swallowing reflexes.
- The spinal accessory nerve: This nerve is tested by evaluating the strength of the trapezius and sternocleidomastoid muscles (e.g. by requesting the individual to shrug the shoulders against resistance and by asking them to turn their head to one side and push their chin against the assessor's hand).
- The hypoglossal nerve: The strength and movement of the tongue muscles are evaluated by testing the individual's ability to protrude the tongue, and also by requesting them to push their tongue against a tongue depressor.

(Brown et al 2020; Hall et al 2022; LeMone et al 2020; Patton & Thibodeau 2019)

Evaluation of motor function

Evaluating motor function involves assessing the individual's gait, posture, muscle strength and tone, balance and coordination. The assessor observes for abnormalities and compares the findings on both sides of the body for asymmetry.

Evaluation of sensory function

Evaluating sensory function involves assessing the individual's ability to perceive various sensations with their eyes closed. Assessment includes testing of sensitivity to touch, pain and temperature or testing of joint motion and position and assessment of discriminative function and vibratory sensation.

Evaluation of reflexes

Evaluation of reflexes involves testing the two types of reflexes to assess the integrity of the motor and sensory systems.

The superficial reflexes

These include the upper abdominal, lower abdominal, gluteal and plantar reflexes. The abdominal and gluteal reflexes are evaluated by applying a stimulus to the skin surface (e.g. stroking with a finger or pointed object and observing for muscle contraction). The plantar reflex is evaluated by stroking the sole of the foot, with one continuous movement from the heel to the toes. Normally, the big toe curls downwards in response to this stimulus. An abnormal response, Babinski's sign, when there is dorsiflexion of the big toe and fanning of the other toes, indicates upper motor neurone disease (Brown et al 2020; Hall et al 2022; LeMone et al 2020).

The deep tendon reflexes

These include the biceps, triceps, quadriceps and Achilles tendons. Deep tendon reflexes are elicited by using a percussion hammer and observing the response, as follows:
- The biceps reflex is tested with the arm partially flexed at the elbow and the palm down. When the hammer is applied to the biceps tendon, the elbow should flex.
- The triceps reflex is tested with the arm partially flexed at the elbow and the palm directed towards the body. When the hammer is applied to the triceps tendon, the elbow should extend.
- The quadriceps reflex is tested with the knee flexed. When the patellar tendon is struck with the hammer, the knee should extend.
- The Achilles reflex is tested with the knee flexed. When the Achilles tendon is struck with the hammer, the foot should plantar flex.

(Brown et al 2020; Hall et al 2022; LeMone et al 2020)

Neurovascular assessment

Neurovascular assessment includes skin assessment (colour, temperature, oedema), palpation and assessment of pulses, sensation, motor function and pain.

Extremities should be palpated for swelling and assessed for pain, an appropriate colour, warmth, symmetry in shape and size, and capillary refill should be less than 2 seconds (immediate). Pulses should be strong and equal. For lower limbs, popliteal, posterior tibial and dorsalis pedis pulses should all be present and assessed for strength and equal amplitude. Assessment findings are used to support a diagnosis and determine or modify nursing care interventions (Berman et al 2021; Crisp et al 2021; Hall et al 2022; LeMone et al 2020).

(See Clinical Skill 35.2.)

Radiographic examination

X-ray

Plain X-ray films of the skull may be performed to detect fractures, to aid in the diagnosis of pituitary tumours or to detect congenital abnormalities. X-ray films of the spine may be performed to detect trauma to the vertebral column or to aid in the diagnosis of conditions that cause motor or sensory impairment (LeMone et al 2020).

Computerised tomography scan

Computerised tomography (CT) (see Figure 35.7) is commonly used to diagnose intracranial and spinal cord

CLINICAL SKILL 35.2 Neurovascular assessment

Please adhere to the policy and procedures of the facility/organisation prior to undertaking the skill. Ensure this skill is in your scope of practice.

NMBA Decision-making Framework considerations (refer to NMBA Decision-making framework for nursing and midwifery 2020):	**Equipment:**
1. Am I educated? 2. Am I authorised? 3. Am I competent? If you answer 'no' to any of these, do not perform that activity. Seek guidance and support from your teacher/a nurse team leader/clinical facilitator/educator.	Neurovascular assessment chart

PREPARE FOR THE SKILL

(Please refer to the Standard Steps on pp. xviii–xx for related rationales.)
Mentally review the steps of the skill.
Discuss the skill with your instructor/supervisor/team leader, if required.
Confirm correct facility/organisation policy/safe operating procedures.
Validate the order in the individual's record.
Identify indication and rationale for performing the activity.
Assess for any contraindications.
Locate and gather equipment.
Perform hand hygiene.
Ensure therapeutic interaction.
Identify the individual using three individual identifiers.
Gain the individual's consent.
Assess for pain relief.
Prepare the environment.
Provide and maintain privacy.
Assist the individual to assume an appropriate position of comfort.

PERFORM THE SKILL

(Please refer to the Standard Steps on pp. xviii–xx for related rationales.)
Perform hand hygiene.
Apply PPE: gloves, eyewear, mask and gown as appropriate.
Ensure the individual's safety and comfort throughout skill.
Promote independence and involvement of the individual if possible and/or appropriate.
Assess the individual's tolerance to the skill throughout.
Dispose of used supplies, equipment, waste and sharps appropriately.
Remove PPE and discard or store appropriately.
Perform hand hygiene.

Skill activity	**Rationale**
Assess the limb distal to the surgery/injury	
Compare affected limb with unaffected limb assessing both limbs for (document affected limb only): • Colour > Visually check colour, document as pink, pale/white or cyanotic, dusky, cyanotic, mottled or purple/black. • Temperature > Check temperature with superficial touch, document as warm, cool or hot. • Pulses > Palpate for presence of peripheral pulses distal to injury. > Document pulses as strong, weak, absent.	Obtains a baseline prior to surgery. Assesses the vasculature and nerve supply to a traumatised limb. Monitors limb status so that permanent damage or complications are avoided by identifying indicators of problems early and intervening. Limb assessed as normal if limb pink in colour, warm to touch, capillary refill of 1–2 seconds, swelling full, strong pulse, normal sensation. Limb assessed as inadequate arterial supply if pale/white or cyanotic in colour, cool to touch, capillary refill >2 seconds, swelling hollow or prune-like.

CLINICAL SKILL 35.2 Neurovascular assessment—cont'd

• Sensation > Touch and assess visual limb surfaces for presence and type of sensation. Document as normal, decreased sensation, loss of sensation, numbness, tingling or pins and needles. • Motor function > Active movement or passive movement. • Pain > Assess pain on movement of limb and document pain score: 0 (no pain), 10 (worst pain). • Swelling and ooze > Visually check for swelling and ooze. > Document swelling as nil, small, moderate.	Limb assessed as inadequate venous return if limb dusky, cyanotic, mottled or purple/black in colour, hot to touch, immediate capillary refill, swelling distended or tense, tissues feel hard. Capillary refill assessment is evaluated by pressing firmly down on the nail bed of fingers or toes for 5 seconds. The nail bed will blanch and the colour should return within 2 seconds once pressure is released. If pulses are not palpable due to plaster casts, assess closely above parameters. Individuals may report changes in sensation if neurovascular compromise is present or may be a result of a nerve block or epidural (this should be documented on the neurovascular chart). Individual assessed as having active movement if able to voluntarily extend and flex an extremity or digit. Individual assessed as having passive movement if assessor is able to extend and flex an extremity or digit. If pulse is not present, document and notify medical officer, observe colour, capillary refill and temperature. Immediately report to medical team if there is any deterioration in neurovascular assessment.

AFTER THE SKILL

(Please refer to the Standard Steps on pp. xviii–xx for related rationales.)

Communicate outcome to the individual, any ongoing care and to report any complications.

Restore the environment.

Report, record and document assessment findings, details of the skill performed and the individual's response.

Report, record and document any abnormalities and/or inability to perform the skill.

Reassess the individual to ensure there are no adverse effects/events from the skill.

(Berman et al 2021; Crisp et al 2021; Hall et al 2022; LeMone et al 2020)

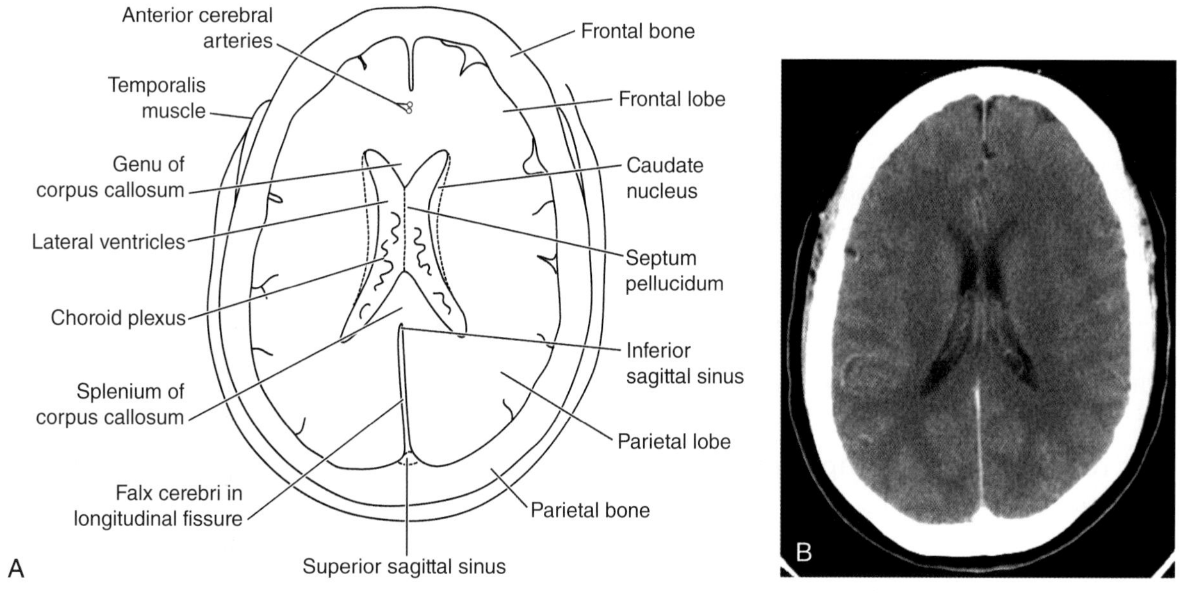

Figure 35.7 A: Line drawing of CT section, **B:** CT image representing structures located at level B

(Rollins et al 2023)

lesions. It is usually non-invasive but a contrast dye is sometimes administered to visualise blood vessels or to define lesions. The individual lies on an X-ray table, with the head immobilised and face uncovered. The head is moved into the scanner, and a moveable frame revolves around it while X-ray films are taken. If a contrast agent is used, the individual may feel warm and experience a transient headache, a salty taste and nausea (LeMone et al 2020; Marieb & Keller 2021).

Myelogram

A myelogram involves fluoroscopy and radiography to evaluate the spinal cord and vertebral column after injection of a contrast medium via lumbar puncture into the subarachnoid space. The individual is positioned to allow the medium to flow through the subarachnoid space. A series of X-ray films are taken, after which the contrast medium may be either withdrawn or allowed to remain in the CSF. Water-soluble agents are allowed to remain, as they will eventually be excreted by the kidneys (LeMone et al 2020).

Angiography

Cerebral angiography involves injecting a radio-opaque contrast medium into an artery for radiological visualisation of the intracranial and extracranial blood vessels. Common injection sites are the carotid or femoral arteries, with X-ray films taken at various intervals after injection of the medium. Cerebral angiography may be performed using either local or general anaesthetic. Digital subtraction angiography is a computer-assisted radiographic procedure for visualising extracranial and intracranial vessels and involves injection of a contrast medium through a catheter into the superior vena cava. Cerebral vessels are visualised on a screen, and pictures taken. Cerebral angiogram is used to diagnose aneurysms, arteriovenous malformations, thrombosis, vasospasm, tumours and haematomas (LeMone et al 2020).

Magnetic resonance imaging (MRI)

An MRI is a non-invasive procedure in which the individual is placed in a strong magnetic field and is subjected to precise computer-programmed bursts of radio pulse waves. The sharpness and detail of the images produced assist diagnosis by providing identification of abnormalities and can detect neurological disorders with structural changes (e.g. stroke, tumour, infection and seizures). MRI is contraindicated in individuals with pacemakers, metallic aneurysm clips and some metallic prostheses (LeMone et al 2020; Marieb & Keller 2021).

Magnetic resonance angiography (MRA)

MRA is used to detect vascular lesions by reconstructing vessels with blood flow. Contrast may be used (LeMone et al 2020).

Positron emission tomography (PET) scanning

PET scanning is a non-invasive nuclear imaging technique used to detect biochemical and physiological abnormalities. The individual is injected with a nuclide that reacts with electrons and produces gamma-ray photons. A scanner detects the gamma rays and codes this data into a computer. Radioisotopes evaluate cellular metabolism, and may show a typical pattern for Alzheimer's disease, and can be used to differentiate tumour reoccurrence from radiation necrosis. The computer then reconstructs cross-sectional images of the tissues being examined (LeMone et al 2020; Marieb & Keller 2021).

Single-photon emission computed tomography (SPECT)

A SPECT scan is similar to a PET scan and can be used to diagnose strokes, brain tumours and seizure disorders.

Carotid duplex study

Identifies carotid artery disease by using soundwaves produced by blood flow to produce an image (LeMone et al 2020).

Electroencephalography (EEG)

An electroencephalogram (EEG) is a recording of the electrical activity of the brain (brainwaves). Surface electrodes are attached to the scalp with a paste and transmit the brain's electrical impulses to a machine that records them as brainwaves on strips of paper. Brainwaves are recorded while the individual is at rest, after hyperventilation, with photic stimulation, after a sensory stimulus and during sleep (see Clinical Interest Box 35.1) (LeMone et al 2020; Patton et al 2019).

Evoked potentials

Evoked potentials are used to measure nerve conduction and diagnose and evaluate neuromuscular disease and nerve damage (LeMone et al 2020).

Electromyogram (EMG)

EMG is used to diagnose neuromuscular diseases by inserting needle electrodes into the muscle to be examined. Recordings measure the electrical activity of skeletal muscles at rest and during contraction (LeMone et al 2020).

Lumbar puncture (LP)

A lumbar puncture (Figure 35.8) may be performed to obtain a sample of CSF for either diagnostic or therapeutic purposes. The diagnostic indications include:

- measurement of CSF pressure
- examination of CSF for the presence of blood or microorganisms
- injection of air, oxygen, or radio-opaque material to visualise parts of the CNS radiologically
- evaluation for signs of blockage of CSF flow.

Therapeutic indications include introduction of spinal anaesthesia for surgery and intrathecal injection of medications.

For the procedure, the individual assumes a lateral position, with their back curled and their knees flexed as close to their chest as possible. The head should be bent forwards

CLINICAL INTEREST BOX 35.1 Care of the individual undergoing an EEG

Individual preparation

- Explain the procedure to the individual, emphasising the importance of cooperation.
- Withhold fluids, foods and medications (as prescribed) that may stimulate or depress brainwaves. These include anticonvulsants, tranquillisers, depressants and caffeine-containing foods (e.g. coffee, tea, cola and chocolate). Medications are usually withheld for 24–48 hours before the test.
- Help the individual to wash their hair before the test.

Individual and family teaching

- The test takes about an hour.
- The test is painless and will be performed while the individual sits in a comfortable chair or lies on a stretcher.
- The electrodes are applied to the scalp with a thick paste.
- During the test, the individual will first be asked to breathe in and out deeply for a few minutes, then to close their eyes while a light is flashed on them and, finally, to lie quietly with eyes closed.
- After the test, the nurse will help the individual wash the paste out of their hair.

(LeMone et al 2020; NSQHS Standard consideration: 'Partnering with Consumers' [action 2.03, 2.04, 2.05, 2.06, 2.07, 2.08, 2.09 & 2.10]; NSQHS Standard consideration: 'Comprehensive Care' [action 5.03])

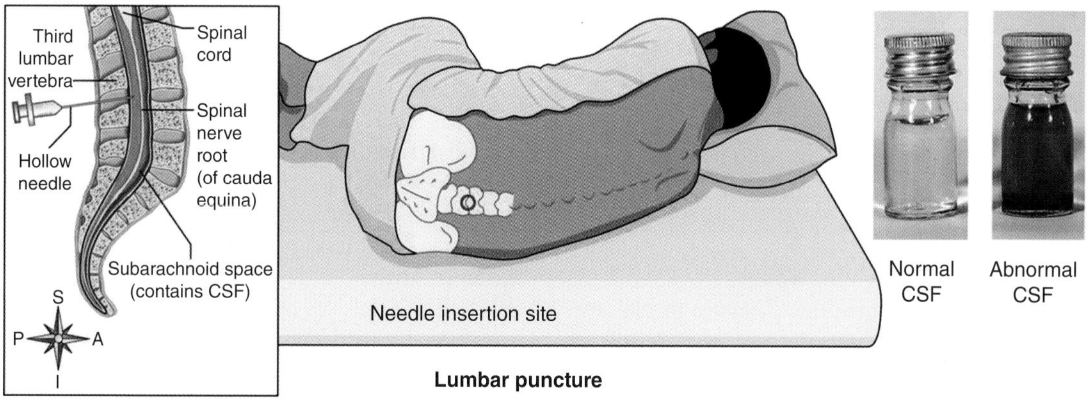

Figure 35.8 Location and positioning for lumbar puncture

CSF, cerebrospinal fluid

(Stein & Hollen 2024)

so that the chin touches their chest (Figure 35.9). After preparation of the site, the medical officer inserts a spinal needle with a stylus (a fine probe) between L3 and L4 or L4 and L5 into the subarachnoid space and fluid is aspirated. If the lumbar puncture is being performed for diagnostic purposes, a manometer may be attached to the needle to measure CSF pressure. Samples of CSF are then collected for visual and laboratory examination. When the procedure is completed, the needle is withdrawn and an adhesive dressing applied over the puncture site (Fowler 2019; LeMone et al 2020; Patton & Thibodeau 2019).

Further investigations—Nerve conduction studies

These studies involve application of an electrical stimulus to peripheral nerves and measurement of their response by means of an oscilloscope (Brown et al 2020; Berman et al 2021; Marieb & Keller 2021).

SPECIFIC DISORDERS OF THE NERVOUS SYSTEM

Disorders of the nervous system may be congenital or genetic, due to multiple causes, degenerative, infectious, or inflammatory, immunological, neoplastic, obstructive or traumatic.

Congenital disorders

Anencephaly

Anencephaly is the failure of normal development of the brain (cerebral hemispheres and cerebellum) and scalp. The precise cause is unknown, and babies with the disorder do not live (Marieb & Keller 2021).

Spinal cord defects

Spinal cord defects include spina bifida, a congenital defect of non-union of one or more vertebral arches

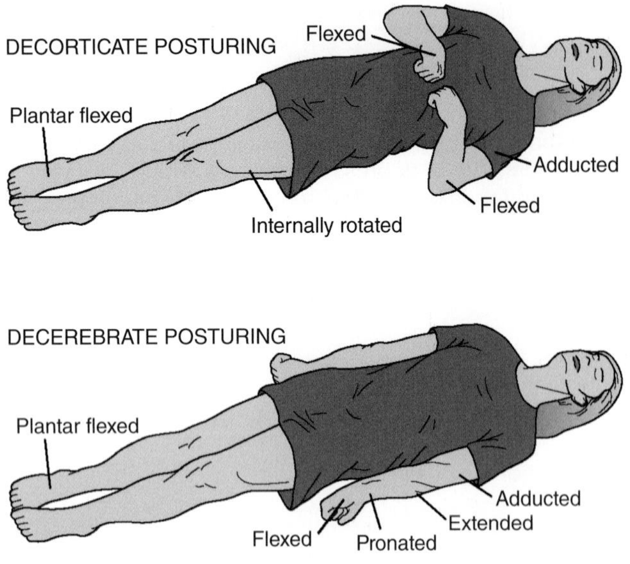

Figure 35.9 Decorticate and decerebrate posture/responses

A: Decorticate posture/response. Flexion of arms, wrists and fingers with adduction in upper extremities. Bilateral extension, internal rotation and plantar flexion in lower extremities,
B: Decerebrate posture/response. All four extremities in rigid extension with hyperpronation of forearms and plantar extension of feet.
(deWit & Kumagai 2013)

allowing protrusion of the meninges, meningocele and myelomeningocele. These conditions are the result of incomplete closure of the neural tube during the first 3 months of embryonic development. Causes are thought to include maternal exposure to viruses, radiation and other environmental factors.

In severe forms, spina bifida involves incomplete closure of one or more of the vertebrae, causing protrusion of the spinal contents in an external sac. In spina bifida with meningocele, the sac contains meninges and CSF. In spina bifida with myelomeningocele, the sac contains meninges, CSF and a portion of the spinal cord or nerve roots. Manifestations of congenital spinal cord defects vary and include a depression, dimple or tuft of hair on the skin over the spinal defect. The more severe defects cause neurological dysfunction such as paralysis of the legs, bowel and bladder incontinence and hydrocephalus (Better Health Channel 2018; LeMone et al 2020).

Hydrocephalus

Hydrocephalus is an excessive accumulation of CSF within the ventricles of the brain. It may result from an obstruction in CSF flow (see Figure 35.7) or from faulty absorption of CSF. The condition can also occur as a result of cerebral injury or disease. In infants, the obvious manifestation of hydrocephalus is abnormal enlargement of the head. Other characteristics include distended scalp veins, thin and fragile scalp skin, downward displacement of the eyes, a shrill high-pitched cry, irritability and abnormal muscle tone of the legs.

A treatment for hydrocephalus is the insertion of a shunt that allows excess CSF to drain to another area of the body. Typical shunt types are a ventriculoperitoneal (VP) shunt, which moves fluid from the ventricles of the brain to the abdominal cavity; a ventriculoatrial (VA) shunt, which moves fluid from the ventricles of the brain to a chamber of the heart; and a lumboperitoneal (LP) shunt, which moves fluid from the lower back to the abdominal cavity. Each shunt has a valve attached. The two most common valves are fixed pressure valves, which are regulated by a predetermined pressure setting, and adjustable pressure valves, which can be adjusted non-invasively by a special magnetic tool (LeMone et al 2020; Medtronic 2023; Wilson & Giddens 2020).

Genetic disorders

Hereditary genetic defects include muscular dystrophy, Huntington's chorea and neurofibromatosis.

Muscular dystrophy

Muscular dystrophy is a group of congenital disorders characterised by progressive wasting and weakness of muscles. There are many different forms and sources of muscular dystrophy, with all of the conditions causing muscle weakness which has a profound effect on the individual's life. Each neuromuscular condition has a characteristic pattern of muscle weakness. It may affect only the muscles around the eyes, throat or legs; however, the severest form may affect all the muscles of the body including the heart. There is no specific treatment. Duchenne's muscular dystrophy is the most common type. It begins to manifest between the ages of 3 and 5 years and is the most severe form. Initially, it affects the leg and pelvic muscles, but there is progressive involvement of all voluntary muscles. Later in the disease, progressive weakening of cardiac and respiratory muscles results in heart or respiratory failure. Early manifestations of Duchenne's muscular dystrophy include a waddling gait, lordosis (increased curvature of the lumbar spine) and marked difficulty rising from a supine to a standing position. As the disease progresses, facial, oropharyngeal and respiratory muscles become involved (Muscular Dystrophy Foundation 2022).

Huntington's chorea

Huntington's chorea is a disorder in which degeneration of the cerebral cortex and basal ganglia causes chronic progressive choreiform movements and mental deterioration. Onset is generally in early middle age, and the individual gradually develops progressively severe choreiform movements and dementia. The movements usually begin slowly, with facial grimacing and jerking arm actions. Over time, the movements become frequent, erratic and violent, affecting the trunk and lower limbs and making speech, swallowing, walking and other basic tasks more difficult. Dementia may be mild at first but eventually severely disrupts the person as the intellectual and emotional symptoms become more advanced (Huntington's NSW 2020; LeMone et al 2020; Marieb & Keller 2021).

Neurofibromatosis

Neurofibromatosis can affect anyone and is one of the most common congenital abnormalities. The condition is usually classified according to which parts of the nervous system are affected. There are three types of neurofibromas: type 1 (NF 1), type 2 (NF 2) and Schwannomatosis. All are characterised by the growth of benign tumours, which can grow anywhere there are nerve cells. In NF 1, multiple cutaneous and subcutaneous nodules of varying size occur. Subcutaneous nodules may attach to the peripheral portion of the nerve, causing pain or pressure and, rarely, sensory loss in the distribution of the affected nerve. Neuromas, which are an overgrowth of subcutaneous tissue, may reach enormous sizes and commonly affect the face, scalp, neck and chest. Neurological symptoms may appear if the tumours cause pressure on the brain or spinal cord as occurs in NF 2 (Children's Tumour Foundation conquering NF 2023).

Disorders of multiple cause

Cerebral palsy

Cerebral palsy comprises a group of neuromotor disorders resulting from prenatal, perinatal or postnatal cerebral hypoxia or damage. The incidence of cerebral palsy is highest in premature infants or in infants who have experienced a difficult birth resulting in cerebral damage. Causative factors include chromosomal abnormalities; prenatal factors such as maternal infections, exposure to harmful chemicals or malnutrition; perinatal factors such as premature birth or instrumental delivery causing cerebral anoxia; and postnatal factors such as trauma, infection or malnutrition causing cerebral damage.

The manifestations of cerebral palsy range from mild muscle incoordination to severe spasticity. The spastic form of the disorder is characterised by rapid alternating muscle contraction and relaxation, muscle weakness and underdevelopment and muscle contraction in response to manipulation. The athetoid form of cerebral palsy is characterised by grimacing, writhing and jerking involuntary movements, which become more severe during stress. Ataxic cerebral palsy is characterised by disturbed balance, incoordination, muscle weakness and tremor. In addition to the range of motor deficits, the individual may experience sensory deficits such as speech, visual or hearing impairment. Intellectual disability accompanies cerebral palsy in about 40% of cases (Cerebral Palsy Alliance 2018; Cerebral Palsy Australia 2023).

Cerebral aneurysm

A cerebral aneurysm is an abnormality (weak spot) of the wall of a cerebral artery that results in a localised dilation. As the aneurysm becomes larger, the wall of the artery becomes weaker and can rupture. If the aneurysm ruptures, blood enters the subarachnoid space or cerebral tissue. Causative factors include congenital defects in the arterial walls, sclerotic changes in blood vessels, hypertension and cerebral trauma. Manifestations of a cerebral aneurysm do not generally appear until the aneurysm ruptures. The most common symptom of rupture is the sudden onset of a severe headache, which may be accompanied by nausea and vomiting, motor deficits, visual disturbances and loss of consciousness. A cerebral aneurysm may be detected before it ruptures if the individual shows signs of oculomotor nerve compression, eyelid ptosis and a pupil that is sluggish or non-reactive (Stroke Foundation 2023a).

Transient ischaemic attacks

Transient ischaemic attacks (TIAs) result in a loss of function to a particular part of the body due to a sudden lack of blood flow to a part of the brain. An episode of cerebrovascular insufficiency is usually associated with partial occlusion of the cerebral artery by an atherosclerotic plaque or an embolus. The attacks, which may last from seconds to hours, are generally considered to be warning signs of an impending thrombotic **cerebrovascular accident (stroke)**, arising from an embolus, thrombus or haemorrhage in the cerebrum. The characteristics of a TIA, which may be caused by micro-emboli or arteriole spasm, are various symptoms of neurological dysfunction followed by a return of normal function. Symptoms include visual disturbances, double or blurred vision, short-term blindness, speech disturbances, slurred or thick speech, swallowing difficulty, staggering or uncoordinated gait, unilateral weakness or numbness, facial numbness or weakness, vertigo and loss of balance, nausea, and vomiting. The difference between a TIA and an ischaemic stroke is that the symptoms of a TIA will completely disappear within 24 hours (Brain Foundation 2023).

Trigeminal neuralgia

Trigeminal neuralgia is a painful disorder of one or more branches of the trigeminal nerve that produces paroxysmal attacks of excruciating facial pain. While the cause is often unknown, the disorder may be associated with other neurological conditions such as aneurysms, cerebral tumours or multiple sclerosis. The individual experiences excruciating burning pain, which generally occurs suddenly in response to a stimulus, such as a draught of cold air, drinking hot or cold fluids, brushing the teeth or speaking or laughing. The frequency of attacks varies from many times a day to several times a month or year (LeMone et al 2020).

Intellectual disability

Intellectual disability is a syndrome of incomplete intellectual development associated with impaired learning and social adjustment. The causes include:

- prenatal factors such as metabolic disorders, chromosomal abnormalities, cranial malformation, maternal infections, malnutrition or anoxia
- perinatal factors such as prematurity, anoxia or intracranial haemorrhage

- postnatal factors such as cerebral injury, CNS infections, anoxia, neoplasms, degenerative diseases, cerebral haemorrhage, nutritional deficiencies and emotional deprivation.

Manifestations include poor motor development, impaired concepts of space and time, learning difficulties, inappropriate behaviour and difficulty with social interactions (Marieb & Keller 2021).

Peripheral neuritis

Peripheral neuritis (polyneuritis) is the degeneration of peripheral nerves, resulting in muscle weakness and atrophy, sensory loss and decreased or absent tendon reflexes. Causes include chronic intoxication (alcohol, arsenic, lead), metabolic and inflammatory disorders (diabetes mellitus, rheumatoid arthritis), nutrient deficiencies (thiamine) and infectious diseases (meningitis or Guillain-Barré syndrome). Manifestations usually develop slowly, beginning with leg pains and numbness or tingling in the feet and hands. As the disease progresses, the individual experiences flaccid paralysis, muscle wasting, pain of varying intensity and loss of reflexes in the legs and arms. Foot drop, ataxic gait and inability to walk will eventually occur (LeMone et al 2020).

Guillain-Barré syndrome

Guillain-Barré syndrome (GBS) is an acute inflammatory disorder that causes the body's immune system to attack part of the PNS, causing what is known as an autoimmune disorder. It is characterised by rapid and progressive neuromuscular paralysis with the first symptoms including decreased function, varying degrees of weakness or tingling sensation, and decreased reflexes distally in the lower limbs that often spreads proximally to include the upper body. In some cases, these symptoms can increase until the muscles are almost totally paralysed, resulting in a life-threatening situation requiring mechanical ventilation due to respiratory dysfunction.

The National Institute of Neurological Disorders and Stroke (2023b) states that most individuals will have good recovery from GBS, although some may continue to have some residual weakness after 3 years.

While there is no known cause of GBS, most individuals who are diagnosed with this condition have a 1–3-week previous history of upper respiratory or gastrointestinal viral infection. Occasionally, surgery may also trigger the syndrome. The disease progression may occur over the course of hours or days, or it may take up to 3–4 weeks. It is confirmed with a lumbar puncture, electromyography and nerve conduction studies.

In GBS, the antiganglioside antibodies attack Schwann cells of the myelin sheath, causing demyelination of the peripheral nerves, which in turn halts nerve conduction. There is no known cure for GBS; however, plasmapheresis (also known as plasma exchange) and high-dose immunoglobulin therapy may be used to treat the complications of the disease. Plasmapheresis causes the Schwann cells to remyelinate, which in turn reduces the severity and duration of the Guillain-Barré episode and in most cases, individuals can expect a full recovery.

When caring for the individual with GBS, the nurse should assess airway and breathing, refer to speech pathology, maintain the individual as nil by mouth until otherwise ordered, ensure adequate analgesia, perform pressure area care, and take steps to reassure the individual (LeMone et al 2020; National Institute of Neurological Disorders and Stroke 2023b).

Prognosis of Guillain-Barré syndrome

GBS can be a devastating disorder because of its sudden and unexpected onset. Most people reach the stage of greatest weakness within the first 2 weeks after symptoms appear, and by the third week of the illness 90% of all individuals are at their weakest. The recovery period may be as little as a few weeks or as long as a few years. About 30% of those with GBS still have a residual weakness after 3 years. About 3% may suffer a relapse of muscle weakness and tingling sensations many years after the initial attack (National Institute of Neurological Disorders and Stroke 2023b).

Bell's palsy

Bell's palsy is a disorder of the seventh cranial nerve that produces unilateral facial weakness or paralysis. An inflammatory reaction occurs in or around cranial nerve VII, resulting in nerve compression and the onset of flaccid facial paralysis. Factors responsible for the inflammatory reaction include infection, prolonged exposure to cold temperature and local trauma. The seventh cranial nerve can also be affected by other conditions such as a cerebral tumour, meningitis or a middle-ear infection. Manifestations are unilateral facial weakness, which is sometimes associated with pain around the angle of the jaw or behind the ear. On the affected side, the mouth droops and the individual is unable to wrinkle the forehead, close the eyelid or smile. There may be excessive watering from the affected eye and drooling of saliva from the affected side of the mouth (Brown et al 2020; National Institute of Neurological Disorders and Stroke 2023a).

Seizure disorders

Seizure disorders may be primary and idiopathic, or secondary and symptomatic of a CNS disorder. The most common type of seizure disorder is epilepsy. Seizures may be focal (partial) or generalised. Focal seizures generally affect a specific body part, and the symptoms of an attack depend on the location of the cerebral focus. For example, the focal motor seizure occurs from a lesion in the motor cortex. Typically, it causes stiffening or jerking in one extremity that is accompanied by numbness or tingling.

Absence seizures only last a few seconds. They generally begin with a brief change in the level of consciousness, which is indicated by a blank stare, eyelid fluttering or head nodding or a pause in conversation. The individual generally retains posture and returns to pre-seizure activity without difficulty. This type of epilepsy usually occurs in childhood and may continue into early adolescence. Some partial seizures may progress to become *generalised seizures*. These are termed 'secondary generalised seizures' (Epilepsy Action Australia 2023).

Although seizures may result from a nervous system disorder, they may be caused by many other factors and are often idiopathic. The common classification of seizures is given in Table 35.3.

The most common generalised seizure is referred to as a tonic–clonic. This type of seizure usually consists of three phases:

1. Aura, which is not always experienced, is a warning of an impending seizure. It is a premonition or sensation (e.g. a specific taste or smell) peculiar to an individual, which may be experienced by the individual immediately before a seizure. The seizure commonly begins with a loud cry, which is caused by air being forced out through the vocal cords that are in spasm.
2. Tonic–clonic phase: The individual then loses consciousness and may fall. The muscles become rigid, then alternate between episodes of muscle spasm and relaxation (tonus and clonus), resulting in jerky spasmodic body movements. Tongue biting, incontinence of urine, laboured breathing, apnoea and cyanosis may occur.
3. Post-convulsive phase: The seizure generally stops within 2–5 minutes, when abnormal electrical conduction in the brain ceases. The individual regains consciousness but may be dazed and confused or fall asleep. Automatisms are more commonly associated with complex partial seizures.

Status epilepticus, a rapid succession of seizures, is a condition in which the individual experiences continuous seizures without regaining consciousness in-between. It is generally accompanied by respiratory distress.

Table 35.4 provides an assessment and rationale for a nursing assessment before, during and after a seizure (LeMone et al 2020). Clinical Interest Box 35.2 provides an outline of teaching for home care of individuals in relation to seizures (Berman et al 2021; Epilepsy Action Australia 2023; Hall et al 2022; LeMone et al 2020).

TABLE 35.3 | Common classification of seizures

Classification	Description
Focal (partial) seizures	About 60% of people with epilepsy have focal (partial) seizures. These seizures can often be subtle or unusual and may go unnoticed or be mistaken for anything from intoxication to daydreaming. Seizure activity starts in one area of the brain and may spread to other regions of the brain. Types of focal (partial) seizures are: • Focal seizure—awareness retained (formerly simple partial seizures) • Focal dyscognitive seizures—awareness altered (formerly complex partial seizures) • Focal seizures evolving to a bilateral convulsive seizure (formerly secondarily generalised tonic–clonic*).
Generalised seizures	Generalised seizures are the result of abnormal activity in both hemispheres of the brain simultaneously. Because of this, consciousness is lost at the onset of the seizure. There are many types of generalised seizures: • absence > typical > atypical absence > absence with special features – myoclonic absence – eyelid myoclonia • tonic–clonic • clonic • tonic • atonic • myoclonic > myoclonic atonic > myoclonic tonic.
Unknown	This a grouping of seizures that cannot be diagnosed as either focal or generalised seizures and are thus grouped as unknown: • epileptic spasm • other.

(Berman et al 2021; Epilepsy Action Australia 2023; LeMone et al 2020)

***Note:** Sometimes a seizure starts as a focal (partial) seizure and then becomes a generalised seizure—almost always a tonic–clonic seizure.*

Most people will only have one or two seizure type(s), which may vary in severity. A person with severe epilepsy or significant damage to the brain may experience several different seizure types.

TABLE 35.4 | Nursing assessments before, during and after a seizure

Assessment	Rationale
What was the individual's level of consciousness? If consciousness was lost, at what point?	Indicates area of brain involved and type of seizure.
What was the individual doing just before the attack?	May suggest precipitating factors.
In what part of the body did the seizure start?	May indicate the site of seizure activity in the brain tissue (e.g. if jerking movements were first observed in right hand, the seizure focus may be in left motor cortex).
Was there an epileptic cry?	Usually indicates the tonic stage of a generalised tonic–clonic seizure.
Were any automatisms such as eyelid fluttering, chewing, lip smacking or swallowing observed?	Often seen in complex, partial and absence seizures.
How long did movements last? Did the location or character change (tonic to clonic)? Did movements involve both sides of the body or just one?	Indicates areas in which focal activity originated.
Did the head and/or eyes turn to one side and, if so, which side?	Helps localise the focus of the seizure. During the seizure, the head and eyes typically will turn away from the side of the epileptogenic focus.
Were there changes in pupillary reactions?	Indicates involvement of the autonomic nervous system.
If the individual fell, was the head hit?	Skull X-ray studies may be needed to rule out subdural haematoma or fracture.
Was there foaming or frothing from the mouth?	Usually indicates a tonic–clonic seizure.

(LeMone et al 2020)

CLINICAL INTEREST BOX 35.2 Health education for home care of individuals affected by generalised seizures

Teaching must be planned around a systematic assessment of the needs of both the individual and their significant others. Significant others need to be included so that they can learn seizure management, care and observations. The importance of safety and maintenance of a patent airway should be stressed. The following recommendations assist the individual and significant others to adjust:

- Correct misconceptions, fears and myths about epilepsy.
- Encourage both the individual and their significant others to express their feelings.
- Provide the name and location of community and national resources (e.g. Epilepsy Australia (http://www.epilepsyaustralia.net)). Facilitate socialisation with others facing the same issues.
- Stress the importance of follow-up care and keeping medical appointments.
- Refer the individual to employment or vocational counselling as needed.
- Review any state and local laws that apply to people with seizure disorders. Usually, a driver's licence can be reinstated after a 2-year seizure-free period and a letter from a medical officer.
- Stress the importance of wearing a medical alert bracelet and always carrying a medical alert card.
- Emphasise the importance of aura identification and plan action to take.
- Emphasise the importance of taking anticonvulsant medication as prescribed, even when seizures no longer occur.
- Avoid physical and emotional stress.
- Help individuals develop a positive focus on life.
- In general, alcohol should be avoided, and caffeine limited.
- Discuss factors that may trigger a seizure (fatigue, abrupt stopping of medication, flashing video games).

(LeMone et al 2020; NSQHS Standard consideration: 'Partnering with Consumers' [action 2.03, 2.04, 2.05, 2.06, 2.07, 2.08, 2.09 & 2.10]; NSQHS Standard consideration: 'Comprehensive Care' [action 5.03])

CRITICAL THINKING EXERCISE 35.2

Maddie, 16 years old, had a seizure. What immediate symptoms would you expect Maddie to exhibit?

Degenerative disorders

Parkinson's disease

Parkinson's disease is a degenerative process of nerve cells in the basal nuclei and substantia nigra. The substantia nigra is an area in the basal nuclei considered necessary for motor control. Although the precise cause of the disorder is unknown, research has demonstrated that a dopamine deficiency prevents affected brain cells from functioning normally. Dopamine is a neurotransmitter that plays a role in the transmission of nerve impulses between synapses. Factors implicated in the development of Parkinson's disease include cerebral atherosclerosis and long-term therapy with drugs such as haloperidol and phenothiazine (LeMone et al 2020; Marieb & Keller 2021; Patton & Thibodeau 2019). Manifestations of Parkinson's disease are related to disturbances of movement: tremor, muscle rigidity and dyskinesia. The most common initial symptom is tremor (e.g. 'pill-rolling' movements of the fingers, and to-and-fro head tremors). Tremors are aggravated by fatigue and stress and decrease when the individual performs a purposeful activity or is asleep. The person experiences difficulty in initiating voluntary movement and loss of posture control, so that walking is with the body bent forwards. The gait consists of short shuffling steps that are slowly initiated. Facial expression becomes mask-like, and the voice is commonly high-pitched and monotone. The person's intelligence is not affected.

Amyotrophic lateral sclerosis

Amyotrophic lateral sclerosis, which is the most common form of motor neurone disease (MND), is a progressive degenerative condition that is generally fatal within 3–10 years after onset. The disease affects the upper and lower motor neurons of the CNS, resulting in progressive muscular atrophy, progressive bulbar palsy, and upper motor neuron deficits. While the cause is unknown, the disease is thought to result from viral, metabolic, toxic, infectious and immunological factors. Manifestations include skeletal muscle weakness and atrophy and impaired speech, chewing, swallowing and breathing. The cause of death is commonly respiratory muscle weakness and bulbar palsy causing respiratory failure (LeMone et al 2020; MND Australia 2024a; MND Australia 2024b).

Alzheimer's disease

Alzheimer's disease is a progressive degenerative disorder that causes cerebral atrophy and dementia. Although the precise cause is unknown, several theories propose that the disorder may result from a genetic factor, immunological dysfunction, a toxin or a virus. People with Alzheimer's disease have low levels of acetylcholine in their brain, which is an important neurotransmitter for memory.

Alzheimer's disease, which affects an estimated 343,000 Australians, is characterised by memory loss and the eventual inability to self-care. Some medications to alleviate the symptoms have been developed, but presently there is no known treatment for the disease (Dementia Australia 2022a & b).

Manifestations of the disease generally occur in three stages:

1. Memory loss, decline in judgment and logic, disorientation, global aphasia, irritability, mood swings and agitation. Aphasia is a communication disorder due to brain damage. It is characterised by partial or complete disturbance of language comprehension, expression or formulation.
2. Neglect of hygiene, inability to carry out deliberate voluntary movements (**apraxia**), inability to recognise the nature or use of objects (agnosia), repetition of a motor or verbal action (perseveration) and seizures.
3. Marked dementia, unresponsiveness, aphasia and apraxia.

Delirium is a common mental disorder affecting older adults. The acute condition is often misdiagnosed as a form of dementia and the underlying cause is therefore missed. The characteristics of delirium are listed in Clinical Interest Box 35.3. A history of the individual's behaviour before delirium developed is essential in early recognition of the condition (LeMone et al 2020).

Immunological disorders

Multiple sclerosis (MS)

Multiple sclerosis (MS) is a disorder characterised by progressive demyelination of nerve fibres in the spinal cord and brain. Patches of demyelination throughout the CNS result in varied neurological dysfunction. The cause is unknown, but the disease is thought to result from viral or immunological factors. Manifestations vary depending on the areas of the CNS that are affected. Some individuals experience mild exacerbations, with long remission periods, while others have frequent relapses, with increasing residual deficits. The most common initial symptoms are fatigue, motor weakness and visual disturbances. Other characteristic changes include numbness and tingling sensations, intention tremor, gait ataxia, paralysis, urinary disturbances and emotional lability. Clinical Interest Box 35.4 provides a teaching plan for the individual as well as their significant others (Brown et al 2020; MS Australia 2023; Patton & Thibodeau 2019).

Myasthenia gravis

Myasthenia gravis is a chronic neuromuscular disorder that affects voluntary muscles and is characterised by fluctuating muscle weakness that is exacerbated by exercise. The disease is considered to be autoimmune in origin, resulting in an acetylcholine-receptor deficiency. The thymus gland is also thought to be involved in the disease because the gland is abnormal and remains active after puberty in individuals with myasthenia gravis.

CLINICAL INTEREST BOX 35.3 Clinical criteria for delirium

Delirium is an acute disturbance of consciousness that is accompanied by a change in cognition. It cannot be accounted for by a pre-existing or evolving dementia. Delirium develops over a short period of time, usually hours to days, and tends to fluctuate during the day. It is usually a direct physiological consequence of a general medical condition:

- There is reduced clarity of awareness of the environment.
- Ability to focus, sustain or shift attention is impaired.
- Person is easily distracted by irrelevant stimuli.
- There is an accompanying change in cognition (memory impairment, disorientation or language disturbance).
- Recent memory is most commonly affected.
- Disorientation is usually shown, with a person disoriented to time or place.
- Language disturbance may involve impaired ability to name objects or ability to write; speech may be rambling.
- Perceptual disturbances may include misinterpretations, illusions or hallucinations.

(Crisp et al 2021; NSQHS Standard consideration NSQHS Standards user guide for health service organisations providing care for patients with cognitive impairment or at risk of delirium; Australian Commission on Safety and Quality in Health Care 2021 'Comprehensive Care' [action 5.27 & 5.28])

CLINICAL INTEREST BOX 35.4 Health education checklist—the individual with multiple sclerosis

In formulating a teaching plan, it is important that the individual's significant others are included. The following aspects may be considered:

- Facilitate access to the Multiple Sclerosis Society of Australia (www.msaustralia.org.au).
- Ensure that the individual understands the clinical course of multiple sclerosis. Dispel any myths.
- Identify strategies to manage symptoms such as dysphagia or altered cognitive responses.
- Plan strategies for preventing complications such as pressure ulcers or depression.
- Identify coping strategies.
- Identify strategies for minimising fatigue.
- Explain how to prevent injury.
- Discuss ways to adapt to sexual dysfunction.
- Develop strategies to control bowel and bladder function.
- Explain benefits of continued physical activity and exercise.
- Identify ways to minimise immobility and spasticity.
- Describe the medication regimen and possible adverse effects.

(NSQHS Standard consideration: 'Partnering with Consumers' [action 2.03, 2.04, 2.05, 2.06, 2.07, 2.08, 2.09 & 2.10]; NSQHS Standard consideration: 'Comprehensive Care [action 5.07, 5.08, 5.09])

Manifestations include progressive weakness of certain voluntary muscles, with some improvement in muscle function after rest. The eye muscles are most commonly affected, with drooping of the eyelids (ptosis) and double vision (diplopia). Other affected muscles include those involved with facial expression, speech, chewing and swallowing. The individual may experience problems with saliva, nasal regurgitation and choking. The shoulder and neck muscles may be affected so that the head tends to fall forwards. Weakened respiratory muscles make breathing difficult and predispose the person to respiratory tract infections (LeMone et al 2020; National Institute of Neurological Disorders and Stroke 2023e).

Infectious and inflammatory conditions

Meningitis

Meningitis is inflammation of the meninges and can be caused by viruses, bacteria or fungi. The inflammation may involve one or all three layers of the meninges. Meningitis often begins when the causative organism enters the subarachnoid space, then the infection spreads because of the open communication over the brain's convexity. The accumulation of exudate from the inflammatory process over the convexities or in the ventricles can obstruct the flow of CSF. Aseptic meningitis is thought to occur from meningeal irritation resulting from encephalitis, leukaemia, lymphoma or the presence of blood in the subarachnoid space. The major manifestations of meningitis are severe headaches, pyrexia, irritability, neck rigidity, photophobia and pain in the back and limbs. Other manifestations are alterations in mental status, altered levels of consciousness and restlessness. Vomiting may occur, and cranial nerve involvement causes visual disturbances, pupil abnormalities, strabismus and vertigo. There may be generalised seizures due to cerebral oedema (LeMone et al 2020; Patton et al 2019; Healthdirect Meningitis 2023).

Encephalitis

Encephalitis is inflammation of the brain tissue caused by viruses, bacteria, fungi or protozoans. Endemic encephalitis begins in a non-human host or reservoir from which the virus is transmitted to humans (e.g. through mosquito bites). After the pathogen gains access to the CNS via the bloodstream or along nerves, the white matter and meninges develop non-suppurative inflammation, and diffuse cerebral oedema results. Initial manifestations are headaches, pyrexia, vomiting, malaise and muscular aches and pains. These are often followed by alterations in the level of consciousness, confusion, motor and sensory deficits, hyperirritability and meningeal signs (LeMone et al 2020; National Institute of Neurological Disorders and Stroke 2023f).

Brain abscess

A brain abscess is a collection of pus, usually occurring in the temporal lobes or the cerebellum. A brain abscess is accompanied by cerebral oedema and congestion. Most brain abscesses develop secondary to a primary source of infection such as mastoiditis or otitis media, or they may develop from a septic focus in the respiratory tract or, less often, from a pelvic or cardiac source. A small percentage result from a penetrating head wound such as a gunshot injury.

Manifestations include headache, pyrexia, vomiting, alterations in the level of consciousness and local or generalised seizures. Other features differ according to the site of the abscess and include motor, sensory and speech disturbances (Brown et al 2020; LeMone et al 2020).

Myelitis

Myelitis is the term that applies to a group of infective and non-infective processes that affect the spinal cord. Myelitis can be due to viruses, occur secondary to meningeal inflammation or be of unknown aetiology. The most common viral diseases causing myelitis are poliomyelitis and herpes zoster. Manifestations include a sudden onset of motor paresis, accompanied by other neurological deficits such as loss of sensory and sphincter functions (National Institute of Neurological Disorders and Stroke 2023f).

Herpes zoster

Herpes zoster is a viral disorder that causes inflammation of the posterior root ganglia. The condition develops from reactivation of the varicella virus, the virus responsible for chickenpox. There is also evidence of a relationship between herpes zoster and certain systemic infections, neoplasms and immunosuppressive therapy. Manifestations include mild to severe neuralgic pain in the affected nerve root distribution. The pain, which may be burning, tingling, dull or sharp, may occur with or be followed by skin reddening and eruption of vesicles. The vesicles become pustules and develop a crust within 1–2 weeks. If infection or ulceration accompanies the vesicles, permanent scarring may result.

Occasionally, herpes zoster involves the cranial nerves, especially the trigeminal or oculomotor nerve. Trigeminal involvement causes eye pain and, possibly, corneal damage and impaired vision. Oculomotor involvement may result in conjunctivitis or ptosis. Rarely, herpes zoster leads to generalised CNS infection. Post-herpetic neuralgia can persist for months or years, and the skin may remain hypersensitive to touch (LeMone et al 2020).

Poliomyelitis

Poliomyelitis is an acute infectious disease caused by one of the three poliomyelitis viruses, which generally enter the body through the mouth or nose, multiply in the bloodstream and travel to the CNS. The viruses are then spread along neural pathways and destroy cells in the anterior horns of the spinal cord. The brainstem may also be damaged. The incidence of acute anterior poliomyelitis has decreased dramatically in the Western world since the introduction of vaccination in 1955.

The virus may cause only a minor illness, or there may be signs and symptoms of viral meningitis and paralysis. The extent of paralysis depends on the location of the affected neurons. The initial manifestations of paralytic poliomyelitis include pyrexia, headaches, vomiting, irritability and pains in the neck, back, arms and legs. About 5–7 days after onset, the individual experiences weakness of various muscles, paraesthesia, hypersensitivity to touch and resistance to neck flexion. If the disease affects the brainstem, the muscles involved in swallowing, chewing and ventilation are also affected (LeMone et al 2020).

Neoplastic and obstructive disorders

Tumours of the nervous system may be benign or malignant, and primary or metastatic. Tumours may arise in the brain tissue, the meninges, the skull, in the peripheral and cranial nerves or in the spinal cord. Brain tissue (cerebral) tumours include astrocytomas and glioblastomas. Meningiomas usually arise from the arachnoid layer of the meninges and do not invade the brain. Skull tumours, which are rare, may be either osteomas (benign) or sarcomas (malignant). Peripheral and cranial nerve tumours include acoustic neuromas, schwannomas and neuroblastomas. Spinal cord tumours may be either extradural or intradural.

Manifestations of nervous system tumours are related to invasion or compression of surrounding neural structures. Brain tumours may produce symptoms as a consequence of increased ICP (e.g. from cerebral oedema). The neurological manifestations of a brain tumour depend on the location of the tumour and its rate of growth. The clinical features associated with a brain tumour include headaches, vomiting, papilloedema (swelling of the optic disc and distension of the retinal vessels), personality or behavioural changes, seizures, visual or hearing defects, dizziness, ataxia and hemiparesis. Manifestations of spinal cord tumours are related to spinal cord compression and include pain, paraplegia (paralysis of the lower extremities and lower trunk) or quadriplegia (paralysis in which all four limbs are affected, also known as tetraplegia), which may be slowly progressive or acute (Brown et al 2020; LeMone et al 2020). All parts below the point of lesion in the spinal cord are affected.

Traumatic disorders

Despite being well protected by bone, meninges and CSF, the brain and spinal cord are frequently injured. Serious cerebral or spinal cord damage can result from a variety of factors such as motor vehicle accidents, sports accidents and penetrating injuries, such as gunshot wounds. Acquired brain injury (ABI) or cerebral injury may be classified as concussion, contusion, laceration, haematomas, and tentorial herniation. Traumatic brain injury (TBI) is a type of acquired brain injury caused by a blow to the head or contrecoup injury, usually with some loss of consciousness. As a result, the brain may be torn, stretched, penetrated, bruised or become swollen (Brain Injury Australia 2016; LeMone et al 2020). (See Case Study 35.1.)

Concussion

Concussion results from a blow to the head and is characterised by a loss of consciousness for less than 5 minutes and memory loss of events preceding and following the injury. Other features include headaches, confusion, dizziness, visual disturbances, vomiting and irritability (LeMone et al 2020; Marieb & Keller 2021).

Contusion

Contusion is bruising of the brain that disrupts normal nerve function in the bruised area and which may be associated with haemorrhage or oedema. Manifestations include drowsiness, confusion, behavioural changes, loss of consciousness, hemiparesis, unequal pupil response and decorticate or decerebrate posturing. With **decorticate** posturing, the individual demonstrates hyperflexion of the upper extremities and hyperextension of the lower extremities. The upper extremities are rigidly flexed at the elbows and at the wrists. The legs also may be flexed (Figure 35.9A). With **decerebrate** posturing, both the upper and the lower extremities are hyperextended (Figure 35.9B). Decerebrate neurological reactions are severely impaired and occur in those individuals in whom cerebral functioning has ceased (Curtis al 2019).

The Westmead Post-Traumatic Amnesia Scale (WPTAS) is used to measure the period of post-traumatic amnesia following a closed head injury caused by either oedema or haemorrhage. The scale consists of seven orientation questions and five memory items that are designed to objectively measure the period of post-traumatic amnesia (PTA). An individual is said to be out of PTA if a perfect score is obtained for all questions 3 days in a row. Once the duration of PTA is determined, the severity of injury can be classified according to the time the individual was in PTA (Department of Psychology, Macquarie University nd; Scope 2015).

CASE STUDY 35.1

John, a 22-year-old construction worker, presented to emergency after falling 3 metres, hitting his head on the concrete below

1. As the Enrolled Nurse in the emergency department, what would you assess for first and which tool would you use?
2. What is the minimum score possible on the Glasgow Coma Scale?
3. What is the maximum score possible on the Glasgow Coma Scale?
4. How specifically will you ask the questions to establish a Glasgow Coma Scale score for John?
5. What scan may be ordered to determine if there has been any trauma to the head and spine?
6. What clinical risks does John present?
7. What may clear or blood-stained fluid leaking from nose or ears indicate?
8. What are other signs and symptoms of CSF leak?

Laceration

Laceration is tearing of the brain tissue, followed by intracerebral bleeding. Manifestations include prolonged unconsciousness, immediate neurological deficits and deterioration of the individual's condition (LeMone et al 2020).

Haematomas

Haematomas are collections of coagulated blood and, in the brain, may be epidural, subdural or intracerebral. An epidural haematoma results from haemorrhage in the epidural space between the skull and the dura mater. A subdural haematoma results from an accumulation of blood in the subdural space, between the arachnoid and dura mater. An intracerebral haematoma is a collection of blood within the brain tissue.

Manifestations of cerebral haematomas vary according to the location and whether the haematoma develops rapidly or slowly. Typically, an epidural haematoma causes immediate loss of consciousness, followed by a lucid interval that eventually gives way to a rapidly progressive decrease in the level of consciousness. Accompanying features include hemiparesis, severe headaches, unilateral pupil dilation and signs of increased ICP (decreasing pulse and ventilation rate, increasing systolic blood pressure). Manifestations of a subdural haematoma may not occur until days after the injury. Common features include headaches, drowsiness, confusion, slow responses and seizures. Pupillary changes and motor deficits commonly occur. Manifestations of intracerebral haematoma include neck rigidity, photophobia, nausea and vomiting, dizziness, decreased ventilation rate and seizures (LeMone at al 2020).

CRITICAL THINKING EXERCISE 35.3

Alex, 21 years old, presented to emergency complaining of a severe headache and stiff neck. On examination, you notice he is febrile, has a rash on his torso and a dislike of bright lights. He is diagnosed with meningitis. What are common symptoms of meningitis in older children and adults?

> **CRITICAL THINKING EXERCISE 35.4**
>
> Hypertension is a precursor to stroke. Explain whether this statement is true or false.

Cerebral herniation

Increased pressure in the cranial cavity can cause damage to the brain through hypoxia, ischaemia and infarction. Unrelieved or untreated raised pressure results in cerebral herniation. When pressure builds up in one area of the brain, brain tissue will begin to move into an area of lower pressure.

Tentorial herniation occurs when part of the temporal lobe herniates through the tentorial hiatus. Typical signs of this form of herniation are pupil dilation and hemiplegia.

Tonsillar herniation or 'coning' occurs when part of the cerebellum and/or brainstem herniates through the foramen magnum. Typical signs of this type of herniation are neck rigidity, dysfunction of the cardiac and respiratory drive and abnormal posturing. Irreversible brain damage and death can occur rapidly (LeMone et al 2020).

Spinal cord damage

Spinal cord damage may occur from traumatic injuries as a result of motor vehicle or sports accidents, gunshot or stab wounds or falls from high places. Fractures and dislocations can occur anywhere along the spinal column and, if the spinal cord is injured, may result in temporary or permanent damage (LeMone et al 2020).

Peripheral nerve damage

Peripheral nerve damage can result from pressure, compression, constriction or traction on a nerve, or as a consequence of skeletal fractures, lacerations or penetrating wounds. Nerve damage can also result from an injection of a toxic or metabolic substance into the nerve. The peripheral nerves most commonly injured are the radial, axillary and ulnar nerves and the brachial plexus. Manifestations include loss of motor function, loss of sensation and muscle atrophy. Depending on which nerve is damaged, there may be foot drop, wrist drop, limited range of motion or paralysis (Marieb & Keller 2021).

CARE OF THE INDIVIDUAL WITH A NERVOUS SYSTEM DISORDER

Although specific nursing actions and medical management vary depending on the particular nervous system disorder, the main aims of care are as follows:

- Promote a clear airway.
- Maintain fluid and nutritional status.
- Prevent and manage alterations in elimination.
- Promote effective communication.
- Promote safety.
- Promote mobility.
- Prevent complications of immobility.

> **CRITICAL THINKING EXERCISE 35.5**
>
> A person who has suffered a small stroke in the right hemisphere is referred to the speech pathologist, occupational therapist and dietitian. Give a rationale for each referral.

- Provide psychological support.
- Assess neurological status.
- Provide a suitable environment.
- Provide pre- and post-diagnostic test care.
- Promote rehabilitation and independence.

Each individual presents specific nursing problems for which an individualised nursing care plan must be developed, implemented and evaluated (LeMone et al 2020).

Promoting a clear airway

Disorders of the nervous system may affect the individual's ability to breathe normally, to cough effectively or to prevent the tongue from obstructing the airway. Altered levels of consciousness, decreased motor function or disrupted cranial nerve function may impair the individual's ability to maintain a clear airway. To ensure a patent airway, the individual's nose, mouth and respiratory tract must be clear, allowing adequate oxygen and carbon dioxide exchange.

With a conscious individual:

- The individual should be assisted into a position that will promote effective breathing. A sitting or upright position provides better lung expansion, which improves breathing and lessens the risk of respiratory tract infection.
- The individual is instructed to take deep breaths hourly and to cough and expectorate mucus frequently. Chest physiotherapy (e.g. percussion) may be necessary to help mobilise secretions.
- If the individual's ability to chew and swallow is impaired, care must be taken when food, fluids or oral medications are being consumed.
- Suction equipment should be readily available if the individual is at risk of choking or unable to expectorate secretions effectively.
- Active or passive range-of-motion (ROM) exercises and 2–4-hourly position changes help to mobilise respiratory tract secretions.
- An adequate fluid input is provided to keep respiratory tract secretions moist.

With an unconscious individual:

- The individual should be nursed in a lateral recumbent position to promote drainage of secretions and to prevent the tongue from obstructing the airway. Positioning on alternate sides 2-hourly should be carried out to prevent pooling of secretions in the lungs.
- Oronasopharyngeal suction should be performed to keep the upper airway free of accumulated secretions. Mouth and nasal care should be performed 2–4-hourly for the same purpose (information on oronasopharyngeal suctioning is provided in Chapter 25).

- Chest percussion and postural drainage may be prescribed to help remove retained secretions, particularly if the cough reflex is impaired.
- The individual may require mechanical assistance for adequate ventilation. A tracheostomy or endotracheal tube may be inserted, and mechanical ventilation provided (information on tracheostomy care and mechanical ventilation is provided in Chapter 25).
- Eye care is essential for the unconscious individual. If the individual's corneal reflex is absent, keep the eyes moist with artificial tears and protect the eye with a protective shield. These should be ordered by a medical officer (LeMone et al 2020).

Maintaining nutritional and fluid status

An individual with a neurological disorder may have deficits that interfere with an adequate intake of food and fluid, such as:

- altered level of consciousness
- altered mental status
- diminished or absent swallowing or gag reflex
- inability to feed themself; for example, if there is paralysis of the arm(s)
- fear of choking
- paralysis of the muscles of mastication and/or the tongue
- loss of appetite due to altered sensory function (e.g. sight, smell, taste).

Information on assisting the individual to meet nutritional and fluid needs is provided in Chapter 26 and Chapter 30. Specific nursing activities to assist the individual with a nervous system disorder include:

- Providing appropriate devices to facilitate the cutting and eating of food.
- Ensuring that suction equipment is readily available should it be needed (e.g. if the individual's swallowing or gag reflexes are impaired).
- Assisting the individual who is unable to feed themselves.
- Placing the food into the unaffected side of the mouth if the individual has any facial weakness. If able to feed themself, the individual should be advised to feed in this manner.
- Preparing food for the individual who has motor deficits (e.g. cutting meat, spreading butter, pouring fluids).
- Redirecting the individual's attention to eating if they become distracted or are unable to concentrate at mealtimes.
- Assisting with the care of the individual who is being provided with nutrition and fluids by alternative methods (e.g. tube feeding or total parenteral nutrition).
- Keeping a record of fluid input and output if the individual has difficulty in feeding themselves or swallowing, or if they are receiving dehydrating medications or intravenous solutions to reduce or prevent increased ICP.

(LeMone et al 2020)

Preventing and managing alterations in elimination

Many disorders affecting the nervous system can result in constipation, retention of urine or incontinence. Factors that contribute to altered patterns of elimination include loss of sphincter control, diminished awareness of the need to empty the bladder or bowel, altered levels of consciousness and impaired mental status, with resulting incontinence (Hall et al 2022; LeMone et al 2020). (Information on the prevention and management of constipation, retention of urine and incontinence is provided in Chapter 31 and Chapter 32.)

Promoting effective communication

Disorders of the nervous system may affect the ability of individuals to express themselves verbally or non-verbally, and the ability to understand the spoken or written word. (General information on communication can be found in Chapter 10.) The ability to communicate may be impaired by factors that include:

- damage to the speech centres in the brain
- damage to the temporal lobes, which hinders the perception and interpretation of stimuli
- damage to the cranial nerves responsible for movement of the lips, tongue, pharynx and larynx
- limited motor function that hinders non-verbal communication actions (e.g. facial expressions and gestures)
- visual or hearing deficits
- altered levels of consciousness or mental status.

The two major terms used to describe communication deficits are **dysphasia** (difficulty in speaking and communicating as a result of inability to coordinate and arrange words in their correct order) and **aphasia** (loss of the ability to communicate) (Berman et al 2021; Brown et al 2020; Hall et al 2022).

Aphasia

Aphasia is subdivided into three major classifications:

1. Expressive aphasia (Broca's aphasia): Inability to express oneself verbally or in writing. The degree of difficulty can range from mild hesitancy in flow of speech to limitation of expression to 'yes' and 'no'. The ability to understand the spoken and written word remains intact.
2. Receptive aphasia (Wernicke's aphasia): Inability to understand the spoken word. Although the individual hears the sounds of speech, comprehension of speech is impaired. The individual can speak but makes many errors when using words and is often unaware of the imperfect messages. The ability to comprehend the written word is also impaired.

3. Global aphasia: A combination of both expressive and receptive aphasia. The individual neither understands what they hear or read, nor can they convey their thoughts in speech or writing.

The loss or impairment of the ability to communicate is devastating and frustrating to the individual and to their significant others, often resulting in fear and depression. Although the speech therapist will be the key person in the treatment of an individual with a communication problem, the nurse must be aware of prescribed therapy so that it can be continued when the speech therapist is not with the individual. The nurse should assume a calm, reassuring and supportive manner that conveys a sense of acceptance of the individual's behaviour. Table 35.5 provides guidelines that can be used when working with an individual with aphasia.

Communication with the unconscious individual is very important because, although the individual appears to be completely unaware of their environment, it is impossible to determine their awareness of any stimulus. Many individuals have recovered from unconsciousness and given accurate details of events or conversations that took place in their presence while they were unconscious. Therefore, the nurse should assume that some stimuli will penetrate the complexities of unconsciousness. Stimuli can be provided by talking to the individual, by touch and by playing a radio or CDs. The individual should be told what the nurse will be doing—orient the individual to time, place and person and describe the surroundings. Coma arousal is a technique whereby the unconscious individual is continuously exposed to a variety of stimuli, such as sounds, touch and smells in an attempt to increase the level of consciousness (Berman et al 2021; Crisp et al 2021; LeMone et al 2020).

Promoting safety

The individual with a nervous system disorder is often susceptible to injury because of factors such as impaired consciousness or awareness, reduced mobility, impaired motor and sensory functions and reflexes. The individual is most at risk of skin breakdown, physical injuries or infection.

Maintaining skin integrity

The nurse should assess the individual for potential skin problems and implement nursing measures in accordance with the National Safety and Quality Health Service Standard 'Comprehensive Care'. This standard describes the systems and strategies that prevent individuals from developing pressure injuries and the best practice management if a pressure injury occurs (ACSQHC 2021a). Nursing measures to prevent skin breakdown from pressure, extremes of temperature and physical trauma are as follows:

- The skin is kept clean and dry to prevent irritation and possible breakdown. Very dry skin should be lubricated with a suitable oil or cream to prevent cracking and breakdown.
- A protective cream or lotion may be applied to the genital area and buttocks if the individual is incontinent. Wet or soiled linen must be replaced immediately.
- The individual's position is changed every 2–4 hours to protect the skin from irritation and prolonged pressure. Pressure-relieving aids may be used.

TABLE 35.5 | Assisting the aphasic individual

Expressive aphasia	Receptive aphasia
Stimulate conversation and ask open-ended questions.	Speak slowly and distinctly, using a common vocabulary and simple sentences.
Allow the individual time to find the words to express themselves.	Stand within the individual's line of vision, so that lip movements can be observed.
Be supportive and accepting as the individual deals with the frustration of finding the right words.	Use simple gestures as an added cue.
Accept self-expression (e.g. pointing or gestures).	Repeat or rephrase any instructions if they are not understood.
Provide charts or books with pictures of common objects so that the individual can point when they cannot say the word.	Speak in a normal voice.
Reassure the individual that speech skills can be relearned, given time.	Divide any tasks into small units, working with the individual to accomplish the task.
Give praise for achievements and progress.	Use pointing and touch to express ideas. Eliminate background distractions.

(Brown et al 2020)

- The skin is assessed every 2 hours for colour, temperature, dryness and the signs of impaired circulation. Any signs of skin breakdown are reported immediately so that appropriate actions can be implemented to prevent further deterioration.
- Precautions must be taken to avoid injury to the skin by hot, cold, sharp or rough objects. The individual is always moved correctly and gently to avoid damage to the skin.

(Berman et al 2021)

Preventing physical injuries

An individual who has impaired motor, sensory or intellectual function must be protected from accidents and injuries in accordance with the National Safety and Quality Health Service Standard 'Comprehensive Care'. This standard describes the methods and strategies to reduce the incidence of individual falls and the best practice management if a fall should occur (ACSQHC 2021a). Protective strategies include:

- maintaining the bed in a low position when not providing direct care at the bedside
- using alarms that are triggered when the individual attempts unsafe activities (e.g. standing from chair unaccompanied)
- accompanying the individual when ambulating if they are unsteady or disoriented
- providing walking aids and handrails as a means of support and to promote greater safety
- providing an uncluttered environment and adequate lighting
- placing the individual's requirements, including the call bell, within reach
- supervising individuals who are at risk of falling while performing the activities of daily living.

Preventing infection

An individual with a nervous system disorder that impairs mobility, motor function or level of consciousness is prone to infection. When a person is ill, the body's natural defence mechanisms are stressed and therefore less able than usual to resist the invasion of pathogenic microorganisms. The two most common types of infection that may occur are urinary tract infection due to urinary stasis or catheterisation, and respiratory tract infection resulting from inadequate lung expansion, pooling of secretions in the lungs, the presence of an artificial airway or mechanical ventilation.

The National Safety and Quality Health Service Standard 'Preventing and Controlling Infections' describes the systems and strategies to prevent individuals within the healthcare system acquiring infections such as a urinary tract infection (ACSQHC 2021a). Strategies to prevent a urinary tract infection include ensuring that:

- The individual receives an adequate fluid input.
- Whenever possible, an external urinary drainage device or intermittent catheterisation is used rather than an indwelling catheter.
- If an indwelling catheter is unavoidable, measures to prevent cross-infection are implemented. These measures include maintaining a sterile closed drainage system, performing meatal and perineal care, maintaining dependent drainage, maintaining strict aseptic care and using correct handwashing technique, which is the most effective way of preventing cross-infection. (Further information on maintaining an indwelling catheter is provided in Chapter 31.)

Measures to prevent a respiratory tract infection include ensuring that:

- When possible, the individual is nursed in a sitting or upright position to promote maximal lung expansion.
- The individual performs 4-hourly deep breathing and coughing exercises.
- If necessary, suction is used to remove oral and nasopharyngeal secretions.
- Aseptic techniques are implemented when caring for an artificial airway.

Promoting mobility and preventing the complications of immobility

Many nervous system disorders impair physical mobility through motor deficits, cerebellar dysfunction, alterations in sensory perception and changes in conscious or mental status. Prolonged lack of physical exercise and movement can lead to many complications, including pulmonary stasis, urinary stasis, venous stasis, decubitus ulcers, constipation and contractures. Impaired mobility varies from reductions in range of motion, or unsteady gait, to total immobility. Maintaining muscle tone and preventing orthopaedic disabilities are of prime importance when caring for an individual with impaired mobility. To prevent functional loss:

- Active or passive range-of-motion exercises should be performed every 4 hours.
- The individual should be repositioned every 2 hours to maintain correct body alignment. Weak or paralysed body parts must be carefully positioned to prevent deformity. Limb splints are often used to maintain joints in normal anatomical position. These must be checked regularly to detect any areas of pressure.
- Specific exercises, such as lifting hand weights, may be prescribed to strengthen a weakened limb.
- As soon as the individual's condition permits, balancing and sitting exercises are implemented. If the individual has been immobile for a prolonged period, it is necessary to progress slowly to prevent orthostatic hypotension.
- Once the individual can balance and sit, transfer activities are started (e.g. from bed to chair).
- When the individual can stand and balance in an upright position, ambulation is started.
- For the individual who is unable to ambulate, wheelchair mobility may be achieved.

The individual's age, severity of illness, other neurological deficits, chronic conditions or complications contribute to progress. The individual's attitude and motivation are also important factors in regaining mobility. Frequent assessment provides evaluation of the individual's needs so that rehabilitation can progress towards the greatest level of independence. More information on preventing the complications of immobility is provided in Chapter 28 (LeMone et al 2020).

Providing psychological support

Many individuals who have a nervous system disorder will suffer neurological deficits resulting in loss of independence, mobility, speech or sensory function. As a result, the individual's body image and self-concept may be greatly altered, and they may experience emotional lability, depression, anxiety, frustration or hostility. The individual may undergo personality changes, which may be functional or organic in origin. They may require a lengthy period to regain what were once automatically performed skills involved in the activities of daily living, or they may have to come to terms with the realisation that some skills may never be regained. The emotional shock to an individual who experiences paralysis can be devastating. The nurse has an important role in providing emotional and psychological support for the individual and their significant others. Some of the key aspects related to supporting the individual are as follows:

- During the period of dependence, it is important that dignity is preserved. Sensitivity is needed when dealing with any problems associated with loss of control (e.g. incontinence or loss of social restraint).
- Positive feedback should be provided for accomplishments no matter how minor they may appear.
- Adequate information about the disease process and its management should be provided, and the individual should be encouraged to participate in decision-making regarding care.
- Individual needs should be anticipated to decrease frustration. As much self-care as practicable should be allowed, as a return to independence is the ultimate goal of care. The individual's significant others should be allowed to be involved in care if they so wish.
- The individual and their significant others should be encouraged to express their feelings and anxieties. If the individual is experiencing a communication problem, appropriate methods of communicating should be developed. Time, patience and understanding are necessary to allow them to come to terms with the effects and implications of the disease.
- The individual should be encouraged to participate in activities of interest that will help to promote a feeling of self-worth. The occupational therapist and physiotherapist generally assist the individual to find activities that interest them and that will also provide exercise for weak or paralysed muscles.

(LeMone et al 2020)

Providing a suitable environment

The immediate physical environment should be adapted to meet the individual's specific needs. Items should be arranged to promote safety (e.g. adequate lighting, the call bell within easy reach and the bed adjusted to a suitable height). If the person is experiencing sensory deprivation (a lack of sensory input from the environment), the nurse can provide multisensory stimuli. Sensory input can be provided by talking to the person, playing a radio or recordings of the voices of the individual's significant others, by touch and by reality orientation. Reality orientation is a process of making the individual aware of their environment (e.g. the date, time, people, place and objects).

Conversely, the individual may experience sensory overload, particularly if critically ill and the condition requires the use of equipment such as mechanical ventilation or a cardiac monitor, or if they are receiving the constant stimuli of nursing care. Sensory overload occurs when sustained multisensory experiences are perceived as confusing or irritating by the individual. The manifestations of sensory overload are confusion, disorientation, restlessness, agitation, panic and possible hallucinations. Every effort should be made to control and moderate the intensity of stimuli (e.g. reducing tactile and environmental stimuli).

When the individual is to be discharged from hospital, the physical home environment should be evaluated, and the delivery of any necessary equipment arranged so that the activities of daily living can be accomplished and independence maintained. The physiotherapist and occupational therapist arrange for the home use of ambulatory equipment and identify special needs and alterations in the individual's environment that could be beneficial to support their independence (LeMone et al 2020).

Providing diagnostic test care

Preparation of the individual for, and care after, diagnostic tests is part of the nurse's role (see Chapter 15). The nurse must refer to the healthcare institution's policy manual for information about preparation of the individual for specific diagnostic tests. Preparation includes a general explanation of the procedure to reinforce the information provided to the individual by the medical officer. Other preparation may include dietary or fluid restrictions, administration of prescribed medications, assisting the individual into a specific position, skin preparation and measurement of baseline vital and neurological signs.

Post-procedural care may include assessing vital and neurological signs, measuring and recording fluid input and output, administering prescribed medications, and assessing the individual for signs and symptoms such as headaches, back pain, neck rigidity, nausea or vomiting, elevated temperature or voiding difficulty (LeMone et al 2020).

Promoting rehabilitation and independence

Rehabilitation is an integral part of care and is a dynamic process in which the individual is assisted to achieve optimal potential. Throughout the individual's illness, all care is directed towards the maintenance of optimal function and prevention of complications to promote as much independence as possible. Rehabilitation of an individual with a nervous system disorder includes helping with relearning the activities of daily living, management of neuromuscular and impaired perception and communication deficits, bladder and bowel retraining and educating the individual and their significant others in preparation for discharge from hospital (Brown et al 2020; LeMone et al 2020). (Information on rehabilitation is provided in Chapter 40.)

CARE OF THE UNCONSCIOUS INDIVIDUAL

Consciousness is defined as a state of awareness of self and the surroundings and documented as level of consciousness (LOC). Consciousness implies an ability to perceive sensory stimuli and to respond appropriately to them. Unconsciousness is defined as an abnormal state in which the individual is unresponsive to sensory stimuli. There are degrees of unconsciousness that vary in length and severity, ranging from a brief episode of unconsciousness in the form of fainting to a prolonged and deep coma (LeMone et al 2020).

Causes of impaired consciousness

Impaired consciousness arises from widespread damage to both cerebral hemispheres or from disruption of the reticular activating system in the upper brainstem. Loss of consciousness may result from a cerebral tumour, abscess, haemorrhage, haematoma, laceration, bruising or ischaemia, or from metabolic processes that depress or interrupt the function of both cerebral hemispheres (e.g. hypoxia, hypoglycaemia or toxic agents) (LeMone et al 2020).

Outcome of unconsciousness

The ultimate outcome of unconsciousness varies from full recovery of brain function, through a wide range of disabilities, to irreversible coma and death. The development of sophisticated monitoring techniques and life-support systems has increased the survival rate for comatose individuals with severe brain damage. A small percentage of individuals emerge from deep coma to a state of wakefulness without awareness, never regaining any recognisable mental function.

Irreversible coma or persistent vegetative state is used to describe a chronic condition occurring after severe cerebral damage. It is characterised by intact autonomic functions, generally intact reflexes, presence of a sleep–wakefulness cycle, spontaneous eye opening to verbal stimuli, no localising motor responses to verbal stimuli and no intact cognitive functions or awareness of self or of the environment (LeMone et al 2020).

Brain death

Brain death is a state of irreversible brain damage characterised by absence of cognitive functions and awareness of self and the environment, inability to maintain vital functions and the absence of isoelectric activity on EEG. In brain death (or brainstem death), the higher cortical functions cease, consciousness and awareness are lost, as is voluntary control of movement and all brainstem function. Some functions are not completely dependent on the integrity of the brainstem (e.g. heart rate continues, though this is usually for a limited time as the individual requires ventilatory support). If brainstem function can be shown to have ceased, then there is no prospect of recovery. The basic criteria for diagnosing brain death usually include:

- no pupillary response
- no corneal response
- no vestibulo-ocular reflex
- no motor response in cranial nerve distribution
- no gag or tracheal response
- no respiratory response to hypercapnia
- apnoea
- irreversible coma
- absence of brainstem reflexes
- isoelectric electroencephalogram (ECG)
- no spontaneous movements.

Before considering a brain death diagnosis, there is a need to exclude that brain dysfunction is the result of structural or metabolic disease, rather than the result of depressant drugs, alcohol, poisoning or hypothermia (Australian Government Organ and Tissue Authority 2021; LeMone et al 2020).

Brain death is a controversial legal, ethical and medical dilemma, but it is considered ethical and legal to terminate life support in individuals diagnosed as brain dead.

Management of an unconscious individual

When an individual is unconscious a high standard of care must be provided, with the objectives of maintaining and restoring body function and preventing complications. Medical management involves establishing a patent airway and providing adequate ventilation, controlling ICP and establishing the cause of unconsciousness and, if possible, reversing it. Nursing care of the unconscious individual requires the following practices, as described below:

- monitoring neurological function
- positioning
- meeting hygiene needs
- meeting nutritional and fluid needs
- meeting elimination needs
- promoting safety
- preventing complications
- providing sensory stimulation
- management of the individual with impaired motor function.

Maintaining a patent airway

With the absence of cough and swallowing reflexes, secretions accumulate in the posterior pharynx and upper trachea. An oral artificial airway may be sufficient to maintain patency, or tracheostomy or endotracheal intubation and mechanical ventilation may be necessary. To prevent airway obstruction:

- The individual is positioned on alternate sides every 2–4 hours to prevent secretions accumulating in the airways on one side. The neck should be maintained in a neutral position.
- Dentures and partial plates are removed.
- Nasal and oral care is provided to keep the upper airway free of accumulated secretions and debris.
- Oronasopharyngeal suction equipment may be necessary to aspirate secretions.
- Chest percussion and postural drainage may be prescribed to assist in the removal of tenacious secretions.

(LeMone et al 2020)

Monitoring neurological function

The individual's neurological signs are monitored at intervals determined by their condition. The results are documented and compared with previous assessments. Information on assessment of neurological function is provided earlier in this chapter.

Positioning

The individual is generally nursed in a lateral position with a small pillow placed under the head and neck to maintain the head in a neutral position. The upper arm is positioned on a pillow to maintain the shoulder in alignment, and the upper leg is supported on a pillow to maintain alignment of the hip. The individual's position is changed so that they lie on alternate sides every 2–4 hours. If hemiplegia is present, the individual may be positioned on the affected side for brief periods, but care must be taken to prevent injury to soft tissue and nerves, oedema or disruption of the blood supply. Because vasomotor tone is decreased in the affected areas, such adverse effects can develop rapidly from improper positioning. If the correct position is maintained, secretions are able to drain from the individual's mouth, the tongue is less likely to obstruct the airway and postural deformities can be prevented (LeMone et al 2020).

Meeting hygiene needs

Care of the skin involves keeping it clean and dry and protected from damage. Areas of the skin, particularly over the bony prominences, should be assessed regularly for the signs of impaired blood circulation and irritation that contribute to the formation of decubitus ulcers. Dry skin may be lubricated with a suitable cream or lotion to prevent cracking and breakdown, and a water-repellent substance may be used to protect the skin against excreta or perspiration. The male should receive a facial shave as part of daily hygiene care; the individual's nails are kept short and clean; and the hair is brushed, combed and washed as necessary.

Care of the mouth involves cleansing all areas at 2–4-hourly intervals to prevent a build-up of plaque, development of caries and development of a focus of infection. To prevent aspiration of fluid while oral hygiene is being performed, the individual's head is turned to one side and suction equipment made available throughout the procedure. The lips are lubricated with a suitable water-based substance.

Care of the nose involves cleansing the nostrils to keep them free of dried mucus. Cottonwool-tipped applicators and saline solution may be used to remove mucus and dried crusts, and a thin coating of cream may be applied to the rim of the nostrils.

Care of the eyes involves swabbing the eyes with moistened cottonwool to remove secretions, the instillation of artificial tears (or antibiotic eyedrops if prescribed) and protecting the eyes from corneal abrasions. If the eyelids do not close fully, the use of eye shields or pads may be necessary to protect the corneas (LeMone et al 2020). (See Chapter 34 for more information on care of the eye.)

Meeting nutritional and fluid needs

The nutritional and fluid needs of the individual must be regularly assessed and met to maintain body function, support tissue repair and combat infection. The dietitian prescribes a nutritional program based on consideration of the individual's energy needs, requirements for tissue repair, loss of fluid and basic life functions. Methods of administering nutritional and fluid support to the unconscious individual include total parenteral nutrition, and enteral feedings administered via a nasogastric, nasojejunal or gastrostomy tube. Parenteral nutrition is only used if there is a long-term gut absorption problem since the aim is to normalise gut function as soon as possible. Fluid input may be restricted to a specific amount of fluid in a 24-hour period. The purpose of fluid restriction is to control increased ICP by keeping the individual slightly under-hydrated. As fluid input is correlated with output, an accurate input and output record must be maintained (LeMone et al 2020). (See Chapter 30 for more information on nutrition.)

Meeting elimination needs

Because an unconscious individual is incontinent, an external urinary drainage appliance or an indwelling catheter (IDC) may be used to manage urinary drainage. Both methods are used to keep the skin dry since urinary incontinence can quickly lead to skin breakdown. Urinary drainage devices also enable accurate calculation of urinary output. Long-term IDC is avoided whenever possible due to risk of infection. Frequent checks and meticulous skin care is preferable. (Information on care of the individual with a urinary drainage device is provided in Chapter 31.)

Constipation and faecal impaction are common complications in an unconscious individual because immobility and lack of a normal diet inhibit peristalsis. A program is established whereby aperients and rectal suppositories are administered to promote regular bowel evacuation. The frequency of bowel actions and the amount and nature of the faeces are documented (see Chapter 32) (LeMone et al 2020).

> **CLINICAL INTEREST BOX 35.5**
> **Altered consciousness and taking temperature**
>
> Temperature should never be taken orally in individuals with altered conscious state. For an oral temperature reading to be taken safely and accurately, the individual must be able to close their lips completely and understand the importance of not biting the thermometer. Measure temperature via the tympanic or axillary routes; of these, tympanic is more accurate and therefore preferred.
>
> *(LeMone et al 2020; NSQHS Standard consideration: 'Recognising and Responding to Acute Deterioration [action 8.02, 8.04, 8.05])*

Promoting safety

Providing and maintaining a safe environment is of prime importance because an unconscious individual is unable to perceive or react to safety hazards. Clinical Interest Box 35.5 suggests alternative routes for measuring temperature when an individual is in a state of altered consciousness.

Preventing complications

Because the unconscious individual is not mobile, they are at risk of developing any of the complications associated with immobility (muscle contractures, decubitus ulcers or venous, pulmonary or urinary stasis) (LeMone et al 2020). Information on preventing these complications is provided in Chapter 28.

Providing sensory stimulation

The extent to which an unconscious individual may be aware of what is happening to and around them cannot usually be determined; the nurse should therefore assume that the brain is receiving some sensory input. When the duration of coma extends into weeks or months, it may seem meaningless to keep explaining each activity to an individual who gives no sign of comprehension. However, on regaining consciousness some individuals have been able to describe accurately events that happened to and around them while they were unconscious. Although they were unable to communicate their feelings, they were able to discriminate between the gentle caring manner of some people and the inattentive ways of others. Some individuals have reported that they longed for someone to talk to them rather than about them.

The nurse should therefore act as though the individual is conscious and demonstrate respect for them as a person. All activities should be explained to them, privacy during procedures should be ensured and they should be treated with dignity. Family members and friends should be encouraged to talk to and touch the unconscious individual. They should be encouraged to perform certain activities for the individual, such as combing the hair or applying skin lotion. Other sensory stimuli can be provided by playing a radio or music, or by placing perfumed flowers in the room.

Recovery from unconsciousness is a gradual process that tends to vary with each individual. Rehabilitation after a prolonged period of unconsciousness includes protecting the individual from orthostatic hypotension. When able to tolerate a vertical position, an ambulation program is developed, unless neurological deficits make it infeasible (Berman et al 2021; Crisp et al 2021; LeMone et al 2020). (Information on rehabilitation nursing is provided in Chapter 40.)

Management of the individual with impaired motor function

Disturbance of motor function is common among individuals who experience disorders of the brain, spinal cord or peripheral nerves, such as cerebral haemorrhage, spinal cord injury or peripheral neuritis. While this chapter addresses the care of an individual who has experienced a stroke or a spinal cord injury, the principles of care can be applied to individuals who experience impaired motor function from other causes. Some terms relating to impaired motor function are:

- Paresis: Incomplete paralysis or muscle weakness.
- Paralysis: Loss or impairment of the ability to move part(s) of the body. Paralysis may be complete or incomplete, spastic, or flaccid, symmetric or asymmetric, temporary or permanent.
- **Hemiplegia:** Unilateral paralysis, or paralysis of one side of the body. Because nerves cross in the pyramidal tract before descending to the spinal cord, damage to one side of the brain causes hemiplegia on the opposite side of the body.
- **Paraplegia:** Paralysis of the lower limbs and, sometimes, paralysis of the lower trunk and sphincters. Paralysis may be complete or incomplete, spastic, or flaccid, temporary or permanent.
- **Quadriplegia** (tetraplegia): Paralysis of the arms and legs and of the body below the level of injury to the spinal cord.

(Brown et al 2020; LeMone et al 2020)

Stroke

A stroke, also known as a cerebrovascular accident or brain attack, is one of the leading causes of death in the Western world, and each year many thousands of individuals survive a stroke but are left with permanent disabilities. A stroke is a sudden impairment of cerebral circulation, which causes cerebral infarction. The two types of stroke are ischaemic and haemorrhagic. In an ischaemic stoke, cerebral blood flow is suddenly impaired by a thrombus or embolus. In a haemorrhagic stroke, the rupture of a cerebral blood vessel causes bleeding into the subarachnoid space or brain tissue.

Manifestations of a stroke vary depending on the artery involved, and consequently the area of brain it supplies, and the severity of damage to cerebral tissue.

Table 35.6 lists the clinical features resulting from specific cerebral artery occlusion or rupture. If the stroke occurs

TABLE 35.6 | Manifestations of cerebrovascular accidents according to vessel involved

Vessel	Manifestations
Middle cerebral artery (MCA)	Hemiparesis or hemiplegia (contralateral to lesion) Aphasia (if left hemisphere lesion) Sensory impairment (same side as hemiplegia) Homonymous hemianopia Deterioration in conscious level from confusion to coma Headaches Inability to turn eyes towards the affected side Denial or lack of recognition of a paralysed extremity (if right hemisphere lesion) Possible Cheyne–Stokes breathing
Anterior cerebral artery (ACA)	Hemiparesis or hemiplegia of leg and foot (contralateral to lesion) Paresis of the arm on the side of hemiplegia Gait dysfunction Expressive aphasia Mental status impairments: • Confusion • Perseveration • Apathy • Amnesia • Short attention span • Slowness Deviation of eyes and head towards the affected side Urinary incontinence
Posterior cerebral artery (PCA)	Peripheral signs: • Homonymous hemianopia • Memory deficits • Dyslexia • Several visual defects • Perseveration Central signs: • Hemiplegia or hemiparesis • Pupillary dysfunction • Intention tremor • Diffuse sensory loss • Nystagmus
Internal carotid artery (ICA) (may show any or all the signs associated with middle cerebral artery and anterior cerebral artery disease)	Hemiparesis with facial asymmetry (contralateral to lesion) Paraesthesia on same side as hemiparesis Hemianopia Repeated attacks of visual blurring or blindness in the ipsilateral eye Dysphasia (intermittent) if dominant hemisphere involved
Posterior inferior cerebellar artery (PICA)	Dysphagia Dysarthria Loss of sensation on ipsilateral side of the face Loss of sensation on contralateral side of the body Horizontal nystagmus Ataxia Vertigo Nausea and vomiting Ipsilateral Horner's syndrome (miotic pupils, ptosis and facial anhidrosis (inadequate perspiration)) Paralysis of larynx and soft palate
Anterior inferior cerebellar artery (AICA)	Horizontal nystagmus Sensory impairment Deafness and tinnitus Nausea and vomiting Facial paralysis Horner's syndrome Ataxia

Continued

TABLE 35.6 | Manifestations of cerebrovascular accidents according to vessel involved—cont'd

Vessel	Manifestations	
Vertebral–basilar system (may show any of the signs of the PCA, PICA or AICA occlusion)	• Dysarthria • Dysphagia • Vertigo • Nausea • Syncope • Memory loss, disorientation	• Ataxic gait • Double vision • Tinnitus • Nystagmus • Facial paresis • Drop attacks

(Brown et al 2020)

in the left hemisphere, it produces symptoms on the right side of the body. If it occurs in the right hemisphere, the left side of the body is affected.

A thrombotic stroke, the most common type, is associated with atherosclerosis, which causes narrowing of the lumen of arteries. A thrombus forms in one of the cerebral arteries, occluding the vessel and resulting in cerebral ischaemia. An embolic stroke occurs when an embolus, which may be part of a thrombus, fat or other substance, is carried to the brain and occludes a cerebral blood vessel. A haemorrhagic stroke, which is often associated with hypertension, occurs when a cerebral blood vessel ruptures, spilling blood into the brain tissue. Rupture of an artery may result from a degenerative change in the arterial wall, or from an anatomical defect such as an aneurysm (Brain Foundation 2023; Stroke Foundation 2023a). (See Case Study 35.2.)

CASE STUDY 35.2

Mr Ng is a 65-year-old male who has been admitted to the neurology unit following a haemorrhagic stroke. He initially presented by ambulance after a sudden onset of severe headache and right-sided weakness. He has a history of hypertension and was on antihypertensive medication. Mr Ng was confused on arrival and had a blood pressure of 220/100. On initial presentation to the emergency department the following assessment data was obtained:

- GCS 13/15 (E4 V3 M 5)
- PEARL 4
- Respiratory rate 18 breaths/minute
- Blood pressure 220/100 mmHg
- Heart rate 56 beats/minute, regular
- T 37.5°C
- Right hemiplegia

1. Detail how you would perform your physical assessment of the individual.
2. What risk factors does Mr Ng have in relation to his stroke and how do the risk factors contribute to stroke?
3. What are some indications of dysphagia?
4. What is your management plan for Mr Ng? What medical interventions will be required?

Risk factors

Educational programs have been developed to inform the general public about stroke and prevention. Many factors have been identified as predisposing a person to a stroke and, by increasing public awareness, those at risk can seek medical advice to have any pre-existing conditions managed, thus reducing the risk of stroke. Risk factors include a history of:

- atherosclerosis
- hypertension
- family history of stroke
- heart disease
- diabetes mellitus
- smoking
- alcohol
- sedentary work with little exercise
- obesity
- elevated cholesterol and triglyceride levels.

(Brain Foundation 2023)

Manifestations of a stroke

In all cases of stroke, areas of the brain are deprived of an adequate oxygen supply. If the blood supply is impaired for an extended period, the involved cerebral tissue may become necrotic, resulting in permanent neurological deficits. In instances of ischaemia, temporary neurological impairment may result. The particular type and degree of neurological deficits depend on the area of the brain involved (see Table 35.6). Table 35.7 lists a comparison of manifestations associated with right- and left-sided hemiplegia.

Care of the individual who has had a stroke

Medical management involves control of cerebral oedema and subsequent increased ICP, surgical intervention if indicated and drug therapy. For example, thrombolytic medication such as tissue plasminogen activator (TPA) may be given to individuals experiencing a non-haemorrhagic stroke. Nursing care of the individual involves:

- managing the acute phase
- meeting basic needs
- preventing complications

TABLE 35.7 | Manifestations of stroke

Left-sided stroke	Right-sided stroke
Right-sided hemiplegia (left stroke)	Left-sided hemiplegia (right stroke)
Aphasia—expressive, receptive or global	Spatial–perceptual deficits
Intellectual impairment	Tends to be distractible, impulsive behaviour
Slow behaviour	Appears to be unaware of deficits, poor judgment
Defects in right visual fields	Defects in left visual fields

(Brown et al 2020)

- providing psychological support
- promoting rehabilitation.

Care during the acute phase

The acute phase begins when the individual is admitted and continues until their condition is stable. Nursing care is directed towards maintaining a patent airway and monitoring vital and neurological signs.

Maintaining a patent airway: This involves positioning the individual on their side, administering oxygen as prescribed and suctioning secretions from the airway. Care must be taken when performing oronasopharyngeal suction because suction applied for longer than 15 seconds at a time may increase ICP.

Recording fluid input and output: This information should be kept to monitor kidney function and to evaluate fluid and electrolyte balance.

Vital and neurological signs: These signs should be assessed frequently (e.g. every 15–30 minutes) to detect changes in the individual's condition. Information on neurological assessment is provided earlier in this chapter. If the individual is unconscious, the principles of care described previously should be incorporated (LeMone et al 2020).

Treatment

The type of treatment depends on the severity and cause of the stroke and is changing with medical advancement occurring all the time.

TPA is the treatment for ischemic stroke. It is important that the individual be evaluated and treated by a specialised stroke team within 3 hours of the start of the symptoms. TPA breaks up blood clots and can restore blood flow to the damaged area (Stroke Foundation 2023b; Stroke Recovery Association NSW 2023d).

Endovascular thrombectomy (also called mechanical thrombectomy or endovascular clot retrieval) is a minimally invasive procedure. The procedure is performed 6–24 hours after the individual was last known to be well and if clinical and CT perfusion or MRI indicate the presence of salvageable brain tissue. A neuro-interventionist performs an angiogram by passing a catheter into the brain to the site of the blocked blood vessel. Various techniques are then available to remove the clot including stent retrievers (Stroke Foundation 2023b).

Care after the acute phase

Detailed information about the nursing measures necessary to meet the individual's basic needs for hygiene, safety, elimination, nutrition and fluids, psychological support, mobility and rehabilitation is provided elsewhere in this text. Clinical Interest Box 35.6 provides some suggestions that can facilitate self-care after stroke.

The main aims of care for an individual who has experienced a stroke are to:

- Assist in meeting hygiene needs.
- Monitor vital and neurological signs.
- Maintain muscle tone and prevent contractures.
- Prevent skin breakdown.
- Prevent venous stasis (thrombus and embolus formation).
- Prevent and manage alterations in elimination (e.g. incontinence, retention of urine, constipation).
- Maintain nutritional and fluid status.
- Establish an adequate means of communication.
- Promote reorientation of a confused individual.
- Enhance self-concept and body image.
- Institute a rehabilitation program aimed at achieving an optimal level of independence.

(Brown et al 2020; LeMone et al 2020; Stroke Recovery Association NSW 2023a)

Rehabilitation

Rehabilitation of the individual begins on admission to hospital and continues for as long as necessary including after discharge home. In some healthcare institutions, the individual may be transferred to a rehabilitation unit after the acute phase of their illness. The focus of rehabilitation is directed at helping the individual to relearn lost skills and to become as independent as possible. The individual and their significant others are made aware of the plan and goals of the rehabilitative phase, and their active participation is encouraged. Recovery from a stroke is a slow process; therefore, the nurse must provide support and positive feedback so that the individual does not become

CLINICAL INTEREST BOX 35.6 Devices to facilitate self-care after stroke

The following list identifies useful items that may assist neurologically impaired individuals to perform self-care more easily and safely after a stroke or other disorders.

Eating devices

- Plate guards to prevent food from being pushed off plate
- Wide grip utensils to accommodate weak grasp
- Non-skid mats to stabilise plates

Mobility aids

- Canes, walkers, wheelchairs
- Transfer devices such as slide boards and belts

Bathing and grooming devices

- Shower and bath chairs
- Electric razors with head at 90 degrees to handle
- Grab bars, non-skid mats, hand-held shower heads
- Long-handled bath sponge

Dressing aids

- Velcro closures
- Elastic shoe laces
- Long-handled shoehorn

Toileting aids

- Raised toilet seat
- Grab bars next to toilet

(Independent Living Centre NSW 2017)

discouraged. Rehabilitation of the individual includes:

- encouraging participation in their own care as much as possible
- teaching them to perform the activities of daily living with regard to ways of compensating for any disabilities
- teaching and assisting with performance of transfer activities (e.g. bed to chair)
- assisting in the regaining of any lost communication skills
- encouraging expression of feelings, to decrease anxiety and to allow for correction of any misunderstood information
- developing a bladder and bowel retraining program (if necessary).

(Stroke Recovery Association NSW 2023c)

More information on rehabilitation nursing is provided in Chapter 40.

Planning for discharge

Discharge planning is directed at facilitating the transition from the healthcare institution to the home environment. Discharge planning involves assessing the individual and the family, identifying specific needs, planning to implement ways of meeting those needs and evaluating the discharge process and the results. After the individual is discharged home, they and the family must have contact with support services, such as the district nurse, whom they can rely on for continued help and support (Stroke Foundation 2023a; 2018b; Stroke Recovery Association NSW 2023b).

CRITICAL THINKING EXERCISE 35.6

Ben sustained a spinal cord injury following a fall. What are the signs and symptoms of spinal cord injury?

SPINAL CORD INJURY

Injuries involving the spinal cord result most often from motor vehicle accidents, falls, sporting and industrial accidents and firearm or stab wounds. Injuries to the vertebral column and spinal cord result from forces applied directly or indirectly to the head, neck or trunk. Apart from direct tearing of the spinal cord, the main damage is caused by haemorrhage, oedema and disruption of the blood supply to the cord. Additional compression can result if bony fragments or disc material press on the spinal cord.

Manifestations of spinal cord damage depend on the degree and site of the injury. Complete spinal cord transection causes a total loss of motor and sensory function below the level of injury. With cervical cord transection, there is paralysis of all four extremities (quadriplegia/tetraplegia). There are varying degrees of arm and ventilatory paralysis, depending on the injury level. With thoracic cord transection, down to the level of the second lumbar vertebra, there is paralysis of the lower extremities (paraplegia). There is often some loss of intercostal muscle function and loss of bladder and bowel function. With transection in the region of lumbar vertebrae there is loss of a combination of sensory, motor, bowel and bladder function.

Complete cord transection results in immediate flaccid paralysis, loss of sensation and loss of reflexes below the level of injury. As paralysis subsides, reflexes usually return and flaccidity changes to involuntary spastic movements. Recovery of any motor or sensory function is rare when there has been complete paralysis of these functions for several days. With incomplete spinal cord injuries, degrees of motor and sensory deficit below the level of damage vary. The individual may experience temporary paralysis, with function returning when any oedema subsides (LeMone et al 2020; Spinal Cord Injuries Australia 2023a).

Damage to the spinal cord and nerve roots results from:

- compression by displaced bone or ligaments, extruded disc or haematoma formation
- excessive stretching, crushing, shearing or severance of neural tissue
- swelling in response to bruising or compression
- impaired capillary circulation and venous return.

There are four possible vectors (forces) that can be applied to the spinal column to cause injury:

1. Flexion: Excessive flexion (hyperflexion) tends to produce compression of the vertebral bodies, with disruption of the posterior ligaments and the intervertebral discs. Hyperflexion injuries are caused by hyperflexion of the head and neck, as in sudden deceleration of a vehicle
2. Extension: Excessive extension (hyperextension) usually causes fractures of the posterior elements of the vertebral column and disruption of the anterior ligaments. Hyperextension injuries are caused by hyperextension of the head and neck, as may occur in a rear-end vehicular accident
3. Rotation (lateral flexion): Excessive rotation is most likely to produce rupture of the ligaments, fracture and fracture dislocation of the vertebral facets. Rotational injuries are caused by extreme lateral flexion or rotation of the head and neck
4. Compression: Compression can result in fractures of the vertebral body and arch, and rupture of the supporting ligaments. Compression injuries are caused by vertical pressure as occurs when a person falls from a height and lands on their feet or buttocks.

(Spinal Cord Injuries Australia 2023a)

Classification of spinal cord injuries

Spinal cord injuries can be classified by the type of injury and by syndromes:

- Concussion: Severe shaking of the spinal cord that causes temporary loss of function lasting about 24–48 hours.
- Contusion: Bruising of the spinal cord, which includes bleeding into the cord.
- Laceration: An actual tear in the spinal cord.
- Transection: Severing of the cord—may be complete or incomplete.
- Haemorrhage: Bleeding into or around the cord. Escaped blood is an irritant to the delicate tissue.
- Anterior cord syndrome: Due to injury of the anterior part of the spinal cord and associated with flexion injuries and fracture dislocations of the vertebrae. Manifestations include loss of pain and temperature sensation and motor function below the level of the injury. The sensations of light touch, position and vibration remain intact.
- Posterior cord syndrome: A rare syndrome in which the senses of position and vibration are involved.
- Central cord syndrome: Due to injury and/or oedema to the central cord in the cervical region (e.g. as a result of hyperextension injuries). Manifestations include a greater loss of motor function in the upper limbs (rather than the lower), bladder dysfunction and varying degrees of sensory impairment.
- Brown-Séquard syndrome: Results from open penetrating wounds that produce transverse hemisection of the cord. Manifestations include loss of pain and temperature sensation on the side opposite the injury, and loss of motor function, light touch, position, and vibratory sensation on the side of the injury.

(Brown et al 2020)

Manifestations of spinal cord injury (SCI)

Generally, the degree of damage to the spinal cord at any level is described as incomplete or complete transection. Incomplete transection of the cord produces loss or impairment of sensation and motor function that reflects the specific nerve tracts that have been damaged. Complete transection of the cord results in permanent loss of voluntary movement, sensation, reflex and autonomic function below the level of injury.

Spinal shock

Spinal shock is an immediate response to an acute spinal cord injury and is the temporary suppression of reflexes controlled by the segments below the level of injury. After a period that may vary from hours to months, the spinal neurons gradually regain their excitability. Subsequent return of some function results from decompression of the cord as oedema resolves (Brown et al 2020; Spinal Cord Injuries Australia 2023a).

Functional loss from spinal cord injury

The different functions and dysfunctions associated with spinal cord injuries at specific levels are listed in Table 35.8. The effects of spinal cord injury on sexual response vary depending on the level and degree of injury. Sexual function is controlled by spinal levels S2, S3 and S4. Knowledge of the physiology of alterations in sexual response after spinal cord injury is incomplete, and significant individual differences exist. People with complete loss of sensation in the genitalia may still experience orgasm in response to sensations produced by stimulation of other areas of the body in which sensation is intact. Sexual pleasure can also be increased by psychological stimuli, such as memory, sight, sound and odour. Physical stimulation of the genitalia may produce reflex erection of the penis and vaginal lubrication, even though there is no sensory awareness of stimulation (LeMone et al 2020; Spinal Cord Injuries Australia 2023c).

Care of the individual with spinal cord injury

Management of the individual at the scene of the accident is critical to the ultimate neurological outcome. The basic objectives of first aid management at the scene are to:

- Prevent death from asphyxia.
- Prevent further spinal cord damage from torsion, flexion, or extension of the unstable spine.
- Transport the individual rapidly and safely to an appropriate facility.
- Subsequent management of the individual involves emergency department care, early management, post-acute and long-term management.

TABLE 35.8 | Spinal cord injury—functional loss

Level of injury	Motor function	Sensory function	Bladder/bowel function	Ventilatory function
C1–C4	Loss of all function from the neck down.	Loss of sensation from the neck down.	No bladder or bowel control.	Loss of independent ventilatory function.
C5	Loss of all function below the upper shoulders.	Loss of sensation below the clavicles.	No bladder or bowel control.	Phrenic nerve is intact, but the intercostal muscles are non-functional.
C6	Loss of all function below the upper arms.	Loss of sensation below the clavicles, but some arm and thumb sensation.	No bladder or bowel control.	Phrenic nerve is intact, but the intercostal muscles are non-functional.
C7	Incomplete quadriplegia. Loss of motor control to parts of the arms and hands.	Loss of sensation below the clavicles but some arm and hand sensation.	No bladder or bowel control.	Phrenic nerve is intact, but the intercostal muscles are non-functional.
C8	Incomplete quadriplegia. Loss of motor control to parts of the arms and hands.	Loss of sensation below the chest and part of the hands.	No bladder or bowel control.	Phrenic nerve is intact, but the intercostal muscles are non-functional.
T1–T6	Loss of function below the mid-chest.	Loss of sensation from the mid-chest down.	No bladder or bowel control.	Independent phrenic nerve function; some intercostal muscle impairment.
T6–T12	Loss of function below the waist.	Loss of sensation below the waist.	No bladder or bowel control.	No interference to ventilatory function.
L1–L2	Loss of most control of the pelvis and legs.	Loss of sensation to the lower abdomen and legs.	No bladder or bowel control.	No interference to ventilatory function.
L3–L4	Loss of control of part of the lower legs and feet.	Loss of sensation to part of the lower legs and feet.	No bladder or bowel control.	No interference to ventilatory function.
L5–S5	Loss of control of parts of the hips, knees, ankles and feet.	Loss of sensation to parts of the lower limbs and perineum.	May or may not be loss of bladder and/or bowel control.	No interference to ventilatory function.

(Brown et al 2020)

Initial management

On arrival of the individual in the accident and emergency department, the medical officer assesses the individual, and X-rays are taken to determine the extent of the injuries. The medical officer develops a plan of care that may include immediate surgery or a non-surgical approach with traction and immobilisation and insertion of a nasogastric tube, indwelling urinary catheter and intravenous infusion. Generally, glucocorticoid steroids are prescribed to reduce cord swelling (LeMone et al 2020).

Early management

After initial assessment and stabilisation of the individual, they are admitted to the intensive care or spinal unit. An individual with less severe injuries may be admitted to a general ward. Medical management will depend on the type of spinal cord injury and any associated injuries. Treatment may be surgical, non-surgical or a combination of both approaches. Surgical management may take the form of decompression laminectomy, fusion of vertebrae, open or closed reduction of fractures or dislocations or the insertion of rods. Non-surgical management involves immobilisation of the spine (Figure 35.10) using skeletal tongs with traction, halo traction, a cervical collar or a device designed to maintain thoracic or lumbar alignment, such as a fibreglass body jacket (LeMone et al 2020).

Nursing care of the individual with a spinal cord injury

Nursing management of spinal cord injury will vary according to the individual's injury and whether a surgical or non-surgical approach is selected. However, the major

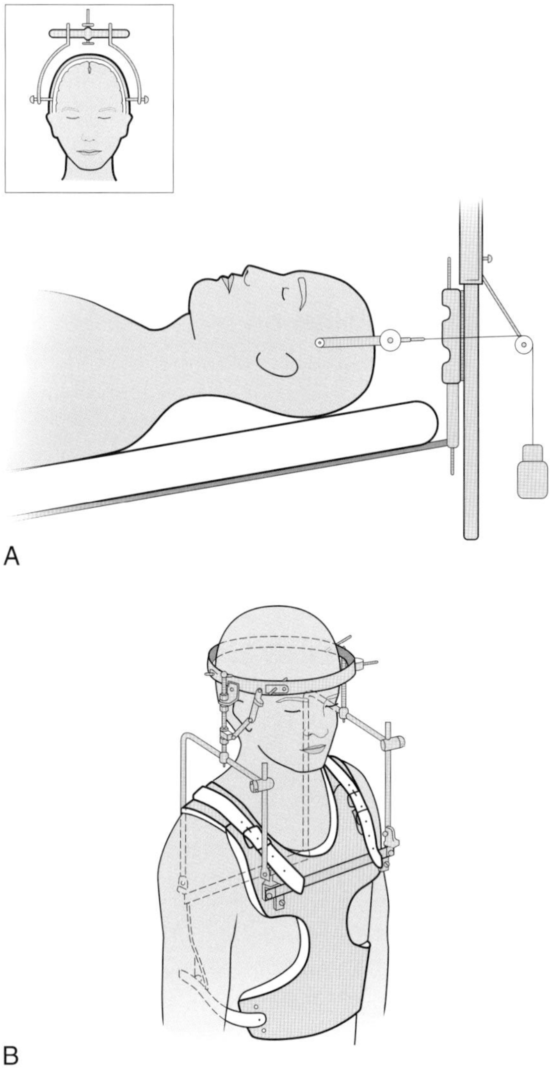

A

B

Figure 35.10 Immobilisation of the spine

A: Cervical traction with tongs. The inset shows the position of the tongs on the bone structure of the skull, **B:** Halo traction and vest.

aspects of care are directed towards maintaining respiratory function, immobilisation and alignment of the spine, preventing complications, meeting basic needs, providing psychological support and rehabilitation.

Respiratory care

An individual with a spinal cord injury can develop varying degrees of respiratory difficulty, depending on the level of spinal injury. The individual will require a plan of care directed at preventing pulmonary complications. Intubation and mechanical ventilation will be required if there is impairment of respiratory muscle function. The program of care includes:

- regular assessment for indications of inadequate ventilation
- chest physiotherapy at least every 4 hours
- maintenance of a patent airway
- use of an incentive spirometer to promote lung expansion.

(LeMone et al 2020)

Immobilisation and alignment of the spine

After alignment of the spine has been achieved, immobilisation serves to maintain alignment and promotes healing at the site of injury. For most thoracic, lumbar or sacral injuries, the individual remains confined to bed, with the back positioned and supported to achieve hyperextension of the spine at the site of injury. A bed with a firm mattress and steel base and correctly positioned pillows is necessary to maintain the prescribed posture (LeMone et al 2020).

Skeletal traction

When the injury involves dislocation or fracture-dislocation of the cervical or high thoracic spine, skeletal traction may be used to accomplish alignment and immobilisation (see Figure 35.10). Skeletal traction may be achieved by means of cervical tongs, such as Crutchfield tongs, or by the halo device. The halo device may also be incorporated with the use of a body vest or jacket to stabilise the spine, thereby allowing the individual to be ambulatory. When skeletal traction is used, the individual may be nursed on a firm mattress and fracture board, or on a special bed such as a Stryker frame.

After skeletal traction has been established, pain is decreased, and the individual's comfort is enhanced. Turning can be carried out using a special technique (as described in Chapter 19) to allow for skin care and a change of position. Management of the individual in cervical skeletal traction includes:

- Checking the traction equipment every 2–4 hours to ensure safety and integrity of the treatment.
- Inspecting, cleansing and dressing the pin sites according to the institution's policy (e.g. every 4–8 hours).
- Changing the individual's position every 2 hours to prevent the complications of immobility. The 'log-rolling' technique or the Stryker frame is used to turn the individual to maintain the vertebral column in neutral position.
- Using various devices (e.g. pillows, a foot board, a cervical roll) to maintain good body alignment. When the individual lies supine, the arms and legs are positioned in extension with support to maintain the feet in dorsiflexion. The hands are placed in a functional position and a cervical roll is used to maintain hyperextension of the neck. When the individual is in a lateral position, the arms and legs are positioned in extension, and pillows are placed to support this position.

(LeMone et al 2020)

Preventing complications

Because prolonged immobility can lead to various complications, specific preventative measures must be implemented. (Information on preventing the complications associated with immobility is provided in Chapter 28.)

Meeting basic needs

Individuals with impaired motor and sensory function require assistance to meet their needs for hygiene, safety, elimination, nutrition and fluids, temperature regulation and pain relief (LeMone et al 2020; Spinal Cord Injuries Australia 2023b). Information on assisting individuals to meet these basic needs is provided in other chapters.

Providing psychological support

A severe spinal cord injury has a devastating effect on the individual and their significant others, and they will experience a range of emotional responses, from the time of injury and through the rehabilitation process. The individual will have to adapt to the loss of motor function and sensory deprivation, both of which severely threaten self-concept and body image. It is important that the nurse is aware of the impact that the injury has on the individual's emotional and psychological equilibrium. The nurse must be sensitive to the emotional and psychological response of the individual to the injury and be supportive as they deal with the impact of the injury. The nurse can help to support the individual by:

- establishing a climate of trust
- accepting behaviour, without being judgmental
- encouraging expression of feelings
- listening empathetically and attentively
- allowing the individual to make decisions and maintain control
- providing information as necessary
- supporting a positive self-concept and self-esteem
- informing the individual that it will take time to adjust to the disability.

(LeMone et al 2020; Spinal Cord Injuries Australia 2023d)

(See Nursing Care Plan 35.1.)

Promoting rehabilitation

In most instances of spinal cord injury, the individual will require long-term rehabilitation. Rehabilitation after spinal cord injury is a lifelong process of learning to live with a disability. The individual and family, together with the healthcare team members, contribute to the development of the rehabilitative plans. (Information on rehabilitation is provided in Chapter 40.)

CRITICAL THINKING EXERCISE 35.7

Following on from the example in Critical Thinking Exercise 35.6: How would you explain spinal shock to Ben's family?

NURSING CARE PLAN 35.1

Mrs Smith, a 65-year-old woman, was at home when she suddenly experienced weakness on the right side of her body and difficulty speaking. On presentation to emergency, Mrs Smith had slurred speech, facial droop, and weakness on the right side. Mrs Smith was diagnosed with an ischemic stroke.

Assessment: On presentation to the ward post-acute phase, Mrs Smith, 65, is assessed. She is alert, orientated to time and person; however, she is confused to place. Pupils equal and reacting to light (PEARTL), severe right-sided weakness in both arm and leg. Right-sided facial droop.

Issue/s to be addressed: Impaired physical mobility related to right-sided hemiparesis.
Impaired nutrition related to right-sided facial droop.
Impaired communication.
Impaired orientation.

Goal/s: Mrs Smith will remain free of complications of immobility and impaired gap reflexes, and assistance will be provided to communicate effectively and reorientate.

Care/actions	Rationale
Positioning	
Encourage independence and minimise risk of pressure injury.	Encourages independence during transfer and positioning. Position prevents contractures, relieves pressure. Prevents adduction of the affected shoulder with a pillow placed under the axilla.
Physiotherapy and exercise program.	Assists to strengthen muscles used to transfer and mobilise. Provides full range of motion four or five times a day to maintain joint mobility. Prevents venous stasis. Regains balance.
Provide education regarding transfer, positioning, nutrition, mobilisation, and safety to decrease falls risk.	Decreases falls risk and anxiety.

NURSING CARE PLAN 35.1—cont'd

Skin integrity.	
Ensure the skin is checked for non-blanching redness, oedema, localised heat and integrity after repositioning.	Monitors for pressure injuries. Documents skin integrity each shift.
Assist with nutrition	
Observe patient for coughing, dribbling, or pooling of food in one side of the mouth. Consult with speech pathologist. Ensure patient is sitting upright when eating and drinking. Advise patient to take smaller boluses of food. Provide thicker liquids and pureed diet.	Decreases risk of aspiration and choking.
Communication	
Provide emotional support and understanding. Avoid completing patient's sentences. Speak slowly and give one instruction at a time. Provide communication boards if required.	Improves communication.
Reduce risk of pressure injury related to immobility.	
Ensure moisture is removed from the skin caused by urinary and faecal incontinence. Orientate. Provide clear and concise information. Repeat information. Use visual cues.	Reduces risk of impaired skin integrity related to incontinence. Improves orientation.
Circulatory care	
Ensure graduated compression stockings or intermittent pneumatic compression (SCDs) are used until fully mobile.	Facilitates venous return from the lower extremities and prevent venous stasis and venous thrombosis.
Assess both lower extremities for skin colour, temperature, skin condition, oedema and Homans' sign (pain in calf with passive dorsiflexion of the foot).	Reduces peripheral oedema.
Administer anticoagulant.	Prophylaxis assists in prevention of venous thromboembolism (VTE).
Evaluation: Mrs Smith can reposition herself with minimal assistance. Nutritional requirements met. Skin integrity observed and documented each shift. Calves assessed each shift. Orientated to time, place and person.	

(Berman et al 2021; LeMone et al 2020)

Progress Note 35.1

23/11/2024
1100 hrs

Nursing: Subdural haemorrhage 5/11/24. Neuro: GCS 14/15. Alert, confused to month orientated to year. Mild weakness to left arm and leg, full power right side. cranial nerves II–XII intact, proprioception intact, normal sensation. Vitals: afebrile, temp, pulse, resp rate, saturations and BP within SAGO chart limits. Pain score 3/10 this morning—given 1 g paracetamol at 0830 hrs with good effect. Pain score at 1045 was 0/10. Intake: Tolerating full ward diet and some free fluids. IV fluids discontinued this morning when IV antibiotics ceased. Output: IDC removed at 0600 hrs. For trial of void. Has not passed urine yet, no palpable bladder nor complaints of discomfort voiced. Medical officer requested bladder scan at 1200 hrs if not voided prior. Bowels not opened yesterday or today. Mr Brown stated would like aperients this evening if bowels not open today. General: Needs assistance of one other person to get out of bed. Walked to shower with assistance of two people using walk belt. Showered with assistance. Cleaned teeth. Pressure points intact. Mr Brown taken for a walk by physio. TEDs in situ with non-slip socks. Family in attendance at time and shown how to help Mr Brown roll on to side to get out of bed. Planned transfer to rehabilitation unit on 25/11 to increase mobility and independence. Family aware of pending transfer.

B Woodward (WOODWARD), *Student Enrolled Nurse*

DECISION-MAKING FRAMEWORK EXERCISE 35.1

Lynelle is a student Enrolled Nurse on an acute neurological unit where she is caring for Mrs Jones, a 64-year-old female.

Mrs Jones has been admitted following a fall and has since been diagnosed with Parkinson's disease following a history of tremors and an unsteady gait.

Mrs Jones did not receive her anti-parkinsonian medication following lunch since she was having a CT scan. When assisting Mrs Jones to the toilet post the evening meal, Lynelle notices that Mrs Jones is more unsteady on her feet. She states she is tired. Her tremors are more noticeable than earlier in the shift.

Using the decision-making framework answer the following questions:

1. Lynelle decides Mrs Jones is too unsteady to walk with the assistance of only one person to the toilet. What alternatives should Lynelle consider to assist Mrs Jones?
2. What hospital policies should Lynelle refer to?
3. Does Lynelle have the required level of education to administer the medication that was missed?
4. Who should be informed regarding the missed medication and what documentation should be completed?

Summary

The nervous system is a complex system, responsible for communication within the body and between the body and its environment. It is divided into two primary divisions: the central nervous system and the peripheral nervous system.

Nervous tissue is commonly described as grey and white matter. The grey matter is composed of cells and the white matter is made up of fibres. Neurons are the primary components of nervous tissue, which are bound together by neuroglia. Neurons have two functional properties: irritability and conductivity. This means that neurons are able to respond to a stimulus, convert it into an impulse and transmit the impulse to other neurons, muscles or glands. Impulses are transmitted through spaces, called synapses, between neurons.

The central nervous system consists of the brain and the spinal cord. The brain is a large organ composed of the cerebrum, diencephalon, brainstem and cerebellum. Each part of the brain has specific functions. The spinal cord lies within a canal inside the vertebral column, extending from the base of the skull to the first or second lumbar vertebra. The spinal cord receives sensory impulses, conveys motor impulses and is the centre through which reflex actions take place. The meninges are three membranes that cover the brain and spinal cord to protect them against physical injury. Cerebrospinal fluid is a clear watery fluid produced in the ventricles of the brain, which circulates in the subarachnoid space surrounding the brain and spinal cord. It protects the brain and spinal cord and provides a medium for the exchange of nutrients and waste products.

The peripheral nervous system consists of 12 pairs of cranial nerves and 31 pairs of spinal nerves. The nerves of the peripheral nervous system may be sensory, carrying impulses to the brain and spinal cord, or motor, carrying impulses away from the brain and spinal cord, or mixed. The motor nervous system is divided into somatic and autonomic nervous system divisions. The autonomic nervous system division is composed of the sympathetic nervous system and the parasympathetic nervous system. It is the section of the peripheral nervous system concerned with the involuntary activity of the body. Sympathetic nerves have a stimulating effect on most organs, while parasympathetic nerves tend to slow down body processes.

Normal function of the nervous system may be impaired as a result of congenital disorders, inflammatory

Summary—cont'd

or infectious conditions, trauma, neoplasia, degenerative conditions or metabolic and endocrine disorders. The major manifestations of nervous system disorders are headaches, sensory changes, motor changes, reflex changes, altered states of awareness or consciousness and seizures. Disorders of the nervous system can be classified as those occurring from congenital or hereditary defects, from multiple causes, degenerative disorders, immunological disorders, infectious or inflammatory conditions, neoplastic or obstructive disorders and trauma.

Diagnostic tests used to assess nervous system function include the neurological examination, radiographic examination, magnetic resonance imaging and electroencephalography. Care of the individual with a nervous system disorder includes promoting a clear airway, maintaining fluid and nutritional status, preventing and managing alterations in elimination, promoting effective communication, promoting safety, promoting mobility, preventing the complications of immobility, providing psychological support, assessing neurological status, providing a suitable environment and promoting rehabilitation.

Review Questions

1. Identify five signs and symptoms of acute subdural haemorrhage and discuss why older individuals are at risk for chronic subdural haematoma.
2. What is brain death? What are the criteria for declaring an individual clinically brain dead?
3. Name one test that is performed to diagnose a brain tumour.
4. What does a Glasgow Coma Scale (GCS) of 15 indicate?
5. What is the blood–brain barrier and what is its role in protecting the brain? What substances can cross the blood–brain barrier?
6. What is the difference between the sympathetic and parasympathetic nervous systems?
7. What is the central nervous system and what are the main components?
8. What is aphasia and what are the three main classifications?

Evolve® Answer guide for the Review Questions, Critical Thinking Exercises, Decision-making Framework Exercises and Critical Thinking Questions in Case Studies is hosted on Evolve: http://evolve.elsevier.com/AU/Koutoukidis/Tabbner.

References

Agency for Clinical Innovation, 2013. Adult neurological observation chart education package. Available at: <https://aci.health.nsw.gov.au/__data/assets/pdf_file/0018/201753/ACI-Adult-neurological-observation-chart-education-package.pdf>.

Applegate, E., 2011. *The anatomy and physiology learning system*, 4th ed. Saunders, St Louis.

Australian Commission on Safety and Quality in Health Care, (ACSQHC), 2021a. National safety and quality health service standards, 2nd ed. ACSQHC, Sydney. Available at: <https://www.safetyandquality.gov.au/publications-and-resources/resource-library/national-safety-and-quality-health-service-standards-second-edition>.

Australian Commission on Safety and Quality in Health Care, (ACSQHC), 2021b. Recognising and responding to acute deterioration. Available at: <https://www.safetyandquality.gov.au/standards/nsqhs-standards/recognising-and-responding-acute-deterioration-standard>.

Australian Government Organ and Tissue Authority, 2021. Best practice guideline for offering organ and tissue donation in Australia. Available at: <https://www.donatelife.gov.au/for-healthcare-workers/clinical-guidelines-and-protocols/best-practice-guideline-offering-organ-and-tissue-donation-australia>.

Banasik, J.L., Copstead, L.E.C., 2019. *Pathophysiology*, 6th ed. Elsevier Inc, St. Louis.

Berman, A., Fandsen, G., Snyder, S., Levett-Jones, T., et al., 2021. *Kozier and Erb's fundamentals of nursing: Concepts, process and practice*, 5th ed. Pearson, Melbourne.

Better Health Channel, 2018. Spina bifida. Available at: <https://www.betterhealth.vic.gov.au/health/condition-sandtreatments/spina-bifida>.

Brain Foundation, 2023. Stroke. Available at: <http://brainfoundation.org.au/disorders/stroke/#whatisastroke>.

Brain Injury Australia, 2016. Brain injury. Available at: <https://www.braininjuryaustralia.org.au/brain-injury-2>.

Brown, D., Edwards, H., Buckley, T., et al., 2020. *Lewis's medical-surgical nursing*, 5th ed. Elsevier, Sydney.

Cerebral Palsy Alliance, 2018. Signs and symptoms of cerebral palsy. Available at: <https://www.cerebralpalsy.org.au/what-is-cerebral-palsy/signs-and-symptoms-of-cp/>.

Cerebral Palsy Australia, 2023. My CP Guide. About cerebral palsy (CP). Available at: <https://www.mycpguide.org.au/about-cp>.

Children's Tumour Foundation conquering NF, 2023. Neurofibromatosis Type 1 (NF1) Healthcare professionals. Available at: <https://www.ctf.org.au/page/105/gps-healthcare-professionals>.

Crisp, J., Douglas, C., Rebeiro, D., et al., 2021. *Potter & Perry's fundamentals of nursing*, Australian and New Zealand edition, 6th ed. Elsevier, Chatswood.

Curtis, K., Ramsden, R., Ramon, Z., et al., 2019. *Emergency and trauma care for nurses and paramedics*, 3rd ed. Elsevier, Australia.

Dementia Australia, 2022a. Principles for a dignified diagnosis of dementia. Available at: <https://www.dementia.org.au/information/for-health-professionals/dementia-essentials/principles-for-a-dignified-diagnosis-of-dementia>.

Dementia Australia, 2022b. Help sheets. Available at: <https://www.dementia.org.au/resources/help-sheets#about-dementia>.

Dempsey, J., Hillege, S., Hill, R., 2014. *Fundamentals of nursing and midwifery: A person-centred approach to care*, 2nd ed. Lippincott Williams & Wilkins, Sydney.

deWit, S.C., Kumagai, C.K., 2013. *Medical-surgical nursing*, 2nd ed. Saunders, St. Louis.

Epilepsy Action Australia, 2023. Understanding epilepsy. Available at: <https://www.epilepsy.org.au/about-epilepsy/understanding-epilepsy>.

Epilepsy Action Australia, 2023. What do you wish people knew about epilepsy? Available at: <https://www.epilepsy.org.au/about-epilepsy/what-do-you-wish-people-knew-about-epilepsy>.

Fowler, G., 2019. *Pfenninger & Fowler's procedures for primary care*, 4th ed. Elsevier, US.

Hall, H., Glew. P., Rhodes, J., 2022. *Fundamentals of nursing and midwifery: A person-centred approach to care*, 4th ed. Lippincott Williams & Wilkins, North Ryde.

Hall, J.E., Hall, M.E., 2021. *Guyton and Hall textbook of medical physiology*, 14th ed. Elsevier Inc., St. Louis.

Healthdirect Meningitis 2023. Available at: <https://www.healthdirect.gov.au/meningitis>.

Huntington's NSW, 2020. What is Huntington's disease (HD)? Available at: <https://huntingtonsnswact.org.au>.

Jain, S., Iverson, L., 2023. Glasgow coma scale. National Library of Medicine.

LeMone, P., Bauldoff, G., Gubrud-Howe, P., et al., 2020. *Medical–surgical nursing: Critical thinking for person-centred care*, 4th ed. Pearson, Melbourne.

Leonard, P.C., 2020. *Quick & easy medical terminology*, 9th ed. Elsevier, St Louis.

Macquarie University, Department of Psychology, nd. The PTA Protocol. Available at: <https://www.mq.edu.au/about/about-the-university/our-faculties/medicine-and-health-sciences/departments-and-centres/department-of-psychology/the-pta-protocol>.

Marieb, E., Keller, S., 2021. *Essentials of human anatomy and physiology*, 13th ed. Pearson, London.

Mayo Clinic, 2023. Vasovagal syncope. Available at: <http://www.mayoclinic.org/diseases-conditions/vasovagal-syncope/basics/definition/con-20026900>.

Medtronic, 2023. About hydrocephalus. Available at: <https://www.medtronic.com/au-en/patients/conditions/hydrocephalus.htmlMND>.

MND Australia, 2024a. About MND. Available at: <https://www.mndaustralia.org.au/mnd-connect/what-is-mnd>.

MND Australia, 2024b. What is motor neurone disease? Available at: <https://www.mndaustralia.org.au/mnd-connect/what-is-mnd/what-is-motor-neurone-disease-mnd>.

MS Australia, 2023. What is multiple sclerosis (MS)? Available at: <https://www.msaustralia.org.au/what-is-multiple-sclerosis-ms>.

Muscular Dystrophy Foundation, 2022. What is MD? Available at: <https://mdaustralia.org.au/what-is-md>.

National Institute of Neurological Disorders and Stroke, 2023. NINDS Anencephaly. Available at: <https://www.ninds.nih.gov/health-information/disorders/anencephaly?search-term=cephalic>.

National Institute of Neurological Disorders and Stroke, 2023a. Bell's palsy. Available at: <https://www.ninds.nih.gov/health-information/disorders/bells-palsy?search-term=bells>.

National Institute of Neurological Disorders and Stroke, 2023b. Guillain-Barré syndrome. Available at: <https://www.ninds.nih.gov/health-information/disorders/guillain-barre-syndrome?search-term=guillian%20barre>.

National Institute of Neurological Disorders and Stroke, 2023c. Headache. Available at: <https://www.ninds.nih.gov/health-information/disorders/headache?search-term=headache>.

National Institute of Neurological Disorders and Stroke, 2023d. Meningitis. Available at: <https://www.ninds.nih.gov/health-information/disorders/meningitis?search-term=meningitis>.

National Institute of Neurological Disorders and Stroke, 2023e. Myasthenia gravis. Available at: <https://www.ninds.nih.gov/health-information/disorders/myasthenia-gravis?search-term=myasthenia>.

National Institute of Neurological Disorders and Stroke, 2023f. Encephalitis. Available at: <https://www.ninds.nih.gov/health-information/disorders/encephalitis>.

Nursing and Midwifery Board of Australia (NMBA), 2020. Decision-making framework for nursing and midwifery. Available at: <https://www.nursingmidwiferyboard.gov.au/Codes-Guidelines-Statements/Frameworks.aspx>.

Patton, K.T., Thibodeau G.A., 2018. *The human body in health & disease*, 7th ed. Elsevier Inc., St. Louis.

Patton, K., Thibodeau, G., Hutton, A., 2019. *Anatomy & physiology*, Adapted international edition. Elsevier, US.

Patton, K., Thibodeau, G., 2019. *Structure & function of the body*, 16th ed. Elsevier, US.

Patton, K.T., Bell, F.B., Thompson, T., Williamson, P.L., 2024. *The human body in health & disease*, 8th ed. Elsevier Inc., St. Louis.

Rebeiro, G., Wilson, D., Fuller, S., 2021. *Fundamentals of nursing: Clinical skills workbook*, 4th ed. Elsevier, Chatswood.

Rollins, J.H., Long, B.W., Curtis, T., 2023. *Merrill's atlas of radiographic positioning and procedures*, 15th ed. Elsevier Inc., Mosby.

Scope, 2015. Westmead post-traumatic amnesia (PTA) scale. Available at: <http://www.scopevic.org.au/wp-content/uploads/2015/05/19.WestmeadPTA.pdf>.

Spinal Cord Injuries Australia, 2023a. Recent spinal cord injury: What to expect. Available at: <https://scia.org.au/resource-hub/?keys=recent-spinal-cord-injury-what-to-expect>.

Spinal Cord Injuries Australia, 2023b. Daily living skills. Available at: <https://scia.org.au/resource-hub/?keys=daily-living-skillsSpinal Cord Injuries Australia, 2023c. Sexuality and fertility. Available at: <https://scia.org.au/health-and-wellbeing/sexuality-and-fertility>.

Spinal Cord Injuries Australia, 2023c. Sexuality and fertility. Available at: <https://scia.org.au/health-and-wellbeing/sexuality-and-fertility>.

Spinal Cord Injuries Australia, 2023d. What to expect. Available at: <https://scia.org.au/what-to-expect>.

Stein, L.N.M., Hollen, C.J., 2024. *Concept-based clinical nursing skills*, 2nd ed. Elsevier Inc., St. Louis.

Stroke Foundation, 2023a. Haemorrhagic stroke. Available at: <https://strokefoundation.org.au/about-stroke/learn/what-is-a-stroke/haemorrhagic-stroke-bleed-in-the-brain>.

Stroke Foundation, 2023b. Living clinical guidelines for stroke management. Available at: <https://informme.org.au/guidelines/living-clinical-guidelines-for-stroke-management>.

Stroke Recovery Association NSW, 2023a. Daily living and social aspects. Available at: <https://strokensw.org.au/about-stroke/living-well-after-stroke/daily-living>.

Stroke Recovery Association NSW, 2023b. Going home – What now? Available at: <https://strokensw.org.au/about-stroke/living-well-after-stroke/going-home-what-now>.

Stroke Recovery Association NSW, 2023c. Rehabilitation. Available at: <https://strokensw.org.au/about-stroke/recovery/rehibilitation>.

Stroke Recovery Association NSW, 2023d. Types of treatment. Available at: <https://strokensw.org.au/about-stroke/initial-stroke-what-now/treatment>.

Wilson, S.F., Giddens, J.F., 2020. *Health assessment for nursing practice*, 7th ed. Elsevier, St Louis.

Recommended Reading

Assistive Technology Australia, 2020. What is assistive technology? Available at: <https://at-aust.org/home/assistive_technology/assistive_technology

Australian Commission on Safety and Quality in Health Care, (ACSQHC), 2021. Preventing and controlling healthcare-associated infection. Available at: <https://www.safetyandquality.gov.au/publications-and-resources/resource-library/national-safety-and-quality-health-service-standards-second-edition

Australian Commission on Safety and Quality in Health Care, 2021. NSQHS Standards user guide for health service organisations providing care for patients with cognitive impairment or at risk of delirium. Available at: <https://www.safetyandquality.gov.au/publications-and-resources/resource-library/nsqhs-standards-user-guide-health-service-organisations-providing-care-patients>.

Cancer Council Australia, 2023. Brain cancer. Available at: <http://www.cancer.org.au/about-cancer/types-of-cancer/brain-cancer.html>.

Parkinson's Australia, 2022. About Parkinson's. Available at: <https://www.parkinsons.org.au/about-parkinsonscognitive-impairment-or-risk-delirium>.

Stroke Foundation, 2023. Ischaemic stroke. Available at: <https://strokefoundation.org.au/about-stroke/learn/what-is-a-stroke/ischaemic-stroke-blocked-artery>.

Stroke Foundation, 2023. Haemorrhagic stroke: Available at: <https://strokefoundation.org.au/about-stroke/learn/what-is-a-stroke/haemorrhagic-stroke-bleed-in-the-brain>.

Stroke Foundation, 2023. Living clinical guidelines for stroke management. Available at: <https://informme.org.au/guidelines/living-clinical-guidelines-for-stroke-management>.

Online Resources

Cerebral Palsy Alliance. Signs and symptoms of cerebral palsy: <https://www.cerebralpalsy.org.au/what-is-cerebral-palsy/signs-and-symptoms-of-cp>.

NSW Health. Adult neurological observation chart: <http://www.aci.health.nsw.gov.au/__data/assets/pdf_file/0018/201753/AdultChartEdPackage.pdf>.

CHAPTER

36

Endocrine health

Christine Standley

Key Terms

acromegaly
adrenal glands
adrenaline
adrenocorticotrophic hormone (ACTH)
aldosterone
antidiuretic hormone (ADH)
calcitonin
congenital adrenal hyperplasia (CAH)
corticosteroids
cretinism
diabetes insipidus (DI)
diabetic nephropathy
diabetic retinopathy
euglycaemia
exophthalmos
follicle stimulating hormone (FSH)
gender dysphoria (gender identity disorder)
gestational diabetes mellitus (GDM)
glucagon
glucocorticoids
gonadocorticoids
growth hormone (GH)
homeostasis
hormone
hyperadrenalism
hyperglycaemia
hypergonadism
hypersecretion
hyperthyroidism
hypoglycaemia
hypogonadism
hypopituitarism
hyposecretion
hypothalamus
hypothyroidism
insulin
latent autoimmune diabetes in adults (LADA)
luteinising hormone (LH)
mature onset diabetes of the young (MODY)
melatonin
mineralocorticoids
myxoedema coma
negative feedback
noradrenaline
oestrogen
oxytocin
pancreas
pancreatic islets (islets of Langerhans)
parathyroid gland
phaeochromocytoma
pineal gland
pituitary gland
progesterone
prolactin (PRL)
syndrome of inappropriate anti diuretic hormone (SIADH)
testosterone
thymosin
thymus gland
thyroid gland
thyroid hormones—triiodothyronine (T3) & thyroxine (T4)
thyroid stimulating hormone (TSH)
thyrotoxicosis
type 1 diabetes mellitus (T1DM)
type 2 diabetes mellitus (T2DM)

Learning Outcomes

At the completion of this chapter and with further reading, learners should be able to:

- Define the key terms.
- Describe the location and basic anatomy of each endocrine gland including factors promoting hormone synthesis and release.
- Define and explain the actions of endocrine hormones.
- Identify and describe the pathophysiology of disorders associated with the endocrine system.
- Identify the signs and symptoms of each endocrine disorder.
- Explain the rationale behind each diagnostic test utilised to assess endocrine health.
- Assist in the planning and implementation of nursing care for the individual with an endocrine disorder.

CHAPTER FOCUS

The endocrine system consists of several small glands that secrete hormones. Hormones act like chemical messengers that promote different physiological processes such as metabolism, growth, fluid balance and reproduction. Overproduction or underproduction of hormones can have widespread effects on other systems in the body. An understanding of hormone function and the effects of hormone imbalances provide healthcare professionals the ability to identify and care for individuals with endocrine disorders (Crawford 2023).

LIVED EXPERIENCE

For as long as I can remember, I'd always been a problem sleeper. It was not uncommon for me to average only 4–5 hours of broken sleep each night. I always felt hot and hungry, yet I was thin no matter how much I ate. In my early teens, I could easily raise a sweat especially when excited or being even mildly active. For this reason, I avoided all sports except swimming. I would still sweat but being in the water, no-one would notice. In my final year of secondary college, my greatest concern was not my end of year exams but rather the fact that I hadn't yet menstruated. While my girlfriends complained of pelvic pain and swollen breasts, I was secretly envious and wondered if, in fact, I was female at all.

Andrea, primary school teacher

I knew that Andrea hadn't got her period, before we married. She'd told me that she'd undergone some tests and would likely need to take some medication to help her fall pregnant. She rarely slept and would often sleep on the couch rather than disturb me with her frequent tossing and turning in bed. She also never liked to cuddle saying that she felt too hot and would begin to sweat if I was anywhere near her. What really worried me was that she seemed to get irritated over minor issues to the point where she would begin to tremble and become short of breath since she couldn't get her words out quick enough. When we finally decided to begin our family, we went to see a GP who confirmed that Andrea's thyroid gland was overactive and was the cause of all her symptoms. Within 2 weeks, Andrea had her thyroid surgically removed, was prescribed thyroid replacement hormone and now all her symptoms seem to have disappeared. She no longer feels hot all the time, does not appear overly stressed or agitated and has 6–8 hours of uninterrupted sleep per night. Oh, and we're now the proud parents of two young children.

Matthew, Andrea's partner of 15 years

INTRODUCTION

Endocrine glands and hormones

The endocrine system is a cellular communication system involving the secretion of hormones by eight major endocrine glands. **Hormones** are chemical messengers that regulate, integrate and direct cellular activities. Once secreted, they are transported through the blood to a target organ where they stimulate specialised cellular activity (Waugh & Grant 2022). Figure 36.1 illustrates the location of the eight major endocrine glands. Hormones produced by endocrine glands are either steroids or proteins that can only act on target cells with special receptors unique to each hormone. Each hormone that binds to its unique receptor initiates a response that may take minutes to days. This is a relatively slow process in comparison to the nervous system, where the effects of neurotransmitters can incite a response in milliseconds (Crawford 2023).

The effects of some hormones are diverse, while others are tissue specific. Major body functions controlled by the endocrine system are reproduction; growth and development; maintenance of body fluids and electrolytes; maintenance of blood nutrients; and cellular metabolism and energy regulation (Crawford 2023). Most of our hormones are continuously secreted at a rate determined by the degree of glandular stimulation controlling their release. This may be enhanced or depressed by blood-borne stimuli, neural or nervous input, or other hormones. Some hormones exert control over other endocrine glands and other hormones by influencing their action, metabolism, synthesis and transport. The activation or inhibition of hormone production relies on **negative feedback** to maintain **homeostasis**. Disruption of the body's homeostasis (i.e. the body's ability to maintain stable, internal, physiological functioning) presents as hormonal imbalances and endocrine pathologies (Waugh & Grant 2022). Figure 36.2 identifies the endocrine glands, the hormones they produce, their target cells or organs and hormonal actions.

The pituitary gland

The **pituitary gland**, or hypophysis, is approximately the size of a pea. It is positioned at the base of the brain in the sella turcica, a depression in the sphenoid bone. The pituitary gland is connected to the **hypothalamus** via a stalk-like structure called the infundibulum that contains both blood vessels and nervous tissue. The pituitary gland is comprised of two lobes—the anterior

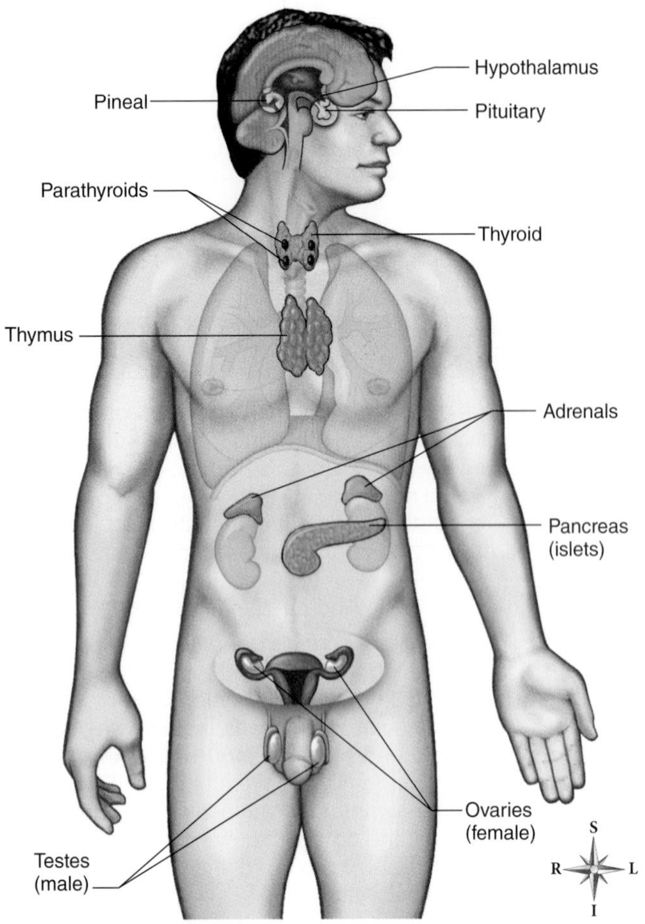

Figure 36.1 Location of the major endocrine glands
(Harding et al 2023)

lobe or adenohypophysis, which is made up of glandular tissue, and the posterior lobe or neurohypophysis, which is made up of neural tissue. The activity of the anterior lobe is controlled by releasing factors secreted by the hypothalamus. The hypothalamus instructs the anterior pituitary to increase or inhibit the production of hormones. On the contrary, the posterior pituitary does not produce any hormones but rather releases or stores specific hormones (ADH and oxytocin) under hypothalamic control. A series of complex, regulatory, glandular functions are controlled by the pituitary gland and therefore the pituitary is often referred to as the 'master' gland' (Figure 36.3) (Crawford 2023).

The anterior lobe of the pituitary gland, or adenohypophysis, produces and releases the following hormones into the bloodstream:

- **Growth hormone (GH)** is a metabolic hormone concerned with body growth, particularly that of skeletal muscles and long bones.
- **Thyroid stimulating hormone (TSH)** is responsible for controlling the growth and activity of the thyroid gland.
- **Adrenocorticotrophic hormone (ACTH)** reacts with receptor sites on the adrenal cortex to stimulate the secretion of cortical hormones, primarily cortisol.
- **Prolactin (PRL)**, also referred to as lactogenic hormone, stimulates the female mammary glands to secrete milk after the birth of a baby.

(Crawford 2023)

The following gonadotrophic hormones control the growth, development and function of the ovaries and testes.

- **Follicle stimulating hormone (FSH)** stimulates the maturation of the ovarian follicle and ovum and the secretion of oestrogen in females, and in males stimulate the seminiferous tubules to produce sperm.
- **Luteinising hormone (LH)** triggers ovulation and stimulates ovarian production of oestrogen and progesterone (the corpus luteum which forms after ovulation secretes progesterone) in females, and stimulates the testes to secrete testosterone in males.

(Crawford 2023)

The posterior lobe of the pituitary gland stores and releases two hormones, which are synthesised in under hypothalamic control:

- **Oxytocin** stimulates contraction of the uterus, initiates childbirth and causes the ducts of the mammary glands to contract and expel breast milk.
- **Antidiuretic hormone (ADH)** stimulates the kidney tubules to reabsorb water, resulting in decreased excretion of water in the urine.

(Crawford 2023)

TSH, ACTH, FSH and LH are trophic hormones that affect the activity and secretion of hormones from other endocrine glands. To this effect, changes in the pituitary gland's function or health have widespread consequences. For example, if the anterior pituitary does not produce sufficient TSH, as which occurs in the autoimmune condition **Hashimoto's disease**, the thyroid gland will not produce sufficient thyroid hormones and the person will develop symptoms of **hypothyroidism**. If left untreated, hypothyroidism can escalate to a life-threatening condition known as **myxoedema coma** (Norman 2022; Waugh & Grant 2022).

The pineal gland

The **pineal gland**, also called pineal body or epiphysis cerebri, is a small cone-shaped structure situated in the roof of the third ventricle of the brain The pineal gland is made up of neurological cells and specialised secretory cells (pinealocytes). These cells produce a hormone called **melatonin** that is secreted directly into the cerebrospinal fluid and transported to the blood. Melatonin controls our 'body clock' and is thought to establish our sleep patterns (Crawford 2023). A rare neoplasm of the pineal gland (pinealoma) may obstruct the flow of cerebrospinal fluid causing hydrocephalus, or fluid in the brain (Favero et al 2021).

The thymus

The **thymus gland** is positioned in the chest behind the sternum. It is large in infants and children, reaching its

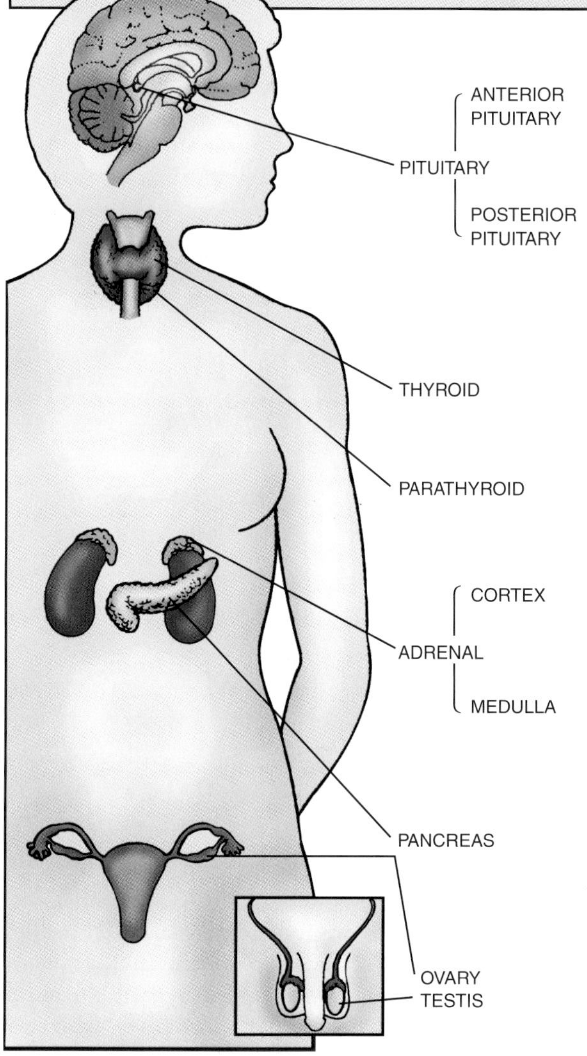

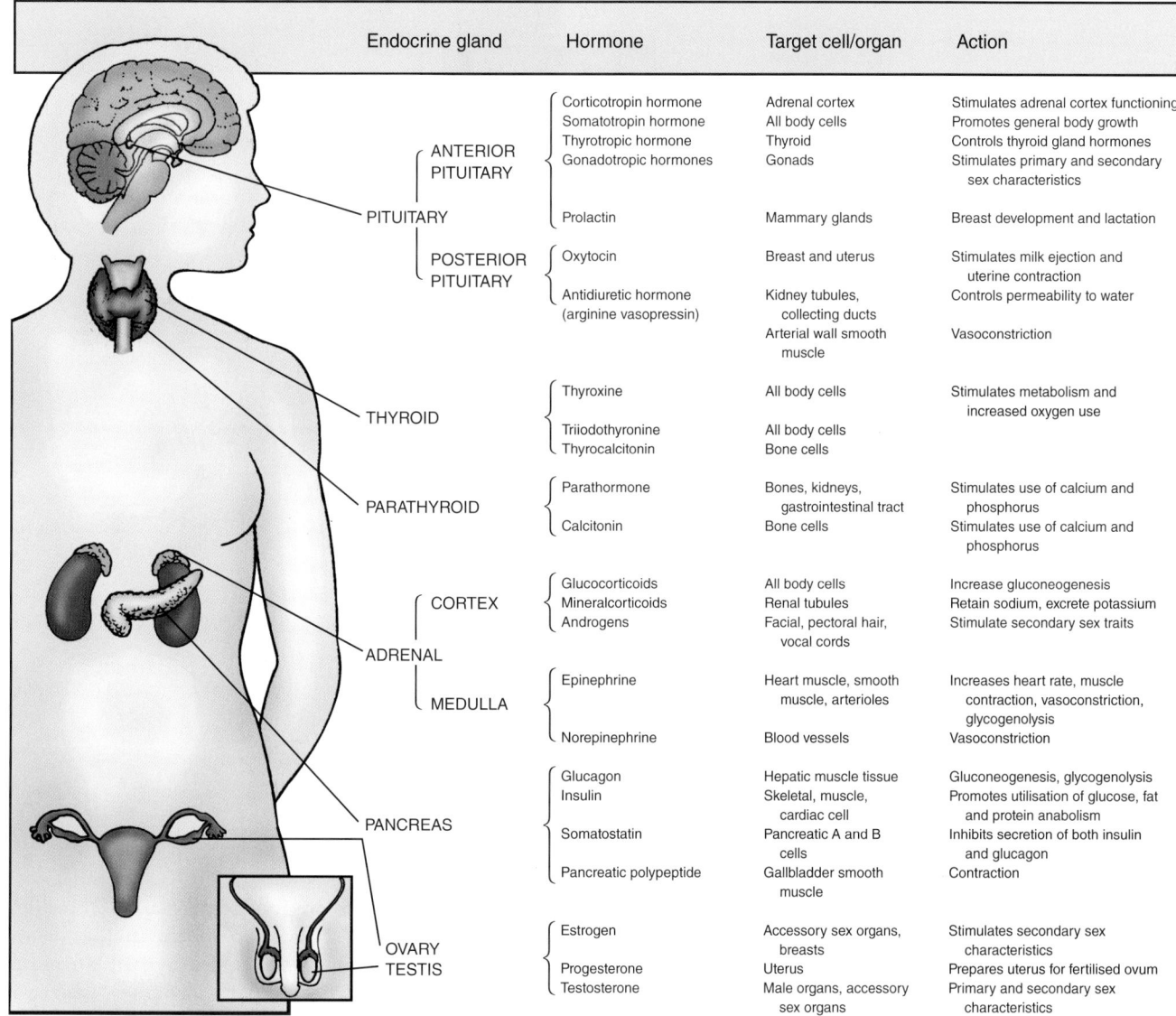

Endocrine gland	Hormone	Target cell/organ	Action
PITUITARY – ANTERIOR PITUITARY	Corticotropin hormone	Adrenal cortex	Stimulates adrenal cortex functioning
	Somatotropin hormone	All body cells	Promotes general body growth
	Thyrotropic hormone	Thyroid	Controls thyroid gland hormones
	Gonadotropic hormones	Gonads	Stimulates primary and secondary sex characteristics
	Prolactin	Mammary glands	Breast development and lactation
PITUITARY – POSTERIOR PITUITARY	Oxytocin	Breast and uterus	Stimulates milk ejection and uterine contraction
	Antidiuretic hormone (arginine vasopressin)	Kidney tubules, collecting ducts	Controls permeability to water
		Arterial wall smooth muscle	Vasoconstriction
THYROID	Thyroxine	All body cells	Stimulates metabolism and increased oxygen use
	Triiodothyronine	All body cells	
	Thyrocalcitonin	Bone cells	
PARATHYROID	Parathormone	Bones, kidneys, gastrointestinal tract	Stimulates use of calcium and phosphorus
	Calcitonin	Bone cells	Stimulates use of calcium and phosphorus
ADRENAL – CORTEX	Glucocorticoids	All body cells	Increase gluconeogenesis
	Mineralcorticoids	Renal tubules	Retain sodium, excrete potassium
	Androgens	Facial, pectoral hair, vocal cords	Stimulate secondary sex traits
ADRENAL – MEDULLA	Epinephrine	Heart muscle, smooth muscle, arterioles	Increases heart rate, muscle contraction, vasoconstriction, glycogenolysis
	Norepinephrine	Blood vessels	Vasoconstriction
PANCREAS	Glucagon	Hepatic muscle tissue	Gluconeogenesis, glycogenolysis
	Insulin	Skeletal, muscle, cardiac cell	Promotes utilisation of glucose, fat and protein anabolism
	Somatostatin	Pancreatic A and B cells	Inhibits secretion of both insulin and glucagon
	Pancreatic polypeptide	Gallbladder smooth muscle	Contraction
OVARY TESTIS	Estrogen	Accessory sex organs, breasts	Stimulates secondary sex characteristics
	Progesterone	Uterus	Prepares uterus for fertilised ovum
	Testosterone	Male organs, accessory sex organs	Primary and secondary sex characteristics

Figure 36.2 Location of endocrine glands with the hormones they produce, target cells or organs, and hormonal actions
(Lough 2024)

maximum size at puberty, then decreasing in size and function throughout adulthood (Waugh & Grant 2022). The gland produces the hormone **thymosin**, which promotes the growth of lymphoid tissue in the body and aids in the body's immune response. While endocrine dysfunction of the thymus gland is uncommon, congenital thymic hypoplasia results in defective cellular immunity making the individual more susceptible to infections (Crawford 2023).

The thyroid gland

The **thyroid gland** lies in the front of the neck, just inferior to the larynx, and consists of two lateral lobes on either side of the trachea. The lobes are joined by a central mass called the isthmus, which lies anteriorly across the trachea. It is highly vascular, which presents a high risk of bleeding when surgically removed. The thyroid gland is the largest pure endocrine gland in the body and produces two main hormones: **thyroid hormone** and **calcitonin** (Crawford 2023).

Thyroid hormone is comprised of two iodine-containing amine hormones: **thyroxine (T4)**, making up 95% of total thyroid hormone, and **triiodothyroxine (T3)**, making up 5% of thyroid hormone. Thyroid hormones contain large quantities of iodine, which is derived from an individual's diet, stored in the thyroid gland and simultaneously produced by the follicles of the thyroid gland. When iodine levels are low, the thyroid is unable to

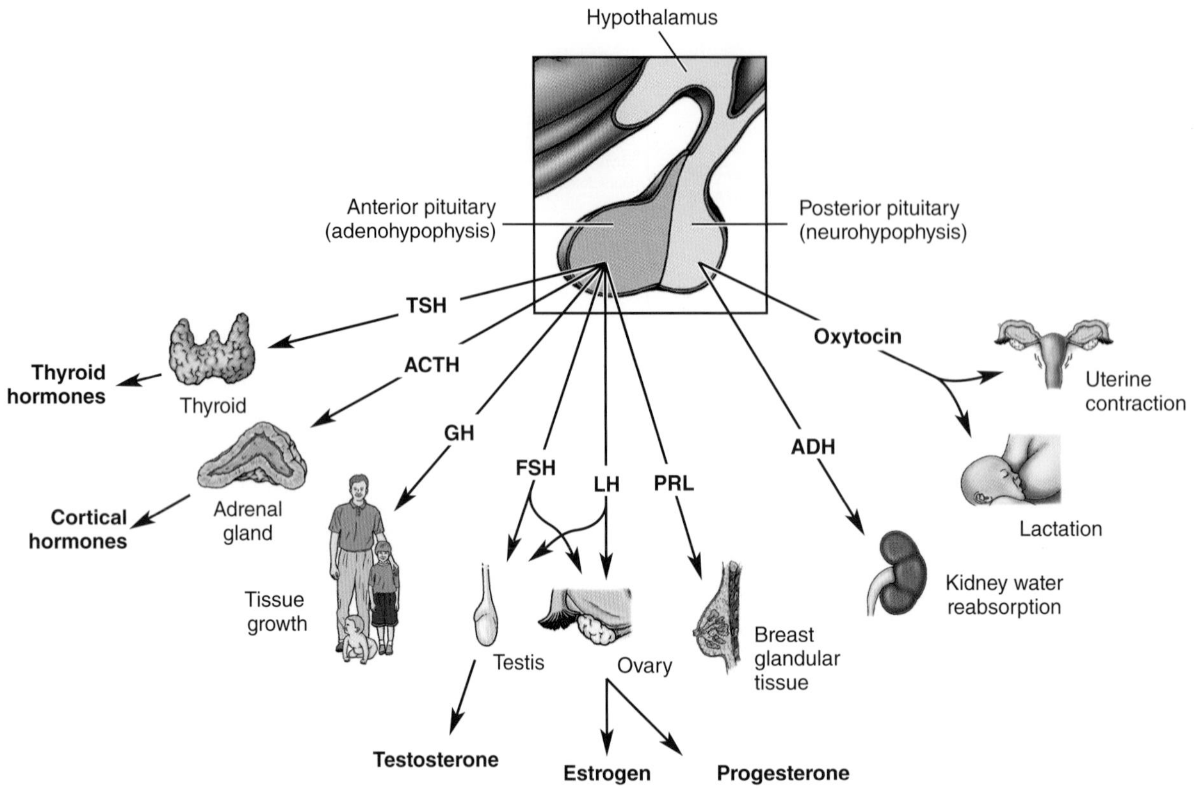

Figure 36.3 The pituitary gland, pituitary hormones and target organs
(Modified from Herlihy, B., Maebius, N.K., 2007. The human body in health and illness, *3rd ed. Saunders, St Louis)*

manufacture thyroid hormone. Thyroid hormone largely controls cellular metabolism, growth and development and therefore affects virtually every cell in the human body. Thyroid hormones influence:

- growth and physical development
- neural and mental development
- the rate at which nutrients are metabolised in the body (metabolic rate)
- body temperature and heart rate
- menstruation and fertility
- sleep.

(Crawford 2023; National Institute of Diabetes and Digestive and Kidney Diseases [NIDDK] 2021b)

Calcitonin, also referred to as thyrocalcitonin, is produced by the parafollicular cells (C cells) of the thyroid gland. Calcitonin decreases blood calcium levels by inhibiting the action of osteoclasts in breaking down bone and decreasing the amount of calcium reabsorbed in the kidneys. In humans, the role of calcitonin is relatively insignificant. For example, individuals who have had thyroid surgery or a thyroidectomy are not adversely affected by the loss of calcitonin secretion. However, individuals with skeletal disorders such as **Paget's disease** (a bone disease where the old bone tissue is replaced with fragile, misshapen new bone tissue) may be prescribed calcitonin to reduce bone turnover and ease bone pain (Parthasarathy 2020; Waugh & Grant 2022).

The parathyroid glands

The **parathyroid glands** are four small glands embedded in the posterior surface of each lobe of the thyroid gland. The parathyroid glands produce **parathyroid hormone (PTH)**, also referred to as parathormone, which is primarily responsible for the regulation of blood calcium and phosphate levels. Parathormone release is triggered by falling blood calcium levels and is antagonistic to calcitonin. Parathormone raises the blood calcium levels by stimulating the release of calcium and phosphate from bones. PTH also enhances the reabsorption of calcium, promotes the excretion of phosphate in the urine and promotes renal activation of vitamin D which assists in calcium absorption in the gut (Waugh & Grant 2022).

The pancreas

The **pancreas** is a large gland located behind the stomach and surrounded by the spleen, liver and small intestine (see Chapter 32). It is approximately 15 cm long and is divided into a head, body and tail. The pancreas has two main functions. It is an enzyme secreting exocrine gland that produces and secretes digestive enzymes into the small intestine, and it also functions as an endocrine gland producing and releasing the hormones **insulin** and **glucagon** which help regulate blood glucose levels (Crawford 2023; Miller 2022). Scattered within the pancreas are small clusters of endocrine cells known as **pancreatic islets** or **islets of Langerhans**. The islet's beta (β) cells produce the hormone insulin, and the alpha (α) cells produce the hormone glucagon. Insulin and glucagon are antagonistic but work together to maintain optimal blood glucose levels (Crawford 2023).

The roles of insulin and glucagon in blood glucose regulation are illustrated in Figure 36.4.

When the hypothalamus detects a rise in the blood sugar level, it signals the pancreatic beta (β) cells to produce insulin. Insulin lowers blood glucose by increasing the uptake of glucose into cells for cellular metabolism. Insulin is essential for cellular metabolism and, without it, cells would be unable to access glucose—their preferred source of energy. Insulin also promotes the storage of glucose as glycogen in the liver, muscle and adipose cells, and blocks the conversion of the liver's glycogen stores back into glucose (glycogenolysis) thus preventing the blood sugar from becoming too high (Miller 2022).

In contrast, glucagon is released in response to decreasing blood glucose and prevents the blood glucose level from becoming too low. Glucagon raises blood glucose levels by stimulating the breakdown and reconversion of the stored glycogen back into glucose (glycogenolysis) and inhibits glycogen synthesis and the storage of glucose in the liver (Miller 2022).

The adrenal glands

The paired **adrenal glands** sit one on top of each kidney. Each gland is surrounded by a capsule comprised of an outer cortex and an inner medulla. The cortex and medulla synthesise different hormones (Crawford 2023).

The adrenal cortex

The cortex is divided structurally and functionally into three zones. Each zone is responsible for the secretion of a class of steroid hormones, known as **corticosteroids**. The adrenal cortex, and therefore the production of corticosteroids,

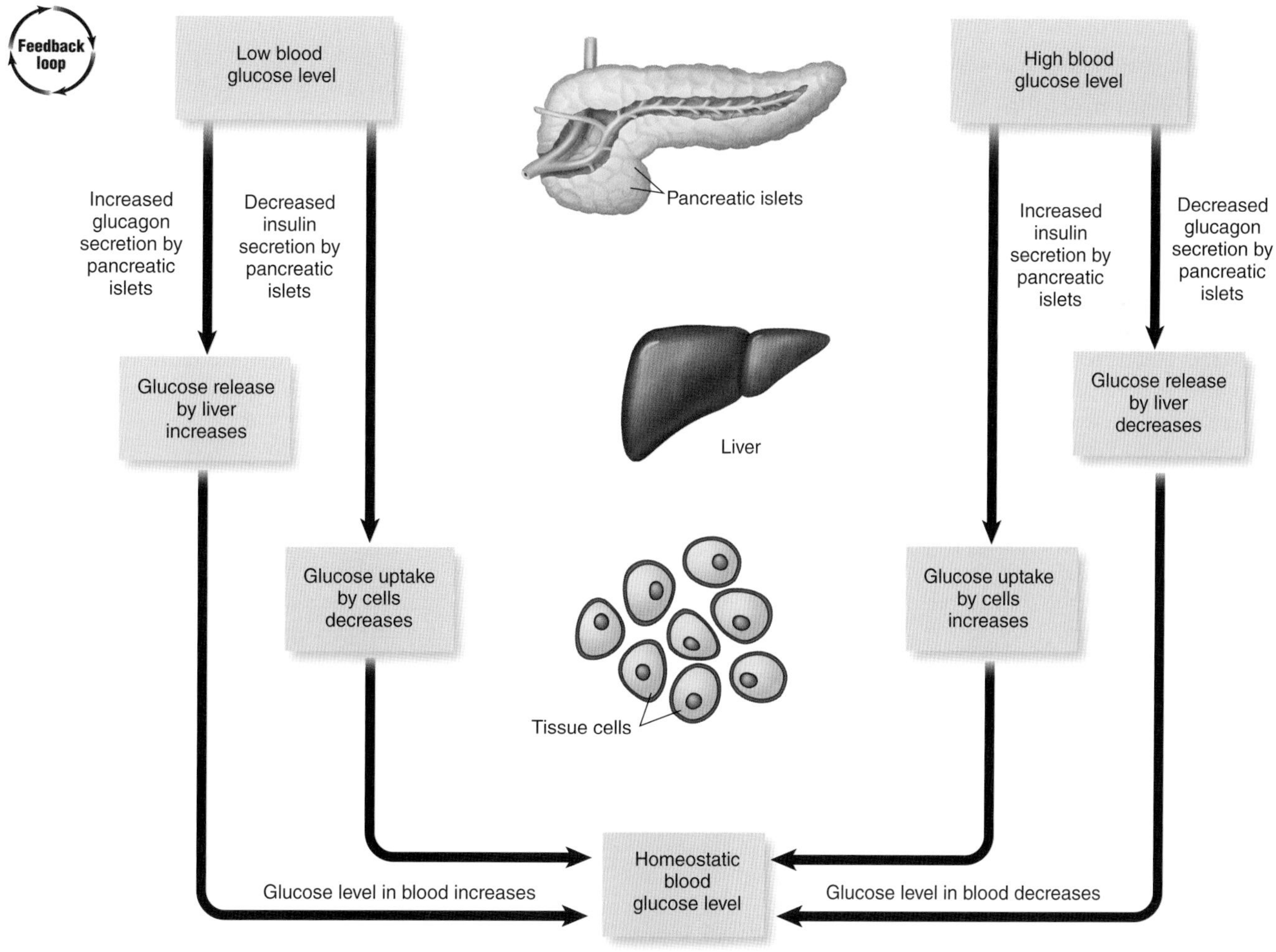

Figure 36.4 Regulation of blood glucose levels—insulin and glucagon
(Williamson et al 2022)

are under the influence of ACTH released by the anterior pituitary gland (Waugh & Grant 2022).

The classes of corticosteroid hormones synthesised and released by the adrenal cortex are as follows:

- **Mineralocorticoids**: Primarily **aldosterone**, which promotes the reabsorption of sodium ions and the elimination of potassium ions in the kidneys. Aldosterone regulates both water and electrolyte balance in the body.
- **Glucocorticoids**: Include cortisone, hydrocortisone (cortisol) and corticosterone promote the following:
  - protein, fat and carbohydrate metabolism
  - the body's response to stress
  - inhibition of inflammatory and immune responses
  - enhancement of the effects of catecholamines, TH and GH.
- **Gonadocorticoids**: (sex hormones—androgens and oestrogens) are concerned with the development of secondary sexual characteristics and the function of the reproductive organs. Both male and female hormones are produced by the adrenal cortex, regardless of gender. These gonadocorticoids released by the adrenal cortex are relatively weak and in low concentration compared with the hormones released by the gonads.

(Banasik 2022)

The adrenal medulla

The medulla, or inner portion of the adrenal glands, produces **adrenaline** and **noradrenaline** which are both hormones and neurotransmitters and very similar in action. Adrenaline (also referred to as epinephrine) and noradrenaline (also referred to as norepinephrine) are also known as catecholamines. When the medulla is stimulated by neurons of the sympathetic nervous system, both adrenaline and noradrenaline are released into the bloodstream (Crawford 2023). The physiological responses to adrenaline and noradrenaline include:

- cardiac and skeletal vasodilation
- visceral and dermal vasoconstriction
- increase in heart rate, cardiac contractility and blood pressure
- dilation of the bronchial tubes
- reduction of peristalsis in the digestive system
- stimulation of the liver to release more glucose into the bloodstream
- dilation of the pupils
- an increase in the metabolic rate.

Adrenaline and noradrenaline prepare the body for 'fight or flight'. They are released when an individual feels threatened or experiences strong emotions such as fear, anger or excitement, and helps the body to cope with stress (Banasik 2022; Crawford 2023).

The gonads

The female gonads are the ovaries, and the male gonads are the testes (see Chapter 37). The gonads produce sex hormones identical to those produced by the adrenal cortex, but in greater concentrations and potency. During and after puberty, the gonads assume a major role in reproductive hormone production (Banasik 2022).

Hormones produced by the ovaries are oestrogens and progesterone. In females, **oestrogens** influence the development of the reproductive organs and the secondary sexual characteristics such as changes in height and body shape. Oestrogen also promotes oogenesis (formation of the egg or ovum) and ovulation and stimulates the lining of the uterus to thicken in preparation for a fertilised ovum to develop. In the later stages, **progesterone** also promotes the thickening of the uterine lining, inhibits uterine contraction and allows implantation of the fertilised ovum (Banasik 2022; Crawford 2023).

The testes produce the androgen **testosterone**, which stimulates the development of male characteristics and the growth and function of the reproductive organs. Testosterone and androgens generally masculinise the human body, irrespective of gonadal sex (Crawford 2023).

Gender dysphoria

Gender dysphoria (or **gender identity disorder**) is characterised by an overwhelming and distressing feeling that an individual had the wrong gender assigned to them at birth, lasting for at least 6 months. Individuals with gender dysphoria may want to be accepted as a member of the opposite sex and may go as far as making changes to their body through surgery and hormone treatment. Presently, the underlying cause of gender identity disorder is unknown. However, in animals, it is known that there are critical periods of time during pregnancy where changes in the amount of oestrogen and testosterone in the developing animal can permanently alter masculine or feminine behaviour. Further research is needed to discover if similar influences are involved in human gender identity disorder. People with gender dysphoria have a normal body appearance and normal hormone levels for their birth gender (Kwong 2023).

It is important for nurses to recognise the difference between gender dysphoria and disorders of sexual development. In gender dysphoria, the gender a person identifies with does not match the gender of their sex at birth. In disorders of sexual development, there is a mismatch between the appearance of the person's genitals and their sex chromosomes (e.g. androgen insensitivity syndrome) (Vora & Srinivasan 2020). The criteria for gender reassignment surgery includes living full time as a person of the opposite gender for a minimum of 1 year, but more often 2 years (Kwong 2023).

ENDOCRINE DISORDERS

Disorders of the pituitary gland

Abnormalities of the pituitary gland are often associated with hypersecretion or hyposecretion of its hormones. Diseases of the pituitary gland, diseases of the hypothalamus, radiation

LIVED EXPERIENCE

The youngest daughter of three, I always hated having my hair tied back in a long ponytail and being dressed in frilly, pink dresses. While my sisters loved playing with their Barbie dolls, I preferred to play in the dirt with my toy dinosaurs. Even as young as four, I remember thinking that I was really a boy and couldn't wait until my 'willy' would grow. The name I was given at birth was Samantha, but I asked all my family and friends to call me Sam for as long as I can remember. In my pre-teen years, Dad didn't seem to mind that I preferred to be dressed in baggy sportswear and have my hair short, but Mum hated it. As I reached puberty, my breasts began to grow and at 13 years I got my period. I was absolutely disgusted and consumed by anxiety. I began to wear tight singlets underneath my t-shirts to hide my developing breasts and cried for 1 week every month when I began to bleed. I couldn't understand why I hated being a girl so much and why I wanted to be treated as the boy I really was. I became so depressed that, unbeknown to my family, I stopped going to school and began to self-mutilate. I even tried to cut my breasts off with a razor blade, but the pain was unbearable. Despite all of this, my parents never seemed to notice that I was so distressed. If they did, they never showed it. Not even my sisters said anything. By 17, it got so bad that I wanted to kill myself. I planned my suicide carefully and even wrote a 'goodbye' letter to my family apologising for any disappointment or pain my suicide might cause. My eldest sister found my letter and confronted me. Had she not done so, I probably wouldn't be here today. She raced me straight to a GP who referred me to a psychologist where my journey towards becoming the man I always was, began. Four years, hormone therapy and multiple surgeries later, I have a deeper voice, full beard, developed muscles and am happily living with my partner, Sally. My family have come to accept me but, to date, my grandfather refuses to even be in my company.

Sam, apprentice carpenter

therapy to the head or neck, trauma or local tumours can interfere with pituitary function and, consequently, the function of other trophic glands like the thyroid, adrenals and gonads. In other words, pituitary problems potentially affect the homeostasis of other hormones, and the effects can be widespread. Individuals with anterior pituitary disorders require professional healthcare to assist them in coping with the physical and emotional changes and help prevent complications involving other organs (Crawford 2023). (Major endocrine disorders are summarised in Table 36.1.)

Hyperfunction of the pituitary gland commonly results from a tumour. Pituitary tumours can create pressure on cerebral structures and cause neurological symptoms such as severe headaches and visual disturbances. In turn, a subsequent excessive secretion of pituitary hormones will result in hyperfunction in the target organs (Crawford 2023). In adults, **hypersecretion** of the anterior pituitary hormones ACTH and GH, results in **Cushing's syndrome** and **acromegaly**, respectively. In females, hypersecretion of prolactin can cause anovulation and failure to lactate. Diseases of the posterior pituitary are rare. Hypersecretion of the posterior pituitary hormone ADH occurs in a condition called **syndrome of inappropriate anti diuretic hormone (SIADH)** (Khardori et al 2022).

Gigantism

Disorders causing hypersecretion of GH are chronic and progressive. These conditions are marked by hormonal dysfunction and skeletal overgrowth, which most commonly appear in two disorders: **gigantism** and acromegaly. Hypersecretion of GH in childhood results in gigantism and begins before epiphyseal closure or fusion of the growth plate in bones. Children with gigantism can grow up to 15 cm each year and may reach a height of 2.4 m. Children with gigantism exhibit delayed sexual development and slow mental development. Radiation therapy, surgical removal of the tumour and drug therapy may be used to reduce the secretion of the GH and slow down excessive growth patterns. With treatment, prognosis for an individual with gigantism is generally good and they avoid most of the complications (Waugh & Grant 2022).

Acromegaly

Acromegaly is the result of GH hypersecretion in adulthood after epiphyseal closure. It is characterised by the breakdown or atrophy of skeletal muscle and the formation of new bone and cartilage. The long bones are unable to grow in length, but the smaller bones of the hands, feet and face grow, which gives the appearance of an enlarged lower jaw, bulging forehead, thickened ears and nose and large hands and feet (Figure 36.5) (Waugh & Grant 2022). Thickening of the tongue may cause the voice to sound deep and hollow and speech may be slurred. Acromegaly is a chronic, progressive, disfiguring disease that often shortens life expectancy since it may lead to respiratory, cerebrovascular and heart disease. Surgery to remove a causative pituitary tumour may lead to hypopituitarism (Crawford 2023; Waugh & Grant 2022).

Prolactinoma

A prolactinoma is a non-malignant, prolactin-producing tumour of the pituitary gland. Hypersecretion of the hormone prolactin often results in gynaecomastia and galactorrhoea (breast swelling and milk production) in both males and non-breastfeeding females. In females, a prolactinoma may lead to irregular or absence of menstrual period, symptoms of menopause, infertility, osteoporosis or alterations in libido. Common causes of this type of tumour are pregnancy, breastfeeding, stress and certain medications (Snyder 2021).

TABLE 36.1 | Summary of major endocrine imbalances

Disorder	Gland or hormone implicated	Homeostatic imbalance
Acromegaly	Pituitary—GH	Hypersecretion in adults
Cushing's disease	Adrenal glands—cortisol	Hypersecretion
Diabetes insipidus	Hypothalamus ADH	Hypersecretion
Type 1 diabetes mellitus	Pancreas—insulin	Hyposecretion/hypoactivity
Type 2 diabetes mellitus	Pancreas—insulin	Resistance or insensitivity to insulin & hyposecretion
Gigantism	Pituitary—GH	Hypersecretion in children
Pituitary dwarfism	Pituitary—GH	Hyposecretion in children
SIADH (syndrome of inappropriate antidiuretic hormone secretion)	Pituitary—ADH	Hypersecretion
Cretinism	Thyroid—TH	Untreated congenital hyposecretion
Hyperthyroidism Graves' disease Thyrotoxicosis	Thyroid—TH, or TSH from pituitary	Hypersecretion
Hypothyroidism: Hashimoto's disease, myxoedema	Thyroid—TH	Hyposecretion
Hyperparathyroidism	Parathyroid—PTH	Hypersecretion
Hypoparathyroidism	Parathyroid—PTH	Hyposecretion
Hypoadrenalism—Addison's disease	Adrenal cortex—cortisol, aldosterone and androgens	Hyposecretion
Primary aldosteronism—Conn's syndrome	Adrenal cortex aldosterone	Hypersecretion
Pheochromocytoma	Adrenal medulla—catecholamines	Hypersecretion
Osteoporosis	Ovary—oestrogen	Post-menopausal hyposecretion
Polycystic ovarian syndrome	Ovary—androgens	Hypersecretion

(Crawford 2023; Waugh & Grant 2022)

SIADH

The syndrome of inappropriate antidiuretic hormone (SIADH) includes excessive ADH secretion from the posterior pituitary which is often unrelated to any other endocrine dysfunction. Individuals with pulmonary problems such as lung cancer, severe pneumonia and other lung diseases may suffer from SIADH. As a result, an individual's pulmonary health needs to be assessed as part of the nursing care and management of SIADH (Banasik 2022; Khardori et al 2022).

Individuals with SIADH produce excessive amounts of ADH, causing significant water retention. The retained fluid lowers blood sodium levels by dilution resulting in hyponatraemia, or low blood levels of sodium. Diagnosis of SIADH includes low serum osmolality and urine hyperosmolality; the symptoms are determined by the severity of ADH release (Khardori et al 2022).

Restricting and monitoring fluid intake, as well as the administration of diuretics, may reduce the underlying cause (strict fluid restriction of 0.5–1 L daily is often prescribed to allow sodium levels to increase slowly). Monitoring urine output (including colour, concentration and volume), weight and blood chemistry are also indicated for individuals with this disorder (Khardori et al 2022).

Hypopituitarism

Hypofunction of the anterior pituitary gland may be caused by a pituitary tumour, infection or secondary to

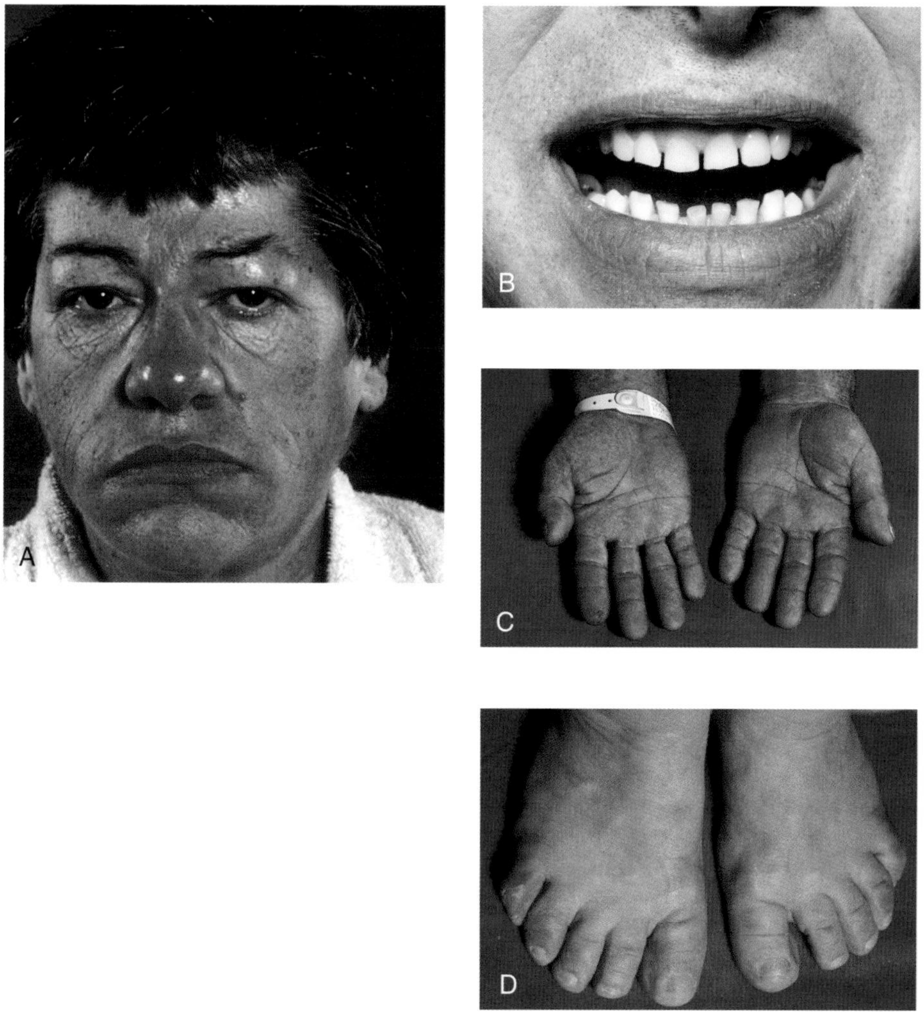

Figure 36.5 Acromegaly

A: Typical facies, **B:** Prognathism and separation of the lower teeth, **C:** Large, fleshy hand, **D:** Widening of the feet.
(Dover et al 2024)

trauma of the hypothalamus. In **hypopituitarism**, there is an absence or deficiency of both GH and gonadotrophins (Cleveland Clinic 2022c). The condition, marked by growth retardation, causes **dwarfism** and a delay in the onset of puberty in children. Hypopituitarism can present in three forms: Fröhlich's syndrome, dwarfism and Sheehan's syndrome. All forms of hypopituitarism share the characteristics of delayed/retarded growth, decreased mentation and impaired sexual development (Crawford 2023; Genetu et al 2021).

Fröhlich's syndrome, also called adiposogenital dystrophy or Babinski-Fröhlich's syndrome, is a rare condition of hypopituitarism caused by a tumour of the hypothalamus. More common in males, this disorder occurs in children and is characterised by uncontrolled hunger, obesity, growth retardation, underdeveloped genitals, excessive daytime sleepiness and occasionally aggression (Pascual et al 2021).

Dwarfism results from **hyposecretion** of GH in childhood and is characterised by proportionately small-statured individuals. Sheehan's syndrome is a form of hypopituitarism caused by necrosis of the anterior pituitary gland following postpartum haemorrhage and shock (Crawford 2023; Genetu et al 2021). Treatment of hypopituitarism varies and depends on the cause and which pituitary hormone(s) are deficient. For this reason, treatment is individualised and commonly involves close monitoring of blood hormone levels and prescription of targeted hormone replacement therapy (Crawford 2023).

Diabetes insipidus

Diabetes insipidus (DI) is a rare condition characterised by polyuria, polydipsia, dilute (hypotonic) urine and life-threatening hyponatraemia. This disease may be neurogenic or nephrogenic in origin. The neurogenic form, also known as central DI, stems from the inability of the hypothalamus to synthesise ADH and the posterior pituitary to release ADH. The nephrogenic form, also known as peripheral DI, is due to the kidney's failure to respond to ADH (Crawford

CASE STUDY 36.1

Ben who is an Enrolled Nurse has just commenced the afternoon shift and is reviewing the documentation of a person in his care. He notes that the client, a bronzed 27-year-old female, has showed no abnormalities during a routine physical examination but is hypotensive at 95/60 mmHg. She tells Ben that she cycles regularly to keep fit. Ben notes that she has had multiple blood and urine tests earlier in the day. Ben asks her how she has been feeling. She tells Ben that recently she has been feeling very thirsty, a little dizzy when she stands up quickly, she has been drinking a lot, urinating large volumes and has developed a craving for salt.

1. What are the clinical terms for the following signs and symptoms? Which common disorder are they typical of?

- Excessive thirst =
- Passing high volume of urine frequently =

Ben asks her whether she has been eating or drinking differently, and she tells him that she has made little change to her diet but has been drinking much more than usual.

'Would you say that you eat a lot of sweets or cakes or sugar?' Ben asks.

'No more than normal but I really crave salt,' she replies.

Ben checks her blood glucose level and finds that random blood glucose level is a little under normal. He also looks at the urinalysis results and finds it is negative for glucose and relatively dilute.

'I'm always drinking and going to the toilet,' she says. 'It's really interrupting my work.'

Ben suspects that there may be an imbalance in the amount of cortisol and/or aldosterone since this is a major hormone of water and sugar balance in the body.

2. What is the rationale behind asking about diet and sugar intake? Do the blood and urine results confirm or rule out your original assumption?

'What do you think it could be?' she asks. Ben explains that the doctor will need to discuss the possible diagnosis, but her blood and urine glucose levels indicate that it probably is not diabetes mellitus, but he cannot be sure. The blood tests indicate that the individual's serum potassium is high at 5.2 mmol/L, her serum sodium level is low at 129 mmol/L, random blood glucose level is a little low and her urine is negative for glucose but dilute. Ben suspects a disorder of cortisol and/or aldosterone secretion since these are the major hormones of water and sugar balance in the body.

3. What are the two major endocrine disorders associated with imbalances in cortisol levels?
4. What are the typical signs or symptoms of these disorders?
5. Given your knowledge about hormone dysfunction, which disorder of cortisol secretion do you think she may be suffering from? Explain your answer.
6. Do you think the information that the individual provided while she was chatting to Ben assisted with your conclusion?

During nursing rounds, Ben revisits this individual and asks her how she is going and she tells him that she is a little anxious about going for a CT scan.

7. Explain the purpose of a CT scan of the abdomen.

2023). Without ADH, the individual exhibits polyuria (passing vast quantities of dilute, colourless urine) with a specific gravity of <1.005. In severe cases, urinary output may be >10 litres/24 hours (see Case Study 36.1). As a result, the individual experiences significant electrolyte imbalance and profound dehydration, despite drinking large amounts of fluid (Khardori et al 2022). Risk factors for DI include family history, brain surgery, major head injury, some medications and a metabolic disorder causing hypercalcaemia or hypokalaemia (NIDDKD 2021a).

Diagnosis

Diagnostic investigations include the following: urinalysis to assess specific gravity, pH and colour; blood tests for electrolytes, osmolarity and ADH; MRI of the hypothalamus, posterior pituitary gland and kidneys to observe any anatomical anomalies; water deprivation test, which involves the denial of fluids for several hours followed by monitoring weight, urine output, urinalysis and blood tests; stimulation test in which fluids with ADH production stimulants are administered intravenously, following which the body's response is measured, and genetic testing (NIDDK 2021a).

Management

Treatment for individuals with diabetes insipidus varies according to cause. In neurogenic DI, if the cause is anatomical, surgery may be performed. In some cases, the individual will be prescribed a lifelong, synthetic form of ADH. If nephrogenic in origin, the individual may be treated with a thiazide diuretic or non-steroidal anti-inflammatory medications. Ironically, treatment with a thiazide diuretic reduces urine output in some people (NIDDK 2021a).

Disorders of the thyroid gland

Hyperthyroidism

Hyperthyroidism is one of the more common endocrine disorders and may be caused by many factors, such as thyroiditis, hypersecretion of TSH or the autoimmune

TABLE 36.2 | Some common signs and symptoms of hyperthyroidism (including Graves' disease) and hypothyroidism

Hypothyroidism	Hyperthyroidism
• Fatigue • Depression • Feeling sensitive to cold • Thinning hair • Muscle stiffness • Stiffness and pain in joints • Slowed heart rate • Decline in the ability to sweat • Constipation • Heavy or irregular menstrual periods • Fertility issues	• Noticeable weight loss • Rapid or irregular heart rate • Nervousness • Difficulty sleeping • Fatigue • Shaky hands • Muscle weakness • Irritation • Tiredness • Frequent bowel movements • Muscle weakness • Goitre

(Banasik 2022; Medical News Today 2023)

condition Graves' disease. An increase in the secretion of the thyroid hormones T_3 and T_4 increases the basal metabolic rate and affects the functions of other body systems. The signs and symptoms of elevated thyroid hormone levels are related to an increase in an individual's metabolic rate (i.e. weight loss, insomnia and heat intolerance). In cases of significant hyperthyroidism (thyrotoxicosis of thyroid storm), the individual often presents with nervousness, cardiac arrhythmias, tremors and anxiety (Crawford 2023; NIDDK 2021b).

Table 36.2 lists the most common signs and symptoms of hyperthyroidism and hypothyroidism.

Graves' disease

Graves' disease is diagnosed by elevated serum levels of TSH receptor antibodies that stimulate the thyroid gland, leading to the production and release of high concentrations of thyroid hormones and potential glandular hypertrophy. Graves' disease is eight times more prevalent in females (Babić-Leko et al 2021; Crawford 2023; NIDDK 2021b) (see Lived Experience at the beginning of the chapter). It often develops following a significant stressful event, illness or shock. Symptoms include voracious appetite with loss of weight, diarrhoea, excessive sweating and extreme thirst. One outstanding characteristic of Graves' disease is **exophthalmos**—a protrusion of the eyeballs due to oedema in the tissues behind the eye that does not resolve even when the hyperthyroidism is corrected (Medical News Today 2023) (Figure 36.6A). An acute complication of Graves' disease is thyroid crisis, also known as thyroid storm or **thyrotoxicosis** (Crawford 2023; NIDDK 2021b). (See Clinical Interest Box 36.1.)

Goitre

An enlarged thyroid gland (**goitre**) may be the result of thyroiditis, thyroid tumour or hyperactivity or hypoactivity. Depending on its size, a goitre may exert

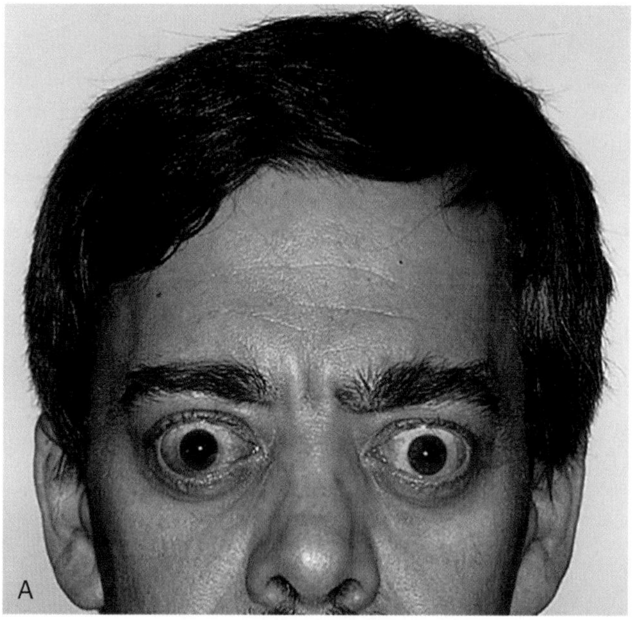

Figure 36.6A Exophthalmos in hyperthyroidism

(From Belchetz, P., Hammond, P., 2003. Mosby's color atlas and text of diabetes and endocrinology. *Mosby, Edinburgh)*

pressure on the trachea and produce dysphagia and/or dyspnoea (Waugh & Grant 2022). A simple or non-toxic goitre occurs in thyroid hypoactivity and is caused by dietary iodine deficiency. Since the introduction of iodised table salt in 1924, the incidence of thyroid hypoactivity in most Western countries has been significantly reduced. Insufficient iodine in the diet results in a range of conditions known as iodine deficiency disorders (IDD). Iodine deficiency is becoming an increasingly common cause of thyroid health problems in Australia (Group 2022). Exophthalmic or toxic diffuse goitre occurs in hyperthyroidism and is characterised by an enlarged

CLINICAL INTEREST BOX 36.1 Thyroid crisis (thyroid storm or thyrotoxicosis)

Thyroid storm or thyrotoxicosis is a sudden, severe form of hyperthyroidism characterised by high fever, tachycardia, tachypnoea and an altered mental state. An individual presenting with thyroid crisis requires immediate medical and nursing attention since this condition can be life-threatening. Thyroid storm can be triggered by emotional stress, infection, trauma, untreated or overtreated hyperthyroidism and post-thyroidectomy. Nursing management involves interventions aimed at lowering body temperature, increasing oxygen levels, rehydration with IV fluids containing glucose and reducing the production of the thyroid hormone.

(Crawford 2023; Medical News Today 2023; NIDDK 2021b)

thyroid, bulging of the eyes and heart palpitations (Figure 36.6A and 36.6B). Thyroid function tests and scans can detect malfunction of the thyroid and treatment may include iodine supplements, hormone replacement or surgery (Crawford 2023).

Hypothyroidism

Hypothyroidism is characterised by a decreased production of thyroid hormones. It may be congenital or develop later in life. Hypothyroidism can also be caused by an autoimmune condition known as Hashimoto's thyroiditis, dietary iodine deficiency or the surgical removal of the thyroid gland. **Cretinism** is the congenital form and typically results from the absence or underdevelopment of the thyroid gland, or from severe maternal iodine deficiency during pregnancy. The signs and symptoms of cretinism are marked depression of metabolic processes and progressive mental impairment. Typically, the infant is overweight, lethargic, has dry thick skin, coarse features, a broad flat nose and a protruding tongue and abdomen. If the disease goes untreated, sexual organs fail to develop and muscle growth is retarded; therefore, it is vital that treatment is started as soon as a diagnosis is made. Lifelong thyroid hormone replacement therapy (THRT) is the primary form of treatment for hypothyroidism (Banasik 2022; Waugh & Grant 2022).

Symptoms of hypothyroidism are the opposite of those of hyperthyroidism (see Table 36.2). The individual is fatigued, drowsy and sensitive to cold, gains weight, has thin nails, brittle hair, bradycardia, low respiratory rate and irregular menstruation Depression has also been linked to hypothyroidism, both causatively and symptomatically. In some cases, depression is misdiagnosed as hypothyroidism. Diagnosis of hypothyroidism may be difficult due to the non-specific nature of the symptoms, which are often diverse and atypical. Hypothyroidism responds well to THRT, and symptoms may disappear after a few months of treatment. Untreated severe hypothyroidism (myxoedema) can be life-threatening (Crawford 2023; Waugh & Grant 2022).

Myxoedema occurs in severe or prolonged hypothyroidism. The name refers to oedema in the dermis of the skin, especially around the eyes, hands and feet (Waugh & Grant 2022). (See Figure 36.7.) If left untreated, myxoedema and myxoedema coma—the decompensated state of severe hypothyroidism in which an individual may lose consciousness—can be life-threatening. Maintenance of vital organ function, and monitoring for increasing severity of signs and symptoms, is a major nursing intervention (Herlihy & Kirov 2022).

Diagnostic tests

A combination of tests is generally performed to evaluate thyroid function, including the following: blood tests that

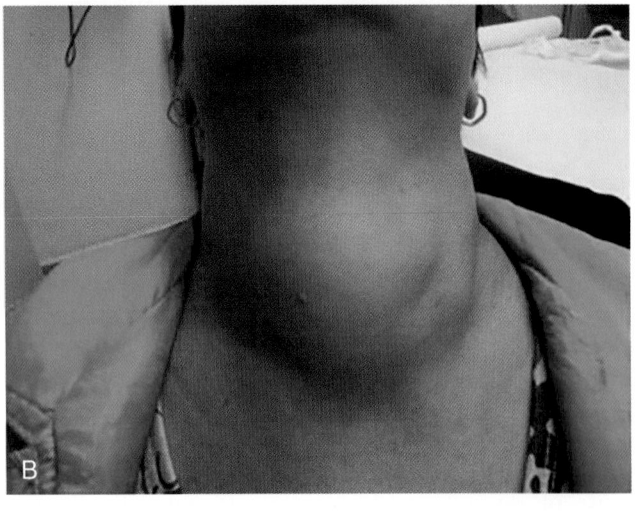

Figure 36.6B Goitre
(Crawford 2023)

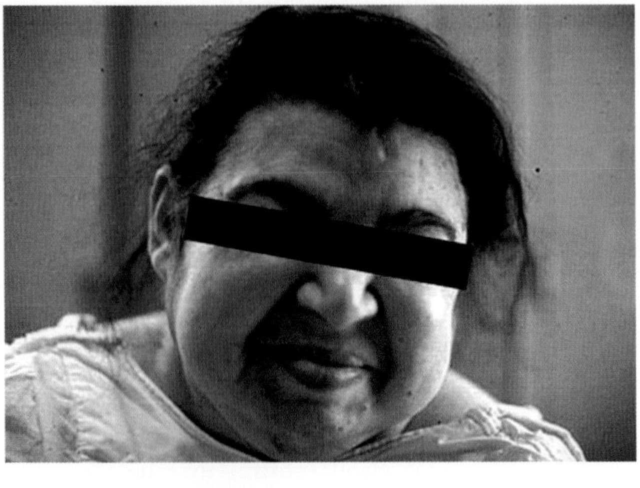

Figure 36.7 Myxoedema
(Khurana & Khurana 2020)

measure the levels of T3, T4, TSH and iodine; radioactive iodine uptake test—an evaluation of thyroid function by measuring the amount of orally ingested radioactive iodine that accumulates in the thyroid gland; nuclear medicine thyroid scan—a procedure that allows for visualisation of the thyroid gland after the administration of a radioactive isotope into the person's vein; and ultrasound of the thyroid utilising soundwaves to evaluate thyroid structure and differentiate a cyst from a tumour (Crawford 2023). If an individual is required to have a thyroid scan, the nurse must review any prescribed or over-the counter medications taken by the individual (especially if they contain iodine) since they may need adjusting (Mayo Clinic 2022b).

The Royal College of Pathologists of Australasia (RCPA) (2017) developed established guidelines for screening of thyroid disease in the general adult population and determined that screening was unnecessary except in the case of 'patients at high risk of developing thyroid disease, or where there is a clinical suspicion based on relevant history, symptoms, test results or signs at presentation'.

Most people with classic hyperthyroidism rarely need hospitalisation. Critically ill individuals, and those with thyrotoxicosis and concurrent illness, require hospitalisation. Management of hyperthyroidism includes assisting the individual and their significant other/s to manage the symptoms of hyperthyroidism until it is controlled with antithyroid medication—medications that slow the heart rate (beta-blockers). Other forms of treatment include radioactive iodine treatment, which destroys the thyroid-hormone-producing cells followed by lifelong thyroid hormone replacement medications, or surgery to remove some or all of the thyroid gland, predominantly in cases of thyroid cancer. An individual who has had a total thyroidectomy requires lifelong hormone replacement (Waugh & Grant 2022).

Nursing intervention includes the assessment and management of the nutritional and emotional status of an individual with hyper or hypothyroidism. Nurses should aim to reassure the individual that emotional reactions they may be experiencing, especially with hypothyroidism, are normal for that condition (Vanderpump 2022).

Disorders of the parathyroid glands

Hyperparathyroidism

Hyperparathyroidism results in an overproduction of PTH and can be caused by hereditary factors, tumours, enlargement of the parathyroid glands or removal during thyroidectomy. Secondary hyperparathyroidism can be caused by renal disease or other conditions such as osteomalacia or rickets. Excessive PTH production leads to hypercalcaemia (excessive calcium in the blood) since the hormone stimulates the reabsorption of calcium from bone, the kidneys and the gastrointestinal system (Crawford 2023). As calcium is drawn from bones, individuals can experience symptoms such as backache, bone curvature and pathological fractures from bone weakness (Waugh & Grant 2022). Renal stones may develop due to excess calcium in the blood. Hypercalcaemia also depresses the nervous system, causing delayed reflexes and weak muscles, and can affect the functioning of vital organs (Crawford 2023).

Hypoparathyroidism

Hypoparathyroidism is an uncommon disorder caused by a deficiency in PTH production, familial hypoparathyroidism, autoimmune disorders or, most commonly, the surgical removal of parathyroid glands during thyroidectomy. In hypoparathyroidism, low serum PTH levels cause hypocalcaemia and hyperphosphataemia (high phosphate levels in the blood), resulting in neuromuscular symptoms ranging from paraesthesia to tetany. Signs and symptoms include muscle spasms, anxiety, hyperreflexia and laryngeal spasm (Crawford 2023). Tetany results from hyperexcitability of nerves and skeletal muscles due to the low serum calcium levels. It begins with tingling in the fingertips, toes and around the mouth. The tingling increases and produces muscle tension and spasms, with consequent adduction of the thumbs, wrists, elbows and toes (carpopedal spasm). The tetany associated with hypoparathyroidism mainly affects the muscles of the face and hands, causing uncontrolled contraction (Cleveland Clinic 2022b).

Diagnostic tests

Diagnosis of both hyperthyroidism and hypoparathyroidism is difficult due to vague symptoms of pain and/or fatigue. One test used to assess parathyroid function is the measure of serum calcium and phosphorus levels (Crawford 2023). An elevated serum calcium level alone is not a definitive diagnosis since blood calcium may be influenced by diet and medication. A 24-hour urine collection measures total calcium in the urine since hyperparathyroidism causes *increased* excretion of calcium in the urine, and hypoparathyroidism causes *decreased* excretion of calcium in the urine. Scans or X-rays show bone changes, and serum antibody parathyroid tests are important in the diagnoses. Testing for hypocalcaemia and hypoparathyroidism involves checking for a positive Chvostek's sign (facial muscle spasm occurring when the facial nerve is tapped) and a positive Trousseau's sign (hand muscle spasm when pressure is applied to the nerves and vessels of the upper arm) (Mayo Clinic 2022a; Waugh & Grant 2022).

Treatment of hyperparathyroidism is directed at the cause and often results in a good prognosis. Surgical removal of tumours or removal of some or all of the parathyroid glands is the preferred treatment in hyperparathyroidism. Even leaving half of one parathyroid gland is all that is required to maintain normal PTH levels (Mayo Clinic 2022a). Treatment of hypoparathyroidism with a form of vitamin D (calcitonin) and calcium supplements will often improve prognosis. Following parathyroidectomy, hypocalcaemia and tetany may occur and are treated with intravenous calcium and PTH as well as vitamin D (Mayo Clinic 2022a).

CRITICAL THINKING EXERCISE 36.1

A series of true events experienced by Stella, mother of three:

I was 35 weeks pregnant and, as usual, I came to the end of my day feeling tired, irritable, nauseous and emotional: all normal pregnancy symptoms! But that night was different. I was experiencing heart palpitations and the nausea and vomiting was worse than usual. I started to shake and despite thinking everything was most probably fine, I felt I should go to emergency at our local hospital just to make sure. To my surprise, I was admitted immediately and began undergoing tests.

During the night, my blood results showed the ________ levels in my blood were very high. The endocrinologists, together with the obstetrics team, decided to deliver my baby the next day by caesarean section.

I underwent an MRI scan soon afterwards that revealed a tumour on two of my parathyroid glands. Two weeks later I was operated on. The following few days were spent in hospital, and I had nurses and doctors giving me 2–3 blood tests daily to ensure that my ________ levels were coming down.

Days later, at home recovering from the operation, I began to experience severe numbing and a pins-and-needles-type feeling in my hands and feet and around my mouth. I woke during the night after my symptoms got worse. Within minutes of waking, I was almost completely paralysed. My face contorted and I had spasms in my hands. Speaking was impossible. I no longer had control over any of my movements. My husband woke to find me unable to speak with my muscles locked. I was rushed to hospital in an ambulance.

My ________ levels had plummeted, which explained what I was experiencing. It was like nothing I'd ever felt before! I was absolutely terrified! Once at the hospital, the nurses set me up with a ________ drip and within 2 hours my body was back to normal. I then went into a deep sleep, much like a person after a severe epileptic fit. I was completely exhausted.

Today, I'm feeling 100% better and take just one ________ tablet to keep my levels in check. I still have 3-monthly check-ups with my endocrinologist. Who would ever have thought ________ plays such an important role in our bodies?

1. Fill in the gaps in the above paragraphs.
2. Given the signs and symptoms Stella experienced, which basic nutrient, vitamin or mineral do you think might be involved? Explain your answer.
3. Which hormone and gland are likely to be the cause of what Stella is experiencing? List the major role and function of this hormone.
4. Based on your answers to questions 1 and 2, explain how a tumour affects this gland.
5. Explain why there was such a change in the serum levels of this particular nutrient, vitamin or mineral following removal of this tumour.
6. What medical terminology (i.e. prefixes) describe under and over function of a gland or deficient and excessive secretion of a hormone?

Disorders of the adrenal glands

Disorders of the adrenal cortex

Hyperadrenalism is a condition characterised by the over-secretion of hormones produced by the adrenal glands, namely corticosteroids, androgens and/or aldosterone. Several major disorders can arise depending on which hormone is excessively produced. These disorders are Cushing's syndrome, Conn's syndrome, primary aldosteronism and congenital adrenal hyperplasia and symptoms will vary according to the presenting disorder. Hyperadrenalism is usually confined to the cortex of the adrenal gland and caused by neoplasms, hyperplasia, or may be iatrogenic (i.e. caused by medical treatment or a medical procedure) (Crawford 2023).

Cushing's syndrome

Hyperfunction that causes increased secretion of cortisol (hypercortisolism) leads to Cushing's disease or Cushing's syndrome. **Cushing's syndrome** occurs when there is an overproduction of corticosteroid hormones regardless of cause. This condition can result from hypersecretion of pituitary ACTH, overuse of corticosteroids, and adrenal or pituitary tumours. Cushing's disease refers to excess endogenous secretion of ACTH. Signs of this condition correspond with hyperglycaemia, abnormal distribution of lipids and protein wasting. Classic characteristics include obesity of the trunk with a pad of fat across the shoulders (buffalo hump), moon face, hirsutism and menstrual irregularities in females, striae (stretch marks) on the breasts, abdomen and legs, muscle wasting, muscle weakness, osteoporosis and skin fragility. (See Figure 36.8.) Persistent hyperglycaemia often develops into type 2 diabetes mellitus. Elevated cortisol levels exacerbate catecholamine effects (i.e. anxiety, palpitations, sweating, headache, stress and hypertension), and can lead to the development of atherosclerosis, ischaemic heart disease and kidney disease (John Hopkins Medicine 2023b).

Cushing's syndrome is relatively rare and most commonly occurs in women aged 20–50 years. A complication of Cushing's syndrome is immunosuppression and an increased susceptibility to infection. Treatment includes surgery, chemotherapy, radiation and corticosteroid suppressing medications (Johns Hopkins Medicine 2023b). (See Clinical Interest Box 36.2.)

Primary aldosteronism

Primary aldosteronism, or **Conn's syndrome**, occurs when the adrenal glands produce excessive amounts of the

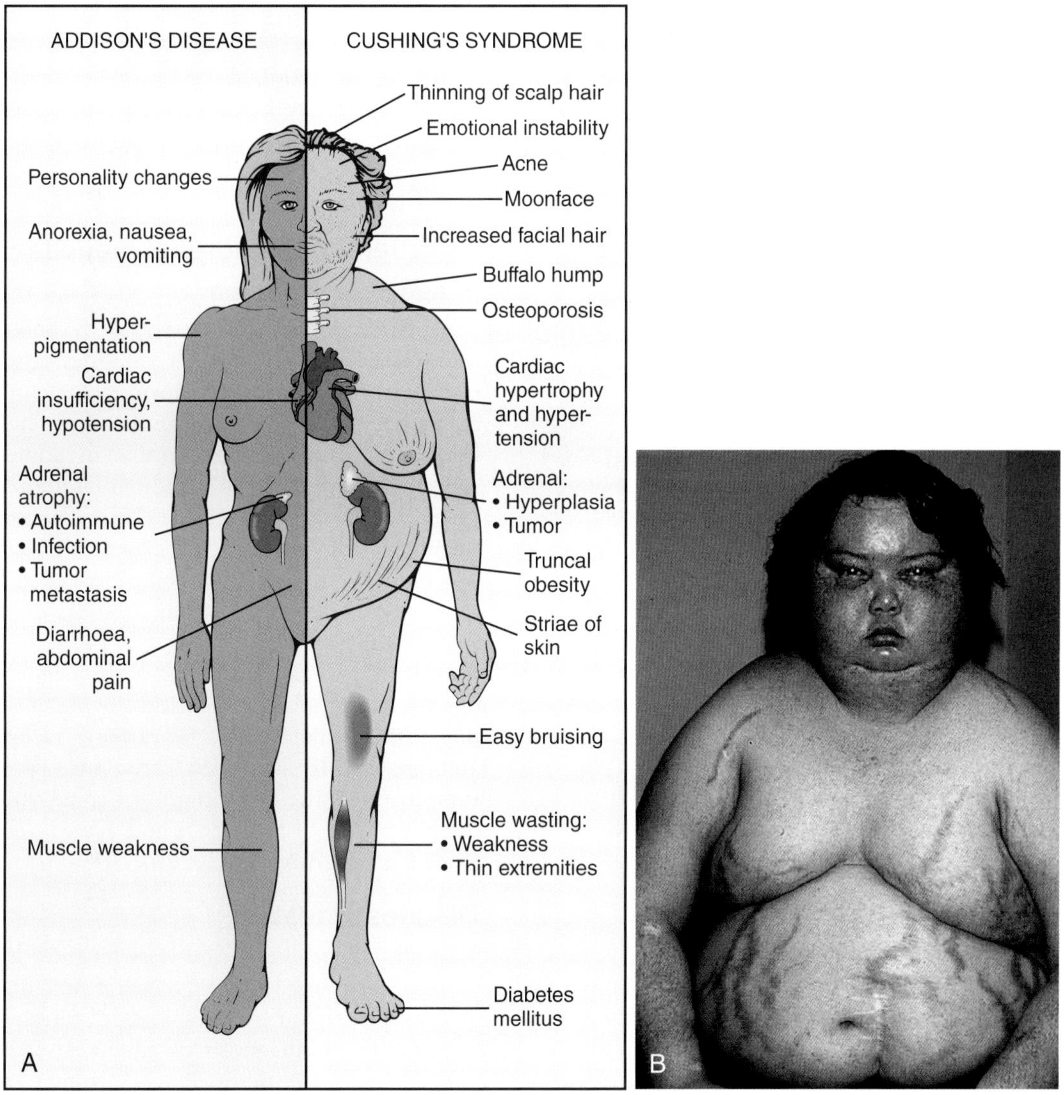

Figure 36.8 Common characteristics in Cushing's disease

A: Comparison of hyperfunction of the adrenal cortex (Addison's disease) and hypofunction (Cushing's syndrome), **B:** Clinical features of Cushing's syndrome called cushingoid features including 'moonface', obesity, and cutaneous striae.

(From Damjanov, I., 2006. Pathology for the health-related profession, *3rd ed. WB Saunders, Philadelphia. Used with permission)*

mineralocorticoid hormone, aldosterone, which plays a major role in controlling blood pressure and blood levels of sodium and potassium (Crawford 2023). The symptoms of Conn's syndrome include hypertension, hyponatraemia, hypokalaemia, muscle weakness, polyuria, polydipsia, metabolic acidosis, and neuromuscular dysfunction (Johns Hopkins Medical 2023c). Given the high incidence of hypertension in Australia (see Chapter 25), alterations of aldosterone function should be considered in the nursing assessment (Crawford 2023).

Adrenogenital syndrome

Adrenogenital syndrome is also known as **congenital adrenal hyperplasia (CAH)** and is an inherited disorder affecting the adrenal glands and genitals. In CAH, there is an excessive production of androgens and a deficiency of cortisol and/or aldosterone (Utiger 2022a). The over production of androgens can cause abnormalities in sexual development and virulisation, while the deficiency of cortisol and/or aldosterone triggers potentially life-threatening hypotension, hypoglycaemia and dehydration. Females with CAH can be born with ambiguous, atypical genitalia (e.g. enlarged clitoris resembling a small penis so that sex determination can be difficult). As the child develops, females may experience hirsutism, especially on the legs, chest and abdomen, a deepened voice and amenorrhoea. In males, CAH can cause penile enlargement and early sexual development. Children with this condition initially appear tall; however, growth slows after puberty, and the children often end up being relatively short as adults (Johns Hopkins Medicine 2023a).

CLINICAL INTEREST BOX 36.2 Cortisone, cortisol and Cushing's syndrome

Hypersecretion, long-term use, abuse or over-administration of corticosteroids may lead to the development of Cushing's syndrome. Corticosteroids have an impact on several vital processes. Their actions include anti-inflammation, immunosuppression, hyperglycaemic and fluid retention. Consequently, corticosteroids are beneficial in the treatment of inflammatory conditions, asthma and in autoimmune conditions such as rheumatoid arthritis and anaphylaxis. Unfortunately, corticosteroids are not selective and taking them can cause adverse reactions. Systemic immunosuppression and the depressed inflammatory response significantly increase the risk of infection, delayed wound healing, hyperglycaemia and hypertension. Nursing interventions must therefore include rigid measures to decrease the risk of infection, promote wound healing, balance blood glucose and control hypertension. Sadly, without treatment, almost half of individuals with Cushing's syndrome die within 5 years of onset.

(Crawford 2023; Johns Hopkins Medicine 2023b; Waugh & Grant 2022)

Disorders of the adrenal cortex—hypoadrenalism

Addison's disease

Hypofunction of the adrenal cortex may be caused by primary insufficiency, resulting in a condition known as **Addison's disease**, or adrenocortical insufficiency. This is a rare condition thought to be due to an autoimmune reaction, infection, acquired immunodeficiency syndrome (AIDS), cancer or adrenal gland atrophy. Up to 90% of the cortex can be destroyed before symptoms become evident. As a result, the disease is often advanced before it is diagnosed. The signs and symptoms are related to a deficiency of corticosteroids and excessive ACTH production. The lack of mineralocorticoids causes hyponatraemia leading to diarrhoea, dehydration, weakness, weight loss and hypotension. Lack of glucocorticoids affects blood glucose levels, leading to hypoglycaemia. An increased ACTH level, due to disturbed negative feedback control, may lead to brown pigmentation or bronzing of the skin and mucous membranes, affecting the palms, elbows, scars, skin folds and areolae (Cleveland Clinic 2022a). Addison's disease may also have profound effects on an individual's mental state, with some exhibiting signs of depression, confusion, or apathy and development of a second autoimmune condition (Cleveland Clinic 2022a; Crawford 2023).

Congenital adrenal hyperplasia (CAH) is often classified together with Addison's disease as general adrenal insufficiency. Like Addison's disease, cortisol and aldosterone are either partially produced or not produced at all. The condition may be classified as 'classic' (congenital, a genetic defect in steroid synthesis) or 'late onset' (early adult onset). Growth and adrenal problems may develop, as in other adrenal insufficiencies. Addison's disease is a chronic condition treated with the synthetic version of cortisol (hydrocortisone) and aldosterone (fludrocortisone) for the rest of the person's life (Cleveland Clinic 2022a).

Disorders of the adrenal medulla

Phaeochromocytoma

Phaeochromocytoma is generally a benign tumour of the adrenal medulla, which causes over-secretion of the catecholamine group of hormones, namely dopamine, adrenaline and noradrenaline—the 'fight or flight' hormones. The incidence peaks in adults between the ages of 30 and 50 years, although it can occur at any age. Phaeochromocytoma may be common amongst family members, and may be associated with a rare group of cancers collectively known as multiple endocrine neoplasias syndrome (MENS) in which tumours develop in two or more endocrine glands (Rare Cancers Australia 2022a; Rare Cancers Australia 2022b). The signs and symptoms of phaeochromocytoma include hypertension, headaches, unexplained diaphoresis (sweating), tachycardia, tremor and anxiety. If diagnosed early, surgery to remove the tumour offers the best prognosis. In advanced cases, there is a higher risk of recurrence and a less favourable outcome (Rare Cancers Australia 2022b).

Diagnostic tests

Typically, blood and urine tests measure levels of adrenal cortical hormones. Blood tests determine the level of serum aldosterone, serum cortisol or serum catecholamines. These tests aid in the diagnosis of adrenal function (e.g. serum cortisol levels are increased in Cushing's syndrome, while decreased serum cortisol levels are seen in Addison's disease). A 24-hour urine collection is often ordered to estimate the total daily free cortisol, aldosterone and catecholamine levels. A CT scan and/or suprarenal venography may also be used to aid in the diagnosis of tumours (Cleveland Clinic 2022a; Crawford 2023).

Surgical removal of the tumour or the dysfunctional adrenal gland (adrenalectomy) may also correct Cushing's syndrome, necessitating lifelong hormone therapy to replace the cortical hormone. Without cortical hormone replacement following adrenalectomy, the individual will develop life-threatening Addison's disease. Clinical Interest Box 36.2 provides an insight into cortisone therapy. Nurses should address the risk of injury and infection by encouraging a balance between rest and activity, promoting skin care and stimulating mental activity. Treatment and nursing care for Addison's disease and CAH includes corticosteroid therapy, and the assessment and management of fluid levels, signs of shock and careful monitoring of symptoms (Cleveland Clinic 2022a; Crawford 2023).

Measurements of blood and urine for catecholamines are the most direct and conclusive tests for disorders of the adrenal medulla like pheochromocytoma. Signs and symptoms such as hypertension, headache, hypermetabolism and hyperglycaemia indicate phaeochromocytoma. Imaging studies can identify the location of the tumour, which can be removed surgically. Treatment and nursing management include lowering blood pressure, blood glucose and heart rate. If surgery to remove the adrenal gland is necessary, the individual will be required to self-administer lifelong hormone replacement therapy (Crawford 2023).

CRITICAL THINKING EXERCISE 36.2

A 25-year-old male under your care presents with diarrhoea, dehydration, weakness, weight loss, hypoglycaemia and hypotension. His serum sodium and glucose levels are low while his serum potassium level is high. You notice that his skin and mucous membranes appear tanned and bronzed and he states that he has recently developed a craving for salty foods. Given what you know about the endocrine system, which endocrine disorder do you think he might have? Is there more than one hormone imbalance that might be responsible for his condition?

Disorder of the gonads

Hypergonadism and hypogonadism

Hypergonadism is a condition of hyperactivity, or overactivity, of the gonads (testes in males or ovaries in females). As a result, there is an overproduction of testosterone and/or oestrogen. Presentation of hypergonadism will differ according to biological sex. In biological males, hypergonadism can cause early baldness, excessive muscle mass, acne and heightened libido. In biological females, hypergonadism can result in increased facial hair, menstrual irregularities, and a deepened voice. In both males and females, this condition can cause precocious puberty (a disorder in which children enter puberty and develop emotionally and physically earlier than expected) (The Aga Khan University Hospital nd).

Hypergonadism can be caused by tumours in the ovaries, life-threatening infections, autoimmune disorders, kidney or liver disease and trauma to the genital, pituitary or adrenal glands. Management ranges from treating the underlying cause (e.g. surgery for tumours or hormone replacement for conditions such as Hashimoto's thyroiditis) (Richardson & Glasper 2021). **Hypogonadism** is a condition characterised by an insufficient production of oestrogen and/or testosterone caused by dysfunction of the ovaries, testes, pituitary gland or hypothalamus. Hypogonadism can occur at any age. It can be present from birth (primary hypogonadism) but go unnoticed for several years or it can develop in adolescence or adulthood (secondary hypogonadism). Children with primary hypogonadism are likely to have a genetic condition called **Turner's syndrome** if female, or **Klinefelter's syndrome** if they are male. Hypogonadism can affect muscles, intellect, bone

CLINICAL INTEREST BOX 36.3 Osteoporosis and oestrogen

Osteoporosis is characterised by an imbalance between bone formation and bone reabsorption, where bone cells called osteoclasts digest bone faster than it can be deposited. Individuals usually become aware of osteoporosis only when the weakened bones break and they are admitted into hospital. Osteoporosis is strongly linked to calcium intake and calcium metabolism regulated by PTH. The onset of menopause in females is closely related to oestrogen and falling levels of oestrogen increases the rate at which bone digestion or breakdown occurs contributing to the development of osteoporosis. The use of hormone replacement therapy (HRT) and dietary supplements helps to address this endocrine imbalance.

(Crawford 2023; Waugh & Grant 2022)

growth, gait, mood, fertility and secondary sexual characteristics. Treatment with testosterone or oestrogen is usually effective (Mayo Clinic 2021).

Endocrine deficiencies of the gonads in the adult biological female are implicated in two common disorders: osteoporosis and **polycystic ovary syndrome (PCOS)** reflecting the strong interrelationship between endocrine organs and hormones (Crawford 2023). Osteoporosis and PCOS are discussed further in Clinical Interest Box 36.3 and Clinical Interest Box 36.4, respectively.

Diagnostic tests

Disorders of the gonads are diagnosed by examining physical features and blood testing, which would show elevated or low levels of the sex hormones, oestrogen and testosterone (Mayo Clinic 2021).

Disorders of the pancreas

Diabetes mellitus

Diabetes mellitus (DM) describes a group of metabolic disorders characterised by abnormal glucose metabolism and elevated blood glucose (hyperglycaemia). There are several types of diabetes mellitus: **type 1 diabetes mellitus (T1DM)**, **type 2 diabetes mellitus (T2DM)** and **gestational diabetes mellitus (GDM)**. T1DM is an autoimmune disorder caused by pancreatic beta-cell (β-cell) failure. A subset of T1DM is a condition known as **latent autoimmune diabetes in adults (LADA)**. Although the cause is the same, T1DM usually presents in children under the age of 14 years, whereas LADA commonly presents after age 35 years. Exposure to toxic substances or viruses are thought to be the environmental triggers of the autoimmune response in susceptible individuals (Banasik 2022). T1DM and LADA are neither curable nor preventable and require lifelong exogenous insulin injections for glycaemic management (Banasik 2022; Miller 2022).

CLINICAL INTEREST BOX 36.4 Polycystic ovarian (ovary) syndrome (PCOS)

Despite the misleading name, polycystic ovarian (ovary) syndrome (PCOS) is a hormonal disorder in females where excessive androgen production is triggered by inappropriate secretion of gonadotrophins. This is perhaps better reflected by the alternative name 'hyperandrogenic anovulation syndrome'. It is the most common endocrine disturbance in women, and is diagnosed in 6–20% of those in reproductive age depending on the diagnostic criteria used.

PCOS develops as a result of ovarian hypersecretion of androgens, with an overall result of increasing testosterone levels. Hyperinsulinaemia (intolerance to insulin) is thought to stimulate this hypersecretion of androgens. Elevated levels of androgens lead to elevated levels of oestrogen and testosterone, which trigger an imbalance in the pituitary gonadotrophins FSH and, especially, LH.

Clinical signs or symptoms of PCOS reflect the interruption of ovulation and the elevated male hormone levels. Various signs or symptoms exhibited by individuals mirror those of other endocrine disorders (especially those of the thyroid, adrenal cortex and gonads generally); thus, nursing assessment of PCOS may be difficult. Manifestations include dysmenorrhoea or amenorrhoea, hirsutism or androgenic alopecia, obesity and infertility. Women with PCOS also appear to be at greater risk of developing hyperglycaemia, cardiovascular disease and type 2 diabetes mellitus later in life.

(Craft et al 2023; Crawford 2023; Endocrine Society of Australia 2023)

T2DM is a progressive disease characterised by an initial insulin resistance, which is compensated by an overproduction of insulin (hyperinsulinaemia). As the pancreatic β-cells become exhausted, sufficient insulin is no longer produced. Obesity, inactivity, poor dietary choices, smoking, heredity and age predispose the individual to insulin resistance, prediabetes and metabolic syndrome. The greatest predictor of T2DM is pre-diabetes and metabolic syndrome. T2DM is more common in adults over the age of 25 years. If the condition occurs before age 25 years, it is referred to as **mature onset diabetes of the young (MODY)** and is more common in families where T2DM is prevalent (Banasik 2022; Miller 2022).

Gestational diabetes mellitus (GDM) occurs in pregnancy in response to the production of placental hormones (human chorionic somatomammotropin, oestrogen and cortisol) and the natural weight gain prompting insulin resistance. Risk factors for GDM include previous history of GDM, giving birth to a child large for gestational age (LGA), obesity, glycosuria, ethnicity, age or a strong family history of type 2 diabetes. Having GDM has consequences for both mother and child during pregnancy, at birth, post birth and in the future. GDM often disappears soon after birth; however, it is not uncommon for the mother to develop T2DM within 5–10 years and the child in their teens or adulthood to develop T2DM (Banasik 2022; Friel 2022).

The following statistics reflect the state of diabetes in Australia in 2021:

- More than 300 Australians develop diabetes every day.
- Almost 1.9 million Australians have diabetes. This includes all types of diagnosed diabetes (almost 1.5 million known and registered) as well as silent, undiagnosed type 2 diabetes (up to 500,000 estimated).
- Total annual cost impact of diabetes in Australia estimated at $17.6 billion (inflation adjusted).
- Diabetes is the seventh most common cause of death by disease in Australia.
- Aboriginal and Torres Strait Islander People are three times more likely to develop type 2 diabetes than non-Aboriginal and Torres Strait Islander People, 4.3 times more likely to be hospitalised with type 2 diabetes, and four times as likely to die from it.
- Around 1.2 million people are hospitalised with diabetes-related conditions every year.
- Around one in six (49,000) females aged 15–49 who gave birth in hospital were diagnosed with GDM.

(Australian Bureau of Statistics [ABS] 2022)

Signs and symptoms

The signs and symptoms of T1DM are relatively pronounced and can be life-threatening. T2DM often goes unnoticed for several years before diagnosis. Signs and symptoms of DM include:

- polydipsia (excessive thirst)
- polyuria (passing large volumes of urine)
- fatigue
- constant hunger
- slow healing wounds
- itching or pigmented skin
- urinary tract or fungal infections
- blurred vision
- unexplained weight loss (T1DM and T2DM)
- gradual weight gain (T2DM)
- dizziness
- leg cramps
- mood swings
- headaches.

(Miller 2022)

Diagnostic tests

- *Glycated haemoglobin (HbA1c):* This is a random blood test that measures the average blood glucose level over the previous 3–4 months. A HbA1c can be measured in mmol/mol or as a percentage. A HbA1c result ≥6.5% (48 mmol/mol) is indicative of a positive result for diabetes whilst a 6.0–6.4% result indicates pre-diabetes.
- *Fasting blood glucose (FBG):* This blood test measures the glucose level after fasting for 8–10 hours. It is

measured in mmol/L (millimoles per litre of blood). An FBG ≥7.0 mmol/L warrants further investigation as it can indicate the presence of diabetes. An FBG of 6.0–6.9 mmol/L indicates pre-diabetes.
- *Non-fasting (or random) blood glucose (RBG):* Also measured in mmol/L, this test measures the blood glucose level at any time of the day regardless of consuming food or fluids. An RBG of ≥11.1 mmol/L indicates diabetes while an RBG of 7.8–11.0 mmol/L is likely pre-diabetes.
- *Oral glucose tolerance test (OGTT):* This test involves taking serial venous blood samples. An FBG is taken before the individual is asked to drink a fluid containing 75 g carbohydrate load, which must be consumed within 5 minutes. Venous blood samples are then taken at 1 and 2 hours after consuming the carbohydrate load. Diabetes is indicated if the FBG is ≥7.0 mmol/L and the 2-hour post carbohydrate load level is ≥11 mmol/L.

(Crawford 2023; Diabetes Australia 2022c; Eyth et al 2022)

Complications of diabetes mellitus

An individual with DM is predisposed to a range of acute and chronic complications related to poor glycaemic control. Acute complications include:
- hypoglycaemia
- hyperglycaemia
- diabetic ketoacidosis
- hyperosmolar hyperglycaemic state (HHS).

(Miller 2022)

Chronic complications include:
- microvascular disease (i.e. peripheral neuropathy, diabetic retinopathy and diabetic nephropathy)
- macrovascular disease (i.e. cardiovascular disease, stroke, heart attack and hypertension).

(Miller 2022)

Nurses need to assess, monitor and help manage both acute and chronic diabetic complications. It is critical that individuals test their blood glucose levels several times per day and try to maintain as close to normal blood glucose ranges as possible. This self-management intervention will help prevent and/or delay both acute and chronic complications. The two main acute complications are hypoglycaemia and hyperglycaemia (Crawford 2023).

Hypoglycaemia

Hypoglycaemia develops when blood glucose levels drop below 4.0 mmol/L. Hypoglycaemia may be caused by the following: administering too much insulin or certain oral glucose-lowering medications; delaying or missing a meal; not eating enough carbohydrates; unplanned physical activity or undertaking more strenuous exercise than usual (Turton 2023). Early signs and symptoms include trembling, weakness, sweating, paleness, hunger, headache, dizziness and mood change. If left untreated, relatively minor hypoglycaemia can progress to confusion and slurred speech. If BGLs continue to drop, hypoglycaemia can become life-threatening as indicated by loss of consciousness, seizures, coma and, ultimately, death. In the case of strenuous physical activity or alcohol intoxication, hypoglycaemia can be delayed for 12 hours, with some people being asymptomatic before suddenly becoming unconscious. Vigilance is therefore critical since this situation can progress rapidly warranting immediate treatment. Late signs and symptoms of hypoglycaemia may include lack of concentration/behaviour change; pins and needles around the mouth; confusion; slurred speech; dysphagia (difficulty swallowing); inability to follow instructions; loss of consciousness and fitting/seizures (Miller 2022; Turton 2023).

Management and intervention

Management of hypoglycaemia within a healthcare facility varies according to organisational procedure and policy, and the person's physical abilities, cognitive state, reason for admission and the medical intervention/treatment the individual is receiving (Turton 2023).

Most healthcare facilities have hypoglycaemia kits containing oral treatment for individuals who are physically able to swallow safely. If an individual is unconscious or has previous/current swallowing difficulties, intramuscular (IM) glucagon or intravenous (IV) glucose can be administered, returning the person to a state of **euglycaemia** (normal blood sugar level) (Crawford 2023; Miller 2022).

If a capillary blood glucose measurement (using a point-of-care blood glucose meter) is less than 4 mmol/L, management protocols dictate that the nurse cease any insulin infusion and instigate treatment according to the person's state of consciousness, which can vary according to the facility's policy and procedures (Miller 2022).

If the individual experiencing hypoglycaemia can swallow, management guidelines advise following the 'Rule of 15':
- Consume 15–20 g of a simple (fast-acting) carbohydrate (e.g. 120–200 mL of orange juice or 6–8 jellybeans).
- Recheck the blood glucose after 15 minutes. If the BGL is >4.0 mmol/L, give the individual a complex carbohydrate such as half a sandwich containing carbohydrate and protein.
- If the level is <4.0 mmol/L, consume a second serve of simple carbohydrate and recheck the glucose in 15 minutes.
- If the BGL remains <4.0 mmol/L after three serves of simple carbohydrate or 45 minutes, urgent medical treatment will be required.
- If available, a glucagon injection can be administered as per manufacturer's instructions.

(Crawford 2023; Miller 2022)

To avoid experiencing hypoglycaemia, individuals and their caregivers should be provided with education regarding strategies for prevention, recognition and treatment of hypoglycaemia (Jarvis 2022). (See Case Study 36.2.)

For individuals who cannot swallow safely, are unconscious, fasting and/or having seizures:
- Cease any insulin infusion, if applicable.
- Check airway, breathing, circulation, disability, exposure (ABCDE).

CASE STUDY 36.2

Anthea, a diabetes nurse educator, introduces 60-year-old Mr Singh to Maddy, the Enrolled Nurse allocated to care for him. Anthea explains that Mr Singh has type 2 diabetes mellitus and that she would like Maddy to assist in educating him about his condition.

Mr Singh feels shy and confused, and says, 'Anthea is nice, but I don't understand what she is trying to teach me about my diabetes. I am having to test my blood sugar level all the time and take all of these tablets.' He shows Maddy a list of medications that Anthea has indicated he may be required to take.

Maddy begins by asking Mr Singh if he knows what his target blood sugar level should be.

Mr Singh cannot remember, so she reminds him.

1. What is the normal blood glucose range before meals for a person with type 2 diabetes mellitus?

'What you mean? I can eat, can't I?' Mr Singh asks.

'Of course you can,' Maddy answers, reassuring him. 'Did Anthea explain to you when you should test your blood?'

'Yes, in the morning before my breakfast. Why?'

2. Explain why Mr Singh needs to test his blood glucose prior to breakfast each day.

He sighs and admits, 'This is not easy. She says I have to do many other things, like watch what I eat. It is too complicated.'

3. What dietary advice would Maddy provide Mr Singh to improve self-management of his diabetes?
4. What sort of changes could Mr Singh make to his lifestyle and habits to improve glycaemic control?

Maddy feels that Mr Singh is overwhelmed, so she comforts him and reassures him that his concerns are normal and that his questions are valid.

5. Other than Anthea, his specific diabetes educator, which other health professionals could Maddy refer Mr Singh to, or at least make him aware of?

Mr Singh smiles and says, 'Thank you, Maddy. You make it easy for me and now I feel much better.'

- If unresponsive, place the individual in the coma position, on their side with head flexed slightly forward.
- Notify medical officer immediately/activate MET response.

(Miller 2022)

If the individual is in a healthcare facility, treatment can include one of two options depending upon IV access and organisational protocol, as follows:

1. For severe hypoglycaemia with no IV access, administer 1 mg of glucagon subcutaneously or intramuscularly (medication order required).
2. For severe hypoglycaemia with IV access, administer 10–25 g of glucose intravenously over 1–3 minutes (medication order required).

After 15 minutes, repeat capillary blood glucose measurement. If blood glucose measurement remains less than 4 mmol/L, seek and follow medical officer's treatment order (Jarvis 2022; Miller 2022).

Hyperglycaemia

Hyperglycaemia occurs when blood glucose levels rise >10 mmol/L. In a person with diabetes, hyperglycaemia may be caused by low insulin levels, a diet high in carbohydrates, lack of physical activity, or stress (infection, pain or surgery being common stressors) (Turton 2023). Without sufficient insulin, glucose and lipids are not able to enter target cells, depriving them of nutrients. This in turn stimulates increased hunger and food intake (polyphagia), glycogenolysis, gluconeogenesis and the release of counter regulatory hormones such as cortisol. Together, these actions will raise the blood glucose level. Polyphagia, polyuria and polydipsia are the three main symptoms of hyperglycaemia and usually occur when the BGL is persistently >10–15 mmol/L (Crawford 2023). If not treated, hyperglycaemia can rapidly progress and become a critical condition known as diabetic ketoacidosis (DKA) or hyperglycaemic hyperosmolar state (HHS), both of which are preventable. DKA is generally associated with T1DM but can occur in people with T2DM in the presence of severe infection or metabolic stress. HHS is more common in people with T2DM and is associated with higher rates of morbidity and mortality (Miller 2022).

Diabetic ketoacidosis is an acute, life-threatening emergency characterised by hyperglycaemia and ketoacidosis. The signs and symptoms include polyuria, polydipsia, BGL >10 mmol/L, hyperketonaemia (≥1.6 mmol/L), glucosuria, ketonuria, and Kussmaul's breathing pattern (i.e. deep, rapid respirations with a sweet, fruity or acetone odour). Hyperglycaemia and hyperketonaemia prompt osmotic diuresis, which causes significant dehydration and serum electrolyte imbalance (Miller 2022).

Hyperosmolar hyperglycaemic state (HHS) is commonly caused by the over-production of cortisol and catecholamines triggered by physical or psychological stress. The production of these hormones increases insulin resistance and promotes glycogenolysis. HHS develops insidiously over several days or weeks rather than hours. HHS is characterised by significantly elevated blood glucose (usually >30 mmol/L), extreme dehydration, electrolyte imbalance and altered level of consciousness. The distinguishing feature of HHS is high serum osmolarity (>320 milliosmoles per kilogram [mOsm/kg] and a normal serum ketone level (0.6–1.5 mmol/L) due to the availability of enough insulin to inhibit ketogenesis (Miller 2022).

Management and intervention In the case of simple hyperglycaemia, consuming more water and administering an individually titrated dose of short-acting insulin may be all that is needed to reverse the hyperglycaemia. If the person goes into DKA or HHS, the hyperglycaemia becomes a medical emergency warranting urgent medical and nursing management (Miller 2022).

Management of DKA and HHS focuses on correcting the fluid and electrolyte imbalances, euglycaemic control, investigating and treating the cause and, in DKA, reversing the hyperketonaemia. Following established protocols/guidelines within the healthcare setting, the management of DKA and HHS includes intravenous infusions of normal saline and short-acting insulin together with electrolyte replacement. The insulin infusion must be titrated against the individual's blood sugar level every hour. Once the BGL returns to normal, the insulin infusion can be ceased, and the individual can return to their regular insulin regime. Initial care is most often in an intensive care unit (ICU) where medical and nursing staff follow established protocols/treatment. Nursing care includes administration of IV fluids, managing the insulin infusion, administering oxygen, identifying and treating the cause, and monitoring vital signs, neurological state, BGL, capillary ketone level, serum electrolytes, fluid balance and central venous pressure. If the individual becomes unconscious, nursing care is aimed at preventing complications of coma (Miller 2022).

Long-term complications

The long-term complications of diabetes are classified as either macrovascular or microvascular (Crawford 2023; Miller 2022).

Macrovascular disease

Diabetes related macrovascular complications are those that affect the larger blood vessels. These complications pose a significant risk factor for cardiovascular disease, myocardial infarction (heart attack), cerebrovascular accident (stroke) and peripheral vascular disease (PVD) (AIHW 2022). The main physiological process in the development of macrovascular disease is atherosclerosis. Atherosclerosis is thought to result from chronic inflammation and injury to the arterial wall in the peripheral and coronary vascular system due to poor glycaemic control. It is a common complication of DM, and in the case of T2DM goes undetected until late in the course of cardiovascular disease. Diabetes also increases the risk of poor outcomes and disability. Peripheral vascular disease is often widespread and characterised by—cold lower extremities, intermittent claudication, diminished or absent pulses, ulcers, infection and gangrene (Crawford 2023; Miller 2022).

Microvascular disease

Diabetic retinopathy affects the retinal blood vessels, which causes them to haemorrhage or leak fluid. Retinopathy occurs in both T1DM and T2DM and is related to the duration of diabetes and degree of glycaemic control. Repeated vitreous haemorrhage may result in retinal detachment or blindness. The risk of glaucoma and cataracts is heightened in those with diabetes. Prevention, screening, early detection and management of eye disease by an ophthalmologist and/or optometrist along with tight glycaemic control is essential to eye health in the diabetic individual. Diabetic retinopathy affects up to 80% of individuals who have had diabetes for ≥20 years and is the leading cause of blindness in those aged 20–64 years. An important consideration in nursing a diabetic individual is the possibility and impact of visual impairment (Crawford 2023; Miller 2022).

Diabetic nephropathy, or diabetic kidney disease, is a progressive condition caused by long-term damage to the capillaries of the glomerulus. Signs and symptoms are often vague until the person develops proteinuria (blood proteins in the urine), uraemia and oedema. Renal function is gradually impaired by glomerulosclerosis (scarring of the kidney's tiny blood vessels) and may progress to chronic renal failure. T2DM-related nephropathy is one of the most common reasons for commencing dialysis. Prevention, screening treatment of impaired renal function, such as urinary tract infections or hypertension, and blood glucose homeostasis reduces the risk of developing diabetic nephropathy (Crawford 2023; Miller 2022).

Peripheral neuropathy occurs when persistent hyperglycaemia damages peripheral blood vessels causing ischaemia, inflammation and degeneration of the peripheral nerves. Initially, the individual will experience tingling, pins and needles or burning of their lower limbs. As the condition worsens, sensation is lost altogether in all limbs and genitalia (Crawford 2023; Miller 2022). (See Figure 36.9.)

Another form of neuropathy is characterised by a decreased sense of spatial awareness (proprioceptive disturbances) and diminished sensation to touch, pain and temperature. These sensory deficits increase the possibility of injury. Diabetic foot disease, due to changes in blood vessels and nerves, often leads to ulceration. Decreased sensation in the feet can lead to the individual not noticing cuts and developing foot infections. If not treated early, these can lead to amputation. Peripheral motor nerve involvement results in muscle weakness and muscular atrophy, which may lead to deformities of the feet (e.g. Charcot's foot). (See Figure 36.10.) Early nursing assessment, education and management is an important part of preventative foot care (Crawford 2023; Miller 2022).

Sexual health

While most people with diabetes are able to lead completely normal sex lives, diabetes may contribute to sexual problems for some. The most common problem is erectile dysfunction

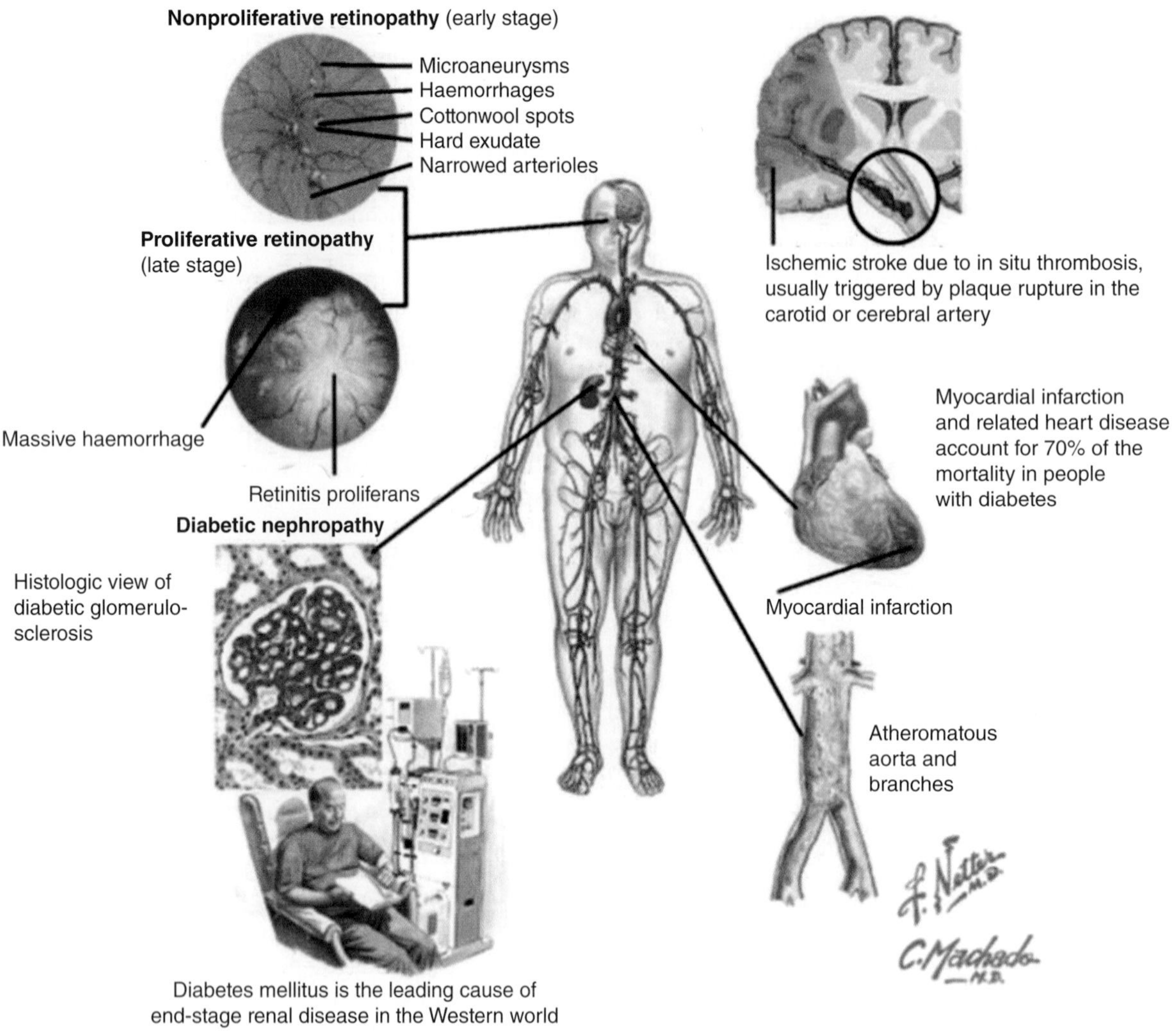

Figure 36.9 Diabetic microvascular and macrovascular complications
(Tchang 2021)

in men (also known as impotence). Reduced blood flow and nerve damage to the penis are generally the underlying reasons for erectile dysfunction. Often, men with diabetes who have the condition also have other related nerve and circulation problems, such as high blood pressure, high cholesterol or heart disease (Diabetes Australia 2023b). Controlling BGLs may assist to prevent impotence associated with diabetes. Possible complications in women include decreased vaginal lubrication and libido, anorgasmia, increased urinary tract infections and vaginitis (Crawford 2023; Miller 2022).

Dental health

The most common oral complications related to diabetes are periodontitis (advanced gum disease) and oral thrush. Symptoms of oral cavity disease include bleeding and swollen gums, halitosis (bad breath), sensitive or loose teeth, dental plaque, recession of the gums and gaps developing between the teeth, which may lead to food becoming stuck. Management includes regular oral health assessment and education on oral hygiene (Turton 2023).

CARE OF THE INDIVIDUAL WITH AN ENDOCRINE DISORDER

The endocrine system's relationship with other body systems is complex and dysfunction of any endocrine gland can be widespread. The possibility that an endocrine disorder may be the cause of illness needs to be considered in a wide range of medical emergencies. Most endocrine disorders result from glandular hyperactivity or hypoactivity and presentation will vary according to the gland affected and the hormone/s it produces (Cleveland Clinic 2022a; Crawford 2023).

Effects of endocrine dysfunction

The medical and nursing management of an individual with an endocrine disorder is dependent upon the type of endocrine disorder and the individual themselves. When developing a plan of care, the nurse must consider the physical and psychological effects the disorder may have on the individual, their carer, family or friends. This

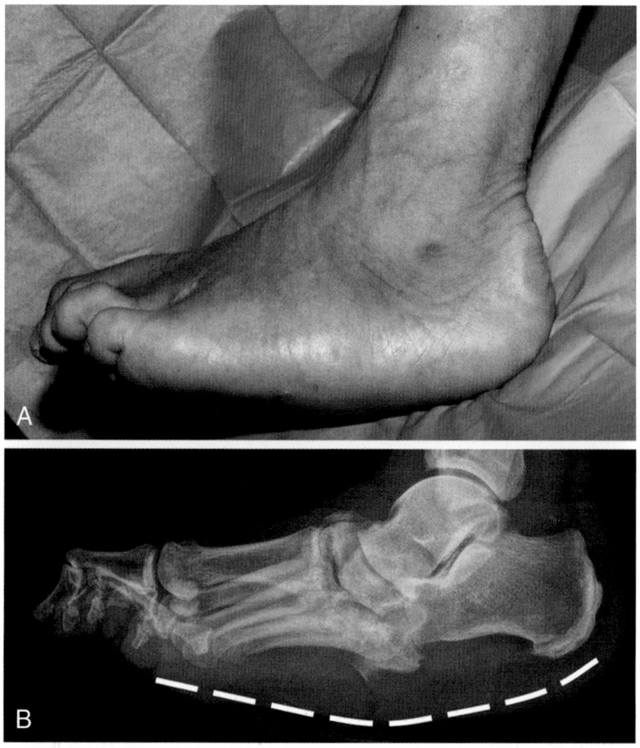

Figure 36.10 Charcot's foot
(Iaquinto & Leslie 2023)

information will allow for the planning and implementation of person-centred care and the involvement of appropriate multidisciplinary healthcare professionals (Crawford 2023).

Lifestyle changes

As a result of an endocrine imbalance, some individuals may need to make lifelong changes to their medication, diet, fluids, physical activity, exposure to stressors and mental health supports. A vast range of supports are available utilising a multidisciplinary team approach to management and care. Individuals with DM must monitor a range of factors including diet, activity, blood glucose levels, eyes, kidneys and feet for the rest of their lives. They are also encouraged to wear a medical alert band that identifies that they have diabetes (Miller 2022).

The prospect of facing major surgery

Surgical removal of a dysfunctional or cancerous gland may be the treatment of choice for some individuals. Those who face major surgery need education and counselling preoperatively and postoperatively to ensure they are adequately informed of the surgical procedure and the impact it may have on the person's future (Crawford 2023; Miller 2022).

Possible postoperative changes

Endocrine surgery may result in an imbalance of hormones. For example, thyroidectomy for hyperthyroidism or hyperparathyroidism may result in the need for lifelong hormone replacement therapy. Individuals will therefore require education regarding the signs and symptoms of both under- and over-functioning glands (Crawford 2023; Miller 2022).

Alterations in nutritional status

Good nutrition is essential to health, and under- or over-nutrition affects a person's health status and response to treatment. All individuals should eat a healthy balanced diet and undertake regular physical activity, not only people with an endocrine disorder or those who are under or overweight. Dietary education should be provided and personalised according to each individual's age, gender, lifestyle, eating habits, cultural preferences, nutritional requirements, endocrine disorder and management plan (Waugh & Grant 2022).

Optimal nutrition may be achieved through collaboration between the individual, their family/friends/carer and healthcare professionals such as doctors, nurses and dietitians. Nurses can identify individuals at high risk of nutritional deficiencies, while dietitians can provide ongoing education and monitoring (Waugh & Grant 2022).

Alterations in fluid and electrolyte balance

Polyuria (excessive production of urine) may occur in DM or posterior pituitary gland disorders such as diabetes insipidus. Loss of fluid may also occur if the individual has diarrhoea, hyperthyroidism or Addison's disease. To address polyuria and increased thirst (polydipsia), individuals with these endocrine disorders may need additional assistance with a nurse in conjunction with medical advice. The nursing care plan includes monitoring intake and output, specific gravity of urine, weight and observing for signs and symptoms of hypovolaemic shock (Crawford 2023; Khardori et al 2022).

Conversely, retention of fluid may occur in disorders such as Cushing's syndrome, hypothyroidism (myxoedema) and SIADH. Stringent fluid intake control for individuals with SIADH is necessary to allow serum sodium levels to increase slowly. Where the effects of aldosterone are compromised or enhanced (e.g. primary aldosteronism), electrolytes and fluids need to be monitored (Khardori et al 2022; Thomas 2021).

Management of discomfort

Many endocrine disorders result in problems related to body temperature regulation. An individual with hypothyroidism is very sensitive to cold, whereas an individual with hyperthyroidism is often intolerant to heat. Other factors that may cause discomfort include pruritus associated with hyperthyroidism or DM; joint pain associated with acromegaly; anxiety and nervousness associated with hyperthyroidism, hypertension; and headache associated with phaeochromocytoma, or apathy and poor concentration with hypothyroidism—all are examples of symptoms promoting discomfort (Crawford 2023; Utiger 2022b).

Reduced independence

Extreme fatigue often accompanies endocrine disorders, and the individual may require assistance to carry out activities of daily living. Certain disorders (e.g. Cushing's syndrome or hyperparathyroidism) may cause alterations in cognitive function and can impact an individual's independence. Individuals who do not manage their blood sugar levels may develop microvascular complications that put them at risk of amputation. This can have major consequences to the individual's ability to drive, travel and/or ambulate unaided (Crawford 2023; Miller 2022).

Altered body image related to physical changes

Endocrine disorders can alter an individual's body image and self-concept in several ways. Body dissatisfaction is an internal process but is often influenced by external factors. Healthcare professionals should be prepared to explain these symptoms and offer support and empathy in the event of changes to self-esteem or behaviours associated with physical changes (Crawford 2023).

Obvious changes in physical appearance can occur in many endocrine disorders. In Cushing's syndrome, individuals may develop a buffalo hump and/or a moon face while people with hyperthyroidism may develop a goitre and exophthalmos (Crawford 2023).

The nursing care plan for an individual with an endocrine disorder needs to focus on providing comfort, psychological support and good nutrition. Person-centred education, specialist psychological management and referrals to support groups should be encouraged (Crawford 2023). A list of organisations and websites is provided in Online Resources later in this chapter.

CRITICAL THINKING EXERCISE 36.3

You are caring for Asmita—a middle-aged woman who has recently been diagnosed with Cushing's syndrome. Cushing's syndrome is associated with an excess of which hormones? What management intervention/s do you think are high in priority when caring for Asmita? Why do you think this is so?

CRITICAL THINKING EXERCISE 36.4

A 38-year-old mother of two has been admitted with an adrenal gland tumour. Considering the role of the adrenal gland, what possible endocrine disorders might they have? List the physical manifestations of each potential disorder. How might you explain what she is experiencing?

Care of the individual with diabetes mellitus

The main aim of diabetes management is to control BGLs, prevent complications and promote self-care. Care of an individual with diabetes involves empowering the individual to regulate BGLs through diet, exercise insulin and/or oral medications, preventing infection and controlling stress. Promoting self-management relies upon education that is supportive and focuses on positive achievements (Miller 2022; Turton 2023). (See Nursing Care Plan 36.1.)

Diet and nutrition requirements

People with diabetes should follow the advice of an accredited practising dietitian. Diet and exercise are the first line of treatment for all types of diabetes since it helps control blood glucose levels and manage cardiovascular and other health risks. Dietitians work with people with DM to provide nutrition therapy, including education to promote glycaemic control and reduce the risk of short- and long-term complications. It is essential that the individual gains an understanding of the principles of the disorder so they can modify and adapt their diet to meet demands during illness, injury, emotional stress or major lifestyle changes. To help manage diabetes, Diabetes Australia (2022c) recommends that individuals:

1. Eat regular meals and healthy snacks spread over the day.
2. Base meals on high-fibre carbohydrate foods such as wholegrain breads and cereals, legumes, vegetables and fruits.
3. Limit the total amount of fat eaten especially saturated fat by choosing lean meats and low-fat dairy foods. Avoid fried takeaway foods, pastries and biscuits.
4. Keep weight within the healthy weight range by matching the amount of food/kilojoules eaten with the amount of kilojoules expended through activity each day.
5. Limit alcohol since it is high in sugar and may interact adversely with some medications. It can also mask or delay hypoglycaemia by up to 12 hours.

(Diabetes Australia 2022a; Diabetes Australia 2022c)

Exercise

A well-planned program of regular exercise and diet is important in maintaining a healthy weight and controlling blood glucose. For a person with diabetes, exercise helps:

- Improve the effectiveness of insulin.
- Maintain a healthy weight.
- Lower blood pressure.
- Reduce the risk of heart disease.
- Reduce stress.

(Diabetes Australia 2022a)

Exercise stimulates the uptake of glucose by muscle cells, lowering blood glucose levels. However, excessive exercise can increase the risk of hypoglycaemia. Individuals

NURSING CARE PLAN 36.1

Assessment: Wendy Long underwent surgical reduction and immobilisation of a left carpal fracture yesterday. No complications from surgery evident at time of report. Client reports a pain score of 3/10 described in left wrist as a dull ache. Client has a past medical history of T2DM and is currently complaining of fatigue, lethargy and is unable to carry out activities of daily living (ADLs) without assistance. Wendy appears unmotivated to mobilise or carry out the normal routine of bathing, dressing and sitting out of bed.

Issue/s to be addressed: Lack of motivation, pain and discomfort, listlessness and inability to maintain ADLs independently, immobility and practising active exercises.

Goal/s: To relieve pain and discomfort, encourage and assist Wendy to maintain daily hygiene activities, encourage mild to moderate active exercise as tolerated to increase energy levels, encourage personal interests and awareness of her surroundings.

Care/actions	Rationale
Discuss with Wendy the need to mobilise (without risk to recovery from surgery to wrist). Plan with Wendy daily ADLs or assistance with ADLs to avoid fatigue.	Education, participation and encouragement may provide motivation to increase mild activity levels even though Wendy may feel too weak or disinterested.
Ensure Wendy has periods of supervised activity alternating with sufficient rest.	To prevent excessive fatigue.
Monitor vital signs before and after activity/exertion and report and note significant changes.	Indicates physiological levels of tolerance to movement.
Increase Wendy's participation in her ADLs as tolerated.	Increases confidence level, self-esteem and activity tolerance level.
Involve Wendy in discussions on strategies to conserve energy during tasks such as bathing (or activities as planned).	Wendy will be able to accomplish more with less energy expended and likely increase her endurance to activities as well as her confidence.

Evaluation: Wendy described her pain level as 1–2 on movement and managed to complete her hygiene this a.m. with very little assistance. She is more receptive to conversation and responds appropriately when encouraged to mobilise. Wendy has managed short frequent walks along with an uninterrupted afternoon rest and now reports feeling less lethargic.

with T1DM and fluctuating or high blood glucose levels (i.e. FBG levels greater than 14 mmol/L and ketonuria) should avoid exercise until their blood glucose has returned to an acceptable level. Exercise in these circumstances can elevate blood glucose and increase ketone production; therefore, careful monitoring is essential (Diabetes Australia 2022a; Dickinson 2023).

Diabetes education is essential for the individual to gain understanding of the relationship between exercise, diet and insulin dosage under varying conditions. Physical activity forms part of CVD risk minimisation. Exercise has the benefit of decreasing cholesterol and triglycerides and reducing the risk of cardiovascular disease. Sedentary behaviour (prolonged sitting) has been linked to heart disease and there is evidence to show it has adverse effects on cardiac health (Diabetes Australia 2022a; Dickinson 2023). For a sample of an entry in progress notes, see Progress Note 36.1.

Medications

Medications should be managed using the principles of medication administration. An understanding of the different types of glucose-lowering medications including their action, duration, administration, storage and disposal will promote empowerment and help improve glycaemic control (Dickinson 2023).

Insulin

Insulin is essential for the normal metabolism of glucose and the regulation of BGLs. There are many types of exogenous insulin used in the management of diabetes mellitus. These insulins vary in time of onset and duration of action (e.g. rapid onset, fast acting, short acting, intermediate acting, long acting or mixed). The type and dose of insulin prescribed can vary according to the time of day, duration and type of activity undertaken, and diet. In people with T1DM, insulin replacement therapy will be lifelong. As soon as possible after diagnosis of DM, an individual is educated to self-manage their insulin injections or diabetic medication and use of the relevant equipment (Dickinson 2023).

Insulin may be administered via an insulin syringe (less commonly used), specialised insulin pens or an insulin pump (continuous subcutaneous insulin infusion or CSII), while

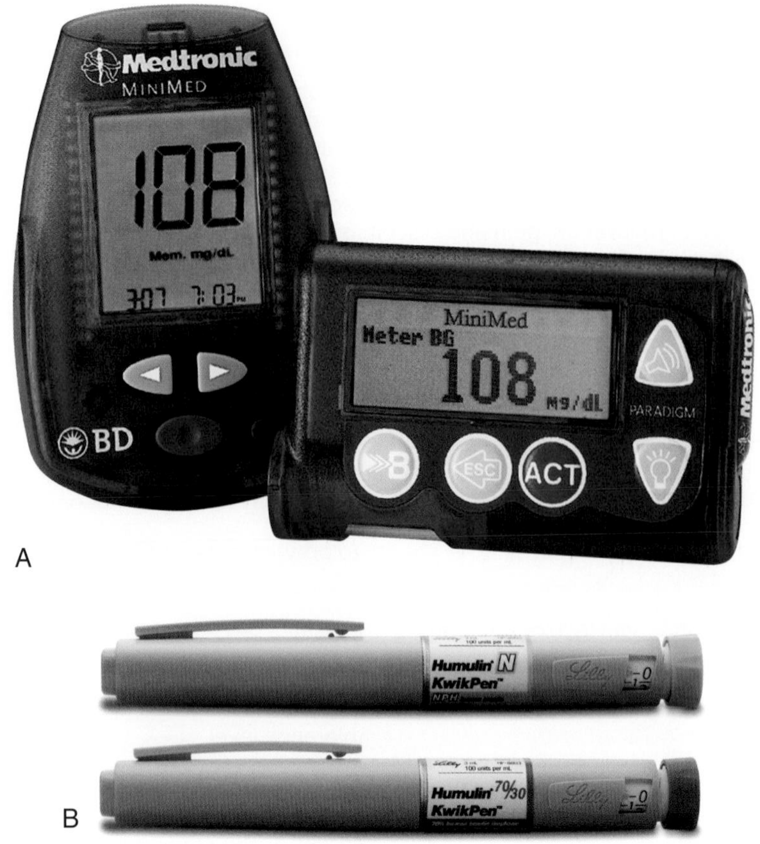

Figure 36.11 A: Paradigm® 515 insulin pump and Paradigm Link™ blood glucose monitor, **B:** Prefilled Kwik Pens, Humulin N and Humulin 70/30

continuous glucose monitors (CGMs) can be used to test and track interstitial glucose levels (Figure 36.11). The abdomen provides the fastest and most consistent rate of absorption and is an easily accessible site; however, individuals are advised to rotate injection sites to prevent tissue atrophy or hypertrophy. Insulin is a high-risk medicine and can cause harm or death if administered incorrectly (Dickinson 2023). See Chapter 20 for further information.

Short-acting insulin may also be delivered subcutaneously via insulin pump, with dosages self-determined and monitored by the individual. Individuals choosing this type of insulin administration need to be motivated, educated and supported by a diabetes educator or other diabetes health professional. Insulin pumps and associated equipment may be subsidised in Australia by the NDSS (NDSS 2022b).

Oral hypoglycaemic agents

Oral hypoglycaemic or oral glucose-lowering medications are often prescribed in the management of T2DM that is unresponsive to diet alone. Different glucose-lowering medications act in a variety of ways to lower blood glucose levels. Some oral hypoglycaemics work by stimulating the pancreas to release insulin, others by reducing insulin resistance and promoting glucose use, or by delaying glucose absorption through the gut (Dickinson 2023; NDSS 2022b; Wexler 2023).

Hygiene and preventing infection

People with diabetes are susceptible to infection since elevated blood glucose provides an ideal environment for bacterial growth and impairs the body's natural defence mechanisms. The individual is particularly at risk of developing urinary tract infections, fungal infections such as *Candida* albicans and infected skin lesions. To minimise the risk of infection, the nurse needs to educate the individual on the importance of glycaemic control, personal hygiene and the need to avoid unnecessary exposure to infection. Skin needs to be clean and free from excessive irritation, friction or pressure. All injuries, however minor, should be cleaned with a mild antiseptic solution, covered with a dressing and reviewed by a healthcare professional if the injury does not heal (Dickinson 2023; Wexler 2023).

Skin cuts or abrasions of the feet commonly occur in people with poor glycaemic control, which can be exacerbated in the presence of impaired circulation and peripheral neuropathy. If a minor injury or lesion goes undetected or untreated, ulceration, infection and gangrene may develop, which in some cases can lead to amputation

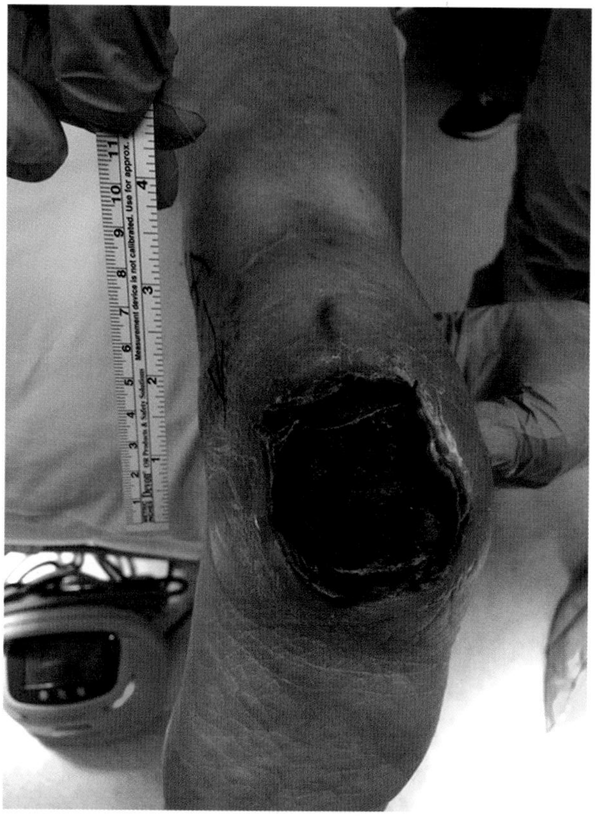

Figure 36.12 Diabetic heel ulceration with necrotic eschar cap and underlying necrosis to the level of bone

(Atway & DiMassa 2020)

(Dickinson 2023) (Figure 36.12). There are more than 4400 amputations every year in Australia as a result of diabetes (Diabetes Australia 2022b). The nurse should also consider that the lesion may be of a different origin. Melanomas of the feet have been misdiagnosed as diabetic foot ulcers. Care of the feet and prevention of foot lesions is of vital importance. National guidelines on the prevention, identification and management of foot complications in DM are available on many websites (NDSS 2022b; Dickinson 2023).

Care of the feet

Considerations for care of the feet for the individual include the following:

- Wear well-fitting socks or stockings, and shoes. Socks should be made from natural fibres with care taken to avoid those with seams.
- Practise daily cleansing, drying and inspection of the feet. Mild soap is recommended, and feet should not be soaked for long periods. After washing, the feet should be patted dry. Dry feet may be gently massaged with lanolin or oil to prevent cracks.
- Consult a podiatrist regularly. Any corns or calluses need professional attention. If toenails require trimming, it is best to file nails rather than use scissors. File straight across the nail to avoid skin damage and help prevent ingrown toenails.
- Keep the feet warm but avoid placing feet near heaters or heat packs. If an electric blanket is used, it should be turned off before the individual gets into bed.
- Never walk barefooted or on hot surfaces.
- Perform daily foot and leg exercises to increase circulation.
- Avoid constrictive clothing (e.g. socks with elasticised tops) and crossing the legs, both of which restrict blood flow to the limbs and feet.
- Seek immediate attention from the podiatrist or medical officer if there is any injury, colour change, infection or discharge of pus or blood.

(NDSS 2022b; Wexler 2023)

CRITICAL THINKING EXERCISE 36.5

Emily, 46 years old, is an active community care worker who has arrived at a medical clinic for assessment. She is concerned by the gradual onset of several symptoms. Emily complains of weight gain, a feeling of 'slowing down', constipation, tiredness, impaired memory and feeling cold despite the warm spring weather. She speaks slowly, occasionally slurring her words. On examination, you record a bradycardia of 52 beats per minute, and note Emily's dry skin, oedematous eyelids and enlarged tongue.

1. What endocrine disorder is Emily likely to be suffering from?
2. Emily started on medication with the aim of normalising her thyroxine blood levels. If these oral thyroid medications cause her to become hyperthyroid, what signs and symptoms would you include as part of her education?
3. What further education might Emily need to assist her in dealing with the condition?

Monitoring blood glucose levels

Blood glucose monitoring provides insight into the effectiveness of the diabetes management plan. The results can provide direct feedback to the individual and caregivers. Capillary blood glucose monitoring is described in Clinical Skill 36.1 and is performed by obtaining a drop of capillary blood, which is applied to a reagent strip and read by one of the many types of blood glucose meters available. Most capillary blood glucose meters provide results that closely resemble the venous blood glucose level, the slight difference being clinically insignificant. A digital display of the glucose level is provided on the screen.

Continuous glucose meters (CGMs) are interstitial glucose monitoring devices that do not require repeated 'finger-pricking'. An interstitial glucose sensor is inserted, and levels can be monitored every 1–30 minutes. The sensor is inserted using an automatic insertion device. Data is sent from the sensor to a transmitter that communicates with an insulin

CLINICAL SKILL 36.1 Measuring blood glucose

Please adhere to the policy and procedures of the facility/organisation prior to undertaking the skill. Ensure this skill is in your scope of practice.

NMBA Decision-making Framework considerations	Equipment:
NMBA Decision-making Framework considerations (refer to NMBA Decision-making framework for nursing and midwifery 2020): 1. Am I educated? 2. Am I authorised? 3. Am I competent? If you answer 'no' to any of these, do not perform that activity. Seek guidance and support from your teacher/a nurse team leader/clinical facilitator/educator.	**Equipment:** Blood glucose meter Reagent strips Tissues or cotton balls Lancet or peripheral blood access Sharps container Disposable gloves Warm washcloth An appropriate chart for documentation

PREPARE FOR THE SKILL

(Please refer to the Standard Steps on pp. xviii–xx for related rationales.)
Mentally review the steps of the skill.
Discuss the skill with your instructor/supervisor/team leader, if required.
Confirm correct facility/organisation policy/safe operating procedures.
Validate the order in the individual's record.
Identify indication and rationale for performing the activity.
Assess for any contraindications.

Locate and gather equipment.
Perform hand hygiene.
Ensure therapeutic interaction.
Identify the individual using three individual identifiers.
Gain the individual's consent.
Assess for pain relief.
Prepare the environment.
Provide and maintain privacy.
Assist the individual to assume an appropriate position of comfort.

Skill activity	Rationale
Assist the individual to wash hands with soap and warm water and dry thoroughly.	Promotes skin cleansing; even the smallest bits of food can alter a reading. Warm water increases the peripheral circulation due to vasodilation, facilitating blood flow at the puncture site. Make sure the site is entirely dry because even water can affect results.

PERFORM THE SKILL

(Please refer to the Standard Steps on pp. xviii–xx for related rationales.)
Perform hand hygiene.
Apply PPE: gloves, eyewear, mask and gown as appropriate.
Ensure the individual's safety and comfort throughout skill.
Promote independence and involvement of the individual if possible and/or appropriate.
Assess the individual's tolerance to the skill throughout.
Dispose of used supplies, equipment, waste and sharps appropriately.
Remove PPE and discard or store appropriately.
Perform hand hygiene.

Skill activity	Rationale
Prepare the blood glucose meter as per the manufacturer's instructions. Check the machine has been calibrated with the test strip. Check the date on the reagent strip and ensure the lid is closed securely.	Blood glucose meters may require recalibration to ensure accuracy of result. Reagent strips may have an expiry date and are affected by moisture in the air.

CLINICAL SKILL 36.1 Measuring blood glucose—cont'd

Insert the reagent strip into the blood glucose meter. Follow manufacturer's guidelines regarding when to insert the strip.	This is generally before the blood is applied to the strip.
Prepare the lancet and place firmly against the soft flesh at either side of the top of the finger. Quickly pierce the finger. If a drop of blood does not appear, gently 'milk' the finger, if necessary, by massaging finger from base towards fingertip, ensuring hand is below heart level.	Ensures the skin is pierced. Reduces discomfort. The fingertip is the most accurate test site because it registers changes in blood glucose more quickly than the rest of the body. There are fewer nerve endings on the sides of the fingers; they are therefore less painful. Increases vasodilation and adequate blood flow for accuracy of result. Excessive squeezing of tissues during collection may contribute to pain, bruising, scarring, haematoma formation, or dilution of the sample with serous fluid.
Allow the blood to drop onto the test strip.	This may differ depending on the monitor. The blood should cover the test strip. Some reagent strips fill from the side.
Apply pressure to the puncture site with tissue or cotton swab for 30–60 seconds or until bleeding has stopped.	Prevents further bleeding after the sample has been obtained and prevents haematoma formation.
Timing is determined by the manufacturer.	Ensures accurate results. Most blood glucose meters display a digital read out.
Read the BGL result from the blood glucose meter.	Note and record result to allow comparison with the individual's normal blood glucose level.
Turn off the blood glucose meter, remove the test strip and dispose of supplies appropriately.	Reduces risk of transmission of infection.

AFTER THE SKILL

(Please refer to the Standard Steps on pp. xviii–xx for related rationales.)
Communicate outcome to the individual, any ongoing care and to report any complications.
Restore the environment.
Report, record and document assessment findings, details of the skill performed and the individual's response.
Report, record and document any abnormalities and/or inability to perform the skill.
Reassess the individual to ensure there are no adverse effects/events from the skill.

(Australian Commission on Safety and Quality in Health Care 2021; Crawford 2023; Dickson 2023; Miller 2022)

pump to administer the required dose of insulin. Newer CGMs can share data with smartphones and can also alert the person if their interstitial sugars are trending low or high (Dickinson 2023; NDSS 2022a). (See Figure 36.11A.)

The frequency of blood glucose monitoring varies according to type of diabetes and glycaemic control. Some people with diabetes can be educated to alter their dose of insulin according to the carbohydrate load of each meal; however, this requires significant education. It is recommended that individuals check their blood sugar level before meals; two hours after a meal; before bed; before, during and after rigorous exercise; and when feeling unwell. For individuals with a CGM, the frequency of interstitial glucose testing can be programmed anywhere from every 1–30 minutes. Whichever device an individual or healthcare facility uses should not be problematic as long as the operator follows the manufacturer's instructions (Australasian Medical & Scientific Limited [AMSL] Diabetes 2023; Dickinson 2023).

The aim of self-management of blood glucose monitoring is to assist the individual to assume more independence. Individuals using blood glucose monitoring benefit from education and advice from a diabetes educator or diabetes nurse educator. (See Clinical Skill 36.1 and Clinical Interest Box 36.5.)

A glycosylated haemoglobin (HbA1c) is another blood sugar level test commonly ordered by a medical officer and analysed in a lab. The HbA1c test identifies the person's average blood glucose level over the past 10–12 weeks. It is used to monitor glycaemic control and to predict risk of long-term diabetes complications (Dickinson 2023).

Performing a urinalysis can identify the presence of glycosuria and ketonuria but is not as accurate as a serum

CLINICAL INTEREST BOX 36.5 Continuous glucose monitoring (CGM)

Continuous glucose monitoring (CGM) links continuous blood glucose measurements to an insulin infusion system driven by a computer, to approximate normal glucose homeostasis. CGM devices measure glucose levels within the body's interstitial fluid. These devices are compact and wearable and measure glucose levels 24 hours a day. Additionally, the device has alarms to let users know if glucose levels are too low (i.e. trending towards a hypoglycaemic episode) or too high. Moreover, CGM devices generally reduce the frequency of daily finger-prick checks. A number of CGM devices work in conjunction with a compatible insulin pump while others send information to a CGM receiver or smartphone. Most of these devices need regular calibration and blood glucose testing about twice a day, as well as confirmation of abnormal sensor readings with a capillary test before corrective action is taken. For some people with diabetes, CGM gives peace of mind since the person is able to see their glucose levels at any time and receive alerts if levels go outside the user's target range.

(Dickinson 2023; NDSS 2022a)

analysis. The presence of glucose in the urine is not always an indication of diabetes. It can also be evident in other disorders such as Cushing's syndrome (Crawford 2023). (See Chapter 31 for further information on urinalysis.)

Education

Personalised diabetes education and shared decision-making allow the nurse to deliver holistic, person-centred diabetes care. Education is an integral part of diabetes self-management. Nurses need to implement a well-planned education program that alleviates anxiety and creates autonomy. This will empower the individual to take control and self-manage their condition. The involvement of family, carers and close friends will assist the individual to adhere to the lifestyle modifications necessary to maintain optimum glycaemic control and good health. A diabetic education program is advantageous because it can help the individual:

- Accept the condition and understand the importance of strict glycaemic control.
- Learn and practise technical skills needed to monitor blood glucose levels and administer medications.
- Understand the importance of diet, exercise, stress management and medication in maintaining normal blood glucose levels.
- Recognise disturbances in blood glucose levels (i.e. hypo and hyperglycaemia) and have the knowledge to self-manage the event to avoid complications.

(Dickinson 2023)

Mobile phone applications are available that make it easier for individuals to record and track blood glucose readings, medications and physical activity. Some applications can identify patterns, set goals and share information with other members of the person's healthcare management team (Dickinson 2023; Miller 2022).

Individuals with DM are encouraged to carry a form of diabetic alert identification, such as a card, bracelet or medallion. Medical data sharing via *My Health Record* is also recommended so that health professionals involved in their care can access the most up-to-date information about their diabetes management. These measures ensure that appropriate care is administered if a medical emergency occurs. Individuals with DM may be referred by their health professional or GP to the NDSS for access to subsidised diabetes products (Australian Digital Health Agency 2023; NDSS 2022c).

CRITICAL THINKING EXERCISE 36.6

Antonio is an obese 64-year-old Hispanic man with a 14-year history of poorly controlled T2DM. Despite his best efforts, Antonio tells you that he is finding it difficult to alter his diet (high in salt, saturated fat and calories) and activity levels (works in an office in front of a computer 5 days per week and occasionally takes his dog for a walk around the block). His doctor has recently told him to take extra care with his feet. He asks you why this is important. What instructions/education would you provide Antonio regarding footcare for people with diabetes mellitus?

Progress Note 36.1

02/03/2024 0950 hrs	Nursing: Wendy supervised with exercise (walk around ward) due to general lethargy and unresponsiveness. Mobilisation completed and Wendy returned to bed. Instructed to call for assistance when bathing or toileting or feeling unwell. Wendy indicated that she felt a bit more capable and energetic and will request assistance only if she is too tired to walk by herself. *S Hope* (HOPE), *EN*

DECISION-MAKING FRAMEWORK EXERCISE 36.1

You are a Diploma of Nursing student who is on clinical placement for the second time. You have just successfully completed the medication administration unit and are caring for an individual who has Graves' disease, a condition that affects the thyroid gland.

Your buddy nurse asks you to administer a patient's medication (an antithyroid tablet) or assist the individual to do so. The buddy nurse will be close by as they will be meeting the care needs of an individual on the other side of the room.

1. Before you undertake this action, do you have the necessary training/education to administer or assist with the administration of oral medication?
2. Since you are still a student nurse what authority do you have with regards to performing medication administration? Do you need assistance? Explain the importance of the proximity of the buddy nurse.
3. You do not feel confident in undertaking this action. Should you go ahead anyway?
4. Given that you have completed stage two in the course (Diploma of Nursing) only a week or so prior to your second clinical placement, explain why you may or may not be competent at this stage of the course to administer medications.

Summary

The endocrine system is made up of several glands that secrete hormones directly into the bloodstream that act as messengers. Hormones have a specific purpose in the body, and hormonal effects are often wide-ranging and lasting. Moreover, hormones influence major body functions as varied as growth, sexual maturation, blood calcium and fluid balance or homeostasis. Under normal conditions endocrine glands and hormones work in harmony to maintain equilibrium in the body's many physiological processes.

Review Questions

1. Describe how the pituitary gland regulates the thyroid, gonads and adrenal glands.
2. Describe gigantism. Does gigantism occur before or after epiphyseal closure? Explain why gigantism differs in signs and symptoms from acromegaly.
3. What is the function of antidiuretic hormone (ADH)? Blood tests of one of your individuals shows they are suffering from hyponatraemia, serum hypo-osmolarity and urine hyperosmolarity. What sort of endocrine imbalance might be occurring? List the gland or glands that are responsible for the imbalances.
4. Explain the difference between diabetes insipidus and diabetes mellitus. List the endocrine glands responsible for these two conditions.
5. Explain the reasons for the following signs and symptoms: hyperactivity, tachycardia and nervousness, all of which are typical of Graves' disease.
6. List three situations that could instigate a thyroid storm or thyroid crisis.
7. The parathyroid glands secrete parathormone (PTH). Explain the action of this hormone. List the name and source of the hormone that is antagonistic to PTH.
8. Describe the main functions of glucocorticoids such as cortisol. List possible health problems that may develop with hypersecretion or the prolonged administration of cortisol.
9. Explain why problems with the adrenal cortex might manifest in body fluid imbalances.
10. Explain why the actions of the adrenal medulla have an identical, but more prolonged influence on your body compared to the sympathetic nervous system.
11. Outline the signs and symptoms expected from a female with an excess of androgens.
12. Describe the two main types of diabetes mellitus (DM).
13. Explain the significance of high levels of ketones in the blood and urine of an individual with T1DM.
14. Describe the best location on an individual's finger to perform a blood glucose test and explain why it is the best location.
15. Match the list of endocrine organs/tissues listed below with their hormones

Gland	Hormone
Pancreas	Adrenaline
Adrenal	TH
Thyroid	GH
Pituitary	Insulin

Evolve® Answer guide for the Review Questions, Critical Thinking Exercises, Decision-making Framework Exercises and Critical Thinking Questions in Case Studies is hosted on Evolve: http://evolve.elsevier.com/AU/Koutoukidis/Tabbner.

References

Atway, S.A., DiMassa, N.V., 2020. Debridement and negative pressure wound therapy. In: Roy, S., Das, A., Bagchi, D., *Wound healing, tissue repair, and regeneration in diabetes.* Elsevier, St Louis.

Australian Bureau of Statistics (ABS), 2022. Diabetes. Available at: <https://www.abs.gov.au/statistics/health/health-conditions-and-risks/diabetes/latest-release>.

Australian Commission on Safety and Quality in Health Care (ACSQHC), 2021. National safety and quality health service standards, 2nd ed. ACSQHC, Sydney. Available at: <https://www.safetyandquality.gov.au/publications-and-resources/resource-library/national-safety-and-quality-health-service-standards-second-edition>.

Australian Digital Health Agency, 2023. My Health Record. Available at: <https://www.digitalhealth.gov.au/initiatives-and-programs/my-health-record>.

Australian Institute of Health and Welfare, 2022. Diabetes: Australian Facts. Available at: <https://www.aihw.gov.au/reports/diabetes/diabetes/contents/summary>.

Australasian Medical & Scientific Limited (AMSL), 2023. Insulin Pump Therapy for Type 1 Diabetes – Tandem®. Available at: <https://www.amsl.com.au/tslim-x2-insulin-pump/>.

Banasik, J., 2022. *Pathophysiology*, 7th ed. Elsevier, St Louis.

Belchetz, P., Hammond, P., 2003. *Mosby's color atlas and text of diabetes and endocrinology.* Mosby, Edinburgh.

Cleveland Clinic, 2022a. Addison's disease. Available at: <https://my.clevelandclinic.org/health/diseases/15095-addisons-disease?>.

Cleveland Clinic, 2022b. Hypoparathyroidism. Available at: <https://my.clevelandclinic.org/health/diseases/22672-hypoparathyroidism>.

Cleveland Clinic, 2022c. Hypopituitarism. Available at: <https://my.clevelandclinic.org/health/diseases/22102-hypopituitarism>.

Craft, J., Gordon, C., McCance, K.L., et al., 2023. *Understanding pathophysiology*, Australia and New Zealand edition, 4th ed. Elsevier, Chatswood.

Crisp, J., Douglas, C., Rebeiro, G., Waters, D., 2021. *Potter and Perry's fundamentals of nursing*, 6th ed. Elsevier, Chatswood.

Crawford, A.H., 2023. Endocrine problems. In: Harding, M. M., Kwong, J., Hagler, D., et al., *Lewis's medical-surgical nursing*, 12th ed. Elsevier, St Louis.

Damjanov, I., 2006. *Pathology for the health-related profession*, 3rd ed. WB Saunders, Philadelphia.

Diabetes Australia, 2022a. Exercise and diabetes. Available at: <https://www.diabetesaustralia.com.au/living-with-diabetes/exercise>.

Diabetes Australia, 2022b. Facts and figures. Available at: <https://www.diabetesaustralia.com.au/facts-and-figures>.

Diabetes Australia, 2022c. Healthy diet for diabetes. Available at: <https://www.diabetesaustralia.com.au/living-with-diabetes/healthy-eating>.

Diabetes Australia, 2023a. Blood glucose monitoring. Available at: <https://www.diabetesaustralia.com.au/managing-diabetes/blood-glucose-monitoring>.

Diabetes Australia, 2023b. Diabetes & sexual health. Available at: <https://www.diabetesaustralia.com.au/living-with-diabetes/preventing-complications/sexual-health>.

Dickinson, J.K., 2023. Diabetes. In: Harding, M.M., Kwong, J., Hagler, D., et al., *Lewis's medical-surgical nursing,* 12th ed. Elsevier, St Louis.

Dover, J., Fairhurst, K., Innes, J., 2024. *Macleod's clinical examination*, 15th ed. Elsevier, St Louis.

Eyth, E., Basit, H., Swift, C.J., 2022. Glucose tolerance test. Available at: <https://www.ncbi.nlm.nih.gov/books/NBK532915>.

Favero, G., Bonomini, F., Rezzani, R., 2021. Pineal gland tumors: A review. Cancers (Basel). doi: 10.3390/cancers13071547.

Friel, L.A., 2022. Diabetes mellitus in pregnancy. Available at: <https://www.msdmanuals.com/en-au/home/women-s-health-issues/pregnancy-complicated-by-disease/diabetes-during-pregnancy>.

Genetu, A., Anemen., Y, Abay., S, et al., 2021. A 45-year-old female patient with Sheehan's syndrome presenting with imminent adrenal crisis: A case report. *Journal of Medical Case Reports* 15(1), 1–5. doi: 10.1186/s13256-021-02827-0.

Griffin, P.A., Potter, P.A., Ostendorf, W.R., Laplante, N., 2022. *Clinical nursing skills and techniques*, 10th ed. Elsevier, St Louis.

Group, D.C., 2022. Iodine in salt: Why is it added? Available at: <https://explore.globalhealing.com/iodine-in-salt>.

Heick, J., Lazaro, R., 2023. *Goodman and Snyder's differential diagnosis for physical therapists: Screening for referral*, 7th ed. Elsevier, St Louis.

Harding, M.M., Kwong, J., Hagler, D., Reinisch, C., 2023. *Lewis's medical-surgical nursing*, 12th ed. Elsevier, St Louis.

Herlihy, J., Kirov, E., 2022. *Herlihy's the human body in health and illness*. Elsevier Health Sciences, Australia.

Herlihy, B., Maebius, N.K., 2007. *The human body in health and illness*, 3rd ed. St Saunders, St Louis.

Iaquinto, J.M., Leslie, M.E., 2023. Neurological foot pathology. In: Ledoux, E., Telfer, S., *Foot and ankle biomechanics.* Elsevier, St Louis.

Jarvis, S., 2022. Hypoglycaemia – emergency treatment and management. Available at: <https://patient.info/doctor/emergency-management-of-hypoglycaemia>.

Johns Hopkins Medicine, 2023a. Congenital adrenal hyperplasia. Available at: <https://www.hopkinsmedicine.org/health/conditions-and-diseases/chongenital-adrenal-hyperplasia>.

Johns Hopkins Medicine, 2023b. Cushing's syndrome. Available at: <https://www.hopkinsmedicine.org/health/conditions-and-diseases/cushing-syndrome>.

Johns Hopkins Medicine, 2023c. Excess of aldosterone: Hyperaldosteronism. Available at: <https://www.hopkinsmedicine.org/health/conditions-and-diseases/adrenal-glands>.

Khardori, R., Ullal, J., Cooperman, M., 2022. Diabetes insipidus. Available at: <https://emedicine.medscape.com/article/117648-overview>.

Khurana, I., Khurana, A., 2020. *Medical physiology for undergraduate students*, 2nd ed. Elsevier, St Louis.

Kwong, J., 2023. Caring for lesbian, gay, bisexual, transgender, queer or questioning, and gender diverse patients. In: Harding, M.M., Kwong, J., Hagler, D., et al., *Lewis's medical-surgical nursing*, 12th ed. Elsevier, St Louis.

Leko, M., Gunjača, I., Pleić, N., Zemunik, T., 2021. Environmental factors affecting thyroid-stimulating hormone and thyroid hormone levels. *International Journal of Molecular Science* 22(12), 6521. doi: 10.3390/ijms22126521.

Lough, M.E., 2024. Endocrine clinical assessment and diagnostic procedures. In: Urden, L., Stacy, K., Sanchez, K., et al., *Priorities in critical care nursing*, 9th ed. Elsevier, St Louis.

Mayo Clinic, 2021. Male hypogonadism. Available at: <https://www.mayoclinic.org/diseases-conditions/male-hypogonadism/symptoms-causes/syc-20354881>.

Mayo Clinic, 2022a. Hyperparathyroidism. Available at: <https://www.mayoclinic.org/diseases-conditions/hyperparathyroidism/diagnosis-treatment/drc-20356199>.

Mayo Clinic, 2022b. Thyroid nodules – Diagnosis. Available at: <https://www.mayoclinic.org/diseases-conditions/thyroid-nodules/diagnosis-treatment/drc-20355266>.

Medical News Today, 2023. What is the difference between hypothyroidism and hyperthyroidism? Available at: <https://www.medicalnewstoday.com/articles/hypothyroidism-vs-hyperthyroidism>.

Miller, B., 2022. Diabetes mellitus – pathophysiology. In: Banasik, J., *Pathophysiology*, 7th ed. Elsevier, St Louis.

Morris, D.C., 2022. *Calculate with confidence*, 8th ed. Elsevier, St Louis.

National Diabetes Services Scheme (NDSS), 2022a. Continuous glucose monitoring. Available at: <https://www.ndss.com.au/wp-content/uploads/fact-sheets/fact-sheet-continuous-glucose-monitoring.pdf>.

National Diabetes Services Scheme (NDSS), 2022b. Looking after your feet. Available at: <https://www.ndss.com.au/wp-content/uploads/fact-sheets/fact-sheet-looking-after-your-feet.pdf>.

National Diabetes Services Scheme (NDSS), 2022c. Medications for type 2 diabetes. Available at: <https://www.ndss.com.au/wp-content/uploads/fact-sheets/fact-sheet-medications-for-type2-diabetes.pdf>.

National Institute of Diabetes and Digestive and Kidney Diseases (NIDDK), 2021a. Diabetes insipidus. Available at: <https://www.niddk.nih.gov/health-information/kidney-disease/diabetes-insipidus#:,:text=Diabetes%20insipidus%20is%20a%20rare,to%20urinate%20frequently%2C%20called%20polyuria>.

National Institute of Diabetes and Digestive and Kidney Diseases (NIDDK), 2021b. Hyperthyroidism (Overactive thyroid). Available at: <https://www.niddk.nih.gov/health-information/endocrine-diseases/hyperthyroidism>.

Nursing and Midwifery Board of Australia, 2020. Decision-making framework for nursing and midwifery. Available at: <https://www.nursingmidwiferyboard.gov.au/Codes-Guidelines-Statements/Frameworks.aspx>.

Pascual, J.M., Prieto, F., Rosdolsky, M., 2021. Craniopharyngiomas primarily affecting the hypothalamus. *Handbook of Clinical Neurology* 181, 75–115. Available at: <https://doi-10.1016/B978-0-12-82063-6.00007-5>.

Parthasarathy, S., 2020. Paget's disease – is it common in South India. *Indian Journal Endocrinology Metabolism* 27(5), 410–420. doi: 10.4103/ijem. IJEM51620.

Rare Cancers Australia, 2022a. Multiple endocrine neoplasia syndromes (MENS). Available at: <https://knowledge.rarecancers.org.au/knowledgebase/cancer-types/199/multiple-endocrine-neoplasia-syndromes?CancerType=&Cat=&Alpha=>.

Rare Cancers Australia, 2022b. Pheochromocytoma. Available at: <https://knowledge.rarecancers.org.au/knowledgebase/cancer-types/208/Pheochromocytoma?CancerType=Pheochromocytoma&Cat=&Alpha=>.

Rebeiro, G., Wilson, D., Fuller, S., 2021. *Potter and Perry's fundamentals of nursing workbook*, 4th ed. Elsevier, Chatswood.

Richardson, E., Glasper, J., 2021. *Textbook of children's and young people's nursing*, 3rd ed. Elsevier Health Sciences, United States.

Royal College of Pathologists Australasia (RCPA), 2017. Thyroid function testing for adult diagnosis and monitoring. RCPA, Sydney. Available at: <https://www.rcpa.edu.au/Library/College-Policies/Position-Statements/Thyroid-Function-Testing-for-Adult-Diagnosis-and-M>.

Shanbrun, L., Tempesta, D., 2023. Endocrine system. In: *Nuclear medicine and molecular imaging: Technology and techniques*, 9th ed. Elsevier, St Louis.

Tchang, B. G., 2021. Diabetes mellitus. In: Leppert, B., Kelly, C., *Netter's integrated review of medicine*. Elsevier, St Louis.

The Aga Khan University Hospital, nd. Precocious puberty. Available at: <https://hospitals.aku.edu/pakistan/diseases-and-conditions/Pages/precocious-puberty.aspx>.

Thomas, C.P., 2021. Syndrome of inappropriate antidiuretic hormone (SIADH) secretion. Available at: <https://emedicine.medscape.com/article/246650-overview>.

Turton, J., 2023. Type 2 diabetes. In: Craft, J., Gordon, C., McCance, K.L., et al., *Understanding pathophysiology*, Australia and New Zealand edition, 4th ed. Elsevier, Chatswood.

Utiger, R.D., 2022a. Congenital adrenal hyperplasia. Available at: <https://www.britannica.com/science/congenital-adrenal-hyperplasia>.

Utiger, R.D., 2022b. Graves' disease. Available at: <https://www.britannica.com/science/Graves-disease>.

Vora, K.A., Srinivasan, S., 2020. A guide to differences/disorders of sex development/intersex in children and adolescents. *Australian Journal of General Practice* 49(7), 417–422. Available at: <https://doi.org/10.31128/AJGP-03-20-5266>.

Waugh, A., Grant, A., 2022. *Ross & Wilson anatomy and physiology in health and illness*, 14th ed. Elsevier, Glasgow.

Wexler, D.J., 2023. Patient education: Foot care for people with diabetes (beyond the basics). Available at: <https://www.uptodate.com/contents/foot-care-for-people-with-diabetes-beyond-the-basics>.

Williamson, P., Thompson, T., Bell, F., Patton, K.T., 2022. *Anatomy & physiology*, 11th ed. Elsevier, St Louis.

Recommended Reading

Babić-Leko M., Pleić N, GunjaČa, I., Zemunik, T., 2021. Environmental factors that affect parathyroid hormone and calcitonin levels. *International Journal of Molecular Science* 23(1), 44. doi: 10.3390/ijms23010044.

Berman, A., Frandsen, G., Snyder, S., Levett-Jones, T., et al., 2020. *Kozier & Erb's fundamentals of nursing*, 5th ed. Pearson, Frenchs Forest.

Brown, D., Edwards, H., Buckley, T., et al., 2020. *Lewis's medical-surgical nursing*, ANZ, 5th ed. Elsevier, Chatswood.

Crisp, J., Douglas, C., Rebeiro, G., Waters, D. (eds.), 2021. *Potter & Perry's fundamentals of nursing*, ANZ edition, 6th ed. Elsevier, Chatswood.

Griffin-Perry, A., Potter, P.A., Ostendorf, W., LaPlante, N., 2021. *Clinical nursing skills and techniques*, 10th ed. Elsevier, St Louis.

Healthline, 2022. Differences between acromegaly and gigantism? Available at: <https://www.healthline.com/health/acromegaly-vs-gigantism#symptoms>.

Hinata, Y., Ohara, N., Komatsu, T., et al., 2022. Central diabetes insipidus after syndrome of inappropriate antidiuretic hormone secretion with severe hyponatremia in a patient with Rathk's cleft cyst. *Internal Medicine* 61(2), 197–203. doi: 10.2169/internalmedicine.6608-20.

LeMone, P., Burke, K., Bauldoff, G., et al., 2020. *Medical-surgical nursing: Critical thinking for person-centred care*, 4th ed, vols 1–3. Pearson Australia, Frenchs Forest.

Ng, X.W., Chung, Y.H., Piston, D.W., 2021. Intercellular communication in the islets of Langerhan in health and disease. *Comprehensive physiology*. doi.org/10.1002/cphy.c200026.

Norris, D.O., Schwartz, T.B., 2022. Endocrine system in Encyclopaedia Britannica. Available at: <https://www.britannica.com/science/endocrine-system>.

Petrosino, M., 2023. Complications of diabetes. Available at: <https://quizlet.com/267687861/complications-of-diabetes-flash-cards/>.

Ride, K., Burrow, S., 2022. Review of diabetes among Aboriginal and Torres Strait Islander people. *Journal of the Australian Indigenous HealthInfoNet* 3(2). Available at: <http://dx.doi.org/10.14221/aihjournal.v3n2.1>.

Snyder, P.J., 2021. Patient education: High prolactin levels and prolactinomas (beyond the basics). Available at: <https://www.uptodate.com/contents/high-prolactin-levels-and-prolactinomas-beyond-the-basics>.

Telfer, M.M., Tollit, M.A., Pace, C.C., Pang, K.C., 2020. Australian Standards of Care and Treatment Guidelines for Trans and Gender Diverse Children and Adolescents, version 1.3. Available at: <https://www.rch.org.au/uploadedFiles/Main/Content/adolescent-medicine/australian-standards-of-care-and-treatment-guidelines-for-trans-and-gender-diverse-children-and-adolescents.pdf>.

Tortora, G.J., Derrickson, B.H., Burkett, B., et al., 2021. *Principles of anatomy and physiology*, 3rd Asia-Pacific ed. Wiley, New Zealand.

Vanderpump, M., 2022. Thyroid disorders and their effect on cognitive function, mood and emotions. Available at: <https://www.markvanderpump.co.uk/blog/posts/thyroid-disorders-and-their-effect-on-cognitive-function-mood-and-emotions>.

Online Resources

American Diabetes Association: <https://diabetes.org>.

Australia and New Zealand Society for Paediatric Endocrinology and Diabetes: <https://anzsped.org>.

Australian Addison's Disease Association: <https://addisons.org.au>.

Australian and New Zealand Bone and Mineral Society: <https://osteoporosis.org.nz/partner/australian-and-new-zealand>.

Australian and New Zealand Endocrine Surgeons: <http://www.endocrinesurgeons.org.au>.

Australian Bureau of Statistics: <https://www.abs.gov.au>.

Australian Diabetes Educators Association: <https://www.adea.com.au>.

Australian Diabetes Society: <https://diabetessociety.com.au>.

Australian Institute of Health and Welfare: <https://www.aihw.gov.au>.

Australian Pituitary Foundation: <https://pituitary.asn.au>.

Clinical Practice Guidelines: <https://www.clinicalguidelines.gov.au>.

Diabetes Australia: <https://www.diabetesaustralia.com.au>.

Diversity Australia: <https://www.diversityaustralia.com.au/lgbtqi>.

National Diabetes Services Scheme: <https://www.ndss.com.au>.

The Australian Thyroid Foundation: <https://www.thyroid-foundation.org.au>.

Transgender Victoria: <https://www.tgv.org.au>.

CHAPTER 37

Reproductive health

Shannon Forsyth

Key Terms

amenorrhoea
balanitis
cervical screening test (CST)
circumcision
contraception
cryptorchidism
dysmenorrhoea
dyspareunia
endometriosis
epispadias
erectile dysfunction (ED)
gamete intrafallopian transfer (GIFT)
hydrocoele
hypospadias
intersex
in vitro fertilisation (IVF)
infertility
intracytoplasmic sperm injection (ICSI)
mastitis
menopause
menorrhagia
metrorrhagia
oligomenorrhoea
oogenesis
paraphimosis
phimosis
polycystic ovary syndrome (PCOS)
priapism
prostate-specific antigen (PSA)
prostatic hyperplasia
prostatitis
spermatogenesis
testicular self-examination (TSE)
testosterone
transurethral resection of the prostate (TURP)
varicocoele
vasectomy
vulvovaginal candidiasis
vulvovaginitis/vaginitis

Learning Outcomes

At the completion of this chapter and with further reading, learners should be able to:

- Define the key terms.
- Describe the physiology of the male reproductive system.
- Describe the physiology of the female reproductive system.
- Consider alterations in health status that affect male and female reproductive systems.
- Discuss factors that influence reproduction.
- Identify factors that may affect sexual and reproductive health.
- Discuss major clinical conditions that may affect sexual and reproductive health.
- Identify diagnostic tests used to assess reproductive function.
- Develop strategies for the management of sexual and reproductive disorders.
- Identify nursing responsibilities in relation to sexual abuse/assault.
- Understand the physical and social implications of sexually transmitted infections.

CHAPTER FOCUS

This chapter identifies key aspects of reproductive health as they affect individuals throughout the lifespan. It will look briefly at the normal anatomy and physiology of the male and female reproductive systems and discuss common alterations that impact on reproductive health. Understanding common diagnostic tests and examinations conducted to assess an individual's reproductive health status will help to define the role of the nurse in identifying individual needs and implementing a management plan.

LIVED EXPERIENCE

I had a basic understanding of reproductive health prior to our fertility journey. My wife and I both underwent various investigations and procedures to determine the cause of our fertility issues, which helped me to really understand the process. Now I have a much deeper grasp on my own reproductive health and am able to take more control and do what I can to improve our reproductive chances.

Sam, 32 years old

THE MALE REPRODUCTIVE SYSTEM

The male reproductive system (Figure 37.1) is composed of the testes, epididymis, ductus deferens, seminal vesicle, prostate gland, penis and urethra. The urethra is shared between the reproductive and urinary systems and allows either urine or semen to pass through the penis.

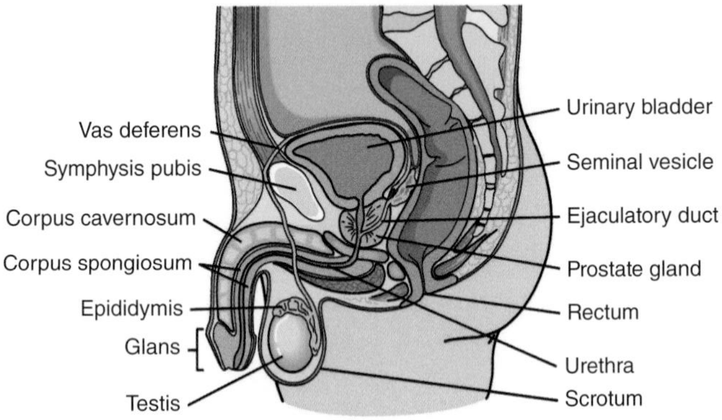

Figure 37.1 Male reproductive system
(Anderson 2023)

Spermatogenesis

Spermatogenesis is the production of sperm cells and occurs in the testes during puberty. In early foetal life, the testes remain suspended in the abdomen, not descending until birth or soon after through the inguinal canal and into the scrotum, where they are suspended in place by the spermatic cords.

The hypothalamus increases release of gonadotropin-releasing hormone (GnRH), which then triggers spermatogenesis. Luteinising hormone (LH) and follicle-stimulating hormone (FSH) are secreted by the anterior lobe of the pituitary gland as a result of GnRH stimulation. With the release of LH, the Leydig's cells located in the testes release testosterone. FSH acts on the Sertoli cells in the seminiferous tubules to stimulate cell division and sperm production.

The mature sperm consists of a head, which contains the genetic material of the cell; a mid-piece, which comprises the mitochondria; and the tail, which helps to propel the cell as it travels through the female reproductive tract (Figure 37.2).

Testosterone

Testosterone has varying effects on the body depending on age and sex. During puberty, testosterone is associated with the development of secondary sex characteristics in males such as hair growth, increase in muscle mass, change in voice and libido, and enlargement of sex organs.

Production of testosterone continues throughout the adult life of the male. Testosterone levels may decrease in older age or as a result of injury, disease or radiation, and after surgeries such as vasectomy.

Testosterone is found in very small amounts in female ovaries, and has a role in growing, maintaining and repairing the female reproductive tissues and bone mass. High levels can be indicative of reproductive conditions that will be discussed later in this chapter.

DISORDERS OF THE MALE REPRODUCTIVE SYSTEM

A majority of disorders affecting the male reproductive system are due to developmental or age-related causes. Early corrective surgery for congenital or structural defects of the genitourinary tract should be considered if the physical

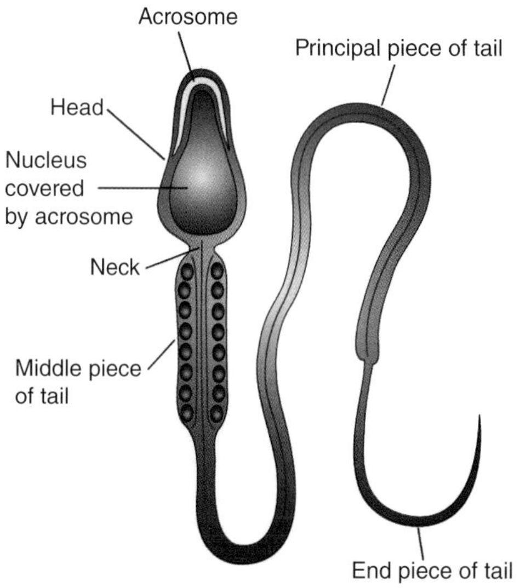

Figure 37.2 Anatomy of a mature sperm cell
(Moore et al 2016)

and psychological impact of the defect is to be significant. Nursing interventions during this time primarily focus on providing support to both the child and the family during the preoperative and postoperative phase. This can be accomplished by providing adequate time to express concerns and fears as well as educating the family and, if appropriate, the child about what to expect before and after the procedure. Utilising relevant and age-appropriate fact sheets can be successful in providing this information.

Genitourinary disorders affect the male reproductive system and are called such due to the shared anatomical structures of the urinary and reproductive systems. Conditions are usually characterised according to the type of alteration, such as:

- alteration in elimination
- alteration in sexual function
- alteration in urethral discharge.

Disorders of the penis

Hypospadias and epispadias

Both **hypospadias** and **epispadias** are congenital defects affecting the urethral opening. Hypospadias is a congenital condition classified according to the position of the urethral meatus, which may be on the underside or dorsal side of the penis (Craft et al 2023). Epispadias is a congenital defect in which there is an exposed or open dorsal urethra. In male epispadias, the urethral opening is on the dorsal surface of the penis. In females, a cleft along the ventral urethra usually extends to the bladder neck (Craft et al 2023). Surgery for both defects involves closure of the abnormal opening and extending the urethra to the normal location (Roen 2022).

Phimosis and paraphimosis

Phimosis is characterised by narrowing of the prepuce orifice, which prevents retraction due to an infection, inflammation or a congenital lesion. The condition predisposes to infection and if present in the adult leads to difficulties during sexual intercourse. Where the condition is complicated by a forcible retraction of the prepuce over the glans penis, inflammation of the prepuce collar can lead to swelling and constriction, a complication called **paraphimosis**. The treatment is **circumcision**.

> **CRITICAL THINKING EXERCISE 37.1**
>
> While circumcision is usually performed as an infant or child, it may be performed as an adult for conditions such as phimosis or balanitis. Would post-surgical management of the circumcised penis be different if performed as an adult?

Balanitis

Balanitis is a common condition characterised by inflammation of the glans penis, which can occur at any age. The condition is more common in non-circumcised males who do not retract the foreskin when cleaning the penis. The common causative organism is *Candida albicans*. It can also develop as a result of an allergic response to chemicals such as latex and soaps, or be an indicator of diabetes. While the condition can cause discomfort, it is easily managed by finding and treating the cause. Treatment may involve circumcision to limit the recurrence of infection.

Peyronie's disease

This condition is characterised by hardening of penile tissue (fibrosis), which sometimes causes a palpable lump or area of scar tissue (plaque). The affected area limits the ability of the erectile tissue in the penis to respond during an erection and can appear as if the penis has a bend. The condition can sometimes occur after an injury to the penis; however, a majority of cases do not have a specific link to an event.

Treatment may include surgery to excise the scar tissue, implantation of a prosthesis to assist with maintenance of a satisfactory erection or plication of the penis (a tuck is put into the lining of the penis on the opposite side to the bend to straighten the penis) (Osmonov et al 2022).

Cancer of the penis

Penile cancer usually presents on the skin surface as a painless wart-type growth or ulcer. If left untreated, the cancer will infiltrate tissues and cause urinary symptoms. Diagnosis of penile cancer involves biopsy of the lesion to confirm the diagnosis, followed by a chest X-ray, CT scan and lymph node biopsy to check for metastases. After confirmation of the diagnosis, management involves surgery and a combination therapy of internal and external radiation and chemotherapy. Surgical procedures can range from circumcision, laser or cryotherapy treatment to partial or total amputation of the penis.

Penile cancer in Australia is rare, with approximately 103 men diagnosed with the disease each year (Cancer Council Australia 2021). There are several risk factors for penile cancer including previous human papillomavirus (HPV) infection, smoking, age, and premalignant lesions/conditions, among others (Cancer Council Australia 2021).

Nursing management of the individual before and after diagnosis is based on providing emotional support and ensuring counselling is readily available. Education should be offered to manage the physical and psychological impact of the related loss of sexual function and the cosmetic impact of a penile amputation.

Erectile conditions

Erectile dysfunction (ED) is possibly one of the most common male sexual conditions in Australia; however, it is likely that a majority of cases go undiagnosed. ED can occur in men of any age, with the incidence increasing as they get older (Brown et al 2020).

ED is characterised as the inability to achieve and maintain an erection sufficient to permit satisfactory sexual intercourse. Causes may be psychological, neurological, hormonal, arterial cavernosal or a combination of these factors (Table 37.1). The condition can be classified as psychogenic, organic, or a mix of the two. Psychogenic factors may include performance anxiety, lack of arousability, relationship difficulties or mental health disorders such as depression and schizophrenia.

The management for a person with ED is dependent on the underlying causation and should include investigations for a chronic disease such as heart disease or diabetes. For most men, a cure for ED may not be possible, although treatment may allow for symptom improvement.

The three main types of treatment include:

1. non-invasive methods such as oral medications (phosphodiesterase-5 [PDE5] inhibitors) and use of external devices including rings and vacuum pumps
2. penile injections
3. surgery such as the insertion of a prosthesis or vascular surgery.

New treatments for erectile dysfunction include the use of low-intensity extracorporeal shock wave therapy, which acts on the blood vessels (Healthy Male 2020). (See Case Study 37.1.)

TABLE 37.1 | Causes of erectile dysfunction (ED)

Cause	Presentation
Psychosocial problems	Performance anxiety Sexual attitudes and upbringing Relationship problems Employment and financial pressures Depression Psychiatric disorders
Nerve function interference	Spinal cord trauma Multiple sclerosis Diabetic neuropathy Prostate or bowel surgery Parkinson's disease Alzheimer's disease
Reduced blood flow	Atherosclerosis
Medication, alcohol and other drugs' interference	Alcohol and drug abuse Drugs such as: • Antihypertensives • Lipidaemics • Antidepressants and psychiatric medications • Prostate medications
Metabolic problems interfering with blood vessel function	Diabetes Hypertension Obesity High cholesterol Sleep apnoea Cigarette smoking
Urological problems	Peyronie's disease Pelvic trauma
Endocrine dysfunctions	Thyroid disease Acromegaly Excessive cortisone Hypogonadism

(Adapted from Andrology Australia 2018a)

Priapism

The condition priapism is characterised by a persistent and painful erection lasting longer than 6 hours, usually only affecting the corpus cavernosum. It is not induced by stimulation of sexual desire. There are two types of priapism:

1. Ischaemic priapism—the most common form, caused by increased blood viscosity that slows blood flow. This type of priapism is considered an emergency as it may lead to permanent damage.
2. Non-ischaemic priapism—less common and usually less painful.

(Sweet & Foley 2020)

CASE STUDY 37.1

Nathan is a 64-year-old man who was diagnosed with diabetes mellitus in his 30s. Five years ago, he started having difficulty achieving and maintaining an erection, which has prevented him from having an intimate relationship with his wife. He saw an article on social media on the weekend about ways to improve his symptoms.

What treatments are available for Nathan?

Priapism may develop due to a complication of diseases such as sickle cell disease, leukaemia, malaria, carbon monoxide poisoning or use of some anaesthetic agents such as papaveretum. Excessive use of drugs to treat ED may also lead to priapism that cannot be resolved through usual methods. A sustained erection leads to a build-up of toxins in the blood, often called 'black blood', which will lead to anoxia and necrosis of tissue. The blood must be aspirated from the blood vessels in the penis in order for the erection to be resolved. If left untreated, a priapism may lead to erectile dysfunction.

Conditions affecting the testes

Cryptorchidism (undescended testis)

Cryptorchidism is the failure of one or both of the testes to descend into the scrotum and can be caused by congenital or acquired factors. Congenital cryptorchidism occurs more commonly in premature males where one or both of the testes fail to descend into the scrotum at birth. It may also be due to hormonal or genetic factors. The rate of cryptorchidism at birth in full-term males is 3–6%, compared to 20–30% of preterm males. The condition is resolved in approximately 75–90% of infants by 1 year of age (Craft et al 2023). Acquired cryptorchidism occurs where the spermatic cord fails to grow at the same rate as the rest of the body and so the shortened cord pulls the testes back into the groin.

The condition is diagnosed by the absence, on palpation, of one or both of the testes in the scrotum. There is believed to be a link between a diagnosis of cryptorchidism and other health conditions such as hernias, testicular cancer and infertility in later life. The condition may be treated with hormone injections or surgery. Surgical placement of the testes in the scrotum (orchiopexy) is recommended before the second year of age to preserve sperm-forming cells that require a lower temperature than that of the abdomen. If the condition is not treated before puberty, there is a risk of atrophy and sterility. The affected testis tends to be smaller and contain more fibrous tissue than the unaffected testis.

Carcinoma of the testes

Testicular cancer is not a common cancer, accounting for approximately 1.2% of all male cancers. However, it is the most common solid tumour cancer in males between the ages of 15 and 35 years (Craft et al 2023). The rate of testicular cancer is reported to have increased by 50% in the past 30 years (Cancer Council Australia 2019a); the reason for this is unknown. However, in a majority of cases treatment is successful and there are very few recorded deaths.

Recognised risk factors for testicular cancer are shown in Table 37.2. There is no proven link between the incidence of testicular cancer and the wearing of tight clothes, hot baths or testicular injuries.

TABLE 37.2 | Risk factors for testicular cancer

Undescended testes (cryptorchidism)	Ten times the chance of developing testicular cancer. The incidence decreases significantly where correction of the undescended testis has occurred prior to 12 months of age.
Previous history of testicular cancer	1 in 25 males with a diagnosis of testicular cancer in one testis will be diagnosed with the condition in the other testis.
Previous history of male infertility	Pre-cancer cells have been found in biopsies taken to diagnose infertility issues.
Familial history	A minor risk where another male member of the family has been diagnosed with testicular cancer.
Down syndrome	A considered increased genetic risk.

(Adapted from Andrology Australia 2018b)

Early diagnosis and improved treatment modalities such as chemotherapy have contributed to improved outcomes for men diagnosed with the condition; the cure rate of testicular cancer exceeds 90% (McCance et al 2019). An early-stage indicator is the presence of a smooth painless lump in the scrotum or a dull ache located in the testes or lower abdomen. Other metastatic symptoms include bowel or urinary obstruction and abdominal pain.

If a lump is detected in the testes, the male who seeks medical advice will have the diagnosis confirmed with an initial physical examination, ultrasound of the scrotum and collection of blood for presence of blood serum markers. Elevated levels of alpha-fetoprotein (AFP) and human chorionic gonadotrophin (hCG) will be detected in males with testicular cancer. Ultrasonography differentiates between a solid and a cystic lesion. Tests to detect potential metastases include chest X-ray and CT scans of the chest, abdomen and pelvis.

Treatment for testicular cancer depends on the type and stage of the cancer. Surgical removal of one or both testicles (orchidectomy) is usually performed for all cases of testicular cancer. The affected testis is then sent to pathology for confirmation of the type and stage of the cancer. Chemotherapy and radiotherapy usually follow surgery to target any remaining cancer cells that may be located in other parts of the body.

Treatment often leads to infertility, which is a major consideration in the management of the male in the pretreatment phase. For the male who may still want children, the option for sperm banking should be discussed. They should also be reassured that the condition should not affect their virility or their ability to achieve an erection. The individual may be referred to support services outside the hospital and should be educated in testicular self-examination. It is recommended that the male individual carry out periodic examinations since there is an increased risk of a second tumour occurring. It is important to reassure the individual that removal of one testis does not necessarily lead to a loss of sexual function and there are options, both medical and surgical, to manage cosmetic abnormalities.

Torsion of testis

Torsion of testis is a condition in which the testis becomes twisted around itself. It is more commonly seen in young athletic males after violent movement or trauma and may also occur due to abnormality of the male anatomy. The twisting results in obstruction of venous blood flow that may lead to infarction. Testicular torsion is a medical emergency and if left untreated, necrosis and total lack of function may occur. The condition may present with severe pain, scrotal swelling, nausea and vomiting. After 6 hours, lasting damage may occur, and if treatment is delayed longer than 12 hours, an orchidectomy may be required (Urology Care Foundation 2022). (See Case Study 37.2.)

Hydrocoele

Hydrocoele is a painless collection of fluid within the tunica vaginalis of the testis from defective or inadequate reabsorption of fluid normally produced within the testis. The condition is fairly common in male infants for whom it is the most common cause of testicular swelling. In infants, the accumulation of fluid is generally due to unhindered drainage from the abdomen, whereas in adults it may be associated with infections, trauma or tumours. The individual may experience a feeling of heaviness or pain associated with increased scrotal size.

Ultrasound and transillumination are diagnostic tests used to differentiate between hydrocoele and other causes, such as tumours. If a hydrocoele is present, transillumination will allow transmission of light through the scrotum. Treatment is not usually required unless there is compromised testicular circulation. However, a scrotal support can be worn to minimise discomfort.

CASE STUDY 37.2

You are working in the emergency department on a Saturday afternoon when Michael presents at triage. It is difficult for him to communicate with you due to severe pain, but he manages to tell you that he was playing football earlier that day and about an hour ago he had a sudden onset of pain in his scrotum, which is also swollen. On examination, it is found that Michael has an asymmetrical high testis, which is also lying horizontally. It is strongly suspected that he has testicular torsion.

What treatment is advised in this scenario, and what nursing care would you provide for Michael?

Varicocoele

A **varicocoele** more commonly affects the left testis and occurs when the valves within the veins prevent blood from draining fully from the testis. This leads to pooling and swelling of the vein above the testis. Varicocoele is often described as a varicose vein of the spermatic cord. The individual describes their symptoms as a 'pulling' sensation, dull ache in the scrotum, pain and/or scrotal swelling. On palpation, the scrotum may be described as feeling like a 'bag of worms'. If left untreated, the condition can lead to a reduced sperm count, atrophy of the testis and infertility. Treatment of a varicocoele can be either by surgery—where the affected vein is ligated—or by an embolisation, which can be performed under local anaesthetic. Post procedure, the individual may require mild analgesics for discomfort and the intermittent use of ice packs to reduce swelling. Wearing a scrotal support can also reduce oedema and discomfort. Strenuous activity should be avoided until after review by the surgeon.

Disorders of the prostate gland

Prostatitis

Prostatitis is a broad term that describes a group of non-inflammatory and inflammatory or infective conditions of the prostate gland, which can have bacterial or non-bacterial origins (Brown et al 2020). It generally develops in association with an obstruction in the urinary tract in elderly males with prostatic hyperplasia, a urinary tract infection (UTI) or a sexually transmitted infection (STI). Clinical manifestations include urinary symptoms such as urgency, frequency, nocturia and dysuria. Bacterial prostatitis is characterised by sudden chills and a moderate to high fever. Pain in the perineum, rectum and lower back during ejaculation may also indicate prostatitis. Diagnosis is based upon urine, urethral and prostatic fluid cultures. Digital rectal examination frequently reveals a tender swollen prostate. Treatment of acute bacterial prostatitis is usually with an appropriate antibiotic and analgesic or, where an abscess has formed, surgical drainage of the pus. Oral antispasmodic agents may provide relief from urinary frequency and urgency. The nurse can support the individual with comfort measures such as salt baths to relax the muscles of the pelvic floor. Stool softeners can reduce pressure on the prostate gland and are administered as prescribed. Fluids should be encouraged to ensure a frequent flow of urine through the urinary tract. Repeated episodes of prostatitis may lead to scarring and thickening of the prostate.

Prostatic hyperplasia

Prostatic hyperplasia is caused by the hormone testosterone that stimulates the growth of the prostate. It becomes more common with age, occurring in 50% of men aged 50, and over 80% of men aged 80 (Healthy Male 2021a). In the majority of males, the condition is benign, referred to as benign prostatic hyperplasia (BPH). Hyperplasia of the prostate can compress the urethra laterally at the neck of the bladder, which can impede urinary flow. Symptoms of BPH may be classified as either noticeable or obstructive (Table 37.3).

Noticeable changes begin as the prostate becomes progressively more enlarged and will eventually require a urology referral for management. An International Prostate Symptom Score (IPSS) is a validated tool used to determine the need for therapy and treatment response (Table 37.4). (See Case Study 37.3.)

The cause of BPH is not well known. There has been some research suggesting there is a genetic or familial link. There has also been research that links increasing age and testosterone to the development of BPH since it is known that the condition occurs in the presence of testosterone.

Diagnosis of the condition is based on the symptoms and may include urinalysis to eliminate UTI, voiding analysis charts, ultrasound, digital examination to detect changes in the surface of the prostate, and blood tests such as a prostate-specific antigen (PSA) test, which measures the level of PSA, a glycoprotein produced by the prostate gland. In the presence of BPH, the PSA levels may be raised. Biopsy of the prostate may also be performed. Biopsies are collected during a transrectal ultrasound (TRUS), which may also be used when there is a strong suspicion of prostate cancer.

Treatment options for BPH range from:

- no treatment
- drug therapies
- natural therapies
- surgical intervention—transurethral resection of prostate (TURP), transurethral incision of prostate (TUIP), open or retropubic prostatectomy.

No treatment may be the best option where the symptoms are mild. It involves close monitoring of the condition. Drug therapy involves the use of medications to relax the muscles in the prostate gland, bladder neck and urethra (alpha-blockers) or the use of medications to block the release of testosterone to help shrink the size of the prostate (alpha-reductase inhibitors). Some men may also try natural therapies or surgery if the condition is severe.

The type of surgery will depend on the size of the prostate, location of the enlargement, whether surgery on the bladder is also needed, and the individual's age and physical condition. The most common surgical management for BPH is **transurethral resection of the prostate (TURP)**. Surgery relieves symptoms quickly, typically doubling the urinary flow within weeks. A fibreoptic scope is passed through the urethra to the prostate. Using a tiny blade or an electric loop, the surgeon pares away the lining of the urethra and bits of excess prostate tissue to expand the passageway.

After a TURP, the individual usually stays in hospital until the prostatic bed stops bleeding and they are able to void normally with minimal haematuria, which can take up to 48 hours. The individual should be educated on the importance of remaining well hydrated after removal of the urinary catheter to ensure they void regularly and do not develop retention due to a micro-clot in the urethral bed. Possible risks should also be discussed prior to surgery, which may include ED, urinary incontinence, UTIs and urethral strictures.

Other approaches to management of the condition, which usually have a shorter stay in hospital and recovery, include:

- laser therapy—green light prostatectomy
- transurethral microwave therapy (TUMT)
- transurethral needle ablasion (TUNA)
- high-intensity focused ultrasound (HIFU)
- electrovaporisation (TVP).

Most of the newer treatment methods are based on destroying, vaporising or dissolving hyperplasia and can be done with little more than a local anaesthetic on an outpatient basis. While less invasive options usually allow individuals to go home on the day of the procedure, there is a possibility that symptoms will return.

TABLE 37.3 | Symptoms of benign prostatic hyperplasia (BPH)

Lower urinary tract symptoms—voiding	• Weak stream • Hesitancy • Intermittency • Abdominal straining • Incomplete bladder emptying
Lower urinary tract symptoms—storage	• Frequency • Nocturia • Urgency • Urinary incontinence
Other	• Perineal pain • Dysuria • Haematuria

(Adapted from Andrology Australia 2018c)

CASE STUDY 37.3

Peter is a 62-year-old man who has presented to his local health clinic with concerns about his ability to pass urine. He reports that over the past month he has frequently had the urge to pass urine through the night but is only passing small amounts and he feels like he hasn't emptied his bladder fully. His urine stream is often weak, and stops and starts. When you question Peter further, he admits that he usually needs to strain to begin urinating and feels the need to pass urine every couple of hours.

Using the IPSS chart provided in Table 37.4, how would you score Peter? Does Peter have a possible hyperplasia of his prostate?

TABLE 37.4 | International Prostate Symptom Score (IPSS)

	Not at all	Less than 1 in 5	Less than half the time	About half the time	More than half the time	Almost always	Score
Incomplete emptying: Over the past month, how often have you had a sensation of not emptying your bladder completely after you finish urinating?	0	1	2	3	4	5	
Frequency: Over the past month, how often have you had to urinate again less than 2 hours after you finished urinating?	0	1	2	3	4	5	
Intermittency: Over the past month, how often have you found you stopped and started again several times when you urinated?	0	1	2	3	4	5	
Urgency: Over the past month, how difficult have you found it to postpone urination?	0	1	2	3	4	5	
Weak stream: Over the past month, how often have you had a weak urinary stream?	0	1	2	3	4	5	
Straining: Over the past month, how often have you had to push or strain to begin urination?	0	1	2	3	4	5	
Nocturia: Over the past month, how many times did you most typically get up to urinate from the time you went to bed until the time you got up in the morning?	0	1	2	3	4	5	
Total Prostate Symptom Score							
	Delighted	**Pleased**	**Mostly satisfied**	**Neither satisfied nor dissatisfied**	**Mostly dissatisfied**	**Unhappy**	**Terrible**
Quality of life (QOL) due to urinary symptoms. If you were to spend the rest of your life with your urinary condition the way it is now, how would you feel about that?							

(Adapted from Ferri 2020. © Copyright 2020 by Elsevier, Inc.)

CRITICAL THINKING EXERCISE 37.2

The average length of stay for the individual who has undergone a TURP is 24–48 hours. What discharge information should you provide?

Prostate cancer

Prostate cancer occurs mainly in males over the age of 50 years, tends to grow slowly and may have metastasised before it is detected. Prostate cancer is the most commonly diagnosed cancer in Australian males. Prostate cancer is very rare in men aged under 40, but the incidence drastically increases with age after 50 (Healthy Males 2021b).

Initially, the person with prostate cancer may be asymptomatic. When symptoms appear, they are often similar to those caused by BPH: difficulty urinating, a weak urine stream, frequent urge to urinate, nocturia, painful or burning urination and haematuria. Because prostate cancer tends to metastasise to the bone, bone pain, particularly in the back, can be another symptom. Usually, the younger the individual, the more aggressive the cancer. The two main methods of diagnosis include digital rectal examination and prostate-specific antigen (PSA) levels. A biopsy may also be taken if there is a high level of suspicion. A procedure called a transperineal ultrasound may be performed to collect biopsies. It involves the insertion of a probe into the rectum and collection of samples, which are viewed in the laboratory and given a grading using the Gleason Score. Aggressive tumours will be rated between 8 and 10.

Treatment

Prostate cancer may be treated by radiotherapy, chemotherapy, hormone therapy (palliative) or by open prostatectomy. Surgery for prostatic cancer is often done for palliative comfort care due to late onset of symptoms. Radiotherapy may be performed to reduce the size of the tumour. Alternatively, hormonal therapy may be used in the short term, which also reduces the size and slows the rate of tumour development. It is usually only successful while the tumour relies on hormone levels to sustain itself; after a time, it will become independent and growth becomes rapid again.

Prostatectomy

There are four types of radical prostatectomy: open, laparoscopic, robotic-assisted and nerve-sparing (Cancer Council NSW 2022a). Open radical prostatectomy is performed through a cut in the abdomen. The procedure can be performed using either a perineal or a retropubic approach. The retropubic approach involves an incision through the lower abdomen to remove the prostate and possibly the pelvic lymph nodes, whereas the perineal approach requires an incision through the perineum (Better Health Channel 2019).

Laparoscopic prostatectomy involves removing the prostate via keyhole surgery where the surgeon watches a screen. The robotic-assisted procedure is a laparoscopic approach which involves the use of a remotely assisted controller-subordinate system—the da Vinci® surgical system (Brown et al 2020). This procedure involves multiple small incisions into the abdominal wall and the introduction of instruments to form a three-dimensional picture to perform the surgery (Cancer Council NSW 2022a). Nerve-sparing prostatectomy is the removal of the prostate and seminal vesicles while trying to preserve nerves that control erections. This is a more suitable procedure for younger men with lower-grade cancers and good erectile function (Cancer Council NSW 2022a).

Nursing management involves supporting the individual prior to surgery and maintenance of hydration and fluid status. An indwelling or suprapubic catheter may be necessary to establish and monitor urinary output. Bowel preparation may include drinking 2–3 L of a cathartic and administration of an evacuant enema. Postoperatively, the nurse should maintain bladder irrigation and drainage and monitor for clots and haemorrhage via a catheter (Brown et al 2020). Post-procedural and discharge education needs to take physical and psychosocial factors into consideration.

Discharge education

After a radical prostatectomy, an indwelling urinary catheter (IDC) may remain in situ for about 2 weeks, so education for the individual should concentrate on care of the catheter. This includes changing or emptying the leg bag and highlighting the importance of maintaining a high fluid intake to reduce the risk of clot formation.

Systemic diseases and ageing

Sexual function declines with age, even in healthy men. The period between sexual stimulation and erection increases, erections are less turgid and ejaculatory force and volume is less. Conditions such as diabetes mellitus, chronic renal failure and cardiovascular disease are believed to be linked to ED (Healthy Male 2020).

A thorough medical, sexual and psychosocial assessment should be undertaken. Urinalysis, full blood count, fasting serum glucose, creatinine, cholesterol, triglycerides and testosterone are recommended laboratory tests. Treatment depends upon the cause. It can include a variety of drug therapies, which may be administered via the oral, transurethral, subcutaneous or intracavernous injection route (Healthy Male 2020).

Surgical procedures

Vasectomy

A **vasectomy** is a surgical procedure commonly performed on males who have children and do not want to father any more. In Australia, approximately 29,000 males have a vasectomy each year (Healthy Male 2021d).

The procedure can be performed under general anaesthesia; however, a majority will be performed under local anaesthesia in a fertility clinic, day procedure unit or a general practice. There are two types of techniques used: scalpel or 'no-scalpel'. The scalpel procedure involves a small incision being made on either side of the scrotum and the ductus deferens being brought to the surface. The 'no-scalpel' technique uses a sharpened instrument to pierce the skin above the vas deferens. Then, a small segment of the ductus deferens is removed and the ends are diathermied to create a seal. This part of the procedure is the same, regardless of which technique is used (Healthy Male 2021).

There is usually no alteration to the male's ability to maintain sexual function or the effectiveness of their erection. Ejaculation is still possible; however, there should be no sperm in the fluid since it will have been prevented from travelling past the epididymis, where it is reabsorbed into the body.

Postoperatively, the male may have minor discomfort and swelling related to the procedure which settles after 24–48 hours. The wound heals quickly without the need for specialised care. The individual should be advised to abstain from unprotected sex until a clear seminal fluid analysis has been completed (between 6 and 12 weeks post procedure), which shows no evidence of sperm in the ejaculatory fluid. In a small number of cases, the procedure may be unsuccessful and the individual may need to undertake further procedures.

ASSESSMENT AND DIAGNOSTIC TESTS

Anxiety and embarrassment may be experienced by the individual during physical examination and discussion of sexual history. A calm insightful approach is required, as is preservation of the person's individuality and dignity throughout. Cultural and religious customs such as circumcision should be considered.

Examination of external genitalia

A complete history of the individual should be collected prior to any procedure. For the male who presents with a condition affecting their reproductive system, this history should concentrate on the presence of urinary problems and symptoms that suggest alteration in normal sexual function. It may be necessary to conduct a physical assessment of the male genitalia and inguinal canal, which may detect or confirm the presence of penile discharge, tenderness, lesions, swelling, lumps or asymmetry.

Testicular examination

Testicular self-examination (TSE) should be performed on a regular basis. The testes are examined for size, shape, symmetry and texture. It is important that both testes are checked at the same time. (See Clinical Interest Box 37.1.)

Digital rectal examination

Digital examination of the prostate involves the insertion of a gloved finger inside the rectum to palpate the prostate. The examination inspects the size, shape and firmness of the prostate through the wall of the rectum.

Prostate-specific antigen test

This test measures the level of **prostate-specific antigen (PSA)**, which is a protein produced by cells of the prostate gland. The test is performed by taking a sample of blood and sending it for analysis. A high PSA is suggestive of a condition affecting the prostate but may not necessarily mean the individual has prostatic cancer. (See Clinical Interest Box 37.2.)

CLINICAL INTEREST BOX 37.1 Individual teaching—testicular self-examination

- Testicular self-examination (TSE) should be done regularly.
- It may be easier to perform this examination after a warm bath or shower when the skin of the scrotum is relaxed.
- Stand in front of a mirror and check for any swelling on the skin of the scrotum.
- Check both testes at the same time.
- Use the palm of the hand and support the scrotum (Note: It is not unusual for one testis to be slightly larger than the other).
- It is important to be familiar with the feel of the texture and size of the testis so you are able to detect changes.
- Roll one testis gently between the thumb and fingers to feel for lumps or swellings.
- Repeat with the other testis. The surface of the testis should feel smooth and firm.
- Use the thumb and fingers to feel along the epididymis for any swelling.
- A testicular self-examination should not be painful.
- See your doctor if you notice any pain, discomfort or changes.

(Adapted from Healthy Male 2021c)

CLINICAL INTEREST BOX 37.2 PSA testing

Most research suggests PSA testing is not indicated in males of 75 years or older unless there is a known diagnosis of cancer.

Results of the PSA test are usually given in ng/mL with levels of total PSA >4.0 ng/mL considered to be abnormal. The test may be repeated every 1–3 months if an abnormal result is reported.

(Hechtman 2019)

Transrectal ultrasound (TRUS)

In a TRUS, a small probe that emits and picks up high-frequency soundwaves is inserted into the rectum. The reflected waves are detected and a visual image displayed on a monitor. The test is useful following suspicious findings on a digital rectal examination or PSA test; however, it is not recommended as a standalone screening tool. It is also used to guide biopsies in sampling abnormal areas of the prostate.

Biopsy

Biopsies of the prostate gland are usually performed in combination with the TRUS to detect abnormal cells. A needle is inserted through the perineal skin and a quantity of prostate tissue is aspirated. Biopsy specimens of tissue are sent for cytological examination.

Urethral culture

A small swab is inserted 3–5 cm into the urethra to obtain a specimen for microbiological analysis. A preliminary result of findings for this test will usually be available within 24 hours of collection, with a more definitive result after 48 hours.

Semen analysis

A sample of semen is obtained and the sperm examined for motility, morphology, quantity and quality. The test requires the individual to provide a fresh sample of ejaculatory fluid, which is sent for analysis as soon as possible after collection. Results of semen analysis are usually available within 24 hours.

Urological tests

A series of tests may be performed to evaluate the urinary tract. These include cystoscopy, intravenous pyelogram, urine flow studies, urogram and ultrasound.

Blood samples

Specific blood tests include hormone levels for infertility, AFP and hCG. For testicular cancer, blood urea nitrogen (BUN), creatinine and urea, to evaluate renal function, are tested.

NURSING INTERVENTIONS IN MALE REPRODUCTIVE HEALTH

The male individual with a condition affecting his reproductive system would be expected to experience concerns about sexual function, fertility, urinary problems and other effects of the condition they are diagnosed with. The nurse should be aware of these concerns and provide supportive services such as counselling in their approach to care and the promotion of a healthy lifestyle.

THE FEMALE REPRODUCTIVE SYSTEM

The female reproductive system (Figure 37.3) functions to secrete hormones, produce ova, receive sperm and allow for fertilisation, implantation, development and birth of offspring. The female reproductive system consists of essential and accessory organs (Brown et al 2020).

The external structures of the female reproductive system include the mons pubis, labia majora, labia minora, Bartholin gland and clitoris. The area between the anus and vaginal opening is referred to as the perineum. Internal reproductive structures include the vagina, uterus, cervix, fallopian tubes and the ovaries.

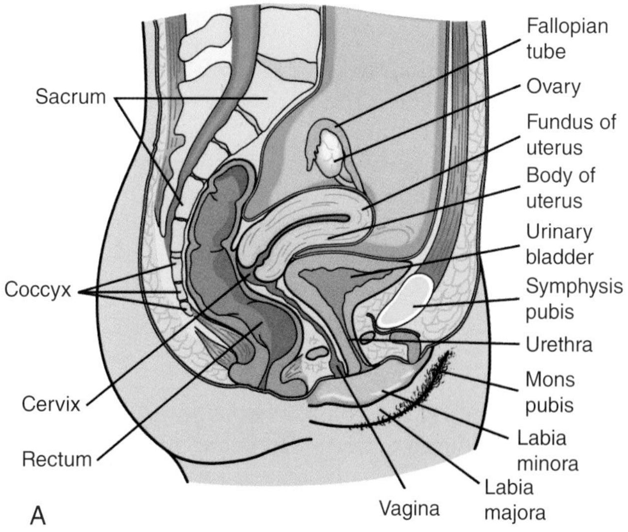

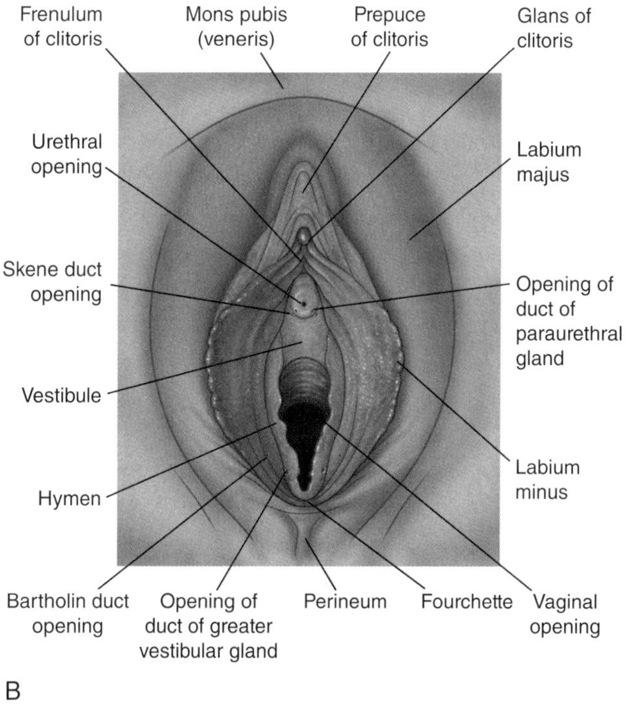

Figure 37.3 A: Female reproductive system, **B:** Female external genitalia

*(**A:** Anderson 2023; **B:** Drake et al 2020)*

Oogenesis

The ovaries function to produce ova (**oogenesis**) and hormones. Production of ovarian hormones begins at puberty. Oestrogen influences the development of the female secondary sexual characteristics including changes in the breast, development of pubic and axillary hair, onset of menses and widening of the pelvis. Oestrogen is also responsible for preparing the uterus for the implantation of a fertilised ovum. (See Clinical Interest Box 37.3.)

Mammary glands

Mammary glands are accessory glands of the reproductive system. The breast is a complex structure composed of a glandular and ductal network, fat, connective tissue, fascia, blood vessels, nerves and lymphatic vessels (Figure 37.4).

CLINICAL INTEREST BOX 37.3 Oogenesis

In utero, the foetus is thought to have 6–7 million oocytes. This number decreases to 1–2 million by the time of birth, and no further oocytes will be produced.

By puberty, the number of oocytes has reduced to 300,000. Of this number, only 400 are believed to be released during a lifetime. Pre-menopause, the number of oocytes drops further until nil remain by menopause.

(Blackburn 2018)

Each breast contains 15–20 lobes that radiate around the nipple and are separated from each other by adipose tissue. Within the lobes are lobules that contain clusters of milk-producing cells called alveoli. Lactiferous ducts drain the alveoli into openings in the nipple. Breast development at puberty is influenced by ovarian hormones. The mammary glands have the function of synthesising, secreting and delivering milk to the newborn and older baby. After cessation of lactation, the breast will return to its normal 'resting' stage, although the time it takes to return varies between individuals.

The menstrual cycle

The menstrual cycle consists of a series of cyclical changes occurring at regular intervals involving the reproductive organs. The average menstrual cycle is about 28 days but may vary from 24 to 35 days (Figure 37.5) and has three phases: follicular, ovulatory and luteal. Hormones produced during the menstrual cycle are summarised in Table 37.5. If fertilisation of an ova occurs, the hormone hCG is produced, which stimulates the corpus luteum to maintain progesterone levels until the foetus is capable of producing its own hormones. (See Clinical Interest Box 37.4.)

DISORDERS OF THE FEMALE REPRODUCTIVE SYSTEM

Common symptoms

The symptoms most commonly observed in a female with a disorder of the reproductive system include bleeding, pain,

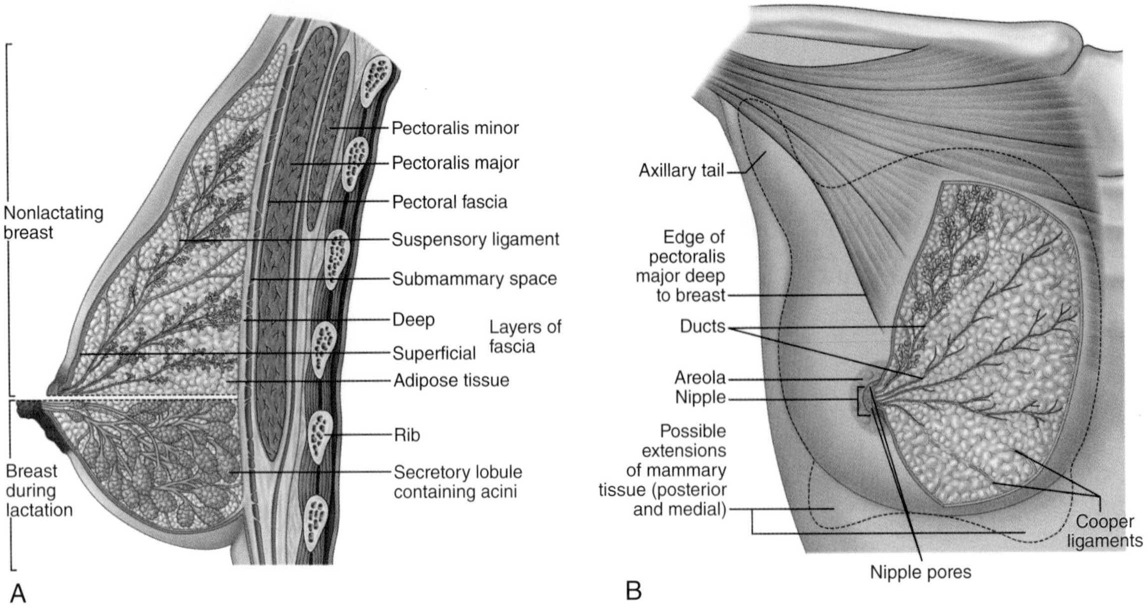

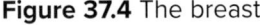

Figure 37.4 The breast

A: Sagittal section, **B:** Anterior section

(Standring 2021)

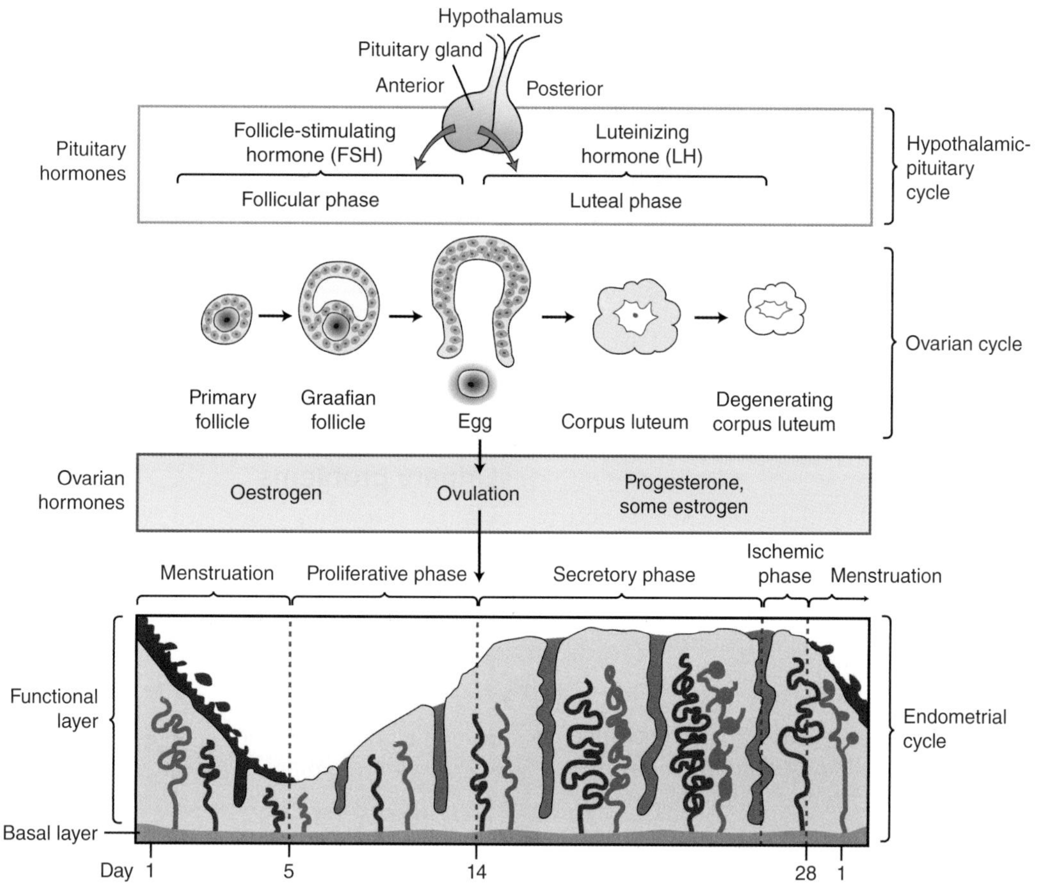

Figure 37.5 The menstrual cycle
(McKenry et al 2006)

TABLE 37.5 | Hormones affecting the menstrual cycle

Hormone	Secreted from	Function
FSH	Anterior pituitary	Stimulates growth of follicle Stimulates oestrogen secretion from developed follicle
Oestrogen	Ovaries	Development of endometrium Stimulates LH secretion
LH	Anterior pituitary	Increase triggers ovulation Development of corpus luteum Stimulates progesterone secretion
Progesterone	Ovaries (corpus luteum)	Thickens endometrium Inhibits LH and FSH

(IVF Australia 2023)

vaginal discharge, pruritus, urinary problems and breast changes.

Bleeding abnormalities

Amenorrhoea is the absence of menstrual bleeding in women. It is normal before puberty, during pregnancy and after menopause. Primary amenorrhoea is considered as the failure of menstruation to occur by the age of 14–16 years. Secondary amenorrhoea generally results from anovulation due to hormonal dysfunction after menarche. In women of reproductive age, a diagnosis of amenorrhoea will usually only be made after first eliminating pregnancy as a possible aetiology.

CLINICAL INTEREST BOX 37.4 hCG levels

Blood hCG levels are often used to confirm pregnancy, with levels doubling about every 48 hours for the first 10–12 weeks. It can be detected as early as one week after conception. There is a wide range of hCG levels between individuals, making it difficult to use to estimate gestational age. In cases of a pregnancy complication, hCG levels may be higher or lower than usual and repeat testing will help to monitor the viability of the pregnancy where necessary.

(Lab Tests Online 2022)

Oligomenorrhoea is a condition where menses occurs at intervals longer than 35 days apart. Common reasons may be due to the lead-up to menopause, following childbirth or after cessation of a pregnancy due to miscarriage or termination. It may also be a symptom of an underlying condition and should be investigated.

Menorrhagia is excessive and/or prolonged bleeding associated with erosive lesions, endometrial hyperplasia, bleeding disorders or neoplasms (tumours). Postmenopausal bleeding may result from the administration of oestrogen (hormone replacement therapy [HRT]), from an oestrogen-producing ovarian neoplasm, uterine hyperplasia, carcinoma or vaginitis. **Metrorrhagia**, or intermenstrual bleeding, can occur at the time of ovulation, or it may be due to factors such as hormonal imbalance or neoplasms.

Pain

Pain may occur as **dysmenorrhoea** (painful menstruation), which is the most commonly experienced type of pain in women. Quantifying the prevalence of dysmenorrhoea in the community is difficult due to the variability of pain perception among women surveyed, but it is estimated that a significant percentage of the population experiences it to some degree (Armour et al 2020). Pain may be described as intermittent cramping, lower abdominal pain, or pain radiating to the back, thighs and groin. Dysmenorrhoea can have a primary cause where pain occurs with no underlying pathological pelvic disease and may appear 6–12 months after menstrual cycles have begun. Secondary dysmenorrhoea occurs when there are underlying pelvic conditions such as endometriosis, uterine fibroids or pelvic inflammatory disease (PID).

Pain may also occur in the lower back due to menstruation, infection, inflammation or neoplasm and may be due to conditions such as torsion of an ovarian cyst or a ruptured ectopic pregnancy. If blood from the ruptured fallopian tube tracks to the diaphragm and stimulates the phrenic nerve, shoulder-tip pain may be evident.

Sexual intercourse may result in pain (**dyspareunia**), which can be the result of conditions such as vaginal or vulval infections, endometriosis, neoplasms or PID. Decreased vaginal lubrication may also cause dyspareunia. Symptoms can therefore vary in location, type and severity.

Vaginal discharge

Normal vaginal discharge should be clear or white. An offensive odour or changes in the consistency, colour or amount of discharge may be suggestive of an underlying problem of the vagina or cervix.

Pruritus

Pruritus (itchy skin) is an irritating symptom suggestive of inflammation, vaginal infection or possibly contact dermatitis.

Urinary problems

Urinary problems associated with female reproductive problems are common and often present as dysuria, urinary frequency or stress incontinence. Causes can include infection, neoplasm and cystocele.

Breast changes

Changes may occur in breast tissue, which may present as pain or tenderness in the breast, a discharge from the nipple, inversion of the nipple or the presence of lumps.

Vulval and vaginal changes

The adult vagina is generally resistant to infections due to the presence of a characteristic normal flora that creates an environment unsuitable for the growth of most microorganisms. When the normal balance of the vagina's pH is disturbed, which may occur with certain medications, diseases and debility, it becomes predisposed to infections.

Vulvovaginitis (vaginitis)

Vulvovaginitis (vaginitis) is inflammation of the vulva and vagina. Causes of vulvovaginitis include infection, vaginal mucosal atrophy, vulval atrophy, chemical irritants and poor personal hygiene. Haemophilus vaginitis is caused by the bacterium *Haemophilus vaginalis*. STIs such as gonorrhoea, chlamydia and trichomoniasis can appear as vaginitis but may also be asymptomatic.

Vulvovaginal candidiasis

Vulvovaginal candidiasis (vaginal thrush) is caused by an overgrowth of a yeast-like fungal organism. In 80–95% of cases, the causative organism will be *Candida albicans* (Family Planning NSW 2020). The condition is characterised by pruritus, vaginal and vulval redness, a thick, white or creamy vaginal discharge and vulval pain including superficial dyspareunia and external dysuria. Treatment may include the use of anti-fungal medication, probiotics and good hygiene practices.

Predisposing factors include diabetes mellitus, pregnancy, broad-spectrum antibiotic therapy and the use of oral contraceptives. It is estimated that up to 75% of women will experience vulvovaginal candidiasis at least once in their lifetime (Family Planning NSW 2020). Half of these women will have more than one episode and 5% will be diagnosed with recurrent thrush, which is classified as four or more episodes in a 12-month period (Family Planning NSW 2020).

CRITICAL THINKING EXERCISE 37.3

Vulvovaginal candidiasis (vaginal thrush) can develop due to various conditions. Identify the main causes of vaginal thrush and what education you would provide to individuals on how to prevent thrush.

Genital herpes

Genital herpes is an infection caused by the herpes simplex virus (HSV) type 1 or type 2 and is transmitted through vaginal, oral or anal sex. HSV type 1 is more commonly seen on oral mucosa; if it is identified in the genitals, symptoms are usually less severe than type 2. Genital herpes (HSV type 2) is characterised by flu-like symptoms, dysuria and painful blisters in the genital area within 2–10 days of exposure. (See Case Study 37.4.) Treatment is generally episodic, used only when lesions occur, to help reduce the length and severity of symptoms. Suppressive therapy can be used if symptoms are frequent and cause significant distress.

Individuals should be educated on symptomatic management including regular saline baths, topical anaesthetic, sitting in warm water to pass urine (to reduce pain) and analgesia. Contact tracing for genital herpes is not routinely recommended due to the ubiquity of the virus and the potential for long dormant periods. It is not a notifiable disease and people are not required to inform future partners of their diagnosis. Condom use is encouraged, and people should be advised to avoid sexual intercourse when symptoms are present to reduce risk of transmission. There do not need to be blisters present to transmit genital herpes; however, transmission is less likely when a person is asymptomatic (Family Planning NSW 2020).

CASE STUDY 37.4

Charlotte is 18 years old and has only recently become sexually active. After a one-night stand at a party 3 weeks ago she has presented to the sexual health clinic with a history of red and itchy vulva, and dysuria. On examination, Charlotte's vulva appears red and inflamed, and there are multiple small blisters as well as lesions present. A doctor also examines the patient and a diagnosis of genital herpes is made.

1. Should Charlotte try to contact the person she had a one-night stand with?
2. What tests would the doctor order to confirm diagnosis of Charlotte's condition?
3. How would Charlotte's condition be managed and what considerations need to be made for Charlotte's future sexual activity?

Genital warts

Genital warts are caused by particular types of the human papillomavirus (HPV) and are transmitted through vaginal, oral and anal sex. The warts appear at the vulval forchette, inside the vagina, on the cervix and on the anus in females. In males, warts can be found under the foreskin, on the shaft and base of the penis and on the anus. Warts may appear as firm, painless, and flesh or white-coloured lumps. They may have an irregular cauliflower-like surface or be flat, pigmented and pedunculated. The main method of treatment is performed by clinicians using liquid nitrogen cryotherapy directly on the wart/s. There are also topical creams, paints or gels that can be used by the person.

Almost all cases of genital warts are caused by HPV (Cancer Council Australia 2019b). HPV is the leading cause of cervical cancer and is also responsible for some anal, penile, vaginal, vulval and oropharyngeal cancers (Cancer Council Australia 2019b). Since the introduction of the HPV vaccine in 2007, there has been a significant reduction in the prevalence of genital warts in Australians under 26 years of age (Family Planning NSW 2020).

Disorders of the internal reproductive organs

Pelvic inflammatory disease (PID)

Pelvic inflammatory disease (PID) is any acute, sub-acute, recurrent or chronic infection of the uterus and uterine tubes that can extend into the pelvic cavity. Causative organisms of PID include *Neisseria gonorrhoeae* and *Chlamydia trachomatis*. Symptoms of PID may include abdominal and pelvic pain, abnormal vaginal discharge, dyspareunia, intermenstrual bleeding, or post-coital bleeding.

Immediate treatment of suspected PID is recommended due to risks of ectopic pregnancy, infertility and pelvic pain if treatment is delayed. Treatment includes antibiotics and appropriate analgesia. Follow-up should occur within 48–72 hours of treatment initiation to ensure compliance and assess effectiveness. Sexual partners should be tested for STIs and treated as appropriate.

Nursing care of the woman with PID includes education to ensure regular perineal hygiene is observed, regular changing of pads where vaginal discharge is present and counselling about the potential complications of PID, which include chronic abdominal pain, future ectopic pregnancy and infertility (Family Planning NSW 2020).

Disorders of the uterus

Endometriosis

Endometriosis is a common condition affecting more than 11% of women (Endometriosis Australia 2022). It is characterised by the presence of tissue similar to endometrium growing outside the lining of the uterus. While it usually affects the reproductive organs, it has also been found in the bowel, bladder, muscle, joints, lungs and brain. The cause is unknown, but research suggests some factors that may contribute include family history, retrograde (backwards) menstruation and metaplasia (Jean Hailes 2023a).

The symptoms of endometriosis depend on the location of the tissue affected. Pain is the most common symptom but it is not indicative of the severity of the condition. Other symptoms include dysmenorrhoea, dyspareunia, menorrhagia, dysuria, diarrhoea and constipation, bloating, tiredness, mood changes and vaginal discomfort. Some women experience little or no symptoms.

Treatment for endometriosis is dependent on the individual and takes into account the symptoms, severity and the woman's wishes to become pregnant or have children. Pain management for endometriosis involves medications such as non-steroidal anti-inflammatory drugs (NSAIDs) and hormone therapy. The aim of using hormonal therapy such as the combined oral contraceptive pill is to suppress the growth of endometrial cells and to stop any bleeding (Jean Hailes 2023a). Progestogens are another hormonal therapy that can help decrease pain. Laparoscopic surgery or a laparotomy to remove endometriosis tissue and repair any damage can be performed to reduce symptoms and improve fertility.

Endometrial tissue is destroyed using a variety of techniques, including vaporisation or excision. Hysterectomy is rarely recommended as a first line treatment option since it may not cure the progression or symptoms of the disease. (See Case Study 37.5.)

CRITICAL THINKING EXERCISE 37.4

A laparoscopic hysterectomy may be performed when non-surgical options have been unsuccessful in treating endometriosis and the woman does not want any more children. Length of stay in hospital is usually 2–3 days. How would you care for the woman post procedure and what education would you provide prior to discharge?

CASE STUDY 37.5

Maddison presents to your clinic with a history of irregular menstrual cycles with heavy bleeding, dyspareunia and occasional post-coital bleeding. She is 22 years old, but due to her symptoms a cervical diagnostic co-test has previously been conducted and the results were NAD: no HPV detected and no abnormal changes to the cells of the cervix. An STI test which was done at the same time was also negative.

What could be a possible diagnosis for Maddison? How would this diagnosis be confirmed and what treatment options does she have available?

Pelvic organ prolapse

Pelvic organ prolapse is characterised by the downward displacement of pelvic organs, mostly the uterus, urinary bladder or rectum into the vagina. Most women are asymptomatic and do not require any intervention.

Uterine prolapse occurs when muscles and ligaments that suspend the uterus become stretched, damaged or weakened through sustained forces brought about by events such as pregnancy, hysterectomy and chronic constipation. The collapse can be either a complete collapse, where it protrudes outside the body, or partial (Table 37.6). (See Clinical Interest Box 37.5.)

Risk factors for uterine prolapse include:

- pregnancy and childbirth
- menopause
- obesity
- chronic coughing, constipation and straining
- heavy/repetitive lifting
- genetic conditions
- previous pelvic surgery
- spinal cord and other muscle atrophy conditions
- familial or racial history.

(Jean Hailes 2023)

TABLE 37.6 | Stages of uterine prolapse

Stage	Results
I	Descent of the uterus into the upper half of the vagina.
II	Descent of uterus nearly to the opening of the vagina.
III	Protrusion of the uterus outside the vagina.
IV	The uterus is completely outside the vagina.

(Adapted from Better Health Channel 2021)

CLINICAL INTEREST BOX 37.5 Clinical scenario: Uterine prolapse

My experience of uterine prolapse began after the birth of my second child with a heavy sensation in my pelvic floor as if things were falling down. This was accompanied by discomfort and some incontinence when lifting heavy weights at the gym or from the pressure of sneezing or coughing. I saw my GP first and was referred to pelvic floor physiotherapy for prolapse. Luckily, the prolapse was only Grade 1 and I was able to work to increase the strength and coordination of my pelvic floor and did not require any surgery. Even though the Grade 1 prolapse has remained, I am back to lifting weights at the gym and am now symptom free.

Stress incontinence is a common symptom experienced by women and may lead to urinary tract infections. Where the posterior aspect of the urinary bladder protrudes into the uterus (cystocele), there may be a feeling of pelvic pressure, and where the rectum herniates into the uterus (rectocele), there is often a feeling of rectal fullness, faecal urgency and incomplete defecation.

Management of the condition may be conservative or surgical. Where the condition is managed conservatively, the woman may be required to perform a series of pelvic floor exercises to strengthen the pelvic floor muscles. Exercises consist of regular tightening then relaxation of muscles surrounding the entrance of the vagina, urethra and anus. Each time the muscle is tightened it is held for 5–10 seconds and then relaxed. The exercise is repeated a number of times and the woman is encouraged to repeat the exercises several times a day. If a woman is struggling to perform or hold pelvic floor exercises, a referral to physiotherapy may be beneficial.

Surgical repair of uterine prolapse is performed by laparoscopic surgery. The uterus or bladder is pulled back into the correct position and reattached to supporting ligaments (Better Health Channel 2021). Procedures such as a hysterectomy using either the vaginal or the abdominal approach may also be considered depending on the circumstances.

Disorders of the ovaries

Ovarian cysts

Ovarian cysts are usually non-cancerous and develop in women of reproductive age when an ovarian follicle fails to burst and release the mature egg, resulting in the accumulation of a fluid-filled sac. Cysts can be either single or multiple small cysts developing to approximately 8–10 mm in diameter (Sweet & Foley 2020). In many cases, the cysts remain asymptomatic; however, if they rupture, they can cause severe abdominal pain and bleeding. Other symptoms may include haemorrhage, ovarian torsion and compression of abdominal and pelvic organs, depending on size. Diagnosis can be made by pelvic examination, ultrasound, CT scan, MRI scan and possibly a blood test for tumour markers. Generally, the cysts resolve without the need for treatment, but a small number of women may require surgery (laparoscopy and/or laparotomy) (Sweet & Foley 2020).

Polycystic ovary syndrome

Polycystic ovary syndrome (PCOS) is a common hormonal condition affecting 8–13% of women of reproductive age, and is more common in high-risk categories such as Aboriginal and Torres Strait Islander women (Jean Hailes 2023b). PCOS is often associated with the presence of multiple, large cysts in the ovary, which may cause health complications if left untreated. Most symptoms associated with PCOS are caused by increased androgen levels in the body causing hyperandrogenism. Insulin is also believed to play a part in developing PCOS. There are many symptoms that present in different ways (see Table 37.7). The management focuses on treating the physical symptoms; however, a healthy lifestyle is one of the most important aspects of successful management. Medical therapies for PCOS include the oral contraceptive pill, insulin-sensitising medications such as metformin, gonadotropins, testosterone-lowering medications, weight-loss medications, antidepressants and anti-anxiety medications (Jean Hailes 2023b).

TABLE 37.7 | Symptoms related to PCOS

Periods and fertility	• Amenorrhoea • Irregular, infrequent or heavy periods • Cysts on ovaries • Difficulty becoming pregnant • Some health challenges during pregnancy
Hair and skin	• Hirsutism (excess facial and/or body hair) • Acne • Alopecia (hair loss) • Darkened skin patches • Weight gain
Mental and emotional health	• Mood changes • Anxiety • Depression • Poor body image • Low self-esteem
Related health conditions	• Sleep apnoea • Increased risk of diabetes and cardiovascular disease • Earlier onset of sexual health challenges

(Adapted from Jean Hailes 2023b)

Tumours of the female reproductive system

Ovarian cancer

Ovarian cancer is the ninth most common cancer in Australian women (Cancer Council Australia 2023a). It is most commonly diagnosed in women over the age of 50 years; however, it can occur in women of any age (Ovarian Cancer Australia 2023). Tumours affecting the ovaries can vary in size, diversity and occurrence (see Table 37.8).

Diagnosis of ovarian cancer is definitively made only after surgery during which biopsies are performed to determine the presence of cancer cells. The woman may have a transvaginal ultrasound (TVU) and blood taken to detect the presence of the tumour marker CA125. It may be possible to detect irregularity on palpation of the abdomen or physical examination if the tumour is large. TVU, which involves the use of a probe inside the vagina to detect the presence of a tumour, and other imaging tests such as abdominal X-rays, CT scans or magnetic resonance imaging (MRI) are occasionally used.

TABLE 37.8 | Types of ovarian cancer

Type	Clinical behaviour
Epithelial	Most common type of ovarian cancer. Accounts for about 90% of cases. Starts in the epithelial layer of the ovary, fallopian tube or peritoneum. Mostly occurs over the age of 60.
Germ cell	Begins in the egg producing (geminal) cells. Rare type, about 4% of tumours. Usually occurs under the age of 40.
Stromal cell (or sex cord-stromal tumours)	Rare cancer, less than 8%. Begins in hormone producing cells in the ovaries. Usually occurs between 40 and 60 years of age.

(Ovarian Cancer Australia 2023)

Ovarian cancer is difficult to diagnose due to its vague presentation and can sometimes be diagnosed prior to the presence of any symptoms.

Symptoms of ovarian cancer include:

- abdominal and pelvic pain
- increase in abdominal size or persistent abdominal bloating
- urgency and frequency of urination
- feeling of fullness after eating
- changes in bowel habits
- unexplained weight loss or gain
- unexplained bleeding
- excessive fatigue
- back pain
- pain or bleeding during or after sex
- indigestion and nausea.

(Ovarian Cancer Australia 2023)

Treatment for ovarian cancer initially involves a laparotomy where biopsies are taken and sent for analysis to confirm diagnosis. On confirmation of cancer, the surgeon will remove the affected ovary. Where the tumour has spread to affect other structures, it may be necessary to perform a partial or total hysterectomy. Surgery may then be followed by chemotherapy or radiotherapy.

Cervical cancer

Cervical cancer is the growth of abnormal cells in the lining of the cervix. Human papilloma virus is the leading cause of cervical cancer. The introduction of the Cervical Screening Program in 1991 has seen the incidence of cervical cancer deaths halved (Australian Institute of Health and Welfare 2022). The National HPV Vaccination Program in 2007 has also impacted the reduction in HPV in Australia. (See Clinical Interest Box 37.6.)

Cervical cancer may be one of two types: a squamous cell carcinoma, which accounts for approximately 70% of cases, or an adenocarcinoma. It begins as a change in the cells covering the cervix and, if not treated, eventually involves the epithelial layer. Invasive carcinoma extends beyond the surface, involving the body of the cervix and may spread via the lymphatic system to surrounding structures. Clinical signs of cervical cancer do not appear in the early stages. Later manifestations include intermenstrual bleeding, heavier or longer periods, post-coital bleeding, dyspareunia, abnormal vaginal discharge and postmenopausal bleeding (Cervical Cancer Australia 2023b).

Screening for cervical cancer involves a routine 5-yearly cervical screening test (CST), unless an individual is symptomatic, in which case a 'co-test' can be done early as part of the investigative process. The cervical screening test screens for the presence of HPV, while the co-test screens for HPV as well as any changes to the cells of the cervix. Diagnosis is performed by colposcopy and biopsies are taken. The stages of cervical cancer are described in Table 37.9. Treatment of the early stages of cervical changes or cancer may be possible by performing a large loop excision of the transformation zone (LLETZ) or cone biopsy. Removal of cervical tissue by a LLETZ

CLINICAL INTEREST BOX 37.6 National HPV vaccination program

The HPV vaccine is currently offered to all children aged 12–13 through the school-based National Immunisation Program, and is free for anyone aged between 12–25 years old. The vaccine provides long-lasting protection against nine types of HPV if it is given prior to infection. It is most effective if administered prior to commencement of sexual activity; however, a person may still benefit from the vaccine after sexual debut.

(HPV Vaccine 2023)

TABLE 37.9 | Cervical cancer stages

Stage	Description
Stage 1	The cancer is found only in the tissue of the cervix.
Stage 2	The cancer has spread outside the cervix to the upper two-thirds of the vagina or other tissue next to the cervix.
Stage 3	The cancer has spread to the tissue on the side of the pelvis (pelvic wall) and/or the lower third of the vagina.
Stage 4	The cancer has spread to the bladder or rectum (stage 4A), or beyond the pelvis to the lungs, liver or bones (Stage 4B).

(Cancer Council Australia 2023b)

procedure is the most common treatment for precancerous cells. A cone biopsy is used to remove a larger section of the cervix if early-stage cancer is suspected.

Endometrial cancer

The benign form of endometrial cancer presents as fibroids, which grow in the wall of the uterus. They are usually asymptomatic and, as the woman enters menopause, the fibroids tend to get smaller. If they cause heavy bleeding, they may need to be surgically treated. Other presentations may be endometriosis and endometrial hyperplasia.

The usual management for women who have malignant neoplasms (cancers) is surgical intervention with a combination of chemotherapy and radiotherapy to eliminate any remaining cancer cells. The typical surgical procedures include:

- hysterectomy with bilateral salpingo-oopherectomy
- pelvic lymphadenectomy (if late-stage disease present).

Vaginal vault brachytherapy may also be performed for endometrial cancer. This involves insertion of small hollow tubes inside the vagina through which small amounts of radioactive agents are administered. The treatment takes approximately 30 minutes to perform.

Hysterectomy is the surgical removal of the uterus and may also involve the removal of other structures depending on the extent of infiltration or damage to reproductive organs. Prior to any woman undergoing a hysterectomy, it is important they are aware they will no longer menstruate or be able to conceive a child. For some, this prospect may bring relief, while for others it may be distressing. A compassionate approach to nursing care is important.

The main five types of hysterectomy operations (see Table 37.10) performed in Australia are:

1. Sub-total or partial hysterectomy: Involves removal of the uterus where the cervix remains intact.
2. Hysterectomy with ovarian conservation: Involves removal of the uterus and cervix, and preservation of the ovaries. Procedure is often referred to as a 'total hysterectomy'.
3. Hysterectomy with salpingo-oopherectomy: Involves removal of fallopian tubes, uterus and cervix and either one or both ovaries.
4. Radical or Wertheim's hysterectomy: Involves removal of fallopian tubes, uterus, cervix, ovaries, nearby lymph nodes and upper portion of the vagina.
5. Hysterectomy with prophylactic bilateral salpingectomy: It is now recommended that fallopian tubes are removed during hysterectomy due to research suggesting that ovarian cancers originate in the tubes.

(Better Health Channel 2022)

With all types of hysterectomy, it is important the woman is fully aware of the procedure to be performed and the implications associated with the surgery. The surgical procedures have a long convalescence postoperatively; the individual is unable to return to normal activities for anywhere between 6 weeks and 3 months. It is also important

TABLE 37.10 | Types of hysterectomy

Surgery	Description of procedure	Advantage	Disadvantage
Vaginal hysterectomy	The uterus is removed through the vagina.	Less pain and shorter healing time. Fewer complications.	Not appropriate for women with adhesions from previous surgeries or conditions such as endometriosis, or those with a very large uterus.
Abdominal hysterectomy	Vertical or horizontal incision is made in the lower abdomen through which the uterus is removed.	Allows good vision of pelvic structures. Allows removal of large uterus, or if adhesions are present.	Greater risk of complications such as bleeding, infection and nerve or tissue damage. Requires a longer hospital stay and recovery time.
Laparoscopic hysterectomy	A laparoscope is inserted into a small incision in the abdomen to view the pelvic organs; three or four other incisions are made through which the surgery is performed. The uterus is removed in small pieces through the incisions, through the vagina or a larger abdominal incision.	Less pain, shorter hospital stay and lower risk of infection than abdominal hysterectomy.	May lead to longer operation time depending on how much of the procedure is performed by laparoscope. Higher risk of damage to urinary tract and other organs.

(The American College of Obstetricians and Gynecologists 2021)

the woman be aware of what to expect in the immediate postoperative phase, such as whether she will have an indwelling catheter, drain tubes or vaginal packing.

A vaginal pack may be inserted after a vaginal hysterectomy and remains in situ for 24 hours. Postoperatively, the nurse is required to assess the volume of discharge from the vagina and if there are any difficulties with voiding. If an indwelling or suprapubic catheter has been inserted during the operation, it may be necessary to commence bladder retraining prior to the removal of the catheter to assist in re-establishing normal bladder sensation and control.

Conditions affecting menstruation

At some time in a woman's life she is likely to experience some form of benign menstrual problem that will often be painful and debilitating. The main menstrual symptoms include dysmenorrhoea, dyspareunia, menorrhagia and pain.

Premenstrual syndrome

'Premenstrual syndrome' is a term used to describe the symptoms experienced by some women in the lead-up to the onset of menstruation. The common symptoms experienced in the 4–7 days before menstruation include transient fluid retention, which may result in oedema in the legs, fingers and abdomen; breast tenderness; headaches; and mood swings.

Menopause

Menopause is often described as the 'change of life' and signals the end of a woman's reproductive life. During menopause, eggs are no longer produced by the ovary and the production of oestrogen and progesterone ceases (Brown et al 2020). In most women, menopause will occur between the ages of 45 and 50 years. Premature menopause occurs from 40 years and may be due to a cessation of ovarian function, after a total hysterectomy or as the result of cancer. A woman is considered to be postmenopausal when 12 consecutive months without a menstrual cycle have elapsed.

The premenopausal woman often describes symptoms such as irregular periods, hot flushes, palpitations, vaginal dryness, tiredness, sleep disturbances, mood swings and crawling sensations on the skin. The woman who believes she is premenopausal can have the diagnosis confirmed with blood tests to determine declining hormone levels. The management of menopause is often determined by the impact of symptoms. Many women try natural therapies or may commence HRT (see Case Study 37.6 and Clinical Interest Box 37.7).

CASE STUDY 37.6

Anna is a 45-year-old woman who has come to your clinic for help with new onset of feeling depressed and crying unexpectedly. She reports that she has been having regular episodes of sweats and chills that started around the same time. Over the past 12 months, her periods have been irregular and she is experiencing menstrual bleeding that is heavier than normal for her. Some months she has missed her period.

1. What tests would be ordered to confirm Anna's medical diagnosis?
2. How could Anna manage her problem non-pharmacologically and pharmacologically?

CLINICAL INTEREST BOX 37.7 Clinical scenario: Menopause

I'd always had normal, regular periods, but this changed in my early 40s when they started to become heavier and irregular. My GP told me it was peri-menopause and I had two endometrial ablation procedures to help with the heavy bleeding. I started menopausal hormone therapy when I was 45 to help with hot flushes and vaginal dryness. I am now 59 and my periods have since stopped, although I still get the occasional hot flush.

Disorders of pregnancy

Spontaneous abortion

Spontaneous abortion (miscarriage) is common, affecting approximately 20% of pregnancies in the very early stages (Brown et al 2020). In the event that the abortion is incomplete and products of conception are retained in the uterus, there is a high risk of infection and this needs to be managed surgically to preserve the integrity of the uterus and to avoid future fertility complications. People should be supported through the grieving process that results from a loss of pregnancy.

Ectopic pregnancy

An ectopic pregnancy occurs where the fertilised ovum implants outside of the uterus, most commonly in the fallopian tubes. Generally, ectopic implantation occurs where the woman has a disorder that slows the passage of the ovum to the uterus, such as scarring, endometriosis or tumours. In the initial stages, the woman's pregnancy will show normal signs of conception, with amenorrhoea and hormonal changes. However, as the foetus develops, spotting and cramping may occur and the fallopian tube can rupture, resulting in severe pain and abdominal swelling. Once the tube has ruptured it is considered a surgical emergency if the woman is to survive the rapid blood loss and shock.

Pre-eclampsia

Pre-eclampsia occurs in a small percentage of pregnancies. The condition usually presents with three characteristic signs: generalised oedema, hypertension and proteinuria.

It usually develops about the 20th week of pregnancy. If detected, mild symptoms may be controlled with little risk to foetus or mother; however, in the event that symptoms become severe, a multidisciplinary approach to management of both mother and baby is required.

Breast disorders

The main disorders affecting the breast are:

- mastitis
- fibrocystic changes
- tumours.

Mastitis

Mastitis is an inflammatory condition of the breast that usually occurs during lactation and breastfeeding (Brown et al 2020). There are many factors that influence the development of mastitis including tight compression on breasts, blocked milk ducts, ineffective use of the baby's oral cavity, or ceasing breastfeeding suddenly. Presentation of the condition includes inflammation, swelling, heat and pain. A woman may report feeling like she has the flu. The infective process may cause abscess formation and cessation of milk flow. Treatment may include soft hand compression on the breast tissue, the use of cold compresses, antibiotics and, where an abscess is present, drainage of fluid (see also Chapter 45).

Fibrocystic changes

Fibrosis of the breast is a benign condition caused by hyperplasia of the fibroblasts in breast tissue. Women between 30 and 40 years are more commonly affected, and the condition is usually detected as a tender or painful mobile lump, often felt just prior to menstruation. The condition is not believed to predispose the woman to cancer.

Cystic changes of the breast occur more commonly in women during the last half of their reproductive life (between 40 and 55 years) and are characterised with single or multiple lumps in the breasts. Each cyst is filled with a thin turgid fluid and, if large, may be visible as a bluish lump under the skin. Each cyst can be drained and the fluid analysed to determine malignancy.

Tumours of the breast

Carcinoma of the breast usually occurs in women over the age of 50 years, although it may also be diagnosed in younger women. The woman may notice an alteration in the size of the breast, dimpling of the skin, a palpable mass or alteration in the shape, retraction of the nipple, a clear discharge and possibly ulceration (Clinical Interest Box 37.8). It should be noted that carcinoma of the breast can also occur in males. An estimated 20,600 people were diagnosed with breast cancer in 2022 and it is the most common cancer in women (Cancer Council Australia 2023c).

Possible causes of breast cancer include:

- increasing age
- familial history
- inheritance of mutation gene (BRCA2, BRCA1)
- exposure to female hormones
- obesity
- excessive alcohol consumption
- long-term HRT.

Diagnosis of breast carcinoma will initially involve a physical examination of the breast and armpits, a diagnostic mammogram and possibly an ultrasound of the breast tissue. More definitive or invasive tests may be conducted to confirm diagnosis which include:

- fine-needle aspiration
- core biopsy
- open biopsy
- hormone tests
- lumpectomy.

> **CLINICAL INTEREST BOX 37.8**
> **Symptoms of breast cancer**
>
> - Lump or thickening in breast or under arm
> - Sore nipples
> - Changes in size or shape of breast
> - Discharge from nipple
> - Inversion of nipple
> - Sores, ulcers, or redness around nipple
> - Dimpling of breast tissue
> - Rash or redness of the breast
> - Persistent, unusual pain in one breast only
>
> *(Cancer Council NSW 2022b)*

Care of the individual with a breast disorder

Surgical treatment of breast carcinoma may include a total mastectomy where the entire breast is removed along with lymph nodes from the axilla. Alternatively, a more conservative approach may be taken—breast-conserving surgery, where the bulk of the breast tissue is conserved. Surgery is usually accompanied by radiotherapy and chemotherapy to eliminate any remaining cancerous cells.

Breast surgery may cause issues with body image, sexuality and feelings of femininity. While reconstructive surgery may be performed, this is often not an option until several months after the mastectomy. Reconstructive surgery involves the formation of a breast mound, nipple and areola. A prosthetic in the woman's bra may be used in the interim to give the appearance of a normal breast. Hormone therapy may be indicated to reduce the size of the breast lump prior to attempting a surgical approach.

A sample of an entry into progress notes has been provided, which documents the care of a patient recovering from a mastectomy (see Progress Note 37.1).

Preoperative preparation

As with any surgical procedure, it is important that the woman is fully aware of the risks and benefits of the surgery she is undergoing and is provided with adequate emotional support. It is advisable that the woman be referred to a breast support nurse, psychologist and advised of any local support networks.

Breast prostheses are available in a range of styles. A soft, lightweight prosthesis is recommended initially while the incision is healing and until tenderness has decreased, if the woman chooses to wear one.

Postoperative care

Physical postoperative care includes providing pain relief, promoting comfort, care of the wound, prevention of complications, exercise recommendations and continued emotional support. The woman should be encouraged to perform a series of post-mastectomy exercises to prevent shortening of the muscles and contracture of joints. Gentle exercise also decreases oedema and helps to maintain range of movement in the arm.

> **CRITICAL THINKING EXERCISE 37.5**
>
> In the surgical management of conditions such as breast cancer, lymph glands are usually removed, either as an axillary clearance where between five and 30 nodes are removed, or sentinel removal, where only 1–2 nodes closest to the cancer are taken. The development of lymphoedema should be considered. What kind of exercises should be performed to avoid lymphoedema in the postoperative individual?

ASSESSMENT AND DIAGNOSTIC TESTS

The performance of a physical examination for any woman can cause anxiety and embarrassment. For this reason, it should be a priority for every nurse to approach the situation with sensitivity and be mindful of creating a calm and comfortable experience for the woman (see Chapter 15). The presence of a female nurse during the examination by a male practitioner is mandatory in most health facilities; if not, the woman should be offered a female staff member to accompany her. Consideration should also be given to addressing social and cultural aspects when performing a physical examination.

External examinations

Hysterosalpingogram

A hysterosalpingogram (HSG) is an X-ray of the cervical canal, uterine cavity and interior of the fallopian tubes. It usually involves the use of a radio-opaque dye, which is injected through the cervix.

Ultrasonography

Ultrasonography uses high-frequency soundwaves to obtain a visualisation of the pelvic organs. It is commonly used to evaluate symptoms of PID or to monitor pregnancy.

Breast examination

A clinical breast examination involves a thorough physical examination of the whole breast area, including breast tissue, nipples, armpits and the chest wall up to the collarbone. Most of the breast tissue in men (a potential site for malignancy) is located behind the nipple, whereas women have a larger area of breast tissue. While a clinical breast examination can be valuable, it is also important to encourage men and women to be breast aware. Regular self-examination of the breasts means that individuals are more likely to notice any abnormal changes at an earlier stage.

Inspection

Inspect the breasts for size and symmetry. Note breast shape and any masses, flattening, retraction or dimpling. Each breast is inspected in four quadrants including the tail of Spence (Figure 37.6). The nipples are inspected for size, shape, colour, discharge and the direction they point.

Palpation

Palpation of the breast may be an uncomfortable experience for some women and has a relatively low sensitivity. If clinically indicated, palpation of all four quadrants of the breast including the tail of Spence is required and may help to identify any suspicious lumps/tissue.

Using the pads of the first three fingers, compress breast tissue gently against the chest wall, noting tissue consistency. Palpation is performed systematically in one of three ways (Figure 37.7):

1. a back-and-forth technique with the fingers moving up and down each quadrant

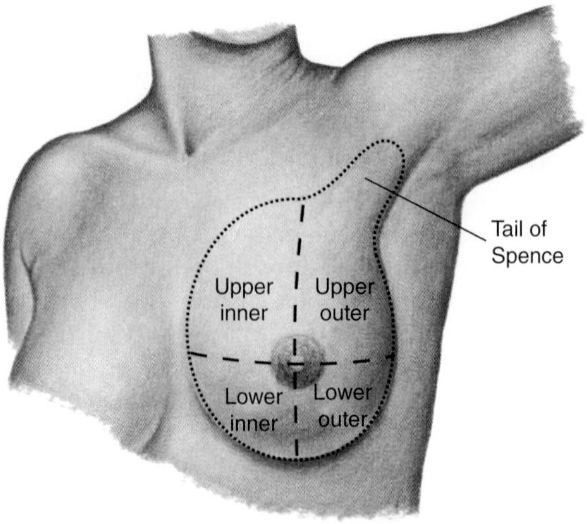

Figure 37.6 Quadrants of the left breast and axillary tail of Spence
(Stewart et al 2023)

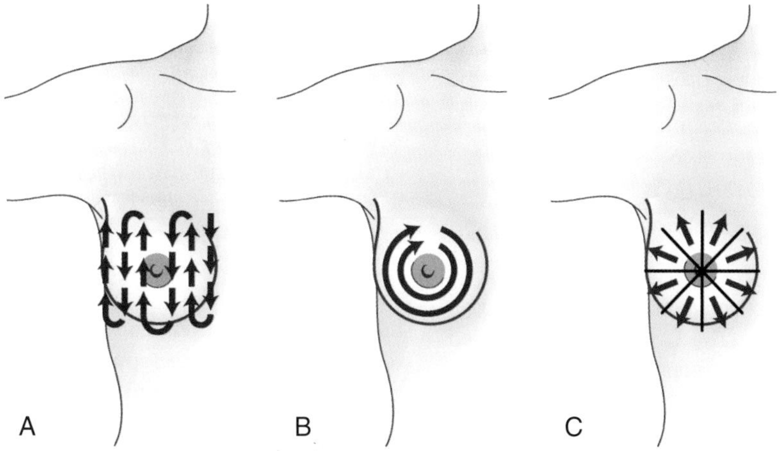

Figure 37.7 Various methods for palpation of breast
A: Palpate from top to bottom in vertical strips, **B:** Palpate in concentric circles, **C:** Palpate out from centre in wedge sections.
(Perry et al 2023)

2. clockwise or counterclockwise, forming small circles with the fingers along each quadrant and the tail
3. palpating from the centre of the breast in a radial fashion, returning to the areola to begin each spoke.

Family Planning NSW (2018) recommends the following guidelines for the early detection of breast cancer:

- Develop breast awareness strategies for individuals, which include:
  - viewing breasts in the mirror when dressing and undressing
  - feeling breasts while bathing or showering. It is recommended that the woman feels all of her breast from the collarbone to below the bra line and in the armpits as well (Figure 37.8)
  - consulting a healthcare provider if any changes are noticed in the breasts.
- Teach the woman to look for:
  - a new lump or lumpiness, especially if it is only in one breast
  - a change in the size or shape of the breast
  - a change to the nipple, such as crusting, ulcer, redness or inversion
  - a nipple discharge that occurs without squeezing
  - a change in the skin of the breast such as redness or dimpling
  - an unusual pain that does not go away.

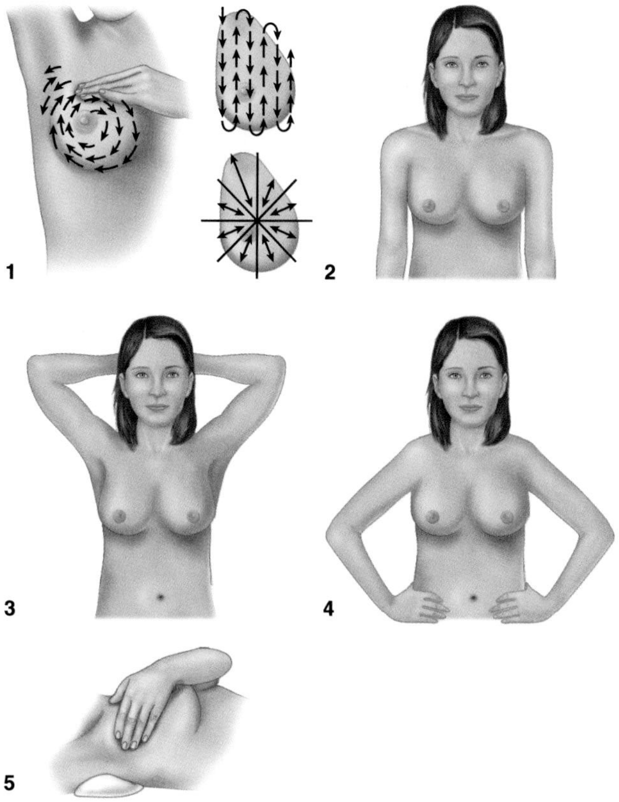

Figure 37.8 Breast self-examination
(Grimm 2025)

Mammography

A mammogram is one of the procedures used to detect or confirm the presence of a palpable lump in the breast. The mammogram is an X-ray, which is usually provided free for women between the ages of 50 and 69 years as part of the BreastScreen Australia program. It is recommended that the test be done every 2 years. Where there is a familial link to the occurrence of breast cancer it may be recommended to commence screening earlier. Mammograms in younger women are often less accurate due to the density of breast tissue prior to menopause. For this reason, younger women are usually screened by MRI if indicated.

Breast ultrasound

Breast ultrasounds are often scheduled for women under 35 years old who have detected an abnormal lump in the breast. The ultrasound allows the medical officer to identify whether the lump is fluid-filled or solid. In the event of a fluid-filled cyst, the medical officer can perform an ultrasound-guided aspiration of fluid for analysis. The procedure is ideal for the pregnant woman who detects a lump because there is little risk to the growing foetus.

Internal examinations and sampling

Cervical screening test

The **cervical screening test (CST)** replaced the Pap test in December 2017 and is more effective at preventing cervical cancers through early detection. The CST is recommended to be performed at 5-yearly intervals in asymptomatic women aged between 25 and 74 years (see Clinical Interest Box 37.9). The sample is collected via vaginal speculum examination of the cervix, and collection of cells is done with a cervical sampler broom. Previously, the Pap smear looked for changes to the cervical cells; however, the new CST looks for the presence of HPV, which can cause those changes. HPV can take 10 or more years to develop into cervical cancer, which is a rare outcome of HPV infection—it is usually cleared from the body spontaneously. Women can be reassured that 5-yearly screening is safe and effective. If HPV is detected, further tests will be performed using the same sample to determine the type of HPV, and if there are any changes to the cells of the cervix. In symptomatic women (i.e. abnormal pain or bleeding), a co-test is recommended, which will automatically check for cell changes to the cervix regardless of HPV infection status (National Cervical Screening Test 2022).

Pelvic examination

Speculum examination can be performed as part of the diagnostic process when initiating investigations into abnormal bleeding, pain or abnormal vaginal discharge. A vaginal speculum is inserted into the vagina to view the cervix and vaginal walls (Family Planning NSW 2020).

Bimanual examination of the pelvis is a useful tool when assessing women with pelvic pain, abnormal bleeding or abnormal vaginal discharge. It is not useful as a screening test for cancer. Ensure the woman has an empty bladder prior to the examination. The medical officer inserts two gloved and lubricated fingers into the vagina and applies gentle pressure to the lower abdomen with their other hand. The cervix, uterus and pouch of Douglas are palpated to identify position, shape, size, mobility, masses, pain or tenderness (Family Planning NSW 2020).

CLINICAL INTEREST BOX 37.9 Individual teaching: Cervical screening test

- A sample of cells from the cervix is used to detect cancer-causing types of HPV. This test replaced the Pap test in 2017.
- It is recommended that everyone with a cervix commence screening at age 25 and continue screening every 5 years until the age of 74, regardless of gender or sexual identity.
- Women who have had a total hysterectomy (including removal of cervix) may still require a cervical screening test (CST). The sample should be taken from the top of the vagina.
- If a woman has had a hysterectomy and cervix remains, routine 5-yearly CST is recommended.
- A woman who is between the ages of 70 and 74 years is eligible for an exit screening test. If the result is negative, she requires no further screening in her lifetime.

(Cancer Council Australia 2023b)

Colposcopy

A colposcopy is performed to assess the nature, extent and severity of changes in the cells of the cervix, noted on the woman's smear test or for investigation of abnormal symptoms. It involves a vaginal speculum examination, where the practitioner inspects the surface of the cervix using a colposcope, which magnifies and illuminates the cervix. It is complemented by cytopathology and histopathology. A biopsy of the cervix may be completed during the procedure.

Cervical biopsy

A cervical punch biopsy is the removal of a small column of cervical tissue. The cervix is compared to a clock face and biopsy tissue labelled accordingly. Cone biopsy is the removal of a cone-shaped piece of tissue from the cervix. Possible complications after the procedure are haemorrhage and infertility due to the removal of mucus-producing glands, and the formation of scar tissue.

Laparoscopy

Laparoscopic procedures are used for a direct visual assessment of the organs in the pelvic cavity including reproductive organs. Laparoscopy involves three or four small incisions into the abdomen and the use of probes and cameras, allowing the surgeon to make a diagnostic examination, take biopsies or possibly to perform surgical procedures.

Diagnostic uterine curettage

A dilation and curettage (D&C) involves the removal of the uterus lining (endometrium). It can be used to obtain a specimen for diagnostic purposes or to remove products of conception that have been retained after a miscarriage or postnatally.

REPRODUCTIVE AND SEXUAL HEALTH PROMOTION

There are a number of national health promotion strategies addressing target health risk areas throughout Australia. Information and education are available in many languages through state, territory and federal health departments.

Strategies cover the prevention of STIs, choosing a suitable contraceptive method and screening for cervical, breast and bowel cancer. The nurse plays an integral part in the promotion of health, education and support of the individual. The nurse should reinforce the medical officer's explanation about any implications for the individual's lifestyle and ensure that the information is understood. It may also be necessary to provide information about fertility control and prevention of STIs.

The nurse should be aware of the changes that occur to the normal reproductive structures and functions throughout the lifespan and be able to identify alterations. It is the role of the nurse to actively promote reproductive and sexual health through individual teaching, education and health-promotion strategies. Individual teaching is implemented by educating individuals about normal developmental changes that occur throughout the lifespan.

Health-promotion strategies and programs should be adapted to local needs, taking into account social, cultural and economic structures.

CONTRACEPTION

A variety of contraceptive options are available for both men and women. The option chosen will be dictated by cultural, economic and personal factors, as well as availability.

Contraception methods available to females prevent ovulation, fertilisation or the successful implantation and development of a fertilised ovum. Women have a number of options available, but there are limited choices for men—namely the use of a condom or a vasectomy procedure.

For most women, selecting and using a method of contraception is a significant decision. It should be noted that no method of contraception is 100% effective. Each method has a number of advantages and disadvantages that should be considered by the individual (see Table 37.11).

Methods of contraception include:

- mechanical barriers
- chemical barriers
- fertility awareness-based methods
- intrauterine devices
- hormonal contraceptives
- sterilisation.

The oral contraceptive pill (OCP) was introduced in Australia over 50 years ago, with Australia being the second country in the world to have access to 'the pill'. The combined oral contraceptive pill (COCP), which is a combination of both oestrogen and progestogen, is one of the most commonly used options. The primary action of the COCP is to prevent ovulation, but it also thickens the cervical mucus, which prohibits sperm penetration. A low-dose alternative is the progestogen-only pill (POP) or 'mini-pill'. The POP works by thickening the cervical mucus to prevent sperm penetration. They are greater than 99% effective with perfect use, but in typical day-to-day use they can be about 93% effective (Family Planning NSW 2023).

There are two types of the intrauterine contraceptive device (IUD): one is copper releasing, and the second, which is more commonly used, is hormone releasing. Both IUDs inhibit sperm migration, interfere with ovum survival and prevent implantation. Additionally, the hormonal IUD causes endometrial changes, such as atrophy, and thickens cervical mucus to prevent penetration of sperm. It can also prevent ovulation in some users. The device must be inserted into the uterus by a trained IUD inserter and once in situ a nylon string approximately 2–3 cm in length protrudes from the cervix. This string is used to remove the IUD when required. The copper IUD can be used as emergency contraception if inserted within 5 days of unprotected sexual intercourse. It is the most effective form of emergency contraception, preventing more than 99% of pregnancies. A copper IUD must be inserted by a trained doctor or nurse.

Contraceptive implants are inserted under the skin of the inner arm and release a steady dose of progestogen to prevent ovulation. The implant is effective for up to 3 years and is easily reversed simply by removing it. The implant used in Australia is called Implanon NXT.

Injectable contraceptives such as Depo Provera have the benefit of providing protection against pregnancy for up to 12 weeks. Unlike other methods of contraception, the effects are not easily reversible, with fertility effects still possible up to 18 months after the injection.

The emergency contraceptive pill (ECP), commonly referred to as the morning-after pill, is designed to be used after unprotected sexual intercourse, a condom has broken or other contraception has been missed.

There are two forms of ECP available in Australia: ulipristal acetate (UPA) and levonorgestrel EC (LNG-EC). UPA is registered for use for up to 120 hours and is slightly more effective than the LNG-EC. LNG-EC is registered for use for up to 72 hours and has limited efficacy if used after 96–120 hours. Both methods work best when taken as soon as possible after unprotected sex and are approximately 85% effective. The ECPs are widely available from pharmacies without a script. It is possible to use LNG-EC more than once in a menstrual cycle, but it is important to note that LNG-EC and UPA should not be used in the same menstrual cycle.

Less commonly used methods of contraception are also available, such as the diaphragm. There is currently only one diaphragm available in Australia (Caya®), which is one size fits all. The diaphragm must be used with lactic acid buffer gel (Caya® gel) every time and must be left in place for 6 hours post intercourse. The gel expires 3 months after opening, and a diaphragm is recommended to be replaced after 2 years. It has been found to be approximately 82% effective.

Alternatively, family planning clinics may discuss the use of devices such as the female condom, dams and vaginal rings. The vaginal ring (NuvaRing®) is another hormone-releasing method. It sits inside the vagina for 3 weeks and the hormones are absorbed through the walls of the vagina. It has a similar method of action to the OCP. After 3 weeks,

TABLE 37.11 | Contraceptive methods

Type	Description	Advantages	Disadvantages/side effects	Convenience	Effectiveness
Male condom	Sheath made of latex or polyurethane. Provides a barrier to prevent sperm entering female reproductive tract.	Offers protection against STIs. Used only as required. High level of effectiveness if used correctly. Easy to use.	Irritation and allergic reactions. May break. May alter sensitivity during intercourse. May affect spontaneity. Pregnancy may result if not used correctly.	Applied immediately before any genital contact. Readily available; no prescription needed. Inexpensive.	88–98%
Female condom	Nitrile loose-fitting sheath. Sits inside the vagina to collect semen.	Offers protection against STIs. Does not interfere with the menstrual cycle. Used only as required. High level of effectiveness if used correctly. Easy to use.	May affect spontaneity. Pregnancy may result if not used correctly. May be difficult to insert and remove. Expensive.	Applied immediately before any genital contact. No prescription needed.	79–95%
Diaphragm	Thin, soft, latex, dome-shaped device that sits in the vagina to cover the cervix.	Does not interfere with the menstrual cycle. Minimal side effects. Can be used with condoms.	May slip out of position. No protection against STIs. High upfront cost. Pregnancy may result if not used correctly.	Applied any time before intercourse. Reuseable devices for up to 2 years. Must be left in place for 6 hours after intercourse. One size.	82–86%
Spermicide	Spermicidal preparations in foam, creams, jellies and vaginal suppositories.	Not recommended as contraceptive.	High failure rate. Associated with mucosal irritation, increasing risk of genital lesions and HIV acquisition.	Not available in Australia.	72–82%
Fertility awareness methods (FAMs)	Based on abstinence from sexual intercourse during the fertile phase of the menstrual cycle. Methods include: rhythm/calendar, temperature measurement, cervical mucus observation.	No disruption to menstrual cycle. No side effects or contraindications. Symptom-based methods are more effective.	Requires commitment to daily awareness and continued vigilance. Infection may alter temperature pattern. No protection against STIs. Affects spontaneity. Unsuitable if irregular or anovulatory cycles.	All methods require considerable motivation and self-discipline. Requires frequent monitoring of body functions.	75–99%

TABLE 37.11 | Contraceptive methods—cont'd

Type	Description	Advantages	Disadvantages/side effects	Convenience	Effectiveness
Levonorgestrel intrauterine device (LNG-IUD)	Device inserted into the uterus to prevent pregnancy. Releases low dose of hormone daily. Inhibits sperm migration. Interferes with ovum survival. Prevents implantation. Causes changes to endometrium. Thickens cervical mucus.	High level of effectiveness. Reversible. Long-acting. Can be used in breastfeeding women. Reduces menstrual bleeding. Can help with endometriosis and adenomyosis pain.	Procedure required for insertion. May be expelled from the uterus. Can be difficult to remove. No protection against STIs. May have unpredictable bleeding pattern for 3–6 months after insertion. Hormonal side effects. Risk of ovarian cysts.	One-time insertion. May remain in place for up to 5 years. Inexpensive over time.	99.7–99.9%
Copper intrauterine device (Cu-IUD)	Device inserted into the uterus to prevent pregnancy. Releases copper. Inhibits sperm migration. Interferes with ovum survival. Prevents implantation.	Non-hormonal method. High level of effectiveness. Reversible. Long-acting. Can be used in breastfeeding women. Can be used as emergency contraception.	Procedure required for insertion. Possibility for heavier and longer periods. May be expelled from the uterus. Can be difficult to remove. No protection against STIs.	One-time insertion. May remain in place for up to 5 years. Inexpensive over time.	99.5%
Combined oral contraceptive pill	Combination of oestrogen and progestogen. Inhibits ovulation.	High level of effectiveness if used correctly. Predictable menstruation, reduced menstrual bleeding. Can be used to manage polycystic ovary syndrome.	Nausea, weight gain, fluid retention, breast tenderness, breakthrough bleeding, mood changes, loss of libido. Requires a person to take a pill every day. Not advised if some medical conditions present. No protection against STIs.	Must be taken daily regardless of frequency of intercourse. Requires prescription.	93–99.5%
Combined vaginal ring	Combination of oestrogen and progestogen. Inhibits ovulation.	High level of effectiveness if used correctly. Predictable menstruation, reduced menstrual bleeding. Can be used to manage polycystic ovary syndrome.	Expensive. Ring needs to be removed every 3 weeks. Not advised if some medical conditions present. No protection against STIs.	Requires prescription. Can remain in place for 3 weeks including during sex.	93–99.5%

Continued

TABLE 37.11 | Contraceptive methods—cont'd

Type	Description	Advantages	Disadvantages/side effects	Convenience	Effectiveness
Progestogen-only pill	Thickens cervical mucus to prevent sperm penetration.	Few contraindications. Good option for women unable to use methods containing oestrogen. High level of effectiveness if used correctly.	Must be taken at the same time every day. Unpredictable bleeding patterns. Weight gain, mood changes, headaches. No protection against STIs.	Must be taken daily regardless of frequency of intercourse. Not suitable for some women if unable to comply with strict pill-taking schedule. Requires prescription.	93–99%
Depot medroxypro-gesterone acetate (DMPA) injection	Long-acting progestogen in injectable form. Inhibits ovulation, thickens cervical mucus.	Highly effective. Undetectable. Good option for women unable to use methods containing oestrogen.	Menstrual disturbances, weight gain, bone density loss. Cannot be reversed once given. May delay return to fertility for up to 18 months. No protection against STIs.	One injection every 3 months. Requires prescription.	96–99.8%
Etonogestrel implant	Long-acting progestogen in implant form. Implanted under skin of upper arm. Prevents ovulation and thickens cervical mucus.	Continuous contraceptive coverage. Highly effective. No need for action by user once inserted.	Inflammation or infection at site of implant. Menstrual disturbances. Weight gain. Breast tenderness. Requires procedure for insertion and removal.	Effective for up to 3 years. Requires prescription. Implanted by healthcare provider as minor surgical procedure.	99.95%
Emergency contraceptive pill	Emergency measure after unprotected intercourse. Delays ovulation.	Can prevent unintended pregnancy. Can be used up to 3 days after unprotected sexual intercourse.	Nausea, headache, abdominal pain. Altered bleeding pattern.	Should be taken within 72 hours. May require prescription.	Prevent about 85% of expected pregnancies
Permanent contraceptive methods	Vasectomy for the male. Tubal ligation for the female. Designed to prevent fertilisation.	Highly effective. No systemic effects. No changes to menstrual cycle. No alteration to sexual function.	Irreversible. Slight failure rate. Minor discomfort after surgery.	One-time surgical procedure.	99.5–99.9%

(Family Planning NSW 2020; Family Planning NSW nd; Family Planning NSW et al 2016)

the ring is removed and remains out for 1 week where a withdrawal bleed would be expected. A new ring is inserted after the ring-free week.

Termination of pregnancy

Pregnancy termination can be induced, where the pregnancy is actively terminated, or can be spontaneous, often called a 'miscarriage' (Brown et al 2020).

The reasons for an induced termination may include:

- family history of foetal chromosomal abnormalities where the foetus has been determined to have abnormalities
- foetal death in utero when the foetus does not spontaneously terminate
- unwanted pregnancy where, after assessment and counselling, it is determined to be in the best interests of the woman to terminate the pregnancy.

A termination may be performed either surgically or medically. A medical termination is possible when the woman is less than 7 weeks pregnant (Brown et al 2020). There are clinics in Australia that will perform a medical termination up to 9 weeks gestation; these vary between the states and territories. Performed under the supervision of a doctor, it involves taking two doses of a medication called mifepristone. The second tablet is taken 36–48 hours after the first tablet, with the woman experiencing a miscarriage shortly after. A surgical termination involves the use of a suction curette that removes the lining and contents of the uterus (Brown et al 2020). The procedure can be done as a day procedure at a clinic or hospital. The gestation of surgical termination of pregnancy also varies between states and territories in Australia and it is important for the nurse to be aware of the laws that apply in their location.

DISORDERS OF REPRODUCTION

Infertility

Infertility is defined as the inability of a couple to achieve conception after 1 year of unprotected intercourse, or the inability to carry pregnancies to a live birth. It is estimated that one in six couples suffers infertility, with a number undergoing both surgical and medical treatment and lifestyle changes. In many instances, no cause can be determined.

Male factors

Many factors can affect the production, transport or ejaculation of sperm and the process can be interrupted by a number of causes, many of which have been discussed within this chapter. For example, excessive heat or tight clothing can cause an increase in the temperature of the testes and inhibit sperm production (see Table 37.12). Hormonal dysfunction of the anterior pituitary gland or hypothalamus will affect testicular function. Autoimmune factors may also be implicated. Diseases such as coeliac disease, diabetes mellitus and alcoholism may prevent normal spermatogenesis.

TABLE 37.12 | Known causes of male infertility

Type of problem	Causes
Sperm production problems	• Chromosomal or genetic causes • Undescended testes • Infections, inflammation or injury to the testes • Torsion • Varicocoele • Medicines and chemicals • Radiation damage • Abnormal hormonal function
Blockage of sperm transport	• Infections • Prostate-related problems • Absence of vas deferens • Vasectomy
Sperm antibodies	• Injury or infection in the epididymis
Sexual problems (erection and ejaculation problems)	• Retrograde and premature ejaculation • Failure of ejaculation • Infrequent intercourse • Spinal cord injury • Prostate surgery • Damage to nerves • Some medicines • Erectile dysfunction
Hormonal problems	• Pituitary tumours • Congenital lack of LH/FSH (pituitary problem from birth)

(Adapted from Andrology Australia 2018d)

Female factors

Most female infertility problems are the result of ovulation issues. Stress, diet or rigorous athletic training are lifestyle factors that can affect hormonal balance. Conditions affecting the female reproductive system and which may result in infertility in women have been identified and include structural abnormalities, endometriosis and scarring from PID.

Intersex conditions

The term **intersex** is used to describe a wide range of conditions where an individual's innate sex characteristics do not fit the social and medical norms for male or female bodies. These can create risks for, or experiences of, discrimination, stigma and harm. Sex characteristics are described as physical features that relate to sex and include chromosomes, gonads, hormones, genitals, other reproductive anatomy, and secondary features that emerge from puberty (Intersex Human Rights Australia 2021a). Early and unnecessary deferrable interventions such as genital surgery on infants can result in pain, loss of sexual function and sensation, shame, trauma, urinary incontinence and urgency, experiences of violation and sexual assault, a requirement for ongoing medical treatment or repeat surgeries, reinforcement of incorrect sex assignment, loss of choice and loss of autonomy. There is also research to suggest that early exposures to general anaesthetic is associated with developmental delays (Intersex Human Rights Australia 2021b). For some individuals, an intersex condition may not be diagnosed until they have investigations for infertility.

Assessment of infertility

Assessment of infertility in males is based on the collection of a specimen of ejaculatory fluid. The semen analysis looks at the number and quality of sperm produced, which is normally between 15 million and 200 million per millilitre. It also assesses shape and mobility, which can affect fertility. Because the majority of sperm are situated in the first part of the ejaculate, it is important to educate the individual to collect the first part of the specimen. It is also important to educate them on the importance of not having intercourse or masturbating for 2–5 days before the test. Some laboratories will have their own requirements for this.

The first step in assessing the female is to determine if ovulation is occurring. This may be done by the female herself by testing basal body temperature and by examining cervical mucus, or utilising urine ovulation test kits, though these tests are not conclusive.

Diagnostic tests include:

- blood tests for hormone levels
- ultrasound of ovaries to check for ovulation
- hysterosalpingogram to check patency of uterine tubes
- laparoscopy to check for disease of tubes or ovaries
- endometrial biopsy to check if lining is normal.

Treatment options

Treatment will depend upon the cause and could include the use of medications and surgical procedures.

Assisted reproductive technology

Assisted reproductive technology (ART) is the use of laboratory technology for fertilisation of the ova with a sperm. All reproductive clinics engaging in this technology are required to comply with the National Health and Medical Research Council's (NHMRC) *Ethical Guidelines on the Use of Assisted Reproductive Technology in Clinical Practice and Research* (ART Guidelines) (NHMRC 2017). Many ART methods are very costly, both financially and emotionally. Common methods of ART used in Australia are discussed further.

In vitro fertilisation (IVF) has been available for many years and was originally introduced to assist infertile women to become pregnant. The female partner will have undertaken an intensive regimen of fertility drugs to ensure they produce an increased number of eggs, which will be removed during a simple surgical procedure or 'harvest'. The sperm is collected from a fresh specimen of ejaculate produced through masturbation the day of the female egg harvest. The sperm collected from the male is then mixed with the eggs of a female partner to create embryos, one of which is usually implanted in the woman's uterus in the same cycle unless there are contraindications to this such as high risk for hyperstimulation of the ovaries. Excess embryos may be frozen for future use if a number have been fertilised.

Gamete intrafallopian transfer (GIFT) is similar to IVF but the fertilised ova are placed into a functioning fallopian tube.

In the event that it is the male who is the infertile partner in the relationship, **intracytoplasmic sperm injection (ICSI)** is more commonly used. The procedure involves a single sperm being injected into the egg through the outer covering of the egg (zona pellucida). The sperm can either be collected from ejaculate or be removed from the testes or epididymis. The nurse's role through this process is to ensure that the appropriate support is offered, and that the individual or couple is given adequate information and education relevant to their journey and situation.

SEXUAL ABUSE

Sexual abuse can occur at any age and to anyone, regardless of social or ethnic background. Statistically, young women are the most at risk of sexual abuse, but it can also happen to men. It is the responsibility of the nurse, as it is for any healthcare provider, to be alert to situations where sexual abuse may be occurring. For the nurse, information may be gained from the presence of physical symptoms which would be suggestive of abuse, from discussions during the admission and individual assessment. The abuse may be happening currently or may be part of the individual's history.

An adult who has experienced sexual abuse has the right to choose who they disclose that information to (or whether to disclose it at all) and what supports they would like to access. The nurse should be aware of the situation and offer sensitive and respectful care where appropriate and offer to refer to support services as requested.

There is no standard profile to identify a person who has experienced sexual abuse, but a combination of clinical signs and symptoms and/or a pattern of behaviour or injury can arouse suspicion. It is the role of the nurse to be mindful of cultural practices (e.g. circumcision) and certain disease processes that may result in variations from the usual.

Regarding the sexual abuse of children: Each state and territory in Australia has different legislation for mandatory reporting; however, all states and territories mandate nurses (and other health professionals) to report any sexual abuse of a child, suspected or confirmed (Australian Institute of Family Studies 2020). Nurses must be aware of their mandatory reporting requirements in the state or territory in which they work as well as the legal age definition for children, as this may vary.

SEXUALLY TRANSMITTED INFECTIONS (STIs)

Sexually transmitted infections (STIs) (see Table 37.13) are acquired through close body contact or exchange of body fluids (Family Planning NSW 2020). Despite health-promotion strategies, the individual incidence of STIs is increasing.

Given the prevalence of STIs, routine screening for the following high-risk groups is recommended:

- people with multiple sexual partners
- sexually active people under 20 years of age
- people over 24 years of age with an inconsistent history of barrier contraception, or having a new or more than one sex partner during the past 3 months.

STIs can be transmitted via any sexual contact, which may include vaginal, oral and anal sex, and the shared use of devices such as vibrators. Some STIs can also be

TABLE 37.13 | Common STIs in Australia—causative organisms and routes of transmission

STI and responsible organism	Main route of transmission
Viral infections	
Genital herpes (herpes simplex virus type 2 [HSV-2])	Direct skin-to-skin contact during vaginal, anal or oral sex
Genital warts (human papilloma virus [HPV])	Direct skin-to-skin contact during vaginal, anal or oral sex
Hepatitis B virus (HBV)	Unprotected oral, vaginal or anal sex Sharing sex toys Sharing unsterile needles Piercing or tattoo with unsterilised equipment Contaminated blood or blood products Sharing toothbrushes or razors Pregnant mother to unborn baby
Hepatitis C virus	Piercing or tattoo with unsterilised equipment Sharing toothbrushes or razors Pregnant mother to unborn baby Contaminated blood or blood products Unprotected oral, vaginal or anal sex if any open wounds Sharing sex toys Sharing unsterile needles
Human immunodeficiency virus (HIV)	Unprotected vaginal and anal sex Sharing sex toys Sharing unsterile needles Contaminated blood or blood products Piercing or tattoo with unsterilised equipment Transmitted from infected mother to infant during birth
Bacterial infections	
Chlamydia (*Chlamydia trachomatis*)	Vaginal, anal or oral sex
Gonorrhoea (*Neisseria gonorrhoeae*)	Vaginal, anal or oral sex
Syphilis (*Treponema pallidum*)	Vaginal, anal or oral sex
Fungal infections	
Trichomoniasis (*Trichomonas vaginalis* parasite)	Vaginal, anal or oral sex Sharing towels—parasites can survive for a few hours on damp towels
Parasitic infestations	
Pubic lice ('crabs') (*Phthirus pubis* lice)	Any intimate contact—not necessarily sexual
Scabies (*Sarcoptes scabies* mites)	Any intimate contact—not necessarily sexual

(Family Planning NSW 2020)

transmitted from a mother to her baby during pregnancy or birth. Diseases such as human immunodeficiency virus (HIV) and hepatitis are blood-borne viruses (BBV) present in body fluids and can therefore be transmitted through sex.

Some STIs and BBVs are relatively harmless and easily treated but others can be life-threatening. The symptoms of STIs vary with each type but there are some common signs. Nurses should be aware of the symptoms of STIs and be prompted to explore the sexual history of individuals reporting any of the following:

- itchiness, burning or discomfort in the genital or anal area
- pain or discomfort during urination or sexual activity
- unusual discharge of fluid from the vagina or penis
- blisters, sores, ulcers, warts, lumps or rashes anywhere in the genital or anal area.

(Family Planning NSW 2020)

Some STIs may be asymptomatic or might start with mild symptoms that the individual might ignore until they disappear.

Diagnosis

The medical officer confirms diagnosis of an STI or BBV with swabs and/or blood tests.

Human immunodeficiency virus (HIV)

Human immunodeficiency virus (HIV) is a virus that affects the immune system. The individual may be HIV positive for a number of years without showing symptoms, during which time the virus progressively damages the immune system and is able to be spread to other individuals.

HIV infection may be treated with a combination of antiretroviral drugs to stop the virus from replicating, which decreases the viral load. It is recognised that untreated HIV can develop into acquired immune deficiency syndrome (AIDS) after approximately 10 or more years if left untreated. However, anti-HIV medication can stop HIV from progressing to AIDS (Family Planning NSW 2020).

The individual with HIV can present with a variety of complex needs at any time during their illness, each requiring careful nursing assessment. Sexuality issues include concerns with the effect on relationships, the ability to find an accepting partner, the risk of transmission and the impact on decisions in relation to parenting. The individual with HIV is encouraged to maintain a healthy lifestyle and many find alternative therapies helpful.

Due to the effective use of pre-exposure prophylaxis and post-exposure prophylaxis, the incidence of HIV transmission in Australia is low and continues to decrease. HIV remains a notifiable disease in Australia (Family Planning NSW 2020).

Syphilis

Syphilis is an STI caused by the organism *Treponema pallidum* (Ferri 2020). If diagnosed and treated as a primary infection, syphilis is usually controlled. However, if untreated, it has the potential to become a chronic disease, which can have variable lengths of latency and presentation. Tertiary syphilis can present 2 or more years after initial infection. An exacerbation of the infection during pregnancy can lead to transmission to the infant from the mother.

Diagnosis of syphilis is performed with a swab culture of the lesions and blood test. A course of benzathine penicillin is the treatment of choice, with the need for all sexual partners to be treated (Ferri 2020). It is a notifiable disease.

Chlamydia and gonorrhoea

Chlamydia is caused by the bacterium *Chlamydia trachomatis*. Many people remain asymptomatic, which makes diagnosis and treatment difficult to initiate (Ferri 2020). In males, infection can affect the prostate, urethra and testes, and in females, it can affect the cervix, uterus and pelvis. Diagnosis is based on a urethral swab, a high vaginal swab, cervical swab or a clean catch of urine. Chlamydia infection is not notifiable; however, contact tracing for the past 6 months is recommended. Treatment is with antibiotics.

Gonorrhoea is caused by the bacterium *Neisseria gonorrhoea* and can present similarly to chlamydia; however, it tends to be more symptomatic. The rates in relation to gonorrhoea appear to be stable. Diagnosis is based on the presence of a thick, yellow, urethral discharge and dysuria, which develops within a week of infection and is confirmed with a culture swab of the discharge and/or clean catch of urine. Confirmed cases of gonorrhoea are notifiable (Ferri 2020).

Prevention of sexually transmitted infections

The only certain way to avoid sexually transmitted infections is to not have sex, which is not a realistic health promotion strategy. Instead, nurses can reinforce, promote and educate about safer sex practices. Safe sex (using condoms) reduces the risk of STIs, but the risk is not completely eliminated. This is because any intimate contact may spread some STIs.

Education about safe sex practices includes discussing:

- testing for STIs before engaging in sexual activity with a new partner
- the use of good-quality latex condoms, with knowledge of how to use them safely and effectively
- not having sex when alcohol or drugs are impairing judgment.

Education about the prevention of STIs also includes stressing the need for:

- prompt treatment of any infection
- investigation and treatment of anyone who has had sexual contact with an infected person
- avoiding sexual activity during the infective stage of the disease
- avoiding sexual contact with a person known to be, or suspected of being, infected
- those engaging in sexual activity with multiple sexual partners to have periodic health checks and tests for STIs, regardless of other preventative measures employed
- advising that the full course of any prescribed antibiotics must be taken
- implementing the recommended blood and secretion precautions as effective infection control measures.

(Family Planning NSW 2020)

A knowledgeable and skilled nurse will encourage individuals to discuss STIs, inform about modes of transmission and treatments, and encourage regular STI screening. The education that nurses are often in a position to relay helps disseminate accurate information. This can increase the number of individuals who seek early medical advice, and so reduce the damaging physical and psychological effects of STIs. (See Case Study 37.7 and Nursing Care Plan 37.1.)

CASE STUDY 37.7

James is a 19-year-old male who has come to the sexual health clinic where you work and is extremely anxious. After building rapport with James, he discloses that he had unprotected oral and vaginal sex with a female partner at a party last week. He has since developed dysuria and has a yellow discharge from his penis. He was started on a course of oral penicillin a few days ago from his GP for a sore throat. He tells you his GP suspects Strep A infection and a swab was taken. James has not noticed any improvement to his sore throat since starting the antibiotics. He tells you that he is worried about these new symptoms being an STI and he does not know what to do if it is.

What is the possible reason for James' symptoms? How would you proceed and what would you discuss with James in this appointment?

NURSING CARE PLAN 37.1

Assessment: Alexandra is 17 years old and has presented to the local sexual health clinic. Before Alexandra sees the on-call medical officer, it is your responsibility to perform an initial assessment and examination within your scope of practice. She states that she has developed a burning sensation with urination following unprotected sex with a regular 2 days ago. Alexandra takes the OCP and states that she never misses a pill. She recently completed a course of antibiotics for bronchitis and was very unwell, requiring time off work to recover. Alexandra has not discussed the situation with anyone else and does not want to talk about it. She is worried that she could become pregnant or have caught an STI and if that means her partner has been having sex with other people.

Issue/s to be addressed: Management of Alexandra's symptoms.
Maintaining confidentiality between Alexandra and the healthcare team at the clinic.
Possible diagnoses: Post-coital cystitis, chlamydia, or other STI.
Effectiveness of OCP while unwell and on antibiotics.

Goal/s: Provide education and options for treatment dependent on the diagnosis.
Management of symptoms.
Education regarding OCP use and what may contribute to its effectiveness.
Education about safe sex practices.

Care/actions	Rationale
Obtain a brief health history including; alcohol and substance use, smoking, medications, occupation, and medical conditions. Take a full sexual and reproductive health history including: • Menstruation • Sexual partners • Sexual activity • Any previous STIs • Contraception use Ask Alexandra to collect a urine specimen and perform a pregnancy test. Discuss social situation. Discuss the possibility of pregnancy and what she would like to do in the event that she was pregnant. Perform a physical examination including blood pressure, heart rate, temperature.	Determine if any of Alexandra's health history makes her high risk or flags any concerns for you. Identify any concerns about her sexual and reproductive health status. First step to assess for pregnancy although it may be too early to show a positive result. Determine Alexandra's support system. Provide education— opportunity to offer emergency contraception and discuss potential options if she does become pregnant. Obtain a baseline.

Evaluation: Urine test for pregnancy is negative—advise Alexandra that it may still be too early for a test to show a positive result, so the possibility is not eliminated.
Discuss emergency contraception options and effectiveness at preventing pregnancy.
Reassure Alexandra that she does not need to talk to anyone until her results are returned, and that she can come back to the clinic for support with same.
Refer to MO for vaginal examination and specimen collection for STI screen.
Set up appointment for review in 1 week for further follow-up.

Progress Note 37.1

26/02/2024 1130 hrs	Nursing: Handover received at 0700 hours. Mrs Evans is alert and oriented, GCS 15, day 2 post left-sided radical mastectomy with auxiliary clearance. Vital signs are within normal parameters compared to her baseline. Medications administered as per order. Tolerating full diet and free fluids. IV therapy ceased today due to good oral intake. Dressing remains intact and drain in situ, 35 mL drained into drain since midnight. Sutures to remain in situ until 10 days post-op. Reports 7/10 pain at drain site and describes a pulling sensation. PRN analgaesia given with good effect. Independent with self-care and toileting needs and reports she is passing urine and BO × 1. For review by the treating team this afternoon. Appointments with oncologist and radiologist to be attended as an outpatient. Referred to social work for review regarding discharging home and psychological support. *C Andrews* (ANDREWS), *EN*

DECISION-MAKING FRAMEWORK EXERCISE 37.1

Luke is a 21-year-old male who presents to the accident and emergency department where you are working. He is holding a jumper in front of himself and walks with a gait suggesting he is in considerable pain. Luke appears embarrassed to answer questions in the triage area of the A&E.

You take Luke into a private room and he reveals that he took some of his father's medication the previous night before going out to a local nightclub. He states he has a partial erection that has been present for almost 8 hours. Further discussion reveals that he has tried several approaches to get rid of the erection but has only been successful at slightly reducing the swelling. Luke begs you to relieve his discomfort.

1. Is this considered a medical emergency?
2. Is there a protocol for the management of this situation?
3. What are the risks associated with the procedure?
4. Who needs to perform this procedure (EN/RN/MO)?
5. Is the procedure within your scope of practice?
6. How can you assist Luke?

Summary

The function of the male and female reproductive systems is primarily to reproduce. The female role is to produce ova, receive sperm and, after fertilisation (the fusion of a spermatozoon and an ovum to form one cell), development and birth of the baby. The male role is to produce the sperm that will ultimately fertilise the ova, resulting in an embryo.

Conditions affecting both the male and the female reproductive system can limit the ability to reproduce. Remaining alert to symptoms that may suggest an infection or disease and referral for early investigations will go a long way towards preventing these conditions further limiting the reproductive health of individuals.

A large number of both nationally and state-based health-promotion activities exist to provide a resource for information, support and education, and are making a positive impact on the health of all.

A variety of contraceptive options are available for both men and women. Choices concerning reproduction are influenced by physiological, psychological, social, religious, economic and environmental factors.

Nurses who work in the area of sexual and reproductive health should be aware of cultural and religious beliefs as well as individual sexual practices and preferences. Health professionals are actively involved in promoting reproductive and sexual health in a variety of healthcare settings. Nursing management of the individual with a disorder of the reproductive system requires an acute awareness of the importance of providing psychological support as well as skilled clinical interventions.

Review Questions

1. When conducting an individual assessment, you suspect the male individual has an enlarged prostate. What symptoms would confirm your suspicions?
2. Erectile dysfunction (ED) is a condition that can affect males of any age. List the possible causes of ED.

3. When performing a testicular self-examination (TSE), what should a person look for?
4. An individual is due for discharge after a vasectomy. What education is important for this individual?
5. Torsion of the testes can lead to serious complications if not treated quickly. What complications may occur if torsion of the testes is left untreated?
6. Endometriosis can present with severe menstrual symptoms. How would a diagnosis of endometriosis be confirmed and what is the medical management?
7. Discuss the preoperative care for a woman who is scheduled for a radical hysterectomy.
8. What are your responsibilities if you suspect sexual abuse of a child in your care?
9. The pregnant woman should be monitored for the onset of pre-eclampsia in the third trimester. What are the characteristic signs of possible pre-eclampsia toxaemia?
10. What considerations should you have when performing a genital examination?

Evolve® Answer guide for the Review Questions, Critical Thinking Exercises, Decision-making Framework Exercises and Critical Thinking Questions in Case Studies is hosted on Evolve: http://evolve.elsevier.com/AU/Koutoukidis/Tabbner.

References

Anderson, A., 2023. *Mosby's® textbook for medication assistants*, 2nd ed. Elsevier Inc, St Louis.

Andrology Australia, 2018a. Erectile dysfunction. Fact sheet online. Available at: <https://www.healthymale.org.au/files/resources/erectile_dysfunction_fact_sheet_healthy_male_2019.pdf>.

Andrology Australia, 2018b. Testicular cancer. Fact sheet online. Available at: <https://www.healthymale.org.au/files/resources/testicular_cancer_fact_sheet_healthy_male_2019.pdf>.

Andrology Australia, 2018c. BPH prostate enlargement. Fact sheet online. Available at: <https://www.healthymale.org.au/files/resources/bph_prostate_enlargement_fact_sheet_healthy_male_2019.pdf>.

Andrology Australia, 2018d. Male infertility. Fact sheet online. Available at: <https://www.healthymale.org.au/files/resources/male_infertility_fact_sheet_healthy_male_2019.pdf>.

Armour, M., Ferfolja, T., Curry, C., et al., 2020. The prevalence and educational impact of pelvic and menstrual pain in Australia: A national online survey of 4202 young women aged 13–25 years. Available at: <https://pubmed.ncbi.nlm.nih.gov/32544516>.

Australian Institute of Family Studies, 2020. Mandatory reporting of child abuse and neglect. Available at: <https://aifs.gov.au/sites/default/files/publication-documents/2006_mandatory_reporting_of_child_abuse_and_neglect_0.pdf>.

Australian Institute of Health and Welfare, 2022. National Cervical Screening Program monitoring report. Available at: <https://www.aihw.gov.au/reports/cancer-screening/ncsp-monitoring-2022/summary>.

Better Health Channel, 2019. Prostatectomy—for cancer. Available at: <https://www.betterhealth.vic.gov.au/health/conditionsandtreatments/prostatectomy-for-cancer>.

Better Health Channel, 2021. Prolapsed uterus. Available at: <https://www.betterhealth.vic.gov.au/health/ConditionsAndTreatments/prolapsed-uterus>.

Better Health Channel, 2022. Hysterectomy. Available at: <https://www.betterhealth.vic.gov.au/health/conditionsandtreatments/hysterectomy>.

Blackburn, S.T., 2018. *Maternal, fetal & neonatal physiology*, 5th ed. Elsevier, St Louis.

Brown, D., Edwards, H., Buckley, T., et al., 2020. *Lewis's medical-surgical nursing*, ANZ, 5th ed. Elsevier, Chatswood.

Cancer Council Australia, 2019a. Testicular cancer. Available at: <https://www.cancer.org.au/about-cancer/types-of-cancer/testicular-cancer.html#note_1>.

Cancer Council Australia, 2019b. HPV. Available at: <https://www.cancer.org.au/about-cancer/types-of-cancer/what-is-hpv.html>.

Cancer Council Australia, 2021. Understanding penile cancer. Available at: <https://www.cancercouncil.com.au/wp-content/uploads/2021/03/Understanding-Penile-Cancer-2021.pdf>.

Cancer Council NSW, 2022a. Surgery for prostate cancer. Available at: <https://www.cancercouncil.com.au/prostate-cancer/management-treatment/surgery>.

Cancer Council NSW, 2022b. Breast cancer. Available at: <https://www.cancercouncil.com.au/breast-cancer/>.

Cancer Council Australia, 2023a. Ovarian cancer. Available at: <https://www.cancer.org.au/about-cancer/types-of-cancer/ovarian-cancer.html>.

Cancer Council Australia, 2023b. Cervical cancer. Available at: <https://www.cancer.org.au/about-cancer/types-of-cancer/cervical-cancer.html#jump_3>.

Cancer Council Australia, 2023c. Breast cancer. Available at: <https://www.cancer.org.au/about-cancer/types-of-cancer/breast-cancer/>.

Craft, J.A., Gordon, C.J., Huether, S.E., et al., 2023. *Understanding pathophysiology*, ANZ edition, 4th ed. Elsevier, Chatswood.

Drake, R., Vogl, A.W., Mitchell, A., et al., 2020. *Gray's atlas of anatomy*, 3rd ed. Churchill Livingstone, Philadelphia.

Endometriosis Australia, 2022. What is endometriosis? Available at: <https://www.endometriosisaustralia.org>.

Family Planning NSW, nd. Contraception fact sheets. Available at: <https://www.fpnsw.org.au/health-information/individuals/contraception>.

Family Planning NSW, Family Planning Victoria and True Relationships and Reproductive Health, 2016. *Contraception: An Australian clinical practice handbook*, 4th ed. Family Planning NSW, Ashfield.

Family Planning NSW, 2018. Breast awareness. Available at: <https://www.fpnsw.org.au/factsheets/individuals/breast-health/breast-awareness>.

Family Planning NSW, 2020. *Reproductive and sexual health: An Australian clinical practice handbook*, 4th ed. Family Planning NSW, Ashfield.

Family Planning NSW, 2023. Progestogen-only pill (POP or 'mini-pill') factsheet. Available at: <https://www.fpnsw.org.au/sites/default/files/assets/Factsheet_Progestogen-Only_Mini_2023-04.pdf>.

Ferri, F.F., 2020. *Ferri's clinical advisor 2020*. Elsevier, Philadelphia.

Grimm, J., 2025. Oncologic and hematologic problems. In: Silvestri, A.E., Bowser, A.E., Silvestri, L.A., et al., *Saunders comprehensive review for the NCLEX-PN® examination*, 9th ed. Elsevier Inc, Philadelphia.

Healthy Male, 2020. Erectile dysfunction. Fact sheet online. Available at: <https://www.healthymale.org.au/files/resources/9_erectile_dysfunction_csg_healthy_male_2022.pdf>.

Healthy Male, 2021a. Prostate enlargement (BPH). Available at: <https://www.healthymale.org.au/mens-health/prostate-enlargement-bph>.

Healthy Male, 2021b. Prostate cancer. Available at: <https://www.healthymale.org.au/mens-health/prostate-cancer>.

Healthy Male, 2021c. Testicular cancer. Available at: <https://www.healthymale.org.au/mens-health/testicular-cancer>.

Healthy Male, 2021d. Vasectomy. Available at: <https://www.healthymale.org.au/mens-health/vasectomy>.

Hechtman, L., 2019. *Clinical naturopathic medicine*, 2nd ed. Elsevier, Chatswood.

HPV Vaccine, 2023. The HPV vaccine program. Available at: <http://www.hpvvaccine.org.au/the-hpv-vaccine/has-the-program-been-successful.aspx>.

Intersex Human Rights Australia, 2021a. What is intersex? Available at: <https://ihra.org.au/18106/what-is-intersex>.

Intersex Human Rights Australia, 2021b. Bodily integrity. Available at: <https://ihra.org.au/bodily-integrity>.

IVF Australia, 2023. Menstrual cycle. Available at: <https://www.ivf.com.au/planning-for-pregnancy/female-fertility/female-fertility-factors/menstrual-cycle#phase-1-the-follicular-phase>.

Jean Hailes, 2023a. Endometriosis symptoms and causes. Available at: <https://jeanhailes.org.au/health-a-z/endometriosis/>.

Jean Hailes, 2023b. Polycystic ovarian syndrome. Available at: <http://jeanhailes.org.au/health-a-z/pcos>.

Lab Tests Online, 2022. Human chorionic gonadotropin. Available at: <https://www.labtestsonline.org.au/learning/test-index/hcg>.

McCance, K.L., Heuther, S.E., Brashers, V., et al., 2019. *Pathophysiology: The biological basis for disease in adults and children*, 8th ed. Elsevier, St Louis.

McKenry, L., Tessier, E., Hogan, M.A., 2006. *Mosby's pharmacology in nursing*, 22nd ed. Mosby, St Louis.

Moore, K., Persaud, T., Torchia, M., 2016. *The developing human: Clinically oriented embryology*, 10th ed. Saunders, Philadelphia.

National Health and Medical Research Council (NHMRC), 2017. Ethical guidelines on the use of assisted reproductive technology in clinical practice and research (ART guidelines). Available at: <https://www.nhmrc.gov.au/sites/default/files/documents/reports/use-assisted-reproductive-technology.pdf>.

Osmonov, D., Ragheb, A., Ward, S., et al., 2022. ESSM position statement on surgical treatment of Peyronie's disease. *Sexual Medicine* 10(1), 100459–100459. doi: 10.1016/j.esxm.2021.100459.

Ovarian Cancer Australia, 2023. Know ovarian cancer. Available at: <https://ovariancancer.net.au/about-ovarian-cancer>.

Perry, A., Stockert, P., Hall, A., Ostendorf, W., Potter, P., 2023. *Fundamentals of nursing*, 11th ed. Elsevier, St Louis.

Roen, K., 2023. Hypospadias surgery: Understanding parental emotions, decisions and regrets. *International Journal of Impotence Research* 35, 67–71 [Preprint]. Available at: <https://doi.org/10.1038/s41443-021-00508-6>.

Standring, S., 2021. *Gray's anatomy*, 42nd ed. Elsevier, London.

Stewart, R., Dains, J., Ball, J., Solomon, B., Flynn, J., 2023. *Seidel's guide to physical examination: An interprofessional approach*, 10th ed. Elsevier Inc.

Sweet, V., Foley, A., 2020. *Sheehy's emergency nursing*, 7th ed. Elsevier, St Louis.

The American College of Obstetricians and Gynecologists, 2021. Hysterectomy. Available at: <https://www.acog.org/Patients/FAQs/Hysterectomy?IsMobileSet=false#different>.

Urology Care Foundation, 2022. Testicular torsion. Available at: <https://www.urologyhealth.org/urologic-conditions/testicular-torsion>.

Recommended Reading

Australian Bureau of Statistics, 2019. Crime victimisation, Australia, 2016–17: Sexual assault. Available at: <https://www.abs.gov.au/ausstats/abs@.nsf/Lookup/by%20Subject/4530.0,2016-17,Main%20Features,Sexual%20assault,10004>.

Brant, J.M., 2020. *Core curriculum for oncology nursing*, 6th ed. Elsevier, St Louis.

Chalmers, K.J., Elkins, M.R., 2021. Sex and gender in physiotherapy research. *Journal of Physiotherapy* 67(4), 238–239. Available at: <https://doi.org/10.1016/j.jphys.2021.08.015>.

Goerling, E., Wolfe., E., 2022. Chapter 4 – Sex differentiation, anatomy, and physiology, introduction to human sexuality. Open Oregon Educational Resources, pp. 40–59.

Jiang, L., et al., 2022. Long-term follow-up results of testicular torsion in children. *Asian Journal of Andrology* 24(6), 653. Available at: <https://doi.org/10.4103/aja2021127>.

National Cervical Screening Program, 2020. About the test. Available at: <http://www.cancerscreening.gov.au/internet/screening/publishing.nsf/Content/about-the-new-test>.

Quick, C.R.G., Beirs, S.M., Arulampalam, T.H.A., 2020. *Essential surgery: Problems, diagnosis and management*, 6th ed. Elsevier, Edinburgh.

Sweet, V., 2018. *Emergency nursing core curriculum*, 7th ed. Elsevier, St Louis.

Online Resources

Enough Is Enough: <https://enough.org>.

Family Planning NSW: <https://www.fpnsw.org.au>.

Fertility Society of Australia: <www.fertilitysociety.com.au>.

Healthy Male: <https://www.healthymale.org.au>.

IVF Australia: <www.ivf.com.au>.

Jean Hailes: <https://www.jeanhailes.org.au>.

Ovarian Cancer Australia: <www.ovariancancer.net.au>

Urological Cancer Organisation: <www.uco.org.au>.

UNIT 8

Specialised nursing practice

CHAPTER

38

Palliative care

Laura Healey

Key Terms

advance care plan
care of the dying
death and dying
empathic
end-of-life care
existential
family-centred care
generalist palliative care
health directive
intersectionality
loss and grief
multidisciplinary palliative care
palliation
palliative care
person-centred care
specialist palliative care
symptom management
thanatophobia

Learning Outcomes

At the completion of this chapter and with further reading, learners should be able to:

- Define the key terms commonly encountered when discussing palliative care.
- Outline the philosophy and principles that inform the provision of palliative care to people living with a life-limiting illness.
- Describe a multidisciplinary approach to palliative care and the nurse's role within this approach.
- Identify a range of physical and psychosocial symptoms that may occur in the individual who is dying.
- Identify nursing interventions to address physical and psychosocial symptoms.
- Identify nursing interventions to support family and carers.
- Describe grief and the purpose of grief.
- Identify nursing interventions to support grief responses in the individual and family.
- Identify the challenges and opportunities to integrate palliative care principles into nursing practice and discuss how nurses may be supported in providing palliative care.

CHAPTER FOCUS

Palliative care is a whole person holistic approach to care that focuses on quality of life for people living with a life-limiting condition, who have no cure and provides support for them, their family and carers. The aim of palliative care is to help individuals have quality for the remainder of their life by providing symptom management for physical symptoms such as pain, while encompassing emotional, psychosocial and spiritual care to live well. Multidisciplinary teams are required to provide high-quality palliative care and nurses are important members of the multidisciplinary team. Nurses provide whole person-centred and family-centred care to manage symptoms in conjunction with the multidisciplinary team. Central to quality palliative care is an effective and caring nurse–person relationship that facilitates psychological and spiritual wellbeing.

LIVED EXPERIENCE

At the beginning of my career I struggled with silence and being quiet with a person; it felt uncomfortable, ruminating thoughts within me that I wasn't being helpful or productive. Then I moved into medical oncology and my role encompassed palliative care, palliation and end-of-life care. I quickly realised that silence can be healing and comforting and it can help. I decided that my productivity within a situation was not the priority and I shifted focus to the person and/or their family and carers. I realised that being present for them was sometimes all that was needed.

Anne, Registered Nurse, 47 years old

INTRODUCTION

Death and dying is an integral part of life. However, the concepts of death and dying are uncomfortable for most people. Although death is common in older people, it can occur at any age. Care of people and families experiencing death and dying is central to the nursing role (Lind et al 2022). As a result, nurses require knowledge and skills in palliative care. This includes an awareness and understanding by the nurse of others' attitudes, feelings and beliefs about death and dying. Importantly, nurses require an understanding of their own attitudes and feelings about death and dying and how these might influence the nursing care they provide (Cheluvappa & Selvendran 2022; Lind et al 2022).

Individual experience of death and dying in modern Western societies has been influenced by various social changes and medical advances. Age, culture, religion, past experiences and physical health are all factors that influence how individuals perceive death and dying. Understanding that people and families respond very differently to death and dying is essential to quality nursing care and successful relationship building. People's responses to death and dying have been learnt from their family of origin and from the culture they come from (Berger et al 2021; Givler & Maani-Fogelman 2023). Feelings about death and dying can also reflect the individual and family adjusting to their pending loss. Where possible, the nurse builds a trusting, therapeutic relationship with the individual and their family. When the person and their family trust the nurse, they are more likely to disclose their beliefs and feelings about death and dying. The person and the family are the experts about their feelings and beliefs. Open and empathic listening is essential to quality nursing care (Cheluvappa & Selvendran 2022). The range of feelings people can experience during death and dying include sadness, anger and fear, or relief and acceptance of death as a natural event (Cheluvappa & Selvendran 2022). Some people experience considerable fear about death and dying, (**thanatophobia**). Common fears include:

- fear of pain and isolation while dying
- fear of loss of dignity
- fear of the process of dying
- fear of the unknown, of non-existence
- fear of what happens after death.

(Berger et al 2021; Lind et al 2022)

The individual who is dying, as well as their family, need assistance from nurses through all of their emotions and grief. All individuals experience and process their emotions and feelings in various ways. When dealing with death and dying, there are no 'right' or 'wrong' emotions and no correct order to experience them (Berger et al 2021). Some people will express feelings of acceptance and some people will not. This is demanding on the nurse because the nurse is faced with the challenge of tolerating difficult feelings in the person and in themselves. A nurse needs to accept all feelings as valid and be respectful and **empathic** (Cheluvappa & Selvendran 2022).

A person who is facing their own death may ask the nurse difficult questions such as, 'Am I going to die?' or 'Am I dying?' Many nurses, understandably, will be uncomfortable with these questions. The nurse's response depends on many factors, such as:

- Has the person and/or their significant others been informed of the prognosis?
- Does the person have capacity to understand what is happening? Have the significant others requested that the person's prognosis be withheld from them, and is this a reasonable request?

- Are the nurses caring for the person adequately supported by experienced and specialist nurses, and by the multidisciplinary team? Have they been prepared adequately to deal with such questions?

There are no standard answers to questions that may be asked by people who are dying. If a person asks the nurse such a question, this indicates that they trust the nurse (Cheluvappa & Selvendran 2022). Additionally, it implies that they want to talk about how they feel about dying. Not all nurses will feel able to engage in a conversation about the person's feelings about death and dying. Alternatively, they may prefer to refer the person to an experienced nurse, a palliative care nurse specialist or relevant member of the multidisciplinary team such as a counsellor or psychologist (Berger et al 2021). Additionally, the nurse can prepare themselves to improve their understanding of the issues that surround death and dying, and of relevant counselling approaches. For example:

- reading recommended up-to-date, evidence-based literature, particularly in relation to the individual dying in a healthcare setting
- discussing aspects of death and dying and their own feelings and attitudes with experienced nurses, palliative care nurse specialists and bereavement counsellors
- attending in-services, seminars, courses or other related educational forums to broaden skills and knowledge.

Discussing death and dying is still considered by many people to be morbid or in poor taste, and Western culture tends to deny death. This taboo against death associates death with sentiments and actions that are marked by extreme sadness and fear. Yet, not all civilisations and belief systems have this perspective on death. Understanding how the death taboo affects individuals both consciously and unconsciously and emotionally prevents death from being processed in a healthy way (Johnson 2022). Many people in Western culture view death and dying as a private and personal matter; however, it is interesting to observe that attitudes in modern society are shifting. Grief expression is widely regarded as a natural and healthy reaction. This is demonstrated by real world instances such as people's response when large numbers have died as a result of earthquakes, tsunamis and the COVID-19 pandemic.

PALLIATIVE CARE

Palliative care is defined by the World Health Organization (WHO) (2019) as: 'an approach that improves the quality of life of patients and their families facing the problem associated with life-threatening illness, through the prevention and relief of suffering by means of early identification and impeccable assessment and treatment of pain and other problems, physical, psychosocial and spiritual'. The aim of palliative care is to achieve the best possible quality of life for both the person who is dying and for their family. This includes physical and **existential** symptom relief, encompassing holistic, person-centred and family-centred care (Crips et al 2021). 'Existential' relates to an individual's existence and their search for meaning (Wong & Yu 2021).

Without hastening or delaying death palliative care aims to relieve distress or suffering and provide comfort for the remainder of the individual's life and a 'good death'. Palliative care respects the dignity of the person who is dying and their family (Berger et al 2021; Palliative Care Australia 2022). The main focus is on the individual and the family's needs and wishes in accordance with their cultural and spiritual beliefs. Where possible, care is provided in the individual's preferred setting such as their home or in a hospice. Holistic palliative care is dependent upon multidisciplinary teams including nursing, medical and allied health professionals, and on volunteer services.

In a multicultural society, those who provide palliative care must be aware of, and be sensitive to, the ways that people from other cultures see the concepts of death and dying. The social and cultural context of death, which is crucial for those who are grieving, differs vastly across cultures and healthcare staff need to display appreciation and acknowledgment of individual differences and how these may affect individuals' values, beliefs and attitudes (Hayes et al 2020). Cultural competence is important for all health professionals and volunteers to reduce the risk of stereotyping and to respect other cultures, through behaviours, attitudes and policies that facilitate effective relationships with diverse cultures (ACSQHC 2023; Givler & Maani-Fogelman 2023). For example, holy candles, holy images and rosary beads as well as receiving Sacrament of the Sick by a priest are important for some Roman Catholic people who are dying (Swihart et al 2022).

Palliative care is not an alternative to other care but is complementary to, and a vital part of, holistic patient care. Individuals in palliative care will have an active, progressive and advanced disease with little or no prospect of cure (Crisp et al 2021; Palliative Care Australia 2023a). Preparing for **end-of-life care** includes planning and decision-making that may include respect of the wishes of the individual, the family and the community. This planning is documented in an **advance care plan** or **health directive**. Advance care planning is an ongoing process that can be constantly reviewed within a changing clinical context and is a term used to describe the process whereby a person thinks about their preferences for future medical care should they become unable to communicate. Advance care planning promotes open and ongoing communication between the individual, families and healthcare professionals about end-of-life decisions. They are helpful in providing information for alternative or nominated decision-makers to guide care decisions to improve the end-of-life experiences of individuals and families (Austin Health 2021). (See also Chapter 2.)

In some settings where palliative care is provided by non-specialists, **generalist palliative care** is provided. The term describes the care provided to those with a life-limiting illness, their families and carers by generalist healthcare professionals who may consult with palliative care specialists. Alternatively,

specialist palliative care may be provided for individuals with increased complex needs within a funded service that provides particular palliative care expertise in partnership with generalist health practitioners (e.g. in community-based home care) (Palliative Care Australia 2022). Palliative care may also be provided solely by specialist services (e.g. as occurs in many hospices). Clinical Interest Box 38.1 provides examples of palliative care definitions.

Throughout this chapter, the term 'family' is used to represent all people identified by the person who is dying as being significant to them. Family includes partners, relatives, friends, neighbours and anyone else providing support (Palliative Care Australia 2018b). Palliative care involves grief and bereavement support for the family that extends throughout and beyond the duration of the illness.

Who can receive palliative care?

Palliative care is available to anyone who has a condition that is not treatable by curative measures, irrespective of age, gender, class, culture, race and religion or belief system. Palliative care assists individuals to manage symptoms they experience secondary to their illness such as cancer, motor neurone disease and end-stage kidney or lung disease to enhance their quality of life (Palliative Care Australia 2023a). Palliative care is delivered in almost all settings where healthcare is provided, including neonatal units, paediatric services, acute hospitals, general practices, community settings and residential aged-care services (Australian Institute of Health and Welfare 2022). There are also specialised palliative care services to cater for diverse needs; for example, Aboriginal and Torres Strait Islander Peoples, people from culturally and linguistically diverse backgrounds and LGBTQIA+ people (My Aged Care nd). Clinical Interest Box 38.2 provides examples of people with diverse needs.

CLINICAL INTEREST BOX 38.1 Palliative care definitions

Generalist palliative care: All healthcare providers who provide care to people living with a life-limiting condition, their families and carers should have minimum core competencies in the provision of palliative care and understand the palliative approach to care.

Specialist palliative care: People will have different levels of need for palliative care. People with more complex needs should be able to access care provided by specialist palliative care services comprising multidisciplinary teams with specialised skills, competencies, experience and training in palliative care. Palliative Care Australia (PCA) refers to this type of care that is provided by specialist palliative care services as 'specialist palliative care'. PCA has specified service delivery standards for specialist palliative care.

(Palliative Care Australia 2022)

CLINICAL INTEREST BOX 38.2 Care for people with diverse needs

Diverse populations frequently experience ongoing stress that comes from being marginalised. Individuals may also be members of more than one minority group (**intersectionality**) and as a result may face increased barriers to accessing appropriate palliative care.

The literature suggests that traditions and practices as well as the significance of ceremony and practices at end of life have been lost due to colonisation. To encourage the resurgence of these practices and improve culturally responsive care, palliative care needs to be organised in collaboration with the community and decision-makers. It should be mentioned that there are differences in Australia's cultures, customs and practices. It is important to respect and act sensitively and safely within cultural norms during a person's final hours of life.

Alternative expressions for 'death' and 'dying' should be explored as these may make some people uncomfortable. It is crucial to discuss preferred language and information requests with the significant family members and/or replacement decision-makers. By doing this, pertinent information regarding the symptoms, such as pain, that a person with a terminal illness experiences can be shared, as well as strategies for managing those symptoms. The family or community may express particular preferences, such as the use of conventional medicine, room for several visits at once, respect for kinfolk and space for more than one person to spend the night.

Examples of people with diverse needs include:

- Aboriginal and Torres Strait Islander People
- people living with a mental illness
- people living with addictions or substance abuse disorders
- people living with dementia
- people in aged care
- people with disability
- people experiencing homelessness
- culturally and linguistically diverse communities
- lesbian, gay, bisexual, transgender, queer or questioning and intersex people.

(Based on Palliative Care Australia 2022. National palliative care standards for all health professionals and aged care services)

PERSON- AND FAMILY-CENTRED PALLIATIVE CARE

Quality **person-centred care** and **family-centred care** requires nursing relationships that can negotiate mutually agreed goals of care, are sensitive, demonstrate respect for uniqueness and recognise the effects of the intimate and intense nature of caring for individuals and family in end-of-life care (Palliative Care Australia 2018a). This requires that the multidisciplinary team have excellent interpersonal, communication and intercultural skills, are able to listen empathically and tolerate hearing difficult feelings and attitudes that may or may not match their own beliefs (Ogbogu et al 2022). At times, the nurse will not know what to say or how to respond to the person and this can be normal. It is crucial to be honest and appropriate to share this with the individual and family (Stein-Parbury 2021). Importantly, a quality nurse–individual caring relationship can also provide a foundation for joy, remembering and finding meaning in life for the person and their family. (See Clinical Interest Box 38.3.)

MULTIDISCIPLINARY PALLIATIVE CARE

The provision of high-quality **multidisciplinary palliative care** means that individuals and families have access to support from a coordinated multidisciplinary team (WHO 2019). This includes generalist healthcare professionals and those with specialty training in palliative care, medical officers, nurses, allied health workers, counsellors, chaplains and volunteers.

Individuals and their families are encouraged to actively participate in all aspects of their care including care planning and delivery, which helps them feel in control of the quality-of-life and symptom-management decisions, including the decision about where care will be provided. Palliative care can be provided in the person's own home, a specialist inpatient hospice unit, an aged-care residential unit (see Case Study 38.1), a hospital or other healthcare facility (Chang & Johnson 2022; Crisp et al 2021).

CLINICAL INTEREST BOX 38.3
Person-centred palliative care

- Manages distressing symptoms such as pain
- Affirms life and regards dying as a normal process
- Intends neither to hasten nor postpone death
- Integrates the emotional, psychological and spiritual aspects of care
- Offers a support system to help individuals live as actively as possible until death
- Offers a support system to help the family cope during the individual's illness and in their own bereavement
- Uses a team approach to address the needs of individuals and their families, including bereavement counselling, if indicated
- Will enhance quality of life, and may also positively influence the course of illness
- Is applicable early in the course of illness, in conjunction with other therapies that are intended to prolong life, such as chemotherapy or radiation therapy, and includes those investigations needed to better understand and manage distressing clinical complications

(WHO 2019)

CASE STUDY 38.1

Tamara is a 43-year-old woman with metastatic breast cancer. Her most recent scans show that she has developed new lesions within her brain: metastasis. She has been experiencing headaches, vision disturbance and nausea. She has no history of comorbidities; however, she is the main carer for her mother who has dementia. Tamara is an only child with no current support services in place. Radiation therapy has been organised with palliative intent for symptom management and all other therapy was ceased. Tamara has accepted radiation and then will be followed up with palliative care at home. She is processing her terminal diagnosis and is not comfortable to complete an advance care directive at this point.

1. In what ways can a multidisciplinary palliative care team continue to support Tamara at home?
2. What safety issues do you feel are a nursing priority with Tamara wishing to continue to live at home?

Home-based care

Many people wish to die at home (Department of Health and Aged Care 2022). Community-based generalist nursing services, palliative care services and general practice services provide care in partnership with **palliation** individuals and their families to enable this wish to be fulfilled. When a person prefers to die at home, nurses assist family members in providing care and managing symptoms associated with palliation. The nurse may also be required to counsel and teach. For example, teaching a family member how to sponge the person in bed or how to assist them safely to a commode (Berger et al 2021; Crisp et al 2021).

Palliative care team services provide palliative care nurse specialist and medical specialist care, and offer a wide range of other services and supports (Palliative Care Australia 2018b; CareSearch 2021). These include counselling, bereavement support and pastoral care, occupational therapy, physiotherapy, relaxation and music therapy, dietary advice and loan of equipment. Many of these services and supports are offered at a day centre or in the individual's home. Trained volunteers play an important role in providing various forms of assistance, including respite for family members and bereavement support. Clinical Interest Box 38.4 provides an example of when home-based palliative care can help.

Hospice-based care

A hospice is another setting of care where specially trained healthcare personnel care for people who are dying (Crisp et al 2021). Individuals can be admitted to a hospice for assessment and management of uncontrolled or distressing symptoms and return home or as they enter the last stages of their illness and remain in the hospice until death occurs. Some hospice facilities also provide respite care or admission

CLINICAL INTEREST BOX 38.4
Home-based palliative care

Rob, 75 years old, was referred to outpatient, outreach palliative care as he was going home to die. Rob had been diagnosed with aggressive skin cancer that had spread and that he had refused treatment for and wished to die at home. Rob and his family did not know what to expect from his disease trajectory, but they knew that he needed help with pain management and mobility. Rob currently was only managing to weight-bear for pivot transfers and knew this would not be manageable eventually. Rob was visited at home by the palliative care team including physiotherapy and occupational therapy; after an open and honest discussion, a management plan was created and equipment organised. Rob and his family felt they were now better equipped to manage Rob's care at home with support from palliative care, home care and the GP. Rob did not wish to be admitted to the hospice and he died at home with his family as he and his family had hoped for.

for individuals experiencing emotional distress or anxiety. Respite care provides a break for a carer or family member. Hospices are an alternative to inpatient palliative care units in busy mainstream hospitals. Clinical Interest Box 38.5 provides an example of when hospice-based palliative care can help.

Residential aged care

Senior Australians who can no longer live independently at home may reside within a residential aged-care facility or aged-care home. These facilities provide ongoing support and assistance with everyday tasks or healthcare (My Aged Care nd). Residential aged-care facilities will aim to provide the best quality of life for individuals and for many, the residential aged-care facility is their home. For many residents, the staff in the facility will assist with managing their end-of-life care, which may include managing pain and symptoms, emotional and cultural support, communicating with family about decisions with care, and supporting family and friends (My Aged Care nd). Staff can provide a warm, caring environment for a dying resident in an aged-care facility by providing a softly lit, quiet environment, encouraging family to stay with the individual and staying close to the individual and family.

Staff within the residential care facility can engage with other health professionals as required to help support the individual. Health professionals who may be accessed could include general practitioners; medical specialists; palliative care teams; wound specialists; allied health professionals including physiotherapists; psychologists; therapists skilled in music, massage, aromatherapy or colour; and acute medical and nursing teams if necessary (My Aged Care nd).

Clinical Interest Box 38.6 provides an example of how palliative care may be implemented in an aged-care home.

CLINICAL INTEREST BOX 38.5
Michael's story—in hospice care

I did not think I was going to die at 56 with end-stage lung disease. Living with the slow deterioration, I had accepted that I would never get better but dying wasn't in my immediate future. I had a turn at home and knew then that my family could no longer manage, not just physically but mentally too. I was dying and the process was just too much for us all and we needed help. My family contacted the palliative care team and they organised for an admission to the hospice for respite. We all knew I would not be coming home. The relief for everyone meant my family could visit and spend quality time with me, not as the carers they had been, but my loved ones.

Michael, 56 years old, 2 weeks prior to his death from end-stage lung disease

Acute/hospital-based care

Most palliative care is provided in the person's home in a community setting, but as the illness progresses the individual may require admission to an acute inpatient facility. The reasons for admission may include treatment for an acute medical or surgical condition, symptom control, respite for carers or to die (Department of Health and Aged Care 2022). The Australian Commission on Safety and Quality in Health Care undertook a major work into understanding the complexity of issues and barriers affecting the delivery of safe and good quality end-of-life care in acute facilities. The outcomes found need for several changes to the delivery

CLINICAL INTEREST BOX 38.6
Residential care—an Enrolled Nurse's experience of palliative care

I feel end-of-life care is performed very well where I work; we do have experience. We pride ourselves on providing our residents with individualised care. We are normally fortunate to have had time to get to know them and can fulfil their wishes at this important time. They have a private, safe space that family members are invited to come and stay and spend time where everyone is made comfortable. The staff are very adept at symptom assessment and management and addressing any issues appropriately. This encompasses family members also and communicating with them to address any issues, concerns or queries they may have throughout the process. We also help to console them after their loved one has died, acknowledging their grief. It is a privilege to provide care and support to all involved and be part of this stage of an individual's life.

of end-of-life care in acute facilities. The *National Consensus Statement: Essential Elements for Safe High Quality End of Life Care* (Australian Commission on Safety and Quality in Health Care [ACSQHC] 2015) sets out suggested practice for the provision of end-of-life care in settings where acute care is provided. The Consensus Statement aligns with the National Safety and Quality Health Service Standards, and provides recommended practice.

Individuals, as well as their families and carers, no matter where they reside, their circumstances, how old they are, or who they are, should have access to the optimal palliative and end-of-life care available (NSW Health 2019). Each state and territory have their own framework such as the NSW End of Life and Palliative Care Framework 2019–2024 (the 'Framework') and South Australia's Strategic Framework for Palliative Care 2022–2027 to name a few.

CRITICAL THINKING EXERCISE 38.1

In what ways do you think COVID-19 impacted the experience of individuals who were dying and admitted to hospital? How do you think COVID-19 impacted care provided? How might nurses reflect on these challenges and prepare for any future crisis?

SYMPTOM MANAGEMENT

Palliative care affirms life and regards dying as a normal process. It is aimed at managing and reducing symptom burden. The individual may have symptoms that relate to physical, emotional or spiritual concerns (Delgardo-Guay & Harding 2021). Physical comfort is a priority and essential if palliative care work is to be effective (Lind et al 2022). However, emotional or spiritual concerns can affect physical symptoms. Therefore, a holistic approach is necessary in **symptom management**. Symptom management aims to minimise or eliminate symptoms expressed by an individual to improve symptom control and quality of life (Delgardo-Guay & Harding 2021). Symptom management requires comprehensive multidimensional assessment and, possibly, referral to the relevant member of the multidisciplinary team. Many individuals experience multiple symptoms concurrently. Pain is common; however, not all people experiencing palliation report pain.

Excellent communication and discussion with the multidisciplinary team are essential for effective symptom management. Assessment must always precede intervention to establish the causes of the symptoms wherever possible (Delgardo-Guay & Harding 2021). Cultural factors must be included in symptom assessment in order to tailor it to the needs of the individual and their family. Any concurrent additional disorders developing over the palliation episode of care (e.g. infections) are diagnosed and treated as appropriate. Once treatment is initiated, nurses are involved in reviewing and evaluating the effectiveness of the intervention.

Symptoms other than pain commonly experienced by people who are dying (Berger et al 2021) require physical care, psychosocial and spiritual care (Stein-Parbury 2021). Common physical symptom areas to be included in an assessment are changes in body weight, nausea and vomiting, constipation or diarrhoea, fatigue and dyspnoea (difficulty breathing). (See Nursing Care Plan 38.1.) Psychosocial and spiritual care issues include challenging emotions such as

NURSING CARE PLAN 38.1

Assessment: Todd is a 54-year-old gentleman with metastatic colorectal cancer. He is alert and orientated and currently nil by mouth due to a bowel obstruction. You are caring for Todd this afternoon on your shift on the general medical ward. Todd is holding his stomach and complaining of nausea.
Issue/s to be addressed: Nausea assessment and management.
Goal/s: To provide adequate nausea relief and any additional comfort measures.

Care/actions	Rationale
Perform a comprehensive nausea assessment. Determine acute versus chronic episode. Note any precipitating factors such as sweating, pale, tachycardia. Assess and determine any contributing factors such as pain, NG discomfort. Provide education on asking for assistance sooner rather than later. Ensure vomit bag is close to hand and call bell. Encourage regular oral hygiene and especially after any vomit.	Nausea is multifactorial and attempting to understand contributing factors may assist in treatment. Being able to identify precipitating factors may assist in timely treatment. Provides information on efficacy of current treatment. Provides information to determine need for change of anti-nausea medication for adequate management of symptoms. Allows Todd to maintain a consistently acceptable level of nausea control. When vomiting is anticipated, a vomit bag and call bell should be kept close at hand. The call bell allows for communication/help to be summoned and reduces anxiety. The vomit bag provides a simple way to manage vomitus.

Evaluation: Todd has requested something to help his nausea and until then he needs a vomit bag and his call bell. Post administration of additional anti-nausea medication, Todd felt more comfortable and able to rest for a period.

anxiety, depression, fear, grief and loss (Berger et al 2021). Holistic nursing care focuses on meeting the person's treatment and physical care needs and psychosocial and spiritual needs.

An example of how an entry in progress notes might be documented has been provided on the subject of nausea management (see Progress Note 38.1).

Pain

Pain can be a common but complex symptom within palliative care, particularly in an individual with a cancer illness. The international association for the study of pain revised the definition of pain as 'An unpleasant sensory and emotional experience associated with, or resembling that associated with, actual or potential tissue damage' (ISAP 2020). The definition also comments on pain being a personal experience and an individual's report of pain should be respected as it is influenced by biological, psychological and social factors (Raja et al 2020). Modern pain management means that pain should be controlled or managed throughout the illness (Palliative Care Australia 2023b; Hallenbeck 2022). To provide relief from pain and physical discomfort, holistic nursing assessment should be attended and a variety of nursing interventions considered that should include pharmacological and non-pharmacological approaches (Hallenbeck 2022). General measures to manage pain or discomfort include:

- repositioning
- administering analgesia prior to repositioning for 'incident pain'
- pressure-relieving aids
- hot or cold packs
- treating reversible causes such as urinary retention.

(Queensland Health 2019)

The National Strategic Action Plan for Pain Management (Department of Health and Aged Care 2021) supports the 'bio-social' approach to pain assessment, which acknowledges overlapping physical, psychological and environmental aspects of pain. Pain assessment is a core skill of the palliative care team and identifying the type of pain experienced and the cause will guide the intervention for the most effective response and outcome. This assessment can be very challenging when an individual enters the last days and hours of life. Verbal communication can be limited at this time and non-verbal cues need to be observed (Dala 2021). Clinical Interest Box 38.7 provides aspects for pain assessment.

The fundamental treatment for pain in palliative care is with medication (Palliative Care Australia 2023b). There are a variety of analgesics routinely used singularly or in combination. Analgesic drugs include opioids, such as morphine, and non-opioid analgesics, such as paracetamol and non-steroidal anti-inflammatory medications. Pain relief (analgesics) can be given orally, transdermally, rectally or intravenously and as immediate-release or slow-release formulations (Marie Curie 2022b). Adjunct medicines also referred to as 'coanalgesics' may also be prescribed, and this can be typical practice within palliative care. While not classed as analgesics, some drugs have painkilling qualities due to their individual mechanism of action and areas of the pain pathway that they target, especially when prescribed along with analgesics (Marie Curie 2022b). Corticosteroids, anticonvulsants and antidepressants are examples of adjunct drugs used for pain management (Marie Curie 2022b).

Other pain-relieving medical interventions used in palliative care include surgery, radiotherapy and nerve blocks (injection of anaesthetic agent close to a nerve to cause temporary or permanent blockage in transmission of pain). Specifically in a person with cancer, systemic treatment such as chemotherapy, immunotherapy and/or targeted therapy can be considered where appropriate. The benefits must outweigh the burden of these treatments, particularly when there are unwanted severe side effects. The key to effective pain management is to tailor therapy to the individual's pain burden whilst closely monitoring treatment outcomes. To maintain a favourable balance between efficacy and adverse effects, medicines are titrated, switched to another and adjuncts used where appropriate based on these assessments. Moreover, some opioids might be more appropriate for certain people than others, such as older people or people with cancer who may already have or be at risk for impaired renal or hepatic function. When utilising opioids for palliative care, it is important to monitor hydration and renal function (Dala 2021).

CLINICAL INTEREST BOX 38.7 Assessing pain

Assessing pain in palliative care is multifactorial and a 'total' pain assessment is required to review contributing factors other than the underlying disease process, which could include:

- electrolyte disturbance or metabolic disorders (e.g. dehydration, diabetes mellitus, hypercalcaemia, hypokalaemia, hypothyroidism, uraemia)
- structural issues (e.g. musculoskeletal, bone metastasis, nerve compression, nerve injury)
- symptoms—infection, sepsis, hypoxia, nausea, vomiting, constipation and/or urinary retention
- neuromuscular dysfunction (e.g. autonomic neuropathy or myopathy)
- pain—referred pain from cancer or comorbidities such as joint pain from arthritis
- psychosocial distress affecting sleep, mood, ability to perform activities, not able to fully care for oneself
- environment—in hospital or hospice not in their own home
- non acceptance of impending death
- other factors—financial instability, marital issues, family conflict.

(Based on Sinha, A., Deshwal, H., Vashisht, R., 2023. End-of-life evaluation and management of pain. In: StatPearls [Internet]. Treasure Island (FL): StatPearls Publishing. PMID: 33760512)

Nurses must take extreme care when administering opioid medications and educate individuals and family regarding potential side effects and management strategy to increase compliance. The use of suitable opioid dosages, the co-administration of adjunct analgesics, interventions, and the use of drugs to prevent/manage anticipated adverse effects can all help to limit side effects (Dala 2021).

Allied health professionals can also provide effective pain-relieving interventions. For example, physiotherapy techniques such as transcutaneous electrical nerve stimulation (TENS), ultrasound and laser therapy can be helpful in managing pain (Watson et al 2019). Additionally, non-pharmacological complementary therapies, such as massage, aromatherapy and guided imagery, can be valuable and are often combined with medical and nursing care to enhance the effectiveness of pain-relief measures, to promote relaxation and to reduce anxiety. People interpret their pain according to their life experiences, values and beliefs (Pain Australia 2020). Some people view the expression of pain as a sign of weakness or a sign that their condition is deteriorating. Some people are fearful of opiate drugs such as morphine because they believe they will become addicted or that it will hasten their death. Nurses encourage and carry out medication management, including assisting people in managing their own analgesic drugs through health education. Nurses play a crucial role in counselling, supporting and educating individuals and their families about the advantages and disadvantages, risks and benefits of treatment options to enable informed decisions. (See also Chapter 33.)

Symptoms requiring physical care

Nursing care is fundamental in addressing many symptom areas, as identified in Table 38.1. This includes nursing care of activities of daily living, such as hygiene and mouth care; nursing care of continence difficulties; nursing management of mobility difficulties including positioning; and nursing care to maintain skin integrity including pressure care (Harding et al 2023). Individuals are encouraged to eat small nutritious meals frequently or what they can when they can to maintain their energy requirements. Nurses encourage individuals to maintain hydration by drinking or sipping on

TABLE 38.1 | Symptom management

Symptoms	Identification of issues	Nursing care
Pruritus (itching) Diaphoresis (sweating) Pressure areas	Impaired skin integrity Alteration in sensory perception	Assess skin for breakdown. Pressure area care. Keep skin clean and dry. Reduce friction or shearing forces.
Sore and dry mouth	Impaired oral mucous membrane	Assess oral mucosa for breakdown. Regular mouth care/denture care. Hydration.
Continence difficulties	Urinary incontinence Bowel incontinence	Assess urinary and bowel function. Use absorbent pads for urinary incontinence. Consider use of indwelling urinary catheter with multidisciplinary team. Encourage movement as tolerated. Encourage fibre in diet. Encourage fluids as appropriate. Consider use of aperients with multidisciplinary team.
Changes in body weight (anorexia, weight loss) Cachexia (weight and muscle loss)	Imbalanced nutrition: Less than body requirements	Assess the individual for cachexia and/or anorexia. Provide frequent small meals in accordance with the individual's wishes and cultural preferences. Assess the individual for dysphagia (swallowing difficulty). Consider use of antiemetic therapies with the multidisciplinary team.
Constipation or diarrhoea	Alteration in elimination Constipation Diarrhoea	Assess the individual for constipation. Encourage movement as tolerated. Encourage fibre in diet. Encourage fluids as appropriate. Consider use of aperients with multidisciplinary team. Assess the individual for diarrhoea. Assess possible contributing factors. Refer to multidisciplinary team.

TABLE 38.1 | Symptom management—cont'd

Symptoms	Identification of issues	Nursing care
Nausea and vomiting	Nausea and vomiting	Assess the individual for nausea and vomiting. Assess possible causes of nausea and vomiting. Consider use of antiemetic therapies with the multidisciplinary team. Provide mouth care after the individual has vomited.
Weakness	Fatigue	Assess the individual for fatigue. Encourage frequent rests. Time activities to conserve energy.
Dyspnoea including cough	Ineffective airway clearance	Assess the individual for dyspnoea. Position the individual to facilitate airway and improve chest expansion. Administer oxygen and anticholinergic agents as ordered. Refer to multidisciplinary team.
Insomnia	Alteration in sleep patterns	Assess for insomnia, anxiety and fears. Explore the causes of insomnia with the individual. Consider referral to the multidisciplinary team. Encourage warm drink before bed. Listen to the individual and provide emotional support.
Confusion, restlessness	Alterations in consciousness Delirium	Assess for spiritual distress. Assess for delirium and refer to multidisciplinary team. Do not restrain. Provide a calm and quiet environment. Limit the number of people at the bedside. Assess need for pastoral care to aid in distress.

(Lind et al 2022; National Institute of Aging 2022; Department of Health, Victoria nd)

fluids frequently throughout the day. Nurses should always offer the person food and fluids; however, they should be guided by the person's wishes to partake or refuse.

Constipation and diarrhoea may be experienced by individuals and require thorough assessment to identify an individual's normal function and the symptoms they are experiencing prior to treatment (Therapeutic Guidelines 2022; BMJ Best Practice 2022). A common side effect of opioid medications is constipation; therefore, all individuals prescribed these medications should be prescribed aperient medication concurrently.

To minimise fatigue and weakness, coordinate nursing and other care activities in accordance with the individual's wishes to preserve energy. Encourage frequent rest periods, again coordinated around the individual's desired activities (Harding et al 2023). Nausea and vomiting must be assessed to identify the cause prior to treating these symptoms with antiemetic medications. Dyspnoea is a challenging symptom as it causes anxiety in the affected individual and their family. Medical assessment and diagnosis is warranted prior to treatment (Henson et al 2020). Acute medical interventions such as surgery or medication may be necessary depending on the aetiology of dyspnoea. Conversely, in the terminal phases of the illness when the person is near death, dyspnoea is generally not treated because it is a characteristic of dying.

People who are experiencing a terminal illness commonly report insomnia (Nzwalo et al 2020). Nursing assessment is required to ascertain the causes or factors contributing to the person's insomnia. These factors may be physical, social, spiritual or psychosocial reflecting the holistic nature of the symptom. Management will depend on the person's wishes and may include counselling or medication (Nzwalo et al 2020; Stein-Parbury 2021). Complementary therapies may be effective (e.g. relaxation and meditation).

Confusion and alterations in consciousness can occur. These symptoms are more likely in the terminal phases of the illness when the person is near death (Harding et al 2023). A thorough assessment is required to attempt to ascertain the causes of the alteration in consciousness. Management will depend on the cause and contributing factors. Confusion can be exacerbated by pain, constipation, urinary retention and infections; therefore, these problems should be identified and treated where necessary (Harding et al 2023; BMJ Best Practice 2022). Alterations in consciousness are frightening experiences for individuals and their families and nurses need to be skilled at providing emotional support and reassurance in these circumstances. The nurse or family member should stay physically close to the frightened individual and provide verbal reassurance. Nurses encourage family members to participate in care. Where possible, individuals with alterations in consciousness should be nursed in a quiet and calm environment.

Maintaining comfort depends on continuous reassessment of the individual's needs because physical changes can occur particularly quickly in advanced illness and care decisions should be re-evaluated (Coelho et al 2022). Pain can escalate rapidly and, because of fatigue, immobility, inadequate nutrition or emaciation, pressure ulcers can develop in a very short time. During all phases of care, the nurse's ongoing evaluation and surveillance can assist in anticipating and in some instances avoiding escalation of symptoms. Nurses are very well adept at noting changes in condition, contributing factors and if treatment is working or not (Brown et al 2020).

Psychosocial and spiritual care

During a terminal illness, emotions such as anxiety, depression and fear are frequently experienced by individuals and their families (Stein-Parbury 2021; Brown et al 2020). Grief and loss are also part of the response to death and dying. People express grief and loss differently depending on their family and cultural background, and also depending on personal differences (Cheluvappa & Selvendran 2022; Harding et al 2023).

Anxiety is a subjective feeling of unease and is often accompanied with fear, where the cause or the contributing factors are not immediately apparent (Cheluvappa & Selvendran 2022). People are often more specific about what they fear and commonly report fearing pain, meaninglessness or the unknown. Depression can accompany anxiety (Stein-Parbury 2021). These difficult emotions may have a variety of root causes, such as poorly managed symptoms like pain, personal or family problems, or concern for the wellbeing of surviving family members. The ability of the nurse to listen empathically, to establish a trustworthy and respectful connection, and to allow the individual to express sentiments that cannot always be 'cured' is necessary for providing nursing care in relation to psychosocial symptoms and spiritual care difficulties.

A supportive and caring nurse–individual relationship forms the foundation for psychosocial and spiritual care (Cheluvappa & Selvendran 2022; Stein-Parbury 2021). Nurses talk to the individual and their family about their feelings and provide support (Cheluvappa & Selvendran 2022; Stein-Parbury 2021). Nursing interventions are dependent on the nursing assessment findings and could include referral to a member of the multidisciplinary team, such as a counsellor or bereavement counsellor, education to reduce anxiety, and encouragement and ongoing emotional support. Medication management may also be part of the treatment plan, which includes escalation of medication doses and if and where appropriate de-prescribing. As mentioned previously, adjunct medications may be required for adequate control of symptoms and anti-anxiety medications and antidepressant medications should be considered. In quality palliative care, the individual and family are involved in all treatment decisions (Tarberg et al 2022).

Individuals, families, nurses and other members of the multidisciplinary team are involved in finding meaning in the death and dying experience (Brown et al 2020). This is understood as spirituality and may or may not include religion or faith. Nurses and the multidisciplinary team are respectful of the different values, beliefs, spirituality and religions of individuals and families in palliative care (Brown et al 2020).

The spiritual dimension of each person is unique (Stein-Parbury 2021; Brown et al 2020). Spirituality is not necessarily connected to an individual's religious practices and beliefs; it is more complex and encompasses all aspects. If specific rites and practices are fulfilled, an individual is more likely to feel spiritually complete. However, if they are not, an individual may feel anxious and troubled and experience spiritual pain. Some people do not adhere to any one religion. Nonetheless, their sense of self and the purpose of life are connected to their spirituality. Nurses caring for individuals who are facing death may experience them searching for comprehension of these difficulties (Harding et al 2023).

The spiritual dimensions of the individual who is dying may be reflected in a search for meaning in life, or in their suffering, or in their relationship with others (Stein-Parbury 2021). It may be reflected in a need for hope, love or a sense of forgiveness. Not all people who are dying experience the same needs, nor do they feel them with equal intensity. The nurse with expertise will be sensitive to the spiritual needs of each individual and will implement actions to help those needs to be met (Stein-Parbury 2021). Some people meet spiritual needs through the rituals associated with organised religion; others may find comfort and meaning in relationships, reading, music, art or meditation.

As with any aspect of caring for the individual who is dying, the multidisciplinary team identify how to provide spiritual support together with the individual (Marie Curie 2022a; Stein-Parbury 2021). Religious leaders including chaplains, priests, or pastoral care workers may be important people to involve in the person's care. The nurse often supports the individual in identifying the person they would like to speak to and may arrange a referral.

Hope is an important aspect of psychological and spiritual wellbeing (Crisp et al 2021). Effective communication is vital when nursing people who are experiencing loss of hope. Nurses are often confronted by individuals and families who experience a loss of hope during death and dying (Crisp et al 2021; Marie Curie 2022a). Nursing interventions focus on empathic listening. Additionally, nurses express hopefulness to individuals and families through psychosocial support and reassuring individuals and families that the multidisciplinary team will provide expert management of symptoms (Crisp et al 2021). Nurses also express hopefulness by supporting individuals to participate in their lives to the best of their ability. This includes encouraging individuals to attend and participate in family or social events, encouraging humour where appropriate and discussing everyday issues.

Nurses further express hopefulness by supporting individuals and families to feel empowered (Crisp et al 2021). Nurses facilitate empowerment by encouraging self-care and the participation of family members in care (Palliative Care Australia 2018a). Often, family members want to care for the person during the illness and at the time of death. The nurse supports family members to provide care safely, in accordance with the individual's and family's wishes, by providing education regarding the focus of care (e.g. hygiene or pressure care that has been agreed to by the individual and family) (Berger et al 2021). In the home setting, with support and education from visiting nurses, family members provide the specific care required by their loved one (Crisp et al 2021). Empowering relatives supports their understanding of having contributed to a 'good death' for their loved one. This can be a source of comfort for family during bereavement after the person dies. (See Clinical Interest Box 38.8.)

LOSS AND GRIEF

People invariably experience **loss and grief** in response to death and dying (Crisp et al 2021). Loss happens when someone or something can no longer be seen, heard, known, felt or experienced. Loss can be actual or perceived, temporary or permanent. Feelings of loss and grief can apply to many events. In palliative care, losses are generally related to life itself, relationships, health, lifestyle, independence, freedom and future hopes and dreams (Crisp et al 2021). All losses affect self-identity (Leifer 2022). The value that a person places on a loss has an impact on the meaning that person attributes to the loss. As loss and the accompanying pain cannot be measured, it is impossible to compare one person's loss to another's.

Loss of an aspect of the self can be devastating and can severely affect a person's body image and self-esteem (Crisp et al 2021). Grief is a common reaction to the loss of a body part or loss of a physiological function. However, many people adjust to losses throughout their lives and some people gain confidence after coping successfully with loss.

CLINICAL INTEREST BOX 38.8
A caring nurse–individual relationship facilitates discussing feelings about dying

I recently worked a shift caring for a 42-year-old male receiving palliative care within my unit. He was accepting of his death; however, his main distress was the fact that he would leave behind his husband. They had been together for 12 years and married for 5 years. I wanted to help him and his emotional distress so opened the conversation about what I could do to help. After chatting, it became apparent that his husband and family did not get on and this was his concern: What would happen after he was gone? His husband and family were all visiting this day and he expressed that he was not ready for them all to be together. We decided that I would police his visitors at his request to enable him to spend quality time with them all separately.

Sam, Enrolled Nurse, Hospice

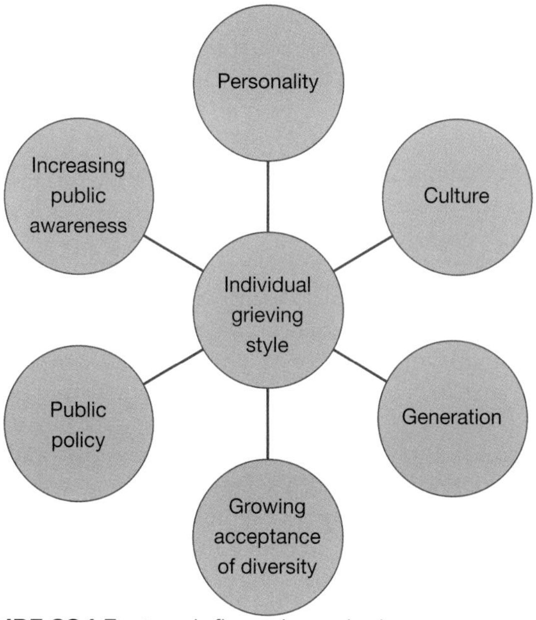

FIGURE 38.1 Factors influencing grieving
(Crisp et al 2021)

Most people experience grief in response to loss. Figure 38.1 illustrates a range of factors that may influence how an individual might grieve. People grieve very differently. Grief can be influenced by a number of factors including:

- Was the deceased's dependency on the bereaved great?
- Were there ongoing disagreements with the deceased that could not be settled?
- Does the person who has lost a loved one have a strong support system?
- What is the meaning of loss to the individual? Have they experienced loss previously?
- Does the bereaved possess effective coping mechanisms? (i.e. their stage of growth and development)
- If they are a young bereaved person, do they need any additional specific intervention?
- Has the bereaved had trouble coming to terms with severe losses in the past?
- Has the person who has lost a loved one ever used drugs, alcohol or had another mental illness?
- Was the deceased a service member or veteran?
- Did the deceased have any cultural and/or spiritual beliefs?
- Are there any socioeconomic status issues affecting the grief process?

(Long 2022)

Grieving is a natural human reaction to loss that is thought to assist an individual cope with the loss. Grief typically entails strong, uncomfortable feelings of loss. Difficult emotions may never completely go away, but they do ease over time. After any great loss, people return to their lives; however, it is likely that they are 'different' (Crisp et al 2021).

A person faced with a serious loss may begin to grieve before the loss actually occurs. For example, older people may experience anticipatory grief as they anticipate the lifestyle changes and losses that old age brings. The process of grieving for a person who is dying is also anticipatory grief. It enables a degree of emotional preparation but, ultimately, the depth of grief is still acute when death eventually does occur (Long 2022). Acute grief is a reaction that begins at the time of a loss (e.g. loss of a person through sudden death or the loss of a limb as the result of an accident).

While people experience grief in different ways, patterns of grieving have been observed and documented (Crisp et al 2021). Theorists often describe grief as a process that involves several stages or phases. The stages are identified according to descriptions of the responses commonly experienced by people as they face a loss. One well-known theory or model of the grieving process is that described in the late 1960s by Dr Elisabeth Kübler-Ross, a psychiatrist and renowned authority on the process of dying, who describes the grieving process as having five stages:

1. denial and isolation
2. anger
3. bargaining
4. depression
5. acceptance.

(Kübler-Ross 1969)

By recognising the stages that a grieving person may experience, nurses are better able to understand what is happening and respond appropriately to that person (Crisp et al 2021). The grieving person may not experience every stage or may experience the stages in a different order. Although grief may be observed to follow a logical sequence, it is not necessarily a linear process. For many people, it is not simply a matter of 'moving on' if and when a previous stage is 'complete'. It is sometimes impossible to differentiate clearly between stages, as a person rarely moves neatly from one to another (Crisp et al 2021). Generally, a person moves back and forth between the feelings of grief until final resolution or acceptance occurs.

The person must be allowed and encouraged to talk and 'work through' their grief (Cheluvappa & Selvendran 2022). The nurse requires a caring, understanding, empathic approach and an ability and willingness to listen. Nurses cannot grieve for the person, lessen the intensity of their feelings or protect or shield people (even children) from the pain of the grief experience (Crisp et al 2021). In caring for a grieving person, the nurse needs to acknowledge the loss, facilitate the expression of thoughts and feelings and support the person as they move through the different feelings of grieving.

Where the person's health is significantly affected by their grieving, the nurse refers them to members of the multidisciplinary team, such as the medical practitioner, bereavement counsellor or psychologist. (See Case Study 38.2.)

CASE STUDY 38.2

John, 70 years old, has heart failure and has agreed to a hospice admission to review his symptoms. John has been in the hospice for over a week and his medications have been optimised; however, he remains very short of breath with limited mobility. Unfortunately, John has been informed that there are no further interventions or medications to be used in his care. John has decided to stay in the hospice and not return home. His family are concerned since they have seen a change in his character and he is angry and his mood has deteriorated. They do not know how to discuss this with John and also do not wish this to be how he dies—angry.

Consider contributing factors to John's anger:

1. Think about how you would begin this conversation with John.
2. Think of other members of the multidisciplinary team who could be consulted to help.

CARE OF THE DYING

Caring of the dying is one of the most demanding tasks nurses face. Nurses frequently care for the dying and are expected to conduct themselves professionally when such circumstances obviously involve intense emotions and a great deal of stress for the nurse (Kostka et al 2021). It can be challenging and stressful, but it can also be immensely rewarding and satisfying. Although a nurse cannot prevent death, there are many things that can be done to make an individual and their loved ones as comfortable as possible in their final days. It is important for the nurse to recognise that a person who is dying is also a living person and that, as long as people who are dying are alive, they have the same needs as anyone else (Berger et al 2021). Because of the dying process, some of those needs assume a greater priority than others. Nurses are very aware of the dying process and provide the individual and family with support and empathy to help the family comprehend and exercise control over their choices and available resources (Leifer 2022). The overall goal of care is the promotion of physical and emotional comfort and spiritual ease. Even during the dying process, the individual should be helped to retain independence. When this is no longer possible, care should be provided in a manner that preserves self-esteem and dignity.

The nurse supports family to maintain a close relationship with the person who is dying right up until the time that death occurs (Berger et al 2021). It is helpful to reinforce that, although the sense of touch may be diminished, the individual may still be able to feel touch and find comfort in this. It is also often helpful to tell family members that hearing may remain intact up until death. If the person who is dying appears to be unaware of their surroundings and not responding, family are advised to speak to them as if they were conscious. It may be comforting for the person who is dying to be able to hear recognised voices or some favourite pieces of music, and relatives may take comfort in providing this solace for their loved one (Berger et al 2021).

CRITICAL THINKING EXERCISE 38.2

You are caring for a 22-year-old woman with metastatic breast cancer who has her 8-month-old daughter and 2-year-old son visiting with her mum. You are similar in age and also have children of similar ages. Reflect on your own beliefs and attitudes and how this affects your thoughts and feelings around this situation. What would change in your life as a result of this prognosis and how would you cope?

Physical care

The dying process is often accompanied by discomfort and nursing problems, including breathing difficulties and alterations in nutrition, hydration, elimination, mobility and sensory perception (Berger et al 2021). Acute or persistent pain may also be experienced by the dying person. The care needs of the person and family are detailed in an advance care directive or health directive; nevertheless, the needs may vary and necessitate reassessment to address common issues and general nursing interventions.

Impaired mobility

When ambulation is no longer possible, maintenance of good body alignment is an essential comfort measure. The individual should be positioned as comfortably as desired, with bedding and pressure-relieving mattresses and devices placed to enhance comfort. Individuals should be gently repositioned every 2–4 hours to promote maximum comfort and prevent muscle soreness, contractures and skin breakdown (Harding et al 2023). Premedication may be required and administered prior to repositioning, turning and performing care. (See Chapter 29.)

Breathing difficulties

The individual may experience shortness of breath and may be unable to cough or expectorate to clear the airway. When possible, the person should be nursed in an upright or semi-upright position to facilitate breathing (Crisp et al 2021). The nurse can also optimise air circulation around the person by using a fan or opening a window. When this is not possible, positioning should be on the side, to prevent aspiration of secretions. Oxygen therapy should not be used routinely for respiratory symptoms in the last days of life since these are usually related to metabolic changes rather than hypoxia. The presence of an oxygen mask and tubing can also be distressing and increase agitation, cause mucosal dryness, irritation and bleeding, and does not necessarily improve feelings of breathlessness (Queensland Health 2019). Suctioning can cause distress and is generally avoided, but oral suctioning may be tolerated and used to remove secretions.

Inadequate nutrition and hydration

If the individual is able to eat and drink, foods and beverages of choice should be provided at the times the individual feels like eating; however, a loss of interest in, and reduced need for food and drink, is a normal part of the dying process. There is minimal evidence that artificial nutrition and hydration are beneficial in the last days of life (Berger 2021; Crisp et al 2021; Queensland Health 2019). Nurses provide regular mouth care to prevent oral complications (Nugent et al 2022). Smaller portions and bland foods may be more palatable if the person is experiencing nausea and vomiting. Death is usually imminent when the individual can no longer eat and drink; therefore, medical interventions, including IV therapy for hydration, are not indicated in palliative care. This can be difficult to accept for families, even when they know the person is dying. It is important to explain that a lack of food and fluid is not responsible for the person's death.

Families may require considerable support and education from nurses when their loved one is no longer able to eat and drink. Uncertainty about the dying person's nutritional requirements is a common and significant cause of distress amongst family/carer(s). Those close to the dying person can be taught how to provide mouth care to help manage any discomfort due to a dry mouth (Queensland Health 2019).

Problems of elimination

Common problems experienced may include constipation, diarrhoea, impacted faeces, retention of urine and incontinence (of urine and faeces) (Williams 2020). Measures that may be implemented to prevent or alleviate these problems include:

- strategically placed protective continence pads, specially designed sheets, or external urinary drainage devices, to prevent discomfort and skin breakdown from urinary incontinence
- maintenance of skin integrity with clean and dry bedding, and removal of soiled sheets and pads in a timely manner
- laxatives to prevent constipation, if fluid or fibre intake cannot be maintained
- rectal suppositories to relieve constipation; careful consideration of risk versus benefit before administration
- a bladder scanner may also be used to diagnose retention in a safe and non-invasive manner
- catheterisation to relieve urine retention or urinary incontinence after obtaining a medical order.

(Queensland Health 2019)

Dry mouth

A clean and moist mouth is extremely important, particularly if the individual is unable to swallow (Berger et al 2021; Williams 2020). Symptoms of a dry mouth do not always indicate dehydration. The most common cause is mouth breathing. Encourage the person to have frequent sips of fluid if possible or provide ice chips (Queensland Health 2019). If the person is unable to manage fluids, use oral hygiene sponges or swabs soaked with water to moisten the person's mouth, tongue and insides of the cheek. Provide lip balm or paraffin for the lips and apply inside the mouth, if needed. Artificial saliva can also be used to relieve symptoms of a dry mouth and prevent associated problems. Avoid using products that exacerbate a dry mouth such as thymol or chlorohexidine (Queensland Health 2019).

Eye problems

Dryness and corneal irritation can occur as a result of decreased blinking reflexes (Berger et al 2021; Williams 2020). Measures to prevent or alleviate eye discomfort include cleansing the eyelids to remove crusts, instillation of artificial tears and instillation of eye lubricant ointment. (See Chapter 34.) Special attention should be given to eye care if the person has indicated a wish to be an eye/corneal donor (Queensland Health 2019).

Skin integrity

If the individual is emaciated and lacks sufficient adipose tissue to support bony prominences, or is unable to move, the risk of developing decubitus ulcers is increased (Berger et al 2021; Williams 2020). The goal of pressure area care during the last days or hours of life is to maintain the person's comfort. To prevent breakdown, the skin should be kept clean and dry, with moisturising lotion applied to counteract any excess dryness. The frequency of repositioning should be determined by skin inspection, assessment and the dying person's individual needs. The use of pressure-relieving aids, cushions, overlays and mattresses can help prevent discomfort and skin problems whilst minimising the need to reposition the person (Berger et al 2021; Queensland Health 2019; Williams 2020). Premedication may be required and administered prior to turning and performing care. (See Chapter 29.)

Altered sensory perceptions

The person who is dying may experience decreasing visual acuity or tactile sensation (Berger et al 2021; Williams 2020). To minimise any anxiety associated with diminished sensory perception, the room should be softly lit, and personal possessions should be placed where they can be easily seen or touched by the individual. Visitors should sit close by and, if the individual's vision is poor, visitors should tell the person who they are. It may be comforting for family to hold their loved one's hand.

The sense of hearing is usually not diminished, so it is important to continue to speak in a conversational tone (Berger et al 2021; Williams 2020). Even if the individual who is dying appears to be unaware of surroundings, all family and personnel should assume that the person is still able to hear. Hearing their favourite piece of music or the voices of their loved ones can provide comfort for some people. For some individuals, relaxation recordings can also be calming. The nurse should attempt to anticipate needs if the patient is unable to talk, and even if there is not a response, individuals should keep trying to communicate and include the dying individual.

Confusion and restlessness

Confusion and restlessness can be caused by physical discomfort such as pain, lack of sleep or retention of urine, or they may be related to medications, such as analgesics, hypnotics and antiemetics (Harding et al 2023). Restlessness may be related to anxiety or fear from a variety of sources. It is important to determine the cause and implement appropriate care. If no cause can be found, or if the individual remains restless and confused, mild sedation may be considered.

In palliative care contexts, death is generally precipitated by failure of one or more of the three major body systems: the central nervous system, the cardiovascular system or the respiratory system (Berger et al 2021; Williams 2020). As a person approaches death, the following physiological changes begin to occur:

- muscle atrophy (loss of muscle tone), which results in relaxation of the facial muscles, difficulty in swallowing, decreased peristalsis, diminished body movement and decreased urine output, with possible incontinence of urine and faeces
- slowing of the circulation, from decreased cardiac contraction, that results in skin mottling, cyanosis of the extremities and cold skin
- changes in vital signs: decreased blood pressure, weaker pulse and changes in breathing. The respirations may become rapid, slow, shallow or irregular. Cheyne–Stokes respiration may occur; this is a cyclical pattern of respirations that gradually become shallower, followed by periods of apnoea (no breathing)
- changes in sensory perception: blurred vision and impaired sense of taste and smell.

(Williams 2020)

Signs of imminent death include loss of reflexes, faster and weaker pulse, noisy breathing due to accumulating secretions in the throat (sometimes called 'the death rattle') and inability to move (Berger et al 2021; Williams 2020). It is important to remember that hearing is usually the last of the senses to fail.

Death occurs when breathing ceases completely and the heart stops (Berger et al 2021; Williams 2020). A central pulse may be palpable for a brief period following cessation of breathing. The pupils become fixed and dilated. This is the time of death.

Family involvement

If appropriate and the death is expected, try to establish with the family if they would like to be present at the time of death and if they wish to be involved in subsequent care. Care after death is discussed in further detail below.

VOLUNTARY ASSISTED DYING

Voluntary assisted dying (VAD), also known as euthanasia, has been practised within Australia since June 2019 in Victoria, followed by Western Australia then Tasmania, Queensland and South Australia in early 2023 and New South Wales in late 2023 (NSW Health 2023).

What does VAD mean for healthcare professionals? An eligible individual may request medical assistance to end their life under voluntary assisted dying. The individual must be suffering from a severe illness, disease or medical condition. They must also be going through tremendous pain and suffering. A person may take or be administered a voluntary assisted dying drug to hasten their death at a time of their choosing if they meet all the requirements and the legal procedures are followed. A qualified physician must write a prescription for the drug.

'Voluntary' implies that the decision must be the subject's own. Only the individual who desires it may request voluntary assisted dying. It is illegal to coerce an individual into requesting voluntary assisted dying. For further information and to keep updated, refer to your state or territory's health department for the latest VAD information relevant to your state or territory. (See also Chapter 2.)

CARE AFTER DEATH

Care after death includes verification and certification of death, notifying and supporting family/carer(s), notifying the coroner (if applicable), care of the deceased and other communication (Queensland Health 2019). A declaration of life extinct or verification of death is the procedure carried out to document the act of establishing death, including recording the time, place and date of assessing when a person has died. Certification of death is a legislated procedure, and a medical practitioner must complete the certificate (Brown et al 2020). The processes that take place after an individual dies are determined by the place and nature of death (expected or unexpected) and other factors such as infectious status or if death occurs following treatment with radioactive substances. Only reportable deaths require referral to the coroner. (See also Chapter 2.) The person's death should also be communicated to other health professionals and providers previously involved in caring for the person (Queensland Health 2019).

Care of the person after death, also referred to as 'last offices' is part of the continuum of care and should be performed with respect and dignity. The protocol for caring for the person after death is often guided by a conversation with the family to determine their wishes, and to observe any cultural and personal requirements and beliefs. If the individual dies within a hospice, hospital or residential aged-care facility, organisational policies and procedures will need to be followed, including completion of all required documentation.

Personal care should be provided after the death has been verified and ideally where possible within 4 hours of the individual dying, to maintain their appearance and condition. Two staff members should be allocated to perform this duty and at least one should be a Registered Nurse or another healthcare worker with the relevant training. Care of the person after death is described in Clinical Skill 38.1.

CARE OF THE BEREAVED

After death has occurred, significant others may experience shock and disbelief, even if the individual's death was anticipated (Crisp et al 2021). Reactions to the death will vary from numbness and immobility, to outbursts of weeping or wailing, or may include expressions of feeling relief or comfort from the fact that their loved one is no longer suffering. The nurse should not discourage bereaved persons from expressing their grief (Cheluvappa & Selvendran 2022). If the nurse is also affected by the death and feels like expressing sadness or crying with the bereaved, this may be appropriate. Alternatively, the nurse may prefer to express their own feelings and grief with a colleague in private.

Family and carer(s) who are present at or after the time of death should be supported according to their individual needs. This includes providing privacy if desired, allowing them to spend time with the person who has died, and support to carry out specific religious or cultural rituals (Queensland Health 2019). Every death and family are different, so discussions with family and carers should be undertaken prior to death to establish how much involvement after death they would like. If the family/significant others were not present at the moment of death, the nurse should ask the family if they wish to view the person. Family members may prefer to view the body later at the funeral directors.

Family/carer(s) may wish to be involved in washing and laying out the deceased. If they wish to be involved in post death care, it is important to sensitively prepare them for changes to the body after death such as rigor mortis (stiffening of the body) and the cooling temperature of the skin. Also discuss any handling and infection control procedures required if they wish to participate in care.

When the family are ready, it is appropriate to direct them to an area where they can sit down and where they can be given the opportunity to discuss their response to the experience (Cheluvappa & Selvendran 2022). If applicable and appropriate, further discussions with the person's family/carer(s) can include corneal and tissue donation and removal of cardiac devices (Queensland Health 2019). Following a death, bereaved family members are required to perform a number of tasks, including gathering the deceased's possessions (if the individual died in a care setting), contacting friends and other family, notifying a funeral director, and planning a funeral or memorial service. The nurse offers assistance in accordance with the family's preferences, including services of social work to support the family if available, and may inform the bereaved about relevant supports available in the community.

SUPPORT FOR THE NURSE

Care of the dying is challenging for nurses (Crisp et al 2021). It can be very satisfying and also demanding, stressful challenging or distressing due to the very personal nature of grief. While this is natural, it is important to acknowledge your concerns and experiences with your colleagues, or contact your employees assistance program (EAP).

Effective self-care strategies are vital to coping with stress and building resilience. A national study of palliative care nurses and doctors in Australia by Mills et al (2018)

CLINICAL SKILL 38.1 Care of the person after death

Please adhere to the policy and procedures of the facility/organisation prior to undertaking the skill. Ensure this skill is in your scope of practice.

NMBA Decision-making Framework considerations (refer to NMBA Decision-making framework for nursing and midwifery 2020): 1. Am I educated? 2. Am I authorised? 3. Am I competent? If you answer 'no' to any of these, do not perform that activity. Seek guidance and support from your teacher/a nurse team leader/clinical facilitator/educator.	**Equipment:** PPE—disposable gloves, disposable apron, protective eyewear Identification labels/tags/name bands Forms—Authority for Removal, Death Certificate, Cremation Certificate (and other forms/checklists as applicable to organisational policy) Washbasin, washcloth, warm water and bath towel Toiletries—mouth care, brush/comb, soap Continence pads Dressings (as applicable) Disposable gown/shroud or clothing according to organisational policy/family/carer(s) wishes Body bag (according to organisational policy) For infectious bodies: Biohazard bags Face mask/shield

PREPARE FOR THE SKILL

(Please refer to the Standard Steps on pp. xviii–xx for related rationales.)
Mentally review the steps of the skill.
Discuss the skill with your instructor/supervisor/team leader, if required.
Confirm correct facility/organisation policy/safe operating procedures.
Validate the order in the individual's record.
Identify indication and rationale for performing the activity.
Assess for any contraindications.
Locate and gather equipment.
Perform hand hygiene.
Ensure therapeutic interaction.
Identify the individual using three individual identifiers.
Gain the individual's consent.
Assess for pain relief.
Prepare the environment.
Provide and maintain privacy.
Assist the individual to assume an appropriate position of comfort.

Skill activity	Rationale
Establish infectious risk.	If the deceased is suspected or has a known infectious disease, then they should be cared for with same precautions as they were in life as this prevents infection and reduces risk of transmission. All staff should be aware of the infectious status of the deceased when organising equipment to prepare the body and when collecting the person for transfer to the mortuary/funeral director. When the deceased has been identified as having/had an infectious disease appropriate care and labelling should be applied (i.e. place an Infectious Disease—Handle with Care label on the outside of the body bag). Remove all disposable PPE and place in biohazard bag and place into a ward clinical waste bin. The mortuary/funeral director is to be notified of infectious status of body at time of collection.

CLINICAL SKILL 38.1 Care of the person after death—cont'd

Review advance care plan/directive for/discuss with family/carer(s) any cultural and/or spiritual/religious rites/preferences that are in line with the deceased's wishes before handling the body. Determine if family/carer(s) wish to be present or help with care of the person.	Respects individuality of person and family/carer(s) and supports their right to having cultural or religious values and beliefs upheld. Provides closure for those who wish to help with body preparation.

PERFORM THE SKILL

(Please refer to the Standard Steps on pp. xviii–xx for related rationales.)
Perform hand hygiene.
Apply PPE: gloves, eyewear, mask and gown as appropriate.
Ensure the individual's safety and comfort throughout use of the skill.
Promote independence and involvement of the individual if possible and/or appropriate.
Assess the individual's tolerance to the skill throughout.
Dispose of used supplies, equipment, waste and sharps appropriately.
Remove PPE and discard or store appropriately.
Perform hand hygiene.

Skill activity	Rationale
Care of the person At time of apparent death: • Lay on back and straighten limbs (if possible). • Place one pillow under the head. • Close the eyes by applying light pressure for 30 seconds. • If the individual had dentures and they were not in the mouth, place them in a labelled denture cup and ensure that they are transported with the person to the mortuary/funeral director. • Cover with appropriate covers.	To maintain the deceased's dignity, ensure the deceased is lying straight prior to rigor mortis which occurs 2–6 hours after death. Supports alignment and helps the mouth stay closed. Closing the eyes maintains dignity, and for tissue protection in case of corneal donation. Helps to retain the shape of the face. To maintain the deceased's privacy and dignity.
Preparation of the person (if not a coroner's case*): • Wash body, unless requested not to do so for spiritual/religious/cultural reasons. • Family/carer(s) may wish to assist with washing. They must be aware of potential infectious risks and, depending on the place of death, wear PPE as instructed. • Clean mouth and teeth or dentures. • Comb and tidy hair. • Use pads to absorb possible leaks from the urethra, vagina or rectum. • Remove tubes such as cannula and catheters. • Cover drain and wound sites with a clean absorbent dressing and secure with an occlusive dressing. • Dress appropriately before they go to the mortuary or funeral directors. This may be in a shroud or personal clothing depending on the place of death, local policy or wishes of the family/carer(s). • Jewellery/belongings—refer to and follow local organisational requirements.	For hygienic and aesthetic reasons. Prevents infection and reduces risk of transmission. The body can continue to excrete fluids after death. To maintain the deceased's dignity and shows respect for the person. To prevent leakage. Invasive devices including cannulas and catheters are removed (except for persons referred to the coroner). Covering/changing dressings controls odours and creates more acceptable appearance. To ensure the deceased's dignity is always preserved.
Identification—refer to and follow local organisational requirements regarding identification labels/tags/name bands.	To meet legal requirements and key contact's wishes and safekeeping of valuables. To ensure correct identification of the deceased.
Offer the family/carer(s) time to be with the deceased as long as they wish prior to transportation to the mortuary/funeral director.	Compassionate care provides family members with meaningful experience during early phase of grief. Ensure privacy and a safe environment.

Continued

CLINICAL SKILL 38.1 Care of the person after death—cont'd

Transfer to mortuary/funeral director organised (as per organisational policy) after completion of: • care of the person or last offices • placement of the person in body bag with label attached to outside of bag • local organisational documentation requirements • verification of death form • medical certificate of cause of death or intention to complete form • cremation certificate (if applicable).	After viewing occurs the person is to be transported to the mortuary/funeral director, in a tag sealed body bag (as applicable to setting/local organisational policy). **Note:** Individuals who are bariatric are transferred to the mortuary on a bariatric bed.

AFTER THE SKILL

(Please refer to the Standard Steps on pp. xviii–xx for related rationales.)
Communicate outcome to the individual, any ongoing care and to report any complications.
Restore the environment.
Report, record and document assessment findings, details of the skill performed and the individual's response.
Report, record and document any abnormalities and/or inability to perform the skill.
Reassess the individual to ensure there are no adverse effects/events from the skill.

**For a Coronial Case, refer to local organisational policy, the MO/RN in Charge for actions to be taken as these will vary to those listed above. (Crisp et al 2021; Hospice UK 2022; Marie Curie 2022c; Perry et al 2022; Queensland Health 2019)*

found that self-care is 'a proactive and holistic approach to promoting personal health and wellbeing to support social and professional roles'. The same study identified that effective self-care involved maintaining a range of personalised self-care strategies within both professional and non-professional contexts and that it is essential to manage barriers and enablers to self-care practice.

Nurses need a network of support to help them cope with these demands. Supports range from personal relaxation activities, support from a professional association like the Australian College of Nursing (ACN), to professional workplace supports such as specialist education and training, critical incident reflection, clinical supervision and counselling (Crisp et al 2021). A debrief session may be beneficial with your line manager and/or other colleagues. If this is not available or does not make you feel comfortable then seek assistance from your general practitioner for a referral to see a counsellor or psychologist. (See Case Study 38.3.) See Chapter 12 for further information on self-care, reflection and debriefing.

CASE STUDY 38.3

Joe, 34 years old, has died from metastatic bowel cancer, 2 days before his 35th birthday. His family want to thank you for all of your care and support during his last days. They comment that you are 'the best' and cared for him better than anyone. Reflect upon this comment and your thoughts in response to this. How will this influence your nursing in the future?

PROGRESS NOTE 38.1

05/02/2024 1545 hrs	Nursing: Care taken over at 1430 hrs and Todd was holding his stomach and complaining of increased nausea. He denies any increased pain; however, comments that if he vomits he gets pain. Reported to RN L Devlin and PRN dose of anti-nausea medication administered. Nausea was reassessed 20 minutes later and had significantly reduced. Todd remains feeling 'seedy' but better. Todd was educated on using his call bell to alert nursing staff if nausea increases and/or if he vomits. Todd has vomit bag as a precaution and his call bell. Discussed with Todd the possible need for a nasogastric tube if his symptoms do not improve since the tube will help reduce the pressure within his stomach that makes him feel nauseated and can increase the risk of vomiting. Further discussion with Todd on oral hygiene to help moisturise oral cavity and keep clean, especially after vomiting. *L Jones* (JONES), *EN*

DECISION-MAKING FRAMEWORK EXERCISE 38.1

You have just commenced working within the medical ward at the Bedford Hospital as an Enrolled Nurse. This is a 30 bed unit that is currently caring for 10 patients awaiting residential aged-care placement, five patients awaiting hospice bed receiving palliative care and 15 medical patients with varying degrees of acuity. The late shift you have arrived for has yourself, a new graduate RN and one casual care worker who holds a Certificate III in aged care. The RN advises you that they will administer the medications, and that you and the casual nurse can attend to the patients' call bells and cares. You discuss this with the nurse unit manager prior to her leaving and she advises you that unfortunately there have been sick calls and they have been unable to fill the roster. This happens routinely and the nightshift have been asked to come in early to assist.

Using the decision-making process address the following:

1. Do you accept this allocation of duties?
2. What (if any) are the issues that could potentially result in you working outside of your scope of practice?
3. Identify the potential and/or actual issues within this scenario.

Summary

Palliative care is a specialty area of nursing. Nurses are valuable members of the multidisciplinary palliative care team and provide care to individuals with a life-limiting illness and their families. Palliative care takes place in many different settings, with many people preferring to die at home. In palliative care contexts, dying is a natural process and people who are dying should be empowered to live life as fully as possible within the limits of their illness. The palliative care team aims to meet physical, psychological and spiritual needs that arise for individuals at the end of their life and to support them and their family. Quality palliative care and symptom management has the person and their family at the centre of care. Nurses are an important part of the multidisciplinary team supporting a 'good death' for individuals in the home and inpatient settings.

Review Questions

1. List three major functions of a multidisciplinary palliative care team.
2. Describe how you could facilitate the care of a palliative patient in the emergency department or acute medical ward.
3. What is an advance care plan and how will this assist a palliative care person as their condition deteriorates?
4. List five non-pharmacological interventions that can be included in the care of a person dying.
5. What factors alert you as the nurse to be aware that an individual is entering the end-of-life phase?
6. Describe five ways you ensure cultural competence in palliative and end-of-life care?

Evolve® Answer guide for the Review Questions, Critical Thinking Exercises, Decision-making Framework Exercises and Critical Thinking Questions in Case Studies is hosted on Evolve: http://evolve.elsevier.com/AU/Koutoukidis/Tabbner.

References

Austin Health, 2021. Advanced Care Planning Australia: Advanced care planning explained. Available at: <https://www.advancecareplanning.org.au/understand-advance-care-planning/advance-care-planning-explained>.

Australian Commission on Safety and Quality in Health Care (ACSQHC), 2015. National Consensus Statement: Essential elements for safe and high-quality end-of-life care. Available at: <https://www.safetyandquality.gov.au/sites/default/files/migrated/National-Consensus-Statement-Essential-Elements-forsafe-high-quality-end-of-life-care.pdf>.

Australian Commission on Safety and Quality in Health Care (ACSQHC), 2023. Action 1.21 Improving cultural competency. Available at: <https://www.safetyandquality.gov.au/standards/national-safety-and-quality-health-service-nsqhs-standards/resources-nsqhs-standards/user-guide-aboriginal-and-torres-strait-islander-health/action-121-improving-cultural-competency>.

Australian Institute of Health and Welfare, 2022. Palliative care services. Available at: <https://www.aihw.gov.au/reports-data/health-welfare-services/palliative-care-services/overview>.

Berger, A.M., O'Neill, J.F., 2021. *Principles and practice of palliative care and supportive oncology*, 5th ed. Lippincott Williams & Wilkins, Philadelphia.

BMJ Best Practice, 2022. Palliative care. Available at: <https://bestpractice.bmj.com/topics/en-us/1020>.

Brown, D., Edwards, H., Buckley, T., et al., 2020. *Lewis's medical-surgical nursing*, ANZ ed, 5th ed. Elsevier, Chatswood.

CareSearch, 2021. Palliative Care in Australia. Available at: <https://caresearch.com.au/tabnid/6456/Default.aspx>.

Chang, E., Johnson, A., 2022. *Living with chronic illness and disability*, 4th ed. Churchill Livingstone Elsevier, Sydney.

Cheluvappa, R., Selvendran, S., 2022. Palliative care nursing in Australia and the role of the Registered Nurse in palliative care. *Nursing Reports* 12(3), 589–596. doi: 10.3390/nursrep12030058. PMID: 35997466; PMCID: PMC9397021.

Coelho, A., Rocha, A., Cardoso, D., et al., 2022. Monitoring and management of the palliative care patient symptoms: A best practice implementation project. *Nursing Reports* 12(2), 365–370. Available at: <https://doi.org/10.3390/nursrep12020035>.

Crisp, J., Douglas, C., Rebeiro, G., et al. (eds.), 2021. *Potter & Perry's fundamentals of nursing*, 6th ed. Elsevier, Chatswood.

Dala, S., 2021. Multidimensional patient assessment. In: Bruera, E., Higginson, J., Von Gunten, C.F., Morita, *Textbook of palliative medicine and supportive care*, 3rd ed. Taylor & Francis.

Delgardo-Guay, O.M., Harding, A., 2021. Multidimensional patient assessment. In: Bruera, E., Higginson, J., Von Gunten, C.F., Morita, *Textbook of palliative medicine and supportive care*, 3rd ed. Taylor & Francis.

Department of Health and Aged Care, 2021. National strategic action plan for pain management. Available at: <https://www.health.gov.au/resources/publications/the-national-strategic-action-plan-for-pain-management>.

Department of Health and Aged Care, 2022. Where is palliative care provided? Available at: <https://www.health.gov.au/topics/palliative-care/about-palliative-care/where-is-palliative-care-provided>.

Department of Health, Victoria, nd. Managing physical symptoms during palliative care. Available at: <https://www2.health.vic.gov.au/hospitals-and-health-services/patient-care/older-people/palliative/palliative-physical>.

Therapeutic Guidelines, 2022. Functional constipation in adults. Available at: <https://tgldcdp.tg.org.au/etgcomplete>.

Givler, A., Maani-Fogelman, P., 2023. The importance of cultural competence in pain and palliative care. In: StatPearls [Internet]. StatPearls. Publishing, Treasure Island (FL). Available at: <https://www.ncbi.nlm.nih.gov/books/NBK493154>.

Hallenbeck, J.L., 2022. *Palliative care perspectives*, 2nd ed. Oxford University Press.

Harding, M., Kwong, J., Hagler, D., 2023. *Lewis's medical-surgical nursing: Assessment and management of clinical problems*, 12th ed. Elsevier Health Sciences, St Louis.

Hayes, B., Fabri, A.M., Coperchini, M., et al., 2020. Health and death literacy and cultural diversity: Insights from hospital-employed interpreters. *BMJ Supportive & Palliative Care* 10(1). Available at: <https://doi.org/10.1136/bmjspcare-2016-001225>.

Hospice UK, 2022. *Care after death*, 4th ed. Available at: <https://www.hospiceuk.org/publications-and-resources/care-after-death>.

Henson, L.A., Maddocks, M., Evans, C., et al., 2020. Palliative care and the management of common distressing symptoms in advanced cancer: Pain, breathlessness, nausea and vomiting, and fatigue. *Journal of Clinical Oncology* 38(9), 905–914. doi: 10.1200/JCO.19.00470. Epub 2020 Feb 5. PMID: 32023162; PMCID: PMC7082153.

International Association for the Study of Pain (ISAP), 2020. IASP announces revised definition of pain. Available at: <https://www.iasp-pain.org/publications/iasp-news/iasp-announces-revised-definition-of-pain>.

Johnson, J., 2022. *Making peace with death and dying*. Monkfish Book Publishing.

Kostka, A.M., Borodzicz, A., Krzemińska, S.A., 2021. Feelings and emotions of nurses related to dying and death of patients – a pilot study. *Psychology Research and Behavior Management* 14, 705–717. doi: 10.2147/PRBM.S311996. PMID: 34113186; PMCID: PMC8187100.

Kübler-Ross, E., 1969. *On death and dying: What the dying have to teach doctors, nurses, clergy, and their own families*. Scribner, New York.

Leifer, G., Fleck, E., 2022. *Growth and development across the lifespan*, 3rd ed. Elsevier, St Louis.

Lind, S., Bengtsson, A., Alvariza, A., Klarare, A., 2022. Registered nurses' experiences of caring for patients in hospitals transitioning from curative to palliative care: A qualitative study. *Nursing & Health Sciences* 24(4), 820–827. Available at: <https://doi.org/10.1111/nhs.12982>.

Long, C., 2022. Care for the dying and those who grieve. In: Fosbre, Chyllia, D., *Varcarolis essentials of psychiatric mental health nursing* – e-Book. Available from ClinicalKey Student (5th edition). Elsevier Limited (UK).

Marie Curie, 2022a. Providing spiritual care. Available at: <https://www.mariecurie.org.uk/professionals/palliative-care-knowledge-zone/individual-needs/spirituality-end-life>.

Marie Curie, 2022b. Pain management in palliative care. Available at: <https://www.mariecurie.org.uk/professionals/palliative-care-knowledge-zone/symptom-control/pain-control>.

Marie Curie, 2022c. Providing care after death. Available at: <https://www.mariecurie.org.uk/professionals/palliative-care-knowledge-zone/final-days/care-after-death>.

Mills, J., Wand, T., Fraser, J.A., 2018. Exploring the meaning and practice of self-care among palliative care nurses and doctors: A qualitative study. *BMC Palliative Care* 17, 63.

My Aged Care, nd. Palliative care. Available at: <https://www.myagedcare.gov.au/support-and-advocacy/end-life-care#palliative>.

National Institute on Aging, 2022. Providing care and comfort at the end of life. Available at: <https://www.nia.nih.gov/health/providing-comfort-end-life>.

NSW Health, 2019. End of life and palliative care framework 2019–2024. NSW Ministry of Health, Sydney. Available at: <https://www.health.nsw.gov.au/palliativecare/pages/eol-pc-framework.aspx>.

NSW Health, 2023. Voluntary assisted dying in NSW. Available at: <https://www.health.nsw.gov.au/voluntary-assisted-dying/Pages/default.aspx>.

Nzwalo, I., Aboim, M.A., Joaquim, N., et al., 2020. Systematic review of the prevalence, predictors, and treatment of insomnia in palliative care. *American Journal of Hospice and Palliative Medicine* 37(11), 957–969. doi: 10.1177/1049909120907021.

Nugent, M.J., Brooke, A., Monks, S., George, N., 2022. Mouth care matters project echo. *BMJ Supportive & Palliative Care*, 12, A19. Available at: <https://doi.org/10.1136/spcare-2021-MCRC.47>.

Nursing and Midwifery Board of Australia (NMBA), 2020. Decision-making framework for nursing and midwifery. Available at: <https://www.nursingmidwiferyboard.gov.au/Codes-Guidelines-Statements/Frameworks.aspx>.

Ogbogu, P.U., Noroski, L.M., Arcoleo, K., et al., 2022. Methods for cross-cultural communication in clinic encounters. *Journal of Allergy and Clinical Immunology* 10(4), 893–900. doi: 10.1016/j.jaip.2022.01.010. Epub 2022 Jan 25. PMID: 35091120; PMCID: PMC8786674.

Pain Australia, 2020. What is pain? Available at: <https://www.painaustralia.org.au/about-pain/pain-australia-what-is-pain>.

Palliative Care Australia, 2018a. National palliative care standards, 5th ed. Available at: <https://palliativecare.org.au/wp-content/uploads/dlm_uploads/2018/11/PalliativeCare-National-Standards-2018_Nov-web.pdf>.

Palliative Care Australia, 2018b. Palliative care service development guidelines. Available at: <https://palliativecare.org.au/wp-content/uploads/dlm_uploads/2018/02/PalliativeCare-Service-Delivery-2018_web2.pdf>.

Palliative Care Australia, 2022. National palliative care standards for all health professionals and aged care services. Available at: <https://palliativecare.org.au/publication/national-palliative-care-standards-for-all-health-professionals-and-aged-care-services>.

Palliative Care Australia, 2023a. What is palliative care. Available at: <https://palliativecare.org.au/resource/what-is-palliative-care>.

Palliative Care Australia, 2023b. Learn more about pain and pain management. Available at: <https://palliativecare.org.au/resource/learn-more-about-pain-and-pain-management>.

Perry, A., Potter, P., Ostendorf, W., Laplante, N., 2022. *Clinical nursing skills and techniques*, 10th ed. Elsevier Inc.

Queensland Health, 2019. Care plan for the dying person: Health professional guidelines. Available at: <https://www.health.qld.gov.au/__data/assets/pdf_file/0023/833315/cpdp-care-plan-hp-guidelines.pdf#:,:text=%E2%80%A2%20Recognition%20that%20the%20person%20is%20in%20the,advocate%20immediately%20after%20death%20is%20dignified%20%26%20respectful>.

Raja, S.N., Carr, D.B., Cohen, M., et al., 2020. The revised International Association for the Study of Pain definition of pain: Concepts, challenges, and compromises. *Pain* 161(9), 1976–1982. doi: 10.1097/j.pain.0000000000001939. PMID: 32694387; PMCID: PMC7680716.

Sinha, A., Deshwal, H., Vashisht, R., 2023. End-of-life evaluation and management of pain. In: StatPearls [Internet]. Treasure Island (FL): StatPearls Publishing. PMID: 33760512.

Stein-Parbury, J., 2021. *Patient and person: Interpersonal skills in nursing*, 7th ed. Elsevier, Sydney.

Swihart, D.L., Yarrarapu, S.N.S., Martin, R.L., 2022. Cultural religious competence in clinical practice. 2022 Nov 14. In: StatPearls [Internet]. Treasure Island (FL): StatPearls Publishing; 2023 Jan–. PMID: 29630268.

Tarberg, A.S., Thronæs, M., Landstad, B.J., et al., 2022. Physicians' perceptions of patient participation and the involvement of family caregivers in the palliative care pathway. *Health Expectations* 25, 1945–1953. doi: 10.1111/hex.13551.

Watson, M., Campbell, R., Vallath, N., Ward, S. and Wells, J. (eds.), 2019. *Oxford handbook of palliative care*. Oxford University Press, USA.

Williams, P.A., 2020. *Fundamental concepts and skills for nursing*, 6th ed. Elsevier Saunders, Philadelphia.

Wong, P.T.P., Yu, T.T.F., 2021. Existential suffering in palliative care: An existential positive psychology perspective. *Medicina (Kaunas)* 57(9), 924. doi: 10.3390/medicina57090924. PMID: 34577847; PMCID: PMC8471755.

World Health Organization (WHO), 2019. WHO definition of palliative care. Available at: < http://www.who.int/cancer/palliative/definition/en>.

Recommended Reading

De Boer, M., Reimer-Kirkham, S., Sawatzky, R., 2022. How nurses' and physicians' emotions, psychosocial factors, and professional roles influence the end-of-life decision making process: An interpretive description study. *Intensive & Critical Care Nursing* 71. Available at: <https://doi.org/10.1016/j.iccn.2022.103249>.

Dickerson, S.S., Khalsa, S.G., McBroom, K., et al., 2022. The meaning of comfort measures only order sets for hospital-based palliative care providers. *International Journal of Qualitative Studies on Health and Well-being* 17(1). Available at: <https://doi.org/10.1080/17482631.2021.2015058>.

Graham, N., Gwyther, L., Tiso, T., et al., 2013. Traditional healers' views of the required processes for a 'good death' among Xhosa patients pre- and post-death. *Journal of Pain & Symptom Management* 46(3), 386–394.

Kissane, D.W., Bultz, B.D., Butow, P.N., et al. (eds.), 2017. *Oxford textbook of communication in oncology and palliative care,* 2nd ed. Oxford University Press, Oxford.

MacLeod, R., Mcleod, S., 2019. *The palliative care handbook: Guidelines for clinical management and symptom control*, 9th ed. Hammond Press, Sydney.

Palliative Care Australia, 2023. The dying process. Available at: <https://palliativecare.org.au/resource/resources-the-dying-process>.

Sallnow, L., Smith, R., Ahmedzai, S.H., et al., 2022. Report of the Lancet Commission on the value of death: Bringing death back into life. *The Lancet* 399(10327), 837–884. Available at: <https://doi.org/10.1016/S0140-6736(21)02314-X>.

Tiziani, A., 2022. *Havard's nursing guide to drugs*, 11th ed. Elsevier, Sydney.

Online Resources

Advance Care Planning: <https://www.advancecareplanning.org.au>.

Australian Commission on Safety and Quality in Health Care: End of life care: <https://www.safetyandquality.gov.au/our-work/end-life-care>.

Cancer Council: <https://www.cancer.org.au>.

CareSearch: Palliative Care Knowledge Network: <https://www.caresearch.com.au>.

Clinical Excellence Commission: Last days of life toolkit: <https://www.cec.health.nsw.gov.au/improve-quality/teamwork-culture-pcc/person-centred-care/end-of-life/last-days-of-life>.

Dying with Dignity NSW: <https://www.dwdnsw.org.au>.

End of Life Essentials: <https://www.endoflifeessentials.com.au>.

National Association for Loss and Grief (NSW) Inc: <https://www.nalag.org.au>.

Palliative Care Aged Care Evidence: <https://www.palliaged.com.au>.

Palliative Care Australia: <https://palliativecare.org.au>.

PCC4U: <http://www.pcc4u.org>.

CHAPTER 39

Mental health and mental illness

Louise Alexander

Key Terms

constructive coping strategies
consumer
deinstitutionalisation
destructive coping mechanisms
mental health
mental health condition
mental illness
metabolic syndrome
myths
protective factors
recovery
recovery principles
resilience
risk factors
self-concept
stigma
stress
theoretical models
trauma informed care
vulnerability factors

Learning Outcomes

At the completion of this chapter and with further reading, learners should be able to:

- Define the key terms.
- Understand the continuum of mental health and mental health conditions.
- Identify factors that influence the development of mental health.
- Reflect on the causes and impacts of stigma on people with mental health conditions.
- Understand the roles of the mental health nurse and the multidisciplinary team.
- Gain an overview of the care issues involved when consumers experience anxiety or depression, or aggressive, self-destructive, elevated or confused behaviour.
- Develop an awareness of some of the basic legal and ethical issues in the field of mental health nursing.

CHAPTER FOCUS

The term 'individual' will be replaced in this chapter with more contemporary and clinically acceptable terms, such as '**consumer**' (Department of Health 2023) or person with a lived experience (Department of Health 2022). Individuals within the **mental health** system are known as mental health consumers or as a 'person with a lived experience of a mental health issue' (Department of Health 2022). The language we use is very important in healthcare, and perhaps even more so in the mental health context since many consumers with a mental health lived experience have been stigmatised and discriminated against.

Mental health nursing is a specialised field of nursing; however, mental health *literacy* is important for all nurses regardless of their specialty area. One in every five Australians (or 20%) will have a mental illness in any 12-month period and the lifetime prevalence for developing a mental health condition between the ages of 16 and 85 is over 44% (Australian Institute of Health & Welfare [AIHW] 2022). For Australia, mental and substance use disorders were estimated to be responsible for 13% of the total burden of disease in 2015, placing it fourth as a broad disease group after cancer (18%), cardiovascular diseases (14%) and musculoskeletal conditions (13%). There has been a significant increase in reported rates of psychological distress nationally since the COVID-19 pandemic (AIHW 2021), resulting in prioritisation of mental health services and funding at a federal government level (Department of Health and Aged Care 2024). Research indicates that individuals with a mental health condition die between 10–32 years earlier when compared with the general population (Royal Australian College of Psychiatrists [RACP] 2022). It is understood that approximately 80% of this premature death is attributed to the poor physical health of people living with a mental illness (RACP 2022). This is significantly affected by socioeconomic status, access to healthcare and long-term side effects (or iatrogenic effects) of psychotropic medications (Roberts 2019). Iatrogenic side effects of psychotropic medications include a serious cluster of conditions known collectively as metabolic syndrome. **Metabolic syndrome** includes increased waist circumference (or abdominal adiposity), hypertension, insulin resistance, hypercholesterolaemia and low levels of high-density lipoproteins (HDL or the good cholesterol) (Goldberg & Ernst 2018). In addition to the obvious consequences of such conditions on individuals, metabolic syndrome also contributes to non-adherence to medical treatment in persons with a lived experience. Individuals with a mental health condition comprise almost half of all people who die in Australia, and they do so at rates over twice that of Australians without a mental health condition. The leading cause of death in Australia is ischaemic heart disease, followed by Alzheimer's disease.

A variety of educational programs are aimed at preparing mental health nurses (MHNs) to work specifically and effectively with consumers who have a mental health condition. Because of the prevalence of mental illness, a nurse who has not undertaken a course specific to mental health nursing is likely to be required to assist in caring for a consumer with a mental illness. The nurse may be required to work in a mental health unit or ward within a general hospital, or to assist in caring for a consumer who has been admitted to a general medical or surgical ward with a physical illness but who has a concurrent mental health problem. It is therefore important that every nurse has a basic understanding of mental health, mental illness and the principles of care related to consumers who are experiencing a disturbance in mental wellbeing. It is not the aim of this chapter to provide the reader with comprehensive knowledge and skills to care for consumers with a mental health condition. Rather, this chapter aims to introduce nurses to the basic concepts of mental health nursing, some of the theoretical frameworks that underpin mental health care and to raise awareness of some legal and ethical issues that confront MHNs. The texts and Online Resources listed at the end of this chapter provide more detailed information.

LIVED EXPERIENCE

Growing up, I'd never really heard of the condition schizophrenia; all I knew about it was that you must be totally crazy to have it! I first started to notice something was off when I was in high school. I had experimented with some drugs, mainly cannabis, but I found that I was down in the time after I used it, and it gave me some weird thoughts.

I stopped going to parties and doing drugs, but things didn't really get back to normal. When I finished Year 12, I worked in a solicitor's office, doing admin duties. Things were better. I made friends and enjoyed the work I was doing. About 12 months into my job, I started having some weird thoughts. I look back on it now and can't believe that I rationalised it, that I thought it was real, but I did. The solicitor I worked for had a lot of meetings and I had to take notes and attend many of them with her. I guess the best way to describe what was happening was that I felt 'watched' and suspicious of people. Her clients used to look at me funny, and I honestly thought that they were trying to set me up. I believed that the reason I was in these meetings was so the rest of the office could plot against me in separate meetings in the room next door. Sometimes I could even hear them.

The friends that I had made were definitely talking about me behind my back, and I started to avoid going out for drinks when them on a Friday night; they were no longer my friends. Often, we would audio-record client meetings and then I would play back the tapes to take minutes and record details. When I would listen back, I started to hear whispers of people discussing me in the background ... saying rude things about me ... telling me to do stuff. It was so

LIVED EXPERIENCE—cont'd

scary, and I believed every word of it. It all came to a head, and I was admitted to hospital about 2 months after I started hearing the voices on the tapes.

I was diagnosed with schizophrenia. It hasn't been easy. The medication makes me tired and fuzzy, and I've put on so much weight, and now I have diabetes. I've been living with schizophrenia now for 15 years. I still hear voices, but I am better at coping with them now, ignoring them. I don't work anymore, but I do some volunteer work with an animal rescue centre and that brings me great purpose in life.

Jill, 36 years old, living with schizophrenia

INTRODUCTION

Perhaps the most important aspect of understanding mental illness is being able to define the difference between mental illness and mental health. This first section aims to help nurses gain an understanding of mental health and mental illness and the factors that impact on both.

WHAT IS MENTAL HEALTH?

The concept of **mental health** is difficult to define since mental health is much more complex than merely the absence of a mental illness; the two are not mutually exclusive (World Health Organization [WHO] 2022). There are numerous definitions of what constitutes mental health. It has been defined as a state in which people are able to fulfil their own potential and manage recurrent stresses of everyday living in an acceptable way (WHO 2022). It has also been defined as the ability of people to cope well with **stress**, develop and maintain meaningful relationships and social connections and to feel valued (Hercelinskyj & Alexander 2022). Mental health is understood to be a holistic state whereby the individual can realise their abilities, cope in the presence of stress, contribute to their community and maintain physical, spiritual and mental wellbeing (Barkway & O'Kane 2020).

The term '**resilience**' refers to our ability to manage day-to-day stress, restore functioning and overcome challenges or difficulties (Barkway & O'Kane 2020). A lack of resilience is highly correlated with negative health outcomes, in particular mental health challenges (Hercelinskyj & Alexander 2022). Being resilient also includes the impacts that a change or adjustment may have on us, and how we overcome adversity. Being resilient does not make you invulnerable to stress, but it enables you to cope better with stressful situations and restore previous functioning by utilising effective coping strategies (Barkway & O'Kane 2020). One of the important factors of resilience is how you manage this adversity; how you respond can have consequences (good and bad) on your wellbeing. As a student, consider your current studies. How quickly do you 'bounce back' from a poor exam or assessment result? How well do you cope with challenges that occur, and what impacts do these have on your ability to function? Resilience is also often themed with protective and risk factors associated with poor mental health (described later). Sometimes people may use maladaptive coping strategies to manage stress, such as taking drugs, self-harm or overeating. Think about how you manage stressful situations: can you identify maladaptive patterns of coping in your behaviours?

For most people, the experience of a mental health condition is non-linear; it is a continuum with ebbs and flows and can vary in intensity and duration. Accordingly, mental health is a state that can change frequently and that can fluctuate depending on specific circumstances. Touhy and Jett (2009) captured the concept of fluctuation in this definition:

Mental health is like a violin with strings of interaction, behaviour, affect (mood) and intellect. All this together may produce a pleasant or stimulating melody, or they may be discordant and irritating. The tune constantly changes. No-one is entirely mentally unhealthy, and no-one is always fully mentally healthy.

The terms 'mental health' and 'mental illness' are often used interchangeably but they should not be; the difference between the two needs to be clear (Foster et al 2020). The American Psychiatric Association (APA) (2022) defines **mental illness** or mental disorder as an illness or a syndrome with psychological or behavioural manifestations and/or impairment in functioning due to a social, psychological, genetic, physical/chemical or biological disturbance. One of the major 'tipping stones' for diagnosis is the impact the condition has for the person living with it. For example, many people claim to have obsessive-compulsive disorder (OCD) because they like order; however, OCD is far more complicated than this and overuse or inappropriate use of terms such as this can trivialise the condition for people who are impacted by it. This point also highlights the difference and complexity between *traits* and *disorder.*

Table 39.1 illustrates some differences between mental health and mental illness.

Development of mental health

The development of mental health conditions is likely a multifactorial interplay between environmental factors and biological characteristics. As Table 39.2 represents, **risk factors** and **protective factors** play a significant role in how an individual will cope with a mental health challenge. According to Foster et al (2020) the factors that influence

TABLE 39.1 | Some differences between mental health and mental illness

Signs of mental health	Possible signs of a mental health condition
Happiness	***Major depressive episode***
Finds life enjoyable. Can see in objects, people and activities the possibilities for meeting their needs. Can manage the day-to-day changes in life successfully.	Anhedonia (loss of interest or pleasure in all or almost all usual activities or pastimes). Dysphoria: Describes mood as low, depressed, sad, hopeless, discouraged, 'down in the dumps'. Weight changes (loss or gain of 5%). Sleep pattern changes (insomnia or hypersomnia). Feelings of hopelessness, excessive guilt or helplessness. Suicidal ideation. Concentration issues.
Moods may fluctuate; however, a happy or elevated mood is not that which consistently interferes with sleep, concentration or how other people may connect.	***Bipolar disorder (manic episode)***
	Experiences persistently elevated, expansive or irritable mood. Decreased need for sleep but remains energetic. Increase in goal-directed activity. Issues maintaining concentration (easily distracted). Talkative. Pressured speech. Grandiosity (inflated self-esteem). May present with psychotic features (hallucinations, delusions, thought disorder).
Control over behaviour	***Control disorder: Under-socialised, aggressive***
Can recognise and act on cues to existing limits. Can respond to rules, routines and customs of the group to which they belong. Has appropriate opportunities for control.	Shows repetitive and persistent pattern of aggressive conduct in which the basic rights of others are violated. Experience of legal difficulties. Avoidance of social situations. Is impulsive. Behaves in socially unacceptable manner.
Appraisal of reality	***Schizophrenia***
Has an accurate picture of what is happening around them. Good sense of the consequences of both good and bad that will follow their acts (judgment). Can see the difference between the 'as if' and the 'for real' in situations.	Delusions. Hallucinations. Thought disorder. Disorganisation in thoughts. Negative symptoms.
Effectiveness in work	***Adjustment disorder with work (or academic inhibition)***
Within limits set by abilities can do well in tasks attempted. When meeting mild failure persists until determines whether they can do the job and adopts healthy coping strategies to manage stress.	Shows inhibition in work or academic functioning whereas previously there was adequate performance. Struggles with imposed limits. May have issues exercising control of behaviour.
Healthy self-concept	***Dependent personality disorder***
Sees self as approaching their individual ideal; as capable of meeting demands. Has a reasonable degree of self-confidence that helps them to be resourceful under stress.	Passively allows others to assume responsibility for major areas of life because of inability to function independently. Lacks self-confidence (e.g. sees self as helpless or stupid). Requires others to make important or trivial decisions for them.

TABLE 39.1 | Some differences between mental health and mental illness—cont'd

Signs of mental health	Possible signs of a mental health condition
Satisfying relationships	***Borderline personality disorder***
Experiences satisfaction and stability in relationships. Socially integrated and can rely on social supports. Manages relationships and behaviours effectively.	Shows patterns of unstable and intense interpersonal relationships. Has chronic feeling of emptiness. Fear of real or imagined abandonment. Impulsiveness. Engages in risk-taking behaviour. Mood fluctuations. Self-harm attempts or suicidal ideation.
Effective coping strategies	***Substance dependence***
Uses stress-reduction strategies that address the problem, issue or threat (e.g. problem-solving, cognitive restructuring). Uses coping strategies in a healthy way that does not cause harm to self or others.	Repeatedly self-administers substances despite significant substance-related problems (loss of employment, family and social networks). Uses substances as a way of coping with daily stress or adverse events.

(APA 2022; Halter 2023; Hercelinksyj & Alexander 2022)

TABLE 39.2 | Risk and protective factors associated with the prevention, exacerbation and development of mental health conditions

Risk factors	↔	Protective factors
Harmful drug and alcohol use	Prenatal environment	Emotional intelligence (and emotional regulation)
Poverty and homelessness	Genetics	Positive relationships with peers and family
Isolation and poor, or few, interpersonal relationships	Self-esteem	Engagement in sport, leisure, religious or community activities
Unemployment (or underemployment)	Temperament	Opportunities to make decisions and take risks
Low levels of education and/or scholastic engagement		Access to and engagement in education
Abuse and neglect (experiences of trauma)		Problem-solving skills
School/community violence		Social and gender equality
Poor physical health/chronic health condition		Financial security and housing security
Minority group (e.g. racial, religious, sexuality etc.)		Workplace satisfaction
Poor conflict resolution skills		Suitable and appropriate role models
Family discord or conflict		Impulse control
Poor coping mechanisms in response to stressful situations (e.g. using violence, illicit substances etc.)		Self-regulatory skills, such as healthy coping mechanisms
Lack of opportunities to exert control over one's life		Access to quality healthcare

(WHO 2022; Hercelinskyj & Alexander 2022)

the development of mental health relate to three main areas: inherited characteristics, nurturing during childhood and life circumstances.

Inherited characteristics

It is believed by some theorists that the ability to maintain a mentally healthy and positive outlook on life is in part connected to a person's genetic makeup, just as inherited flawed genes are thought to predispose particular people to illnesses such as schizophrenia and depression.

Nurturing during childhood

Nurturing during childhood relates primarily to the relationships that develop between children, their parents and their siblings. It is thought that positive relationships, those that promote feelings of being loved, secure and accepted, facilitate the development of children into mature and mentally healthy adults. It is thought that negative relationships may result when children experience maternal deprivation, parental rejection, serious sibling rivalry and early communication failures. Such relationships are more likely to result in a poor sense of self-worth and a lower level of mental health (Hoffnung et al 2022). The quest for a sense of self begins in childhood; children who have positive nurturing experiences are more likely to have a stronger sense of identity than those who have negative nurturing experiences (Hoffnung et al 2022).

Life circumstances

Life experiences can influence mental health from birth onwards. Positive life experiences include pleasurable times and success at school and with friends, a good job, financial security and good physical health. Negative experiences include poverty, poor physical health, abuse, domestic violence or discord, unemployment and unsuccessful personal relationships (CDC 2021). More recently, mental health researchers are understanding the significant role that trauma plays in the development, exacerbation and continuation of adverse mental health experiences. Many serious mental health conditions have trauma as an aetiological factor and understanding this plays an important role in treatment (Hercelinskyj & Alexander 2022). Mental health care now operates under a model called **trauma informed care**. This means we operate under the assumption that most people with a lived experience of a mental illness have a trauma history. Trauma informed care requires that we understand how trauma impacts a person and seek to establish a professional relationship that encompasses safety, trust, choice, collaboration and empowerment (Hercelinskyj & Alexander 2022).

Different people will react to childhood experiences and life circumstances in different ways; this is what makes us unique as human beings. Some, despite negative circumstances, will develop positive strategies for coping and will not develop a mental health condition. Generally, it is people who have not achieved a strong sense of identity who are more prone to mental health challenges, or poorer outcomes with a diagnosis (Polacsek, Boardman & McCann 2022). Perhaps this is most clearly understood when considering the mental health of Aboriginal and Torres Strait Islander populations. It is not difficult to imagine how the effects of colonisation, the removal of children from their families, the loss of traditional lifestyle and cultural practices and the resulting social disruption may impact negatively on mental wellbeing. These experiences can result in what is known as 'transgenerational trauma' and be passed on to future generations. It is generally understood that the difficulties involved in belonging and adjusting to two different cultural contexts can make it difficult to establish a strong sense of identity.

Many disparities exist between Aboriginal and Torres Strait Islander Peoples and non-Aboriginal and Torres Strait Islander People's mental health and the Australian Government has made this a priority area of concern. In Australia, Aboriginal and Torres Strait Islander People experience psychological distress at rates 2.7 times higher than non-Aboriginal and Torres Strait Islander People and suicide is rated the second leading cause of death in Aboriginal and Torres Strait Islander males (AIHW 2018). In fact, suicide rates in Aboriginal and Torres Strait Islander populations in Australia are of particular concern. The rate of suicide deaths in Aboriginal and Torres Strait Islander populations is six times higher than in non-Aboriginal and Torres Strait Islander People, and 90% of Aboriginal and Torres Strait Islander People have been personally touched by suicide (ABS 2018).

Nurses working with Aboriginal and Torres Strait Islander People can better empathise and not negatively judge behavioural signs of a mental health condition if they recognise that it often stems from deep mental anguish and spiritual sorrow relating to the effects of European invasion (Hungerford et al 2020). Given that rates of mental health conditions in Aboriginal and Torres Strait Islander communities are disproportionately higher than in other demographics, mental health care in this population is an important health practitioner consideration (Hercelinskyj & Alexander 2022).

Risk (or vulnerability) and protective factors

Risk or, as they are also known, **vulnerability factors**, are those circumstances that increase a consumer's vulnerability or susceptibility to develop a mental health condition or worsen an existing condition (Hercelinskyj & Alexander 2022). While the presence of these factors does not equate to a certainty of developing a condition, they are a good predictor of a consumer's susceptibility in developing a mental health issue. Given that risk or vulnerability factors may predispose or increase the likelihood a consumer will develop a mental health condition, there are, in contrast, several factors that can aid in the prevention of a mental health condition. Individuals may experience only one risk factor that may significantly impact on their mental health, or they may experience many. For example, homelessness is unlikely to be experienced in isolation from poverty and unemployment. Similarly, financial security is often experienced in addition to secure housing. Table 39.2 outlines the different risk and protective factors associated with the exacerbation (or worsening) and the prevention of mental health challenges.

What is a mental illness?

Not only is it difficult to arrive at a precise definition of mental health, but it is also difficult to succinctly define mental illness because it is often related to what a given society considers is 'normal' or acceptable behaviour and, as with mental health, mental illness is a matter of degree. Despite this, the APA (2022) has defined a mental illness as a condition that results in notable disturbance in cognition, emotional regulation or behaviour that is clinically significant. These disturbances manifest in psychological and behavioural dysfunction that cause the individual distress or impairment in their occupational and social functioning (APA 2022). This dysfunction will often present in **behaviour** that the person exhibits. For example, believing that people are trying to kill them (paranoia) or avoiding certain situations where they may be observed by others (anxiety).

In addition to behaviours exhibited, an individual may experience feelings that are suggestive of mental illness. For example, feeling like they no longer want to live (suicidal ideation) or feeling that they are worthless (depression). It is also important to note that it is normal for people to experience symptoms of mental illness from time to time, but this does not mean they have a mental health issue. For example, anxiety about having to do a class presentation is perfectly normal. Activities with high stakes are often anxiety provoking, but this is not the same as having an anxiety *disorder* because there are several criteria a person must meet over certain time periods to be diagnosed with one. This is why the language we use is so important. As previously stated, people will often say 'Oh, I have OCD!' because they like things tidy or neat, without really considering that it is a clinically significant and distressing condition associated with obsessions and compulsions that are often ritualistic and not simply a desire for order or cleanliness.

What society considers 'normal'

People tend to evaluate the behaviour of others based on their own social, cultural, ethical and behavioural standards. Therefore, behaviour that is regarded by one person as acceptable and 'normal' may be perceived by another person as totally unacceptable. In addition, what is accepted as 'normal' in a society may change over time and what is deemed socially unacceptable in one society may be acceptable in another. For example, homosexuality was previously considered a diagnosable clinical health condition but is now no longer classified as a mental health condition (McGuire 2022). When a person's behaviour is in question, it is appropriate to ask 'Who is qualified to decide whether this behaviour is acceptable or not?' and 'What is the meaning and relevance of this behaviour in relation to the context in which it is occurring and to the person's society, religion and culture?'

In every society and cultural group, there are different interpretations of certain behaviours and events. For example, in Western psychiatric terms, visual or auditory hallucinations (images or sounds that are seen or heard by a consumer but by no-one else) are viewed as abnormal and a sign of mental illness, whereas in some cultures these happenings are viewed as experiences of symbolic and spiritual importance and those experiencing them may be revered as visionaries rather than mentally ill (Kitafuna 2022). As a nurse, it is important to demonstrate respect and cultural competency when working with people from other cultures and religions.

A matter of degree

Anxiety, fear, anger, sadness and the need to be alone are feelings commonly identified in mental health conditions, but they are normal feelings experienced at different levels of intensity by most people at various times. Depending on the intensity of the emotions, people may not feel as mentally healthy as they do at other times but will not necessarily be classified as mentally unwell. It is when the feelings are exaggerated and extend over longer periods of time than deemed normal that the person is likely to seek professional help and be diagnosed as having a mental health condition. For example, a diagnosis of a depressive disorder is likely when sadness or feelings of being 'down in the dumps' become deep, long-lasting feelings of despair that the person cannot escape from without professional help. The ramifications of these negative feelings can impact on the consumer's ability to function at school or work, and in interpersonal relationships. Mental health conditions therefore designate changes from normal mental functioning that are sufficient to become, and be diagnosed as, a clinical disorder. Broadly, a **mental health condition** can be defined as a state in which a consumer exhibits disturbances of emotions, thinking and/or action, but it can be defined in a multitude of ways.

There is no clear line that divides mental health from mental illness, although explicit diagnostic criteria is useful in identifying mental states that deviate from the 'norm'.

Table 39.3 provides some areas of comparison between the two, but it should be noted that while these are general traits that mentally healthy people or people experiencing a mental health challenge tend to share, different types of mental health conditions manifest with different effects and with different levels of intensity. In addition, mentally healthy people may experience more than one type of mental dysfunction at different periods in their lives. You may be able to relate to some of these experiences in Table 39.3. One thing to consider is the permanency of these experiences; however, are they transient, or do they occur frequently? For some consumers, more than one mental health condition may occur concurrently, or over time, or a consumer may develop a substance misuse disorder in addition to a mental health condition (known as dual diagnosis). For example, while depression and anxiety are very different conditions, they often occur together. Similarly, gambling

TABLE 39.3 | Areas of comparison between mental health and mental illness*

Attribute	The mentally healthy person	The person experiencing a mental health challenge
Self-concept	Accepting of self and others. Able to develop talents and potential to fullest extent. Adequately in touch with self and able to use the personal resources identified. Acknowledges personal strengths and limitations.	Poor self-image, low sense of self-worth and unable to recognise talents, so cannot achieve personal potential. Lacks confidence and feels inadequate. Tends not to recognise personal strengths and limitations.
Relationships	Able to form close, meaningful and lasting interpersonal relationships. Can communicate emotions and can give and receive. Can accept authority. Can share with people and grow from the experiences. These factors often mean the presence of a strong social support network that aids coping in times of stress.	Inability to cope with stress can result in disruption, disorganisation, inappropriate responses and unacceptable behaviour that make it difficult to meet the expectations of others in work or social environments. This means that there may be an inability to establish or maintain meaningful relationships. These factors may result in a limited social support network.
Outlook on life	Optimistic and positive view, sense of purpose and satisfaction. Is able to set and achieve realistic goals.	Tends to a pessimistic negative view of present and future, or it may be unrealistic.
Coping and adaptation	Able to tolerate stress and return to normal functioning after stressful events (is resilient). Can cope with feelings such as frustration and aggression without becoming overwhelmed.	Can feel overwhelmed by even minor levels of stress and may react with maladaptive behaviour (such as self-harm or other internalising behaviours). Does not return to previous functioning in the event of a stressful situation (poor resilience).
Judgment/decision-making	Uses sound judgment to make decisions and is able to problem-solve. Can learn the consequences of behaviour and apply it to new situations.	May display poor judgment and avoid problems rather than attempting to solve them. May be unable to apply previous learning to a new situation; lacks understanding of the consequences of actions.
Characteristics/traits	Can delay gratification.	May feel an urgency to have personal wants and needs met immediately and may demand immediate gratification.
Level of functioning	Accepts responsibility for own actions. Can function effectively and independently.	May act irresponsibly, be unable to accept responsibility for own actions and may blame others for outcomes (projecting or externalising behaviours). May exhibit dependency needs because of feeling inadequate.
Perceptions	Able to differentiate between what is imagined and what is real because can test assumptions by considered thought. Can change perceptions considering new information.	May be unable to differentiate reality (e.g. hearing voices or seeing spirits that others cannot).

**It should be noted that these are general points only. Different types of mental health conditions manifest with different effects and while there are traits that mentally healthy people tend to share, many mentally healthy people may experience several areas of dysfunction at different periods in their lives. Mental health conditions may occur as a temporary inability to cope; they may occur episodically with long periods of mental health in-between; or they may occur as a chronic condition that is constantly present.*

(Foster et al 2022; Halter 2023; Hungerford et al 2020; Steele 2023; Hercelinskyj & Alexander 2022)

disorder is also commonly associated with a diagnosis of major depressive disorder.

Signs and symptoms of a mental health condition

Symptoms of a mental health condition occur on a continuum and range from minimal to severe. A person usually receives a diagnosis of having a mental health condition when the level of psychological distress causes them to seek professional help or when others perceive that they need professional psychiatric help. It is important to recognise that in relation to the differences between mental health and mental illness, there is a 'grey' area into which all consumers may enter from time to time. Those with a severe and long-term mental health condition may dip back into relative mental health and reality-based living for a while and, similarly, sometimes the stresses of everyday living are so overwhelming that the well-adjusted 'normal' person may experience marked irrational thoughts, feelings and actions. The concept of recovery is important in this context and is discussed later in this chapter. As in the case of physical illness such as diabetes, heart disease or cancer, anyone can develop a mental health condition. A mental health condition is not the fault of the person affected, and the cause may be related to a combination of biological, psychological and sociocultural factors, or an interplay of all these factors simultaneously. This randomness and unpredictability of mental illness is also supported by how commonly it occurs. One in every five Australians, or 20% of the population, reported a mental health condition in 2021, and the lifetime prevalence of developing a mental illness is 44% (AIHW 2022).

Symptoms of a mental health condition are dependent on the condition itself. For example, the symptoms of schizophrenia are very different to those of depression; however, there is a subtle overlap of symptoms (e.g. negative symptoms of schizophrenia have similarities with major depression). There are over 350 mental health conditions, and each has its own set of symptoms and threshold criteria (APA 2022).

Some common symptoms of a mental health condition may include changes in personal habits, social withdrawal and changes in behaviour, mood and thinking. While particular symptoms occur with specific disorders, there are warning signs that may indicate the presence of a mental health problem. As with cultural differences, genetics and trauma, diverse experiences can also increase mental health risks and vulnerabilities. Clinical Interest Box 39.1 provides an overview of lesbian, gay, bisexual, transgender, queer, questioning and intersex (LGBTQIA+) considerations. Clinical Interest Box 39.2 provides examples of early warning symptoms of mental health conditions that may occur in children, adolescents and adults.

Who is most at risk of developing a mental health condition?

Anyone can develop a mental health condition, but some groups of people in society are particularly at risk.

CLINICAL INTEREST BOX 39.1
LGBTQIA+ considerations

- Individuals who identify as lesbian, gay, bisexual, transgender, intersex, queer or questioning demonstrate concerning and significantly higher rates of mental health conditions than their heterosexual counterparts.
- Considered a minority, LGBTQIA+ individuals have higher rates of suicide, suicide behaviours and self-harm.
- LGBTQIA+ individuals are impacted by discrimination, isolation and social rejection, and these all affect mental health and wellbeing.
- Rates of depression, anxiety and psychological distress are significantly higher in individuals who identify as LGBTQIA+ as are suicidal ideation (thoughts).
- There are specific issues related to the mental health of identifying as LGBTQIA+ and these include the impacts of high rates of suicide in this community, resulting in friends being 'bereaved by suicide', which increases suicide rates further; the impacts associated with 'coming out' and the fear of (or actual) rejection by family and friends and the subsequent impacts on mental health; difficulties in 'belonging' and being true to their gender identity in the face of discrimination; and higher rates of substance use in the LGBTQIA+ community and the effects this has on mental health.

(Hercelinskyj & Alexander 2022; LGBTIQ+ Health Australia 2023)

Clinical Interest Box 39.3 identifies groups of people at greater risk of poorer mental health. It is well established that most mental health diagnoses (75%) occur before the age of 24 years (Mental Health Foundation 2022). This highlights both the importance and impact of mental illness on an individual during their formative years.

Many people from all age groups and of different social, educational and cultural backgrounds cope with highly stressful events and accumulative stressors.

Classification of mental health conditions

There are more than 260 classified forms of mental illness. These include:

- neurocognitive disorders (e.g. dementia, delirium)
- substance-related and addictive disorders (e.g. alcohol abuse or dependence, drug abuse or dependence)
- anxiety disorders (e.g. phobias, panic disorder)
- obsessive-compulsive and related disorders
- schizophrenia spectrum and other psychotic disorders (e.g. schizophrenia, schizophreniform disorder)
- trauma and stressor-related disorders (e.g. post-traumatic stress disorder (PTSD)

CLINICAL INTEREST BOX 39.2 Warning signs and symptoms of a possible mental health condition

People may have one or two of these or other symptoms at any one time. This does not necessarily mean there is cause for alarm, but it is advisable they see their GP. A combination of multiple symptoms is a strong signal that professional assessment and help should be sought as soon as possible.

In younger children:

- Decline in standard of performance in schoolwork or activities that does not pick up again over time.
- The child is not managing or coping with tasks as expected at their developmental age (or they regress).
- Suggestions from teachers that there may be a learning difficulty, a behavioural problem or a problem making friends (issues with social skills).
- Bullying.
- Hyperactivity.
- Persistent crying, waking at night or nightmares.
- Persistent disobedience or aggression.
- Frequent temper tantrums.
- Excessive anxiety (e.g. preoccupation with fears of burglars, barking dogs or parents getting killed).
- Constant fighting with other children, and reports from school of the child being 'angry or disruptive'.
- Refusal to go to school.
- Refusal to go to bed, inability to sleep or a need to sleep with, or close to, parents.
- Decreased interest in playing.
- The child tries to stimulate themself in various ways (e.g. hair pulling, rocking of the body, head banging).
- The child constantly says things that indicate low self-esteem (e.g. 'I'm stupid', 'I never do anything right', 'No-one likes me', 'I'm too skinny', or too fat, too tall, too ugly, etc.).
- The child is preoccupied with fire (or sets fires).
- The child is physically aggressive to people or animals.
- Regression of toilet training.

In older children and adolescents:

- School refusal, skipping school, changes in performance.
- Frequently asks or hints at the need for help.
- Fears or phobias that interfere with normal activities.
- Substance misuse.
- Change in sleeping/eating/hygiene habits.
- Isolating self from others excessively.
- Exhibits violence to others or bullies others.
- Inability to cope with problems (poor resilience) and usual daily activities.
- Excessive complaints about physical aches and pains.
- Emergence of bizarre or unusual behaviour or thoughts.
- Defiance of authority, truancy, theft and/or acts of vandalism.
- Intense fear of weight gain, frequent exercising, weight loss and dieting behaviours.
- Frequent outbursts of anger.
- Demonstrates ritualistic behaviours (e.g. preparing for bed, a meal or going out) using routines that are exact, precise and never vary.
- Provocatively sexual behaviour that is not appropriate.
- Participates in mutilating or killing animals.
- Persistent and prolonged low mood (a major concern, especially if accompanied by poor appetite or thoughts and talk of death or signs of self-harm).

In adults:

- Confused thought processes.
- Prolonged periods of sadness/low mood and apathy or prolonged periods of excessive happiness.
- Feelings of extreme highs and lows.
- Persistent irritability.
- Excessive anxiety/worrying.
- Unrealistic or excessive fears.
- Strange or grandiose ideas.
- Social withdrawal.
- Marked changes to eating/sleeping/hygiene or other habits.
- Strong feelings of anger/outbursts of violent behaviour.
- Increasing inability to cope with usual activities of everyday life.
- Denial of anything being wrong even considering obvious problems.
- Numerous unexplained physical ailments.

CLINICAL INTEREST BOX 39.2 Warning signs and symptoms of a possible mental health condition—cont'd

- Substance misuse.
- Delusions or hallucinations.
- Thoughts/talk about suicide or homicide (professional help needed immediately).

(APA 2022; National Alliance on Mental Illness 2023; Hercelinskyj & Alexander 2022)

CLINICAL INTEREST BOX 39.3 People at risk of mental illness

Anyone can develop a mental illness, but people at particular risk include:

Life stages

- Adolescents: Face a period of enormous physical, psychological and social change. Some adolescents may not have sufficient resources to cope with the demands placed on them at this challenging stage of life and to complete the developmental tasks necessary to move successfully from adolescence to adulthood. We know that resilience plays an important role in protecting people from mental health conditions, and resilience development is important in childhood. Erik Erikson's theory of personality development (Erikson & Erikson 1997) is useful to explore in relation to life stages and developmental tasks. Childhood is a particular period of vulnerability to abuse and neglect, both of which increase the likelihood of mental illness developing
- New parents: Face a multitude of stressors (things that trigger a stress response) as well as many pleasures connected with a new baby. Stressors may include conflict over the acceptance of the pregnancy (is the pregnancy planned/wanted?), transition from being a couple to being parents, sleep deprivation, loss of financial income, a baby's constant demands and anxiety about the infant's welfare.
- Women: Face factors such as a disadvantaged status in society, internal conflict arising from decisions about whether to pursue a career, become a homemaker or try to achieve both, or being subjected to domestic violence or abuse. These are social factors that may possibly predispose some women to mental illness.
- Men: May face difficulties in expressing concerns about their mental health for fear of being judged. Men account for 75% of all suicide deaths in Australia.
- Older adults (male and female): May face many stressors, including loss of work role status because of retirement, reduced income, fear of declining physical and mental abilities, relocation, death of a partner and/or friends and siblings of similar age. The effect of these multiple losses may accumulate and leave some older adults at risk of mental illness.

Populations

- Refugees and migrants: May experience a grief reaction on leaving their homeland, friends and family to live in a country where the cultural practices, values and beliefs are different and where they may be considered to be of low status and worth. It may be difficult for some migrants to work successfully through their grief because of language barriers, the stress from job and financial uncertainty, and lack of support from relatives and friends left behind. Some refugees and migrants may experience problems of adjustment, racism, isolation and loneliness, each of which may contribute to mental illness. In some cases, refugees have experienced torture and trauma in their country of origin, which creates a high risk of developing a post-traumatic stress disorder.
- Aboriginal and Torres Strait Islander Peoples
- Homeless people
- Unemployed people
- Individuals who identify as LGBTQIA+
- Physically or intellectually impaired persons: Factors such as isolation, lack of meaningful relationships, social restrictions caused by disabilities, poor self-esteem and negative stigmatising community attitudes towards people with disabilities are all aspects of experience that can elevate the risk of mental illness, particularly anxiety and depression.

Individual risk factors

- Alcohol and other drug use
- Physical health
- Genetics
- Temperament
- Discrimination and racism

Continued

CLINICAL INTEREST BOX 39.3 People at risk of mental illness—cont'd

Community-level risk factors

- Social exclusion
- Discrimination
- Bullying
- Poverty
- Regional and remote communities

(Australian Institute of Family Studies 2022; Foster et al 2022; Hungerford et al 2020; Steele 2023)

- dissociative disorders (dissociative identity disorder, formerly multiple personality disorder)
- mood disorders (e.g. depression, bipolar disorder)
- personality disorders (e.g. antisocial personality disorder, dependent personality disorder, borderline personality disorder)
- sexual and gender identity disorders
- feeding and eating disorders
- sleep–wake disorders
- sexual dysfunctions
- disruptive, impulse-control and conduct disorders
- paraphilic disorders.

(APA 2022)

Diagnosis

The American Psychiatric Association's (2022) *Diagnostic and Statistical Manual of Mental Disorders*, Fifth Edition (DSM-5-TR) is a respected and influential classification system under which mental health conditions are determined according to the symptoms experienced and the clinical features of the condition. The International Classification of Disease (ICD) is produced by the WHO and is mainly used in Europe. It also assists with diagnosis and classification. In Australia, New Zealand and the USA, the 5th edition of the DSM (DSM-5-TR) (APA 2022) is most commonly used.

There are many categories of classification, but mental health conditions are mainly classified within the following areas:

- thought disorders, such as schizophrenia and psychosis, which disrupt the ability to think and perceive things clearly and logically and can impair a person's perception of reality
- mood disorders, which affect how a person feels and can result in persistent low mood (depression) or cycles of low and elevated moods (bipolar disorder)
- behavioural disorders, which involve people acting in potentially self-destructive ways, including eating disorders such as anorexia nervosa and bulimia
- personality disorders, which involve pervasive patterns of internal experience that deviate considerably from what others experience
- mixed disorders, which have components of two or more of the other categories.

(APA 2022)

Diagnosis according to the DSM-5-TR (APA 2022) has the benefit that consumers may feel great relief when they have a diagnosis that helps them make sense of what is happening to them, and a medical diagnosis can guide clinical treatment. Diagnostic labels can also help with funding (e.g. NDIS funding, which usually necessitates a diagnosis for financial support of treatment). But this diagnostic system has a disadvantage in that a diagnosis can also be a label that has negative connotations (e.g. a label of schizophrenia or a personality disorder is associated with significant social **stigma**). The impacts of stigma on consumers experiencing a mental health condition are significant and range from reduced self-esteem and delay in treatment-seeking behaviour to treatment and medication non-adherence and suicide (Hercelinskyj & Alexander 2022; Ross et al 2018). Diagnostic labels describe certain types of behaviour, but they indicate very little about the nature or causes of the experience.

MHNs develop nursing diagnoses in response to the consumer's experience, emotions and behaviours. Nursing care responds holistically to the consumer's biological, psychosocial, spiritual and environmental needs and specifically addresses the consumer's feelings and behavioural responses to those feelings, many of which are common across several different medically classified conditions. Examples of some nursing diagnoses commonly used in mental health nursing are provided in Clinical Interest Box 39.4. An example of a progress note for an individual who presents with psychotic symptoms is provided in Progress Note 39.1.

A mental health condition can be categorised as temporary, episodic or chronic/enduring, according to the way it manifests:

- Temporary: A temporary inability to cope (e.g. a single experience of depression; the condition is isolated and non-recurring).
- Episodic: An illness that occurs episodically (e.g. recurrent episodes of a disabling condition such as bipolar disorder [once known as manic-depression] or schizophrenia). For many people living with bipolar disorder, it is very common to have multiple episodes of a mood illness during their lifetime. While the condition is disabling when it occurs, the person affected can often enjoy a comparatively normal life for much, if not most, of the time.

CLINICAL INTEREST BOX 39.4 Examples of identification of issues by nurses used in mental health nursing

- Impaired social interaction: Insufficient or excess quantity or ineffective quality of social interactions.
- Ineffective coping: Inability to form a valid appraisal of the stressors, inability to use available resources. Inability to 'bounce back' after adversity (lack of resilience).
- Chronic low self-esteem: Long-standing negative feelings about self or own capabilities.
- Self-care deficit: Impaired ability to perform or complete activities of daily living (e.g. hygiene, toileting, nutrition).
- Imbalanced nutrition, less than body requirements: Intake of nourishment insufficient to meet the body's metabolic needs.
- Powerlessness: Perception that one's own actions will not significantly affect an outcome. A perceived lack of control over a current situation.
- Disturbed thought processes: Disruption in cognitive abilities and activities.
- Disturbed sensory perceptions: Alteration in the amount or patterning of incoming stimuli accompanied by a diminished/exaggerated/distorted/impaired response to the stimuli (often used for consumers who are experiencing delusions, hallucinations or illusions or have impaired awareness of self/environment).
- Impaired verbal communication: Diminished, delayed or impaired ability to understand or transmit verbal messages.
- Dysfunctional grieving: Prolonged unsuccessful use of strategies and responses by which people attempt to work through the process of grieving.
- Risk for injury: Potential for injury because of environmental conditions interacting with the consumer's adaptive and defensive resources.
- Risk for self-directed violence, risk for other-directed violence: Existence of the potential for a consumer to be physically, emotionally or sexually harmful to self or others.
- Risk for suicide: Potential for self-inflicted life-threatening injury.

(Foster et al 2022; Hungerford et al 2020; Steele 2023)

- Chronic/enduring: A constant disabling and unrelenting illness that is extremely challenging for the affected person and their family to deal with (e.g. chronic schizophrenia or bipolar disorder or irreversible dementia can be disabling).

Although use of the terms 'psychosis' and 'neurosis' to describe particular illnesses is no longer favoured, nurses need to be aware of the meanings associated with each since the terms are still used in some contexts. The terms are out of favour because symptoms ascribed to each condition can occur in the other, and this causes confusion. The term 'psychosis' refers to experiences that are so marked and incapacitating that the person who is afflicted experiences altered sensory perceptions (hallucinations), unusual or bizarre thoughts (delusions), and speech or behaviour that is disorganised. Psychosis can occur as a result of illicit substance use, such as methamphetamine misuse and alcohol withdrawal. Psychosis is typically seen in schizophrenia (and associated schizophrenia spectrum disorders), mania and sometimes in severe depression (Hercelinskyj & Alexander 2022). Clinical Interest Box 39.5 provides explanations and examples of delusions and hallucinations.

Unlike people experiencing a psychotic disorder, those with what used to be termed a 'neurosis' tend to have insight into their condition. For example, a person who has an obsessive-compulsive disorder may experience persistent and intrusive thoughts (obsessions) about personal cleanliness (APA 2022) and are usually aware that this experience is not 'normal' but cannot control the intrusive thoughts. To decrease the level of anxiety the person may wash their hands hundreds of times a day, even if their hands become red and raw (compulsion to act). When they are extreme, such thoughts and acts may be so unusual and disrupt the person's life to the degree that, to the observer, the person is experiencing a mental health condition. Unlike those experiencing a psychotic disorder, the affected person is usually aware that the behaviour is not consistent with other people's experiences (there is insight into the behaviour and the illness). Despite their condition, people who have what was once classified as a neurosis can often continue to function in society, whereas a person who is psychotic may not function effectively (Foster et al 2022). Nursing diagnosis should always be developed through the lens of a consumer-centred approach, which respects the consumer's social and individual experience of their illness. They remain the expert of their experiences and illness and this expertise needs to be respected by healthcare professionals.

Theoretical models and causation of mental illness

Historically, the medical profession was prominent in the care of people with mental health conditions and, as a result, there has been, and still is, a strong focus on identifying physical causes of mental illness. However, others have looked at psychological, sociocultural, interpersonal and human development factors and there are now many

CLINICAL INTEREST BOX 39.5 Delusions and hallucinations*

Delusion: a fixed false thought or belief that is not reality based or true, is not consistent with the person's level of education and development or cultural background and is not amenable to reason. It is categorised as a thought disorder.

Type	Example
Somatic delusions (a false belief involving a body part or function)	A young man who believes he is pregnant with an alien baby.
Nihilistic delusions (false feeling that the self, others or the world is non-existent)	A consumer who believes that she has no circulating blood, because she is in fact dead inside.
Delusions of persecution (over-suspiciousness: the person falsely believes themself to be the object of harassment)	A consumer who believes that his employer is trying to get him sacked from work and has been spying on him during office hours.
Delusions of control (false belief that one is being controlled by an external source)	A consumer who believes her feelings, thoughts and actions are being controlled by the president of the United States who sends messages to her via the television, instructing her on what to do.
Delusions of grandeur (exaggerated beliefs about personal importance or powers)	A consumer who believes he is the prime minister and controls Australia.
Delusions of self-depreciation (beliefs of unworthiness)	A consumer who believes she is ugly and sinful, saying, 'I don't deserve to be loved—look at me—it shows that I am full of sin'.
Delusion of erotomania (beliefs that someone usually of a higher status has romantic feelings for them)	A young man who believes that a news presenter is in love with him and that they are going to marry.

Hallucinations: False sensory perceptions that are not founded on any external stimuli. They may involve any of the five senses. They are most commonly visual or auditory.

Type	Example
Visual hallucination (a false experience of seeing something that others cannot)	A consumer tells you that he sees spirits when he looks out his front window.
Auditory hallucination (a false experience of hearing something others cannot)	A 26-year-old consumer tells you a dead baby communicates with him through crying, 'You are worthless, you don't deserve to live'.
Gustatory (taste) hallucination (a false experience of tasting something that others cannot)	A middle-aged consumer with organic brain syndrome complains of a constant metallic taste in his mouth.
Olfactory hallucination (a false experience of smelling something others cannot)	A 30-year-old consumer states that she smells 'decomposing bodies' in her bedroom, although no-one else can smell anything unusual or unpleasant.
Tactile hallucination (a false sensation of feeling something that is not real touching them)	A middle-aged woman experiencing symptoms of alcohol withdrawal reports someone tickling her toes at night.

**Consumers can experience delusions and hallucinations together. For example, a consumer who claims to hear the voice of a deceased army veteran whenever he walks past a war monument believes that he has been chosen to do the army's work by preaching about war.*

(Hercelinskyj & Alexander 2022; Foster et al 2022)

theoretical models used to explain the presence of a mental health condition. MHNs select concepts from the various relevant models that best explain the consumer's behaviours, problems and needs. They then draw on these concepts as a basis for the consumer's assessment and then for planning, conducting and evaluating care (Foster et al 2022). The following provide very basic examples of a small selection of theoretical models. To work effectively in mental health, however, nurses need a deep and sound understanding of a wide range of models.

The medical or biological model

This model explains a mental health condition as being caused by a physiological 'malfunction' in the body. Physical causes can be separated into acquired and non-acquired factors. Acquired causes include head injury, cerebral infection, and substance misuse. Non-acquired causes include genetic transmission, electrical conductivity changes in the brain or alterations to the production and/or activity of neurotransmitters (Foster et al 2022). There is evidence to support biological explanations. For example, studies indicate that depression and schizophrenia may be linked to abnormal neurotransmitter function, and that genetic factors may be linked to both (Hercelinskyj & Alexander 2022). A medical approach to treating mental health conditions tends to focus primarily on medication and sometimes includes electroconvulsive therapy (ECT), both of which aim to correct chemical imbalance in the body believed to be caused by abnormal neurotransmitter function in the brain. Emil Kraepelin (1856–1926) is a theorist associated with the origins of the medical model.

Psychological and psychodynamic models

The psychoanalytical model, first conceptualised by Sigmund Freud (1856–1939), is possibly the best-known model in this group. Freud's model viewed human personality as developing predominantly within the first 5 years of life and focused mostly on unconscious, non-rational and instinctual parts of human behaviour (Barkway 2020). Freud attributed disrupted behaviour in the adult to developmental tasks that were not accomplished successfully at earlier developmental stages. For example, within this theoretical framework a mental illness may be linked to a failure during adolescence to move successfully from dependence on parents to independence. Freud's mode of treatment was psychoanalysis, which aimed to bring unconscious problems to conscious awareness.

Carl Jung (1875–1961), Melanie Klein (1882–1960) and Erik Erikson (1902–1994) are some of the theorists who expanded on Freud's thinking about the nature of human development and behaviour. Erikson's theory has provided nurses with a developmental model that encompasses the entire lifespan. Erikson studied healthy personalities and focused on human strengths as well as weaknesses, emphasising how people who failed to achieve developmental milestones at various life stages could rectify these failures at later stages (Foster et al 2022).

It was Freud who identified the way humans develop and use defence mechanisms to ward off anxiety that might otherwise be overwhelming and incapacitating (Barkway 2020). Defence mechanisms prevent conscious awareness of threatening feelings and can be a helpful response in adapting to stress, but their overuse can be a sign of maladaptation to stress and an indicator of mental ill-health. They are particularly relevant in understanding stress-vulnerability and stress-adaptation models of health and illness. Stress-vulnerability/adaptation models recognise that throughout life there is a need for everyone to adapt to change (e.g. to adjust to school and then work life, to living with a partner or to becoming a parent or a grandparent and then to retirement and perhaps the death of a spouse). The model views that some people find it more difficult than others to adapt to life's changes and to cope effectively with the stressors that change can bring. When life results in a stressful situation or there is an accumulation of multiple stressors, people who have been unable to develop and establish adequate coping skills and coping resources are at the highest risk of developing a mental illness.

Social and interpersonal models

Social/interpersonal models draw attention to the impact of factors within a person's social environment on mental wellbeing. The basic concept is that negative social factors such as low status, low levels of support, isolation and poverty contribute to and increase the risk of developing a mental illness such as depression (Foster et al 2022).

Interpersonal models encompass the premise that internal conflict within one's personality and particular behaviours may be derived from unresolved conflicts within personal relationships, sometimes during early life experiences. This model also encompasses the premise that a consumer's wellbeing is dependent on the amount of stress experienced and the effectiveness of personal coping strategies in dealing with that stress. Karen Horney (1885–1952), Harry Stack Sullivan (1892–1949) and Hildegard Peplau (1909–1999) are some of the important theorists who have conducted research related to social and interpersonal factors and mental health.

Cognitive behaviour models

Cognitive behaviour models stem from the assumption that behavioural responses are learned. Ivan Pavlov (1849–1936) developed the understanding of learned behaviours when he found that when a bell was repeatedly rung each time dogs were given food the dogs began to salivate just at the sound of the bell. This conditioned reflex was termed 'classic conditioning' and is acknowledged as a form of learning that applies to humans, learning in which a previously neutral stimulus comes to elicit a given response through association. For example, behavioural theorists would suggest that children who observe parents responding to every minor stress with anxiety would soon learn the response and develop a similar pattern of behaviour (Foster et al 2022). According to the behavioural model, this early learning experience would be considered a significant factor in the cause of an anxiety disorder and limited **constructive coping strategies** in later life.

BF Skinner (1904–1990) added to behavioural theory by introducing the concept of operant conditioning. Operant conditioning refers to the use of reinforcers to motivate the repetition of particular behaviours. The use of positive reinforcement (the continual rewarding of desired behaviours) forms the basis of behaviour modification therapy used to help motivate consumers to change undesirable behaviours. It has been effective for consumers with phobias, alcohol dependency and a variety of other conditions (Foster et al 2022).

Aaron Beck was one of the early founders of cognitive behaviour therapy (CBT), now a common and often successful form of psychological treatment. It is based on the view that dysfunctional behaviour is linked to dysfunctional thinking, and that thinking processes are shaped by underlying beliefs. For example, the consumer with depression believes, 'I am no good at anything, I'm worthless, and nobody likes me.' CBT is based on helping consumers recognise, challenge and change dysfunctional thinking. Beck's work has primarily focused on helping people with depression but he has expanded the use of CBT to include working with people who have complex disorders such as borderline personality disorder and schizophrenia, and there are distinct signs of success (Foster et al 2022).

Attachment theory

The role of attachment theory in the development of a personality disorder has been well established in both our *understanding* and *treatment* of personality disorders. In particular, insecure attachment has been associated with maladaptive patterns of behaviour seen in borderline personality disorder (Luyten et al 2021). Attachment theory (which originated from Bowlby and Ainsworth) describes an infant's need to bond with their responsive caregiver in the first 6 months, and how any alteration to this can be detrimental to personality development. There are four hypothesised types of attachment styles: secure, anxious-ambivalent, disorganised and avoidant. Those associated with personality disorders are more commonly seen in disorganised and insecure attachment (Luyten et al 2021).

Best practice in the mental health context combines both psychological and biomedical approaches to treatment, which is also known as 'adjunct therapy'. This premise recognises that a combination of all approaches to care has better outcomes for people experiencing a mental health challenge, rather than one single approach. For example, an individual with depression may take an antidepressant medication in addition (adjunct) to seeing a psychologist regularly. Research indicates that this combined approach to treatment is associated with superior outcomes (Hercelinskyj & Alexander 2022). Mental health, like physical health, is clearly affected by a multitude of factors. Consequently, MHNs and psychiatrists are concerned with all the aspects of people's lives that distinguish them as human beings. The MHN uses knowledge from the psychosocial and biophysical sciences, and theories of stress vulnerability, personality and behaviour to develop a framework on which to base the art of nursing. The MHN is an integral part of the interdisciplinary team required to meet the needs of consumers who have a mental illness.

THE PROVISION OF CARE

The multidisciplinary team

Many people may be involved in assisting a person who is experiencing a disruption or potential disruption to their mental health. Mental health care commonly employs an interdisciplinary team approach to care management. The consumer's care, according to individual needs, is planned and implemented by a team composed of MHNs, psychiatric social workers, occupational therapists, counsellors, clinical psychologists, general or specialist medical officers (depending on the consumer's physical status), psychiatrists, peer workers and pharmacists. Additional team members may be required and, depending on individual needs, these may include a dietitian; a recreational, art, music or dance therapist; complementary healthcare therapist; and a chaplain or other spiritual support person. (See Clinical Interest Box 39.6.)

CLINICAL INTEREST BOX 39.6 Some members of the healthcare team

- The psychiatrist: A consultant physician whose specialty is mental health conditions and who is responsible for diagnosis and treatment. A psychiatrist has the legal power to prescribe and to write treatment orders and, as such, is often the team leader.
- The mental health nurse: A nurse with experience and expertise in clinical psychiatry, who promotes a holistic approach to care.
- The clinical psychologist: A psychologist who has undertaken specialised education in mental health and whose function includes applying and interpreting psychological tests and the implementation of specific therapies such as behaviour modification programs and sexual, marital or family therapy.
- The mental health social worker: A social worker in the field of mental health, whose function includes assisting the consumer to prepare a support system that will help maintain their mental health on discharge into the community from an inpatient facility. A social worker may liaise with employers, contacts in day-treatment centres and those providing training and educational programs. The social worker may also assist the consumer to locate and access sources of financial aid and accommodation.
- Occupational, recreational, art, music and dance therapists: According to their specialist areas of expertise, these various therapists help consumers to gain skills that assist them to cope more effectively, to gain or retain employment, to use leisure time in a way that promotes their mental wellbeing and to express their emotions in healthy ways.

(Foster et al 2022; Hungerford et al 2020; Steele 2023)

It should never be forgotten that the most important member of the team is the consumer, and often consumers know what they need to promote their own recovery. Some consumers have reflected on the times when they have been at their most vulnerable. For example, some consumers who have experienced admissions to acute care settings have identified that what they need most at times of severe mental distress is somewhere they can feel safe and supported, somewhere they can relax, calm their thoughts and for someone to be with them who will listen and really hear them (Hungerford et al 2018). While the consumer may feel the need for medication, many will not want to take any medication, and this requires a balance between accepting the consumer's wishes and ensuring that they are safe. It is also not appropriate or helpful to implement other therapeutic interventions, such as group therapy, recreational therapy or family therapy, until the consumer is feeling less distressed and can collaborate in decisions about what sort of interventions will be most helpful. Skilled helping involves actively listening to the consumer and working collaboratively with the consumer to achieve a process of recovery. (See Chapter 10 for information concerning active listening as a therapeutic measure.) The therapeutic process involves health professionals, including nurses, as facilitators who use their knowledge to help the consumer become more resourceful and self-reliant. This helping relationship needs to be a participative but never a directive process (Foster et al 2022). The model of helping relationships established by Carl Rogers (1961) and the model of skilled helping established by Gerard Egan (1994) are consumer-centred models of caring on which MHNs can reliably base their therapeutic interactions with consumers.

Responsibilities of the mental health nurse

Mental health nursing may be described as an interpersonal process in which the nurse uses the presence of self, interpersonal communication skills and knowledge of physiology, psychology and sociology to help consumers experiencing a mental health challenge. A combined understanding of biological processes and psychodynamic processes is essential for the MHN because many people with a mental health condition have a concurrent physical problem, and the two are often interconnected (Foster 2022). This interplay between physical and psychological conditions is multifaceted. Many of the pharmacological treatments of mental illness can result in the development of serious iatrogenic conditions, such as diabetes, hypertension, hyperlipidaemia and obesity (Hercelinskyj & Alexander 2022). Individuals with physical illness may also be more prone to develop mental illness. For example, those with chronic conditions or individuals with chronic pain are at greater risk of mental health issues.

Another important factor to consider when working in healthcare is the concept of diagnostic overshadowing. Diagnostic overshadowing occurs when a person with a mental health issue who experiences a physical complaint is not taken seriously and their physical complaint is misattributed as part of their mental health condition. For example, the person with schizophrenia who presents with chest pain at the emergency department is treated as someone who is delusional. This is a dangerous phenomenon and plays a role in why people with mental illness die up to 20 years earlier than those without one. Therefore, it is important that the nurse has a rounded understanding of the mental and physical healthcare needs of the consumer in their care.

MHNs are very involved in mental health inpatient services and in community mental health services. They play a major role in education and health promotion, as well as in the provision of continuing care and counselling for people with mental health challenges. For some experienced MHNs, the role may include conducting specific psychological therapies such as CBT, solution-focused therapy and acceptance and commitment therapy.

Nursing care aims to help consumers cope with their experience of a mental health condition, prevent relapse and to promote a return to mental health (as they themselves define it) through a successful rehabilitation program. The primary aims of mental health nursing are to help individual consumers to:

- Identify and clarify their needs and problems and advocate for the consumer.
- Support the consumer to exercise control over their recovery, and to ensure that the consumer is at the centre of their treatment and recovery plan.
- Create a better future for themselves (e.g. empower consumers by developing self-help strategies).
- Provide consumers with holistic, evidence-based, individual and person-centred care that incorporates their family and carers as directed by them.
- Collaborate with consumers and promote active participation in decision-making processes and autonomy.
- Create strategies to enable consumers to move forward (e.g. consumers can become stuck in a particular way of responding to situations).
- Adopt a recovery-focused approach to care by empowering the consumer and their carer to actively participate in this process.

(Adapted from ACSQHC 2021; Department of Health 2013; Australian College of Mental Health Nurses 2022)

Rehabilitation is important for many people who have been discharged from a mental health ward or unit. Some people need minimal support, but others represent a population of chronically unwell consumers who return to hospital periodically over many years and require support in several different areas of their lives. The community MHN and other members of the community mental health team may be involved in:

- primary mental health care
- mental health community teams
- acute community intervention services
- mental health triage
- crisis and assessment teams

- police, ambulance, and clinical early response teams (PACER)
- community care teams
- case management.

(Hercelinskyj & Alexander 2022)

Some of the roles of the mental health nurse in the community may include:

- social skills training
- consumer and family therapy
- medical care for concurrent physical problems
- vocational training and support
- monitoring medication.

(Foster et al 2022)

There are several specialised community services for people experiencing mental health issues that are facilitated by mental health nurses and multidisciplinary teams in the community and inpatient context. These include:

- perinatal mental health services (both public and private)
- older persons' mental health services
- forensic mental health services
- homelessness outreach services
- Aboriginal and Torres Strait Islander mental health services
- child and adolescent mental health services (CAMHS)
- refugee and culturally linguistically diverse (CALD) services.

(Hercelinskyj & Alexander 2022)

Recovery and mental health conditions

The concept of **recovery** has been apparent for the past few decades and is manifest mainly in policy at various levels such as health services management, practitioners and consumer/survivors of healthcare services (Edward et al 2018). Many consumers, some of whom were mental health professionals, began to speak about their experiences of mental illness and their individual journey of recovery, which led to the development of the consumer-recovery movement (Deegan 1988; Lovejoy 1984). In the USA, the consumer-recovery movement was boosted by William Anthony, a rehabilitation expert who challenged the state health system on its vision of recovery that was based on a belief that mental illness was essentially a 'chronic' condition with little hope of getting back to full health (Anthony 2000). According to Anthony (2000), mental health services need to be grounded in the idea that people can recover from mental illness, and that the construction of the service delivery system must be based on this knowledge. From that period, most Western countries adopted an approach to recovery that is based on practices and principles of autonomy and self-determination.

Contemporary mental health nursing care is now based on the **recovery principles** that refer to the person's rights to self-determination and inclusion in community life regardless of their diagnosis of a mental health condition. The implementation of peer support models of recovery in Australia has seen the advancing role of the consumer in sharing their journey of the lived experience in helping those currently experiencing a mental health condition (Davies et al 2014). Recovery principles are based on an approach that hope is central to recovery and that shifting the focus from symptom management and diagnostic labels to one that keeps people well gives their lives value and meaning. Personal and social recovery is the primary focus of contemporary mental health nursing care. In addition to this recovery framework of practice to guide practitioners, most states and territories in Australia now have contemporary mental health legislation that ensures consumers' preferences and wishes form the basis for their treatment which should not be coercive or restrictive.

> **CRITICAL THINKING EXERCISE 39.1**
>
> Describe how a peer support model of recovery is beneficial to a consumer with a mental health condition. What are the evidence-based benefits of this model?

Facilitating development of constructive coping mechanisms

The nurse's role in stress and stress management has some specific points that need to be highlighted here. To recognise and deal with stress, consumers need to be provided with information about and helped to recognise:

- issues and events related to health and illness, and the importance of adhering to sound health practices (e.g. adequate nutrition, sleep, exercise and relaxation) as a way of promoting mental wellbeing
- the dimensions of potential stressors, possible outcomes and the consumer's own established positive and negative coping mechanisms and coping resources
- their existing strengths and how to develop and maximise their abilities in problem-solving, tolerating stress and dealing effectively with interpersonal relationships
- where and how to gain access to additional coping resources (e.g. vocational training, support groups and counselling).

There is a wide variety of activities that consumers may find helpful in promoting coping, but there is no one right or best activity. What works for one person may not work for another. Nurses have a responsibility to provide consumers with information and options, but only the consumer can know what feels appropriate, so the choice of what activities to attempt or to become involved with should ultimately rest with the consumer. Clinical Interest Box 39.7 provides examples of constructive coping strategies, coping resources and **destructive coping mechanisms**.

CLINICAL INTEREST BOX 39.7 Examples of constructive coping strategies, coping resources and destructive coping mechanisms

Constructive coping strategies

- Postpone major life changes
- Resolve personal conflicts
- Take part in enjoyable activities
- Keep work under control
- Seek help
- Practise breathing and muscle relaxation techniques
- Do some research
- Establish good sleeping patterns
- Keep active
- Reduce alcohol and other drugs

Coping resources

- Economic assets
- Established abilities and skills
- Social supports
- Personal motivation
- Physical health, strength and energy
- Positive beliefs about self
- Established problem-solving and social skills
- Social and material resources
- Knowledge and intelligence
- Strong sense of identity
- Cultural stability
- A clear and stable system of values and beliefs
- An orientation towards preventative measures in health

Destructive coping mechanisms

- Always being submissive to others and so failing to get own needs met
- Excessive use of alcohol and/or other drugs or overeating (seeking comfort in substances)
- Self-harm (such as cutting, burning etc.)
- Increase in risk-taking behaviours (e.g. dangerous driving, drink driving, physical altercations etc.)
- Promiscuity (seeking love and acceptance in a way that does not improve self-esteem)
- Overuse of defence mechanisms to cope with unacceptable or ambivalent feelings. Defence mechanisms commonly used in a maladaptive manner (Foster et al 2022) include:
  > Regression: Reverting to behaviour synonymous with earlier developmental stage (e.g. tantrums)
  > Projection: Blaming others for what is happening
  > Denial: Denying there is a problem (e.g. 'I am in control of my anger')
  > Rationalisation: Avoiding dealing with an issue (e.g. 'What does a bit of shouting and banging matter? The children know I would never actually hit them')

(Foster et al 2022; Hungerford et al 2020; Steele 2023; Beyond Blue, www.beyondblue.org.au)

The nurse's role in educating the public and reducing stigma

One particularly important facet of the community MHN's role is educating the public about mental illness to reduce stigma, which for many people with a lived experience of mental illness is the biggest hurdle to overcome (Hungerford et al 2020). There is a general lack of knowledge in the community about what constitutes a mental health condition and about the prognoses of such conditions; this ensures that mental health conditions are often surrounded by mystery, misinformation and stigma (Hercelinskyj & Alexander 2022). Despite positive interventions in recent years, people experiencing a mental health condition remain among the most stigmatised, discriminated against, marginalised, disadvantaged and vulnerable members of society (Foster et al 2022; Hungerford et al 2020).

Review Case Study 39.1, which explores the stigma of mental illness.

CASE STUDY 39.1

The stigma of mental illness

My son Ed was diagnosed with schizophrenia 2 years ago. Getting a diagnosis was such a relief for the family, but Ed has struggled accepting his diagnosis. The nurses have taught us about schizophrenia and now, because we know what to look for, we pick up the early warning signs. Last year Ed started to go to church every day. I was worried because last time he became unwell, religion was a factor. He thought God was talking to him. I also noticed he wasn't sleeping well, so I called his case manager, Beth. She came and assessed him, and we found out he'd stopped taking his medication. I feel more comfortable about looking for the signs of relapse now.

Ed is in a good place now, but the thing that's upset him and us most is the way some people have treated him. He lost his girlfriend and his best mate. That was really hard. After he told his university course coordinator, they told him he should consider leaving his accounting course because of his illness. Even my own sister won't have him babysit his young cousins anymore. Ed now feels it is not safe to tell anyone about it. I understand why he feels that way. How do you think that makes him feel? If it was diabetes that made him ill, I wonder if people would have reacted the same.

Sarah, mother of Ed, age 21

Sarah and Ed's experiences are not dissimilar to other people experiencing mental-health-related discrimination.

1. As an Enrolled Nurse working with Ed and Sarah, what types of support services would you look for?
2. Understanding signs of relapse is very important for consumers living with schizophrenia. What are some of the warning signs you could educate Sarah and Ed about?

Several **myths** about mental health conditions create fear of those affected and this fear serves to increase stigmatising behaviours and attitudes. For example, there is a widely held perception that people experiencing a mental health condition are often out of control, unpredictable and may pose a threat. The truth is that most people with a mental health condition do not behave in this way; however, severe psychological distress is often highlighted in the media, and this links images of dangerous behaviour with mental illness in the minds of the public (Alexander et al 2018). In fact, consumers with a mental health condition are more likely to be victims of crime, rather than perpetrators (Appelbaum 2013; Desmarais et al 2014; Pollack 2013). The notion of perceived dangerousness in relation to mental illness probably stems from the media's propensity to portray individuals with a mental health condition as dangerous and unpredictable and facilitates the isolation and stigmatisation of an already marginalised group (Alexander et al 2018). Overall, violence in society associated with mental health conditions is not significant (Foster et al 2022). The Sane Australia 'StigmaWatch' website monitors misuse, misrepresentation or inappropriate references to mental illness in the media and assists in making the media accountable for perpetuating misleading perceptions and stigma.

The lack of accurate knowledge about mental health conditions that leads to fear, mistrust and sometimes violence against people with a lived experience of a mental health condition and their families can also serve to:

- lower the morale and self-esteem of people with a lived experience
- prevent people with a mental health condition from seeking professional help or remaining adherent to treatment when they do
- result in deaths from suicide, and increases in self-harming actions
- prevent people with a mental health condition from gaining paid employment
- result in social disadvantage and discrimination
- limit the participation of people with a lived experience in community activities and force them into a reclusive lifestyle, further exacerbating their condition
- cause families and friends to turn their backs on an individual with a mental health condition when support is most needed.

The picture is not always as dismal as this. Many mental health care users are themselves excellent ambassadors for people living with a mental health condition. By calling themselves 'consumers' they have empowered themselves to become advocates for other people experiencing mental health conditions. Mental health care users or consumers now have a vital role to play in participating and planning the delivery of mental health services (Hungerford et al 2020). Consumer advocacy groups now exist in every state and territory of Australia and in New Zealand to promote participation of consumers in planning, implementation and evaluation of mental health services. Accordingly, most consumers live and work within a local community, use the same facilities (e.g. shops, library, cinema, sports centres) as everyone else, are accepted by the people within the community and experience no harassment and attract no hostility from the local residents. All nurses can play a part in highlighting and reducing stigma by:

- Acknowledging the person by using respectful language (e.g. never referring to someone as a 'borderline', but rather referring to them as a person with a lived experience of borderline personality disorder).
- Discouraging the use of disrespectful language (e.g. terms such as 'schizo, lunatic, psycho, crazy, nut case or barmy'). The nurse can advocate for people with a mental health condition by alerting someone to the fact that they are expressing a stigmatising attitude. Many people do this automatically without realising the hurt they are causing and the negative impact on the individual with the condition or their family members.
- Emphasising the person's abilities rather than their limitations—this means adopting a strengths-based approach.
- Avoiding representing a successful person with a mental health condition as 'superhuman'.

Mental health first aid

Mental health first aid (MHFA) is a relatively new concept associated with the management of a mental health crisis by 'first responders' until a person capable of managing these types of situations arrives. This type of intervention is akin to the medical management of a patient during a medical emergency (or MET) call; the only difference being, it is psychological management. Individuals working in healthcare environments are often confronted with situations arising from consumers and/or their families in distress and appropriate, sensitive and safe management, based on an understanding of mental health conditions and crisis is important. Examples of a situation that may require MHFA include a threatened or non-fatal attempt at suicide, an incidence or threat of deliberate self-harm, distress related to psychotic symptoms such as acute paranoia, or an anxiety or panic attack. The first responder should remain calm and engage the consumer in a compassionate and gentle manner. The MHFA Australia (2022) website is a useful resource for all nursing and healthcare students. This site contains useful information regarding common mental illnesses, and the management of crisis situations.

CRITICAL THINKING EXERCISE 39.2

There are many reasons why consumers delay seeking treatment for mental illness; however, stigma is one of the major reasons. Discuss the effects of stigmatisation of mental illness, including the implications to:

- the consumer
- mental health practitioners
- society.

In part, it is the way that people with mental health conditions were treated in the past that influences current perceptions of mental illness and the associated stigma. The next section provides a brief overview of historical perspectives relevant to understanding societal attitudes today.

HISTORICAL PERSPECTIVES AND MENTAL HEALTH CARE

In the past, when emotions, thoughts or actions were deemed to be 'abnormal', the terms 'madness' and 'insanity' were linked to those affected. Reasons for the perceived abnormalities were once attributed to a variety of factors such as the influences of magic, witchcraft, possession by the devil or evil spirits, loss of the soul or punishment by the gods. Healing methods included exorcism, magical ritual and incantation (Hercelinskyj & Alexander 2022). Later, it was proposed that an imbalance of 'body humours' was responsible—body humours being blood, black bile, yellow bile and phlegm—and such imbalances were corrected by bloodletting. During the medieval period, beliefs returned to those connected with magic and demonology but also included beliefs that the moon influenced 'madness' (hence the term lunacy). Some of those perceived as 'mad' or 'lunatics' were flogged, tortured and starved, and those whose illness resulted in violent behaviour were shackled in prisons or put out to sea as a means of ridding them from society. Fear and lack of knowledge resulted in significant cruelty.

In the late 19th and early 20th centuries, those with behaviours that were not manageable, who were misunderstood or were simply not acceptable in society were placed in custodial care inside large public mental hospitals or asylums. It can only be imagined how being confined and isolated inside large institutions might have caused feelings of abandonment and rejection. During this period, doctors classified the symptoms of mental illness but had limited understanding of the sources of psychological anguish (Hercelinskyj & Alexander 2022).

Increased understanding of psychological distress was promoted by the psychological, psychosocial and interpersonal theories to explain behaviour espoused by theorists such as Freud, Erikson and Stack Sullivan. The introduction of psychotropic drugs, such as chlorpromazine (Largactil) in the 1950s, helped staff members manage large numbers of consumers with challenging behaviours, who were often accommodated in crowded conditons in the large institutions. In the 1990s (the time known as the decade of the brain), biological, scientific and technological concepts combined to expand on earlier understandings of mental illness (Hercelinskyj & Alexander 2022). As a result, advanced brain-imaging techniques now allow direct viewing of the structure and function of the living brain while it is functioning.

In the latter part of the 20th century, the negative impact of institutionalisation for people experiencing a mental health condition was recognised. This recognition was in part the stimulus that shifted public policy to one of **deinstitutionalisation** and community-based care for people living with mental illness. The push towards community-based mental health services also came from the human rights movement and the philosophy of normalisation for people with disabilities of all kinds. (See Chapter 41 for explanations about the principles of normalisation and people with disabilities.) The discovery of psychotropic drugs in the 1950s also contributed to the current predominance of care in the community because these agents helped to modify challenging behaviours (Hercelinskyj & Alexander 2022).

Mental health care today

Mainstreaming of mental health care has resulted in the provision of psychiatric care to consumers in general hospitals with an inpatient mental health unit, hostels and other residential care facilities, and sometimes in forensic centres for individuals with mental health conditions who have committed crimes. Under contemporary mental health legislation, community care is now a common mandate of treatment, and in Australia it is recognised that treatment should only occur in the least restrictive of environments. This means that all efforts should be made so that a person with a mental health issue is able to be treated in the community rather than an inpatient setting. The current emphasis is on inclusion and collaboration with consumers and for this to occur effectively, treatment should not be compulsory.

Nurses may meet with consumers in a variety of community settings, including:

- the consumer's home
- the consumer's foster home
- community care units
- special residential units
- day and drop-in centres
- general practitioner clinics
- boarding houses
- on the street (homeless consumers).

Current healthcare policy promotes not admitting people to an inpatient setting unless essential and, when it is necessary for consumers to be admitted, they must be discharged back into the community as early as possible. Ideally, community-based mental health services provide appropriate networks of supports and resources for those who need it. The aim of service providers is to ensure that there are caring interventions aptly suited to assist each person to rehabilitate successfully and to cope well in society. The policy of community-based care has enabled many of those who once lived in psychiatric institutions to resettle successfully in the community and to be well supported. It is important to remember that the environment in which the consumer is seen affects the therapeutic relationship. In community settings, the MHN enters the home of the consumer as a guest, engaging with the consumer on a more relational and contextual basis.

While there are still many problems for people with a lived experience and health professionals to contend with and resolve, there is now more cause for optimism in relation to mental illness than in the past. Success rates for the treatment of many common mental health conditions such as anxiety, major depression and schizophrenia now equal or exceed the success rates for many other medical conditions (Hungerford et al 2020).

While this chapter does not aim to inform the nurse about the range of treatments available to assist consumers with specific conditions, the next section provides a summary of possible nursing responses to some common emotional and behavioural problems that challenge consumers with a mental health condition. The terminology used in mental health care, some of which is contained in the next section, is extensive and different from terms used in other areas of nursing. Some of the more common terminology is defined in Table 39.4.

CARE OF CONSUMERS WITH SPECIFIC EMOTIONAL OR BEHAVIOURAL CHALLENGES

Here, we address some of the more common mental states that consumers being cared for may experience. Information is provided on caring for a person who is anxious, depressed, aggressive, displaying self-destructive behaviour, hyperactive, confused or disoriented. It is important to note that these are common experiences for any person admitted to a hospital setting, not only someone diagnosed with a mental health condition.

The consumer experiencing anxiety

Anxiety disorders are the most diagnosed mental health conditions (Hercelinskyj & Alexander 2022). Anxiety is an internal feeling usually experienced as an unpleasant or uncomfortable emotion and is frequently associated with conflicts and frustrations. While a certain mild degree of anxiety can be beneficial when it stimulates motivation and energy, severe anxiety can be devastating and is the basis of many mental health conditions. Formal anxiety disorders include conditions such as:

- Separation anxiety disorder (excessive anxiety response to separation from a caregiver such as a mother, usually seen in small children).
- Selective mutism (consistent failure to speak in certain situations where the expectation is a verbal interaction—e.g. at school, when meeting new people).
- Specific phobia (severe anxiety response to a situation or object such as spiders, heights etc.).
- Social anxiety disorder (significant anxiety associated with socialisation).
- Panic disorder (the physiological response to severe anxiety, also known as a 'panic attack').
- Agoraphobia (extreme fear of situations that usually involve open or closed spaces—e.g. fear of riding in an elevator, leaving home, public transport etc.).
- Generalised anxiety disorder (severe anxiety and worry resulting in physiological response such as sleep disturbance, poor concentration and restlessness). Generalised anxiety disorder is the correct diagnostic term for what most people would call 'anxiety disorder'.

(APA 2022)

Anxiety differs from fear in that anxiety attacks the person at a deeper level than fear, and the source of the anxiety may be unknown. Sometimes, in extreme anxiety, a person may experience panic attacks that result in markedly disturbed behaviour. The person may be unable to process what is happening in the environment and may lose touch with reality. During a panic attack, behaviour may be erratic, uncoordinated and impulsive. There are three different forms of panic attack: 'out of the blue' attacks, which are not brought on by a trigger; situation-bound attacks, which are brought on by exposure to a trigger; and situation-predisposed attacks, which are comparable to situation-bound, but which do not happen every time the person is exposed to a trigger.

Anxiety invades the very centre of a person's being. Severe anxiety is profound and persistent and can erode and destroy a person's sense of self-esteem and self-worth that contribute to a sense of being fully human (Foster et al 2022).

Anxiety is experienced in a wide variety of situations and is generally the result of a threat to a person's self-esteem or physical integrity. Threats to self-esteem include factors such as interpersonal difficulties, change in job status, social or cultural group pressures, a change in role or confusion over one's identity. Threats to physical integrity include factors such as decreased ability to perform the activities of daily living (e.g. as a result of injury or illness) or lack of basic requirements such as food, shelter and clothing. Mild and moderate levels of anxiety can alert the person to the fact that something is wrong and may be the stimulus to take appropriate action. For example, a looming deadline for an assignment can cause anxiety that results in the person getting their assignment finished. Severe levels of anxiety interfere with problem-solving abilities, so that those affected have difficulty finding effective solutions to problems. For example, someone who experiences panic attacks may use unproductive relief behaviours to avoid the attacks from occurring, such as refraining from leaving the house to avoid the risk of a panic attack when driving the car, at work or at the supermarket. This is an example of avoidant behaviour, which is common to anxiety disorders. Unproductive relief behaviours perpetuate the cycle of anxiety (Hercelinskyj & Alexander 2022).

Whether the source is known or unrecognised, anxiety can produce physiological responses, behavioural changes

TABLE 39.4 | Terms associated with mental health conditions

Term	Description
Addiction	Physical or emotional dependence, or both, on a substance, such as alcohol or illicit or prescription drugs.
Affect	Current, observable state of emotion, feeling or mood such as sadness, anger or elation. The visual representation of a mood.
Aggression	Forceful behaviour that may be physical or verbal, as well as subtle manipulation.
Akathisia	A condition of excessive restlessness that causes a person to move about constantly, fidget or pace. This can be a side effect of certain medications (such as some antipsychotics) used in psychiatry.
Amnesia	Loss of memory of events for a period of time that may range from a few hours to many years.
Anhedonia	Reduced or complete inability to feel pleasure from activities previously enjoyed. This condition is often seen in consumers with depression. For example, a consumer who previously enjoyed walking their dog no longer feels any pleasure when they do it now.
Anxiety	A feeling of apprehension, dread or unexplained discomfort associated with a sense of helplessness, arising from internal conflict. Heightened anxiety is seen in a number of mental health conditions and is the most common mental health condition.
Apathy	Lack of feeling, emotion, concern or interest, which is seen in depression.
Asylum	A place of safety or sanctuary, a refuge from the stresses of life. Historically, the term 'asylum' was associated with institutions that provided custodial care for people with a mental illness. Unfortunately, they were often associated not with the real meaning of asylum but with mistreatment and cruelty.
Autism	A developmental disorder seen in childhood characteristic of issues with communication (both reciprocating and responding to communication) and impaired social interactions. Autism occurs across a spectrum with varying degrees of impact.
Behaviour	Any human activity, either physical or mental. Some behaviour can be observed while other behaviour can only be inferred.
Behaviour modification	A method of changing or controlling behaviour through the application of techniques based on the principles of classical conditioning.
Bipolar disorder	A type of mood disorder that causes alternating periods of low and high moods. Usually, a consumer will experience a combination of depression and mania, but these are not rapid. For example, mania may last weeks, followed by depression a month later (which may last months). Bipolar disorder is not associated with rapid daily changes in mood states from low (depression) to high (mania). Consumers will, however, often experience rapid changes of aroused mood states such as elevated, irritable, excited and hostile in a short space of time.
Body image	The conscious and unconscious attitudes a person has towards their body (e.g. feelings about size, function and appearance). Eating disorders such as anorexia nervosa and bulimia nervosa are associated with issues with body perception.
Catatonia	A state characterised by muscular rigidity and immobility (stuporose type) and which, at times, is interrupted by episodes of extreme agitation (excited type) and is usually associated with schizophrenia. Catatonia is rarely seen now due to improvement in psychotropic medications and prompt mental health care.
Compensation	A process by which a person makes up for a deficiency in their self-image by strongly emphasising some feature of themself that they regard as an asset.
Compulsion	An uncontrollable persistent urge to perform an act repetitively to relieve anxiety. For example, compulsively washing hands or checking door locks. Compulsive behaviour often accompanies obsessions and may be directly linked to them. Compulsive behaviour is seen in obsessive-compulsive disorder.

Continued

TABLE 39.4 | Terms associated with mental health conditions—cont'd

Term	Description
Confabulation	The fabrication of experiences or situations recounted in a plausible way to fill in and cover gaps in the memory. Used most often as a defence mechanism and most commonly by people with head injuries, dementia, amnesic disorders or alcoholism, especially those with Korsakoff's syndrome (a severe dementia caused by alcohol dependency).
Confusion	A cluster of abnormalities constituting disturbances of judgment, orientation, memory, affect and cognition.
Consumer	An individual with a lived experience of a mental health condition.
Coping mechanisms	Any effort directed towards stress management. They can be unconscious (defence) mechanisms that protect the consumer against anxiety, or conscious attempts to solve a problem that is creating stress.
Deinstitutionalisation	A shift in the location of treatment from large public hospitals to community settings. This occurred in the 1990s in Australia, and the focus on mental health legislation remained that consumers be treated in a least restrictive environment (e.g. in their home, not in hospital).
Delusion	A fixed false belief held despite evidence to the contrary. A delusion of grandeur is a false belief that one has great prestige, power or money, which may be manifested in the belief that the consumer is a famous person. A delusion of persecution is a consumer's belief that they are in danger, being harassed, are under investigation or are at the mercy of some powerful force. A somatic delusion is a belief that one's body is changing and responding in an unusual way. Delusions are commonly seen in schizophrenia and mania.
Dementia	A mental health condition characterised by a gradual onset of usually irreversible cognitive impairments.
Depression	A mood state that may be mild or short-lived or more severe and persistent. The latter, a mood disorder, is characterised by extreme sadness, persistent low mood, feelings of hopelessness, low self-worth and little or no conviction that things can ever improve.
Disorientation	Lack of awareness of the correct time, place or person.
Electroconvulsive therapy (ECT)	A therapeutic procedure in which an electric current is briefly applied to the brain to produce a seizure. This is used in treatment of severe symptoms that do not respond to other measures; most used in the treatment of depression and bipolar disorder.
Hallucination	A false sensory experience that is not the result of an external stimulus; may be visual, auditory, tactile, gustatory or olfactory. Commonly seen in schizophrenia and mania.
Hyperactive	Excessively or unusually active.
Illusion	Misperceptions and misinterpretations of real external stimuli. For example, mistaking a piece of fluff on the carpet for a spider.
Labile	Subject to frequent or unpredictable changes: the term is commonly used with reference to emotions and the individual may oscillate (for example) between happy, irritable and excited in quick succession. Labile mood is often seen in mania and borderline personality disorder.
Mania	A mood characterised by an intense feeling of elation or irritability, often accompanied by increased goal-directed activity, rapid speech and poor judgment. Mania is a condition only seen in bipolar disorder and schizoaffective disorder.
Mood disorder	A group of disorders in which the predominant feature is disturbance in mood. Conditions include depression and bipolar disorders.
Negative symptoms	A cluster of symptoms seen in schizophrenia consisting of social withdrawal, apathy, alogia (loss of speech), anhedonia and affective restriction. Negative symptoms are best understood to be a removal of behaviours seen in healthy individuals.

TABLE 39.4 | Terms associated with mental health conditions—cont'd

Term	Description
Obsession	A persistent thought, idea or impulse that cannot be eliminated from consciousness by logical effort (e.g. 'germs contaminate my hands'). Obsessions are seen in obsessive-compulsive disorder.
Obsessive-compulsive disorder	A condition with a foundation in anxiety characterised by intense, unwanted and distressing recurrent thoughts (obsessions) and repeated behaviours (compulsions) that are beyond the affected person's ability to control.
Panic	A period of sudden intense anxiety, often associated with feelings of impending disaster and accompanied by strong physiological symptoms, including shortness of breath, pounding heart or palpitations and dizziness.
Paranoia	A serious personality distortion in which the person is markedly suspicious and mistrusting of others and may be convinced that they wish to harm them. Paranoia is commonly seen in schizophrenia.
Phobia	An intense fear of some situation, person or object, so that the danger is magnified out of proportion and may result in a panic. Examples include fear of spiders, heights or needles.
Positive symptoms	A cluster of symptoms only seen in schizophrenia that include delusions, hallucinations, thought disorder, agitation and paranoia. Positive symptoms are best understood as experiences added onto a healthy person.
Psychosis	An acute state in which a person's mental capacity to recognise reality, communicate and relate to others is impaired. Psychosis includes the presence of delusions, hallucinations and disorganisation of thinking and behaviour. Psychosis is a state seen in schizophrenia and mania, and can occur in the presence of illicit drugs and severe depression.
Psychotic	A person who is psychotic experiences delusions and hallucinations that cause disorganised thinking, unusual behaviours and a loss of touch with reality. Psychosis is an acute presentation often present in schizophrenia, mania and some illicit substance-intoxicated states.
Recovery	A meaningful and individual process that is non-linear and different for every consumer. Not simply symptom amelioration.
Schizophrenia	A complex condition that results in hallucinations and delusions, distorted thinking and negative symptoms. Schizophrenia is classified as a severe mental illness and can be associated with significant impairment in functioning.
Self-harm	Harmful actions towards oneself where there is intention to harm but not die. Examples include cutting, burning and scratching. Commonly seen in borderline personality disorder and dysphoric emotional states.
Suicide	An act of intentionally causing one's own death.
Suicidal ideation	Thoughts of suicide (or thinking about suicide) with an intention to end one's life.
Tardive dyskinesia	A side effect of some antipsychotic medications (usually first generation, typical agents) that manifests with a variety of involuntary muscle movements including those that affect the face, jaw and tongue, the trunk and the extremities of the body. The involuntary movements are often irreversible. They are also referred to as extrapyramidal side effects.

(Foster et al 2022; Halter 2023; Hungerford et al 2020; Steele 2023; Hercelinskyj & Alexander 2022)

and emotional reactions. The type and extent of response depends on the level of anxiety experienced. Table 39.5 lists some physiological and other responses to different levels of anxiety. Emotional reactions are usually apparent in the person's descriptions of their experience. For example, they may state that they feel apprehensive, irritable, angry, depressed, helpless, on edge, unable to concentrate or remember things or they may feel detached from events and the environment. The person may experience angry outbursts or a tendency to cry frequently.

Other conditions with a foundation in anxiety (but which are not recognised as specific anxiety disorders) include:

- post-traumatic disorder—condition associated with the experience and re-experiencing of a traumatic

TABLE 39.5 | Physiological and other responses to anxiety

Mild anxiety	Moderate anxiety	Severe anxiety	Panic level of anxiety
Slight discomfort Restlessness, irritability or mild agitation Mild tension-relieving behaviour (e.g. foot or finger tapping, lip chewing, hair twisting, fidgeting)	Voice tremors Change in voice pitch Difficulty concentrating Shakiness Repetitive questioning Loss of appetite Diarrhoea/constipation Memory impairment (e.g. interference with recall of events/facts) Chain smoking Increased use of alcohol or other substances Somatic (bodily) complaints (e.g. urinary frequency and urgency, insomnia) Increased respiration rate Increased pulse rate Increased muscle tension that may lead to backache or headache More extreme tension-relieving behaviour (e.g. pacing, banging hands on table, constant wringing of hands)	Feelings of dread or impending doom Confusion and bewilderment Purposeless activity, lack of coordination of movements and actions Worsening of somatic complaints (e.g. dizziness, nausea, headache, sleeplessness) Hyperventilation Tachycardia Elevated blood pressure Sweating Facial pallor Dry mouth Difficulty in breathing Withdrawal from interpersonal interactions Disturbances in sexual function Loud and rapid speech Intense tension-relieving behaviour that may include threats and demands	Feelings of absolute terror; fear that death may result Immobility or severe hyperactivity or flight Dilated pupils Chest pains/palpitations Severe dizziness Unintelligible communication or inability to speak Severe tremors Sleeplessness Extreme psychomotor activity may lead to exhaustion Severe withdrawal (e.g. agoraphobia) Hallucinations and delusions may occur, and the person may lose touch with reality

(Foster et al 2022; Halter 2023; Hungerford et al 2020; Steele 2023; Hercelinskyj & Alexander 2022)

incident (e.g. witnessing or being the victim of a violent crime, or a soldier who returns from a conflict/war)
- obsessive-compulsive disorder—high levels of anxiety related to an obsession (e.g. fear of germ contamination), which is only relieved through a compulsion (e.g. excessive hand-washing).

Specific treatment and care of a person experiencing anxiety depends on the level of anxiety experienced and the effects on the consumer, but generally, interventions are directed towards reducing intense anxiety to a more manageable level and helping the person to develop self-help strategies to prevent overwhelming anxiety. Cognitive behavioural therapy (CBT), for example, helps consumers develop strategies for controlling their anxiety and reducing the incidence of panic attacks (Hercelinskyj & Alexander 2022). Minor tranquillisers such as diazepam (Valium) and lorazepam (Ativan) are sometimes prescribed short term to suppress the consumer's feelings of anxiety but, since these medications do not cure the condition and there are problems with dependence, long-term use is not appropriate (Hercelinskyj & Alexander 2022). Antidepressants are generally well tolerated, safe and effective in the ongoing treatment of anxiety, with proven clinical efficacy (Hercelinskyj & Alexander 2022). Examples used for the long-term treatment of anxiety include the selective serotonin reuptake inhibitors (SSRIs) fluoxetine (Lovan, Prozac) and sertraline (Zoloft). In addition to these medications, beta-blockers such as propranolol (Inderal) and atenolol (Tenormin) are also used to treat the physiological impacts of anxiety, such as tachycardia (Hercelinskyj & Alexander 2022). More recently novel agents such as serotonin and norepinephrine reuptake inhibitors (SNRI) have also demonstrated efficacy (Hercelinskyj & Alexander 2022). These include the antidepressants duloxetine (Cymbalta) and venlafaxine (Effexor).

General care of the consumer with anxiety involves:
- establishing and maintaining a trusting relationship
- managing acute symptoms such as hyperventilation
- attempting to identify the cause (stressors) of the anxiety and encouraging the consumer to take effective action
- facilitating open and honest communication about the consumer's anxiety and/or problems
- identifying existing coping mechanisms and coping resources
- discussing with the consumer ways of resolving conflicts
- providing information about, and teaching, constructive coping strategies that can help to manage stress.

The most common coping mechanisms taught and encouraged for the consumer with anxiety are:
- problem-solving
- assertiveness

- positive self-talk
- stress and anger management
- communication skills
- skills for establishing and maintaining relationships
- conflict resolution
- time management
- community living skills.

(Foster et al 2022; Hungerford et al 2020)

An understanding of the types and levels of anxiety and defensive patterns of behaviour used in response to anxiety is basic to effective mental health nursing care. Hildegard Peplau was a nurse theorist whose conceptual model of anxiety provides a firm basis on which nurses can plan interventions for consumers experiencing anxiety. Nurses would benefit from reviewing the work of Peplau (1991) and other psychiatric nursing texts to enhance their knowledge of the relationship between anxiety and mental illness and the range of treatment options available.

Care during a panic attack

Care during a panic attack can take the form of:

- Remaining with the person during the attack and speaking in a calm, confident voice using short and simple sentences.
- Ruling out that the person is experiencing a cardiac incident.
- Asking the person to take slow deep breaths and to breathe in and out through their nose. Place their hand on their diaphragm to focus their attention on their breathing and reduce the breath rate to 10 per minute until the anxiety recedes.
- Explaining to the person to cup their hands around their mouth and to breathe into their hands can assist in preventing fainting from hyperventilating.
- Following the panic attack, explaining to the person what they have experienced is a panic attack; reassure the person that they can get help to manage panic attacks.
- Referring the person to their general practitioner for a full physical assessment to rule out a physical cause.

(Hungerford et al 2020; Foster et al 2022)

In addition, strategies to help tolerate and decrease the effects of anxiety can be taught, although these address the effects rather than the cause of anxiety. These strategies include complementary therapies such as visualisation techniques, guided imagery, meditation and relaxation training.

The consumer experiencing depression

Depression is an emotional state that most people experience at one time or another. It can manifest anywhere along a continuum from intermittent feelings of sadness to a persistent deep sense of unending despair accompanied by hallucinations and delusions (Hungerford et al 2020). Often, at the onset of depression, the mood begins with a feeling of sadness that may be described as 'feeling down in the dumps'. As depression worsens, sad feelings deepen until those affected feel gloomy and dejected much of the time. At this level of depression people may describe the experience with statements such as 'I have no joy in my life anymore' or 'I just feel unhappy'. They will often describe feeling no pleasure in undertaking previously pleasurable activities (such as going to the movies with friends)—this is known as anhedonia. For some people, the depressed mood can deepen even further until there is a persistent feeling of utter desolation. Severely depressed people have a sense of hopelessness about the past and the present, and the future looks black and bleak. The heavy feelings of despondency, wretchedness and acute misery are relentless. People affected feel desperately low and worthless, and this experience is accompanied by a sense of despair so profound that they do not believe the feelings will ever lift (Foster et al 2022).

Feelings of sadness and even intense grief, such as might be felt at the death of a loved one, are normal reactions to the various losses encountered by most people during their lives. Sadness and depression in such cases may be transitory, with the person moving through a grieving process and recovering successfully after the loss. Sometimes, recovery after a significant loss does not occur and the person moves into a level of persistent and severe depression that does not resolve without professional assistance. Bereavement is a differential diagnosis for major depressive disorder and is associated with the usual symptoms of depression in addition to feelings of emptiness and loss (APA 2022). Bereavement is also usually associated with intensity reduction over time that may peak when the individual thinks or reminisces about their lost loved one. For many people with depression, there is no catalyst for their despair, however, and bereavement is categorised by a loss.

Feelings of depression are so common that depression is sometimes known as the 'common cold' of psychiatry. It can occur at any age, even in very small children. Children with parents diagnosed with a depressive disorder have a higher risk of experiencing depression than others, and certain events may predispose young people to develop depressive symptoms (Steele 2023). These events include:

- loss of parents through divorce
- death of other individuals close to them (e.g. grandparents, siblings, other relatives or friends)
- death of a loved pet
- moving to a new neighbourhood or town
- academic difficulties or failure
- physical illness or injury that entails a stay in hospital.

Depression has a wide range of signs and symptoms, but even so, some people are able to hide their depression from others. Clinical Interest Box 39.8 lists the common signs and symptoms of depression. For some people, depression may also be accompanied by anxiety. Some people experience alternating moods of depression and elation that can be disruptive to their lives. The periods of elation may be accompanied by significant increase in goal-directed activity and insomnia. Such conditions are categorised as bipolar disorders, whereas mood disorders that have only the one dimension of depression without periods of elation are termed unipolar (Foster et al 2022).

CLINICAL INTEREST BOX 39.8 Signs and symptoms of depression

Signs and symptoms of depression vary according to the severity of the low mood but may include:

- non-verbal cues (sad facial expression, crying, slumped posture, lack of eye content, mask-like facial features)
- disturbed sleep patterns (e.g. insomnia or sleeping for much longer periods than usual)
- self-criticism and expressions of guilt feelings
- low self-esteem that may result in thoughts of self-harm or self-destruction
- indecisiveness and poor concentration
- psychomotor retardation or marked reduced mental or physical activity (slow dragging gait, slowed speech pattern and slow, flat, lifeless, colourless verbal responses, lack of concern and apathy about maintaining personal appearance)
- psychomotor agitation (some people with depression experience significant anxiety that may manifest as restlessness, pacing or constant walking or constant purposeless movements such as pulling at hair or wringing of hands)
- appetite disturbance—marked loss of weight or weight gain
- loss of energy
- loss of sexual libido
- headaches, chest pains, gastrointestinal disturbances and other physical manifestations
- increased consumption of substances such as nicotine, alcohol and illicit substances
- anhedonia (inability to feel any pleasure when participating in activities that previously were pleasurable)
- delusions and/or hallucinations.

Signs that may be associated with depression in children and adolescents include:

- frequent, vague, non-specific physical complaints such as headaches, muscle aches, stomach aches or tiredness
- frequent absences from school or poor performance in school
- efforts to run away from home (or talk of this)
- outbursts of shouting, complaining, agitation, unexplained irritability or crying
- complaints of being bored
- lack of interest in playing with friends
- reckless behaviour
- extreme sensitivity to rejection or failure
- increased irritability, hostility or anger
- difficulty with relationships
- substance misuse
- fear of death.

(Foster et al 2022; Hungerford et al 2020; Steele 2023)

Care of a depressed consumer is directed first towards addressing immediate safety needs in those at risk of self-harm or suicide. Suicide is the deliberate act of inflicting harm to oneself where the intention is to die. Self-harm, on the other hand, is self-inflicted injury (such as cutting, scratching or burning) where there is no intention to die. This may require hospitalisation and frequent or constant observation of those so seriously depressed as to be actively contemplating suicide. Antidepressant medication, when necessary, is started immediately, but the symptomatic relief is not generally achieved for up to 6 weeks after therapy starts. Other specific interventions include consumer, family, group, cognitive and behavioural psychotherapy (Hercelinskyj & Alexander 2022). The major goals are to lift the consumer's mood, improve self-esteem, identify and reduce the impact of any major identified stressors, promote the development of constructive coping mechanisms, assist the consumer to regain interest and motivation in life and to address any concurrent problems associated with physical health. General care involves:

- ensuring the consumer is safe
- establishing and maintaining a trusting relationship
- helping the person, when the acute phase is resolved, to recognise and express emotions (e.g. through verbal and non-verbal communication)
- helping the consumer to set realistic, achievable goals
- encouraging the consumer to establish and maintain social contact and interpersonal relationships
- encouraging visits by family or significant others, to reduce any feeling of isolation
- promoting physical health and wellbeing (e.g. adequate exercise, sleep and nutrition)
- providing information concerning measures that may reduce and help manage stress
- identifying existing coping mechanisms and coping resources
- promoting recovery
- assisting the consumer to develop and enhance constructive coping mechanisms, including decision-making and problem-solving skills.

(Hercelinskyj & Alexander 2022)

Table 39.6 outlines nursing interventions and care for the consumer with depression.

TABLE 39.6 | Key nursing interventions and principles of care for consumers with depression

Action	Rationale
Accept consumers as they are and adopt a strengths-based recovery focus.	People with depression may have low self-image. Focusing on an individual's strengths promotes supported decision-making and empowerment. A strength-based approach is also aligned with contemporary mental health recovery frameworks in Australia.
Promote the consumer's own decision-making; minimise dependency.	Indecisiveness is a symptom of depression and can mean that consumers struggle to make even the most basic decisions. Supported decision-making is important in empowering individuals to take control over their health, engender independence and improve self-esteem.
Avoid presenting consumers with decisions to make when they are not yet ready to make decisions for themselves.	At the height of a depressive illness, it is best to simply present situations to the consumers that do not require a decision (e.g. 'It's time to come for lunch', 'It's time to have your shower', 'Here is a cup of tea'). However, it is important to collaborate with consumers and involve them in decision-making and as the consumer progresses in their recovery this becomes even more important. Research strongly supports the notion that people involved in making decisions about their care have improved outcomes.
Spend time (brief but frequent) with withdrawn and isolative consumers, even when this feels uncomfortable.	Therapeutic silence is an important skill of a mental health nurse. Withdrawn consumers remain aware of their surroundings and, even if they do not acknowledge the presence of the nurse or communicate in any way, they can be reassured by that presence. Spending time with the consumer communicates the consumer's worth as a person. It may be that the consumer will learn to be comfortable with the nurse and eventually initiate dialogue. A therapeutic relationship is more than 'talking', and sharing silence and space are also important aspects of a caring relationship.
Involve consumers in activities in which they can experience success.	People can feel good about themselves in many ways. Accomplishment is one way to develop a sense of self-worth.
Avoid reinforcing hallucinations or delusions.	While hallucinations and delusions are not commonly seen in depression, they can occur and are usually contextualised to grief or burden and denigration (i.e. they continue to make the person feel worthless and useless and guilty for existing). Validating and acknowledging the distress these experiences cause without concurring in them is important. For example, acknowledging distress is an important response: 'Simon I can imagine how frightening it must be to think that your mum is trying to hurt you'.

(Steele 2023)

People who are depressed are often very vulnerable and this may be, in part, why they often withdraw and isolate themselves. This can make it very challenging for the nurse needing to establish effective communication. Clinical Interest Box 39.9 provides some strategies for promoting effective communication with consumers who have depression.

Depression is a major problem in older adults and may also be accompanied by excessive worry, focus on physical ailments, anxiety and ill-placed guilt. Symptoms of depression in the older age group are relatively common but often go undetected and untreated. This may be because sadness is considered a normal response to the losses associated with ageing, such as physical decline, loss of social role and loss of a spouse, and it may not be recognised when normal sadness and grief have developed into clinical depression requiring treatment. Depression is not a normal part of the ageing process and should always be treated. The age of the person experiencing depression should never factor into *if* it is treated, only *how*. It is important to be aware that men over the age of 85 years have the highest suicide rate in Australia; this exceeds all other age groups and is more than three times the national average (AIHW 2023a). In addition, the complexities of physical illness, the side effects of medication and the symptoms of dementia may combine with symptoms of depression, making diagnosis of what is happening complex and difficult (Foster et al 2022). It is very important for nurses working with older consumers, particularly those with dementia, to be alert for and report changes such as unusual expressions of sadness, increasing focus on physical health, voicing the wish to die, decrease in appetite, reduced enjoyment, loss of interest in activities or other symptoms that may indicate the presence of depression. Clinical Interest Box 39.10 lists some issues relating to the mental health of older adults.

CLINICAL INTEREST BOX 39.9 Strategies for promoting effective communication with consumers who have depression

Acceptance

Spend time with the consumer and accept the person without judgment. People who have depression are not always able to express feelings and may express them through behaviour that is unusual or even bizarre. The nurse should be careful not to make or imply any criticism of the consumer's behaviour because people with depression usually have low self-esteem and are particularly vulnerable to feelings of disapproval that may be interpreted as rejection.

Openness and honesty

Because people with depression are less able than others to tolerate disappointment, the nurse should be truthful at all times and never make promises that for any reason might not be kept. Nor should the nurse offer false reassurance.

It is important for the nurse to develop a trusting relationship with the consumer, and this will only be achieved with honesty. For example, a consumer may wish to share something private with the nurse but not want the nurse to tell anyone else about what is disclosed. The nurse builds trust by telling the consumer that significant information will need to be shared with other members of the healthcare team. The consumer learns to trust the nurse as a professional whose main concern is shown to be the consumer's own best interest.

Empathy

Any attempts to cheer up a depressed consumer may be perceived as a failure to understand their feelings or difficulties. Inappropriate approaches such as this may cause the consumer to withdraw further from interactions and may increase their isolation and depression.

Empathy means facilitating the consumer to express feelings of pain and inner distress and to respond in a way that indicates recognition and understanding of that pain and distress.

Tolerance

People with depression may be unable to make even the simplest decision (e.g. where to sit, what clothing to select and put on). The nurse needs to understand how low mood slows physical as well as mental responses and that the psychomotor retardation is part of the illness, not a deliberate act. It is impossible for consumers with depression to 'shake themselves out of it' and it is not therapeutic to try to badger people with depression into activity. This is likely to result in further feelings of guilt and inadequacy in the consumer. Tolerance is also required for consumers with depression who experience psychomotor agitation.

Underlying anxiety in the depressed consumer may also manifest as hyperactivity or anger and hostility that may be directed towards the nurse. Consumers sometimes shock themselves at the hostile and sometimes hateful things they say to others during periods of depression. It is a normal response for the nurse to feel some frustration and irritation or even anger towards consumers at times, but the nurse must be mindful that the consumer's behaviour is an outward reflection of inner anguish and that to be therapeutic they must remain patient. To assist in this the nurse must reflect on, and implement, the strategies needed to maintain personal mental wellbeing. This may include discussing feeling responses to consumers with a colleague.

(Foster et al 2022; Hungerford et al 2020; Steele 2023)

CLINICAL INTEREST BOX 39.10 Mental health issues in older adults

- The older person is vulnerable to emotional and mental stress from many losses, including the loss of a spouse, loss of social roles and resources, decreased income and loss of status and socialisation associated with paid employment.
- Physical health problems such as chronic illness, disability, visual problems, falls and incontinence.
- Issues with polypharmacy.
- Disorders common in the older population include depression, paranoid reactions and dementias.
- Depression is the most common emotional disorder in the older population.
- Paranoia may be related to depression and/or neurological disorders. It is also associated with sensory deficits and loneliness.
- Of the dementias, the Alzheimer's type is the most common non-reversible dementia.
- The risk of suicide increases with age, with men aged 85 and over being particularly vulnerable.
- Family carers of people with dementia are more likely than other family carers to experience emotional health problems such as stress, exhaustion and depression.

(Dementia Australia 2022)

CRITICAL THINKING EXERCISE 39.3

Max is a 27-year-old man with a previous diagnosis of schizophrenia. In his teens, Max regularly smoked marijuana and had several episodes of drug-induced psychosis. For the past 18 months, Max has been well, meeting with his psychiatrist and treating team regularly and taking his prescribed medication. He has been working in a warehouse for the past 12 months and has been approached about being the new storeman. While Max is very excited by this opportunity, he is also very nervous and worried about it. His worry about the job interview has impacted his sleeping and more recently he has been skipping doses of the aripiprazole that he has been on for years. Last week, Max became convinced that his neighbour has been breaking into his house when he is at work and tampering with his food. This has prompted him to miss days of work, so he can keep watch on his neighbour and now his boss is upset with him. Max is feeling very stressed and worried. Last night, Max heard the voice of his grandfather telling him to confront his neighbour and 'sort this out like men'. When his neighbour leaves his house in the morning to go to work, Max confronts him about the food tampering and an altercation ensues.

1. Define the terms hallucination and delusion and identify where these phenomena are expressed in Max's case.
2. A risk assessment is an integral role of the mental health nurse. What risks do you think Max may pose?
3. Investigate the recovery framework. Discuss four ways a mental health nurse could support a consumer like Max in their recovery.

The consumer experiencing feelings of anger and hostility

Anger is a feeling experienced by most people at certain times. It generally occurs in response to fear, confusion or frustration. Anger often occurs in response to the anxiety a person feels when a threat is perceived. Most people have little difficulty in handling mild anger, which is experienced as annoyance and usually subsides quickly. Feelings of anger, disappointment and frustration may be expressed verbally or non-verbally (e.g. by swearing or kicking a car when it will not start). When a person is very frustrated, such as when they are unable to attain an important goal, anger may become more intense. A person experiencing intense anger may try to disperse the unpleasant feeling through an angry outburst or an act of aggression. Occasionally, a person may be so consumed by feelings of anger that they become violent and pose a threat to themselves and to others nearby.

Nurses may encounter anger while providing nursing care (e.g. a person whose health is disrupted becomes frustrated, and frustration can lead to anger). Sometimes people express their anger through verbal or physical abuse towards others, including staff members. Therefore, it is important that nurses are aware of the reasons why a person may be angry, of their own responses to outbursts of angry feelings and of how to help a consumer to express anger in an appropriate manner. Anger may be the result of various stressors. Some of the factors that may cause anger or aggression in people who are in hospital for any reason include:

- a feeling of loss of control and/or independence, particularly evident when the consumer has no insight into their illness and is compulsorily (or involuntarily) detained
- a sense of isolation from family and familiar environment
- a feeling of loss of identity or individuality
- feelings of fear and discomfort because of inadequate privacy
- anxiety about the possible outcomes of illness (e.g. altered body image).

Some of the specific risk factors leading to a potential for aggression in consumers with mental illness have been identified as:

- a diagnosis of an illness with paranoid features (paranoia can lead to fears that induce aggressive acts aimed at defending against a perceived threat—for example, the belief that someone is plotting against you or trying to harm or kill you can lead to lashing out at that person defensively)
- substance misuse
- deterioration in family and/or social relationships
- a previous history of aggression or violence and declared threats of violence
- developmental history of exposure to aggression and violence
- non-adherence to a medication regimen
- failure to learn to delay gratification of wants (e.g. extreme frustration when need is not met immediately)
- failure to learn alternative strategies other than aggressive responses
- unresolved conflicts
- hostility to authority
- denial of aggressive behaviour
- lack of remorse.

(Foster et al 2022)

Aggressive outbursts may occur when a person is unable to find a solution to a problem that is causing fear, confusion or frustration. Aggressive action may be directed towards the person or object perceived as the source of the frustration, or at other persons or objects in the vicinity. Displacement is a defence mechanism whereby a consumer discharges pent-up feelings, such as anger, on a person or object other than the one that aroused the feelings (Halter 2021). Approaches for dealing with anger and hostile behaviour in the mental health care environment are outlined in Table 39.7. Nurses may apply the principles of these approaches, when necessary and appropriate, in any healthcare setting.

TABLE 39.7 | Approaches for dealing with anger and hostile behaviour in the mental health care environment

Action	Rationale
Accept the consumer but make it clear that certain behaviours are not acceptable and provide alternatives for expressing anger.	This is a non-judgmental approach that informs the consumer that they are accepted as a person but that certain aspects of their behaviour are not appropriate.
Acknowledge the person's anger and their right to their feelings.	This demonstrates respect and acceptance of the consumer. Use terms such as 'I can see that you're really frustrated right now...'
Be careful not to cite policy in response to anger.	Most individuals react poorly to being told a 'policy says no' or being told to 'calm down'.
Validate feelings of anger.	Acknowledge the consumer's anger: 'Sarah, I can see that you are really upset at the moment. It's very frustrating when you feel like no-one is trying to help you'.
Allow expression of the anger in appropriate safe ways (e.g. voicing angry feelings verbally, discharging anger in non-destructive acts such as not damaging property or person).	Anger is self-limiting and it may be better to let it run its course than to forcibly try to stop an angry person. Attempting to stop the person's expression of anger can restimulate the aggressive feelings and lead to a continuance of displayed anger.
Try to remain calm (self-talk and relaxation techniques such as deep breathing and muscle relaxation can help with this). Provide psychological containment by staying in the same calm 'gear' and avoiding any tendency to retaliate or placate.	Anger should always be met with calm, despite how difficult this can be. Consumers need their feelings to be acknowledged and understood; retaliation and appeasing do not achieve this.
Be aware of your body language—try not to communicate threatening non-verbal signals (e.g. keep your hands in a low position) and avoid trying to touch a consumer who is agitated.	Raised hands may be interpreted as a threatening gesture, particularly by consumers who are experiencing paranoia, confusion or disorientation, and such a gesture may be interpreted as indicating a failure to understand the consumer's feelings and point of view. Touching a person who is agitated may be interpreted as threatening, and consumers who are paranoid may already be experiencing heightened fear.
Do not try to defend the person or situation the consumer is feeling angry about.	Simply listen, emphasise and validate. Consider how you would feel in a similar situation. What would make you feel better?
Set limits and be firm and consistent in treatment approaches. Encourage the consumer to take control by raising awareness of options at times of angry feelings (e.g. time-out, walking/talking with nurse, medication). The consumer should also be aware of potential outcomes if self-restraint is not possible (in a non-punitive manner).	A consumer at risk of aggressive outburst is helped to remain in control if limits on what is acceptable are clear and alternative options for dealing with feelings are provided (e.g. exercise, informing and seeking help from a nurse or other therapist when feelings are surfacing). It is important to ensure that all staff are consistent with limit-setting and send the same messages to the consumer.
Later, when the consumer is calm, assist them to explore the immediate cause of the anger and anything that precipitated the aggressive response.	Recognition of triggers can assist with problem-solving and is a useful tool for consumers for when they are discharged.
Help the consumer engage in problem-solving and exploring alternative ways of handling their feelings.	Engaging the consumer in solving their own problems is empowering because it informs the consumer that they can take responsibility for their actions. This is also very important for when consumers are discharged and managing volatile situations by themselves.

TABLE 39.7 | Approaches for dealing with anger and hostile behaviour in the mental health care environment—cont'd

Action	Rationale
Consider negotiating.	Negotiating provides options and helps to empower a person who may feel that they have no choices. 'Betty, I can see that you're really frustrated right now, and I have some medication here for you now. Would you like to take it in a liquid or tablet form today?'
Do not make promises that you cannot keep or enact.	This will damage your therapeutic relationship and will likely result in increasing anger.
Be supportive and provide positive feedback when the consumer controls hostile or aggressive behaviour.	Positive reinforcement is a way of helping people to modify unwanted behaviour.
Accept that some anger may be displaced or projected onto you.	The defence mechanisms of displacement and projection serve to reduce the anxiety and the threat to self caused by the intense emotions. Understanding this helps the nurse to avoid taking the hostility personally.
Avoid multiple staff talking.	This can result in confusion and may make a consumer who is already possibly experiencing decreased cognitive capacity feel even more overwhelmed.
Where possible, see if a staff member (who has an established therapeutic relationship with the consumer) can de-escalate them.	Consumers, like all people, respond best to people they are comfortable with and have an existing positive relationship with. Such staff members are also more likely to have a better understanding of the consumer's individual circumstances.
Do not take unnecessary risks. If a person's anger is not subsiding but is in danger of escalating into destructive or violent acts, take action to protect yourself and others (e.g. duress alarm, remove yourself and others from the area, seek assistance from others).	Workplace safety is very important, and nurses have rights in relation to workplace safety. Apart from the risk of personal harm to the nurse or others, the consumer who causes harm can later feel devastated by what has happened. Such an occurrence can be extremely destructive to the person's self-esteem and to the therapeutic process.
Debrief with colleagues after the incident and seek any additional support that you feel you require.	Dealing with aggression is challenging and can be frightening. Debriefing is a way of relieving the associated stress and can serve to identify ways for nurses to reduce risks and improve responses in the future. Debriefing is valuable in seeing the aspects of the intervention that worked well and those that did not and this can help inform any subsequent de-escalation.

(Foster et al 2022; Halter 2023; Hungerford et al 2020; Steele 2023; Hercelinskyj & Alexander 2022)

Preventing aggression and violence is important for the wellbeing of consumers and others. Assertive behaviour is one constructive way of dealing with anger. To be assertive is to stand up for oneself while considering other people's interests and feelings. It takes time to develop the ability to be assertive when people are in the habit of being subservient or responding to situations they are unhappy with by being aggressive. It is within the role of MHNs to conduct training for consumers who will be helped by developing assertiveness skills.

The consumer who is at risk of self-destructive behaviour

Self-destructive behaviour is that which results in physical harm and, sometimes, in the person's own death by suicide. Self-destructive behaviour includes self-mutilation and any form of suicidal activity. Other self-destructive behaviours may include illicit substance or alcohol misuse, often in response to difficulty in coping with an event or situation.

Deliberate self-harm

Deliberate self-harm results from overwhelming psychological distress and is the deliberate destruction of body tissue without conscious intent of suicide (Hercelinskyj & Alexander 2022). While the intent is not to die with self-harm, it can still occur unintentionally (e.g. an accidental overdose or cutting too deep). Self-harm may occur once, or it may become repetitive. It may or may not be impulsive. It is a behaviour associated with a range of mental health conditions including:

- childhood and physical and sexual abuse
- schizophrenia
- drug-induced psychosis and substance use disorders
- borderline personality disorder
- eating disorders
- cognitive impairment disorders
- depressive and mood disorders
- obsessive-compulsive disorder
- post-traumatic stress disorder.

(Foster et al 2022)

Self-harm may involve skin cutting, severe skin scratching or burning, head banging, self-biting, eyeball pressing, tearing out hair, self-punching or inserting dangerous objects into body orifices such as the vagina or rectum. It may involve skin carving (words, designs, symbols), bone breaking or interfering with healing by picking at wounds. Very rarely, extremely serious acts of self-mutilation occur, such as eye enucleation or amputating fingers, toes or genital organs. Other behaviours that may be considered self-destructive include involvement in unsafe sex, irresponsible gambling or spending, substance misuse, driving recklessly and binge eating (Foster et al 2022; Hungerford et al 2020). The reason for self-mutilation is not totally clear but various explanations are possible. It may be:

- a maladaptive coping mechanism that raises low self-esteem by denying helplessness or powerlessness
- a self-punishing act that helps relieve unconscious feelings of guilt
- risk-taking behaviour that, when overcome, raises self-esteem
- a way to reconnect to feeling real and alive, as opposed to feeling empty or feeling nothing
- a way of releasing endorphins
- a way of releasing tension or anger
- using physical pain to create distraction from emotional pain
- an unspoken request for nurturing and love
- a 'cry for help'.

Nursing skills for helping consumers manage self-harming behaviour include:

- adopting an empathic and non-judgmental attitude
- demonstrating support and using active listening
- encouraging the consumer to share their thoughts and feelings about self-harm
- helping the consumer to identify personal triggers and stressors
- exploring with the consumer adaptive ways to cope with uncomfortable feelings
- gaining the consumer's agreement that they will contact a staff member if they experience negative or overwhelming thoughts concerning self-harm
- demonstrating a sense of calm and safety for the consumer
- staying with the consumer and providing support if they are distressed
- telling the consumer that you will spend time with them when they need emotional support
- encouraging the consumer to engage in their usual activities and self-care where possible
- maintaining a safe environment—removing harmful substances or objects from the consumer and the area
- selecting a room that is close to the nurses' station to keep the consumer safe
- providing safer means to experience physical pain that do not result in disfigurement, such as holding ice to a location on the body the consumer wishes to cut or harm
- following the policies and procedures of the setting regarding observation and medication.

(Foster et al 2022; Hungerford et al 2020; Hercelinskyj & Alexander 2022)

Suicidal behaviour

Suicide is an action where the intention is to result in self-inflicted death, as opposed to self-harm, where the intention is to hurt oneself but not die. Self-destructive behaviour may result from any stress a person perceives as overwhelming and is commonly associated with low self-esteem. Suicide may also be an impulsive act in response to a distressing situation or event where the person has an overwhelming sense of being unable to recover (Hercelinskyj & Alexander 2022). For example, a significant gambling debt that will result in the loss of the family home, or criminal charges that may result in incarceration. When the sense of self-worth is extremely low, self-destructive behaviour reaches its peak and it is at this point that the risk of suicidal behaviour is likely. Suicidal behaviour implies a loss of the ability to see oneself as being of any value or worth at all (Foster et al 2022). Some of the risk factors for suicide are identified in Table 39.8.

It is important to utilise sensitive language when discussing suicide. Acceptable terms include:

- died by suicide
- suicided
- suicide survivor
- took their own life
- bereaved by suicide (e.g. for a family member).

There are also terms to avoid. Most of these are not appropriate because they give the impression that suicide was a desirable goal or have a legal stigmatising connotation. Terms to avoid include:

- successful suicide
- failed suicide attempt

TABLE 39.8 | Suicide risk factors

Variable	Risk categories
Age	Risk generally increases with age, but also at particular risk are young men aged between 15 and 44 years and men over 75.
Cultural heritage	Aboriginal and Torres Strait Islander People experience suicide at rates three times those of non-Aboriginal and Torres Strait Islander People. Aboriginal and Torres Strait Islander People are also more likely to be bereaved by suicide.
Marital status	Higher risk in single, widowed, separated and divorced people. The death of a loved one is a particular risk factor in the older population.
Gender	More common in men than in women (more women engage in suicide behaviour but more males die). Males represent 75% of suicide statistics in Australia.
Physical health	Those experiencing chronic, debilitating, progressive or life-threatening illness. Alcohol and drug misuse/addiction. Sleep disorder/deprivation.
Psychological health	Low self-esteem. Depression. Feelings of hopelessness. Feelings of loneliness and abandonment ('nobody cares'). Experience of significant loss. Unrelenting and distressing hallucinations/delusions. Command hallucinations (auditory hallucinations instructing the person to self-harm). Impulsiveness, hostility and aggression. Bereaved by suicide.
Social health	Social isolation/exclusion or sense of alienation. Poor level of social supports. Conflict with supportive others. Social upheaval (e.g. divorce, accommodation changes). Unemployment and those in low paid, unskilled employment. Poverty and poor living conditions (e.g. homelessness).
History	Suicide behaviours in previous 12 months. Previous suicidal actions. Family history of suicide. Expressed intent. Evidence of planning (e.g. has given away possessions, made a will, said goodbyes). Evidence of preparation (i.e. has the means available—e.g. has a gun, has the pills). Early recovery phase in severe depression.

(Hercelinskyj & Alexander 2022)

- unsuccessful suicide attempt
- committed suicide
- completed suicide.

(Hercelinskyj & Alexander 2022)

Risk assessment is a crucial intervention in estimating a person's intent to self-harm or end their own life, and a formal risk assessment should be conducted whenever a mental state examination is conducted. It should be noted that the successful use of an assessment tool involves the ability to establish effective open and honest communication with the consumer, and expertise in the art of therapeutic communication is perhaps the most important component of the MHN's contribution to care (see Chapter 10).

The first priority in working with a person who is at risk of, or exhibits, self-destructive behaviour is to protect the person from harm. All dangerous or potentially dangerous objects that could be used in an act of self-harm should be removed from the consumer's environment. This includes knives and other sharp implements, matches, glass, phone chargers, items of clothing such as belts, scarves or stockings or anything else that may be used by the consumer to inflict self-harm. Other approaches for working with self-harm and suicidal behaviour are outlined in Table 39.9. While it takes time and experience to become an accomplished MHN, and the care and management of at-risk consumers requires expertise, the principles of care, when

TABLE 39.9 | Approaches for dealing with self-harm and suicidal behaviour in the mental health care environment

Action	Rationale
Engage in an open exploration of suicidal ideas, including the frequency and intrusiveness of the thoughts, the planning and motivation.	Open exploration is an essential component of identifying the level of risk of self-harm. Any statement that alludes to self-harm (e.g. a threat or suggestion made by the consumer that they are thinking about harming themself) should be taken seriously.
Assess the risk factors.	All consumers need a formal risk assessment when in the mental health unit. Risk-minimisation strategies appropriate to the level of risk identified should be put in place (e.g. close observation, removal of objects deemed unsafe, contractual agreement for the consumer to report to the nurse when thoughts of self-harm are likely to be acted on). Mental health care agencies usually have specific guidelines and policies for management of consumers at risk of self-harm.
Be with consumers in a calm, accepting and empathic manner.	Facilitates open and honest communication and the development of a therapeutic relationship.
Engage in therapeutic conversation that facilitates the safe expression of distress and the identification of the underlying issues and concerns.	Helps the consumer to identify the factors (stressors) responsible for wanting to engage in self-harm and will inform as to the measures that are appropriate to facilitate the healing of mental anguish. Therapeutic silence is also powerful. Often, remaining quietly with the consumer without speaking is a powerful tool.
Recognise the opportunity for learning, personal growth and positive change as a potential outcome of the consumer's present experience.	Recognising that positive outcomes are possible stimulates a sense of hope in the nurse, which can be relayed to the consumer. Hope and realistic optimism facilitate recovery.
Work collaboratively with at-risk consumers, their significant others and other health professionals in assessing needs and planning care.	Appropriate interventions may involve different areas of professional expertise (e.g. recreational therapist, psychiatrist, dietitian, psychologist). The consumer's significant others may need to be aware of the strategies required to maintain the consumer's safety and their involvement can be supportive for the consumer.
An appropriately qualified person should negotiate a risk-minimisation plan with the consumer and significant others.	Risk-minimisation plans may involve a contractual agreement, and this needs to be firm and clear. Nurses are advised to work with experienced staff in relation to these before attempting to implement them.
Be clear about the consumer's responsibility for their own safety within the context of the plan.	Consumers need to understand that, within the contractual arrangement, control of the situation is theirs. This is empowering, but consumers also need to feel supported in managing their feelings.
The care plan must be clear to all staff working in the consumer's environment (see Nursing Care Plan 39.1 as an example).	It is a team responsibility to support and protect the consumers and facilitate the success of the contractual arrangement.
Be clear about the availability of support when a person feels unsafe, and ensure the person understands the boundaries that apply.	The consumer needs to be clear about who is available and when they can provide support, and the type of support that is possible. This ensures that the risk of dependency on staff is reduced and the consumer's sense of responsibility in the situation is reinforced.
Mobilise social support.	Social support is important in maximising the consumer's coping abilities. It can also assist the consumer to increase self-esteem (e.g. by promoting relationships with others). For consumers who are at risk but living in the community, arrangements may be made for another person to 'keep the means' (e.g. the consumer's medication), and for people to visit the consumer during times of the day when they are likely to be on their own.
Engage in problem-solving with the consumer.	Helps maximise the consumer's constructive coping strategies and develop others.

TABLE 39.9 | Approaches for dealing with self-harm and suicidal behaviour in the mental health care environment—cont'd

Action	Rationale
The nurse must be aware of personal and team responsibilities and accountability in relation to caring for at-risk consumers.	Consumer safety depends on staff fulfilling responsibilities. Responsibilities include knowing which consumers are demonstrating an increasing risk of self-harm (e.g. increasing alienation) and which are showing signs of improvement (e.g. smiling, interacting with others). The nurse should be aware that signs of improvement can be misleading (e.g. the consumer has decided to end their life and are at peace with this decision and feel a sense of relief).

(Foster et al 2022; Hungerford et al 2020)

NURSING CARE PLAN 39.1

Assessment: Relapse schizophrenia.
Issue/s to be addressed: Disturbed thought process.
Goal/s: To develop trusting relationship with staff.
To be adherent with medication regimen, resulting in improvement in mental state.
For mental state to improve.

Care/actions	Rationale
Establish rapport/therapeutic relationship with Eli.	Trust and collaboration are important factors of the therapeutic relationship. Eli will approach staff when feeling distressed and staff will implement distraction techniques.
Promote need for prescribed medication through psychoeducation.	Engage Eli in a discussion about why he does not want to take his medication. Choice regarding treatment preferences is mandated by most state and territory mental health legislation. Research indicates that consumers who are aware of the common side effects of their medication are more likely to remain adherent. Psychotropic medications have demonstrated efficacy in reducing distress and agitation of psychosis, and Eli has a history of responding therapeutically to psychotropic medication in the past.
Frequent mental state examination (MSE).	Changes in MSE may be indicative of medication adherence and efficacy of medication. Alternatively, decline in MSE may be indicative of non-adherence to medication regimen and/or poor response to specific medication.

Evaluation: Eli has developed a trusting rapport with his primary nurse Paula and seeks out staff when distressed. Eli has taken an active role in decision-making processes and his recovery.
While at times Eli demonstrates a mistrust of medication, he has remained adherent, and his mental state has improved.
Psychoeducation continues to remain important, and frequent discussions about Eli's individual treatment preferences are ongoing.
Daily MSE has indicated an improvement in psychotic symptoms, indicating response to medication.
Assessment: Relapse schizophrenia.
Issue/s to be addressed: Reduced nutritional intake.
Goal/s: To develop trust with Eli so that he is comfortable taking food from staff.
To monitor weight.

Continued

NURSING CARE PLAN 39.1—cont'd

Care/actions	Rationale
Staff continue to engage with Eli and develop a trusting rapport: • Have someone he trusts bring in food. • Observe Eli preparing his own food. • Medication adherence.	If Eli trusts staff, he may feel more secure in eating food from the unit. Not 'forcing' Eli to eat unit food may help alleviate his paranoia.
Monitor hydration/nutrition through observation of hydration levels and weight, in addition to observing eating/drinking behaviours.	To ensure that Eli remains hydrated and is eating regularly. To ensure that Eli is cognisant of the potential for his medication to result in iatrogenic complications such as metabolic syndrome, and to ensure that his weight is controlled. Educate him that due to existing hypertension and hyperlipidaemia, he will need ongoing close monitoring.

Evaluation: Eli has developed good rapport with staff on the unit and he has begun to eat food on the unit. Eli has remained well hydrated and nourished. Continue to monitor weight and provide healthy choice options and education about diet.

(Hercelinskyj & Alexander 2022)

necessary and appropriate, may be applied by others in any healthcare setting to protect consumers.

Deliberate self-harm and suicide are complex issues, and a simple and brief overview has been provided here. Since people with depression and self-harming tendencies may be encountered in every area of nursing, it is recommended that nurses explore the issues further by accessing psychiatric or mental health nursing textbooks and state government policies. See, for example, Suicide Prevention Practice (Queensland Health 2021) or Suicide Prevention Network (Black Dog Institute 2023).

The consumer who experiences elevation of mood

Mood elevation can be a manifestation of a variety of mental health disorders, or caused by the misuse of certain substances, such as cocaine and amphetamines (Foster et al 2022) but is particularly associated with bipolar disorders. Bipolar disorders are a group of mood disorders that manifest with periods of depression and mania, usually interspersed with periods of balanced, or 'normal' mood (Hercelinskyj & Alexander 2022). The elevation associated with mania is quite different from the normal exuberant activity engaged in by most people at various times. Hypomania is a clinical syndrome like, but not as severe as, mania (Hercelinskyj & Alexander 2022). Previously, people who experienced the mood cycles associated with bipolar disorders were said to have a 'manic-depressive' illness.

Mania is characterised by excitability, an increase in goal-directed activities, marked hyperactivity, talkativeness and a decreased need for sleep (APA 2022). The symptoms vary in intensity. In the milder form, people can appear to have excess energy, they may present as the 'life and soul of the party', be able to work long hours and be very productive in work and leisure activities and function on little sleep. If the symptoms increase to the most severe level (where psychosis occurs), people may experience serious impairment in judgment that allows them to behave in ways not usually in keeping with their personalities. For example, a normally shy and quiet woman may become loud, dress in bright and gaudy clothing and become overtly sexually provocative; a normally sensible and frugal young man may run up huge and unmanageable debts on his credit card, drive his car at outrageously dangerous speeds and yell obscenities out of the car window as he narrowly misses other vehicles and pedestrians. Such dangerous and life-threatening behaviours may be of no concern to the affected person if they have psychotic symptoms, because delusional thoughts may make them believe that they are indestructible. For example, the young man above may believe that he is immortal because he is a new god come to save the world. Common symptoms associated with mania are summarised in Table 39.10. People who are experiencing the severe form of mania may need to be admitted to an inpatient unit for treatment, especially if their insight is impaired, which is common.

Treatment includes firm boundary setting, cognitive therapy, counselling and medication. Lithium (a mood stabiliser, or antimanic) is one drug that is effective in treating the symptoms of mania and in reducing or preventing recurrence of the mood fluctuations associated with bipolar disorders. However, lithium and other drugs often cause unwanted side effects and levels in the blood require strict monitoring to prevent lithium toxicity. In addition, some of the feelings of elation and mania are enjoyed, so consumers are understandably not always

TABLE 39.10 | Common symptoms associated with mania

Type	Symptoms
Affective (mood)	Labile, irritable, elation or euphoria. Expansiveness. Humorousness (witty). Inflated self-esteem. Intolerance of criticism. Lack of shame or guilt.
Physiological	Dehydration. Inadequate nutrition. Weight loss. Reduced need for sleep.
Cognitive	Ambitiousness. Denial of realistic dangers. Distractibility and poor attention span. Flight of ideas (jumping from one train of thought to another without pause). Grandiosity (e.g. delusions of grandeur). Illusions. Lack of judgment and impaired decision-making (e.g. unable to evaluate realistic danger and consequences of actions). Looseness of associations. Delusions.
Behavioural	Irritability/argumentativeness/aggressiveness especially if thwarted in achieving what is desired. Excessive spending when unemployed or broke and other forms of irresponsibility. Grandiose acts that may involve excessive risk taking (e.g. overspending, risky sexual behaviours). Increased motor activity and pressure of speech (extreme rapidity). Impulsiveness (e.g. making important financial decisions with little thought). Poor or bizarre personal grooming (e.g. unusual and frequent clothing choices, failure to attend to ADLs). May wear bright and ornate clothing (reflect elevated mood). Sexual provocativeness and sexual hyperactivity that is often promiscuous. Excessive involvement in pleasurable activities without regard for negative consequences (e.g. swimming in dangerous conditions, unprotected sexual activity with strangers).

(Foster et al 2022; Hercelinskyj & Alexander 2022; Hungerford et al 2020; Steele 2023)

willing to take the medications that stop the feelings so drastically, and they may seek alternative ways of controlling the illness. Nursing interventions vary according to the level of mania and include:

- maintaining consumer's safety and the safety of others
- maintaining the consumer's biological normality (e.g. meeting rest, nutrition, fluid and elimination needs)
- facilitating activities of daily living (e.g. meeting hygiene needs)
- helping the consumer to regain and maintain self-control
- preserving the consumer's dignity when behaviour is out of character and when it will be a source of embarrassment or humiliation when functioning more normally (a manic episode has a particularly high risk of damage to a person's reputation)
- reducing the amount of stimulation to which the consumer is subjected
- providing a structured daily program that allows opportunities to expend energy in set activities (e.g. physical activity such as using an exercise bike or walking may help to drain excess energy)
- promoting sleep and rest (which may require sedatives such as temazepam).

The overall goals of care are to help lower the consumer's mood to a more stable level, to promote insight and restore functioning. To do this, the MHN must establish and maintain a trusting relationship with the consumer. Attempting to do this can be challenging and frustrating for the nurse, partly because particular unusual speech patterns are common in people experiencing episodes of mania, which impact on the ability to communicate effectively, particularly when consumers are in the acute phase of mania. The speech patterns associated with mania are listed in Clinical Interest Box 39.11.

CLINICAL INTEREST BOX 39.11 Examples of speech patterns associated with mania

Speech pattern	Description
Pressured speech	Rapid and accelerated speech that continues without pauses between words or sentences. The flow of rapid talking continues without regard to others who may be attempting to answer, intervene or add something.
Clang associations	The stringing together of words that rhyme without regard to their meaning. Words are chosen for their sound, not their meaning.
Circumstantiality	Use of long irrelevant descriptions when trying to describe a person, situation or event. The account may include vast amounts of irrelevant and unrelated information and may include lots of repetition.
Loose associations	Lack of a logical relationship between thoughts and ideas that renders spoken communication vague, unfocused (waffly) and diffuse (longwinded).
Flight of ideas	A nearly continuous flow of accelerated speech characterised by abrupt verbal skipping from topic to topic, usually based on chance associations between words.
Tangentially	Constantly diverging in mid-conversation to different and unrelated topics. When describing a situation, frequently losing the train of thought, and not completing descriptions of anything.

(Hercelinskyj & Alexander 2022)

Some of the factors that present challenges to nurses in developing therapeutic relationships are that the consumer may:

- Have a brief attention span.
- Find it difficult to be still, and need to be in perpetual motion.
- Find it difficult to listen to others and constantly interrupt.
- Appear unaware of verbal and non-verbal cues indicating that others wish to speak.
- Continue with a constant stream of speech that is sometimes unintelligible.
- Have confused thinking, with thoughts racing one after the other (this makes it difficult for the consumer to make connections between concepts and so when speaking they may jump rapidly from one subject to another).
- Have diminished awareness of personal space boundaries and tend to invade the 'intimate zone' of others.
- Have little understanding of how overpowering, excessive and confrontational their interactions can feel to others.
- Test the rules and limits set for the therapeutic environment.
- Be insistent on having their own way and may attempt to manipulate people, including the nurse, to achieve this.
- Be consumed by delusional beliefs (e.g. that they are scientist with a new cure for COVID-19 and are on the brink of international recognition for their insights).
- Frequently insult staff or others, use foul or sexually explicit language, taunt and annoy others (when consumers regain insight, they are often devastated by these behaviours).
- Be seductive towards the nurse (among others)—this is because one of the elements of mania is hedonism and people can be hypersexualised.

(Hercelinskyj & Alexander 2022; Halter 2023)

Management includes setting clear limits on behaviour while being supportive but firm. Setting limits involves reinforcing that it is the behaviour and not the person that is rejected. For example, it is preferable to say, 'That sort of language is not accepted in this unit', rather than, 'You are so crude speaking like that'.

The nurse always needs to remain calm, speak clearly and explain what is required simply and firmly but in a caring manner. Staff should be mindful of not mirroring manic behaviour, ensuring they take note of the tone, speed and volume of their speech and voice. All staff must be aware of the limits and rules set for the consumer's behaviour, which must be constantly reinforced to assist the consumer to regain control of their behaviour. It must be remembered that behaviours that appear manipulative, fault finding or exploitative of others' vulnerabilities are the outward expression of inner turmoil, distress, and often serious emotional need. Such behaviour is the consumer's way of trying to gain a sense of control at a time when they have no control of most aspects of their life, including their own thoughts or feelings (Halter 2023). Table 39.11 provides some approaches for dealing with hyperactivity associated with the manic

TABLE 39.11 | Approaches for managing elevation of mood associated with bipolar disorders (manic or hypomanic phase)

Action	Rationale
Use a firm and calm approach.	This helps promote a therapeutic relationship and is reassuring for the consumer and provides structure and control for a consumer who is out of control.
Use short concise explanations or statements.	A short concentration span and confused thinking make it difficult for the consumer to absorb complex information. Avoid providing lengthy discussions as individuals with poor concentration can rarely stay on topic and may become frustrated.
Remain neutral, avoid power struggles and value judgments.	Avoids provoking hostility or combativeness. Consumers can use inconsistencies and value judgments as justification for arguing and escalating mania. Nurses need to operate on the notion of unconditional positive regard.
Maintain a consistent approach (e.g. provide a consistent and structured environment and keep expectations the same).	This provides the framework that assists the consumers to regain a feeling of control. Clear and consistent limits and expectations minimise the potential for consumers to misunderstand discussions, and ensures equal treatment.
Firmly redirect energy into appropriate and constructive channels, provide an outlet for physical energy in a non-stimulating environment (e.g. use of a punching bag in a quiet area).	Helps in establishing constructive mechanisms for coping with excess energy. Can help release pent-up hostility and relieve muscle tension.
Decrease environmental stimuli whenever possible (e.g. avoid loud music, noises, bright lights, people).	Limits distractions that can elevate consumers further, and impacts on concentration levels.
Provide structured solitary activities—tasks that take minimal concentration are best. Avoid groups and stimulating activities.	Solitary activities are best until distractibility is settled, and the consumer can comfortably tolerate being part of a group. This may also be best for other consumers who may find the consumer with mania challenging.
Spend one-on-one time with the consumer, especially when psychotic or anxious.	Provides reassurance and gives the message that the consumer is a worthwhile person. As mania and mood elevation settles, provide time for exploration of issues.
Encourage frequent rest periods. Provide high-calorie fluids and finger foods frequently throughout the day. Daily, monitor the consumer's sleep pattern, food and fluid intake and elimination pattern (constipation is a common problem).	It is important that the consumer's physical wellbeing is maintained during the time they are not concerned with it themselves.
Provide the consumer and the family with explanations and written information about the illness and the treatment plan (it is particularly important that the consumer and family, if appropriate, understand the information concerning medication).	Information is important for consumers and carers to facilitate decision-making. Consumers who understand their medication, its effects and side effects have higher rates of medication adherence and reduced incidences of relapse.
Ensure consumer and family or significant others understand how to access the supportive services in the community.	Knowing about community supports includes information about accessing help in a crisis, which can be reassuring. Information about support groups and activities aimed at prevention are helpful in promoting coping mechanisms and recovery.

(Foster et al 2022; Hercelinskyj & Alexander 2022; Hungerford et al 2020; Steele 2023)

phases of bipolar disorders, but the principles apply to consumers experiencing excessive or mood elevation from any cause.

Bipolar disorders and any disorder in which mood and behaviour elevation is a serious problem can be potentially devastating for consumers and their families. It is an important part of the MHN's role to ensure that everyone affected understands about the illness causing the behaviour and is aware of what can and cannot be done to control the illness, and what services and supports are available to help them to cope.

CRITICAL THINKING EXERCISE 39.4

Raj is a 33-year-old married father of three boys. Raj has experienced significant periods of depression since he was a university student but has responded well to treatment and maintains his visits with his psychologist. Raj has also had periods where he was 'high' or very happy but because these experiences were so wonderful and he could be productive in his job as a manager in IT, he didn't see the need to ask for help. As a busy parent and IT consultant Raj has found his sleep disturbed in the past, but nothing like what is happening now. Raj hasn't slept the last two nights and he is consumed by his new idea to open up an internet café. Yesterday Raj left his three small children unattended at home to look for a property. He brought his idea up with his wife Sita, who thinks it is ridiculous. Sita becomes very concerned when she learns that Raj has gone to the bank and applied for a $100,000 personal loan. Outline the different symptoms Raj is exhibiting that may suggest he is experiencing a manic episode. What risk factors are present?

Consumers experiencing confusion or disorientation

A person may become confused or disoriented for a variety of reasons, including as a result of delirium or dementia, or from the toxic effects of alcohol and some prescribed medications or illicit drugs. The effect in each case is a significant marked change in cognitive abilities from the consumer's previous level of functioning. Cognitive functioning includes the mental processes of memory, reasoning, judgment, orientation, problem-solving, decision-making, the acquisition of knowledge and the ability to use and comprehend language. Some causes of cognitive dysfunction are reversible, others are not. Delirium, for example, is a syndrome that involves a disturbance to a person's state of consciousness, which is accompanied by changes in cognition, almost always due to an identifiable cause that can in most cases be rectified. Dementia, on the other hand, is a progressive, irreversible and disabling condition in which changes in cognitive function are caused by gradually increasing, permanent damage to the brain. The focus here is on caring for those with progressive dementia.

Dementia is one of the most common causes of confusion and disorientation, with over 400,000 people in Australia currently identified as having the illness (Australian Institute of Health & Welfare 2023b). It is a condition normally associated with older consumers but, although the risk of dementia does increase with age, more than 27,000 of those identified as having dementia are under age 65 (Dementia Australia 2022a). Alzheimer's disease (AD) is the most common form of the illness, but all types of dementia share similar symptoms and require similar interventions. Dementia is currently the second leading cause of death in Australia, and the leading cause of death for women (Dementia Australia 2022b). Dementia is associated with high rates of diagnosed comorbid mental illness in residents of aged-care facilities (affecting up to 50% of dementia sufferers) (Dementia Australia 2022b). The symptoms depend on the sequence in which areas of the brain are damaged by the disease process, so the progression of symptoms varies in different people. Symptoms change and increase in severity over the duration of the illness, which in the case of AD can be 3–20 years, the average span being 7–10 years (Dementia Australia 2022c). Symptoms include:

- Gradual memory loss.
- Increasing loss of language and communication skills.
- Progressive decline in ability to perform routine tasks despite having intact physical functioning (in the early stages of dementia this may mean difficulty with coordination when preparing a meal or when shopping and handling money, or when driving a car. Later this extends to include difficulty with tasks such as dressing, eating and bathing).
- Impaired judgment, abstract thinking.
- Difficulty in concentrating and learning new information or skills.
- Changes in behaviour (e.g. wandering, incessant walking, constant repetition of words, confabulation).
- Changes in personality and mood (up to two-thirds of people with AD have symptoms of depression, and about 20% exhibit aggression).
- Hallucinations and delusions (hallucinations are experienced by about 16% of people with AD, delusions by about 30% and they are often paranoid in nature).
- Loss of initiative.
- Altered sleep–wake patterns.
- Loss of bladder and bowel continence (usually later stage).

(Dementia Australia 2022c)

Caring for the consumer with dementia

Care interventions for a consumer with dementia are dependent on the consumer's abilities, and the focus of care should be on what the consumer can still do, rather on abilities lost. General care interventions are listed in Table 39.12 and in Clinical Interest Box 39.12. (See Chapter 24 for more information.)

TABLE 39.12 | Information for nurses and for consumers with dementia and their family carers

Information that nurses need to know	Information that nurses need to give people with dementia and their family carers
• Short-term memory loss is a primary symptom in the early stages of dementia of the Alzheimer's type. Memory loss later becomes global and affects short- and long-term memory. • Certain medications, especially in combination, can cause increased confusion and agitation. • Safety in the home and in healthcare settings is a primary concern because consumers with dementia are at increased risk of falls and other injuries from the combination of sensory effects, medications, memory loss and age-related factors.	• Teach consumers (in the early stages of the illness) and their families about the disorder and explain the progression of the illness and prognosis so that expectations are realistic. Consumers with dementia (especially those with young-onset disease) can choose and plan what they want to do with their lives in light of their prognosis, and can deal with any legal matters while cognition allows (e.g. make a will, advance directives). • Teach the family carers actions and precautions to reduce the consumer's risk for falls or other injury. • Instruct the family how to observe for non-verbal signs of pain and discomfort (e.g. groaning, cold clammy skin, holding body part, changed vital signs).
• Consumers may be unable to communicate pain or emotional distress; the nurse needs to assess consumers regularly and monitor closely for physical and mental concerns, including concurrent depression, which can exacerbate the symptoms of dementia. • Sundowning syndrome (evening agitation associated with a busy time of day and resulting from consumer fatigue) may lead to challenging behaviours. Planned activities for consumers are helpful in preventing agitated behaviour at this time. • A structured environment with minimal changes is critical because it reduces consumer anxiety, confusion and agitation. • Consumers with AD may occasionally confabulate (attempt to fill memory gaps with unrelated information), which is not considered lying. • Consumers who confabulate may need gentle validation of their sense of what is true, or they may be gently redirected to another topic because confronting them with reality may result in confusion and distress. • Intake of nutritional supplements, herbs and over-the-counter medications may interfere with the consumer's prescribed medications. • Consumers cared for at home may resist outside help and place undue demands and stress on the family carer. • Stressors that can provoke consumer anxiety or confusion should be identified and modified or avoided as much as possible (e.g. loud music, cluttered rooms). • Potential elder abuse may be a result of family carer strain, and consumers and carers need to be evaluated if abuse is suspected. Carers need to be made aware of all available supports and respite services in the community to reduce strain when people with dementia are cared for at home.	• Teach the family about sundowning syndrome and offer strategies to reduce fatigue, confusion and agitation (sometimes family carers themselves discover helpful strategies that they can pass on to professional carers, as the 24-hour/day care they provide often makes them experts in dementia management and care). • Teach the family about changes in condition (e.g. exacerbation of confusion, signs of depression) that are signs of health problems separate to dementia. Ensure awareness of who to contact for help and advice. • Teach strategies that promote the consumer's existing memory and connectedness with others (e.g. validation, reminiscence, environmental cues, familiar songs, pictures, pets etc.). • Ensure awareness of correct medication regimen, possible side effects and importance of following the medical officer's directions for administration. • Ensure awareness of discussing use of non-prescribed drugs (e.g. herbal remedies) with the medical officer to avoid side effects when combined with prescribed medications. • Suggest that the consumer remain under care of one medical officer to provide consistent care and clear medication regimen. This avoids the risks of adverse drug interactions from incompatible medications and polypharmacy (multiple medications). • Teach the family about confabulation and stress that it is not lying, and that it is best to validate the person's belief of what is true. Stress that it can be distressing to challenge the person's view of reality. For example, if the person says they had egg, bacon and mushrooms for breakfast, it is best not to contradict them even if you are certain that they only had porridge. • Teach to identify stressors (anxiety triggers) in the home environment, and offer realistic solutions. • Explain the benefits of outside help when the help comes from skilled and reliable carers who can bond with the person with dementia. • Encourage the family carer to take advantage of respite and other services that will reduce the strain of caring for someone with dementia. Be aware that carers have high rates of depression themselves and consider providing details for support services for them. Encourage family members to share the caregiving responsibilities.

Continued

TABLE 39.12 | Information for nurses and for consumers with dementia and their family carers—cont'd

Information that nurses need to know	Information that nurses need to give people with dementia and their family carers
• Access current resources available on the internet and in the library.	• Stress the importance of 'time-out' for the family carer to recharge personal batteries, and the importance of maintaining their own health. This includes attendance to preventative strategies such as routine health checks, mammograms, and flu injections. • Inform family carers about how to access current information via the internet and libraries, and from agencies such as Dementia Australia. (There are dementia information centres in many areas of Australia, many of which offer consumer and family carer support groups, among other services. Many also offer educational programs for family and professional carers.)

(Dementia Australia 2023; Fortinash & Holoday Worret 2011)

CLINICAL INTEREST BOX 39.12 Interventions appropriate for consumers experiencing confusion or disorientation

Appropriate care for the confused or disoriented consumer includes:

- a safe, consistent, pleasant and familiar environment
- freedom from physical/emotional/spiritual pain
- a calm, relaxed, caring and non-challenging atmosphere
- a stable and familiar staff
- staff who have appropriate expertise and are compassionate
- skilled communicators (expertise in communicating with cognitively impaired consumers)
- tactful use of humour
- frequent contact and interaction with staff/family
- contact with pets if desired (especially the consumer's own pets)
- opportunities to socialise
- a structured, individualised routine (as close to the consumer's familiar routine at home as is possible)
- the presence of the consumer's own familiar belongings (e.g. personal objects)
- therapeutic activities/programs to promote cognitive stimulation (e.g. reminiscence therapy, music therapy)
- nutritious diet/adequate hydration, including pleasurable snacks
- adequate periods of rest and sleep
- high standard of hygiene/personal grooming
- effective use of well-maintained visual/hearing/sensory aids
- adequate daily exercise
- access to a pleasant and safe outdoor area
- maintenance of treatments ordered by the medical officer.

(Foster et al 2022; Hungerford et al 2020; Steele 2023)

Reality orientation is a form of rehabilitation used to orientate confused or cognitively impaired consumers by promoting or maintaining their awareness of person, time and place. It is recognised as unrealistic to expect to orientate people in the later stages of dementia to present time reality, but some of the principles of reality orientation are appropriate and helpful (Foster et al 2022). Helpful aspects include:

- calling the consumer by their preferred name every time they are approached
- stating your name each time you start an interaction with the consumer
- maintaining a normal day–night cycle (e.g. opening curtains and blinds during the day and closing them at night and encouraging the consumer to dress in their own clothes during the day, rather than in nightwear)
- leaving the furniture and the consumer's belongings in the same place, as rearranging objects in the environment adds to confusion

- encouraging the consumer to wear their spectacles and/or hearing aids, as not wearing them adds to sensory confusion
- maintaining a routine and a sense of order in daily activities
- ensuring that the environment is designed to minimise confusion (e.g. using distinctive colours or pictures on bathroom or toilet doors to help the confused person identify these areas, and ensuring adequate lighting in all areas to minimise the effect of shadows that might confuse perceptions of what is seen)
- using a notice board to display information about the date and place that is consistently maintained to give residents an opportunity to remain orientated to dates, times and important events.

Consumers who have temporary confusion or who are in the early stages of dementia and are seeking to maintain orientation to time and place may benefit from the following interventions:

- telling the person, the date and time each morning and repeating the information as appropriate during the day
- having the day and date displayed in large bold letters on a board and having the person change it accordingly each day
- reminding the person of holidays, birthdays and other special events
- providing cues to reinforce verbal information (e.g. clocks with clear and large numbers, large calendars)
- discussing current affairs (e.g. items in the newspaper or on television news).

(Foster et al 2022)

A key to providing quality care is to find a way to connect with consumers who have dementia. This is different from simply communicating, which can be one-sided, with the nurse talking and the consumer largely passive. Connecting involves the nurse or other carer having to develop skills and spend time and effort establishing connection. The use of validation therapy, reminiscence and remotivation therapy promotes connection and these therapies are highly appropriate for use with consumers who have dementia (Halter 2021). (How to communicate effectively with consumers who have dementia and the use of appropriate therapies such as validation and reminiscence therapy are outlined in Chapter 10.) Recreational, occupational and complementary therapies can also be therapeutic in promoting cognitive, sensory and physical stimulation and can provide opportunities for staff to connect with consumers.

Managing challenging behaviours in confused consumers

Many of the behaviours that people with dementia exhibit are a direct result of the illness and so need to be considered as 'normal' symptoms of the condition, rather than abnormal behaviours. Behaviours that fall into this category include aimless wandering, becoming lost, muddled actions and conversations, disturbances in sleep–wake cycles and, especially with some particular types of dementia (e.g. Pick's disease), loss of emotional control and aggressive reactions (Foster et al 2022). Other behaviours, such as unusual outbursts of physical or verbal aggression, dressing or disrobing publicly or refusing to bathe, eat or attend activities previously enjoyed, can be due to a range of influences that can exacerbate the normal effects of the illness. The reason for the behaviour—the core of the problem—may be related to a variety of issues including:

- a change in the environment (e.g. too noisy, too busy, causing feelings of being overwhelmed)
- the person's physical condition (e.g. too hot or cold, clothing uncomfortable, pain or discomfort)
- hallucinations or delusions (may create fear and anxiety)
- provocation by another resident
- the way a particular staff member interacts with the person (e.g. being loud or bustling or rushing the person).

Whatever the consumer's behaviour, it is important for the nurse to respond quietly, calmly, confidently and kindly. This kind of response is often enough to modify the behaviour. The use of psychotropic medications for managing challenging behaviour is best avoided because these agents tend to have little effect on problem behaviour associated with dementia, particularly of the Alzheimer's type, and they may cause serious side effects more difficult to deal with than the behaviour itself (Foster et al 2022). As dementia is often associated with older persons, the risk of polypharmacy is greater when introducing psychotropic medications. In addition to this, the sedation common to most psychotropic medications (which is usually a desired effect) make the risk of falls in older persons greater. When behaviour is not acceptable the nurse should firmly let the person know that this is the case, and behaviour that is appropriate should be praised.

Care by staff who fully understand the effects of the dementia illness and have appropriate expertise in communicating with confused people is important to the consumer's sense of wellbeing, and it is clear that disruptive behaviour is less likely in residential care settings when the principles of dementia care management are followed (Foster et al 2022). The appropriate interventions for consumers with challenging behaviour are outlined in Clinical Interest Box 39.13.

It should be noted that, while many of these principles apply to caring for consumers who are confused or disoriented from causes other than progressive dementia, the approach for reversible confusion or temporary disorientation may include strategies to assist the person with progressive dementia to remain orientated to reality.

Dementia is one of the most complex and disabling conditions. It presents huge challenges to nurses and to the many family carers who tend loved ones with dementia at home. Table 39.12 provides a summary of some of the

CLINICAL INTEREST BOX 39.13 Nursing responsibilities for managing challenging behaviour

- Maintain a calm environment and respond to the situation calmly.
- Remain neutral, do not attribute blame, never 'tell off' the consumer in any way.
- Avoid the use of restraints, including chemical restraints; in particular, physical restraints tend to increase agitation and confusion.
- Try to identify the cause.
- Observe and keep a record of when the behaviour occurs, the type of behaviour, the consumer's mood and where and with whom the behaviour occurs. This helps to identify triggers for the behaviour that in many cases suggest how the cause can be eliminated.
- Assess the person.
- Is there a physical or emotional trigger for the behaviour? Is the consumer or resident unwell, in pain, overtired, overstimulated, bored, anxious, embarrassed, or feeling ignored, misunderstood or patronised?
- Is the consumer or resident reacting to an unpleasant incident or is the behaviour associated with:
  - A change?
  - A disturbing memory?
  - A particular person or occurrence?
  - A situation or request that is culturally inappropriate?
  - Delusions or hallucinations?
  - The memory of a traumatic past experience stimulated by the current situation?
- Consider all the facts together—ask:
  - Does the behaviour always happen in the same place or in similar surroundings?
  - Is it new behaviour?
  - How was this situation (e.g. daily shower) managed when the consumer lived at home?
  - Does it occur with a particular person in particular circumstances?
  - Is it connected with a particular staff member, relative, friend or other resident?
  - What does the consumer say, if anything, about the behaviour?
  - Can the family carer provide any insights into the behaviour?
- Use a team approach to problem-solving.
- It may take time and several different ideas may need to be implemented before certain problem behaviours are resolved. If one nurse finds a successful intervention, this should be documented appropriately and shared with all team members.

Redirection

Redirection involves distracting the consumer from the situation causing the behaviour. For example, the nurse may distract the consumer who is upset and shouting at another resident without obvious cause by saying, 'I don't know what's wrong but I think we should get away from here—let's go for a walk outside.' The consumer who is jumping up from the meal table and upsetting other consumers by saying, 'This food is bad, it tastes like poison' may be directed if the nurse responds, 'I can see you're upset, how about you come with me, you can leave that food, let's go and find something else to eat' or 'Let's leave that then, let's get something else to eat later on—can you come and help me water the plants outside and then we'll eat later?'

Triggers

The following example is an illustration of how identifying a trigger can help to reduce challenging behaviour and how different strategies may need to be tried until a successful way of stopping the behaviour is found.

Mrs Peters, 72 years old, who has dementia and is living in a residential care facility, was generally happily confused but on some days would be very agitated, pace about, bang on tables and sometimes swear and shout out abuse such as 'Get away, you cow' at the top of her voice. On these days she would often start crying for no apparent reason and the staff found it difficult to console her or to establish what was upsetting her. On the last two occasions of being so upset, she became physically aggressive and even succeeded in biting one of the nurses.

After keeping a detailed record of when and where the behaviour occurred it was realised that it was on certain days of the week that corresponded with when a particular nurse was on duty. This was a surprise, as the nurse was respected for her compassion and skill in dementia care nursing, but it was soon confirmed that the challenging behaviour was triggered by the nurse's presence. It was only after consulting with Mrs Peters' sister that the cause became clear. The nurse bore a close resemblance to a next-door neighbour who had reversed her car over and killed Mrs Peters' much adored labrador dog over 40 years previously.

The problem was discussed at a team meeting. It was decided that the nurse should not be responsible for Mrs Peters' personal care and that she should attempt to reinforce her own identity with Mrs Peters. When the nurse next came on duty, she wore her hair differently and made a point over the next few weeks of consistently introducing

CLINICAL INTEREST BOX 39.13 Nursing responsibilities for managing challenging behaviour—cont'd

herself and showing Mrs Peters her name badge. She managed to tell Mrs Peters about herself; she even used photographs of her family, her home and her holidays to assist the process of trying to reinforce her real identity. This seemed to be effective on most occasions, although Mrs Peters sometimes continued to respond with agitation and aggression towards the nurse she believed had killed her pet dog.

Mrs Peters one day yelled at her, 'Get out, dangerous bitch.' The nurse quickly said, 'I'm so sorry, I was so careless, I never meant to hurt your dog. I am so sorry, please forgive me.' With this, Mrs Peters acknowledged the apology with a firm quick nod of the head, walked to her chair and with a sigh sat down. This seemed to settle what for Mrs Peters might have been unfinished business. The nurse continued to use this approach whenever Mrs Peters was agitated and eventually the agitation and aggressive response to the nurse stopped.

(Halter 2021)

information that nurses need to know and some of the information that nurses need to teach to family carers.

Dementia care, while not always acknowledged as such, is a specialty area of nursing, requiring a high level of integrated skills. It is predominantly a condition of the elderly, who often have multiple other concurrent health issues that the nurse must be knowledgeable about. Consumers living with dementia are often not able to explain their feelings or their needs; the nurse therefore needs high-level observation and communication skills to provide quality care. The nurse also needs to be able to support the family carers of people with dementia, who are often devastated by what has happened to their loved ones. Carers live with observing the cognitive decline in functioning in their loved one, until they are no longer recognised at all. Dementia, like all mental health conditions, is associated with considerable carer burden and burnout, and nurses need to be cognisant of this.

Though this section has briefly highlighted some of the many issues relating to dementia care, it is recommended that nurses undertake specialist courses to enhance their knowledge and skills in this area. Organisations such as Dementia Australia provide up-to-date information relevant to people with dementia, their families and health professionals. All caring needs to be undertaken with an understanding of the legal and ethical issues that relate to mental health nursing. The next section adds some specific points to the general legal and ethical principles impacting on mental health nursing.

LEGAL AND ETHICAL ASPECTS OF MENTAL HEALTH NURSING

The provision of healthcare for consumers experiencing a mental health condition is governed by government mental health Acts. Each Australian state and territory has its own Act and these Acts are periodically revised. The nurse who is involved in mental health nursing has a responsibility to be aware of the relevant current Acts in the geographical area of their employment. Information about legal issues may also be accessed from government departments responsible for the health of the community such as the Department of Health and Human Services (Victoria) or its equivalent in other states and territories.

Mental health Acts provide guidelines and directions regarding the provision of mental health care (e.g. criteria for determining criteria for compulsory admission to hospital), and regulations and requirements regarding the periodic review of consumers experiencing mental illness. The information here is based on the law as it relates to mental health consumers in the state of Victoria, but the principles apply to laws across Australia.

Legal issues relating to informal and formal admission

Treatment in a mental health care facility or by a community mental health care team may take the form of informal or formal admission. Informal (voluntary) admission is when a consumer chooses to receive treatment and is the most preferred modality of treatment. Treatment may be at personal request or based on the advice of family or a health professional, and the consumer is able to withdraw from treatment or leave the healthcare facility whenever they choose.

Formal (compulsory) admission is when the request for admission usually comes from a source other than the person experiencing a mental health condition, who may be deemed unable to make an informed decision. A consumer may be referred for admission if they pose imminent danger to themselves or others or if they require treatment but are too confused, distressed or disorganised to seek voluntary admission. The consumer is examined by a number of healthcare professionals during the process of compulsory admission to ensure that they meet appropriate admission criteria, and that they cannot be treated in a less restrictive environment, such as in the community. The purpose of having different clinicians providing assessment also ensures that the consumer receives an objective assessment that is not biased. Carers are also encouraged to take an active role in the process and many Acts now have provisions to include carers in any decision-making at the consumer's request.

In a crisis situation, it may be a team of professionals based in the community, such as a crisis assessment and treatment team (CATT), that is called to assist. The team can request formal (compulsory) admission for a consumer.

As soon as a consumer no longer meets all admission criteria, they must be discharged from their compulsory status, or what is termed formal detention. There are strict guidelines governing who should review formal consumers and how often they should be reviewed. Consumers have the right to appeal their detainment as a community mental health patient or an inpatient in a facility. Nurses working in the mental health field need to have a thorough understating of the mental health Act that relates to their state or territory.

Treatment orders and issues of consent

Mental health consumers who are admitted compulsorily to a mental health service are sometimes treated under a community treatment order (CTO) while living in the community. The CTO may require that the person lives in a particular place to facilitate treatment, and may stipulate which psychiatrist will provide treatment, where and how often treatment should be expected and how long the order will last. It may also stipulate other specific conditions under which the consumer may remain in the community while receiving treatment. All formal consumers, whether treated in the community or in a hospital, are legally obliged to accept recommended treatment, and treatment can be enforced against the consumer's will if necessary. This is a last resort, however, and all efforts to engage the consumer in voluntary treatment should be taken. It is in everyone's best interest for formal and informal consumers alike to be given all relevant information connected with any treatment, and informed consent should be gained whenever possible. The right of formal and informal consumers to seek a second opinion must be respected.

The mental health Acts in each state and territory have clear guidelines concerning issues such as informed consent to treatment, the way treatments may be administered (e.g. electroconvulsive therapy) and the use of restraint, including the use of seclusion as a therapeutic measure. It is an offence to restrain or seclude someone if it is not conducted within the requirements of the mental health Act applicable to where the practice occurs, and the mental health service can be prosecuted and fined if an offence is committed.

Legal issues and electroconvulsive therapy

Electroconvulsive therapy (ECT) is a prescribed treatment and as such it is regulated under the different mental health Acts and regulations in each state. The use of ECT may be indicated when the consumer has an increased risk of suicide, has not responded to psychotropic medication, or has had an adverse reaction to medication. It is also indicated when the consumer has had a previous history of a good response to ECT (Hercelinskyj & Alexander 2022).

ECT involves the consumer being given a light general anaesthetic and muscle relaxant medication. A regulated electrical current is passed through the brain until a seizure occurs (a therapeutic 'fit'). This has previously been referred to as 'shock treatment'. A course of ECT involves a series of treatments. Informed consent must be gained whenever possible for any form of treatment, but there are some issues specific to ECT.

Further information about ECT and the law can be located in the mental health Act for the relevant state or territory. References and websites for accessing legal information are provided in the Online Resources at the end of this chapter.

ETHICAL ISSUES AND DILEMMAS

Ethical issues and dilemmas abound in mental health nursing. It is sometimes a challenge to balance the consumer's right to autonomy, the rights of others and the legal concepts relevant to nursing care. Some of the areas that may give rise to ethical concerns include:

- informed consent/refusal of treatment
- seclusion and other forms of restraint
- inclusion of carers and confidentiality
- consumer confidentiality versus the need to prepare/warn/protect other parties
- consumer autonomy (self-reliance and choice issues) as opposed to paternalism
- boundary issues in the nurse–consumer relationship.

Within these areas are situations that may give rise to the nurse experiencing conflicting or troublesome feelings. For example, enforcing medication or treatment that is refused, or needing to restrain a consumer by enforced seclusion, may give rise to feelings of guilt, concern or distaste. Or the nurse may be torn between a consumer's right to confidentiality and the importance of informing a family carer about a consumer's diagnosis, such as the risk of violence if the consumer has voiced threats when they do not want their diagnosis, feelings or voiced intentions revealed.

It can also be discomforting and confusing trying to balance establishing and maintaining a trusting and helping relationship while maintaining the appropriate professional boundary with certain consumers, and this can cause ethical dilemmas, particularly for nurses new to psychiatric nursing (Foster et al 2022). Nurses must practise within professional codes of practice and the law, and consistently remain aware of the ethical principles of beneficence (do good), non-maleficence (do no harm), autonomy (consumer self-determination) and those of justice, fairness and equity when caring for consumers. Whenever ethical concerns arise where the decisions about what to do are not clear, nurses should raise the issues and discuss them openly with colleagues (see also Chapter 2). Nurses considering a career in mental health nursing are advised to access further information concerning ethical issues in mental health care.

Progress Note 39.1

17/10/2023 1725 hrs	Nursing: Eli is a 33-year-old man admitted via ED following referral from GP requesting psych assessment for psychotic symptoms. Eli describes ongoing increasing feelings of suspicion towards partner (Heidi). He believes that Heidi is being unfaithful. Social: Landscape gardener. Lives with his partner Heidi. Heidi describes recent decline in social contacts with friends and an insistent belief that she is having an affair with his friend, Earl. Eli recently had an argument with a long-term client of his, an elderly man for whom he has been mowing lawns for several years. He saw a car parked in the driveway that he is convinced is Earl's. He also believes that he needs to plant olive trees in people's gardens because these are biblical plants and has recently had several significant arguments with clients who don't want them. One man he mows for threatened to hit him if he planted any olive trees on his property. P/H: Past history of schizophrenia, one admission in the past, managed by community team for past 3 years. Past medical history includes hypertension and hyperlipidaemia. Maintained with aripiprazole 10 mg/day with good effect, but Heidi believes Eli has stopped taking his medication as she found several tablets in the toilet last week. Heidi states that he is also avoiding eating food from the house and notes that in the past, he has had paranoia about food contamination. Heidi believes Eli has lost weight. Appearance & behaviour: Dishevelled man, average height who is overweight. Poor eye contact. Appears hypervigilant, frequently looking towards door and requiring ++ reassurance no-one else is listening to our conversation. Generally cooperative with interview process; however, distracted at times. Mood: Congruent; however, anxious at times. Rated mood 5/10, when asked to elaborate, 'well how would you feel if your wife was having an affair with your best mate?' Describes ongoing insomnia related to rumination about wife and an inability to sleep next to 'the cheating cow'. Stated he sleeps on the couch in spurts because it's so uncomfortable. Reports significant interpersonal issues with Heidi. Appetite poor. Affect: Blunted. Speech: Disorganised at times. Perception: Denies hearing voices but said that 'he knows' Job from the Bible has told him to leave his wife. Would not elaborate. Denied presence of further perceptual disturbance during interview yet seemed ++ distracted and distressed at one point, muttering to himself, and turning his head. Thought: Themes involving conspiracies and the need to listen to Job to 'keep the Satan quiet' were expressed frequently. Preoccupied with intrusive need to 'stay alert' to catch Heidi with Earl. Paranoid delusions expressed. Thoughts loosely associated and at times difficult to follow. Evidence of thought blocking. Cognition: Intact. Memory good (recent, remote, past). Judgment: Poor. Insight: Impaired. Drug history: States he is a social drinker. Denies use of illicit drugs. Risk: Risk of interpersonal violence directed towards his clients, as evidenced by recent threats and arguments. Eli is also quite paranoid, hypervigilant and suspicious of others. Risk of nutritional deficits as evidenced by paranoia re. food contamination. *P Alberta* (ALBERTA), *EN*

DECISION-MAKING FRAMEWORK EXERCISE 39.1

You are an Enrolled Nurse working in the acute mental health unit when the nurse in charge goes on her lunch break. Before she leaves, she tells you that you will need to do the 15-minutely observations for the consumer who is currently in seclusion. She tells you she will just sign the sheet when she comes back. While you have seen many RNs do this, as an EN you know that you are not permitted under your jurisdiction's mental health Act to sign off these observations. This nurse has been working in this unit for over 10 years.

Using the decision-making framework:

1. Do you undertake the observations? Why or why not?
2. Consider the legal requirements of clinical observations in seclusion. Is it acceptable for someone to sign off on something they never did?
3. How would you approach this situation with the nurse?

Summary

Many Enrolled Nurses (ENs) may wish to follow a career in the specialty area of mental health nursing, and those who remain in other fields may be required to assist in the care of consumers experiencing a mental health challenge (e.g. when they are being cared for in general hospitals or in residential care facilities).

There is no clear dividing line between mental health and mental illness; rather, mental wellbeing is represented on a continuum, and no-one is entirely mentally unhealthy or fully mentally healthy at all times. The ability to remain mentally healthy depends on a wide range of interrelating factors, including those that are physiological, psychological and sociocultural. There are many theoretical models to explain the development of mental illness, on which MHNs base their clinical practice. These include the biological (medical) model, psychological/psychodynamic, social/interpersonal, cognitive–behavioural and stress vulnerability/adaptation models.

Mental health conditions can be diagnosed and formally classified according to the presenting symptoms. A diagnosis can guide treatment but also places a label on the person that can be a source of stigma, which can be one of the most difficult aspects of mental illness for consumers to cope with. It is a primary role of the MHN to educate the public about mental illness to reduce stigmatising attitudes, which are in part based on historical factors.

MHNs, who work as members of a multidisciplinary team, develop nursing diagnoses and focus care on the feelings of consumers and the behavioural manifestations of mental distress that they display. The development of a trusting, helping relationship is essential to being able to work therapeutically with consumers experiencing a mental health condition and in promoting the healing process. Assisting consumers to develop constructive coping mechanisms is an important component of the therapeutic relationship, as is supporting effective rehabilitation of consumers living in the community, where currently most mental health care takes place.

This chapter has not provided detailed information about mental illness, but it has provided a brief overview of some issues and suggestions appropriate to the care of consumers who are anxious, depressed, aggressive, self-destructive, elevated or confused. The nurse interested in working in the wonderfully challenging area of mental health nursing is advised to access more information about manifestations of mental anguish, models of care and the legal and ethical issues that relate to this dynamic field of nursing.

Review Questions

1. Describe the concepts associated with mental health.
2. Describe the concepts associated with mental illness.
3. Describe four factors that can be considered indicators of mental illness.
4. Identify four groups of people in society that are at particular risk of developing a mental illness and why.
5. Identify four early warning signs of mental illness in children and in preadolescents.
6. Explain the primary characteristics of thought disorders, mood disorders and behavioural disorders and give an example of each.
7. How can nurses reduce stigma about mental illness?
8. Define the terms *hallucination*, *delusion* and *confabulation*.
9. Define the following four terms and indicate when they are experienced: akathisia, anhedonia, anxiety and apathy.
10. Outline five skills the EN could use when working with a consumer who has an elevated mood (mania).
11. Outline four strategies for promoting effective communication with consumers who have depression.
12. Identify 10 interventions necessary to provide quality care for people with dementia in an aged-care residential facility. Consider the environment, the staff and nursing care activities.

Evolve® Answer guide for the Review Questions, Critical Thinking Exercises, Decision-making Framework Exercises and Critical Thinking Questions in Case Studies is hosted on Evolve: http://evolve.elsevier.com/AU/Koutoukidis/Tabbner.

References

Alexander, L., Rinehart, N., Hay, M., et al., 2023. Nursing students' attitudes and experiences with mental illness: A cross sectional study. *Teaching & Learning in Nursing* 18(1), 72–77. Available at: <https://doi.org/10.1016/j.teln.2022.09.011>.

Alexander, L., Sheen, J., Rinehart, et al., 2018. The role of television in perceptions of dangerousness. *The Journal of Mental Health Training, Education and Practice* 13(3), 187–196. doi: 10.1108/JMHTEP-02-2017-0006.

American Psychiatric Association, 2022. *Diagnostic and statistical manual of mental disorders*, 5th ed. Text revision. American Psychiatric Association, Washington, USA.

Andrews, G., Dean, K., Genderson, M., et al., 2013. *Management of mental disorders*, 5th ed. CreateSpace Independent Publishing Platform.

Anthony, W.A., 2000. A recovery-oriented service system: Setting some system level standards. *Psychiatric Rehabilitation Journal* 24(2), 159–168.

Appelbaum, P.S., 2013. Public safety, mental disorders, and guns. *JAMA Psychiatry* 70(6), 565–566.

Australian Bureau of Statistics (ABS), 2018. Intentional self-harm in Aboriginal and Torres Strait Islander people. ABS cat. no. 3303.0. Available at: <https://www.abs.gov.au/ausstats/abs@.nsf/Lookup/by%20Subject/3303.0~2018~Main%20Features~Leading%20causes%20of%20death%20in%20Aboriginal%20and%20Torres%20Strait%20Islander%20people~2>.

Australian College of Mental Health Nurses, 2022. What mental health nurses do. Available at: <https://acmhn.org/what-mental-health-nurses-do>.

Australian Commission on Safety and Quality in Health Care (ACSQHC), 2021. National safety and quality health service standards, 2nd ed. ACSQHC, Sydney. Available at: <https://www.safetyandquality.gov.au/sites/default/files/migrated/National-Safety-and-Quality-Health-Service-Standards-second-edition.pdf>.

Australian Institute of Family Studies (AIFS), 2022. Understanding the mental health and help-seeking behaviours of refugees. Available at: <https://aifs.gov.au/resources/short-articles/understanding-mental-health-and-help-seeking-behaviours-refugees#:~:text=For%20a%20range%20of%20reasons,is%20low%20and%2For%20problematic>.

Australian Institute of Health and Welfare (AIHW), 2018. Mental health services in Australia. Australian Government. Available at: <https://www.aihw.gov.au/reports/mental-health-services/mental-health-services-in-australia/report-contents/summary-of-mental-health-services-in-australia/prevalence-and-policies>.

Australian Institute of Health and Welfare (AIHW), 2022. Prevalence and impact of mental illness. Available at: <https://www.aihw.gov.au/mental-health/overview/mental-illness>.

Australian Institute of Health and Welfare (AIHW), 2023a. Suicide and self-harm monitoring. Available at: <https://www.aihw.gov.au/suicide-self-harm-monitoring/summary/suicide-and-intentional-self-harm>.

Australian Institute of Health and Welfare (AIHW), 2023b. Dementia in Australia. Available at: <https://www.aihw.gov.au/reports/dementia/dementia-in-aus/contents/summary>.

Barkway, P., O'Kane, D., 2020. *Psychology: An introduction for health professionals*. Elsevier.

Black Dog Institute, 2023. Suicide prevention network. Available at: <https://www.blackdoginstitute.org.au/education-services/suicide-prevention-implementation/network>.

Centre for Diseases (CDC), 2021. About mental health. Available at: <https://www.cdc.gov/mentalhealth/learn/index.htm>.

Davies, K., Gray, M., Butcher, L., 2014. Lean on me: The potential for peer support in a non-government Australian mental health service. *Asia Pacific Journal of Social Work & Development* 24(1–2), 109–121. doi: 10.1080/02185385.2014.885213.

Deegan, P.E., 1988. Recovery: The lived experience of rehabilitation. *Psychosocial Rehabilitation Journal* 11(4), 11–19.

Dementia Australia, 2022a. What is younger dementia? Available at: <https://yod.dementia.org.au/about-younger-onset-dementia>.

Dementia Australia, 2022b. Dementia statistics. Available at: <https://www.dementia.org.au/statistics#:~:text=Dementia%20is%20the%20second%20leading%20cause%20of%20death%20of%20Australians.&text=Dementia%20is%20the%20leading%20cause%20of%20death%20for%20women.&text=In%202022%2C%20there%20are%20up,almost%201.1%20million%20by%202058>.

Dementia Australia, 2022c. Diagnosis dementia. Available at: <https://www.dementia.org.au/information/diagnosing-dementia>.

Department of Health, 2013. A national framework for recovery-oriened mental health services: Guide for practitioners and providers. Available at: <https://www.health.gov.au/sites/default/files/documents/2021/04/a-national-framework-for-recovery-oriented-mental-health-services-guide-for-practitioners-and-providers.pdf.>.

Department of Health, Victoria, 2023. Lived experience. Available at: <https://www.health.vic.gov.au/mental-health-reform/lived-experience>.

Department of Health, Victoria, 2022. Working with consumer and carers. Available at: <https://www.health.vic.gov.au/mental-health/working-with-consumers-and-carers>.

Department of Health and Aged Care, 2024. About mental health. Available at: <https://www.health.gov.au/topics/mental-health-and-suicide-prevention/about-mental-health#mental-health-during-the-covid19-pandemic>.

Desmarais, S.L., Van Dom, R.A., Johnson, K.L., et al., 2014. Community violence perpetration and victimization among adults with mental illnesses. *American Journal of Public Health* 104(12), 2342–2349.

Edward, K.L., Munro, I., Welch, A., Cross, W. (eds.), 2018. *Mental health nursing: Dimensions of praxis*, 3rd ed. Oxford University Press, Melbourne.

Egan, G., 1994. *The skilled helper: A problem management approach to helping*. Brooks Cole, Pacific Grove.

Erikson, E., Erikson, J., 1997. *The life cycle completed.* WW Norton, New York.

Evans, K., Nizette, D., O'Brien, A., 2017. *Psychiatric mental health nursing*, 4th ed. Elsevier, Sydney.

Fortinash, K.M., Holoday Worret, P.A., 2011. *Psychiatric nursing care plans*, 5th ed. Mosby, St Louis.

Foster, K., Marks, P., O'Brien, A., Raeburn, T., 2020. *Mental health in nursing – Theory and practice for clinical settings.* Elsevier.

Goldberg, J.F., Ernst, C.L., 2018. *Managing the side effects of psychotropic medications*, 2nd ed. American Psychiatric Association, Washington, DC.

Halter, M.J., 2021. *Varcarolis' foundations of psychiatric-mental health nursing*, 9th ed. A clinical approach. Elsevier, USA.

Hercelinskyj, G., Alexander, L., 2022. *Mental health nursing*, enhanced edition, 1st ed. Cengage.

Hoffnung, M., Hoffnung, R.J., Seifert, K.L., et al., 2022. *Lifespan development*, Australasian Edition, 5th ed. Wiley, Singapore.

Hungerford, C., Hodgson, D., Clancy, R., et al., 2020. *Mental health care: An introduction for health professionals*, 4th ed. Wiley, China.

Jakopac, K.A., Patel, S.C., 2009. *Psychiatric mental health case studies and care plans.* Jones & Bartlett, USA.

Kitafuna, K.B., 2022. A critical overview of mental health-related beliefs, services and systems in Uganda and recent activist and legal challenges. *Community Mental Health Journal* 58, 829–834. Available at: <https://link.springer.com/article/10.1007/s10597-022-00947-5>.

LGBTIQ+ Health Australia, 2023. Available at: <www.lgbtiqhealth.org.au>.

Lovejoy, M., 1984. Recovery from schizophrenia: A personal odyssey. *Hospital & Community Psychiatry* 35(8), 809–812.

Luyten, P., Campbell, C., Fonagy, P, 2021. Rethinking the relationship between attachment and personality disorder. *Current Opinion in Psychology* 37, 109–113. Available at: <https://doi.org/10.1016/j.copsyc.2020.11.003>.

McGuire, J., 2022. "We are not ill" – A history and analysis of LGBT pathologization. Review YOUR Review 9. Available at: <https://link.springer.com/chapter/10.1007/978-981-19-0460-8_26>.

Mental Health Foundation, 2022. Children and young people: Statistics. Available at: <https://www.mentalhealth.org.uk/explore-mental-health/statistics/children-young-people-statistics#:~:text=50%25%20of%20mental%20health%20problems,and%2075%25%20by%20age%2024.&text=10%25%20of%20children%20and%20young,at%20a%20sufficiently%20early%20age>.

National Alliance on Mental Illness, 2023. Available at: <www.nami.org>.

Peplau, H.E., 1991. *Interpersonal relations in nursing: A conceptual framework of reference for psychodynamic nursing.* Springer, New York.

Polacsek, M., Boardman, G.H., McCann, T.V., 2022. Self-identity and meaning in life as enablers for older adults to self-manage depression. *Issues in Mental Health Nursing* 43(5). Available at: <https://doi.org/10.1080/01612840.2021.1998263>.

Pollack, H., 2013. Reality-based mental health reform. *Washington Monthly* 45(3–4), 15–20.

Queensland Health, 2021. Suicide prevention practice. Queensland health guideline. Available at: <https://www.health.qld.gov.au/__data/assets/pdf_file/0027/1125864/qh-gdl-967.pdf>.

Roberts, R., 2019. The physical health of people living with mental illness: A narrative literature review. Charles Sturt University. Available at: <https://www.equallywell.org.au/wp-content/uploads/2019/06/Literature-review-Equally-Well.pdf>.

Rogers, C., 1961. *On becoming a person.* Houghton Mifflin, Boston.

Rosenstreich, G., 2013. LGBTI people: Mental health & suicide. National LGBTI Health Alliance. Available at: <https://www.beyondblue.org.au/docs/default-source/default-document-library/bw0258-lgbti-mental-health-and-suicide-2013-2nd-edition.pdf?sfvrsn=2>.

Ross, A.M., Morgan, A.J., Jorm, A.F., Reavley, N., 2018. A systematic review on the impact of media reports of severe illness on stigma and discrimination, and interventions that aim to mitigate any adverse impact. *Social Psychiatry and Psychiatric Epidemiology* 54, 11–31. Available at: <https://doi.org/10.1007/s00127-018-1608-9>.

Royal Australian College of Psychiatrists, 2022. Physical health & mental illness. Available at: <https://www.ranzcp.org/practice-education/guidelines-and-resources-for-practice/physical-health/physical-health-and-mental-illness>.

Steele, D. 2023. *Keltner's psychiatric nursing*, 9th ed. Elsevier.

Touhy, T.A., Jett, K.F., 2009. *Ebersole and Hess' gerontological nursing & healthy aging*, 3rd ed. Mosby, St Louis.

World Health Organization (WHO), 2022. Mental disorders. Available at: <https://www.who.int/news-room/fact-sheets/detail/mental-disorders>.

World Health Organization (WHO), 2012. Risks to mental health: An overview of vulnerabilities and risk factors. World Health Organization. Available at: <http://www.who.int/mental_health/mhgap/risks_to_mental_health_EN_27_08_12.pdf>.

World Health Organization (WHO), 2015. Mental health: A state of well-being. Available at: < http://www.who.int/features/factfiles/mental_health/en>.

Recommended Reading

American Psychiatric Association, 2013. *Diagnostic and statistical manual of mental disorders*, DSM-5, 5th ed. American Psychiatric Association, Washington, DC.

Evans, J., Brown, P., 2012. *Videbeck's mental health nursing*, 1st Australian ed. Lippincott Williams & Wilkins, Philadelphia.

National Health and Medical Research Council, 2012. Clinical practice guideline for the management of borderline personality disorder. Available at: <https://www.nhmrc.gov.au/about-us/publications/clinical-practice-guideline-borderline-personality-disorder>.

Nursing and Midwifery Board of Australia (NMBA), 2016. Enrolled nurse standards for practice. Available at: <http://www.nursingmidwiferyboard.gov.au/Codes-Guidelines-Statements/Professional-standards.aspx>.

Online Resources

Alcohol & Drug Foundation: <https://adf.org.au/reducing-risk/aod-mental-health>.

Australian and New Zealand College of Mental Health Nurses: <www.anzcmhn.org>.

Beyond Blue: <https://www.beyondblue.org.au>.

Black Dog Institute: <https://www.blackdoginstitute.org.au>.

British Psychological Society: <www.bps.org.uk>.

Department of Health & Aged Care: <https://www.health.gov.au/topics/mental-health-and-suicide-prevention>.

Head to Health: <https://headtohealth.gov.au>.

Headspace: <http://www.headspace.org.au>.

Mental Health First Aid: <mhfa.com.au>.

SANE Australia: <https://www.sane.org>.

World Health Organization, 2015: <http://www.who.int/topics/mental_health/en>.

CHAPTER

40

Rehabilitation

Sally Moyle

Key Terms

adaptation
choice
community
decision-making
disability
education
empowerment
habilitation
independence
person-centred goals
rehabilitation
team

Learning Outcomes

At the completion of this chapter and with further reading, learners should be able to:

- Define the key terms.
- Recognise the terminology used in rehabilitation nursing to describe the individual's level of functioning.
- Explain the philosophy of rehabilitation.
- Outline the functions of each member of the rehabilitation team.
- Describe the process of adjustment to disability.
- Recognise a person-centred approach to nursing care of the individual who requires rehabilitation.
- Develop a plan of care for a person experiencing disability within the context of their environment.
- Examine the effects of interactions between the individual, carers/family, health professionals and community context in the rehabilitation process.
- Demonstrate problem-solving skills appropriate to the discipline by identifying potential issues involved in assessment and nursing care for a person with a disability.

CHAPTER FOCUS

Rehabilitation is a dynamic process which, to be effective, must occur as a collaborative process involving all members of the rehabilitation team, of which the individual is the most important. Effective rehabilitation enables the individual to achieve optimal physical, emotional, psychological, social and vocational potential to maintain dignity and self-respect. Rehabilitation empowers the individual to make informed choices about healthcare and achieve a level of wellness that is acceptable to that individual. The rehabilitation nurse provides care and employs education and supportive strategies based on rehabilitation philosophy, goals and concepts. Rehabilitation is a process of functional improvement that involves the individual, family, community and healthcare provider. Optimal function is achieved when the uniqueness and wholeness of the individual is recognised. The focus of this chapter is to introduce the nurse to the processes of rehabilitation and the many facets of rehabilitation that can be practised in any care setting.

LIVED EXPERIENCE

I was so frightened when I heard that James had been hurt badly in an accident when he was riding his bike and was hit by a car. At the start, I didn't think that he would ever do anything for himself again, but there have been so many improvements, some of them just small, but I count them all the same. We would go for a bike ride together with our children every Sunday morning to the park, but we can't do that anymore and we're the ones who now need to help look after him.

Sara, wife to James, 42, who suffered multiple fractures and an acquired brain injury following a cycling accident 6 months previously

INTRODUCTION

Rehabilitation is a complex process with a range of dimensions including motivation; adaptation to change; coping with stress; adjustment to altered circumstances, body capabilities and/or appearance; and regaining independence and wellness.

The basic aim of rehabilitation nursing is to limit the effects of disability and impairment in individuals with particular conditions. It begins with immediate care to minimise the effects of damage and to prevent complications in the stage immediately after an accident or the onset of illness. It continues through the time individuals are receiving restorative care and it often necessitates helping them to adapt to a permanently changed situation and a new kind of life. Rehabilitation nursing includes a wide range of activities to collaborate with other members of a rehabilitation team for the following:

- Retrain physically damaged individuals to walk again.
- Retrain cognitively damaged individuals to communicate effectively orally or in writing.
- Help individuals adapt to impairment in a way that enables them to care for their own needs, such as showering, dressing and eating and using ordinary toilet facilities.
- Promote individuals' abilities to manage ordinary everyday modes of travel.
- Teach individuals how to put on, remove and care for different types of prosthetic appliances (e.g. an artificial limb or eye).
- Provide support to the individual and help them adjust emotionally to their change in function.

(McQuillan 2020; Ralston et al 2022; Steinmetz & Benzel 2021)

The rehabilitation process comprises the following stages:

- assessment
- goal setting: short-term, medium-term and long-term
- development of a plan to achieve goals
- evaluation of progress.

(Ignatavicius et al 2021; Ralston et al 2022)

Clinical Interest Box 40.1 describes this process in more detail.

Rehabilitation also takes place in mental health nursing and includes minimising impairment in function and preventing relapse in individuals who experience recurrent problems with mental health. Clinical Interest Box 40.2 indicates the main characteristics of the rehabilitation process.

CLINICAL INTEREST BOX 40.1 What is rehabilitation?

At its core, rehabilitation is about:

- maximising a person's abilities and independence
- restoring lost function
- preventing new or further functional loss
- working with other healthcare professionals.

CLINICAL INTEREST BOX 40.2 The rehabilitation process

- Assessment: The individual must first be assessed by the rehabilitation team prior to planning for their treatment. This assessment will involve all aspects of their health, including physical, social, emotional and psychological aspects.
- Goal setting: Goal setting will focus on both long-term and short-term goals and will be personalised to the individual.
- Development of a rehabilitation plan: The rehabilitation plan will be developed by the rehabilitation team in conjunction with the individual.
- Implementation: Implementation of the rehabilitation plan will involve the rehabilitation team and the individual. It will be consistently reassessed in order to ensure it is relevant to the individual and their goals.
- Evaluation of progress: Evaluation of the individual's progress will occur at regular intervals during their rehabilitation and any changes deemed necessary will be implemented into their rehabilitation plan.

Rehabilitation services can be delivered using a number of models of care including multidisciplinary and interdisciplinary teams, inpatient, outpatient, domiciliary and community-based rehabilitation services. All models include, to a varying extent, a **team** of people comprising the individual, their family, allied health and nursing professionals and specialist rehabilitation doctors, working collaboratively to achieve the individual's goals.

Categories of individuals requiring rehabilitation

A person may experience a **disability** of acute or chronic onset at any stage of the lifespan. Those conditions requiring rehabilitation can be categorised as follows:

- acute onset (e.g. stroke, head injury, myocardial infarction)
- gradual onset/relapsing course (e.g. multiple sclerosis, rheumatoid arthritis, motor neuron disease, Parkinson's disease)
- acute onset/constant course (e.g. spinal cord injury, burns)
- gradual onset/progressive course (e.g. heart failure, some cancers, HIV, respiratory conditions).

(Brown et al 2020; Chang & Johnson 2022; Cifu 2020)

Rehabilitation services have four target groups:

1. individuals who cannot go home from hospital without a return of, or improvement in, function
2. individuals discharged after an acute admission who require continuing care as an outpatient
3. people living with congenital or acquired disability or progressive illness with the goal of preventing the need for hospitalisation
4. people who are ageing and experiencing the functional losses associated with multiple chronic diseases.

(Gutenbrunner et al 2020; Tijsen et al 2019)

Rehabilitation programs may be developed and implemented for an individual who is experiencing any of the conditions listed in Clinical Interest Box 40.3.

In many situations, complete rehabilitation is achieved; but in others, complete recovery of function is not possible, and the individual faces a permanent disability or impairment. (See Chapter 41 for definitions of these terms.) When this happens, individuals must be helped to accept and adapt to and compensate for the existing or progressive impairment in order to establish an optimal level of **independence** and quality of life.

Adaptation implies the ability to adapt oneself or to modify behaviour and expectations in line with changing circumstances. Adaptation is a mechanism that affects the whole being—physically, socially and psychologically—and is a necessary process of normal life. However, in times of trauma or when facing disability, individuals may find it beyond their capabilities to adapt to circumstances without professional assistance. For a clearer understanding of adaptation, it is recommended that the reader refer to Sister Callista Roy's work, *The Roy Adaptation Model*, first published in 1984.

People involved in rehabilitation include children, adolescents, adults or older people; therefore, it is important for the nurse involved in rehabilitation nursing to apply relevant theoretical knowledge of the social, physical and psychological stages of development (Cifu 2020).

CLINICAL INTEREST BOX 40.3 Conditions frequently requiring rehabilitation

- Spinal cord injury
- Cancer
- Burns
- Joint replacement
- Brain injury
- Multiple sclerosis
- Guillain-Barré syndrome
- Heart failure
- Myocardial infarction
- Alzheimer's disease and other dementias
- Parkinson's disease
- Airway disease
- Organ transplantation
- Renal impairment
- Psychiatric or emotional disturbances

(Brown et al 2020; Chang & Johnson 2022; Cifu 2020)

The meaning of habilitation and rehabilitation

Habilitation, rather than rehabilitation, is a term that refers to the process in which a person who is born with an impairment is helped to achieve optimal independence and function by learning new skills that empower them to make choices and have degrees of control. Long-term habilitation programs are necessary for individuals born with conditions such as spina bifida, Down syndrome or intellectual or physical impairment.

One function of rehabilitation is to address long-term problems such as chronic health problems and degenerative diseases. Although there may be no cure for such conditions, a rehabilitation program can improve the quality of life. In this sense, rehabilitation is directed towards the maintenance of optimal function and prevention of complications, or towards retaining the greatest amount of function and independence that the individual desires for as long as possible.

Rehabilitation begins at the onset of illness or accident and continues until it is decided by the individual, in consultation with the rehabilitation team, that the optimal level for that particular individual has been attained. The rehabilitation process may extend over a period ranging from a few weeks to several months or years.

Rehabilitation programs are conducted in a variety of settings, including acute care hospitals, specific rehabilitation institutions, day clinics, outpatient settings, the home and in the **community** (Crisp et al 2021; Hayton & Dimitriou 2019; Wade 2020).

PHILOSOPHY OF REHABILITATION

A philosophy is a broad statement of basic related principles, concepts and beliefs. A philosophy of rehabilitation offers a framework from which the rehabilitation process can be developed. Although rehabilitation teams devise their own philosophy, philosophies of rehabilitation are generally based on the premise that rehabilitation recognises the worth and uniqueness of the person as a valuable human resource, and that rehabilitation programs must be a major integral component of care offered by health services. Rehabilitation necessitates the participation and coordination of all health team members through constant communication with the individual and significant others to develop a comprehensive rehabilitation plan acceptable to, and agreed to by, the individual. The individual receiving rehabilitation must be viewed as an active team member, and the process must actively involve the family and significant others in the individual's life. By doing this, the rehabilitation process adopts a person-centred approach.

Rehabilitation is concerned with the whole person and includes the sociocultural aspects of the person's life, sexuality, job, vocation, religion, community role and family and home. Rehabilitation aims to achieve the highest level of empowerment and independence possible for the individual and is person-centred and goal focused (Chang & Johnson 2022; Jesus et al 2022).

Person-centred goals and empowerment

Goal setting can be seen as a way to give control back to individuals and make empowerment real. As individuals reach goals, the nurse must help the individual to realise that their achievements are due to their own abilities. The nurse can guide the individual so that they are empowered in **decision-making**, taking control, and accepting that progress is due to their own effort. This knowledge will help them maintain the motivation to continue to strive for more independence. Person-centred goal planning in individuals with spinal cord injuries has been found to facilitate increases in independence and gains in physical, social and psychological functioning (Rose et al 2019).

In healthcare, **empowerment** is defined as an educational process designed to help individuals develop the knowledge, skills, attitudes and self-awareness required to effectively assume responsibility for their health-related decisions. Empowerment is an approach that aims to establish the individual's autonomy and self-control and enables groups or individuals to change after being given the skills, resources, opportunities and authority to do so (Chang & Johnson 2022; Pekonen et al 2020). Traditionally, individuals have been regarded as passive recipients of care, with healthcare providers being considered the experts. This view differs from the modern paradigm of empowerment in which the individual should become an expert in their own healthcare. This approach allows individuals to acquire skills and knowledge for improving their overall health status and focuses on health promotion, individuals' abilities rather than disabilities, and wellness rather than illness.

A partnership between team members and the individual transfers power and builds on the person's self-esteem and self-worth. Often individuals in rehabilitation experience feelings of poor self-esteem and a sense of worthlessness. They can be grieving for what they perceive as a loss of independence and lifestyle. **Person-centred goals** can assist in identifying what is important to that individual. The individual may not always set the goals at the level the team believes they should be able to achieve. It is not an effective use of resources if therapists aim for the individual to walk 100 metres if the person only wants to walk around the house or only wants to be able to walk to the letterbox. The goals must be realistic, and the individual must have a desire to reach them. Clinical Interest Box 40.4 discusses how to set effective goals. One of the most effective ways the nurse can empower the individual is to offer **choice**. Asking the individual what they would 'normally' prefer to do, and then allowing it to happen, is a step towards empowerment. The rehabilitation nurse should include the individual's own beliefs, wishes and goals in the delivery of

CLINICAL INTEREST BOX 40.4 Goal setting

Goals are an important component in the rehabilitation care of an individual. Goals are often set using the SMART acronym as follows.

- Specific
- Measurable
- Attainable
- Relevant
- Time-bound

It is also important that large goals are broken down into smaller goals or steps in order to maintain the individual's motivation.

care; therefore, goal setting should be a collaborative process between the individual and the healthcare team (Cifu 2020; Rose et al 2019).

The importance of the individual feeling in control of what is happening, what is being planned and of decisions that affect their life cannot be emphasised strongly enough. Person-centred rehabilitation is precisely that—rehabilitation planned together with an individual and their carers, families and friends, around their goals, needs and existing circumstances. There is great skill involved in empowering the individual. This sense of control is facilitated when the individual participates in determining their own rehabilitation goals.

It is important for nurses working in the area of rehabilitation to keep in mind that throughout the process of rehabilitation the individual and the family are often facing markedly changed circumstances and may be struggling to adapt to what has happened. This may also be a time when an individual's choices may not be guided by rehabilitation-orientated goals and can lead to ethical concerns regarding risk of harm to the individual versus maintaining the individual's autonomy (Gutenbrunner et al 2022; Rose et al 2019).

ADJUSTMENT TO DISABILITY

The process of adjustment as it relates to disability is similar to that in dying. (See Chapter 38 for more information on loss, grief and dying and palliative care.) Disability involves loss and is accompanied by an adjustment process as the individual and significant others learn to come to terms with the disability and its implications. The grieving process gradually occurs as the impairment increasingly impacts on the individual's level of function (Forber-Pratt et al 2019). The individual may experience loss of:

- sensation
- skin integrity
- a body part
- ability to walk
- use of an arm
- bowel and/or bladder control
- sexual function
- ability to speak, read, write and comprehend
- memory
- ability to relate to other people and the environment
- self-image, sense of self-worth, self-esteem, sexuality
- independence.

The person whose disability has only occurred recently generally experiences four stages in adjustment during the rehabilitation process:

1. Acute disorganisation: The individual may express feelings of extreme anxiety, fear and disbelief that such an event has occurred.
2. Assessment: The individual begins to assess what has happened and begins to recognise and identify changes in function and ability. They may experience anger, depression, denial and bargaining. The individual may hope for a spontaneous recovery or a medical miracle and tends to resist activities designed to help regain function from impairment (Forber-Pratt et al 2019).
3. Mourning: The individual continues to experience anger and depression; however, there is a new awareness of the losses involved. The individual begins to accept the changed probable future and no longer denies or ignores the disability. Eventually the individual begins to participate more fully in the rehabilitation program.
4. Re-entry: The individual resolves the depression of the mourning process and begins to experience more positive feelings about the self and the future. They recognise that the disability does in fact exist and are keen to find means to adapt their personal lifestyle to the disability.

It is important for nurses to understand that each person will have an individual timetable for adjusting and adapting to living with a disability. Thus, while some people adjust in a relatively brief time, others will take much longer. There is no normal period of time before a person finally accepts and adjusts to a disability. It must not be forgotten that the family also goes through a process of grieving and adjustment, including experiencing feelings of overwhelming shock, helplessness, denial, disbelief, sadness, anger and anxiety (Kitzmuller et al 2019). The rehabilitation team plays an important role since it supports the individual and family during the process of adjustment and adaptation. Progress Note 40.1 displays documentation of an individual who is having difficulty adjusting and displays anxiety in relation to their change in independence and level of function.

CRITICAL THINKING EXERCISE 40.1

Discuss the emotional and psychological effects an individual may have following a decline in their physical level of function and how this may then affect their participation in their rehabilitation program.

CRITICAL THINKING EXERCISE 40.2

Discuss why it is so important that an individual has sufficient social and emotional support during rehabilitation and following their discharge. Who can assist the individual with this support?

THE REHABILITATION TEAM

Effective rehabilitation involves person-centred care planning with the individual, family or significant others and the whole healthcare team. The special needs of the individual determine the fields of expertise that are represented in the rehabilitation team. An interprofessional team is required and consists of members from various disciplines, each with a vital role to play. Clinical Interest Box 40.5 identifies some of the people who might be included in a rehabilitation team. Which team members are included depends on the specific needs of the individual e.g. a non-English-speaking person would need an interpreter to be included).

Members of the rehabilitation team

The individual

It is essential that the individual who requires rehabilitation be viewed as a pivotal team member. The other team members must help motivate the individual to be actively involved in the rehabilitation process, however slow it may be. Unless the individual is encouraged, a lack of motivation and cooperation with prescribed therapy may result. It is important that each small achievement is positively reinforced (e.g. recognised, praised or rewarded). At all stages of rehabilitation, the rest of the team must consider the individual's strengths and weaknesses and the social and cultural influences that affect adjustment to disability (Yun & Choi 2019). The team must be aware of how the individual perceives the illness and the impact of the disability that has occurred.

A disturbance of an individual's body image—for example, paralysis resulting from a cerebrovascular accident—is difficult to accept. The initial reaction is usually one of shock, followed by denial. As the individual gradually realises what has happened and that life may never be the same again, they may experience depression, anger or guilt (Stott et al 2021). Self-esteem and self-worth are threatened (see Chapter 39 and Chapter 41). While there is inevitable dependency initially, the overall aim of rehabilitation is to help the individual regain optimal quality of life. The motivation of the individual is crucial, and it is essential that the individual be regarded as the most important team member, who must be encouraged to participate actively in all aspects of the rehabilitation process. The individual must be involved in planning the personal rehabilitation program with the team. The individual must learn in detail about the disability that has been experienced and ways of accomplishing the desired goals. The team must inform the individual as to what options are available so that the person can choose the best options for a successful outcome (Rose et al 2019).

CLINICAL INTEREST BOX 40.5
Members of the rehabilitation team

- The individual
- The individual's family/friend(s) or significant other(s)
- Nurse
- Case manager
- Counsellor (possibly an expert in grief and loss counselling)
- Physiotherapist
- Occupational therapist
- Speech therapist
- Social worker
- Dietitian
- Podiatrist
- Prosthetist/orthotist
- Psychiatrist
- Psychologist
- Chaplain or other religious/spiritual support person
- Teacher/educator (essential for children undergoing long-term rehabilitation)
- Medical officer (often the team's clinical director)

(Brown et al 2020; Crisp et al 2021)

The family or friends

The family, or significant others, are recognised as a potential support system for the individual. Members of the family are evaluated to determine their ability to help with the rehabilitation process. All families, or significant others, cannot contribute in the same way or to the same degree. In some instances, the individual can return home and receive excellent care and support, while in other situations, the family may be unable or unwilling to help care for the person. Since each situation presents different problems, individual evaluation is essential.

The family, or significant others, need to understand and/or be involved with the rehabilitative goals that the individual develops with the team, and the methods selected to meet these goals. Partners, family members or supportive friends need to understand that their greatest contribution may be to allow the individual to be as independent as possible. This may be difficult for them at times, as their natural instinct may be to assist and 'do for' their loved one. In addition, those supporting the individual can be instructed in how to assist with specific therapy, thus enabling them to feel that they are playing a vital role in rehabilitation.

It is important to understand that when illness or disability occurs, family life is interrupted and altered. The effects of illness have significant implications for the family as well as for the individual. Plans for the rehabilitation process should, therefore, also address the needs of the family as well as those of the individual (Kokorelias et al 2019).

The nurse and the team must remember that a spouse or partner can become depressed if their loved one faces permanent lifestyle changes. It is important to inform the spouse or significant other that this is a normal reaction and encourage the person to seek assistance from a medical officer or team psychologist. Another concern with family occurs when ageing carers assisting relatives with disabilities in the home environment themselves become ill and are no longer able to provide care for their dependent relatives. People who have been cared for by their loved ones in the community for many years are sometimes suddenly faced with a crisis because that carer has become ill. This often limits the amount of support that the carer has for transition back into the community, and placement of the individual they cared for may be an issue if the carer cannot resume a level of functioning that enables a return to the role of carer.

The nurse

Rehabilitation nursing is a specialty area of practice requiring specialised knowledge, skills and attitudes.

The skills of the rehabilitation nurse include:

- communication
- listening
- facilitating
- enabling
- coordination
- leading
- collaboration
- empowerment
- liaison
- advocating
- educating
- planning.

The goal of rehabilitation nursing is to assist people with disability and chronic illness to attain maximal functional ability, maintain optimal health, prevent and minimise disability and adapt to an altered lifestyle (Chang & Johnson 2022; Ralston et al 2022). Goals of rehabilitation nursing include maximising:

- potential
- learning
- ability
- quality of life
- family-centred care
- wellness
- culturally competent care
- community reintegration.

Nurses are in a prime position to promote these things because they spend more time with the individual than any other member of the rehabilitation team, and therefore play a pivotal role in assessing, planning, implementing and evaluating care. A nursing assessment includes an evaluation of the extent to which the individual's physical and psychosocial needs are met.

In rehabilitation, a Registered Nurse (RN) makes a nursing assessment and develops a nursing care plan to meet the needs of the individual, taking into account the person's goals, both short and long term. An Enrolled Nurse (EN) provides care under the direction of the RN. In many settings, nursing is the only component of the rehabilitation team represented throughout the entire 24 hours of each day. Nurses are therefore responsible for reinforcing the health education of other team members—such as the physiotherapist and occupational therapist—throughout this time, so that there is continuity of the rehabilitation program. The rehabilitation nurse's role includes preventing complications that would impede the restoration of optimal functioning; therefore, attention to potential problems as well as actual problems is necessary (Gutenbrunner et al 2022).

The effective rehabilitation nurse understands the short- and long-term goals of the individual and the rehabilitation program. The nurse has a pivotal role in the multidisciplinary team and is aware of the need to liaise and communicate closely with all team members to achieve coordinated and effective outcomes for the individual. This often means that the nurse's role needs to be flexible and amenable to change. The nurse requires a full understanding of the role and function of each team member and needs to recognise when to refer to the expertise of others as the individual's needs indicate.

Individuals react and respond in various ways to personal health conditions and the rehabilitation program. The nurse must be able to assess accurately, monitor and educate the individuals and their significant others throughout the process, so that the individual's goals and the rehabilitation goals can be achieved successfully. The nurse works in a partnership with the individual, assisting them to make informed choices and have control over the process. At times, the nurse might find it difficult to empower the individual, especially if they are despondent and in the early stages of denial. It is essential that the nurse takes time to build rapport and trust. Advocacy for the person is vital for this trust to develop. The nurse should be responsive to the individual's rights and be able to advocate for the individual in team discussions. The nurse's role involves being an educator, not only for the individual but also for the family, carers and other staff. This **education** will involve teaching rehabilitative techniques, preventing complications and promoting a healthy lifestyle. The nurse will act as a resource for information and clarification and know when to call in other professionals to assist.

Many clinical skills are employed when working as a rehabilitation nurse. Depending on the individual person, skills employed may include pain and continence management, preventing pressure areas, wound management and behaviour management. While the rehabilitation nurse needs to acquire excellent general nursing knowledge, there may be a necessity to refer to more advanced trained rehabilitation nurses specialising in neurological, orthopaedic, cardiac/pulmonary, oncology, renal, gerontic or paediatric rehabilitation nursing. The rehabilitation nursing team members among them commonly have a skill mix that meets the needs of the individual (Gutenbrunner et al 2022).

Rehabilitation nursing takes place in any specialty or clinical environment where the aim is to maximise independence and minimise the impact of disability in individuals with particular impairments. Therefore, many nurses, including those who have not specialised in rehabilitation nursing, are involved in the rehabilitation process. However, should a nurse choose to make rehabilitation nursing a career focus, there are many different specialty areas of rehabilitation nursing, including orthopaedics, burns, spinal injury, head injury, amputation, cardiac and stroke rehabilitation (Brown et al 2020).

The case manager

The case manager can be of any discipline. It is a popular role for the rehabilitation nurse with advanced training. The case manager develops a formal, written, comprehensive needs assessment that includes a formal review of evaluations performed by other members of the rehabilitation team. The case manager assists the individual and the service provider in planning and program development that meets the individual's needs as identified and prioritised in the assessment. The case manager's role and function will vary depending on the practice setting. The case manager may be employed in an institutional setting such as a hospital or rehabilitation facility, or they may work in the insurance industry, such as the Transport Accident Commission (TAC) or a health insurance organisation.

The physiotherapist

Physiotherapists evaluate the individual's physical capabilities and limitations in a collaborative assessment process. The physiotherapist administers therapies designed to correct or minimise deformity, increase strength and mobility or alleviate discomfort or pain (Ignatavicius 2021; Killingback 2022). The physiotherapist has a person-centred approach. Treatments include the use of specific exercises, heat, cold, hydrotherapy and electrophysical therapy. A physiotherapist is also involved in educating the individual and their family or significant others and other team members in correct methods of positioning, transferring and mobilising so that what is taught in therapy sessions can be carried over to day-to-day activities and reinforced by the nurse.

Physiotherapy will help with weak or tight muscles, stiff joints, poor coordination, balance, stair practice, walking and general fitness along with everyday functional activities such as rolling in bed, sitting, standing up and reaching forward/using hands.

The occupational therapist

Occupational therapists are concerned with assisting the individual to achieve independent performance in the activities of daily living (ADLs). They also assess the need for, and provide, adaptive devices (e.g. aids such as specially designed cutlery or making a splint for someone's hand so they can grasp their cutlery to feed themselves).

The occupational therapist usually assesses the individual's home in preparation for transition back into the community. This is done in conjunction with the individual and family on the pre-discharge home visit. Home modifications may be required to an individual's home to ensure the individual's safety and enhance their ability to mobilise and function as independently as possible despite any physical limitations. Equipment may need to be provided to ensure that the home environment is safe and conducive to the individual's independence level. Modifications may be minor, such as installation of a handrail, or major, such as structural alterations to enlarge space in a toilet and bathroom if a wheelchair or lifting machine needs to be accommodated. The occupational therapist may also be involved in teaching someone with memory problems strategies so that, for instance, they can remember to purchase everything they need at the supermarket (Chang & Johnson 2022).

The speech pathologist/therapist

Speech pathologists, otherwise referred to as speech therapists, are also involved in the individual's goal-setting process. They are concerned with assessing, diagnosing and treating aphasia, which encompasses communication and language disorders, such as the formation and perception of speech, the ability to articulate words and to understand and initiate speech, retraining reading and writing skills following a stroke, or teaching someone how to speak after a traumatic brain injury (Chang & Johnson 2022; Willis 2020). As part of the rehabilitation process a speech therapist may be required to assist a person to relearn communication skills. Communication deficits present a real problem for affected individuals, and much reassurance and counselling are often required. The individual who cannot speak may feel hopeless and frustrated. Often, depending on the area of brain affected by a brain injury, the individual can understand fully but cannot articulate. Technical devices may need to be used to assist the individual to communicate with others. If both areas of the speech centre are damaged, global aphasia may occur, in which the person cannot speak or understand the spoken word. How to empower this individual is a challenge.

A speech pathologist may also be involved in the management of an individual with dysphagia in which their swallowing abilities are impaired (e.g. after a stroke). The speech pathologist liaises closely with the nurse, dietitian and family to achieve safe swallowing strategies for the individual. In consultation with the individual, a videofluoroscopy may be required to ascertain the extent of the swallowing deficit. (See Clinical Interest Box 40.6.) Often, the individual and family will resist the strategy of thickened fluids to prevent aspiration; therefore, in-depth education and counselling are required so that informed choices, including a full understanding of the risks, can be made. It is the individual's choice as to whether treatment strategies are followed.

CLINICAL INTEREST BOX 40.6 Videofluoroscopy—a diagnostic test to identify dysphagia

Videofluoroscopy is a modified barium swallow conducted by the speech pathologist and radiologist to determine the extent of dysphagia and to identify if the individual is at risk of aspiration. The test allows for the viewing of the oral cavity, laryngopharynx and cervical oesophagus. The person swallows small amounts of a liquid puree or solid mixed with barium. As the individual manipulates the bolus in the oral cavity and swallows, the fluoroscopic study is recorded on videotape. Videotaping of the swallowing study allows clinicians to have repeated viewing and slow-motion analysis.

(Labeit et al 2022)

The social worker

Social workers are concerned with counselling and assisting individuals and their families who are experiencing personal problems as a result of illness or injury. A social worker acts as an advocate by liaising with existing community groups and resources and assists the individual and the family to deal with social, domestic, financial and emotional implications of the illness or condition. The social worker engages in discharge planning and often accompanies the occupational therapist and individual on the pre-discharge home visit. The social worker communicates with the community services that may be required to assist the individual when discharged home or, if alternative placement is required, the social worker would assist in this process (Jellema 2021).

Social workers assist individuals and their carers to deal with the emotional impact of illness, traumatic injury and disability and the adjustment to hospitalisation. Social workers help individuals and carers to adjust to life changes and challenges, deal with grief and loss, explore emotions, thoughts and behaviour, improve relationships and plan for the future.

Social workers provide counselling to individuals and families, assist individuals with financial, accommodation, legal and other problems, run groups to provide support for carers, participate in discharge planning and link individuals to community support services for assistance post discharge.

The dietitian

Dietitians are concerned with assessing nutritional needs and planning ways to meet those needs (Chang & Johnson 2022). As part of the rehabilitation process, the individual may require specific dietary restrictions or modifications, and a dietitian collaborates closely with the individual to plan an appropriate diet. The dietitian also plays a key role in ensuring that all those involved with the individual's care understand the importance of a specific diet for the person's recovery. Nutritional screening is also important for persons over the age of 65.

The podiatrist

Podiatrists are concerned with assessing, preventing and treating disorders of the feet. As part of the rehabilitation process, an individual may be required to relearn how to ambulate (e.g. after a cerebrovascular accident). To mobilise, the feet must be in good condition, with no skin lesions or nail disorders, and the podiatrist plays an important role in maintaining the health and integrity of the skin and toenails. In collaboration with the individual, the podiatrist determines appropriate footwear for safe mobilisation.

The prosthetist/orthotist

Prosthetists are concerned with assessing an individual's need for prosthesis, such as an artificial limb. After assessment, a prosthetist designs and supplies an appropriate prosthesis. Generally, a temporary prosthesis is provided and trialled before a permanent one is supplied. Modifications to an existing prosthesis may be made by a prosthetist who also checks at regular intervals to ensure that the prosthesis is meeting the individual's needs (Figure 40.1). Some individuals may need to be fitted with splints or braces to correct deformities or provide added support. Such mechanical devices are called orthoses, and include braces

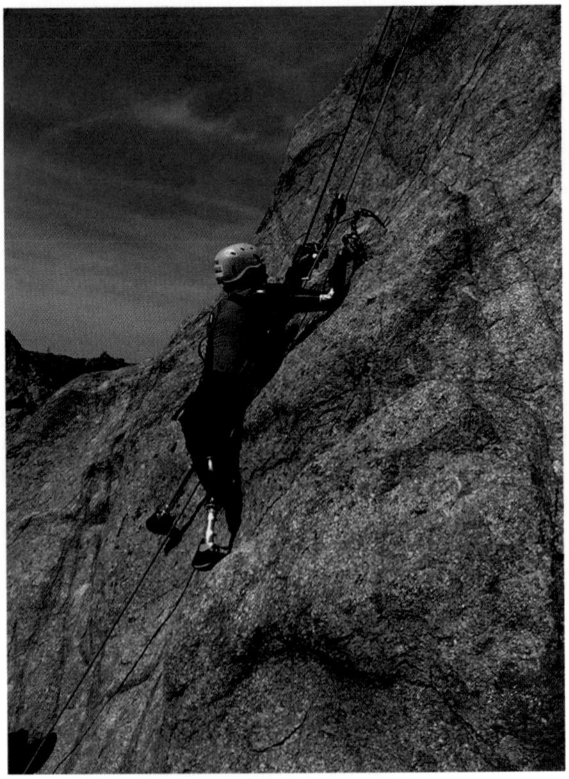

Figure 40.1 Some prostheses are specifically designed for activities

(Pendleton and Schultz-Krohn 2018)

for the neck, arm or leg. These assist with mobilisation and improve the quality of life for individuals (Kubiak et al 2019).

The psychiatrist and psychologist

If the individual is experiencing a psychiatric or emotional problem, either a psychiatrist or a psychologist is generally involved in the rehabilitation process. A psychiatrist is concerned with the causes, prevention and treatment of mental, emotional and behavioural disorders. A clinical psychologist is concerned with the causes, prevention and treatment of individual social problems, especially regarding the interaction between the individual and the physical and social environment. A psychiatrist, clinical psychologist or neuropsychologist may be involved in the rehabilitation of an individual who is depressed as a result of the implications of the disability, or if behavioural problems result from the condition. The psychologist can also assist the rehabilitation team with strategies to manage individuals who have behavioural disturbances that impact on the day-to-day rehabilitation process. These disciplines can also assist the family or significant others if problems of coping and adaptation are identified. Depression can be common in the individual undergoing rehabilitation, especially individuals who have been hospitalised for a prolonged period of time; family members are also vulnerable to depression (Cifu 2020).

The clinical director (medical officer)

The clinical director is commonly a medical officer specialising in rehabilitation medicine and is often the first member of the team to encounter the individual as a response to a referral for rehabilitation intervention. The medical officer is responsible for the medical and/or surgical management of the person and oversees the treatment that involves meeting the physical, emotional and social needs of the individual (Chang & Johnson 2022). These needs must be satisfied to successfully restore the individual's quality of life to maximum potential. The medical officer collaborates with all members of the team and is usually the team leader. They assess the individual's health status regularly and explain the diagnosis and prognosis to the individual and relatives. The medical officer often takes on the role of chairing the case conferences and other meetings, such as team and family meetings. Regular ward rounds are conducted by the medical officer, who also has an active educative role with team members, particularly for more junior medical members of the team.

Case conferences and team meetings

These meetings are held at regular intervals and are the forum at which team members discuss the progress and problems of every individual who is undertaking rehabilitation. During these meetings, the individual's short- and long-term goals are discussed, with each member being aware of, and respecting, the roles of others in accomplishing these goals. Goals must be re-evaluated regularly with the individual, so that the individual and therapists can determine whether they are realistic and/or whether they have been accomplished. All goals should be set with specific timeframes. Specific therapy goals are also set at these meetings. These therapy goals are compatible with the individual's goals but are usually broken up into smaller attainable sequences, with timeframes. For example, William will stand for 3 minutes, with the aid of the tilt table, three times tomorrow. William will increase time on the tilt table in increments of 2–3 minutes until standing for 10 minutes three times a day.

Each team member explains to the other members the procedures and techniques to be carried out. The proceedings are documented in terms that are meaningful and valid for all persons concerned. The individual and/or family may or may not be present at the case conference, depending on the time limitations of the meeting and the individual healthcare facility's policy. Quite often a designated team member meets with the individual and family before or after the meeting to discuss and inform and assist in the decision-making process. Family conferences can be conducted aside from the case conference when more time can be given to the concerns of the individual and their family.

THE PROCESS OF REHABILITATION

The rehabilitation process involves assessing the individual's rehabilitation potential, planning and implementing an appropriate program and continuous evaluation of progress (Cifu 2020; Wade 2020).

Assessment of rehabilitation potential

Assessment of the individual and a realistic evaluation of their rehabilitation potential is the first step towards planning a program. Assessment involves determining the individual's:

- expected level of functional ability
- readiness to participate
- knowledge level
- ability to understand expectations and instructions
- self-efficacy
- self-esteem
- energy levels
- priorities at any point in time.

(Ignatavicius 2021; Salawu et al 2020)

In some instances, assessment can be a relatively simple process, while in others, it is more complicated. For example, it is comparatively easy to assess the rehabilitation potential of a healthy young adult with a fractured femur, while it is more difficult to make an assessment in an elderly person with diabetes who has experienced a stroke.

Assessment may take the form of observation, listening, interview, physical exam and consultation with other team members and/or family.

Assessment of each individual must take into account:

- The nature of the disability. Some conditions affect only isolated areas of the body, while others exert widespread effect. Some disorders cause progressive and diverse impairment of function.
- The overall condition of the individual and their ability to cope with a rehabilitation program. There may be other existing conditions that could influence the choice of rehabilitation measures (e.g. chronic conditions such as arthritis or emphysema may restrict the person's ability to engage in active exercise).
- The motivation of the individual and the understanding of the situation. The individual's motivation should stem from a realistic acceptance of the situation and should not be the result of over-optimism or a refusal to acknowledge limitations.
- The individual's home environment and the ability of the family or significant others to be supportive.

Physical and psychological assessment of the individual is performed to evaluate functional state, so that a suitable program involving both short- and long-term goals can be set (Rose et al 2019; Wade 2020). Assessment includes evaluating muscle function, range-of-joint motion, body alignment and posture, neurological function, cardiopulmonary function, mood and cognition. The assessment should identify both the abilities and the limitations of ADLs and mobility.

A number of tests can be used to assess functional ability and ADLs and include the Functional Independence Measure (FIM) and the Barthel Index. The FIM is an 18-item assessment used to measure the individual's ability to perform ADLs related to self-care, elimination, locomotion, transfers, communication and cognition. The FIM assesses and tracks changes to the individual's level of disability and function during their rehabilitation. (See Clinical Interest Box 40.7.)

Assessment of concerns/alterations to sexual function should also be taken into consideration. (See Case Study 40.1.)

CLINICAL INTEREST BOX 40.7 Functional Independence Measure (FIM)

The FIM instrument is used to assess the severity of an individual's disability and their level of function and then track any changes. It includes the following 18 items:

- eating
- grooming
- bathing
- dressing upper body
- dressing lower body
- toileting
- bladder management
- bowel management
- transfer to bed/chair/wheelchair
- transfer to toilet
- transfer to shower/tub
- locomotion
- stairs
- comprehension
- expression
- social interaction
- problem-solving
- memory.

CASE STUDY 40.1

Emily's experience

Emily, aged 36, was diagnosed with multiple sclerosis (MS) 3 years ago. She is married to Chris and has a 4-year-old son. She continues to work 3 days a week as a school teacher. Recently, she has had a relapse of MS and as a consequence fell and fractured her wrist and needed to stay in hospital for rehabilitation. During the night, the nurse found Emily in her room, crying and unable to sleep. When she asked her what was keeping her awake she said 'nothing' but proceeded to cry.

What are some strategies the nurse could use to facilitate Emily discussing her feelings?

Determining short- and long-term goals

Short-term goals of a rehabilitation program are those that may be achieved in a short period of time. For example, activities such as achieving a standing position, moving from a bed to a chair, managing meals independently, tying shoelaces or formulating a sentence may be set as short-term goals. Long-term goals are those that are expected to take much longer to accomplish and depend on success in achieving the short-term goals. These may include activities such as walking, managing to climb stairs, independence in the ADLs or returning to employment. An example of the use of goals within a plan of care to assist the individual in improving their health and level of function can be found in Nursing Care Plan 40.1.

The value of setting goals is that both the individual and the team know what they are aiming for and will be able to identify when they have achieved a specific goal. As mentioned earlier, the individual and family assist in the

NURSING CARE PLAN 40.1

Assessment: Emma has had a stroke and needs full assistance with ADLs and all mobility. Sometimes in the morning when she is having breakfast in bed, she experiences some trouble swallowing and often coughs. She is experiencing dysphagia and is on a soft diet. She is incontinent of urine and faeces and wears an incontinence pad at all times. Because of this, her skin around her groin is starting to become red and excoriated. She is only able to sit out of bed in her chair for short periods during the day due to fatigue and finds that when she sits out in the morning, she is often too tired to sit out in the afternoon.

Issue/s to be addressed: Dysphagia and coughing, especially at breakfast.
Incontinence and consequent skin excoriation.
Fatigue management.

Goal/s: Emma will not cough while eating her breakfast.
Emma's skin will be intact and healthy, especially surrounding her groin area.
Emma will sit out of bed for 3 hours a day in increments of up to 1 hour, including during the afternoon.

Care/actions	Rationale
Emma will sit out of bed for breakfast.	To decrease the risk of aspiration when eating and to help with the motion of swallowing.
Emma will be toileted every 2 hours and skin care attended to at this time.	To decrease incontinence episodes and to protect her skin from breaking down.
Emma will sit out of bed for each meal, including morning and afternoon tea.	This will give Emma a timetable of sitting out of bed and ensure that she is resting between these times to assist with fatigue management.

Evaluation:
Emma does not cough with breakfast or with any meal.
Emma's groin and skin integrity remains intact.
Emma sits out of bed each day for a minimum of 3 hours.

(Chang & Johnson 2022; Crisp et al 2021)

development of the goals and this assists in empowering the individual and providing a degree of control. If realistic goals are to be set, the entire rehabilitation team must be involved in the planning process and must meet frequently to re-evaluate the situation.

It may be difficult for an individual to maintain a high level of motivation and they may think that little progress is being made and that the set goals are unattainable. They may view the rehabilitation program as tedious, boring, exhausting or painful. As a result, they may become depressed and discouraged. The nurse may help by:

- Being empathic about the situation, which involves trying to understand how the person is feeling.
- Emphasising what progress has been made and expressing honest confidence in the person's ability to make further progress.
- Spending as much time as possible with the person, particularly during activities in which active encouragement is required.
- Ensuring that the individual does not become overtired or attempt to exceed the limits prescribed. Encourage the individual to take one day at a time. Some days will be better than others.
- Encouraging the individual to concentrate on achieving one goal at a time. An over-ambitious program may result in frustration and despair.
- Encouraging the individual to express feelings. A relationship can be established by listening to the individual. This creates a sense of trust so that the person feels able to express concerns and feelings to the nurse (see Chapter 10).

CRITICAL THINKING EXERCISE 40.3

Discuss ways that as a nurse you can encourage and increase an individual's feelings of empowerment during their rehabilitation.

PLANNING AND IMPLEMENTATION

Nursing aspects of rehabilitation

Based on goals set, a collaborative plan of action needs to be developed. The nursing activities involved will depend on many factors such as the individual's age, degree of independence and type of impairment. The overall purpose of rehabilitation is restoration of the individual to optimal functioning or to assist the individual to adjust to a disability after an illness or injury. As a member of the rehabilitation team, the nurse provides support and assists the individual to meet personal physical and psychological needs. Nursing care may include care of the skin, hygiene, nutritional care, continence, sexual health, ADLs, wound management, medication administration, mobility and transfers.

Regardless of the specific impairment, the philosophy and aims of rehabilitation remain the same. The nurse plays a key role in assisting the person to carry out the ADLs and must be aware that the ultimate aim is to achieve the goals that the individual has developed with the team. The achievement of personal goals that the individual has developed is one of the most important aspects of their rehabilitation.

For example, in a program developed for a person who has experienced a stroke and subsequent hemiplegia, one specific long-term goal may be that the person is able to dress themselves. For that goal to be achieved, short-term goals will be set, such as, 'The person is able to sit up in a chair.' The occupational therapist will be involved in teaching dressing and undressing techniques, and the nurse should understand the techniques the person is using so that the teaching of the occupational therapist can be reinforced in day-to-day activity. (See Case Study 40.2.)

Continuity of care is vital for effective rehabilitation outcomes. The individual's day should be planned to maximise the rehabilitation process. It is also important that the nurse working with the individual is aware of the plan and works with them to achieve their goals. There is a tendency to 'get the work done' and, rather than allowing the time for the individual to wash and dress themself, the nurse does it for them because it is quicker than supporting them to do it themselves. It is destructive to the rehabilitation process for the nurse to take over when an individual is attempting to dress themselves (e.g. doing up the buttons on a shirt when a person is making slow progress may save the busy nurse time), but it undermines the importance of the individual's efforts and may deter them from trying in the future.

CASE STUDY 40.2

Mary, a 76-year-old woman, lives by herself and fell over while meeting her friends for lunch. She fractured her hip and required surgery. She was admitted to the rehabilitation unit 4 days after surgery for a reconditioning program.

She is on a combination of antihypertensive and cardiac medications, as well as medication for hypercholesterolaemia and vitamin D deficiency. She also requires the administration of aperients to keep her bowel actions regular. She suffers from occasional urinary incontinence and uses a pad at night. She is able to walk with a frame, and requires assistance with transfers, dressing her lower body and applying her anti-embolic stockings. She is progressing well with her therapy and a home visit identified modifications required for her bathroom, which were attended to. She is ready to be discharged home 2 weeks after admission.

1. Outline the nursing care plan you may be involved in for Mary.
2. List the rehabilitation team members involved in Mary's care and explain why they are included.
3. What education might Mary require before discharge?

In line with the National Safety and Quality Health Service Standards to manage risk, it is important that nurses ensure that any potential harm that can occur to individuals during rehabilitation is minimised, such as harm from falls and malnutrition (ACSQHC 2022).

It is especially important with individuals undergoing rehabilitation to ensure any complications from immobility are prevented, which include:

- decubitus ulcers
- contractures
- foot drop
- venous stasis
- pulmonary stasis
- urinary stasis
- constipation
- postural hypotension
- subluxation of a hemiplegic shoulder
- psychological consequences such as boredom or depression.

(Crisp et al 2021; McGlinchey et al 2020)

(See Chapter 28 for more information concerning mobility.)

Evaluation

Progress towards achieving goals needs to be reviewed regularly and is a collaborative approach between the individual, family and all the team members. Evaluation of progress may take the form of individual self-reporting, physical measurements such as timed walking, range-of-joint movements, quality-of-life indices, and team reports based on observation and interaction with the person. Based on this evaluation, the individual's goals and action plan should be reviewed and amended as required.

Aids to daily living

There are numerous devices to help a person with a disability to perform ADLs. Such devices are invaluable since they make a degree of independence possible. For example, there are long-handled shoehorns to promote independence with dressing (Figure 40.2), long-handled brushes to promote independence with hygiene (Figure 40.3) and devices to promote independence with meals (Figure 40.4) and drinking (Figure 40.5). In addition to aids assisting with ADLs, aids are also available to assist with recreational and vocational activities such as sport wheelchairs, postural support devices including Hi-Lo seating and modifications to commonly used items such as footwear, electronic equipment and workspaces. Nurses should be familiar with the full range of aids available and should be capable of teaching the individual and their family the correct way to use them. A range of available aids are listed in Clinical Interest Box 40.8.

In Australia, there are centres for independent living that provide a wide range of aids to assist with the tasks of

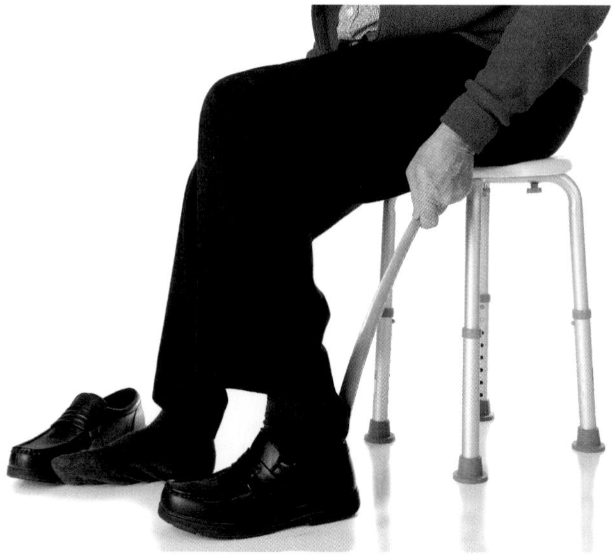

Figure 40.2 *Long-handled shoehorn*

(Wellcome Photo Library)

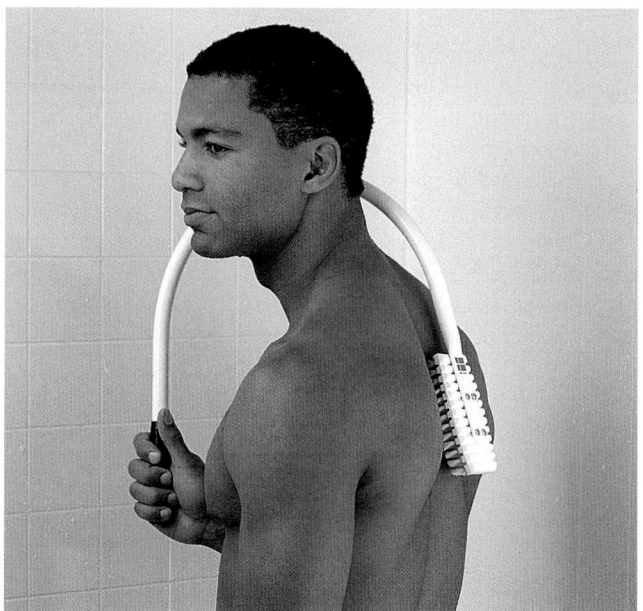

Figure 40.3 *Long-handled brush*

(Patterson Medical USA)

daily living. A variety of community services is available to assist persons with disabilities to remain at home, including community health centres, day hospitals and day centres, drop-in centres, elderly/senior citizens clubs, self-help groups, home nursing services, home meal services and sheltered workshops. Nurses should be aware of the state/territory-specific social welfare services and agencies, most of which can be found in the telephone directory or through an internet search for community services in Australia.

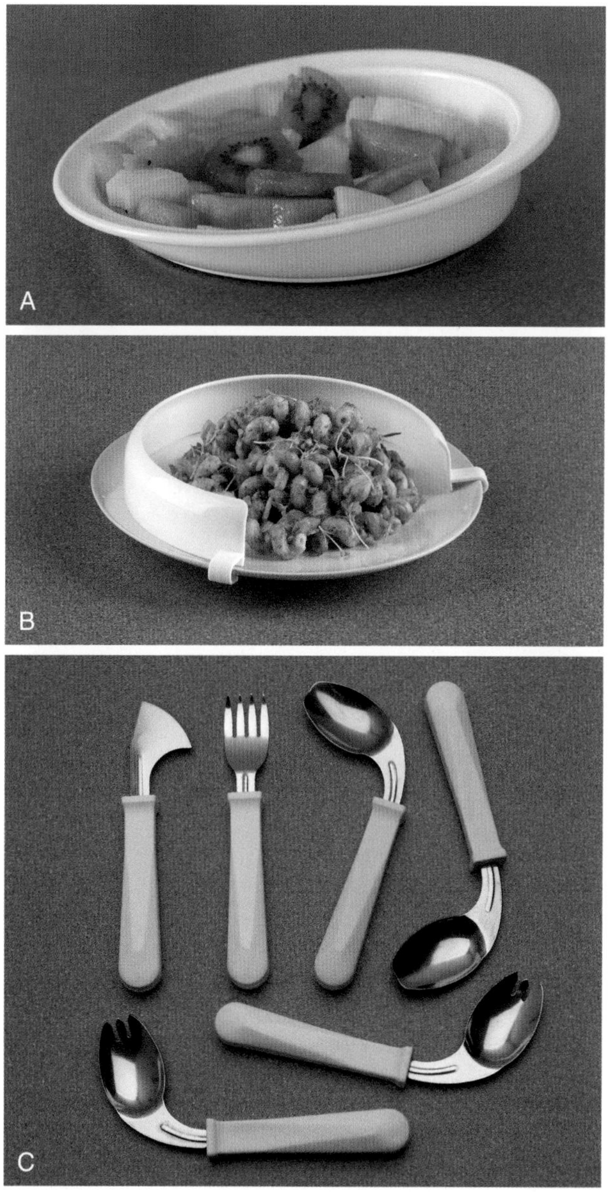

Figure 40.4 Aids to promote independence with eating

A: Scoop dish, **B:** Food guard, **C:** Easy-hold utensils (knife blade cuts in both slicing and rocking).

(Patterson Medical USA)

CULTURALLY RELEVANT CARE

In rehabilitation, nurses can bridge cultural barriers to facilitate and improve outcomes. Outcomes, interactions and responses are influenced by social and cultural factors. Family members or significant others are also interviewed to obtain accurate information as to pre-morbid functional status, personal interests, cultural considerations and discharge plans affecting the rehabilitation admission.

For those individuals from cultures different to that of the nurse, the nurse needs to take into consideration cultural influences—of their own and of the individual—on participation and decision-making. An Australian study

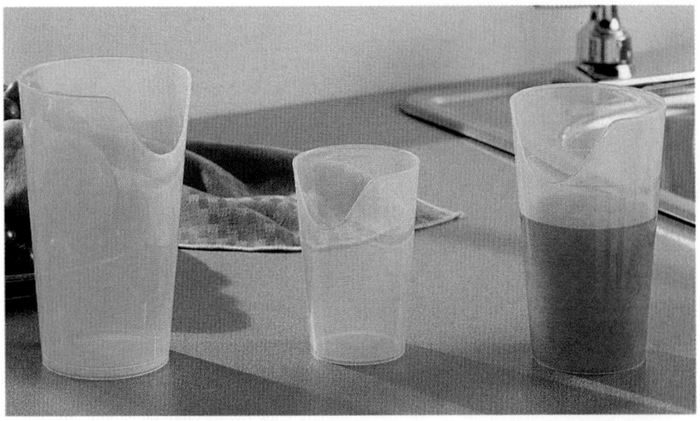

Figure 40.5 Aids to promote independence with drinking

Tumbler with a special cut-out for the nose allows the individual to drink without tipping their head back.

(Patterson Medical USA)

CLINICAL INTEREST BOX 40.8 Aids to independent living

- Suction devices fitted to kitchen utensils or backs of nail brushes for the benefit of a person with the use of only one hand
- Boards with spikes to hold fruit or vegetables to be peeled, or bread to be buttered
- Face washers in the shape of a mitten, with a pocket to hold the soap
- Long-handled tongs for a person who is unable to pick items up by bending or stooping
- Dressing sticks with one end covered by foam rubber to grip the sleeve or shoulder of a garment, making it easier to don and remove
- Various devices to enable socks and stockings to be put on
- Overlapping adhesive fastenings (e.g. velcro) on clothing for people unable to manage other conventional types of fastenings
- Long-handled shoehorns to make bending or stooping unnecessary (Figure 40.2)
- Elastic shoelaces, which do not have to be untied when shoes are removed
- Cuffs which, when placed over the hand, hold a pencil, toothbrush or razor
- Easy-to-turn tap fittings
- Raised toilet seats
- Chairs with an ejector seat, which rises as the occupant leans forward
- Ramps to replace stairways
- Hand grips in bathroom and toilet areas
- Long-handled brushes to enable individuals to perform their own hygiene activities (Figure 40.3)
- Low-level fittings for occupants of wheelchairs (e.g. sinks, stoves, mirrors, light switches)
- Eating and drinking aids (Figure 40.4 and Figure 40.5)
- Walking aids

that focused on the difficulties arising from cross-cultural care found that communication barriers were often a major factor contributing to non-adherence and non-participation in services and self-management strategies and, furthermore, these individuals were also disadvantaged in accessing health services (Brooks et al 2019). See Chapter 13 for further information on culturally appropriate care.

While 65 years of age is traditionally used as the point where the term 'older age' may be applied in the non-Aboriginal and Torres Strait Islander community, Aboriginal and Torres Strait Islander Peoples would regard a person over 45 years as an older person requiring aged-care services. The Aboriginal and Torres Strait Islander population experiences significantly greater morbidity and premature mortality compared with non-Aboriginal and Torres Strait Islander People (Secombe et al 2020; Willis et al 2020). This is a result of, among other things, the increased prevalence of chronic conditions such as cardiovascular disease, diabetes, kidney disease, chronic respiratory disease and cancer. Chapter 14 gives the reader further understanding of issues impacting Aboriginal and Torres Strait Islander Peoples.

DISCHARGE PLANNING

Discharge planning prepares the individual for the transition to another setting, such as from hospital to home. It is the link between hospitals, community-based services, organisations, families and carers. The elements of the discharge planning process should begin on the day of admission. The overall goal of discharge planning is to promote continuous healthcare services to meet the individual's needs (see Chapter 17). Effective discharge planning can decrease the chances that a person is readmitted to the hospital, can help identify care issues and needs and enable appropriate care plans to be developed.

Although discharge planning is a significant part of a person's overall care plan, frequently there is a lack of consistency in both the process and the quality of discharge planning across the healthcare system.

An effective discharge plan depends on the resources available to the individual who is being rehabilitated. Available resources include:

- the family or significant others—the individual's support systems
- home care nursing
- social and counselling agencies
- volunteer community services
- support and special interest groups (e.g. those dealing with multiple sclerosis, diabetes, cancer, heart conditions, arthritis)
- medical supplies and equipment
- adaptation of the home environment for safety and optimal independence.

The individual and the nurse, together with other team members, assist in coordinating and developing the discharge plan, using the steps of the nursing process to achieve the final plan. A discharge planner or continuing care coordinator is sometimes part of the hospital staff and functions as a consultant for the discharge planning process within a health facility, providing education and support to hospital staff in the development and implementation of discharge plans.

CRITICAL THINKING EXERCISE 40.4

Discuss some of the possible roles and functions of the nurse when planning for an individual's discharge following inpatient rehabilitation.

CRITICAL THINKING EXERCISE 40.5

Describe three community services or other resources that could help to facilitate a successful community re-entry for a person following discharge from inpatient rehabilitation.

Progress Note 40.1

31/10/2024 1400 hrs	Nursing: Mrs Jones was observed crying in her room after home visit this morning with the OT. States 'I know everyone is telling me I'm doing fine, but I just don't think that I'll be able to cope at home'. She also stated she 'Needs so much help with showering, and how can she get that help when she lives alone?' Mrs Jones is currently receiving minimal assistance with putting her shoes and socks on, otherwise she is independent with showering and dressing. She was reassured by nursing staff and is currently not crying and watching TV. OT informed and will assess with Mrs Jones tomorrow morning with her personal ADLs and determine any discharge needs. *M Woods* (WOODS), *EN*

DECISION-MAKING FRAMEWORK EXERCISE 40.1

You are working as an Enrolled Nurse (EN) within a neurological rehabilitation ward and have been allocated 12 individuals to care for with a Registered Nurse (RN) under the organisational team nursing policy. This is your second week as an EN and you have never worked in the healthcare system before. At the commencement of your shift, all of your individuals are medically stable. During your shift you notice that one of the people under your care, Mrs Turner, is deteriorating. She had a craniotomy for a subarachnoid haemorrhage following a burst aneurysm 8 days ago and is complaining of feeling generally unwell. When you question her further, she says she feels very tired, dizzy and 'muddled in her head'. You perform a set of observations on her and find she has a temperature of 38.8°C, her blood pressure is 88/60 mmHg, heart rate is 109 beats/min, oxygen saturation level is 96% and respiration rate is 20 breaths/min.

You report these findings to the RN you are working with. You state that you do not know what to do next and do not feel confident providing care to Mrs Turner. The RN tells you that this can often happen to individuals undertaking neurological rehabilitation and asks you to decide on a plan of action and report back to her. You feel unsure of what you need to do and are worried about Mrs Turner's current health status and her potential for deterioration.

Using the decision-making framework:

1. What would you do following this discussion with the RN?
2. When you do not feel confident providing care for someone under your care, what should you do?
3. Who is accountable for the provision of nursing care when working within a team nursing model?

Summary

Rehabilitation is a dynamic process in which individuals are assisted to achieve optimal quality of life by increased function and independence and within the limits of their disability. A disability is any physical, mental, emotional or social impairment that limits a person's ability to perform an activity in the usual manner.

Effective rehabilitation involves the individual, family or significant others and professional members of the healthcare team. As part of the rehabilitation team, the nurse plays a vital role in helping the individual to meet physical and psychological needs as independently as possible. The rehabilitation process empowers the individual to make informed decisions and choices about treatment modalities, care regimens and lifestyle options.

Review Questions

1. Identify and list six types of illness, condition or injury that individuals might experience in which rehabilitation would be essential.
2. What are the main goals of a rehabilitation program and how do these relate to the philosophy of rehabilitation?

3. List four rehabilitation nurse roles.
4. What are the five stages of the rehabilitation process?
5. List three ways a rehabilitation nurse can assist in empowering the individual who has lost the ability to speak but can understand following a stroke.
6. List two activities rehabilitation nurses undertake in collaboration with the rehabilitation team.
7. List three areas of health education that might be helpful for the rehabilitation nurse to provide for an older person who has recently suffered a fractured hip following a fall at home.

Evolve® Answer guide for the Review Questions, Critical Thinking Exercises, Decision-making Framework Exercises and Critical Thinking Questions in Case Studies is hosted on Evolve: http://evolve.elsevier.com/AU/Koutoukidis/Tabbner.

References

Australian Commission on Safety and Quality in Healthcare (ACSQHC), 2022. Comprehensive Care Standard. Available at: <www.safetyandquality.gov.au/standards/nsqhs-standards/comprehensive-care-standard>.

Brooks, L.A., Manias, E., Bloomer, M.J., 2019. Culturally sensitive communication in healthcare: A concept analysis. *Collegian* 26(3), 383–391.

Brown, D., Edwards, H., Buckley, T., et al., 2020. *Lewis's medical-surgical nursing ANZ*, 5th ed. Elsevier.

Chang, E., Johnson, A., 2022. *Living with chronic illness & disability: Principles for nursing practice*, 4th ed. Elsevier, Chatswood.

Cifu, D., 2020. *Braddom's physical medicine and rehabilitation*, 6th ed. Elsevier, Philadelphia.

Crisp, J., Douglas, C., Rebeiro, G., et al. (eds.), 2021. *Potter and Perry's fundamentals of nursing*, 6th ed. Elsevier, Sydney.

Forber-Pratt, A.J., Mueller, C.O., Andrews, E.E., 2019. Disability identity and allyship in rehabilitation psychology: Sit, stand, sign, and show up. *Rehabilitation Psychology* 64(2), 119–129. doi: 10.1037/rep0000256.

Gutenbrunner, C., Nugraha, B., Gimigliano, F., et al., 2020. International classification of service organisation in rehabilitation: An updated set of categories (ICSO-R 2.0). *Journal of Rehabilitation Medicine* 52(1). doi: 10.2340/16501977-2627.

Gutenbrunner, C., Stievano, A., Nugraha, B., et al., 2022. Nursing: A core element of rehabilitation. *International Nursing Review* 69, 13–19.

Hayton, J., Dimitriou, D., 2019. What's in a word: Distinguishing between habilitation and re-habilitation. *International Journal of Orientation and Mobility* 10(1).

Ignatavicius, D.D., Workman, M.L., Rebar, C.R., et al., 2021. *Medical-surgical nursing: Concepts for interprofessional collaborative care*, 10th ed. Elsevier, St Louis.

Jellema, S., Van Erp, S., Nijhuis-van der Sanden, M.W.G., et al., 2021. Activity resumption after acquired brain injury: The influence of the social network as described by social workers. *Disability and Rehabilitation* 43(8), 1137–1144. doi: 10.1080/09638288.2019.1652855.

Jesus, T.S., Papadimitriou, C., Bright, F.A., et al., 2022. Person-centered rehabilitation model: Framing the concept and practice of person-centered adult physical rehabilitation based on a scoping review and thematic analysis of the literature. *Archives of Physical Medicine and Rehabilitation* 103(1), 106–120. doi: 10.1016/j.apmr.2021.05.005.

Killingback, C., 2022. Being more than 'just a bog-standard knee': The role of person-centred practice in physiotherapy: A narrative inquiry. *Disability and Rehabilitation* 44(20). doi: 10.1080/09638288.2021.1948188.

Kitzmuller, G., Mangset, M., Evju, A.S., et al., 2019. Finding the way forward: The lived experience of people with stroke after participation in a complex psychosocial intervention. *Qualitative Health Research* 29(12), 1711–1724. doi: 10.1177/1049732319833366.

Kokorelias, K.M., Gignac, M.A.M., Naglie, G., et al., 2019. Towards a universal model of family centered care: A scoping review. *BMC Health Services Research* 19(564). doi: 10.1186/s12913-019-4394-5.

Kubiak, C.A., Etra, J.W., Brandacher, G., et al., 2019. Prosthetic rehabilitation and vascularized composite allotransplantation following upper limb loss. *American Society of Plastic Surgeons* 143(6), 1688–1701.

Labeit, B., Ahring, S., Boehmer, M., et al., 2022. Comparison of simultaneous swallowing endoscopy and videofluoroscopy in neurogenic dysphagia. *Journal of the American Medical Directors Association* 23(8), 1360–1366. doi: 10.1016/j.jamda.2021.09.026.

McGlinchey, M.P., McKevitt, J.J., et al., 2020. The effect of rehabilitation interventions on physical function and immobility-related complications in severe stroke: A systematic review. *BMJ Open* 10. doi: 10.1136/bmjopen-2019-033642.

McQuillan, K.A., 2020. *Trauma nursing: From resuscitation through rehabilitation*, 5th ed. Elsevier.

Pekonen, A., Eloranra, S., Stolt, M., et al., 2020. Measuring patient empowerment: A systematic review. *Patient Education and Counseling* 103(4), 777–787. doi: 10.1016/j.pec2019.10.019.

Pendleton, H.M., Schultz-Krohn, W., 2018. *Pedretti's occupational therapy: Practice skills for physical dysfunction*, 8th ed. Elsevier Inc, St. Louis.

Ralston, S.H., Penman, I.D., Strachan, M.W.J., et al., 2022. *Davidson's principles and practice of medicine*, 24th ed. Elsevier, Edinburgh.

Rose, A., Rosewilliam, S., Soundy, A., 2019. Shared decision making within goal setting in rehabilitation settings: A mixed methods study. *Clinical Rehablitation* 33(3), 564–574. doi: 10.1177/0269215518815251.

Salawu, A., Green, A., Crooks, M.G., et al., 2020. A proposal for multidisciplinary tele-rehabilitation in the assessment and rehabilitation of COVID-19 survivors. *International Journal of Environmental Research and Public Health* 17(13), 4890. doi: 10.3390/ijerph17134890.

Secombe, P.J., Brown, A., Bailey, M.J., et al., 2020. Critically ill Indigenous Australians and mortality: A complex story. *Medical Journal of Australia* 213(1), 13–14.

Steinmetz, M.P., Benzel, E.C., 2021. *Benzel's spine surgery*, 5th ed. Elsevier, Philadelphia.

Stott, H., Cramp, M., Turton, A. 2021. 'Somebody stuck me in a bag of sand': Lived experiences of the altered and uncomfortable body after stroke. *Clinical Rehabilitation* 35(9). doi: 10.1177/02692155211000740.

Tijsen, L.M.J., Derkson, E.C.C., Achterberg, W.P., et al., 2019. Challenging rehabilitation environment for older patients. *Clinical Interventions in Aging* 14, 1451–1460. doi: 10.2147/CIA.S207863.

Wade, D.T., 2020. What is rehabilitation? An empirical investigation leading to an evidence-based description. *Clinical Rehabilitation* 34(5), 571–583. doi: 10.1177/0269215520905112.

Willis, E., Reynolds, L., Keleher, H., 2020. *Understanding the Australian health care system*, 4th ed. Elsevier, Chatswood.

Yun, E.W., Choi, J.S., 2019. Person-centered rehabilitation care and outcomes: A systematic literature review. *International Journal of Nursing Studies* 93, 74–83. doi: 10.1016/j.ijnurstu.2019.02/012.

Recommended Reading

Agostini, F., Mangone, M., Ruiu, P., et al., 2021. Rehabilitation settings during and after Covid-19: An overview of recommendations. *Journal of Rehabilitation Medicine* 53(1), 2737. doi: 10.2340/16501977.

Chiarici, A., Andrenelli, E., Serpilli, O., et al., 2019. An early tailored approach is the key to effective rehabilitation in the intensive care unit. *Archives of Physical Medicine and Rehabilitation* 100(8), 1506–1514.

Leonardi, M., Fheodoroff, K., 2021. Goal setting with ICF (International classification of functioning, disability and health) and multidisciplinary team approach in stroke rehabilitation. *Clinical Pathways in Stroke Rehabilitation*, 35–56.

Levack, W.M.M., Rathore, F.A., Pollet, J., et al., 2019. One in 11 Cochrane Reviews are on rehabilitation interventions, according to pragmatic inclusion criteria developed by Cochrane rehabilitation. *Archives of Physical Medicine and Rehabilitation*. doi: 10.1016/j.apmr.2019.01.021.

Mahoney, F.I., Barthel, D., 1965. Functional evaluation: The Barthel index. *Maryland State Medical Journal* 14, 56–61.

Min, K., Beom, J., Kim, B.R., et al., 2021. Clinical practice guideline for postoperative rehabilitation in older patients with hip fractures. *Annals of Rehabilitation Medicine* 45(3), 225–259.

Pryor, J., Smith, C., 2000. A framework for the specialty practice of rehabilitation. Rehabilitation Research and Development Unit. ARNA, Sydney.

Phillips, M., Turner-Stokes, L., Wade, D., et al., 2020. Rehabilitation in the wake of Covid-19 – A phoenix from the ashes. *British Society of Rehabilitation Medicine* 1(2), 1–20.

Spruit, M.A., Wouters, E.F.M., 2019. Organizational aspects of pulmonary rehabilitation in chronic respiratory diseases. *Respirology* 24(9), 838–843. doi: 10.1111/resp.13512.

Szczepanska-Gieracha, J., Mazurek, J., 2020. The role of self-efficacy in the recovery process of stroke survivors. *Psychology Research and Behaviour Management* 13, 897.

World Health Organization (WHO), 2001. The international classification of functioning, disability and health. WHO, Geneva.

Zanca, J.M., Turkstra, L.S., Chen, C., et al., 2019. Advancing rehabilitation practice through improved specification of interventions. *Archives of Physical Medicine and Rehabilitation* 1(100), 164–171.

Online Resources

Ability First Australia: <www.abilityfirstaustralia.com.au>.

Association of Rehabilitation Nurses (USA): <https://rehabnurse.org>.

Australasian Faculty of Rehabilitation Medicine: <https://www.racp.edu.au/about/college-structure/australasian-faculty-of-rehabilitation-medicine>.

Australasian Rehabilitation Nurses' Association: <https://www.arna.com.au>.

Australasian Rehabilitation Outcomes Centre: <www.uow.edu.au/ahsri/aroc>.

New Zealand Rehabilitation Association: <http://www.rehabilitation.org.nz>.

CHAPTER

41

Chronicity and disability

Vicki Blair Drury and Ai Tee Aw

Key Terms

chronic disease
disability
equity and access
health promotion
impairment
inclusion
independence
normalisation
self-management
social role valorisation (SRV)

Learning Outcomes

At the completion of this chapter and with further reading, learners should be able to:

- Define the key terms.
- Describe how chronic diseases and disability are defined.
- Identify factors that lead to an increase in long-term conditions.
- Apply an understanding of mental health, lifestyle risk factors and intrinsic motivation to an individual's ability to self-manage.
- Critically examine contemporary models of care for long-term conditions.
- Apply an understanding of supportive holistic care, symptom control and detection of complications in the management of prolonged symptoms following infection with SARS-CoV-2 (long COVID).
- Apply a self-management approach to the management of individuals with long-term conditions and/or disability.
- Identify factors that lead to disability.
- Apply an understanding of mental health issues to the care of a patient with a long-term condition and/or disability.
- Understand what 'mindfulness' involves and how it relates to therapeutic approaches to managing anxiety and depression.
- Apply an understanding of normalisation and inclusion to the management of individuals with disabilities.
- Acknowledge the important role family/carers play in supporting people with disabilities or chronic diseases.
- Identify health promotion strategies that serve to reduce the incidence of disability and chronic diseases in society.
- Identify the importance of educational supports and strategies that serve to reduce the impact of having a disability or chronic disease, including the benefits of early intervention.

CHAPTER FOCUS

Chronic illness and disability affect people across the lifespan irrespective of race, gender or cultural group. However, some conditions are more prevalent in some cultures or races than others. Socioeconomic factors and education have been found to influence illness and mortality (Coste et al 2022; Kivimäki et al 2020), with socioeconomic inequalities evident for most of the chronic diseases (Cambois et al 2020). The ageing population globally means there has also been a significant increase in chronic disease. Chronic diseases are now the leading causes of illness, disability and death in many countries (Gregory et al 2022; World Health Organization 2023). Chronic disease, also known as long-term conditions, encompasses a broad spectrum of diseases. Comorbidity—the co-existence of two or more diseases together—is a common feature of chronic disease. Additionally, comorbid chronic diseases often share similar risk factors that act together to affect individual health status (Aïdoud et al 2023; Zhang & Bierma-Zeinstra 2023).

Although chronic disease and disability are often discussed together, not all people with chronic disease have a disability and not all people with a disability have a chronic disease. While chronic disease is often classified according to major disease groups and risk factors, disability is categorised according to severity.

Chronic disease is defined as a disease that lasts more than 3 months and for which there is no cure. Disability is considered to be a condition that in some way affects a person's ability to carry out day-to-day activities.

This chapter outlines the classification and causative factors of chronic diseases and disabilities. Models of care focus on normalisation and facilitating **independence** through individual empowerment. The theme throughout this chapter is the need for nurses and other allied health professionals to recognise and promote the importance of successful inclusion and acceptance into the community and to work towards improving the quality of life for all people with disabilities.

LIVED EXPERIENCE

Annie, 76 years old, cares for her husband Paul, 80 years old, who was diagnosed with Parkinson's disease at the age of 70. Both Annie and Paul were retired when Paul was diagnosed. At the time of his diagnosis, they had bought a caravan and were in the midst of a trip around Australia. Although Annie and Paul live in Western Australia, their family is dispersed throughout Australia with both their children and their families living in Victoria. Initially, Paul managed his condition with help from Annie; however, over the past few months, Annie has noticed a deterioration in his condition. Paul's movements have become more rigid, his gait is now more unsteady and has resulted in a number of falls. His cognition is declining with poor memory and the inability to concentrate. Paul and Annie have not applied for any assistance since they were travelling; however, with the deterioration in Paul's condition, they have now returned to their family home in Western Australia.

Annie admits she is finding it increasingly difficult to provide the care that Paul needs, and his recent falls have made her realise that his safety is an issue. An assessment by an Aged Care Assessment Team (ACAT) has recommended a home care assessment package to enable Annie to continue to care for Paul at home. Paul now attends a day centre twice a week and, although Annie feels disappointed that she was unable to provide all the care that was needed, she acknowledges that this enables her to 'have some downtime and do some things for herself'. Annie admits that until Paul's Parkinson's disease, she had not realised the challenges of being a full-time carer and now finds she is more tolerant and patient with others with any sort of disability.

Annie, aged 76

INTRODUCTION

Confusion often surrounds chronic diseases due to the numerous definitions used in the literature. **Chronic diseases** are also called long-term conditions, non-communicable diseases, or lifestyle diseases. These definitions do not appropriately define chronic disease because some may be due to communicable factors, such as cervical cancer, and others are determined more by environmental factors rather than behavioural or lifestyle factors (Australian Institute of Health and Welfare 2022c). However, chronic diseases generally extend for a long period, progress slowly and have no cure. The Australian Institute of Health and Welfare (2022a) defines chronic diseases as being characterised by 'complex causality, multiple risk factors, a long latency period, a prolonged course of illness, and functional impairment or disability'. This definition clearly illustrates the complexity of chronic diseases.

The World Health Organization (WHO) asserts that chronic diseases often start at a young age but take many years to evolve and that they require a long-term and systematic approach to management. Examples of chronic diseases include high blood pressure, heart disease, chronic obstructive pulmonary disease, diabetes, macular degeneration, glaucoma, tinnitus, some cancers, Parkinson's disease, Crohn's disease, epilepsy, schizophrenia, bipolar affective disorder, systemic lupus erythematosus and arthritis.

Prevalence, classification and causes of chronic diseases

The WHO categorises causes of death and disability into three large categories: communicable (infectious diseases, including maternal, perinatal and nutritional conditions), noncommunicable (chronic diseases) and injuries. The SARS CoV-2 (coronavirus) pandemic, classified as an infectious disease, that began in 2020 resulted in a number of deaths globally (Msemburi et al 2022; Woolf et al 2021). However, despite the impact of the COVID-19 pandemic on health and mortality, chronic diseases remained the leading cause of death globally (OECD/WHO 2022; Office for National Statistics 2023; Xu et al 2022). During the first year of the COVID-19 pandemic, Australia observed a much lower than expected mortality, with death rates hitting historic lows. Numerous causes of mortality fell, but respiratory illness deaths were particularly significant in their decline. Australia's experience was distinct from that of many other nations that had notable increases in mortality that were primarily caused by COVID-19 deaths. Despite the pandemic, in 2022, the top five causes of death in Australia were ischaemic heart disease, dementia, cerebrovascular diseases, cancers and respiratory diseases (Australian Bureau of Statistics 2022). Chronic disease impacts on the individual, the community and the country. Chronic diseases cause premature death, decreased quality of life and place financial burdens on families and communities.

Chronic diseases are often classified according to disease types, with cardiovascular diseases (mainly heart disease and stroke), cancer, chronic respiratory diseases and diabetes being the main classifications. However, vision and hearing impairments and genetic diseases also account for a significant portion of the global disease burden. Other chronic diseases include mental disorders, bone and joint disorders and oral diseases (World Health Organization 2022).

The causes of many chronic diseases are well known and reported widely in various media from medical literature to daily newspapers. The three most significant modifiable behavioural factors influencing chronic diseases are poor nutrition, lack of exercise and tobacco use. These behavioural risk factors are more common in the lower socioeconomic areas, as well as in rural and remote places. At the societal level, access to healthcare, immunisation programs and a hygienic environment can foster good health and lower the chance of acquiring or worsening chronic diseases. In addition, building design, access to green space, advertising exposure, the availability of healthy food, portion sizes of prepared food and the convenience of pre-packaged, calorie-dense food are all environmental elements that contribute to overweight and obesity, which are risk factors for the emergence of chronic conditions. These factors affect blood pressure, lipid control, blood glucose and body mass index and, combined with non-modifiable risk factors of age and heredity, explain why there has been a global increase in chronic diseases (World Health Organization 2022). (See Figure 41.1.)

Long COVID

The novel viral infection with the severe acute respiratory syndrome coronavirus-2 (SARS-CoV-2) that causes COVID-19 disease was first reported as a pneumonia of unknown origin in December 2019 (Sharma et al 2020). The current outbreak of COVID-19 has been classified by the World Health Organization as a global pandemic as the virus evolved rapidly in less than 6 months causing widespread mortality. By 24 April 2020, in Italy—the most affected European country—there had been 192,994 confirmed COVID-19 related infections and 25,969 deaths (Indolfi & Spaccarotella 2020). Singapore reported its first

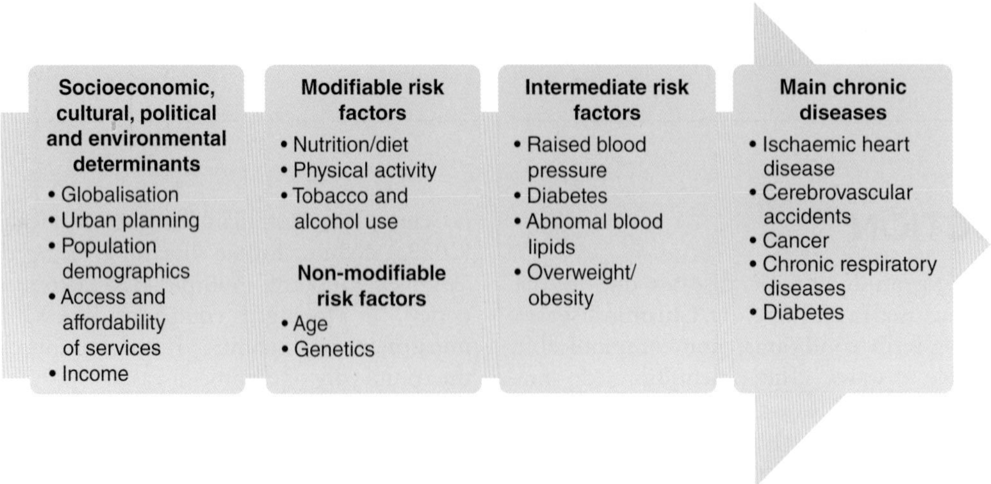

Figure 41.1 Risk factors for chronic diseases
(das Neves Júnior et al 2023)

confirmed case of COVID-19 infection in January 2020. Shortly after, the Republic of Singapore diagnosed over 800 cases, which translates to approximately 137 cases per million population (Ng et al 2020). In Australia, by 2022 almost 6 million cases of COVID-19 had been confirmed since the start of the pandemic (Australian Government 2023a).

SARS-CoV-2 is spread via direct contact and aerosol transmission of respiratory droplets and has a median incubation period of 5.1 days (Guan et al 2020). A recent study found that SARS-CoV-2 lasts in aerosols for up to 3 hours and remains detectable for up to 72 hours on plastic and stainless-steel surfaces (Balaji et al 2020). Close contact with sick people and comorbidity are factors that contribute to the rapid transmission of the disease (since the virus has an airborne transmission mechanism. The main types of detection and identification of SARS-Cov-2 are:

- molecular analysis for the detection of virus RNA (PCR)
- rapid detection of virus antigen by immunochromatography (rapid-test)
- various methods for the detection of virus antibodies by immunoassays.

(Majumder & Minko 2021)

SARS-CoV-2 (COVID-19) is an infectious viral pneumonia to which the human population has low or no preexisting immunity. Newly identified people with COVID-19 may experience a mild and self-limiting illness with upper respiratory tract symptoms and non-life-threatening pneumonia or severe pneumonia with acute respiratory distress syndrome that begins with mild symptoms and then progresses rapidly to respiratory failure requiring intensive care management (Cascella et al 2022).

The most common presenting symptoms in the general population are fever, cough, dyspnoea and myalgias or fatigue. The current proposed mechanism for cell entry is via the angiotensin-converting enzyme-2 (ACE-2) receptor found in the lungs, endothelium, heart, kidneys and gastrointestinal system. Thus, most older adults may have some form of organ damage occurring due to SARS-CoV-2 including acute respiratory disease syndrome, acute kidney injury, cardiac injury and liver dysfunction. This likelihood of having multiple comorbidities places older adults at an even greater risk of increased mortality from SARS-CoV-2 (Beyerstedt et al 2021; Cascella et al 2022).

In all age groups, chest computed tomography (CT) imaging of people with SARS-CoV-2 revealed ground glass opacities (Liu & Liu 2020). Infection with COVID-19 can leave a lingering trail of changes that on CT scans of the lungs shows pleural thickening, indicative of pulmonary fibrosis (Akbarialiabad et al 2021). Another remarkable finding is the high proportion of people with COVID-19 in general, but especially in the severe cases, with leukopenia and lymphopenia. People with severe COVID-19 disease had more prominent laboratory abnormalities including lymphopenia and leukopenia because the number of T-cells was significantly decreased, especially T helper cells in individuals with severe forms of COVID-19.

Several acute viral infections are known to induce immune and inflammatory responses and lead to long-term sequelae. The mechanisms underlying autoimmune diseases may offer some conceptual models relevant to individuals with pre-existing chronic medical conditions. People with chronic medical diseases, such as cardiovascular disease, diabetes and hypertension, are regarded as a high-risk group that is more vulnerable to infection with COVID-19. Epidemiologic evidence has shown that over 94% of hospitalised people diagnosed with COVID-19 had at least one comorbidity (Richardson et al 2020). Moreover, people with chronic diseases have a higher risk for developing serious complications from COVID-19, such as organ damage, respiratory failure and cardiac arrest (Guan et al 2020; Zaim et al 2020).

Long COVID is a multisystem condition that has had, and continues to have, a significant impact on the global economy, society and healthcare systems. It is a multisystem disease marked by continuing, persistent symptoms that may linger for weeks or months after COVID-19 infection. Symptoms may fluctuate over time or develop into newly diagnosed chronic illnesses such as heart disease, diabetes, renal disease and neurological problems (AIHW 2022b). Recent studies estimate that 1 in 10 people who have had COVID-19 will experience long COVID, defined as ongoing symptomatic COVID-19 symptoms lasting more than 4 weeks. Post-COVID-19 syndrome, which is also long COVID, is defined as symptoms after 12 weeks that are not explained by alternative diagnosis (Davis et al 2023). People with long COVID reported turning to a vast range of over-the-counter medicines, remedies, supplements, complementary and alternative therapies, and dietary changes to manage relapsing and remitting symptoms (Brown et al 2022). In December 2020, the National Institute for Health and Care Excellence (NICE) published guidelines on symptom management of people with long COVID. The variability of symptoms accompanying long COVID syndrome is very high. It includes the following three definitions:

1. acute COVID-19: the first 4 weeks of symptoms
2. ongoing symptomatic COVID-19: symptoms from 4 to 12 weeks
3. post-COVID-19 syndrome: symptoms for more than 12 weeks.

(Davis et al 2023)

The disease mechanisms causing long COVID are unknown, and there are no evidence-based treatment options at this stage. Clinical guidelines focus on symptom management, and various treatment options are being evaluated. Some people who had an apparently 'mild' COVID-19 infection (whether confirmed or suspected) continue to suffer from persistent symptoms, including fatigue, cognitive impairment, neuropathy and paraesthesia, chest pain and palpitations, muscle and joint aches and shortness of breath (Davis et al 2023; Ziauddeen et al 2022).

For people with COVID-19 infection, treatment is focused on supportive care. For the mild and moderate disease, self-monitoring and confinement of the individual at home is required with the aim of symptomatic treatment and rest. Laboratory and imaging tests are not required. Good hydration and bed rest until the fever subsides are also recommended. If there are any other symptoms apart from fever, symptomatic treatment such as antiemetics, expectorants antidiarrhoeal drugs are recommended. Antibiotics may be administered only on clinical, imaging or laboratory evidence of co-infection with bacterial pneumonia. Administration of dexamethasone or other corticosteroids is not recommended (Tsang et al 2021).

In all cases of asymptomatic, mild or moderate disease, the therapeutic approach becomes more intensive in individuals with underlying chronic diseases or immunosuppression. In these cases, close monitoring of individuals and daily communication with attending physicians, good hydration and monitoring of temperature and oxyhemoglobin saturation with an oximeter at least twice a day are essential. It is also recommended to take antipyretic drugs in the case of fever, to continue treatment of the underlying disease, to administer other symptomatic drug therapy and to use antibiotic therapy on clinical and paraclinical evidence of bacterial lung infection (Tsang et al 2021). For moderate to severe disease, the Australian Government has recommended to start early antiviral drug therapy for seniors, Aboriginal and Torres Strait Islander Peoples and those over the age of 18 with chronic diseases (Australian Government 2023b).

CONCEPTUAL MODELS OF CHRONIC CARE

Several models of care have been developed that focus on a broader framework integrating individual, community and organisational goals to manage chronic diseases. The most significant of these is the Chronic Care Model (CCM) developed by Wagner in 2001 (Reynolds et al 2018). This model remains the foundation of most chronic disease models today and identifies individuals' empowerment, self-management support and organising community and organisational resources to meet the individuals' needs as the key principles required to improve chronic disease management. Despite evidence that the model remains effective (Ansari, Harris, Hosseinzadeh et al 2022), it was identified that it excluded health promotion and preventative healthcare strategies, which were viewed as integral to effective sustainable chronic disease management. This has resulted in expanded models of this framework that now include social determinants of health and the inclusion of preventative healthcare strategies (Barr et al 2003).

In 2019, the WHO Global Action Plan for the Prevention and Control of Non-communicable Diseases 2013–2020 was extended by the World Health Assembly to 2030. The assembly also called for the creation of an implementation roadmap from 2023 to 2030 to speed up the prevention and control of non-communicable diseases. This roadmap encourages initiatives to reach nine global goals that will have the most effect on non-communicable disease prevention and management. The WHO asserts that governments must take action to meet the increasing burden of chronic diseases and provide guidelines that countries can use to improve health service delivery and management of chronic diseases (World Health Organization 2022). In 2002, the WHO joined with the MacColl Institute to adapt the CCM to a more globally appropriate model. The resultant framework was the Innovative Care for Chronic Conditions Model (see Figure 41.2), which focused on improving care for people with chronic conditions at three levels:

1. the macro level concerning policies and the environment
2. the meso level involving organisations and the community
3. the micro level comprising individuals and their families.

(Reynolds et al 2018)

While each level of this framework is important, the macro level is essential for the development of programs and providing leadership at both the meso and micro levels. It is at the macro level that partnerships are developed, and human and material resources are provided for the sustainability of programs (Reynolds et al 2018). At the meso level, it is essential to improve continuation of holistic care and facilitate healthcare and community organisations working together. At the micro level, individuals need to be empowered to become active participants in their own care.

Healthcare staff need to be informed and take on a supportive and educative role in care. Chronic disease self-management acknowledges that the person with a chronic disease must cope not only with the disease and the effects of the disease but also with the impact on their quality of life (Drury 2021). There is evidence to support the idea that individuals affected by trauma or chronic disease go through four phases of adaptation. Following the onset and diagnosis of a chronic disease, individuals go through these phases that outline a predictable path individuals take in order to define a new self and a new life. Like Kubler-Ross's work on stages of death and dying, the Fennell Four-Phase Model offers a framework for comprehending this crucial process (Fennell et al 2021; Pederson et al 2020). See Clinical Interest Box 41.1 and Clinical Interest Box 41.2 for examples of the adjustments and adaptations that individuals with chronic disease face.

DISABILITY

Historically, the term **disability** was medically or diagnostically focused; however, over time this has evolved to one that is functionally focused, thus making an important distinction between two concepts—functional limitation and disability. Disability thus becomes something that occurs outside of a person, rather than something a person has. The functional limitation is influenced by numerous

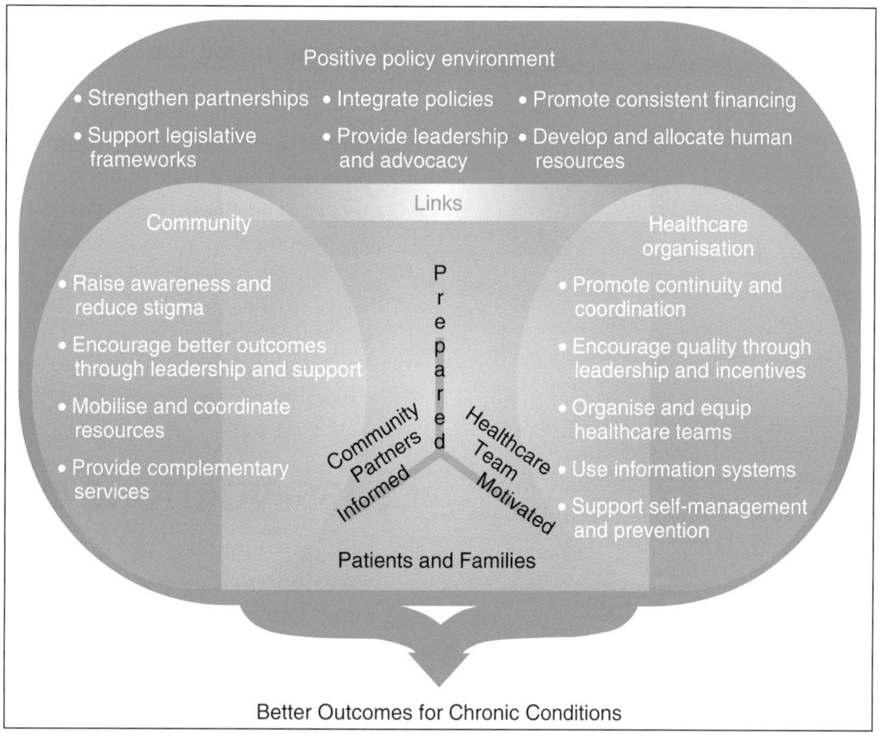

Figure 41.2 Innovative Care for Chronic Conditions Model

(Epping Jordan et al 2004)

CLINICAL INTEREST BOX 41.1 Phases of adjustment to living with a chronic disease

Crisis phase

- Sense of dismay and urgency to find treatment.
- May use drugs and/or alcohol to cope.
- Seek alternative interventions.
- Blame self or others.
- Fear and anxiety.

The goal of this phase is for the person to regain a sense of control. The healthcare team assists the person to manage physical and psychological symptoms and offers support. The healthcare team must help the person turn negative thoughts into positive thoughts and empower them to regain control.

Stabilisation phase

- Acute phase of the illness has passed and there is an awareness that this is now a chronic condition.
- Friends and family may retreat.
- Feelings of isolation and helplessness.

The goal of this phase is for the person to restructure their life. The healthcare team assists the person to understand what they can do and helps them to achieve their goals.

Resolution phase

- Coming to terms with the chronic disease.
- Learning to live with the consequences of the disease.
- Heightened sense of control and empowerment.
- Renewed sense of self.

Integration phase

- Accepting that the disease has provided positive life experiences.
- Sense of pride in achievements.

(Pederson et al 2020)

factors such as the environment, functional ability, life experiences and age. This new definition views disability as a matter of degree: the person is more or less disabled based on the intersection between the individual, their functional abilities and the many types of environments with which they interact.

The WHO's framework for evaluating health and disability at both the individual and population levels is the International Classification of Functioning, Disability and Health (ICF). The WHO defines disabilities as 'an umbrella term, covering impairments, activity limitations and participation restrictions. An **impairment** is a problem in

CLINICAL INTEREST BOX 41.2 Adjustments and adaptations to living with a chronic disease

- Loss of roles
- Changes to health status
- Loss of identity
- Lifestyle changes
- Financial adjustments

(Livneh 2022; Van Wilder et al 2021)

body function or structure; an activity limitation is a difficulty encountered by an individual in executing a task or action; while a participation restriction is a problem experienced by an individual in involvement in life situations' (World Health Organization 2021).

PREVALENCE AND CAUSES OF DISABILITIES

The WHO estimates that around one in six people globally experience some form of significant disability (World Health Organization 2021). It has been found that disability and poverty are interwoven due to the impact poverty has on nutritional status, access to health services, living and working conditions and sanitation while, conversely, disabled people are often forced into poverty due to the challenges they encounter accessing education, health services and social activities (Friedman 2022; Pinilla-Roncancio & Alkire 2021). During the COVID-19 epidemic, a significant portion of persons with disabilities endured higher rates of financial hardship than non-disabled adults (Friedman 2022; Mitra & Turk 2022). People with disabilities who experience financial difficulty may experience long-lasting effects on their general wellbeing, physical and mental health, and quality of life. The global ageing population and the rise in chronic disease incidence will further increase the number of people living with disabilities.

CLASSIFICATIONS OF DISABILITY

Classifying disability is complex. Although it is acknowledged that all people with disabilities do not have the same desires nor confront the same challenges, policy-makers and clinicians need a system of classification that enables the organisation of disabilities into categories, enabling the application of universal codes. These codes are then used for a range of purposes, including tracking prevalence of disabilities, reimbursement of costs and assisting with making decisions about services. In Australia, disabilities are categorised according to the type and cause (Table 41.1), and according to the level of restriction

TABLE 41.1 | Classification of disability according to type and cause

Disability	Description	Example
Intellectual	Appearing in the developmental period (age 0–18 years) and associated with impairments of mental functions, difficulties in learning and performing certain daily life skills and limitations of adaptive skills in the context of community environments compared with others of the same age	Down syndrome, autism, attention deficit hyperactivity disorder
Physical	Conditions that are attributable to a physical cause, or impact on the ability to perform physical activities	Paraplegia, quadriplegia, muscular dystrophy, motor neurone disease, neuromuscular disorders, cerebral palsy, absence or deformities of limbs, spina bifida, arthritis, back disorders, ataxia
Acquired brain injury	Disabilities arising from damage to the brain acquired after birth	Stroke, brain tumours, alcohol and drug abuse
Neurological	Impairments of the nervous system occurring after birth, includes epilepsy and organic brain syndrome	Alzheimer's disease, multiple sclerosis, Parkinson's disease, epilepsy
Deafblind	Dual sensory impairments associated with severe restrictions in communication and participation in community life	Usher syndrome, rubella, cerebral palsy

TABLE 41.1 | Classification of disability according to type and cause—cont'd

Disability	Description	Example
Vision	Blindness and vision impairment that is not corrected by glasses or contact lenses	Age-related macular degeneration, myopic dystrophies, retinitis pigmentosa, glaucoma, Fuch's dystrophy
Hearing	Includes deafness, hearing impairment, hearing loss	Ménière's disease, age-related hearing loss, Usher syndrome, acoustic neuroma, rubella, mumps
Speech	Speech loss, impairment and/or difficulty in being understood	Neurological disorders, brain injury, intellectual disabilities, drug abuse, cleft lip or palate
Psychiatric	Symptoms and behaviours that impair personal functioning in normal social activity	Schizophrenia, affective disorders, anxiety disorders, addictive behaviours, personality disorders, stress, psychosis, depression and adjustment disorders

(Adapted from National Disability Service 2022)

TABLE 41.2 | Classification of disability according to restriction

Level of restriction	Example
Profound	A person is unable to perform self-care, mobility and/or communication tasks, or always needs assistance.
Severe	A person sometimes needs assistance with self-care, mobility or communication.
Moderate	A person does not need assistance, but has difficulty with self-care, mobility or communication.
Mild	A person has no difficulty with self-care, mobility or communication, but uses aids or equipment.

(Australian Bureau of Statistics 2019a)

TABLE 41.3 | Classification of disability according to area affected

Type	Example
Sensory	Vision impairment
	Hearing loss
Physical	Arthritis
	Paralysis due to spinal cord injury
	Acute pain
Psychological	Schizophrenia
	Dementia
	Depression
Intellectual	Intelligence quotient (IQ) score below 70

(Adapted from National Disability Service 2022)

incurred (Table 41.2). In addition, disabilities are described according to whether limitations or restrictions are sensory, physical, psychological or intellectual (Table 41.3) (National Disability Services 2022). Multiple or complex disabilities generally refer to the co-existence of two or more conditions, for example, a physical and intellectual disability. In addition, it has been found that many people with disabilities have comorbid chronic diseases (Eva & Pathak 2023; van den Bemdet al 2022).

The unique meaning of disability

Disability is a subjective experience. An injury to the leg that results in permanent inability to bend the knee or stand for long periods of time might be a serious anxiety-provoking disability for a person working as a nurse or as a tradesperson. The impact of the same disability on an elderly person who lives alone and spends most of their time watching television and rarely going out of the house may be quite different. Many people learn to adapt so well with their disability that it becomes inconsequential. These people often say that they can do everything an able-bodied person can do; they just do it differently. A disability places a restriction or functional limitation on the person.

Therefore, a disability is not something that a person has, but is, instead, something that occurs outside of the person; the person has a functional limitation.

CONCEPTUAL MODELS OF DISABILITY

Conceptual models of disability have struggled for years with whether disability should be viewed through a medical lens or a social lens. In isolation, neither of these models provided an adequate framework for supporting people with disabilities. In 2001, the WHO endorsed the International Classification of Functioning, Disability and Health (ICF), which provides a framework for measuring health and disability at both individual and population levels. The ICF definition of disability, referred to as the biopsychosocial model, evolves from the medical and social model and incorporates the idea that anyone might become disabled (van der Veen et al 2022). This framework views disability not as something that a person has but as a functional limitation that occurs outside of the person. Disability occurs as a result of the interaction between a person, their functional ability and the environment. Therefore, a disability may be minimised by designing environments to accommodate varying functional abilities and providing individualised solutions.

In 2014, the WHO global disability action plan 2014–2021 'Better health for all people with disability' was adopted by the World Health Assembly. This action plan, based on recommendations from the WHO and the World Bank report on disability, has three aims: (i) to remove barriers and improve access to health services and program; (ii) to strengthen and extend rehabilitation, habilitation, assistive technology, assistance and support services, and community-based rehabilitation; and (iii) to strengthen collection of relevant and internationally comparable data on disability and support research on disability and related services (World Health Organization 2015).

Adjustment

Adjustment to a disability is dependent on numerous factors, and most people also transition through a number of phases before accepting their disability (see Clinical Interest Box 41.3).

It is important to recognise that adjustment to disability may be short and relatively uncomplicated, but commonly it can be a long and difficult process involving extensive rehabilitation and a process of grieving. While individuals respond differently, it is helpful to recognise that in the initial period after illness or accident, when individuals are first facing disability, they may be extremely stressed. This stress may result in behaviours that the person does not usually display, including:

- hostility or anger at themselves, their families or primary carers and the professional staff who aim to support them
- rebelliousness (e.g. refusing care, refusing to get up or shower)
- refusal to socialise, shunning visitors, even close family and friends (this may be due to embarrassment at changed appearance or abilities, or fear of rejection)
- depersonalisation (avoiding or disowning self or parts of self, which may be demonstrated by a refusal to acknowledge, talk about, or look at an altered body part, such as a stoma, a stump or a burned area)
- refusal to participate in activities.

(See Table 41.4.)

CLINICAL INTEREST BOX 41.3 Phases in adjusting to a disability

Shock

- Feeling emotionless
- Sense of unreality

Denial

- A sense that the situation is not happening
- A coping mechanism that allows the individual time to adjust

Anger

- Withdrawal
- Isolation
- Hostility
- Self-blame
- Grief for loss of roles or changes to self-image

Acceptance

- Does not mean the individual is happy with the status quo
- Accepts the disability
- Takes back control over life
- May benefit from speaking to others in similar situations

(Livneh 2022)

Mental health

People with long-term health conditions are two to three times more likely to develop a mental health condition such as depression or anxiety. Similarly, people with mental health conditions are at a higher risk of developing chronic diseases such as diabetes and hypertension (Sporinova et al 2019). Almost 40% of people with cancer and over 20% of people with cardiovascular disease or diabetes will have a comorbid mental health issue (De Hert et al 2022; Pearson-Stuttard et al 2022). Although some degree of sadness and feelings of loss are normal, depression and acute anxiety are not normal and will exacerbate the symptoms and impede management of the chronic disease.

Nurses working with individuals with chronic diseases and/or disabilities need to be able to recognise the clinical manifestations of an anxiety disorder and depression, assess the person and refer appropriately.

Anxiety is a response to an internal or external threat. It can have behavioural, emotional, cognitive and physical symptoms (Chand & Marwaha 2022). Anxiety can be positive or negative, depending on the duration and degree

TABLE 41.4 | Factors affecting adjustment to disability

Factor	Example
Amount and quality of support	Good social support is associated with better functioning.
Acceptance of disability	Acceptance of the disability is important if the person is to move into a phase of adjustment and reintegration.
Degree of impairment	The greater the impairment the more difficult the adjustment and acceptance.
Emotional reactivity	Personal beliefs promote adaptation.
Attitudes and behaviours of others	Stigma and non-acceptance by others affect the confidence and self-esteem of the person with a disability and may prevent acceptance of the disability.
Psychological resilience	Interventions promoting resilience of individuals with a chronic disease or disability will increase positive outcomes.
Access and affordability of health services	Access and affordability to health services promotes better outcomes.

(Alonso-Sardón et al 2019; Proescher et al 2022; Ogawa et al 2021; Zhang et al 2019; Dunn & Wehmeyer 2022; Bollier et al 2021; Kimet al 2019; Lim et al 2020; World Health Organization nd)

of anxiety. Mild anxiety is when the person is aware that there is something different—for example, a student has an exam tomorrow—and the anxiety helps the person to focus and be motivated to act in a specific way. However, when anxiety causes panic, an inability to process information or problem solve, and physical symptoms such as tightening in the chest and a racing pulse manifest, intervention and management is needed.

Anxiety may be escalated by a lack of information or external stimuli. It is important to ensure that the person is in a quiet area. Mindfulness and relaxation have been found to be successful in helping people manage anxiety. Referral to a mental health professional is important (Jones et al 2022; Komariah et al 2023).

Depression is when a person has feelings of sadness most of the time for more than 2 weeks and has lost pleasure or interest in activities they usually enjoy. Some of the clinical signs of depression include the following:

- decreased enjoyment of previously pleasurable activities
- weight change
- sleep disturbances
- agitation
- tiredness
- feelings of inadequacy or worthlessness
- difficulty thinking or making decisions
- hopelessness, helplessness.

(Hungerford et al 2021; Jones et al 2022)

There is a range of effective treatments for depression including cognitive behaviour therapy, interpersonal therapy and medication. Relaxation and mindfulness exercises may be used as adjuvant therapeutic approaches in managing depression. Referral to a mental health professional is fundamental to treating the depression.

Mindfulness

Mindfulness is a therapeutic intervention that helps a person focus on being in the present moment and teaches them to respond to negative emotions with acceptance and compassion. Mindfulness encourages the person to have a sense of control over their situation and reflect on what is most important (Aytac & Mizrachi 2022). Research has shown that mindfulness has three pillars: intention or knowing the reason that the person is practising mindfulness; attention and being able to focus on the present; and attitude, which is being compassionate towards oneself (Villamil et al 2019).

Mindfulness-based relaxation techniques have been found to be effective in helping people manage chronic disease and disability (Hente et al 2020). The aim of mindfulness is to be in tune with one's own mental, emotional and physical being. Mindfulness is a type of meditation whereby the person focuses on the present moment, usually by being attentive to their breathing, their body and their senses (Komariah et al 2023). Mindfulness techniques are usually taught by trained health professionals. These techniques can be used anywhere, anytime and do not require that the person stop an activity to use the technique (Reina & Kudesia 2020).

Providing care for individuals and their families

Nurses may provide care for individuals with disabilities and their carers in any setting in which care is provided. These include:

- the person's own home
- community houses

- day or drop-in centres
- day clinics
- residential care facilities
- general hospitals
- rehabilitation units
- schools or preschools
- obstetric units (neonates born with a disability)
- respite care accommodation.

Nurses may encounter individuals with a disability who are hospitalised for totally unrelated reasons (e.g. a person who has epilepsy but is hospitalised because they need an appendectomy). Others may be in care to provide respite for a family carer (e.g. a person with multiple sclerosis or perhaps dementia) and some may have only just acquired the disability (e.g. hemiplegia as a result of a cerebrovascular accident or a spinal cord injury due to road trauma). This means that nurses need to adapt the ways they communicate with and respond to individuals according to the type of disability and the specific circumstances.

Clinical Interest Box 41.4 provides some guidelines to aid the nurse caring for individuals with disabilities. Sometimes people with disabilities demonstrate behaviour that even experienced nurses find challenging to manage. There are often complexities involved in managing challenging behaviours—now more commonly known as behaviours of concern—and it is recommended that nurses refer to texts that deal specifically with this issue to enhance their knowledge and expertise. Additional information in managing challenging behaviours is provided in Chapter 39.

The move to community-based service provision

Historically, people with disabilities were institutionalised, segregated from society and from their local communities

CLINICAL INTEREST BOX 41.4 Suggestions to aid relationships between nurses and individuals with disabilities

Keep in mind that:

- In many cases, the individual and the family carer will know more about the disability than the nurse.
- The person with a disability is the same as anyone else, just with particular needs associated with their disability.
- Many difficulties that the person faces are likely to be more to do with societal attitudes than the disability itself.
- It is best to concentrate on what the person can do rather than on the things they are unable to do.
- It is best to let the person guide how and at what pace things should be done.
- Self-responsibility should be handed over to people with disabilities as soon as they are ready.

When communicating:

- Adapt your pace of communication to suit the other person and, when communication ability is impaired, allow time for responses.
- Speak directly to the person—do not use another person as a go-between (e.g. family carer).
- Monitor how much input into the conversation the person with the disability has—be careful that you do not dominate the conversation.
- Take the person's lead, pick up on what the person may prefer to talk about or finds interesting or important. Be alert to signals and act on them (e.g. for a person whose speech is impaired, eye movement towards an object may indicate that the object is wanted).
- Ask the person what help is required, avoid automatically doing things for the person and do not insist on helping and do not assist without asking first.
- Ask if unsure of how to behave towards the person (e.g. if the person has an arm missing or has uncontrolled limb movements, how do they prefer you to place meals or other objects?).
- Respond with understanding and goodwill if the person knocks something over or spills something (e.g. a glass of water). Humour can also be helpful and, when used effectively, can minimise embarrassment.
- Do not be overly concerned if you say something that feels inappropriate (e.g. saying 'Do you want to hop into the shower now?' to a person who has a right leg amputation). Having a disability does not remove a person's sense of humour, and humour can relieve discomfort for both nurse and an individual.
- Whatever the disability, always use age-appropriate language (e.g. speak to the adult person with intellectual or cognitive impairment in the same manner as you would any other adult). (Chapter 34 provides more information on communicating with people who have hearing, vision or cognitive impairment.)

Caring for people in wheelchairs:

- Do not assume that the person in a wheelchair needs assistance.
- Do not try to move the person or wheelchair without first gaining permission.
- Do not hold onto the wheelchair unnecessarily. It is part of the person's body space and the person cannot step away from you.

CLINICAL INTEREST BOX 41.4 Suggestions to aid relationships between nurses and individuals with disabilities—cont'd

- Ensure you are familiar with how a wheelchair is pushed and manoeuvred before taking a person in a wheelchair out and about. This includes knowing how to get it up and down steps, how to tip it backwards, how to use the brake and how the armrests are removed (never lift a wheelchair by the armrests—most are removable) and how it folds up. It is a useful exercise to practise pushing and manoeuvring a wheelchair with a person who does not have a disability sitting in it.

Promoting confidence:

- Reinforce that people with disabilities have the same rights as other people in their community and in society as a whole.
- Reinforce that they have the right to have a say in all decision-making that concerns their lives, their treatment and their general wellbeing.
- Reinforce that it is appropriate to be assertive and persistent in defending their rights, and to be firm but polite when defending their rights to things such as access, independence or privacy.

Encourage people with disabilities to:

- Feel comfortable about asking for assistance when needed and avoid apologising for what they cannot do.
- Feel comfortable in communicating in whatever way is appropriate for them, and about having to repeat things that are not understood or about asking other people to repeat or re-explain things that are unclear.
- Understand that many people have little knowledge of disabilities (e.g. the realities of cerebral palsy), and be tolerant of and polite to people who are unsure of how to respond to them in social situations, or who offer help that is not needed.
- Be prepared for times when they may feel anxious or depressed. Reinforce that such feelings are common and that help is available should they need it.
- Try to create opportunities to instigate the person's contact with positive role models or others who have a similar disability. For example, it may be encouraging to a person who has recently become vision-impaired to talk with a person who has adapted successfully to vision impairment. It may be helpful for people who are hearing impaired to meet with deaf people communicating avidly with sign language.

(Agaronnik et al 2019; Australian Federation of Disability Organisations 2023)

and denied the rights of access to services and opportunities available to the rest of the population. People who entered institutional care facilities often remained there for their entire lives.

Australia went through a process of deinstitutionalisation in the mid-1980s. Although the process of deinstitutionalisation had started in the 1970s, it was with the release of the Richmond Report in 1983 that the process began in earnest. Richmond's recommendations included a government-funded system of community support underpinned by acute hospital services (if needed) and accommodation services. The findings from this report changed the provision of both mental healthcare and disability service provision, initially in New South Wales and then throughout Australia. Subsequently, other services such as foster care for children were also influenced by the findings (Vrklevski et al 2017; Weise et al 2021).

During this process, the asylum network was dismantled. The goal of deinstitutionalisation was not only to assist people with disabilities move into the community but also to develop new services to meet the changed needs this created. For example, dispersed housing in the community has been shown to be a preferable alternative to large-scale institutions for improving the quality of life for people with disabilities (Gooding 2016). The process of deinstitutionalisation now forms the basis of the provision of care for people with disabilities. For people with disabilities, being part of the community is essential to their wellbeing and to improve their quality of life. Unfortunately, the process was not always smooth, particularly for people with severe and profound levels of intellectual disabilities or those with severe behaviours of concern (Vrklevski et al 2017), and while there is some contestation over the success of deinstitutionalisation, there is also a significant body of evidence supporting the positive outcomes in relation to improved quality of life and independence (Belcher 2022).

In Australia, despite the development of a national strategy to achieve **equity and access** for disabled persons, the systems available today continue to be challenged by poor resourcing, overlapping and fragmented responsibilities, inequitable availability of services and poor access to basic services in rural areas (Wakerman & Humphreys 2019). Table 41.5 lists some of the national organisations in Australia that work to address issues concerning the rights of people with disabilities.

TABLE 41.5 | National organisations in Australia concerned with the rights of people with disabilities

Organisation	Role
Australian Human Rights and Equal Opportunities Commission (HREOC)	A commission established in 1986 with specific objectives: to eliminate discrimination against people with disabilities and to promote acceptance and inclusion of people with disabilities into the community.
Disability Services Australia	Provides a range of services, including daytime activity programs and support with accommodation to help bridge the gap between school and adult life.
Australian Council for Rehabilitation of the Disabled (ACROD)	National industry association for disability services, influencing government legislation and funding to promote quality services for people with disabilities.
Action for Carers and Employment (ACE)	National body representing the many state and territory organisations that provide employment assistance and support to people with disabilities in the regular workforce.
Australian Institute of Sport (AIS)	Activities include a program to coach elite athletes with disabilities.
Australian Sports Commission (ASC)	Promotes active lifestyle for all Australians, including those with disabilities. Activities include an education program to train teachers and community leaders to run sports and other outdoor events suitable for people with disabilities.
Australian Sport and Recreation Association for People with an Intellectual Disability (AUSRAPID)	National sporting body that promotes equal access to sport and recreational programs for people with intellectual disabilities.
Other organisations that promote inclusion in sporting activities include Blind Sports Australia, Deaf Sports Australia, Disabled Wintersports Australia (DWA), Riding for the Disabled Association of Australia, Disability Sports Australia.	

(Department of Social Services 2023)

THE PHILOSOPHY OF INCLUSION AND NORMALISATION

The concept of **normalisation** for people with disabilities is not new and has been discussed by governments and organisations for more than 30 years. The principle of normalisation stems from the work of Bengt Nirje and was further defined by Wolf Wolfensberger and identifies a basic philosophy that socially valued roles for people with disabilities should be supported and defended because their social roles as individuals are at risk of being devalued (Wolfensberger et al 1972).

Intrinsic to the concept of normalisation is the belief that all people are capable of growth and development. Normalisation is not concerned with making everyone normal; rather, the goals are to provide equitable access and services for people with disabilities. Wolfensberger (1972) asserts that normalisation should instead be called **social role valorisation (SRV)** since this is more inclusive and values the social roles held by an individual with a disability. The key principle underpinning SRV is that if a person holds valued social roles, that person is more likely to receive from society the good things in life that are available to that society. These include home and family; friendship; being accorded dignity, respect and acceptance; a sense of belonging; an education; the development and exercise of one's capacities; a voice in the affairs of one's community and society; opportunities to participate; a decent material standard of living; at least a normative place to live; and opportunities for work and self-support (Barr et al 2020). Clinical Interest Box 41.5 provides some examples of how the philosophical principles of **inclusion** and normalisation have been, or are still to be, implemented. (See Case Study 41.1.)

CONTINUING CHALLENGES

Despite the many changes that have occurred in the past three decades, there is still stigma attached to both chronic illness and disability. The more profound and obvious the disease or disability, the more significant the social barriers are (Barr et al 2020).

If these challenges are to be overcome, the essential first step is to educate healthcare professionals so that they can:

- influence the physical and social environments in which people with disabilities live and work
- educate the public so that people with disabilities are included
- advocate to governments, service providers or councils for changes in the way current services are provided and suggest affordable improvements that provide easy access.

CLINICAL INTEREST BOX 41.5 Implementation of normalisation and inclusion principles

Education

Significantly increased integration of children with disabilities into mainstream schools.

Arts, sports and recreation

Being inclusive in arts, sports or recreation is about providing a range of options to cater for people of all ages and abilities in the most appropriate manner possible. It is more than including people with disability in regular sport activities; it includes ensuring that an individual chooses to participate in a range of opportunities that take into account:

- their functional ability
- the sport in which they are participating
- the opportunities within their local environment
- their personal preferences.

Drama groups have provided ongoing opportunities for people with disabilities to fully participate in all areas of theatre production including international arts festivals, as well as working with organisations such as the Melbourne Symphony Orchestra.

Employment

Access to employment has improved as a result of stipulated requirements and government schemes.
Employers are required to modify workplaces to facilitate the employment of people with disabilities (e.g. purchasing special equipment, providing wheelchair access) unless doing so causes unjustifiable hardship to the workplace.
Government funding is available to assist with modifications to some business workplaces.
Advertisements for jobs must not discriminate against or exclude a person with a disability from applying for the position provided that they have the ability to do the work.

Transport

The Transport Standards are mandatory standards in Australia and are supported by state legislation such as the *Disability Services Act 2006* (Queensland). The Transport Standards cover premises and infrastructure and apply to public transport operators including bus, coach, train, taxi and aviation companies.

Access to buildings

The Building Code of Australia stipulates that buildings must be designed to facilitate access and meet the needs of people with a range of disabilities. Requirements include:

- doorways wide enough for people using wheelchairs
- appropriate toilet space and facilities
- minimum lighting to meet the needs of vision-impaired people and those who communicate by sign language or lip-reading.

Entertainment

Captioning: In 1982, the Australian Captioning Centre was established to provide captioning services for hearing impaired people. Captioning on film or television provides written on-screen messages about what is being said and what sound effects or music are happening. Australian legislation requires that captions are provided for news, current affairs and prime-time television programs. In 2001, captioning was introduced in major cinemas around the country, but at the time of writing not all films are yet captioned.

(Francisco et al 2020; Collins et al 2022; Maguire-Rosier 2016; Dimov et al 2022; Macleod et al 2022; Australian Building Codes Board 2022; Australian Communications and Media Authority 2023)

CASE STUDY 41.1

Grace is 42 years old. She was born with a brain injury as a result of birth trauma. Her parents have been her primary carers since birth. Grace requires a high level of physical assistance. For example, every day of her life her father has lifted her from her bed in the morning and carried her to a recliner chair in the lounge and later returned her to bed the same way. Each day her mother has prepared Grace's food and assisted Grace with her meals. Because of the difficulties Grace has with chewing and swallowing her food, mealtimes have always been a lengthy process. Personal care routines such as showering and dressing are provided by her parents. Sometimes Grace resists and yells out. Grace is incontinent of urine and her parents fit her with disposable pads every morning and change them frequently during the day. They take care of the pressure areas that sometimes develop.

Continued

CASE STUDY 41.1—cont'd

After leaving her special developmental school at 17 years old, Grace began attending a day centre 3 days each week. She was taken there in a community bus specially designed to accommodate her wheelchair. Activity at the centre revolved mostly around the staff meeting the hygiene, toileting, medication, mobility and nutritional needs of the two dozen or more people with severe or profound disabilities who also attended. The staff reported that Grace spent a lot of her time there simply dozing.

On the days she is at home, Grace has many things surrounding her that give her pleasure. She has a box containing many different pieces of material. She enjoys the feel of the different textures, especially the velvet and silk. Other times she holds on to colourful toys and, although she has a profoundly limited vocabulary, she is able to express her pleasure in her favourite television programs and music. Grace also enjoys being with her mother in the kitchen and sitting on the outside veranda watching people walk past the house. Many of the neighbours greet her cheerfully.

Grace's parents have been anxious for some time about their future ability to care for her, but now Grace's mother has fallen and fractured her hip. Her father is exhausted and cannot manage to care for Grace alone. Grace has been admitted to a residential care unit, where most of the residents are elderly and have dementia. There is nowhere else available at the moment.

1. What might Grace's mother and father be feeling about this situation? What could be done to help them?
2. What might be the impact of this move on Grace? How might she be feeling? How can staff help ease the transition to her new accommodation and situation?
3. What other support services could you refer both Grace and her parents to?
4. What are Grace's rights? What are the risks of those rights being infringed?
5. What can staff do to ensure that her rights are not infringed?
6. How can staff create a stimulating and pleasurable environment for Grace?
7. What does social role valorisation or normalisation mean to Grace?

APPROACHES TO MANAGEMENT OF INDIVIDUALS WITH CHRONIC CONDITIONS OR DISABILITIES

Assessment

Assessment of the individual is integral to the development of effective nursing care plans. People with chronic conditions and/or disabilities should always be assessed holistically, placing the person at the centre of the assessment. (See Nursing Care Plan 41.1 and Progress Note 41.1.)

A multidisciplinary approach to assessment is generally required. Depending on the age and type of disability the person is experiencing, assessment may involve a range of professionals including but not limited to teachers, doctors, occupational therapists, speech pathologists, social workers, psychologists and nurses.

The purpose of assessment is to identify the abilities, strengths and specific needs of an individual so that appropriate care may be planned. The overarching goal is to ensure support that allows the person to live life as near as possible to the way they desire. The assessment process should consider all aspects of the person's life including:

- physical needs
- health and medical needs
- financial support
- spiritual and emotional support needs
- cultural needs
- learning needs
- behavioural support needs
- need for meaningful work
- recreation and leisure needs
- transport issues
- accommodation needs
- support networks (family and community)
- impact of the person's environment.

The team may assess the individual using a variety of methods, such as observation, interviewing and testing. A checklist may be used to help identify activities that can be performed independently by the individual, and those for which assistance is required. When assessment is complete, the team, collaboratively with the individual or family carer, can plan the care to be implemented following the principles of person-centred planning.

The extensive types of disability, and the fact that many individuals will have multiple disabilities, means that after the assessment process nurses may determine a broad range of nursing diagnoses for each person. Clinical Interest Box 41.6 identifies some common issues that need to be considered for a nursing assessment of individuals with disabilities. The list is by no means exhaustive and not in any particular sequence. The degree of relevance and nursing response will vary with each person and each situation.

Planning and implementing care

Using the information obtained from the assessment process, a care plan or treatment plan is developed to meet the individual's needs. Central to development of a program is the concept of helping the individual to achieve as much independence as possible (Table 41.6). The aim of professional support is to facilitate the person living as independently as possible and assisting them to engage in

NURSING CARE PLAN 41.1

Mrs Carter is a 70-year-old with comorbid type 2 diabetes and rheumatoid arthritis. She lives independently at home with her husband. Pain and stiffness due to the rheumatoid arthritis limit her ability and motivation to be physically active. Her social activities are limited to family, and she rarely leaves the house unless accompanied by her husband. Due to an increase in her pain and stiffness she has been admitted to hospital for assessment. The Registered Nurse asks you, the Enrolled Nurse, to complete the admission assessment on Mrs Carter. Mrs Carter informs you that the pain and stiffness in her hands has made washing and dressing difficult lately. With more probing you discover that eating has also become difficult since Mrs Carter is finding it difficult to use normal utensils. She currently rates her pain and stiffness as 7 out of 10.

Assessment: Self-care deficit: impaired ability to perform activities of daily living for oneself such as showering, dressing and feeding related to pain and stiffness.

Issue/s to be addressed: Able to perform activities of daily living—showering and dressing—with assistance.

Goal/s: Mrs Carter will be able to self-care using modified equipment and appropriate aids.

Care/actions	Rationale
Educate Mrs Carter on how to pace activities.	Rheumatoid arthritis causes fatigue and understanding this will help Mrs Carter modify behaviours.
Assess and manage chronic and acute pain: Pillow supports, warm compresses, pain medication, relaxation.	Improving comfort level will enable Mrs Carter to self-care.
Refer to an occupational therapist for assessment and advice on assistive aids.	To identify what aspects of the task Mrs Carter needs assistance with and to determine what aids will meet her needs (buttonhooks, long-handled shoehorns, hand-held shower etc.).

Evaluation: Mrs Carter is able to perform self-care activities consistent with her ability.

CLINICAL INTEREST BOX 41.6 Nursing considerations related to the needs of individuals with chronic disease or disabilities

Psychological needs

- Impaired adjustment
- Ineffective individual coping
- Self-concept disturbance (incorporating body image/self-esteem/role performance/personal identity)
- Hopelessness
- Powerlessness
- Altered sexuality pattern
- Impaired social interaction

Physical needs

- Impaired physical mobility
- Impaired verbal communication
- Self-care deficit (incorporating hygiene/dressing and grooming/toileting)
- Sleep pattern disturbance
- Altered patterns of elimination (incorporating urinary/bowel)
- Potential for impaired tissue integrity
- Potential for falls/injury

(Chang & Johnson 2021; Gutenbrunner et al 2022)

activities that enhance their quality of life while encouraging them to develop effective interpersonal relationships and make informed choices.

Evaluation

Evaluation must be performed continuously to assess progress in achieving the goals of care. Continuous evaluation is also needed to identify whether there are potential risks that have not been considered previously and to confirm that safe, holistic care is maintained.

Person-centred care

Person-centred care views individuals and their significant others as equal partners in the planning and provision of services. Unlike other models of care, this model places the person at the centre of their own care and considers the needs of the individual (Phelan et al 2020). The concept of person-centred care originates from the counselling approach developed by Rogers in the late 1940s. Person-centred care believes that all people have a personal responsibility and choice in decisions and that no-one should make decisions for another person. Rather than give advice, the role of the clinician is to maintain an 'attitude of positive regard'; that is, to be non-judgmental and supportive. More recently, the inclusion of other strategies such as motivational interviewing has strengthened this model. Clinical Interest Box 41.7 outlines the principles

TABLE 41.6 | Stages in the development of a care plan for a person with a disability or chronic disease

Stage	Action
Identify a person's capabilities	What are the person's strengths and weaknesses? What does the person need assistance with? Focus on what the person can do rather than what they cannot do.
Establish common goals	Assist the person to set SMART goals. • **S**pecific • **M**easurable • **A**ttainable • **R**elevant • **T**ime-bound Set small goals to develop a sense of achievement. Ensure family and significant others are aware of the goals.
Identify and prioritise skills that need to be developed	What skills does the person need? What resources are needed? How can the family/significant others assist?
Determine the most effective teaching strategies	How will the person learn the new skills? • Experientially? • Practically? • Vicariously?
Determine the most effective interventions to meet social, educational and other needs	What does the person want to achieve? How can this be achieved?

(Drury 2021)

CLINICAL INTEREST BOX 41.7
Principles of person-centred care

- Develop a rapport and get to know the person and caregiver.
- Responsibility and decision-making are shared.
- Individual's preferences are respected.
- Provision of accurate and easy-to-understand information so that individuals can make informed choices.
- Care is coordinated and integrated, working seamlessly to improve a person's outcomes.
- The environment supports staff in the provision of person-centred care.

(McCormack et al 2021)

of person-centred care and Table 41.7 provides a list of some of the core skills and knowledge required by nurses to support individuals to self-manage.

Motivational interviewing and assessing readiness to change behaviour

In a model of care where the person is regarded as being an equal, it is essential that the clinician does not 'tell a

TABLE 41.7 | Core knowledge and skills essential for healthcare professionals to provide self-management support

Skill	Ability
Assessment skills	Able to assess: • Readiness for change • Risk factors • Support systems • Self-management ability • Strengths and weaknesses
Behaviour change skills	• Motivational interviewing techniques • Understanding models of behaviour change • Able to assist the individual with goal setting, problem-solving and developing action plans
Organisational skills	• Able to work in multidisciplinary teams • Applies evidence to practice • Sound knowledge of community resources

(Drury & Aw 2020; Drury et al 2017)

person what to do'. As previously mentioned, the role of the clinician is to support the person while encouraging the person to explore issues preventing behaviour change. Prochaska and DiClemente's model of behaviour change describes a process of behaviour change that occurs over time, with individuals moving through five stages, from pre-contemplation to maintenance (Prochaska & Norcross 2001). This model is a useful way of identifying whether a person is ready and motivated to modify or change behaviours (Drury 2021).

Prior to moving to discuss a plan of action and intervention, the clinician should ascertain the individual's readiness to change. If the individual is not in the preparation or action phase, then motivational interviewing strategies may be used to explore reasons preventing change. Table 41.8 outlines the phases in the stages of change model.

Motivational interviewing

Motivational interviewing (MI) strategies have become the 'gold standard' communication method of working with individuals who are reticent about making changes considered necessary for optimal health (Self et al 2022). Based on the principle that most people do not enter into relationships with clinicians motivated to make changes or modify their behaviour, the role of the clinician, therefore, is to assist the individual to explore their ambivalence about making the behaviour change. There are four phases in MI:

1. engaging
2. guiding
3. evoking
4. planning.

(Self et al 2022; Williams 2023)

See Table 41.9 for more detail.

Motivational interviewing may take a number of sessions and a considerable amount of time. Unfortunately, in the real world, clinicians do not always have unlimited time nor do individuals always return for appointments. Therefore, it may be more useful to use brief MI strategies since these are designed to be used in a single session of approximately 45 minutes. Using the same communication strategy as that used in MI, the clinician works through seven stages to encourage the individual to explore ambivalence:

1. Build rapport—establish a therapeutic relationship and encourage the individual to openly share. Be non-judgmental and empathetic. This may help you

TABLE 41.8 | Phases in the stages of change model

Phase	Description
Pre-contemplation	The individual does not intend to change behaviour within the next 6 months. In this phase, the individual lacks motivation but also may lack the knowledge and skills to make any changes.
Contemplation	During this phase, the individual is considering making changes within the next 6 months; however, they are hampered by ambivalence and tend to focus on the barriers and challenges that will be encountered rather than the positive effects.
Preparation	The individual is preparing to take action within the next month and has usually developed a plan and may already have initiated some actions.
Action	The individual is actively taking action to modify and change behaviour. Relapse is a real concern at this stage and ongoing support is essential.
Maintenance	The individual has made the changes and the risk of relapse is decreasing as time goes on. At this point, the individual will usually state they are confident they can continue the new behaviour.

(Del Rio et al 2021; DiClemente & Graydon 2020; Prochaska & Norcross 2001)

TABLE 41.9 | Phases in motivational interviewing

Phase	Clinician's role
Engaging	Assess the individual's stage of change. • **O**pen-ended questions • **A**ffirmations • **R**eflective listening • **S**ummarise the discussion
Guiding	Explore the attitudes and values held by the individual. Encourage the individual to identify costs and benefits of changing or not changing behaviour. Assist with goal planning and set goals that are measurable and achievable in a short space of time.
Evoking	At this stage, the individual is motivated to change behaviour. Ask the individual to identify reasons for making the change and then reinforce the change with these statements. Affirm all positive action. Encourage the individual to reflect on the change.
Planning	Identify and set measurable and achievable goals.

(Miller & Rollnick 2012; Williams 2023)

to understand whether the person plans to make any changes and where they are in the stages of change model.
2. Open the discussion—allow the person to discuss their concerns by inviting them to tell their story. Use open-ended questions and probing to elicit further information.
3. A typical day—ask the person to describe a typical day to you from the time they get up in the morning. This often helps the individual to identify and explore issues that are a problem or triggers for behaviours that need changing.
4. The good things and the less good things—encourage the person to talk about the good things and the less good things. The terminology here is important since speaking of the less good things rather than 'concerns' allows the person to identify problem areas without feeling that these behaviours are being labelled as problematic. Use open-ended questions to probe further and affirmation when the person identifies good coping skills.
5. Provide information—avoid giving advice. Ask if the person would like information about specific issues and provide it if wanted. Use reflective listening and paraphrase to ensure you heard the correct message.
6. The future and the present—this strategy can be used if the person is concerned about a particular behaviour. Ask the person how they would like things to be different in the future.
7. Explore concerns—this essential step is where you listen to the person and facilitate them thinking about changing behaviour.

(Gillam & Yusuf 2019)

As goal-directed and focused types of counselling approach, both MI and brief MI require training and practice. It is essential that any clinicians using this approach have received appropriate training from a qualified person and receive adequate supervision while they become proficient in its use (Garrison et al 2023). Referral to clinicians trained in MI should be organised if ability to provide competent MI counselling is outside the clinician's scope of practice.

Self-management for individuals with chronic diseases and/or disability

The origins of self-management of chronic disease are in Lorig's seminal work with those suffering from arthritis in the USA in the 1970s. **Self-management**, also called self-care, is a theory-based approach to healthcare that recognises the central role played by the individual in health promotion, disease prevention and successful management of illness. It is the ability to manage the disease process, the emotional consequences of living with the disease and the changes that occur to daily living as a consequence of the disease. Evidence in the literature shows that education programs incorporating self-management skills can enhance health outcomes (Riegel et al 2021). Self-management is both a process whereby training is provided to people with chronic illness and an outcome that indicates when people with chronic health problems achieve the skills and knowledge to manage the medical, emotional and role aspects of their illness (Drury & Aw 2020).

Previous development of many self-management programs has focused on the major chronic illnesses existing in industrialised societies (e.g. arthritis, diabetes, chronic obstructive pulmonary disease and heart disease). In more recent times, however, there has been a move to facilitate self-management principles into programs for people with disabilities, with evidence suggesting statistically significant positive outcomes (Bringmann 2020; Fisher et al 2023).

Disease self-management programs can be delivered to groups or individuals by health professionals or lay people, via face-to-face format or interactive technology such as the internet or telephone. Each of these methods of delivery requires healthcare professionals to learn new skills and refine existing skills (Schopp & Rhoda 2021).

Integral to self-management is the support and advocacy provided by healthcare professionals that empower the individuals to make informed choices and actively participate in the management of their disease or disability. This involves a partnership between the person and the healthcare provider where the person is the manager of the daily consequences of the disease and the healthcare professional is the coach (Schopp & Rhoda 2021). This model is similar in principle to person-centred care whereby the healthcare professionals share information with the person and caregivers, understand the person's values and goals and help them to create a care plan that meets their goals. Self-management support involves three steps:

1. defining the issues or problems
2. setting goals and developing problem-solving strategies
3. active sustained follow-up.

(Schopp & Rhoda 2021)

The main difference in this model is that the person is acknowledged as being the expert in managing their disease and the healthcare professional is the expert in the disease and disease process. Thus, the person takes an active role in determining care and setting goals. Despite the role of the healthcare professionals being described as providing support to the person by assisting them to make informed choices, set their own goals and develop problem-solving skills, it has been found that they remain in a position of power and therefore, in many instances, collaboration between healthcare professional and the individual is limited (Salemonsen et al 2020).

Experts in self-management programs suggest that core knowledge and skills essential for healthcare professionals to provide self-management support can be centred on assessment and behaviour change skills and organisational strategies (Schopp & Rhoda 2021).

Establishing a rapport with the person and eliciting information about their challenges and successes are components of effective self-management support (Seabra et al 2023). Assessing the individual for readiness to change and exploring the consequences of current behaviour and any ambivalence towards change are the first steps in self-management support (Drury & Aw 2020).

Ambivalence is at the core of change, and it is essential to acknowledge that not all people are ready or willing to change. The role of the healthcare professional is not to tell the individual they must change but rather help them explore their ambivalence and behaviours, provide information, and help them understand their lifestyle and concerns in the hope that they will become intrinsically motivated to make changes. The interpersonal relationship that develops must provide the individual with a safe and supportive place to do this.

CRITICAL THINKING EXERCISE 41.1

Joyce is a 62-year-old overweight woman diagnosed 2 years ago with osteoarthritis. She works full-time as a receptionist in a busy medical clinic and is mother to two grown-up children who are working but live at home. Her husband is a fly-in fly-out worker and is on a 2-1 roster, which means he is away for 2 weeks and then home for a week. She has constant pain, which she has managed with physiotherapy, NSAIDs and steroid injections. However, recently the pain has worsened, and she is now finding it difficult to sleep at night. She acknowledges her diet is unhealthy and is heavily loaded with sugar, fats and carbohydrates. She also tells you that she has been using medicinal cannabis, which she buys illegally from a local person, to help manage her pain. She has come into the surgery to have a consultation with her GP for a team care management plan. The doctor has requested the nurse take her vital observations including weight, height, waist measurement and a BMI be calculated. She appears upset and reticent to be weighed, saying she is in a hurry and needs to get home. As the nurse in the surgery, you realise you have limited time to effectively explore the issue with her. What brief motivational interviewing strategies might you use that could get Joyce to consider the consequences of her behaviour?

Provision of services

The federal, state and territory governments in Australia fund a range of services for people with disabilities and their family carers, including:

- family support services, such as respite care and community-based respite care
- domiciliary support, such as help with cleaning, house and garden maintenance and Meals on Wheels
- personal care support
- home modification and provision of equipment
- independent-living skills programs
- pre-vocational training, vocational placement and employment support
- social support, including recreational and culturally specific activities
- community-based accommodation and support (fe.g. support available to people with a disability living at home or in other accommodation in the community)
- counselling in the areas of sexuality
- education and training for carers, individuals and their families
- behaviour management programs and specialised training in this area
- specialist assistance from professionals such as psychiatrists, psychologists, speech therapists and occupational therapists
- case management (both short- and long-term), providing individual support, advocacy and monitoring
- a person's disability allowance
- carer's allowance (small regular financial payment to assist with additional expenses).

(Department of Social Services 2023)

These services aim to assist people with disabilities to achieve as much independence as possible by promoting and supporting family and community acceptance and involvement, by providing sufficient support services and by offering a range of accommodation options.

As highlighted earlier, there is now much greater acceptance of the importance of family living and of participation in community life than previously. The well-being and the quality of life of people with disabilities depends on recognition and acknowledgment of their rights, promotion of community acceptance and the implementation of programs that appropriately promote education, provide training for employment, develop independent skills in activities of daily living and promote enjoyment of life. Professional support is primarily directed towards enabling a person with a disability to achieve as much independence as possible, through interventions and by providing support that promotes independent living and vocational capacities. Planning and implementation of appropriate educational and vocational programs is performed on an individual basis and takes into account any associated physical, sensory or emotional effects of the disabilities.

Basic principles that should guide the provision of services include:

- A collaborative approach between health professionals: the individual and the family should be consulted to decide what is needed, what will be of most help and how that help should be implemented for maximum benefit.
- Identification of the individual's and family's strengths and capabilities.
- Recognition and validation of emotions, needs and concerns.

These principles should be kept in mind when assessing, planning, implementing and evaluating care.

NATIONAL DISABILITY INSURANCE SCHEME AND NATIONAL DISABILITY INSURANCE AGENCY

The National Disability Insurance Scheme (NDIS) is the most major overhaul of social and disability services in Australia since the implementation of Medicare in 1984. The NDIS has attracted substantial funding from the federal and state governments as well as backing from a variety of interest groups and is hailed as the cornerstone of Australia's disability services. The NDIS was introduced in 2013 in Australia and provides Australians under the age of 65 with the support and services they need to live a fulfilled life (Carey et al 2021). Prior to its introduction, services were poorly coordinated, with funding sources divided between local, state and federal governments, often leading to inadequate service provision. The aim of the NDIS was to overcome these shortcomings and provide sustainable long-term care and support for individuals with disabilities from birth to 65 years (Carey et al 2021). However, to fulfil its stated goals, the scheme's deployment is exceeding the ability of service consumers, service providers and the body in charge of administering it, which poses a threat to its success. According to research, problems with the scheme's execution can be partly ascribed to how the policy was designed and partially to how it was implemented, both of which made little use of the lessons learned from similar reforms (Olney & Dickinson 2019). The National Disability Insurance Agency (NDIA) is an independent statutory agency whose role is to implement the NDIS (Olney & Dickinson 2019). Therefore, while the NDIA provides assessment services and funding, it does not provide services. Services are provided through a range of government and non-government organisations, and people with disabilities and their carers can choose their providers and the services they want, thus tailoring disability support packages to individual needs (Buckmaster & Clark 2019).

Under the NDIS, a care plan is developed that is individualised and provides appropriate support services. This plan is reviewed annually, and changes made according to the individual's goals and support needs (Buckmaster & Clark 2019).

CAREGIVERS OF PEOPLE WITH CHRONIC DISEASE OR DISABILITY

The role of family carers providing care to people with a disability or chronic illness is recognised as an indispensable part of the provision and sustainability of the health and social care systems in England, Australia and Asian countries. In 2019, 10.8%% of the Australian population, or 2.65 million people, identified as carers. Of these, 12.3% (of all females) were women and 9.3% (of all males) were men. More than 235,000 carers were under the age of 25 (Australian Bureau of Statistics 2019b). The support provided by carers is often extensive, covering a range of activities from eating and bathing to assisting with healthcare, financial management and property maintenance.

There are many reasons for taking on a caring role. The most given reason for taking on caring roles was a sense of family responsibility (70.1%). Compared to non-carers (25.6%), 50% of all carers (50.2%) resided in homes with equivalised gross incomes in the lowest two quintiles. The next most common reason was a feeling the carer could provide better care than anybody else, followed by a feeling of emotional obligation to undertake the role When the person being cared for was an older person (aged 65 years and over), it was more likely that no other friends or family were available to take on the caring role (Australian Bureau of Statistics 2019b).

Carers Australia has successfully placed the needs of carers on the political agenda for over 25 years. The primary role of Carers Australia is advocacy, which has been fundamental to the *Carer Recognition Act 2010*, the National Carer Strategy Action Plan (2011–2014) and the Carer Supplement.

Family and carers of people with chronic disease and/or disabilities are often expected to provide care and support 24 hours a day. Unpaid caregiving is almost always a deeply interpersonal practice that resonates with the most troubling preoccupations of both caregivers and those being cared for regarding living, self and dignity. Caregiving is relational and reciprocal and is an embodied experience for both the caregiver and receiver. Caring acts are centred on physical acts of touching, embracing, steadying, lifting, toileting and so on. Caring has to do with sensibilities of empathy, compassion, respect and love. Those sensibilities involve cognitive and emotional and moral processes that underwrite the actual practices of giving and receiving care. Unlike nurses, family carers do not get breaks between shifts or get to go home after finishing their work. Even when respite is available, the responsibility is permanent, 7 days a week, often lifelong and often falling primarily on one family member (Sherman 2019).

For many, the responsibility begins with the birth of a child with a chronic disease such as cystic fibrosis or a disability such as a hearing impairment. Parents in this situation are faced with an unplanned lifetime of giving full-time care that interferes with their ability to give as much time as they would like to their other children or to conduct their lives as previously planned. They are faced with coping with the situation as they deal with the grief associated with lost expectations about their baby and the future. For others it begins at the stage of life when caring responsibilities are expected to reduce (e.g. the parent caring for an adolescent offspring who has an acquired brain injury or has developed serious mental illness). Caregiving responsibilities may also begin in older age when a spouse develops a chronic disease, such as dementia or chronic obstructive pulmonary disease.

Families caring for adolescents face particular challenges impacting on daily life including internal factors such as changing family roles and relationships, and external factors such as service discontinuity, where forfeiting of a desired option may be necessary. Also, teenagers with intellectual disabilities have significantly more health problems than the rest of the population and many encounter difficulties accessing the services they need (Alsharaydeh et al 2019; Franklin et al 2019). Challenges such as these mean that family routine in the adolescent years is dynamic rather than static. Families use multiple strategies to accommodate these challenges, which are underpinned by their beliefs, values and resources. Professionals working with families caring for an adolescent with disability need to be aware of these in order to support families effectively to sustain a meaningful family routine during the adolescent years (Franklin et al 2019). Some professionals find the families they support considering relinquishing or actually relinquishing the care of the adolescent to the state (Shrier 2021). The professional must ensure the family has an understanding of the ramifications of this decision.

The impact of caring: Lifestyle changes and loss

Whenever the carer role begins, it is often associated with great lifestyle changes and many losses, including:

- loss of the ability to continue with a career or paid employment
- loss of income and financial security
- loss of status and socialisation that often accompanies a paid work position
- lost hopes and dreams of what the future will bring
- loss of freedom and socialisation
- loss of a normal or expected relationship (e.g. loss of companionship or a sexual partner when physical and cognitive functioning are profoundly affected).

(Bastawrous et al 2015; Neri et al 2016)

Despite the seriousness of their situation, many people caring for family members with disabilities gain pleasure, a sense of satisfaction and feelings of personal fulfilment from the role they have undertaken.

The grief associated with loss cannot be ignored and one of the greatest and most difficult challenges confronting people with long-term conditions or disabilities is coming to terms with the loss. Often, despite the losses being significant, the grief surrounding them will largely go unnoticed. The person may not be aware that they are grieving as they struggle to manage the complexities of their new life. Although it is acknowledged that people experience loss in unique and individual ways, the common responses to loss identified by Kübler-Ross in her seminal work are applicable to the loss and grief experienced in chronic illness and disability (Kübler-Ross & Kessler 2005). These stages are denial, anger, bargaining, depression and acceptance. These stages help us understand where a person may be in relation to accepting and living with their chronic illness or disability, but they are not prescriptive; that is, not everyone experiences all stages and the stages are not always linear. Grief and loss are a unique experience. Individuals experiencing these emotions need support from a range of health professionals. To help the person move forward and develop positive coping strategies, professional counselling may be critical at this time. Referral to a general practitioner, a psychologist or a counsellor should all be considered at this stage.

Support for primary (family) carers

It is essential that nurses and other professionals acknowledge and credit family carers as having the primary caregiving role, and carefully assess how to best enable and facilitate their ongoing coping abilities. Some family carers prefer to cope independently; some prefer a regular visit from a nurse or other team member; others may view such visits or other interventions as an invasion of privacy. Some simply need the reassurance of having a contact to call when information or assistance is needed. Others need a significant amount of support when supporting people with complex health needs or in managing challenging behaviours (Statler 2023; Zajdel et al 2023). The amount and type of support may vary in terms of its frequency or intensity but whenever and whatever services are implemented they should be determined in collaboration with the primary carer. There are key times when additional services or support may be needed. These include:

- at the time of diagnosis or identification of a disability
- during the care of a preschool child with a disability
- when educational needs and the person's potential need to be determined or reviewed
- before transition from child to adult services or from adult to aged-care services
- when the person is unwell
- when the primary carer is unwell
- when the person's general functioning declines and care needs increase.

(Zajdel et al 2023)

The opportunity for primary carers to take short-term breaks using respite services should be integrated into care planning. Even though such breaks do not resolve the stresses and strains of full-time caring, they may have a positive influence on the ability of the primary carer to continue the carer role in the long term. However, some family carers feel guilty about putting a dependent loved one into respite care and choose not to take much-needed breaks. Even so, demand for respite services sometimes exceeds supply (Groenvynck et al 2021).

One of the significant issues facing primary carers is what will happen to the dependent loved one if they should get sick or die. This is particularly worrying for parents who have spent a lifetime caring for dependent children with limited-service support. As resources and services experience higher demand with shrinking budgets, families often carry the added burden of planning for ongoing care, in particular in the area of accommodation, because of the ongoing shortage of appropriate accommodation for people with disabilities.

Whenever possible, individuals, families and carers need to develop a plan in advance to ease this worry, but this can be a complicated matter. The current shortage of suitable accommodation options for young people already results in young people with disabilities living in aged-care facilities. This situation is not likely to improve in the near future. In future years, the current older generation of family carers will need to relinquish care of adult children with disabilities and thus demand for appropriate accommodation and care will increase significantly. There is a very real possibility that, unless action is taken now, many people with disabilities will be left without a suitable home and without appropriate care and support. It is essential that professionals such as nurses continue to advocate for appropriate resources for people with disabilities. In addition, based on the assessment of the family needs made by the nurse, grief counselling for the family and caregivers may help relieve caregiver burden and compassion fatigue.

Caring for people with profound or multiple disabilities is challenging. The nurse needs to make an informed assessment of needs, plan sensitive and timely interventions, and demonstrate respect for the individual. It is also of vital importance the nurse acknowledges and shows empathy for the role of the primary carer. These attributes are at the heart of excellent nursing care for people with disabilities.

HEALTH PROMOTION: DISABILITY PREVENTION

Several **health promotion** strategies have been implemented with the aim of reducing the number of people who are born with or acquire a disability (see Clinical Interest Box 41.8).

Prevention of disability needs to be a priority. Currently, it is estimated that one in nine (11.6%) of people aged 0–64 and one in two (49.6%) of people over 65 years have a disability (Australian Bureau of Statistics 2019b). It is difficult to determine exactly how many of these disabilities were preventable; however, it is known that many of these injuries occur in preventable situations such as traffic accidents, or are sporting injuries, or are due to the misuse of illicit substances.

Many of these causes of acquired brain damage, and some other congenital or acquired disabilities, could be minimised by health and safety education programs and/or programs that promote and support a healthy lifestyle.

CLINICAL INTEREST BOX 41.8 Strategies for health promotion/disability prevention

- Vaccinations: Promoted to prevent serious illness that can lead to a range of impairments (e.g. vaccination against the COVID-19 virus is important because of the risk of severe illness or death from the virus).
- Road safety campaigns and swim safe campaigns: Aimed to reduce the number of disabilities caused by road accidents, diving accidents and near-drowning accidents.
- Safe sex campaigns: Aimed to reduce the incidence of AIDS and sexually transmitted infections that can cause disability.
- Safety in the workplace and safety in the home programs: Aimed to reduce avoidable injuries to employees, children and adults.
- Anti-smoking campaigns: Aimed to reduce the physical impairment caused by damage to the lungs and other organs from smoking.
- Education of pregnant mothers about the dangers of smoking for the unborn infant: Aimed to reduce the risk of brain damage and intellectual disabilities in children. Education programs for pregnant mothers have also focused on the importance of healthy nutrition and the elimination of alcohol and other drugs.
- 'SunSmart' campaigns: Aimed to reduce disability caused by skin cancer.

(Germani et al 2022; Rural Heath Information Hub 2023)

An important role for nurses, particularly those working in community settings, is the prevention of additional illness in people with disabilities by ensuring their ongoing access to routine health screens. This is sometimes difficult, perhaps due to a physical disability preventing a person achieving the correct position for a particular health screen, such as a mammogram or a cervical screening test, or a person with an intellectual disability giving consent for these procedures. This does not mean that health screening should be put in the 'too hard basket'. Consultation between medical officers, radiographers, physiotherapists, nurses and, especially, the person with the disability is needed to establish a way in which tests can be successfully managed.

ABUSE AND ADVOCACY

Unfortunately, despite all the information and support available for caregivers, people with disabilities and chronic diseases are still subject to abuse, neglect, exploitation and risk. There are legislative frameworks such as the International Convention on the Rights of Persons with a Disability and the *Disability Discrimination Act* that exist to

TABLE 41.10 | Types of abuse

Types of abuse	Examples
Physical	Bodily harm caused by hitting, pushing or similar actions
Emotional	Saying hurtful words, shouting or threatening a person
Financial	Misappropriation of finances by a trusted person
Sexual	Forcing a person to partake in or watch sexual acts
Neglect	Not responding to the needs of the person (e.g. not assisting with toileting)
Abandonment	Leaving a person alone for long periods without planning for their care

(Legano et al 2021; Nagaratnam & Nagaratnam 2019)

protect people with disabilities and chronic diseases against abuse. Abuse can take many different forms (Nagaratnam & Nagaratnam 2019). (See Table 41.10.)

In Australia, there are mandatory reporting laws related to suspected abuse in children. This means that if a person working in a mandated profession, such as nursing, policing or teaching, suspects, on reasonable grounds, that a child is being abused they have a responsibility to report it (Australian Government 2020). Elder abuse, however, often goes unreported due to shame and fear of the consequences (e.g. being placed in a nursing home) (Dow et al 2020).

Advocacy is considered to be a core competency of all nurses and involves knowledge and experience as well as confidence. Most nursing codes of ethics identify the nurse's responsibility to protect the rights of individuals and be a voice for the individual (Nsiah et al 2019). Advocacy involves listening skills, problem-solving, communication and being objective (Abbasinia et al 2020). Advocacy, therefore, includes ensuring individuals are informed of their choices, protecting people's rights and supporting the person's autonomy (Gerber 2018). Being an effective advocate involves:

- assessing the needs of the individual
- identifying what the individual's goals are
- providing information and helping the individual to make ethical choices
- communicating the individual's choices to the healthcare team
- evaluating the outcome of the advocacy and the individual's decision.

(Abbasinia et al 2020; Shoemark 2021)

Advocacy is a professional responsibility of all nurses and is viewed as one of the tenets of nursing. As healthcare professionals, it is our responsibility to know and understand the legislation we work under. It is also essential that people with disabilities understand their own rights. If you have concerns regarding a person in your care, you should refer the issue to a more experienced staff member.

Progress Note 41.1

21/10/2024 1500 hrs	Nursing: Mrs Carter has been assessed by the occupational therapist (OT), who has advised her of some assistive devices that may help her perform her ADLs. The OT will organise to have Mrs Carter's home assessed for bathroom modifications. Medications given as per medication sheet. Pain relief was given an hour prior to showering with good pain management. Mrs Carter was provided with a shower chair and a bath glove for showering, which she found helpful. Mrs Carter states her pain has decreased to a manageable 4 out of 10.

K Marter (MARTER), *EN*

DECISION-MAKING FRAMEWORK EXERCISE 41.1

You are the EN allocated to care for Mrs Green who is in the palliative care unit in the final stages of pancreatic cancer. During a conversation, she voices her concerns regarding how her husband will manage when she dies. In addition to atrial fibrillation, her husband has been diagnosed with long COVID and suffers with shortness of breath, fatigue, headaches and often an inability to concentrate at times. His atrial fibrillation is stable and both rhythm and rate controlled; however, since developing long COVID he often has episodes of palpitations that make him anxious. Their only son lives an hour's drive away and Mrs Green tells you that he is unable to care for her husband. Mrs Green asks you for advice and wants to know if you can help her husband manage.

1. How would you approach this scenario?
2. What suggestions could you make to allay Mrs Green's fears and support her?

Summary

This chapter has provided a brief overview of chronic disease and disability focusing on normalisation and individual empowerment.

Chronic disease and disabilities are becoming more common globally as societies confront the challenges of ageing populations. The impact of a chronic disease and/or disability on an individual's life may vary from mild to profound. Experiences are subjective and the meaning of impairment is unique to each person.

Although the focus of service provision for people with chronic diseases and/or disabilities has shifted from institutionalised and acute care to community-based primary care, allowing many to live independently or semi-independently in their own environments, there is still a long way to go before service provision meets need.

The philosophy of person-centred care, where the person is supported to self-manage and is provided with the resources and support to make informed choices, means that nurses and other healthcare professionals must take on the role of support and advocate. This support role provides advice, assessment and access to empower people to take control.

Review Questions

1. Identify the ways in which disabilities may be classified.
2. Define the terms 'medical model', 'social model' and 'biopsychosocial model of disability'.
3. Define the levels of restrictions that are used to categorise the assistance needs of people with disabilities.
4. Explain what is meant by the terms 'social role valorisation' and 'normalisation'.
5. Identify the nursing considerations related to caring for a person with a chronic condition.
6. Identify actions that can help to prevent chronic conditions.
7. List the principles of person-centred care.

Evolve® Answer guide for the Review Questions, Critical Thinking Exercises, Decision-making Framework Exercises and Critical Thinking Questions in Case Studies is hosted on Evolve: http://evolve.elsevier.com/AU/Koutoukidis/Tabbner.

References

Abbasinia, M., Ahmadi, F., Kazemnejad, A., 2020. Patient advocacy in nursing: A concept analysis. *Nursing Ethics* 27(1), 141–151.

Agaronnik, N., Campbell, E.G., Ressalam, J., Iezzoni, L.I., 2019. Communicating with patients with disability: Perspectives of practicing physicians. *Journal of General Internal Medicine* 34, 1139–1145.

Aïdoud, A., Gana, W., Poitau, F., et al., 2023. High prevalence of geriatric conditions among older adults with cardiovascular disease. *Journal of the American Heart Association*, e026850.

Akbarialiabad, H., Taghrir, M.H., Abdollahi, A., et al., 2021. Long COVID, a comprehensive systematic scoping review. *Infection*, 1–24.

Alonso-Sardón, M., Iglesias-de-Sena, H., Fernández-Martín, L.C., Mirón-Canelo, J.A., 2019. Do health and social support and personal autonomy have an influence on the health-related quality of life of individuals with intellectual disability? *BMC Health Services Research* 19(1), 1–10.

Alsharaydeh, E.A., Alqudah, M., Lee, R.L.T., Chan, S.W.-C., 2019. Challenges, coping, and resilience among immigrant parents caring for a child with a disability: An integrative review. *Journal of Nursing Scholarship* 51(6), 670–679.

Ansari, R.M., Harris, M.F., Hosseinzadeh, H., Zwar, N., 2022. Implementation of chronic care model for diabetes self-management: A quantitative analysis. *Diabetology* 3(3), 407–422.

Australian Building Codes Board, 2022. Access for people with a disability. Available at: <https://ncc.abcb.gov.au/editions/2019-a1/ncc-2019-volume-one-amendment-1/section-d-access-and-egress/part-d3-access-people>.

Australian Bureau of Statistics, 2019a. Disability, ageing and carers, Australia: Summary of findings. Available at: <https://www.abs.gov.au/statistics/health/disability/disability-ageing-and-carers-australia-summary-findings/latest-release#disability>.

Australian Bureau of Statistics, 2019b. Disability, ageing and carers, Australia: Summary of findings. Available at: <https://www.abs.gov.au/statistics/health/disability/disability-ageing-and-carers-australia-summary-findings/latest-release>.

Australian Bureau of Statistics, 2022. Causes of death, Australia. Available at: <https://www.abs.gov.au/statistics/health/causes-death/causes-death-australia/latest-release#:,:text=Media%20releases-,Key%20statistics,the%20leading%20cause%20of%20death>.

Austraian Communications and Media Authority, 2023 Available at: <https://www.acma.gov.au/compliance-priorities>.

Australian Federation of Disability Organisations, 2023. Communication with people with disabilities. Available at: <https://www.afdo.org.au/resource-communication-with-people-with-disabilities>.

Australian Government, 2020. *Mandatory reporting of child abuse and neglect*. Available at: <https://aifs.gov.au/resources/resource-sheets/mandatory-reporting-child-abuse-and-neglect>.

Australian Government, 2023a. *Australia's health 2022: Data insights*. Government Printing Press, Canberra.

Australian Government, 2023b. *Updated eligibility for oral COVID-19 treatments*. Australian Government, Canberra.

Australian Institute of Health and Welfare (AIHW), 2022a. Chronic disease. Available at: <https://www.aihw.gov.au/reports-data/health-conditions-disabilitydeaths/chronic-disease/overview>.

Australian Institute of Health and Welfare (AIHW), 2022b. Long COVID in Australia –a review of the literature (Vol. PHE318). AIHW, Canberra.

Australian Institute of Health and Welfare (AIHW), 2022c. National Strategic Framework for Chronic Conditions: Reporting framework. Australian Government, Canberra.

Australian Nursing and Midwifery Council, nd. Communication skills. Available at: <https://www.nmsupport.org.au/students-and-graduates/communication-skills>.

Aytac, S., Mizrachi, D., 2022. The mindfulness framework for implementing mindfulness into information literacy instruction. *The Reference Librarian* 63(1–2), 43–61.

Balaji, T.M., Varadarajan, S., Raj, A.T., Patil, S., 2020. The SARS-CoV-2 virus may remain viable on oral appliances for up to 3 days. *Journal of Contemporary Dental Practice* 21, 597.

Barr, O., Conway, M., Melby, V., 2020. Person-centred support for people with learning disabilities. In: McCormack, B., McCance, T., Bulley, C., et al (eds.), *Fundamentals of person-centred healthcare practice*. Wiley-Blackwell, London.

Barr, V., Robinson, S., Marin-Link, B., et al., 2003. The expanded chronic care model. *Hospital Quarterly* 7(1), 73–82.

Belcher, J.R., 2022. Deinstitutionalization and the development of community mental health. *Research Handbook on Mental Health Policy*, 161–171.

Beyerstedt, S., Casaro, E.B., Rangel, É.B., 2021. COVID-19: Angiotensin-converting enzyme 2 (ACE2) expression and tissue susceptibility to SARS-CoV-2 infection. *European Journal of Clinical Microbiology & Infectious Diseases* 40, 905–919.

Bollier, A., Sutherland, G., Krnjacki, L., et al., 2021. Attitudes matter: National survey of community attitudes toward people with disability in Australia. Centre of Research Excellence in Disability and Health, Victoria.

Bringmann, K.P., 2020. *Using strengths to self-manage a life with visual impairment – a qualitative interview study.* (BA (BMS)), University of Twente, Netherlands.

Brown, K., Yahyouche, A., Haroon, S., et al., 2022. Long COVID and self-management. *Lancet (London, England)* 399(10322), 355.

Buckmaster, L., Clark, S., 2019. The National Disability Insurance Scheme: A quick guide – May 2019 update.

Cambois, E., Brønnum-Hansen, H., Hayward, M., Nusselder, W.J., 2020. Monitoring social differentials in health expectancies. *International Handbook of Health Expectancies*, 45–66.

Carey, G., Malbon, E., Blackwell, J., 2021. Administering inequality? The National Disability Insurance Scheme and administrative burdens on individuals. *Australian Journal of Public Administration* 80(4), 854–872.

Cascella, M., Rajnik, M., Aleem, A., et al., 2022. Features, evaluation, and treatment of coronavirus (COVID-19). *StatPearls [Internet]*.

Chand, S., Marwaha, R.A., 2022. Anxiety. *StatPearls* (Vol. Jan). StatPearls Publishing, Treasure Island, Florida.

Chang, E., Johnson, A., 2021. *Living with chronic illness and disability: Principles for nursing practice*. Elsevier Health Sciences.

Collins, A., Rentschler, R., Williams, K., Azmat, F., 2022. Exploring barriers to social inclusion for disabled people: Perspectives from the performing arts. *Journal of Management & Organization* 28(2), 308–328.

Coste, J., Valderas, J.M., Carcaillon-Bentata, L., 2022. The epidemiology of multimorbidity in France: Variations by gender, age and socioeconomic factors, and implications for surveillance and prevention. *PloS One* 17(4), e0265842.

das Neves Júnior, T.T., de Queiroz, A.A.R., de Carvalho, E.A., et al., 2023. Clinical and sociodemographic profile of users with chronic diseases in primary health care. *Enfermería Global* 22(1), 271–282.

Davis, H.E., McCorkell, L., Vogel, J.M., Topol, E.J., 2023. Long COVID: Major findings, mechanisms and recommendations. *Nature Reviews Microbiology* 21, 133–146.

De Hert, M., Detraux, J., Vancampfort, D., 2022. The intriguing relationship between coronary heart disease and mental disorders. *Dialogues in Clinical Neuroscience* 20(1), 31–40.

Del Rio Szupszynski, K.P., de Ávila, A.C., 2021. The transtheoretical model of behavior change: Prochaska and DiClemente's model. *Psychology of Substance Abuse: Psychotherapy, Clinical Management and Social Intervention*, 205–216.

Department of Social Services, 2023. Disability and carers. Available at: <https://www.dss.gov.au/disability-and-carers>.

Department of Social Services, 2023. National Disability Representative Organisations. Available at: <https://www.dss.gov.au/our-responsibilities/disability-and-carers/program-services/consultation-and-advocacy/national-disability-peak-bodies>.

DiClemente, C.C., Graydon, M.M., 2020. Changing behavior using the transtheoretical model. *The Handbook of Behavior Change*, 136.

Dimov, S., Devine, A., Shields, M., et al., 2022. Improving Disability Employment Study (IDES): Methods of data collection and characteristics of study sample.

Dow, B., Gahan, L., Gaffy, E., et al., 2020. Barriers to disclosing elder abuse and taking action in Australia. *Journal of Family Violence* 35, 853–861.

Drury, V., 2021. Models of care. In: Chang, E., Johnson, A. (eds.), *Living with chronic illness and disability: Principles for nursing practice.* Elsevier Health Sciences.

Drury, V., Aw, A.T., 2020. Nursing care: Chronic illness and disability. In: Koutoukidis, G., Stainton, K. (eds.), *Tabbner's nursing care: Theory and practice*, 8th ed. Elsevier Health Services, Australia.

Drury, V.B., Aw, A.T., Shiow, L.H.P., 2017. Self-management of vision impairments. In: Martz, E., *Promoting self-management of chronic health conditions: Theories and practice*, pp. 440–464. Oxford University Press.

Dunn, D.S., Wehmeyer, M.L., 2022. Positive psychology and disability. In: Wehmeyer, M.L., Dunn, D.S. (eds.), *The positive psychology of personal factors: Implications for understanding disability*, pp. 15–26. Lexington Books/ Rowman & Littlefield.

Epping-Jordan, J., Pruitt, S., Bengoa, R., Wagner, E.H., 2004. Improving the quality of health care for chronic conditions. *BMJ Quality & Safety* 13(4), 299–305.

Eva, J., Pathak, Y., 2023. Global trends in growth of chronic diseases. In: *Applications of functional foods and nutraceuticals for chronic diseases*, pp. 3–16. CRC Press.

Fennell, P.A., Dorr, N., George, S.S., 2021. Elements of suffering in myalgic encephalomyelitis/chronic fatigue syndrome: The experience of loss, grief, stigma, and trauma in the severely and very severely affected. *Healthcare (Basel)* 9(5), 553. doi: 10.3390/healthcare9050553. PMID: 34065069; PMCID: PMC8150911.

Fisher, K.R., Purcal, C., Blaxland, M., et al., 2023. Factors that help people with disability to self-manage their support. *Disability & Society*, 1–19.

Francisco, M.P.B., Hartman, M., Wang, Y., 2020. Inclusion and special education. *Education Sciences* 10(9), 238.

Franklin, M.S., Beyer, L.N., Brotkin, S.M., et al., 2019. Health care transition for adolescent and young adults with intellectual disability: Views from the parents. *Journal of Pediatric Nursing* 47, 148–158.

Friedman, C., 2022. Financial hardship experienced by people with disabilities during the COVID-19 pandemic. *Disability and Health Journal* 15(4), 101359.

Garrison, A., Fressard, L., Mitilian, E., et al., 2023. Motivational interview training improves self-efficacy of GP interns in vaccination consultations: A study using the Pro-VC-Be to measure vaccine confidence determinants. *Human Vaccines & Immunotherapeutics*, 2163809.

Germani, A.C.C.G., de Mello Cahú, F.G., Miranda, F.E.S., et al., 2022. Health promotion to people with disabilities: Case report from two university extension projects. *Research, Society and Development* 11(1), e56111124956–e56111124956.

Gillam, D.G., Yusuf, H., 2019. Brief motivational interviewing in dental practice. *Dentistry Journal* 7(2), 51.

Gregory, G., Zhu, L., Hayen, A., Bell, K.J., 2022. Learning from the pandemic: Mortality trends and seasonality of deaths in Australia in 2020. *International Journal of Epidemiology* 51(3), 718–726.

Groenvynck, L., de Boer, B., Hamers, J.P., et al., 2021. Toward a partnership in the transition from home to a nursing home: The TRANSCIT model. *Journal of the American Medical Directors Association* 22(2), 351–356.

Guan, W.-j., Liang, W.-h., Zhao, Y., et al., 2020. Comorbidity and its impact on 1590 patients with COVID-19 in China: A nationwide analysis. *European Respiratory Journal* 55(5).

Gutenbrunner, C., Stievano, A., Nugraha, B., et al., 2022. Nursing – a core element of rehabilitation. *International Nursing Review* 69(1), 13–19.

Hente, E., Sears, R., Cotton, S., et al., 2020. A pilot study of mindfulness-based cognitive therapy to improve well-being for health professionals providing chronic disease care. *The Journal of Pediatrics* 224, 87–93. e81.

Hungerford, C.L., Donna, D., Clancy, R., et al., 2021. *Mental health care: An introduction for health professionals.* John Wiley & Sons.

Indolfi, C., Spaccarotella, C., 2020. *The outbreak of COVID-19 in Italy: Fighting the pandemic*, vol. 2, pp. 1414–1418. American College of Cardiology Foundation, Washington DC.

Jones, J.S., Beauvais, A.M., 2022. *Psychiatric mental health nursing: An interpersonal approach.* Jones & Bartlett Learning.

Kalav, S., Bektas, H., Ünal, A., 2022. Effects of Chronic Care Model-based interventions on self-management, quality of life and patient satisfaction in patients with ischemic stroke: A single-blinded randomized controlled trial. *Japan Journal of Nursing Science* 19(1), e12441.

Kim, G.M., Lim, J.Y., Kim, E.J., Park, S.M., 2019. Resilience of patients with chronic diseases: A systematic review. *Health & Social Care in the Community* 27(4), 797–807.

Kivimäki, M., Batty, G.D., Pentti, J., et al., 2020. Association between socioeconomic status and the development of mental and physical health conditions in adulthood: A multi-cohort study. *The Lancet Public Health* 5(3), e140–e149.

Komariah, M., Ibrahim, K., Pahria, T., et al., 2023. Effect of mindfulness breathing meditation on depression, anxiety, and stress: A randomized controlled trial among university students. *Healthcare (Basel)* 11(1), 26. doi: 10.3390/healthcare11010026. PMID: 36611488; PMCID: PMC9819153.

Legano, L.A., Desch, L.W., Messner, S.A., et al., 2021. Maltreatment of children with disabilities. *Pediatrics* 147(5).

Lim, K.K., Matchar, D.B., Tan, C.S., et al., 2020. The association between psychological resilience and physical function among older adults with hip fracture surgery. *Journal of the American Medical Directors Association* 21(2), 260–266. e262.

Liu, J., Liu, S., 2020. The management of coronavirus disease 2019 (COVID-19). *Journal of Medical Virology* 92(9), 1484–1490.

Livneh, H., 2022. Psychosocial adaptation to chronic illness and disability: An updated and expanded conceptual framework. *Rehabilitation Counseling Bulletin* 65(3), 171–184.

Macleod, K., Kamruzzaman, L., Musselwhite, C., 2022. Transport and health equity, social inclusion and exclusion. *Journal of Transport & Health* 27, 101543.

Majumder, J., Minko, T., 2021. Recent developments on therapeutic and diagnostic approaches for COVID-19. *The AAPS Journal* 23, 1–22.

McCormack, B., McCance, T., Bulley, C., et al., 2021. *Fundamentals of person-centred healthcare practice*. John Wiley & Sons.

Miller, W.R., Rollnick, S., 2012. *Motivational interviewing: Helping people change*. Guilford Press.

Mitra, M., Turk, M.A., 2022. COVID-19 and social determinants of health among people with disabilities. *Disability and Health Journal* 15(4), 101378–101378.

Msemburi, W., Karlinsky, A., Knutson, V., et al., 2023. The WHO estimates of excess mortality associated with the COVID-19 pandemic. *Nature* 613, 130–137.

Nagaratnam, K., Nagaratnam, N., 2019. Elderly abuse and neglect. In: Nagaratnam, N., Nagaratnam, K., Cheuk, G., (eds.), *Advanced age geriatric care: A comprehensive guide*, pp. 19–24. Springer, Cham.

National Disability Service, 2022. Disability types and description. Available at: <https://www.nds.org.au/disability-types-and-descriptions>.

Ng, A.S.H., Chew, M.H., Charn, T.C., et al., 2020. Keeping a cut above the coronavirus disease: Surgical perspectives from a public health institution in Singapore during Covid-19. *ANZ Journal of Surgery* 90(5), 666.

Nsiah, C., Siakwa, M., Ninnoni, J.P., 2019. Registered nurses' description of patient advocacy in the clinical setting. *Nursing Open* 6(3), 1124–1132.

OECD/WHO, 2022. Health at a glance: Asia/Pacific 2022: Measuring progress towards universal health coverage. OECD Publishing, Paris.

Office for National Statistics, 2023. Monthly mortality analysis, England and Wales: December 2022. Available at: <https://www.ons.gov.uk/peoplepopulationandcommunity/birthsdeathsandmarriages/deaths/bulletins/monthlymortalityanalysisenglandandwales/december2022>.

Ogawa, M., Fujikawa, M., Jin, K., et al., 2021. Acceptance of disability predicts quality of life in patients with epilepsy. *Epilepsy & Behavior* 120, 107979.

Olney, S., Dickinson, H., 2019. Australia's new National Disability Insurance Scheme: Implications for policy and practice. *Policy Design and Practice* 2(3), 275–290.

Pearson-Stuttard, J., Holloway, S., Polya, R., et al., 2022. Variations in comorbidity burden in people with type 2 diabetes over disease duration: A population-based analysis of real world evidence. *EClinicalMedicine* 52, 101584.

Pederson, C.L., Gorman-Ezell, K., Brookings, J.B., 2020. Psychological distress among postural tachycardia syndrome patients in the Fennell Crisis phase. *Fatigue: Biomedicine, Health & Behavior* 8(2), 108–118.

Phelan, A., McCormack, B., Dewing, J., et al., 2020. Review of developments in person-centred healthcare. *International Practice Development Journal* 10(3).

Pinilla-Roncancio, M., Alkire, S., 2021. How poor are people with disabilities? Evidence based on the global multidimensional poverty index. *Journal of Disability Policy Studies* 31(4), 206–216.

Prochaska, J.O., Norcross, J.C., 2001. Stages of change. *Psychotherapy: Theory, Research, Practice, Training* 38(4), 443.

Proescher, E., Aase, D.M., Passi, H.M., et al., 2022. Impact of perceived social support on mental health, quality of life, and disability in post–9/11 US military veterans. *Armed Forces & Society* 48(1), 115–135.

Reina, C.S., Kudesia, R.S., 2020. Wherever you go, there you become: How mindfulness arises in everyday situations. *Organizational Behavior and Human Decision Processes* 159, 78–96.

Reynolds, R., Dennis, S., Hasan, I., et al., 2018. A systematic review of chronic disease management interventions in primary care. *BMC Family Practice* 19(1), 1–13.

Richardson, S., Hirsch, J.S., Narasimhan, M., et al., 2020. Presenting characteristics, comorbidities, and outcomes among 5700 patients hospitalized with COVID-19 in the New York City area. *Jama* 323(20), 2052–2059.

Riegel, B., Dunbar, S.B., Fitzsimons, D., et al., 2021. Self-care research: Where are we now? Where are we going? *International Journal of Nursing Studies* 116, 103402.

Rural Heath Information Hub, 2023. Health Promotion and Disease Prevention in Rural Communities. Available at: <https://www.ruralhealthinfo.org/toolkits/health-promotion/1/introduction>.

Salemonsen, E., Førland, G., Hansen, B.S., Holm, A.L., 2020. Understanding beneficial self-management support and the meaning of user involvement in lifestyle interventions: A qualitative study from the perspective of healthcare professionals. *BMC Health Services Research* 20(1), 1–12.

Schopp, F., Rhoda, A. (eds.), 2021. *Self-management in chronic illness: Principles, practice, and empowerment strategies for better health*. Springer International Publishing, USA.

Seabra, P., Nunes, I., Sequeira, R., et al., 2023. Designing a nurse-led program for self-management of substance addiction consequences: A modified e-Delphi study. *International Journal of Environmental Research and Public Health* 20(3), 2137.

Self, K.J., Borsari, B., Ladd, B.O., et al., 2022. Cultural adaptations of motivational interviewing: A systematic review. *Psychological Services* 20(1), 7–18. doi: doi.org/10.1037/ser0000619.

Sharma, A., Tiwari, S., Deb, M.K., Marty, J.L., 2020. Severe acute respiratory syndrome coronavirus-2 (SARS-CoV-2): A global pandemic and treatment strategies. *International Journal of Antimicrobial Agents* 56(2), 106054.

Sherman, D.W., 2019. A review of the complex role of family caregivers as health team members and second-order patients. *Healthcare (Basel)* 7(2), 63. doi: 10.3390/healthcare7020063. PMID: 31022837; PMCID: PMC6627519.

Shoemark, T., 2021. Identifying barriers to patient advocacy in the promotion of a safety culture: An integrative review. *ACORN* 34(2), e36–e42.

Shrier, P., 2021. How can we decide? When ought a person with disabilities be moved from their home to full-time residential care? *Journal of Disability & Religion* 25(2), 132–158.

Sporinova, B., Manns, B., Tonelli, M., et al., 2019. Association of mental health disorders with health care utilization and costs among adults with chronic disease. *JAMA Network Open* 2(8), e199910–e199910.

Statler, M., 2023. The long good-bye: Supporting caregivers of patients with Alzheimer's disease. *Lynchburg Journal of Medical Science* 5(1), 50.

Tsang, H.F., Chan, L.W.C., Cho, W.C.S., et al., 2021. An update on COVID-19 pandemic: The epidemiology, pathogenesis, prevention and treatment strategies. *Expert Review of Anti-infective Therapy* 19(7), 877–888.

van den Bemd, M., Schalk, B.W., Bischoff, E.W., et al., 2022. Chronic diseases and comorbidities in adults with and without intellectual disabilities: Comparative cross-sectional study in Dutch general practice. *Family Practice* 39(6), 1056–1062.

van der Veen, S., Evans, N., Huisman, M., et al., 2022. Toward a paradigm shift in healthcare: Using the International Classification of Functioning, Disability and Health (ICF) and the capability approach (CA) jointly in theory and practice. *Disability and Rehabilitation*, 1–8.

Van Wilder, L., Pype, P., Mertens, F., et al., 2021. Living with a chronic disease: Insights from patients with a low socioeconomic status. *BMC Family Practice* 22, 1–11.

Villamil, A., Vogel, T., Weisbaum, E., Siegel, D., 2019. Cultivating well-being through the three pillars of mind training: Understanding how training the mind improves physiological and psychological well-being. *OBM Integrative and Complementary Medicine* 4(1), 1–28.

Vrklevski, L.P., Eljiz, K., Greenfield, D., 2017. The evolution and devolution of mental health services in Australia. *Inquiries Journal* 9(10).

Wakerman, J., Humphreys, J.S., 2019. Better health in the bush: Why we urgently need a national rural and remote health strategy. *Medical Journal of Australia* 210(5), 202–203.

Weise, J., Mohan, A., Walsh, J., Trollor, J.N., 2021. Salutary lessons from the delivery of mental health services to people with intellectual disability – A historical perspective from intellectual disability mental health experts in New South Wales, Australia. *Journal of Mental Health Research in Intellectual Disabilities* 14(1), 70–88.

Williams, L., 2023. Motivational interviewing. In: Cooper, D., *Alcohol use: Assessment, withdrawal management, treatment and therapy: Ethical practice,* pp. 363–380. Springer.

Wolfensberger, W.P., Nirje, B., Olshansky, S., et al., 1972. *The principle of normalization in human services.* Books: Wolfensberger Collection 1. Available at: <https://digitalcommons.unmc.edu/wolf_books/1>.

Woolf, S.H., Chapman, D.A., Lee, J.H., 2021. COVID-19 as the leading cause of death in the United States. *Jama* 325(2), 123–124.

World Health Organization, nd. Quality of care. Available at: <https://www.who.int/health-topics/quality-of-care#tab=tab_1>.

World Health Organization, 2015. WHO global disability action plan 2014–2021: Better health for all people with disability. WHO, Geneva.

World Health Organization, 2021. Disabilities. Available at: <https://www.afro.who.int/health-topics/disabilities>.

World Health Organization, 2022. Noncommunicable diseases. Available at: <https://www.who.int/news-room/fact-sheets/detail/noncommunicable-diseases>.

World Health Organization, 2023. Global health estimates: Life expectancy and leading causes of death and disability. Available at: <https://www.who.int/data/gho/data/themes/mortality-and-global-health-estimates>.

Xu, J., Murphy, S., Kochanek, K., Arias, E., 2022. Mortality in the United States, 2021. *Data Brief, no 456.* Available at: <https://www.cdc.gov/nchs/data/databriefs/db456.pdf>.

Zajdel, M., Swan, T., Robinson, T., et al., 2023. Stress, coping, and physical health in caregiving. *Translational Issues in Psychological Science.*

Zaim, S., Chong, J.H., Sankaranarayanan, V., Harky, A., 2020. COVID-19 and multiorgan response. *Current Problems in Cardiology* 45(8), 100618.

Zajdel, M., Swan, T., Robinson, T., et al., 2023. Stress, coping, and physical health in caregiving. *Translational Issues in Psychological Science* 9(2), 123–136. Available at: <https://doi.org/10.1037/tps0000349>.

Zhang, Q., Shan, X., Ling, Y., et al., 2019. Psychosocial predictors of adjustment to disability among patients with breast cancer: A cross-sectional descriptive study. *Journal of Nursing Research* 27(2), e15.

Zhang, Y., Bierma-Zeinstra, S.M., 2023. Diagnosis, risk factors for OA development and progression, OA prevention, and recognizing comorbidities. *Osteoarthritis health professional training manual,* pp. 39–53. Elsevier.

Ziauddeen, N., Gurdasani, D., O'Hara, M.E., et al., 2022. Characteristics and impact of Long Covid: Findings from an online survey. *PLoS One* 17(3), e0264331.

Recommended Reading

Boeykens, D., Sirimsi, M.M., Timmermans, L., et al., 2023. How do people living with chronic conditions and their informal caregivers experience primary care? A phenomenological-hermeneutical study. *Journal of Clinical Nursing* 32(3–4), 422–437.

Brown, K., Yahyouche, A., Haroon, S., et al., 2022. Long COVID and self-management. *Lancet (London, England)* 399(10322), 355.

Garcimartín, P., Astals-Vizcaino, M., Badosa, N., et al., 2022. The impact of motivational interviewing on self-care and health-related quality of life in patients with chronic heart failure. *Journal of Cardiovascular Nursing* 37(5), 456–464.

Heaton-Shrestha, C., Torrens-Burton, A., Leggat, F., et al., 2022. Co-designing personalised self-management support for people living with long Covid: The LISTEN protocol. *PloS One* 17(10), e0274469.

Horsell, C., 2023. Problematising disability: A critical policy analysis of the Australian National Disability Insurance Scheme. *Australian Social Work* 76(1), 47–59.

Magee, C., Murphy, T., Turley, M., et al., 2018. 19 stories of social inclusion–Ireland: Stories of belonging, contributing and connecting.

Online Resources

Australian Human Rights Commission: <https://humanrights.gov.au>.

Dementia Australia: <https://www.dementia.org.au>.

Australian Government, Department of Health and Aged Care: <https://www.health.gov.au>.

Department of Health (WA): <https://www.health.wa.gov.au>.

Northern Territory Health: <https://health.nt.gov.au/homepage>.

Health Vic: <https://www.health.vic.gov.au>

NSW Health: <https://www.health.nsw.gov.au>.

SA Health: <https://www.sahealth.sa.gov.au>.

Tasmanian Dept of Heath: <https://www.health.tas.gov.au>.

Queensland Health: <https://www.health.qld.gov.au>.

Kidsafe—Child Accident Prevention Foundation of Australia: <https://kidsafe.com.au>.

Ministry of Health NZ: <https://www.health.govt.nz>.

Multiple Sclerosis Australia: <https://www.msaustralia.org.au>.

National Disability Insurance Scheme: <https://www.ndis.gov.au>.

National Disability Services: <https://www.nds.org.au>.

SANE Australia Mindfulness: <https://www.sane.org/information-and-resources/facts-and-guides/mindfulness>.

United Nations: <https://www.un.org/en>.

World Health Organization: <https://www.who.int>.

CHAPTER

42

Acute and perioperative care

Lise Martin

Key Terms

acute kidney injury (AKI)
anaesthesia
cellulitis
deep vein thrombosis (DVT)
diverticulitis
Guillain-Barré syndrome (GBS)
informed consent
intraoperative
perioperative
postoperative
preoperative
pulmonary embolism (PE)
scope of practice
sepsis
septic shock
surgery
venous thromboembolism (VTE)

Learning Outcomes

At the completion of this chapter and with further reading, learners should be able to:

- Define the key terms.
- Identify the impact of an acute illness or injury on the individual and family.
- Describe nursing interventions to support healthcare of individuals with an acute illness or injury.
- Demonstrate critical thinking and problem-solving approaches in undertaking individual care.
- Contribute to the development and implementation of nursing care plans for the individual with an acute health illness, injury or requiring surgical intervention.
- Describe the nature of the operative experience and outline the phases it entails.
- Describe the individual care roles of the perioperative nurse.
- Describe the general physiological, psychological and local responses to surgical intervention.
- Describe the various classifications of surgical procedures.
- Define informed consent and discuss the role of the nurse in ensuring consent.

CHAPTER FOCUS

Enrolled Nurses (ENs) work in the acute care setting as valued, skilled members of the multidisciplinary team (MDT), and are moving into highly acute clinical areas such as cardiac and respiratory units, emergency departments and neonatal care, areas once only reserved for Registered Nurses (RNs) (McKenna et al 2019). The increasing **scope of practice** of ENs, however, has not been without its challenges, and not all healthcare organisations and individual state and/or territory government health departments have embraced their expanding scope of practice, which can in some settings limit their value and skill.

Perioperative nursing encompasses the care of an individual who is undergoing a surgical procedure, and takes place from the time the decision is made to have surgery through to recovery from the procedure. Throughout the perioperative period it is essential that there is a flexible multidisciplinary team approach to ensure continuity of individual care from admission, throughout the surgical experience to recovery at home. It is important for the nurse to be familiar with the types of surgery an individual is likely to undergo in order to plan and implement adequate individualised care and to provide appropriate physiological and psychological support.

This chapter explores the role of the EN working in the acute care and perioperative environments and its challenges.

LIVED EXPERIENCE

An older person had been admitted to the acute care ward after a fall at home. Imaging on initial presentation revealed no fractures. On day two, the older person expressed relentless pain despite the administration of both regular and PRN analgesia as charted over the preceding 24-hour period. Vital observations were stable and it was assumed by many that the older person was simply experiencing pain from the initial fall at home and that this would resolve in time. After undertaking a primary and secondary survey and gathering both subjective and objective data, I discovered the older person had left upper abdominal pain that they described as a severe grabbing pain. Further conversation with them revealed that they had in fact fallen in the hospital bathroom on day one of admission. The older person had failed to advise nursing staff for fear of being placed in a nursing home. Subsequently investigation revealed two fractured ribs and pneumonia.

A case conference was organised so the older person, their family and the multidisciplinary team could work together to formulate a plan of care plan for the person to recover well and return to their own home.

As a nurse working in the acute care setting, I've found that my core nursing knowledge and my critical thinking and problem-solving skills are used extensively in practice, and are so important when assisting an acutely unwell person in a person-centred and holistic way.

Tania, Enrolled Nurse

INTRODUCTION

Hospital care

Acute care is a broad term that encompasses a range of healthcare domains and settings to which an individual may be admitted for planned or unplanned care for a medical illness, surgery or for diagnostic purposes (Crisp et al 2021). When discussing acute care, most people will automatically assume care takes place in a hospital; in many cases, this is where care commences—in the ED. Length of hospital stay and outcomes may vary. Some individuals require only short-term care and are then discharged home, while others require a longer period of convalescence in hospital. Once discharged home, some individuals will engage in follow-up services through outpatient clinics provided by the hospital. For others, follow-up care through their local GP will be sufficient.

Length of hospital stay may also be influenced by the needs of the individual. While some individuals only require admission to one area of a hospital before they are discharged home, others may require several different services within the facility. An individual admitted for a surgical procedure, for example, will be transferred to theatre, possibly followed by the need for admission to an intensive care unit (ICU) or high-dependency unit (HDU) before reaching a surgical or medical ward. There may also be further need for transfer to a sub-acute or rehabilitation setting for follow-up care before the individual is ready to be discharged home to their usual place of residence.

Australian hospitals may organise their services in order to help attract individuals and/or contain their costs by reducing the number of inpatient beds available, increasing throughput of individuals through outpatient services such as EDs and day procedure units, changing the skill mix of staff on varying units and restructuring the hospital management. Innovative outpatient services such as nutrition classes, diabetes outreach programs and birthing centres have been formed to improve overall hospital care (Berman et al 2020).

Individuals across the lifespan who are critically ill and may be at high risk of actual or potential life-threatening conditions, will require specialised care. Critical care is a broad term incorporating subspecialty areas such as intensive care, high-dependency care, emergency care and coronary or cardiothoracic care (Aitken et al 2019).

ICUs provide critically ill individuals with life-saving treatments, with the support of technology and access to immediate nursing and medical staff. In Australia, the nursing ratio for ICUs is usually 1:1 and may include close invasive monitoring and/or respiratory support (Aitken et al 2019). HDUs provide a level of care between ICU and the general wards. The staffing ratio for an HDU is usually 1:2, as these individuals still require close monitoring, but not the intensive, complex care required to remain in ICU. HDUs may be part of either the ICU environment or a step-down unit in a dedicated area. Care within either critical care environment is based on workload; complexity of the care, both psychological and physical; and the overall acuity of the individual (Aitken et al 2019).

Most wards in hospitals are specialised, and individuals may be admitted to a particular ward according to their individual needs. Specialty areas may include respiratory, cardiothoracic, vascular, neurological, burns, oncology, haematology, gastrointestinal, renal, trauma and/or orthopaedics, general surgical and medical, and, in some instances, paediatrics, midwifery and/or gynaecology, special care nursery or neonatal care, and mental health. When an individual is admitted to acute care, the aim is to allocate a bed on the most appropriate ward; however, this is not always possible.

Home care

Treating individuals with an acute illness or injury at home is becoming more common. Services such as hospital in the home (HITH), post-acute care and district nursing have the ability to offer safe clinical care to individuals within their own environment. Individuals are still admitted by the primary hospital as HITH is a hospital substitution program. Individuals who can be treated in the home must be referred, usually via the ED if initial presentation, or via the ward to shorten the individual's length of stay. Clinical conditions that may not require a stay in hospital but do require some form of acute intervention may include:

- cellulitis
- deep vein thrombosis (DVT)
- urinary tract infections (UTIs)
- pneumonia
- exacerbation of chronic obstructive pulmonary disease (COPD).

HITH services are provided by a combination of visiting specialist nurses, other health professionals and family or carers for individuals who require further acute treatment post a length of stay in hospital. Such services include burns dressings, anticoagulation therapy, administration of long-term intravenous antibiotics via a peripherally inserted central catheter (PICC) or the administration of chemotherapy (Crisp et al 2021; NSW Health 2018).

Post-acute care is short-term care provided to safely reduce the individual's length of stay in hospital. Unlike HITH, to be eligible for post-acute care support, the individual's support must be assessed as requiring short-term, community-based assistance for recuperating in the community. Short-term community-based supports include community nursing, personal care such as hygiene and home care such as grocery shopping and cleaning. These services are provided for a finite period of time as the individual recuperates. Any longer-term care requirements are referred to the council, district nurse or GP (Victorian Government 2021).

District nursing provides short- and long-term care to assist individuals requiring some form of clinical intervention or management. The goal is to prevent the number of acute admissions to hospital or reduce the length of hospital admissions by providing community support. District nursing is provided by either a private agency or via regional or rural hospitals.

ACUTE NURSING: SCOPE OF PRACTICE

The Australian healthcare system is under constant and increasing pressure. It is estimated that by 2066 Australia's population will likely reach somewhere between 37.4 and 49.2 million people (ABS 2018). The Nursing and Midwifery Board of Australia (NMBA) is responsible for defining the practice and behaviour for nurses and midwives in Australia. Historically, the RN was viewed as the assessor, planner and evaluator of care, while the Enrolled Nurse (EN) worked under the supervision of the RN. The EN and RN standards for practice include the core standards that provide the framework for assessing the practice of nurses in Australia and provide clarity regarding supervision, delegation and role relationships between the EN and RN (NMBA 2016a & b). These standards reflect educational, practical, professional and reflective demands of ENs and RNs as we move further into the 21st century.

For an EN, scope of practice may be determined by the acute care environment they are working in at any given time. It is therefore essential that the EN considers several factors before undertaking any particular clinical skill to determine their suitability for the task required.

Considerations around scope of practice for the EN must always include:

- the qualification they hold
- any additional current training competencies achieved
- policies and procedures of the organisation where the skill is to be performed.

RNs, at times, may not understand the scope of practice of ENs, which is primarily related to educational variations, such as upskilling, leading to different levels of enrolled nursing ability and, as such, this can create confusion. Uncertainty of roles may also lead to medical staff becoming frustrated with the variations in scope. Role definition has also led to uncertainty among other healthcare professionals in recognising the roles and scope of nurses, and the introduction of Assistants in Nursing (AINs) has also contributed to the ENs' confusion regarding their own scope of practice (McKenna et al 2019).

All nurses must work within their scope of practice and as an active member of the interdisciplinary healthcare team. Great emphasis is placed on the importance of team work in the acute care setting, yet this can be difficult to achieve when a blurring and discrepancy of roles exists, or may not be fully understood.

CHARACTERISTICS AND IMPACT OF ACUTE ILLNESS/INJURY

The impact of an acute illness or injury will vary according to the nature, severity and the duration of the illness or injury, and whether there are any associated life-altering changes due to short- or long-term physical or psychological disability, such as pain, amputation, paralysis or post-traumatic stress disorder. Socioeconomic impact includes financial burdens, lifestyle changes or adjustments to usual roles. Individuals' own attitudes and beliefs of illness can also be a factor relating to the impact of acute illness (Berman et al 2020).

The individual

Acute illness or injury can occur suddenly, with often (but not always) severe symptoms. In many cases, the acute illness or injury has a short-term duration and resolves with residual effect, and the individual returns to their previous level of functioning. Sometimes, however, there is a resolution of the acute illness or injury, with a remaining residual effect. An example may include the occurrence of an acute brain injury that results in a residual cognitive deficit. In this case, the initial acute illness or injury may have long-term consequences, including an increase in subsequent hospitalisations possibly due to complications or ongoing manifestations of the initial illness or injury. An individual's quality of life may also be negatively impacted, if their self-concept and self-esteem is affected. It is important that nurses support the individual's right to self-determination and autonomy as part of person-centred care, encouraging them to participate in their decision-making and maintain a feeling of control in their care. Participating in making healthcare decisions and receiving education regarding their current condition encourages the individual to take on responsibility for their own health during their course of stay and on discharge (Berman et al 2020). Involving the individual in decisions related to their care is included in the National Safety and Quality Health Service (NSQHS) Standards. Individuals must be respected and engaged in the care they receive. The 'Partnering with Consumers' Standard states that all care concerning an individual must be respectful, providing ongoing shared information, working with individuals and their significant others to help plan care; it emphasises the importance of including the individual in all aspects of care (Australian Commission on Safety and Quality in Health Care [ACSQHC 2021]. During a hospital admission, effective communication is essential for the development of a therapeutic relationship. (Refer also to Chapter 10.)

Once discharged after an acute illness, an individual will need to resume their former role/s and responsibilities. If the time recovering from the acute illness or injury is short, this may be achieved without issue. However, if the recovery is complex, long term or requires ongoing outpatient appointments, then returning to one's former level of functioning may be more difficult. When diagnosed with an acute illness or injury, an individual must adapt to being in a foreign environment. Feelings of mortality, fear, pain and the possible impact their illness or injury may have on their own life and also that of their loved ones may need to be addressed. Post discharge, individuals may report feelings of fatigue, weakness, ongoing pain, sleep difficulties, nightmares and flashbacks, any of which may lead to emotional and behavioural changes impacting on the individual's ability to cope with their new-found lifestyle. Individuals may experience alterations in their role and responsibilities in the family; they may be more dependent on others, which can lead to feelings of resentment (Berman et al 2020). (See Case Study 42.1.)

The family

Person- and family-centred care improve the overall quality of care, especially when an individual is acutely or critically ill (Mol et al 2017). For many cultures, family is central to caregiving. It is important to provide education and encourage families to take an active role in caregiving (Crisp et al 2021). Family members as informal untrained caregivers can assist with the physical, emotional and psychosocial care of the individual (e.g. assisting with activities of daily living [ADLs] and running errands). This may be particularly significant in the care of infants, children (Hockenberry et al 2022) and also for persons with cognitive impairment (Butcher 2018).

The establishment of a positive, genuine and mutually respectful relationship between the nurse, the person being cared for, and their family, is a significant factor for family involvement in care (Crisp et al 2021). It is essential to develop a therapeutic relationship based on trust with both the individual and their family. To achieve this, healthcare professionals must actively listen to the individual, and involve the family in care planning as appropriate (always first and foremost with the individual's consent). Improving overall outcomes for the individual requires support and encouragement from family presence and active involvement to build a trusting relationship. Involving family in the individual's care recognises the knowledge and expertise that the individual and family may have regarding the illness or injury, by respecting the value and level of understanding they may have regarding the different aspects of

CASE STUDY 42.1

Stella's acute care experience

About 2 years ago, Stella started experiencing intense headaches, which culminated one day in her collapsing at work. She worked as a nurse and her nurse unit manager put her in a wheelchair and took her around to the ED of the hospital that she worked in. This was the beginning of 2 months of being admitted and discharged from hospital—in total five times. She had all the tests done—MRI, CT, blood test and even a lumbar puncture—but no doctor could tell Stella why her head felt like it was going to explode. When admitted to the neurological ward, she felt that once the nurses realised that they were caring for a fellow nurse, they treated her differently from other individuals. Procedures and the rationale for these were not explained since it was assumed that Stella understood what was happening. For Stella, one of the scariest experiences was when she had a drug reaction; she thought she was going to die.

On her last admission, one of the nurses looking after her suggested she see an osteopath and get her back and neck looked at. Stella took her advice and achieved some relief. Two years on and what started as an acute episode has turned into a chronic pain issue, resulting in Stella having to change jobs and work part time as the chronic pain causes her constant exhaustion. This has had a major impact on her life and she has had to modify her lifestyle to manage the pain she experiences every day. Stella still has not been told what the actual cause of her pain is.

What impact may Stella's illness and chronic pain have on her life?

the individual's care needs. Communication is without doubt one of the most important factors that can impact quality of care. Effective communication can reduce complaints from both the individual and family members (Mol et al 2017).

In person- and family-centred care, the individual defines their 'family' and communicates how they and their support network will be involved in the overall decision-making, especially if the individual is unable to make informed decisions (Johnson 2016). The individual's family participates to assist with the required care in conjunction with allied health and nursing staff. Additionally, family members should not be made to feel guilty if they cannot or do not wish to participate. It is important that the individual's preferences, values and priorities are primarily respected (Johnson 2016).

For those family members who are able and willing to assist with the care of a loved one, the physical and emotional toll must be recognised and strategies put in place to prevent family burn-out (Mol et al 2017).

The extent of the impact of acute illness or injury on the family may be dependent on three factors: which member of the family is ill, the length and seriousness of the illness or injury, and how the illness or injury may affect the family's cultural and/or social norms. The family may be significantly impacted by factors including role changes; increased stress and anxiety related to the severity of the person's illness or injury; stress and anxiety related to financial strain and employment options; increases in demands based on time away from work or other duties; isolation, loneliness and/or pending loss; and change in social norms, with some (if not all) of these continuing well after discharge (Berman et 2020). (See Case Study 42.2.)

CRITICAL THINKING EXERCISE 42.1

You are looking after Ian, a 45-year-old man, who has been admitted to the cardiothoracic ward post an acute myocardial infarct (AMI). He is recovering post coronary artery bypass graft surgery. Ian is the main income earner in his family and has two young children under the age of 5 years and a supportive wife, Lucy, at home.

1. Identify the physical issues Ian may experience.
2. Identify psychosocial issues Ian may experience.
3. List the ongoing care (including allied healthcare) that Ian and his family may require during his recovery.

CASE STUDY 42.2

Stella's acute care experience: The family's perspective

When Stella started experiencing headaches, I thought nothing of it; she had suffered from migraines since a young age. Then suddenly they escalated and she had to be admitted to hospital multiple times. I can't explain the sense of helplessness I felt as her mother. I felt I should have been able to make it all better. It was very frustrating that the doctors could not give us any answers; they didn't listen to her when she said it wasn't a migraine. One of the worst moments for me was receiving a phone call from my sister who was visiting Stella when she had the drug reaction. My sister thought Stella was going to die. Another moment that stands out for me was being ordered from her room as nurses rushed in. No-one told me what was going on. I found out later she'd been given too much morphine and had a dangerously low respiratory rate. Two years on and I am proud of how Stella deals with the pain; most people have no idea that she has pain every day. It's lucky that I'm a casual worker so I can take time off when Stella needs to be taken to hospital. I don't know what would happen if I had to work full time.

Lisa, mother of Stella

What impact might Stella's illness and chronic pain have on her family?

ACUTE DISORDERS

The following acute disorders are ones that may not have been covered in other chapters.

Cellulitis

Cellulitis is an acute, localised bacterial infection of the dermis and subcutaneous tissue (Dinulos 2021). Cellulitis can occur in intact skin or associated with a wound, such as an ulcer, or furuncles (boils) or carbuncles (a group of infected hair follicles). In more severe forms, it can include tissue necrosis. Cellulitis can be difficult to diagnose, and is therefore sometimes misdiagnosed, resulting in unnecessary exposure to antibiotics and, at times, unnecessary hospitalisation. Inflammatory skin disorders misdiagnosed as cellulitis include vascular eczema, lymphoedema and lipodermatosclerosis (Moran & Talan 2017). Refer to Chapter 29 for more information on skin integrity and wound care.

Clinical manifestations

Clinical manifestations of cellulitis include localised pain, warmth, erythema and swelling. There may or may not be a clear distinction between affected and non-affected skin. Where possible, marking the border with a permanent marker enables observation of the site to determine healing or further spread of infection. Individuals diagnosed with cellulitis may also develop vesicles over the cellulitic area and/or systemic signs of infection including fever, chills, headache, malaise and swollen lymph glands. Cellulitis commonly develops in the lower extremities with only one limb affected. It is rare for an individual to develop cellulitis in both legs (LeMone et al 2020).

Risk factors

Risk factors for developing cellulitis involve both systemic and local factors. Systemic risk factors include obesity, diabetes mellitus, weakened immune system and past history of cellulitis. Local risk factors may include chronic lymphoedema, intravenous drug use, injury to the skin (e.g. a cut, a scratch, or even a surgical wound), or a pre-existing skin condition characterised by the presence of skin breaks (e.g. eczema). Human and insect bites may also carry a high risk of causing cellulitis (Watson & Cherney 2022).

Pathophysiology

Cellulitis usually occurs due to a break or lesion on the skin that allows microorganisms to invade the body; however, in some cases, there is no identifiable skin break or lesion. In adults, the infection is usually caused by a group A streptococcus (*Streptococcus pyogenes*) and *S. auresus* (Dinulos 2021). The infection may possibly spread due to the production of a substance known as hyaluronidase (spreading factor). This substance is produced by the causative agent and breaks down fibrin networks and other barriers that normally localise infection (LeMone et al 2020). When treated appropriately and without delay, cellulitis is rarely fatal; however, any misdiagnosis, delay in treatment, or inappropriate treatment may result in complications including subcutaneous abscesses, necrotising hypodermatitis or fasciitis, septic shock and even death (Tianyi et al 2018).

Medical management

The medical management of cellulitis (when the infection is mild) includes treatment with oral antibiotics that are effective against *Streptococcus* species and *S. aureus*. Antibiotics such as dicloxacillin and cephalexin (both to be used if there is suspected methicillin-sensitive *S. aureus*; MSSA) or clindamycin (should not be used if the suspected cause is methicillin-resistant *S. aureus*; MRSA) should be considered (McCreary et al 2017).

Treatment of severe cases of cellulitis, or those that do not respond to oral antibiotics, should include the use of intravenous antibiotics. Duration of therapy (oral or IV) may be anywhere from 5–14 days, depending on clinical response and severity. Adequate analgesia should be prescribed to assist with the pain (Spelman & Baddour 2023).

Nursing care

A key role of nursing care is to prevent the spread of infection and restore skin integrity. Many individuals with cellulitis are treated at home, so it is important to educate the individual and their significant others about the importance of hygiene and the prevention of further infection, elevating the affected limb to help reduce the swelling, taking analgesia as required and monitoring the site. Individuals should be instructed to see their GP or, if referred to HITH, present to the ED if signs and symptoms worsen. The individual may need the application of a wound dressing if the affected area is open or they are at high risk due to an underlying ulcer. Antiseptic dressings such as silver or honey may be used (LeMone et al 2020). Intermittent cold compresses can be applied to the affected area if required for hot and painful skin. The use of warm compresses has now been contraindicated (Bachi-Ayukokang et al 2019). (See Progress Note 42.1.)

Individual education

Individual education for cellulitis has an emphasis on prevention of future episodes and healing the area (LeMone et al 2020). Refer to Chapter 5 for more information on health promotion.

Venous thromboembolism

Venous thromboembolism (VTE) is an umbrella term that includes both deep vein thrombosis (DVT) and pulmonary embolism (PE). It can result in complications such as post-thrombotic syndrome, pulmonary hypertension, recurrent thrombosis, or death (ACSQHC 2020). VTE is the third most common cause of cardiovascular disease globally and, in Australia, approximately 17,000 people develop VTE each year; the lifetime risk of VTE is 8%, with 1% of those aged 80 years or older experiencing a VTE for the first time (Swannell 2019). In Australia, VTE is estimated to be one of the leading

Progress Note 42.1

09/06/2024 1430 hrs	Nursing: Individual is day 3 of 7 for antibiotic treatment for R lower leg cellulitis. Individual is alert and orientated. Pain 4/10 in right lower leg. Analgesics provided as per medication chart, nil further report of pain. Temp 37.0°C, HR 78 beats/minute, BP 126/78 mmHg. Right lower leg remains swollen, nil further progression of cellulitis—refer to wound chart. Individual showered with minimal assistance this am. Tolerating FWD and fluids. All medications provided as per medication chart. Individual currently sitting out of bed with right leg elevated. For physio and OT review tomorrow. *F Daly* (DALY), *EN*

preventable causes of death in hospital, with modelling of healthcare statistics showing that PE accounts for 7% of all deaths in Australian hospitals every year (ACSQHC 2020).

Refer to Chapter 18 for more information on venous thromboembolism assessment.

Pathophysiology

Venous thrombosis forms on the wall of the vein, resulting in the wall of the vein becoming inflamed and leading to some obstruction of blood flow. It occurs more commonly than arterial thrombus due to lower blood pressure and flow within the veins. These factors lead to vessel damage, venous stasis and increased coagulability of blood, and are known as *Virchow's triad.* Changes in blood flow are usually a result of immobility. Changes in blood composition are in the form of hypercoagulability, which can be due to immobility, inflammation, malignancy or tissue damage (LeMone et al 2020).

Deep vein thrombosis (DVT) originates in the deep veins of the body and usually involves the lower extremities, with approximately 80% originating in the calf. It often extends proximally into the popliteal and femoral veins and is usually asymptomatic. Major complications of DVT are PE increasing the incidence of mortality, and venous insufficiency to the affected limb (LeMone et al 2020).

Pulmonary embolism (PE) is most commonly caused by an underlying venous thrombosis that has migrated to the pulmonary circulation (LeMone et al 2020).

A PE most commonly occurs when a blood clot fragments and loosens from the vein (usually from a DVT), travels along the large veins into the right side of the heart, enters the pulmonary circulation and eventually lodges in the pulmonary artery, occluding the flow of blood to the lungs. Mortality occurs when the mismatch between ventilation (airflow) and perfusion (blood flow) is too great, resulting in cardiac arrest (LeMone et al 2020).

Clinical manifestations

A DVT can be either superficial or deep. It commonly occurs in the lower extremities and can be mistaken for other forms of limb pain such as cellulitis, muscle strain, lymphoedema or contusion. DVTs are often asymptomatic, but clinical manifestations may include unilateral oedema or cyanosis, dull aching pain when walking or tenderness at rest, localised warmth and erythema (LeMone et al 2020). When an individual presents to a doctor or ED with these symptoms a Wells score will help to determine the person's risk of developing a DVT. This score rates the likelihood that the symptoms are the result of a DVT based on past medical history and physical examination (Seladi-Schulman 2018). (For information on prevention of DVTs see Chapter 29.)

The clinical manifestations of PE may include acute onset of pleuritic-type chest pain and dyspnoea, tachycardia, tachypnoea, haemoptysis, hypoxia and symptoms associated with a DVT (Doherty 2017).

Risk factors

Risk factors associated with VTE are shown in Clinical Interest Box 42.1 and Clinical Interest Box 42.2.

CLINICAL INTEREST BOX 42.1 Risk factors associated with developing a VTE

- Advancing age
- Postoperative
- ICU admission
- Recovering from a serious acute illness
- Major surgical procedures—orthopaedic, abdominal, thoracic and genitourinary
- Trauma—primarily fractures of the spine, pelvis, femur and tibia, and spinal cord injury
- Hormone therapy

(LeMone et al 2020)

CLINICAL INTEREST BOX 42.2 Pathological risk factors for developing a VTE

- Previous DVT
- Coagulation disorders
- Cancer, including treatments for pancreatic, breast, lung, ovarian, testicular, bladder, kidney and stomach
- Sepsis
- Obesity
- Pregnancy

(LeMone et al 2020)

Diagnostic tests

Diagnosis of a VTE requires a combination of imaging such as duplex venous ultrasonography (DVT), or computed tomography pulmonary angiogram (CTPA) or ventilation perfusion (VQ) scan (PE); clinical prediction rules or Wells score; and a D-dimer (Doherty 2017; Swannell 2019). A D-dimer—a protein fragment produced as a by-product of a blood clot being dissolved by the body—detects fibrin breakdown that is present in the blood post thrombus formation. The test is used for negative predictability only, but is not definitive in ruling out a VTE without the other two indicators (Michiels et al 2017).

Medical management

Prevention of a VTE is essential. A comprehensive risk assessment is necessary including identifying risk factors related to the individual, illness and/or proposed surgery or injury (see Clinical Interest Box 42.1 and Clinical Interest Box 42.2). A prevention plan should be developed if there is a clear risk of developing a VTE, which should include:

- prophylactic low-molecular-weight (LMW) heparin—Clexane or Fragmin
- mechanical compression—anti-embolism stockings (TEDS) or pneumatic compression devices
- maintaining the person's hydration—IV therapy may need to be considered
- early mobilisation postoperatively—if possible.

(ACSQHC 2018; ACSQHC 2020)

As per the current NSQHS 'Medication Safety' Standard, all inpatient medication charts in acute settings have been standardised to include VTE prophylaxis—pharmacological and mechanical as per a standardised VTE medical risk assessment. The medication charts are called the Pharmaceutical Benefits Scheme Hospital Medication Charts (ACSQHC 2021).

If the individual develops a VTE, treatment is to be commenced immediately. The current treatment regimen includes a combination of anticoagulation therapy and thrombolytic therapy with the aim of preventing the thrombus from growing or fragmenting. The current recommendations are to use anticoagulant therapy for 3–6 months, depending on whether the DVT or PE is no longer present or associated with a non-surgical risk factor. If the DVTs or PEs are recurrent, then longer anticoagulation should be considered, with thrombolysis—clot lysis anticoagulants such as urokinase, alteplase or streptokinase—indicated for a massive (haemodynamically unstable) PE (Swannell 2019).

Individuals with recurrent PEs despite anticoagulation therapy, or who have contraindications to anticoagulant therapy, may need to have an inferior vena cava (IVC) filter inserted. IVC filters can have a significant effect on short-term mortality, especially in persons aged 80+. IVC filters would only be used if there was a clinical need for the person to have one inserted (Zuin et al 2019).

Nursing care

Nursing care for prevention of a VTE includes:

- Early ambulation post surgery.
- Individuals should be advised to stay hydrated.
- Wear lose clothing.
- Exercise calf muscles with intermittent ankle flexion and extension.
- Apply mechanical aids such as sequential compression devices (SCDs) if prescribed.
- Administer LMW heparin if prescribed.
- If the person is to be resting in bed and if mechanical compression is contraindicated, position them to allow for optimal venous return from the lower extremities by placing a pillow below the knee to elevate the calves and feet.
- Monitor for any signs and/or symptoms of a VTE.
- Ensure IV cannulas are changed as per policy and monitored for any signs of inflammation.
- Educate the individual on their management and signs and symptoms of a VTE.

(LeMone et al 2020)

Nursing care if VTE is diagnosed:

- Administer treatment-dose anticoagulants subcutaneously, by IV and/or orally.
- Administer analgesia as prescribed.
- Apply mechanical aids such as sequential compression devices (SCDs) if not contraindicated.
- Encourage mobility if not contraindicated.
- If resting in bed, position individual to allow for optimal venous return from the lower extremities by placing a pillow below the knee to elevate the calves and feet.
- Exercise their calf muscles with intermittent ankle flexion and extension.
- Monitor for any signs and/or symptoms of deterioration.
- Educate the individual regarding their care including prolonged bleeding associated with the anticoagulant treatment and maintaining as much independence as possible.

(LeMone et al 2020)

Individual education

Prior to discharge, the individual should be advised to report any unusual bleeding to their doctor if they remain on anticoagulant treatment. For women, menstrual bleeding may be slightly increased; they should contact their doctor if it increases significantly. Men and/or women should shave with an electric razor to reduce the risk of cuts, and soft-bristle toothbrushes should be used. Medications must be taken at the same time every day to avoid missing a dose and regular blood tests may be required to calculate further doses. Contact sports should be avoided to prevent any risk of internal bleeding or haematomas. Diet should be low in vitamin K, alcohol consumption should be minimal and the individual should ask the pharmacist for advice regarding any over-the-counter medication as all of these can be contraindicated in anticoagulant therapy (Hawes 2018).

> **CRITICAL THINKING EXERCISE 42.2**
>
> You receive handover from the morning nurse on Brooke, who is expected to be discharged this afternoon. Brooke is a 31-year-old female admitted with a DVT who has responded well with treatment and will be transferred to HITH. The nurse handing over reports that this morning Brooke complained of slight back and shoulder-tip pain, which was resolved with 1 g oral paracetamol. All paperwork for her referral to HITH has been completed and Brooke is waiting for her discharge medications before she can leave. When you enter Brook's room, you find her pale and complaining of dyspnoea and chest pain.
>
> 1. What will your first action be?
> 2. What do you think has happened?
> 3. What sign did the morning nurse miss?
> 4. What diagnostic tests need to be done?

Diverticular disease

Diverticula are sac-like dilations or outpouchings of the mucosa and submucosa through the muscular coat of the colon that likely result from a combination of structural and functional factors (Brown et al 2024; Banasik 2022). The term 'diverticular disease' generally refers to diverticulosis, or the presence of multiple non-inflamed diverticula in the colon. The prevalence of diverticulosis increases with age; approximately 30% of the general population at 60 years of age and approximately 80% at 80 years will have diverticula in the colon (Banasik 2022). When diverticula become inflamed or infected, the condition is referred to as **diverticulitis** (Banasik 2022).

Clinical manifestations

Diverticulosis usually has no symptoms. However, the presence of many diverticula may cause a range of symptoms including abdominal pain and bloating, constipation and diarrhoea and flatulence. Symptoms of diverticulitis include sharp pain in the abdomen (most commonly in the lower left side of the abdomen), bloating, constipation or diarrhoea, fever, blood in the stools, nausea and vomiting (Agency for Clinical Innovation [ACI] 2019).

Risk factors

The risk of developing diverticulitis increases with age and a diet low in fibre (DeRanieri 2018).

Pathophysiology

Inflammation and infection occur due to the build-up of undigested food and bacteria collecting in the diverticula, impairing mucosal blood supply and allowing bacterial invasion to occur. In some instances, perforation may occur due to mucosal ischaemia (injury), which could lead to an abscess formation or peritonitis (Flanagan 2018; Herrington 2020).

Diagnostic tests

Diverticula are visible using a barium enema, flexible sigmoidoscopy or colonoscopy. For individuals presenting with signs and symptoms as outlined above, diagnosis of diverticulitis is achieved via abdominal CT with contrast during an acute attack since it will enable visualisation of infection, as well as any perforations and abscesses (Flanagan 2018; Herrington 2020).

Medical management

The goal of treatment in acute diverticulitis is to let the colon rest and inflammation subside. Some individuals can be managed in an outpatient setting with oral antibiotics and a clear fluid diet. If symptoms are severe, the individual is unable to tolerate oral fluids or has comorbid diseases, hospitalisation is indicated (Brown et al 2024). Treatment of diverticulitis involves making the individual nil per oral (NPO) or nil by mouth (NBM) to rest the bowel, and the administration of IV fluids and antibiotics. In cases where persistent vomiting is present, a nasogastric tube may be inserted. The use of anticholinergic medications may assist in the reduction of colonic spasms. For individuals who develop complications such as abscess, fistula or perforation, or with recurrent attacks, surgical intervention may be required (Herrington 2020). Surgery usually involves resection of the involved colon with either a primary anastomosis if adequate bowel cleansing is possible or a temporary colostomy, which is re-anastomosed after the colon heals (Brown et al 2024).

Nursing care

As the individual with diverticulitis is at risk for bowel perforation, vital signs must be monitored 4-hourly or more frequently as clinically required. The abdomen should be assessed at the same time, measuring girth, auscultating bowel sounds and palpating for tenderness. Any changes must be immediately reported to the doctor since they may indicate spread of infection. The individual must rest in bed with limited activity to promote healing. Administer analgesia for pain and intravenous antibiotics for infection as prescribed. The individual may also need to be NBM to rest the gut, so ensure regular mouth care is performed (LeMone et al 2020).

Individual education

On discharge, educate the person about diet, with the additional option of referral to a dietitian, and if a colostomy is required, the person will require education regarding care of the colostomy and, possibly, counselling. Education on the signs and symptoms of diverticulitis and the importance of regular colonoscopies as per the advice of the medical team is also important (LeMone et al 2020).

Guillain-Barré syndrome

Guillain-Barré syndrome (GBS) is a rare acute inflammatory autoimmune disorder of the peripheral nervous system characterised by rapid progressive symmetrical neuromuscular paralysis. GBS often occurs after an individual has had a respiratory or gastrointestinal viral or bacterial infection 1–3 weeks prior to the onset of GBS symptoms (LeMone et al 2020). The incidence of GBS is one or two cases per 100,000 per year; it is more common in males than females, and with increasing age (Brown et al 2024). In severe cases (approximately 20%), GBS can cause paralysis of the respiratory nerves, resulting in the inability of the individual to breathe for themselves, leading to intubation and respiratory support in ICU and, in some instances, death (Ancona et al 2018).

Clinical manifestations

Individuals with GBS will initially complain of decreased motor function, weakness and decreased sensation in their arms and legs, numbness and paraesthesia. This rapidly develops into muscle weakness, commencing distally then travelling proximally, with decreased reflexes and sensations. Cranial nerves may be affected, resulting in dysphagia, difficulty chewing and dysphasia. Level of consciousness and cognition are not affected (LeMone et al 2020). Autonomic nervous system dysfunction causes symptoms of orthostatic hypotension, hypertension and abnormal vagal responses (bradycardia, heart block, asystole). Other autonomic dysfunctions include bowel and bladder dysfunction, facial flushing and diaphoresis. Pain is common, and may be experienced as paraesthesia, muscular aches and cramps, and hyperaesthesia. The most serious complication is respiratory failure, which occurs if the paralysis progresses to the nerves that innervate the thoracic area (Brown et al 2024).

Pathophysiology

The pathophysiology of GBS occurs as an immune response to a preceding viral or bacterial infection—most commonly *Campylobacter jejuni* gastroenteristis, but also human immunodeficiency virus, cytomegalovirus or Epstein–Barr virus. The immune response interferes or cross-reacts with the peripheral nerves' myelin or axon, resulting in either axonal or demyelinating forms of GBS (Vriesendorp 2019).

Diagnostic tests

Diagnosis of GBS is via a lumbar puncture (LP) to check cerebrospinal fluid (CSF) protein levels, which will be elevated in GBS; electromyography, which measures nerve activity via thin-needle electrodes being inserted into the muscles; and nerve conduction studies, which measure nerve conductivity to stimuli using electrodes, which are taped to the skin above the nerves (Mayo Clinic 2023a).

Medical treatment

Individuals diagnosed with GBS may be treated with immunoglobulin (IVIg) or plasmapheresis (plasma exchange). IVIg is a blood product containing healthy antibodies, with high doses blocking the damaging antibodies associated with GBS. Plasmapheresis is when plasma is separated from the person's blood cells and the blood cells are re-transfused back into the body. The returned blood, free from the 'damaged' plasma, will then manufacture more plasma free from the damaging antibodies. Both treatments are administered either simultaneously or one after the other. It can take approximately 6–12 months (sometimes 3 years) for a person to fully recover from GBS depending on complications such as mechanical ventilation or pneumonia (Mayo Clinic 2023a).

Nursing care

Nursing care is aimed at supportive care of body systems until the individual recovers, particularly ventilatory support during the acute phase and preventing complications such as pneumonia and VTEs. It is important that close monitoring of deterioration in airway and breathing is maintained. Autonomic dysfunction is common and usually takes the form of bradycardia and arrhythmias, so blood pressure (BP) and cardiac rate and rhythm should be monitored. Pain assessment and management will also be required. Risk factors associated with immobility should be considered and VTE prophylaxis and pressure area injury prevention care should be implemented (Brown et al 2024). Referral to a physiotherapist to assist with any chest drainage and muscular support will be required. The individual may need to have a nasogastric tube (NGT) inserted if they have dysphagia and provided with enteral nutrition. Care must be taken to watch for any reactions to the IVIg and regular analgesia should be administered if required. Supporting the family and the individual through their progress is required to help relieve stress and anxiety, and encouraging independence through recovery will assist with better long-term outcomes (LeMone et al 2020; Vriesendorp 2019).

Acute kidney injury

Acute kidney injury (AKI) is the sudden reduction of kidney function causing disruptions in fluid, electrolyte and acid–base balances; retention of nitrogenous waste products; increased serum creatinine level; and decreased glomerular filtration rate (GFR) (Banasik 2022). The most common causes of AKI include reduced blood supply to the kidneys due to a significant physical trauma or myocardial infarction; direct damage to the tissue of the kidney, usually due to medications (NSAIDs), radioactive dye or contrast, or sepsis; or obstruction of the urinary tract due to renal calculi, blood clots or enlarged prostate (Kidney Health Australia 2020a). A study in the Kimberley region of Western Australia found that AKI in the Kimberley region is more common by more than one-quarter in Aboriginal and Torres Strait Islander individuals under 45 years of age compared with other non-Aboriginal and Torres Strait Islander individuals, primarily due to lack of resources and diagnoses such as pneumonia, and infections of the skin and subcutaneous tissue (Mohan et al 2019).

Clinical manifestations

Clinically, AKI may progress through phases: oliguric, diuretic and recovery (Brown et al 2024). Signs and symptoms differ according to the underlying cause of the

AKI, which can have effects on other body systems, such as the cardiovascular, respiratory, hepatic and neurological systems. The individual may present with symptoms including (but not limited to) increased oedema in the lower extremities, increased fatigue, dyspnoea, nausea, hypertension, pruritus and nocturia (Kidney Health Australia 2020b).

Risk factors

Risk factors for the development of an AKI relate to acute causes as mentioned above. AKI is usually a short-term disorder and reversible if caught early; however, there are higher risks of developing chronic kidney disease (CKD) and kidney failure in the future (Kidney Health Australia 2020a & b). For more information on CKD, refer to Chapter 31.

Pathophysiology

The causes of AKI are multiple and complex, and categorised as prerenal, intrarenal (or intrinsic) and postrenal causes (Brown et al 2024). AKI can be classified into three categories: prerenal injury, intrarenal injury and postrenal injury (LeMone et al 2021; Banasik 2022):

1. Prerenal injury is the result of hypoperfusion of the kidneys due to processes occurring outside (upstream) of the kidney. Hypoperfusion of the kidneys leads to a decrease in the glomerular filtration rate. Renal hypoperfusion may be the result of volume depletion from hypotension, hypovolaemia or cardiac insufficiency. (See Figure 42.1.)
2. Intrarenal injury results when there is damage to glomerulus, vessels or kidney tubules. This is most often due to prolonged causes (Figure 42.1), infections and toxins that result in inflammation or injury.
3. Postrenal injury is caused by obstruction of normal outflow of urine from the kidney, which may be a result of renal calculi, strictures, thrombosis, benign prostate hypertrophy, malignancies and pregnancy (Figure 42.1). The obstruction causes pressure to increase in the kidney resulting in injury to the kidney.

(LeMone et al 2020; Lough 2023)

Diagnostic tests

Diagnosis of AKI is based on the individual's history and potential cause, clinical presentation and kidney function. When an individual is suspected of having AKI, there are many investigations that may be ordered. These include:

- urinalysis
- blood tests—urea nitrogen, phosphorus, creatinine and potassium, which are renal specific
- GFR—glomerular filtration rate (GFR) can be determined via blood to determine reduced kidney function
- renal ultrasound
- CT, MRI
- renal biopsy.

(Kidney Health Australia 2020; Lough 2023)

Medical management

- Treat the underlying cause and complications until the kidneys recover.
- Admission to ICU may be required if the individual is critically ill.
- Dialysis may be required in severe cases of AKI.

(Lough 2023)

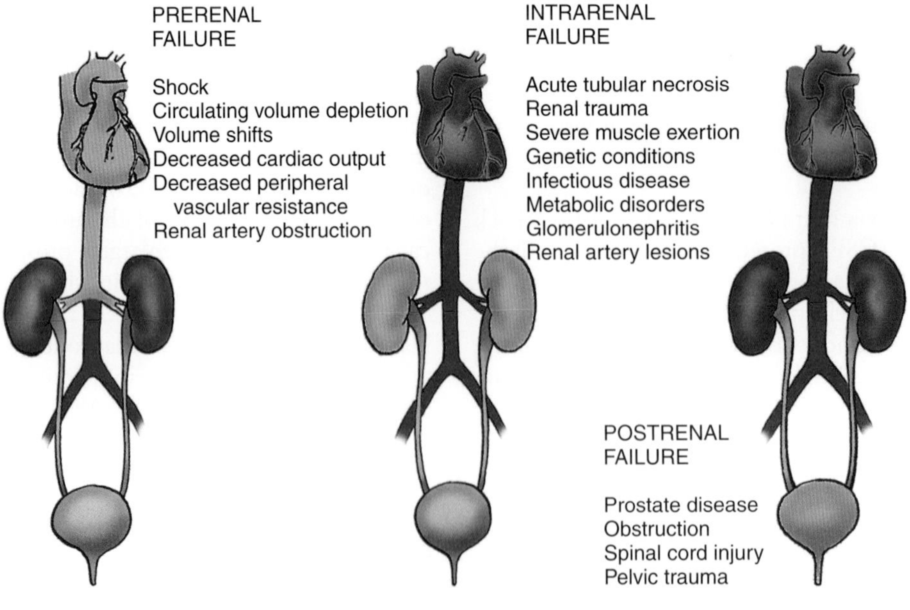

Figure 42.1 Causes of kidney failure
(Black et al 2019)

Nursing care

Close monitoring of individuals with AKI is required since, in the majority of cases, there are underlying issues, causing the kidneys to fail. The individual may be in ICU until they recover. Close monitoring in the ward includes:

- vital signs
- observe for signs of deterioration
- strict fluid balance monitoring and observe for signs of increased swelling to lower extremities and orbital area
- daily weight
- insertion and care of an indwelling catheter (IDC)
- electrolyte monitoring and replacement
- maintain IV fluids
- monitor for signs and symptoms of nausea and anorexia
- educate and reassure the individual and their family.

(LeMone et al 2020; Lough 2023)

Individual education

The individual with AKI needs education on avoiding nephrotoxic agents (especially over-the-counter medications, herbal remedies and vitamins) and regarding infection prevention and any signs or symptoms of relapse. Educate the individual how to monitor their blood pressure, weight and pulse, and continue to maintain a diet low in salt, protein and potassium. The individual will need to be monitored by their GP for any signs of relapse and future kidney disease (LeMone et al 2020; Lough 2023). (See Table 42.1.)

Sepsis and septic shock

Sepsis is a life-threatening complication caused by the body's response to infection, leading to damage of the body's tissues and organs. Severe sepsis, or a delay in treatment, can lead to **septic shock**, resulting in severe sudden hypotension, organ failure and death (Mayo Clinic 2023b; The George Institute 2018). Annually in Australia there are more than 55,000 cases of sepsis, with more than 8700 cases of sepsis-related deaths. Furthermore, up to 50% of adults who are treated for sepsis will experience a residual effect of either disability or impaired function (ACSQHC 2022b). While sepsis can affect anyone, it is the very young, the elderly, those in high-risk groups including Aboriginal and Torres Strait Islander People, and those who are immunocompromised who are most at risk (ACSQHC 2022a).

All healthcare professionals play a vital role in the early detection of sepsis. Recognising and responding to the acute deteriorating individual is included in the NSQHS Standards. The intention of the standard ensures prompt and appropriate action is taken once acute deterioration is recognised in an individual and that the health service must have processes in place for healthcare professionals (doctors and nurses) to detect the physiological signs of acute deterioration (ACSQHC 2021). The 'Sepsis Clinical Care' Standard (2022a) was developed by the ACSQHC in partnership with The George Institute for Global Health to help assist in early detection of sepsis. The aim of the clinical care standard is to focus on key areas of care where quality improvement is needed most. The quality statements and indicators contained in the clinical care standard aim to help support the delivery of evidence-based clinical care by assisting health professionals to consider the question 'Could it be sepsis?' (ACSQHC 2022a).

Hospitals in Australia, in line with state health departments, have developed sepsis pathways for paediatrics and

TABLE 42.1 | Differences between acute kidney injury (AKI) and chronic kidney disease (CKD)

	Acute kidney injury	Chronic kidney disease
Health history	Recent presentation of acute illness and causative factor	Usually not diagnosed until there is severe damage to the nephrons. Underlying medical history of diabetes, hypertension, glomerulonephritis, polycystic kidney disease, reflux nephropathy or previous kidney damage.
Clinical examination	Oedema in the lower extremities and orbital area, dyspnoea, decreased urine output, nausea and anorexia	Most signs and symptoms related to uraemia: hypertension, anaemia, leukopenia, anorexia, nausea, vomiting, hiccups, peripheral neuropathy, seizures, bone tenderness, muscle weakness, glucose intolerance, dry and itchy skin.
Creatinine Urea Haemoglobin	Elevated Elevated Usually normal	Elevated in later stages of CKD. Elevated in later stages of CKD. Decreased in later stages of CKD.
Renal ultrasound	Will diagnose potential obstruction	Kidneys appear small and shrunken with decreased cortical width.

(LeMone et al 2020)

TABLE 42.2 | Clinical manifestations of septic shock

Early (warm) septic shock	Late (cold) septic shock
Increased temperature >38°C, warm to touch and flushed ± chills Normotensive to hypotensive Tachycardia and pulse thread Tachypnoea and deep breaths Alert, orientated and anxious Urine output normal Weakness and lethargy Nausea, vomiting and diarrhoea	Normal to decreased temperature <36°C, cool and oedematous Hypotensive Tachycardia and dysrhythmias Tachypnoea with dyspnoea and shallow breaths Lethargic, drowsy ± unconscious Oliguria to anuria

(LeMone et al 2020)

adults, which are available in emergency and ward departments (see Online Resources).

Clinical manifestations

Clinical manifestations include increased or decreased fever, peripheral oedema, normotension to hypotension, tachycardia, tachypnoea, nil to severe alterations in mental state and hot flushed or pale skin (Mayo Clinic 2023b). (See Table 42.2.)

Risk factors

Sepsis can happen to anyone with an infection—fungal, viral or bacterial. Individuals at higher risk are older persons, pregnant women, children <1 year, persons with chronic diseases causing immunocompromise—diabetes, COPD, CKD or cancer—and those with weakened immune systems (Mayo Clinic 2023b).

Pathophysiology

Sepsis develops when there is an overwhelming release of inflammatory mediators in response to an infection, resulting in an immune-inflammatory cascade. In other words, it is a dysregulated inflammatory response to how the body usually deals with infection (Arwyn-Jones & Brent 2019; Jacobi 2022). Sepsis can develop in severity, with the added complication of organ dysfunction, and blood clots can develop in the organs including the brain, heart, kidneys, upper and lower extremities, including fingers and toes. Multi-organ failure and tissue death results (Mayo Clinic 2023b; Jacobi 2022) and severe coagulopathy leading to disseminated intravascular coagulation (Al-Khafaji 2020). (See Table 42.3.) If an individual remains hypotensive in spite of adequate fluid resuscitation, the individual is said to have progressed into septic shock (Mayo Clinic 2023b; Jacobi 2022).

Diagnostic tests

The diagnostic tests for sepsis are the same as those for investigating the cause of an infection, to ensure the best possible treatment. These include:

- blood samples: blood cultures, clotting profile, full blood exam, liver function (LFT), and urea and electrolytes. (How to perform venipuncture is described in Clinical Skill 42.1).
- urine sample: midstream urine (MSU) or catheter specimen urine (CSU)
- wound swab
- respiratory secretions: sputum, nasopharyngeal aspirate
- imaging: MRI, CT, X-ray, ultrasound.

(Mayo Clinic 2023b; Jacobi 2022)

Medical management

The European Society of Critical Medicine, in conjunction with the International Sepsis Forum and the Society of Critical Care Medicine, developed 'The Surviving Sepsis Campaign: International Guidelines for Management of Sepsis and Septic Shock 2021'. The aim of the campaign is

TABLE 42.3 | Signs of multiple organ dysfunction syndrome (MODS) in sepsis

Body system	Clinical manifestation
Central nervous system	Altered mental function and level of consciousness; encephalopathy and peripheral neuropathy
Urinary	Acute oliguria
Endocrine/metabolic	Hyperglycaemic without the presence of diabetes, fever and chills
Respiratory	Hyperventilation and respiratory alkalosis; acute respiratory distress syndrome
GIT/digestive	Paralytic ileus, no bowel sounds; liver failure (increased liver enzymes and bilirubin, coagulopathy, buildup of toxins and ammonia)
Cardiovascular	Decreased cardiac output, decreased perfusion, hypotension, dysrhythmias

(Al-Khafaji 2020)

CLINICAL SKILL 42.1 Venipuncture

Please adhere to the policy and procedures of the facility/organisation prior to undertaking the skill. Ensure this skill is in your scope of practice.

NMBA Decision-making Framework considerations (refer to NMBA Decision-making framework for nursing and midwifery 2022):	Equipment:
1. Am I educated? 2. Am I authorised? 3. Am I competent? If you answer 'no' to any of these, do not perform that activity. Seek guidance and support from your teacher/a nurse team leader/clinical facilitator/educator.	Disposable gloves Protective eye wear Diposable collection tray Tourniquet Vacutainer access device/21–23 G Needle and syringe/butterfly 21–23 G with vacutainer attachment Pathology test tubes Sharps container Alcohol wipes Dressing (e.g. pressure dot, cottonwool and tape or bandaid) Completed pathology request form and pen Biohazard specimen transport bag

PREPARE FOR THE SKILL

(Please refer to the Standard Steps on pp. xviii–xx for related rationales.)
Mentally review the steps of the skill.
Discuss the skill with your instructor/supervisor/team leader, if required.
Confirm correct facility/organisation policy/safe operating procedures.
Validate the order in the individual's record.
Identify indication and rationale for performing the activity.
Assess for any contraindications.
Locate and gather equipment.
Perform hand hygiene.
Ensure therapeutic interaction.
Identify the individual using three individual identifiers.
Gain the individual's consent.
Assess for pain relief.
Prepare the environment.
Provide and maintain privacy.
Assist the individual to assume an appropriate position of comfort during the activity.

PERFORM THE SKILL

(Please refer to the Standard Steps on pp. xviii–xx for related rationales.)
Perform hand hygiene.
Apply PPE: gloves, eyewear, mask and gown as appropriate.
Ensure the individual's safety and comfort throughout skill.
Promote independence and involvement of the individual if possible and/or appropriate.
Assess the individual's tolerance to the skill throughout.
Dispose of used supplies, equipment, waste and sharps appropriately.
Remove PPE and discard or store appropriately.
Perform hand hygiene.

Skill activity	Rationale
Place tourniquet about 10 cm above intended puncture site (above the elbow or wrist joint) and clip ends together and tighten firmly, so that two fingers can fit under comfortably. Palpate the distal pulse to ensure the artery is not occluded.	Helps to distend vein. Prevents discomfort due to tourniquet being too tight. Helps prevent complications.

Continued

CLINICAL SKILL 42.1 Venipuncture—cont'd

Locate the vein by palpating using the index and middle fingers of your dominant hand. Use distension methods (drop and dangle, heat pack). Once the vein is located, release tourniquet.	Palpating for the vein enables assessment of the vein through touch (bouncy and full of blood). Facilitates filling of the vein and distension. Facilitates refill of the vein.
Skill activity	**Rationale**
Cleanse the area with an alcohol wipe using circular motion (inner to outer) from the intended puncture site for 30 seconds and wait 30 seconds for the area to dry. Reapply tourniquet. Stabilise the vein by anchoring (stretching) the skin below the insertion site with your non-dominant hand. Insert needle tip with bevel up into the vein. The needle should be parallel to the vein and above it with the angle of insertion approximately 15–30 degrees. Once the tip of the needle is in the vein, remove your anchor and attach the tubes one by one to the vacutainer and fill each tube with blood. Release the tourniquet once you are getting flow to prevent haemolysis.	Prevents the introduction of microorganisms and ensures proper antiseptic preparation of skin. Enables the smooth entry into the vein and prevents the vein from moving around. Going in too deep can lead to puncturing the vein all the way through and causing a haematoma. Haemolysis can interfere with an accurate result.
Once the required tubes are filled and removed from the vacutainer, the tourniquet is also released. Support the insertion site with the cotton ball (do not push down) and withdraw the needle. Apply pressure to the puncture site and ask the individual to continue to put pressure on the site if able. Discard sharp immediately into the sharps container.	Prevents discomfort to the site. Prevents excessive bleeding and a haematoma from forming. Complies with infection control and WHS legislation.
Invert tubes, as per recommendation from manufacturer. Label and sign the tubes of blood and verify the individual's details. Sign the pathology form and place form and tubes in the required pathology biohazard bag.	Mixes blood with additives, avoids incorrect results/re-collections. Abides by organisational guidelines and ensures the correct results for the correct individual. Enables proper transporting of tubes.
Check the puncture site to ensure the bleeding has stopped and change the cotton ball if required and apply tape. Inform individual to notify you of any further bleeding, pain at the site or if a haematoma forms.	Prevents complications from the procedure.
Send blood specimens to pathology in a timely manner.	Ensures blood tests are as fresh as possible for accurate results.

AFTER THE SKILL

(Please refer to the Standard Steps on pp. xviii–xx for related rationales.)
Communicate outcome to the individual, any ongoing care and to report any complications.
Restore the environment.
Report, record and document assessment findings, details of the skill performed and the individual's response.
Report, record and document any abnormalities and/or inability to perform the skill.
Reassess the individual to ensure there are no adverse effects/events from the skill.

(Carter & Notter 2024; Crisp et al 2021; Tollefson & Hillman 2021)

to decrease mortality and morbidity associated with sepsis by providing health professionals with guidelines for the early recognition and treatment of sepsis (Evans et al 2021; Society of Critical Care Medicine 2021).

Sepsis is a medical emergency and treatment of sepsis should begin within the first hour of diagnosis. This includes:

- measuring the person's lactate level
- obtaining blood cultures before administering antibiotics
- commencing broad-spectrum antibiotics
- commencing fluid resuscitation with crystalloid solution for hypotension or high lactate level
- commencing vasopressors if hypotension not resolved or continues (maintain mean arterial pressure of >65 mmHg).

Once the causative pathogen has been identified, antimicrobials should be reassessed to provide a more targeted approach to treatment. The person's condition must be monitored closely to ensure they are responding to treatment and to determine when medications can be reduced. Signs of multiple organ dysfunction syndrome (MODS) should be treated accordingly and the person may need to be admitted to ICU for close monitoring and critical intervention (Evans et al 2021).

DECISION-MAKING FRAMEWORK EXERCISE 42.1

You are performing a ward round with Toni, the RN you have been allocated to work with. One of the individuals under your care, Jesse, has an IV antibiotic due to be given. Jesse has a PICC inserted in their right arm, which is being used to administer the IV antibiotic. You are new to this ward and have never cared for a PICC line or administered medications via one. While you have the required knowledge to give the medication, from your education, you do not have the confidence to go ahead with the procedure on your own. Toni insists that hospital policy is that you, as an EN, can administer medications via a PICC, which you have not had time to look up.

Using the decision-making framework, determine if you are able to give this medication and include the rationale for your answer. (See Clinical Interest Box 42.3 for CVAD information and Clinical Skill 42.2 for Central Venous Access Device management.) (See Case Study 42.3.)

CLINICAL INTEREST BOX 42.3 Central venous access device (CVAD) management

Indications for the insertion of a central venous access device (CVAD):

- administration of vesicant or highly irritating medications: Certain chemotherapeutic agents, high doses of potassium
- administration of large volumes of intravenous fluids or blood products: Severe hypovolaemia or haemorrhage
- long-term access for prolonged use of treatment: Chemotherapy, antibiotics, total parenteral nutrition
- long-term access for frequent or prolonged use: Blood sampling, apheresis, haemodialysis
- monitoring of central venous pressure (CVP).

Types of CVADs include:

- Non-tunnelled central venous catheter (CVC) inserted in the internal jugular, subclavian or femoral veins (not recommended for children). The tip of CVCs rests in the distal end of the superior vena cava near its junction with the right atrium.
- Percutaneously or peripherally inserted central catheter (PICC), inserted in the basilic or brachial veins of the upper arm.
- Vascath (specialised central catheter): Contains two large bore lumens—one for blood out and one for blood in. Usually inserted in the subclavian vein for plasmapheresis, plasma exchange or dialysis.
- Tunnelled cuffed CVAD (Broviac or Hickman), usually inserted in the internal jugular or subclavian vein. Subcutaneous skin granulates around the cuff, which sits just below the skin, to prevent accidental dislodgement and acts as a mechanical barrier to infection.
- Implanted ports: Consist of a surgically implanted central venous catheter connected to a reservoir or port. The catheter tip lies in the desired vein. The port lies in a surgically created subcutaneous pocket on the upper chest or arm. It consists of a titanium or plastic reservoir covered with a self-sealing silicone septum.

Complications include:

- infection (most common complication)
- occlusion
- migration of the tip of the CVAD, resulting in infiltration or extravasation
- bleeding and haematoma after insertion
- temporary nerve damage or pain
- dysrhythmias
- arterial puncture
- air embolism.

Refer to Chapter 20 for more information on medication administration.

(Brown et al 2024; The Royal Children's Hospital Melbourne 2020)

CLINICAL SKILL 42.2 Central venous access device (CVAD): Monitoring and management

Please adhere to the policy and procedures of the facility/organisation prior to undertaking the skill. Ensure this skill is in your scope of practice.

NMBA Decision-making Framework considerations (refer to NMBA Decision-making framework for nursing and midwifery 2022):

1. Am I educated?
2. Am I authorised?
3. Am I competent?

If you answer 'no' to any of these, do not perform that activity. Seek guidance and support from your teacher/a nurse team leader/clinical facilitator/educator.

Equipment

Dressing change:
- Sterile gloves
- Disposable gloves
- Sterile dressing pack
- Occlusive dressing
- Solution (as per healthcare facility policy, usually 2% chlorhexidine and 70% alcohol)
- Sterile bungs/caps
- Stabilisation device
- Extra sterile gauze squares
- Waste bag

Catheter removal:
- Sterile gloves
- Disposable gloves
- Sterile dressing pack
- Occlusive dressing
- Solution (as per healthcare facility policy, usually 2% chlorhexidine and 70% alcohol)
- Extra sterile gauze squares
- Suture remover
- Scissors
- Specimen container
- Completed pathology request form and pen
- Biohazard specimen transport bag
- Waste bag

PREPARE FOR THE SKILL

(Please refer to the Standard Steps on pp. xviii–xx for related rationales.)

Mentally review the steps of the skill.
Discuss the skill with your instructor/supervisor/team leader, if required.
Confirm correct facility/organisation policy/safe operating procedures.
Validate the order in the individual's record.
Identify indication and rationale for performing the activity.
Assess for any contraindications.
Locate and gather equipment.
Perform hand hygiene.
Ensure therapeutic interaction.
Identify the individual using three individual identifiers.
Gain the individual's consent.
Assess for pain relief.
Prepare the environment.
Provide and maintain privacy.
Assist the individual to assume an appropriate position of comfort during the activity.

PERFORM THE SKILL

(Please refer to the Standard Steps on pp. xviii–xx for related rationales.)

Perform hand hygiene.
Apply PPE: gloves, eyewear, mask and gown as appropriate.
Ensure the individual's safety and comfort throughout skill.
Promote independence and involvement of the individual if possible and/or appropriate.
Assess the individual's tolerance to the skill throughout.
Dispose of used supplies, equipment, waste and sharps appropriately.
Remove PPE and discard or store appropriately.
Perform hand hygiene.

CLINICAL SKILL 42.2 Central venous access device (CVAD): Monitoring and management—cont'd

Skill activity	Rationale
Open a sterile dressing pack and place any additional equipment within easy reach.	Prevents cross-infection. Prevents the introduction of microorganisms.
Dressing change	
Don disposable gloves and gently peel back old dressing towards the insertion site, anchoring the catheter. Remove stabilisation device (if present). Inspect for signs of infection. Measure length of catheter from the insertion site to the tip.	Prevents cross-infection. Prevents the dislodgement of the catheter. Assesses for complications, which may need further management. Identifies external catheter migration.
Remove gloves, perform hand hygiene (as per policy) and don sterile gloves. Cleanse skin with appropriate cleaning solution as per hospital guidelines. Wait for cleaning solution to dry. Place stabilisation device onto the skin in the correct place (if PICC line). Apply occlusive dressing over the catheter insertion site including the stabilisation device (if used).	Prevents the introduction of microorganisms and ensures asepsis. Prevents cross-contamination. Ensures full antisepsis has been achieved. Secures the catheter to prevent dislodgement. An occlusive dressing allows the area to breathe by preventing moisture under the dressing, preventing infection. Allows monitoring for any signs of infection.
Catheter removal	
Confirm medical order for removal of central catheter. Position the individual in a supine position. Don disposable gloves and gently peel back old dressing towards the insertion site, anchoring the catheter. Remove stabilisation device (if used). Inspect for signs of infection.	Abides by legal and organisation guidelines. Reduces the risk for air embolism during catheter removal. Prevents cross-infection. Prevents the dislodgement of the catheter. Used generally on PICC lines. Assesses for complications, which may need further management.
Remove gloves, perform hand hygiene (as per policy) and don sterile gloves. Cleanse skin and visible portion of catheter with cleaning solution in an outward circular motion as per hospital guidelines. Wait for solution to dry. Remove any sutures. Ask the individual to perform the Valsalva manoeuvre. (If unable to comply, remove during expiration.) Place a piece of sterile gauze over the insertion site and gently remove the catheter from the vein in one smooth motion, leaving the gauze in situ once removed. Place the tip of the catheter on the sterile field of the dressing tray. Check the site for any excess bleeding or exudate before covering with an occlusive dressing. **Note:** If the tip is to be sent to pathology, cut the tip with sterile scissors and place tip in a sterile specimen container.	Prevents the introduction of microorganisms and ensures asepsis. Prevents cross-contamination. Ensures full antisepsis has been achieved. Reduces the risk of air embolism during catheter removal. Do not force catheter, as it may break apart. If any resistance, stop the procedure, cover with a sterile dressing and inform the nurse in charge/doctor. Reduces the risk of contamination. Prevents post-removal air embolism and the introduction of microorganisms. The doctor may want to test for any microorganisms.
Label and sign the container and verify the individual's details. Sign the pathology form and place form and specimen container in the required pathology biohazard bag.	Abides by organisational guidelines and ensures the correct results for the correct individual. Enables proper transporting of specimen.
Send specimen container to pathology in a timely manner.	Ensures specimen is as fresh as possible for accurate results.

Continued

CLINICAL SKILL 42.2 Central venous access device (CVAD): Monitoring and management—cont'd

AFTER THE SKILL

(Please refer to the Standard Steps on pp. xviii–xx for related rationales.)
Communicate outcome to the individual, any ongoing care and to report any complications.
Restore the environment.
Report, record and document assessment findings, details of the skill performed and the individual's response.
Report, record and document any abnormalities and/or inability to perform the skill.
Reassess the individual to ensure there are no adverse effects/events from the skill.

(Crisp et al 2021; The Royal Children's Hospital Melbourne 2020; Tollefson & Hillman 2021)

CASE STUDY 42.3

Septic shock

Sandra, a 28-year-old with acute myeloid leukaemia, was admitted to the ward. Sandra had undergone a bone marrow transplant which had yet to take, and was neutropenic. Sandra started spiking temperatures of 38°C or more. As per protocol, the medical officer ordered blood cultures each time this happened, which kept coming back negative. Despite empirical antibiotic therapy as per the recommended neutropenic protocol, this continued for 2 days before Sandra deteriorated very suddenly and was taken to the ICU in septic shock. The source of the sepsis was eventually found to be the tip of the Hickman catheter, which showed a Gram-negative bacillus. Sandra finally recovered after spending over a month in the ICU and another 4 months on the ward before being discharged.

Identify some of the ongoing issues that Sandra may face.

Nursing care

The best treatment for sepsis is prevention, which all nurses must aim to achieve by being diligent with correct handwashing and aseptic technique, and the use of standard and additional precautions. Early detection of the signs of sepsis is also important. Goals of care should be discussed with both the affected individual and their family. Many individuals with multiple organ failure will not survive. Counselling and support for the individual (if awake) and their family should be provided, with palliative care if indicated (LeMone et al 2020).

PERIOPERATIVE CARE

Perioperative nursing encompasses the care of an individual who is undergoing a surgical procedure. The perioperative period comprises the preoperative, intraoperative and **postoperative** phases. Perioperative nurses are RNs and ENs who fulfil the roles of circulating nurse (scout), instrument nurse (scrub), anaesthetic and post-anaesthesia recovery nurse (see Table 42.4). The responsibilities of these nurses are specialised and multifaceted. The principal aim is to ensure that holistic, safe, clinically effective, evidence-based care and support is given to the individual throughout their perioperative experience. The perioperative nurse provides this care alongside other members of the multidisciplinary team, in an environment that is challenging, changing and fast paced. The nurse acts as the individual's advocate and provides continued and effective communication with the individual, their significant others and the surgical team. The nurse undertakes efficient assessment and intervention, maintains accountability for their own practice, documents care and emphasises individual safety in all phases (Crisp et al 2021; Sutherland-Fraser et al 2022).

In Australia, professional standards, guidelines and policy statements for perioperative nursing are set by the Australian College of Perioperative Nurses (ACORN). ACORN's ongoing focus is to 'advance safe, quality perioperative nursing care for Australians' (ACORN 2023). The World Health Organization (WHO) developed the Surgical Safety Checklist (SSC), which has been adapted in Australia and across the world to promote a multidisciplinary approach to surgical safety (WHO 2009; Sutherland-Fraser et al 2022).

SURGERY

Undergoing surgery is a unique experience that may expose an individual to numerous stressors. The anticipation of having a surgical procedure may incite fear and anxiety. Some individuals associate having surgery with pain, disfigurement, loss of independence and even death. It is important for the perioperative nurse to quickly establish rapport with individuals, listening to them so that their concerns are heard and relieved. In the perioperative environment the individual is at their most vulnerable and reliant on the skills and knowledge of the multidisciplinary team (MDT) to achieve an optimal outcome.

TABLE 42.4 | Role responsibilities of the perioperative nurse

Anaesthetic nurse	• Identifies individual and adheres to 'surgical safety checklist' (SSC) • Collaborates with and assists the anaesthetist during preparation, induction, maintenance and emergence phases of the anaesthesia • Anticipates and provides equipment/supplies for routine and emergency anaesthetic procedures • Assists the individual to maintain a clear airway • Individual assessment and monitoring • Assessment/documentation of fluid balance • Assists with individual transfer and positioning before and after surgery • Individual advocate, especially when anaesthetised • Evaluates effectiveness of planned care • Collaborates with post-anaesthetic care unit (PACU) staff to provide individual care
Circulating (scout) nurse	• Identifies individual and adheres to SSC • Anticipates the needs of the surgical team before/during surgery • Monitors any breach in aseptic technique and initiates corrective action • Performs the surgical count with the instrument nurse • Correct handling and labelling of surgically removed human tissue and implanted items • Advocates for the anaesthetised individual • Documentation of intraoperative nursing care
Instrument (scrub) nurse	• Identifies individual and adheres to SSC • Prepares the instruments and equipment needed in the operation • Anticipates the needs of the surgical team before/during surgery • Adheres to and maintains aseptic technique throughout the procedure • Monitors any breach in aseptic technique and initiates corrective action • Performs the surgical count with the circulating nurse • Correct handling of surgically removed human tissue and implanted items • Documentation of intraoperative nursing care
Post-anaesthetic nurse	• Individual assessment, observation, monitoring and airway management • Performs resuscitation • Management of acute pain, nausea and vomiting • Management of the individual's fluid balance • Documentation of nursing care during the immediate postoperative period • Prompt acting on and reporting of changes in the individual's condition to anaesthetist/surgeon • Provision of a comprehensive individual handover to the nurse caring for the individual in the receiving unit

(Sutherland-Fraser et al 2022)

The purpose of surgery

Surgery is performed for a variety of reasons:

- Cosmetic—performed to improve the individual's appearance and/or physiological functioning. For example, a breast reduction or a rhinoplasty.
- Curative—to eliminate or repair a condition or disease. For example, the removal of a malignant tumour.
- Diagnostic—surgical exploration to confirm a diagnosis; tissue may be removed for further diagnostic testing
- Explorative—to examine and/or determine the extent of a disease. For example, an arthroscopy to inspect the inside of a knee joint to determine the extent of cartilage damage from a meniscal tear.
- Palliative—alleviates or reduces the intensity of disease symptoms. For example, the removal of a tumour pressing on a nerve causing pain. The surgery will not cure the disease (e.g. metastatic cancer); however, the individual may benefit from pain relief.
- Preventative—surgery is aimed to remove a possible threat to life before it occurs. An example may include a mastectomy in an individual with a family history of breast cancer, or the removal of benign polyps in the colon that may have the potential to turn into a malignancy.

(Crisp et al 2021)

Classifications of surgery

Surgery is classified under the descriptors of risk and urgency. Surgery may be classified as minor (e.g. the excision of a skin lesion or an endoscopy/colonoscopy), intermediate (e.g. a hernia repair, laparoscopic cholecystectomy, arthroscopy or tonsillectomy) or major/complex (e.g. a total abdominal hysterectomy, joint replacement or colonic resection) (Queensland Health 2021). Surgery may be a carefully planned event (elective surgery) or may arise with unexpected urgency (emergency surgery) (Brown et al 2024). The classification of surgery for each individual may change, depending on the time lapse between identification of the need for surgery, any increase in symptoms and the time surgery occurs.

Responses to surgical intervention

Any surgical procedure comes with a degree of risk. Various factors may increase an individual's risk during surgery. Knowledge of any pre-existing risk factors allows the nurse to appropriately plan individualised care. Some of these risk factors may include:

- Age—the very young and the elderly are at increased risk during surgery due to their physiological status being either immature or declining. Physiological changes associated with the ageing process may have an effect on the ability of an older adult to tolerate surgery. The presence of pre-existing comorbidities, and the duration of the surgical procedure may also be influencing factors (Potter et al 2023).
- Nutrition—the need for adequate nutrition is intensified by surgery; normal tissue repair and resistance to infection is dependent on sufficient nutrients.
- Obesity—the bariatric (obese) individual is at an increased surgical risk of complications including reduced ventilatory and cardiac function, acute kidney injury and an increased risk of VTE. There is also a greater susceptibility to wound infections and poor wound healing due to the structure of fatty tissue, which contains deficient blood supply (Rothrock 2023).
- Fluid and electrolyte balance—the body responds to surgery as a form of trauma; the more extensive the surgery, the more severe the stress. The degree of fluid and electrolyte imbalance is influenced by the severity of the stress response evoked.

Physiological responses

In response to surgical invasion, the body mobilises defences to maintain homeostasis. Most of these mechanisms are generally favourable to survival and healing. If, however, the mechanisms are prolonged or uncontrolled, they may contribute to the development of complications. Table 42.5 outlines the physiological responses to the stress of surgery.

Local responses to tissue injury

After injury, local inflammatory reactions occur to promote healing. A surgical incision, even though created under sterile and controlled conditions, still constitutes injury or insult. The inflammatory response begins with the creation of a surgical wound, and the normal sequence of tissue replacement and wound healing must occur to ensure tissue recovery. The physiology of wound healing

TABLE 42.5 | Physiological responses to the stress of surgery

Response	Purpose
Increased peripheral vasoconstriction and blood coagulation	Prevents excessive blood and fluid loss
Increased rate and strength of heart beat, and dilation of the coronary arteries	Maintains cardiac perfusion and oxygenation
Increased reabsorption of sodium ions from the kidneys, causing retention of sodium and water	Maintains blood volume, blood pressure and cardiac output
Decreased peristalsis in the gastrointestinal tract	Reduces metabolic activity which is non-essential in the short-term emergency
Relaxation of smooth muscle that promotes dilation of the bronchioles	Improves gas exchange and tissue oxygenation
Increased breakdown of protein	Increases the availability of amino acids for repair of tissues
Proliferation of connective tissue	Promotes wound healing
Increased circulation of glucose and mobilisation of stored fat	Provides required energy
Increased basal metabolic rate	Provides required energy and nutrients for the tissues

(Rothrock 2023; Potter et al 2023; Brown et al 2024)

involves a specific sequence of events and is discussed in Chapter 29, as are influences on healing and the specific care of wounds.

Psychological responses

The physiological and psychological reactions to surgery and anaesthesia may elicit a stress response. Factors that may influence an individual's susceptibility to stress include age, past experiences with illness and pain, and current health. As a result of psychological stress related to surgical intervention, the individual may experience any of the following:

- Anxiety, which may be related to the procedure itself, or to associated factors, including changed social circumstances, loss of independence or privacy, separation from family/support people, financial hardship or prolonged recovery time.
- Fear of anticipated pain, concern of disfigurement or decreased function, dread of death, panic of waking up under anaesthetic.
- Grief associated with loss of health or a body part, self-image change, altered function or presence of a scar.
- Hope may be the individual's way of coping. Some surgeries such as those that repair (e.g. plastic surgery for burn injury), rebuild (e.g. total hip replacement) or extend and save life (e.g. organ transplant, repair of aneurysm) can be anticipated hopefully.

(Brown et al 2024)

See Table 42.6 for information about medications with special implications for the individual undergoing surgery.

PREOPERATIVE CARE

The **preoperative** phase begins whenever surgical intervention is first considered, and ends when the individual is transferred to the operating table. This phase may be of short duration if the individual is taken directly to an operating room from the emergency department or transferred soon after admission to a surgical unit. The duration depends

TABLE 42.6 Medications with special implications for the individual undergoing surgery

Drug class	Effects during surgery
Antibiotics	Antibiotics potentiate (enhance action of) anaesthetic agents. If taken within 2 weeks before surgery, aminoglycosides (gentamicin, tobramycin, neomycin) may cause mild respiratory depression from depressed neuromuscular transmission.
Antiarrhythmics	Antiarrhythmics (e.g. beta-blockers such as metoprolol [Lopressor]) can reduce cardiac contractility and impair cardiac conduction during anaesthesia.
Anticoagulants	Anticoagulants, such as warfarin (Coumadin), alter normal clotting factors and thus increase risk of haemorrhaging. Discontinue at least 48 hours before surgery. Aspirin is a commonly used medication that alters clotting mechanisms.
Anticonvulsants	Long-term use of certain anticonvulsants (e.g. phenytoin [Dilantin] and phenobarbitone) alters metabolism of anaesthetic agents.
Antihypertensives	Antihypertensives, such as beta-blockers and calcium channel blockers, interact with anaesthetic agents to cause bradycardia, hypotension and impaired circulation. They inhibit synthesis and storage of noradrenaline in sympathetic nerve endings.
Corticosteroids	With prolonged use, corticosteroids, such as prednisone, cause adrenal atrophy, which reduces the body's ability to withstand stress. Before and during surgery, dosages are often temporarily increased.
Insulin	Individuals' need for insulin changes after surgery. Stress response and IV administration of glucose solutions often increase dosage requirements after surgery. Decreased nutritional intake often decreases dosage requirements.
Diuretics	Diuretics such as furosemide (Lasix) potentiate electrolyte imbalances (particularly potassium) after surgery.
Non-steroidal anti-inflammatory drugs (NSAIDs)	NSAIDs (e.g. ibuprofen) inhibit platelet aggregation and prolong bleeding time, increasing susceptibility to postoperative bleeding.
Herbal therapies: ginger, ginkgo, ginseng	These herbal therapies have the ability to affect platelet activity and increase susceptibility to postoperative bleeding. Ginseng is reported to increase hypoglycaemia with insulin therapy.

(Potter et al 2023; Brown et al 2024)

on a number of factors, such as the amount of time required to prepare the individual adequately for surgery. The preoperative phase may begin with the individual as an outpatient in a designated pre-admission clinic, where preoperative investigations are undertaken prior to the individual's surgical admission.

In Australia, day surgery is well established. It is common practice for an individual, depending on the type of surgery to be performed, to be admitted for same-day surgery. In this instance, the individual is admitted in the early or late morning depending on the time of the operation or procedure. The individual is prepared for and undergoes surgery, is recovered from the anaesthetic and is cared for in the day surgery unit (DSU) after the procedure. The individual is then discharged home on the same day, provided they are safe to do so.

Day surgery is suitable for less complex surgical procedures or invasive techniques for which some anaesthesia is required (e.g. endoscopy). These units are staffed by both RNs and ENs. The advantages of day surgery to the individual and their relatives may include the following: reduction in cross-infection risk compared with individuals who remain in hospital; decreased risk of thromboembolism associated with early ambulation; less anxiety for the individual as an overnight stay in hospital is avoided, particularly in the case of children for whom minimal separation from parents is beneficial, and for the older individual who may become disoriented when subjected to unfamiliar surroundings for extended periods of time. Financial benefits may include the need for less time off work and less stress for relatives saving time, travel and, in some cases, the need for accommodation to visit an inpatient in hospital (Sutherland-Fraser et al 2022).

In contrast to day surgery, individuals who are going to be admitted to the hospital for postoperative inpatient care are usually admitted on the day of surgery known as a day of surgery admission (DOSA). The admission process is usually carried out in an admission clinic (sometimes this is the DSU) where the DOSA individual will wait until they are taken into theatre. Following the surgical procedure, the individual will initially be transferred to the post anaesthetic care unit (PACU), which is often referred to as 'recovery', before being transferred to the appropriate ward.

Overall length of stay in hospital after surgical procedures is generally decreasing. With the practice of earlier discharge comes the implication that individuals may go home with complex medical and nursing needs and will require suitable follow-up with visiting nurses, or involvement in a 'hospital in the home' or a 'rehab in the home' program. (See Chapter 40 for further information on rehabilitation.) Follow-up at home must be available for continuity of care to occur.

Regardless of the type of surgery or the intended length of stay in hospital, all individuals undergoing a surgical procedure require preoperative preparation and education. The overall aim of preoperative preparation is to ensure that the individual is in optimal physical and psychological condition prior to undergoing surgery. It is essential to gather appropriate data concerning the individual's health status through gathering baseline observations and a detailed and accurate history. Nursing assessment is based on data collected and includes the identification of both actual and potential problems/issues that may be faced by the individual throughout any phases of the perioperative period. Although certain aspects of preoperative preparation are similar for most surgical procedures, other factors are specific, depending on the individual's condition and the type of operation to be performed. (See Nursing Care Plan 42.1.)

Preoperative preparation requires input from many members of the multidisciplinary team and includes:

- providing information
- teaching activities (e.g. deep breathing and coughing techniques, and leg exercises)
- examination of the individual by the anaesthetist and surgeon
- performing laboratory tests and diagnostic studies
- gaining the individual's informed consent
- preparation of the individual both psychologically and physically.

NURSING CARE PLAN 42.1

Sahra, 29 years old, is a recent arrival in Australia from Somalia. Sahra is booked for a cone biopsy of the cervix due to a cervical screening test result showing moderate changes. On arrival, it was apparent that Sahra was severely distressed and fearful. With careful questioning it became clear that Sahra thought a much more invasive surgery was to be undertaken.

Assessment: Preoperative emotional/psychological assessment.

Issue/s to be addressed: Anxiety, fear of surgery related to misinformation/misunderstanding and cultural issues.

Goal/s: Individual to verbalise reduced anxiety, a clear understanding of, and acceptance/informed consent to, the surgical procedure.

Care/actions	Rationale
Encourage individual to verbalise cause of anxiety.	To ensure the understanding of the assessing nurse.
Explain and describe in simple terms the exact nature of the surgical procedure using diagrams if required.	To enhance communication and aid in the understanding and informed consent of the individual.

Evaluation: Preoperatively with follow-up in PACU.

Providing information

The treating medical team will assess and inform the individual about the details of the surgical procedure to be undertaken. The information given to the individual and, as appropriate, to their significant others should include:

- preoperative procedures to be performed and the reasons for them (e.g. restriction of food and fluids, cessation of smoking or preparation of the operation site)
- immediate preparation (e.g. insertion of an intravenous [IV] cannula, the administration of pre-medication and the induction of anaesthesia, and what sensations may be experienced)
- details of the recovery phase in the post-anaesthetic care unit (PACU) before returning to the intensive care unit (ICU), high-dependency unit (HDU), DSU or the ward
- postoperative situations to be expected (e.g. the presence of an IV infusion or wound drain, and why these are necessary)
- postoperative activities (e.g. deep breathing and coughing, early mobilisation and why they are important)
- anticipated pain or discomfort, and options for how this will be managed
- any additional information specific to the operation to be performed.

The information must be provided in such a way that the individual can understand it, and it should be repeated if necessary. This is essential since anxiety about hospitalisation and/or the surgical procedure may influence the individual's ability to process and retain information.

Medical history

Individuals will present for admission with varied health and illness backgrounds. Some may have chronic illness, others a recent diagnosis that may or may not be related to the reason for the surgical admission. Existing conditions may have an impact on the individual's post-surgical recovery, and likewise the surgical procedure may have an impact on the severity or management of any pre-existing condition. See Table 42.7 for an outline of common medical conditions that may increase the risk of surgery. The nurse needs to be aware of potential challenges to an optimal recovery, in order to plan and implement effective care in all phases of the perioperative experience. The nurse also needs to be aware of the effect that an individual's currently prescribed medications may have on their ability to cope with the stresses of surgery and recovery.

Physical examination

The anaesthetist and a medical officer each perform a thorough physical examination of the individual (Sweitzer 2023). The anaesthetist pays particular attention to the individual's cardiovascular and respiratory systems to evaluate the general level of function and to identify any problems that may cause difficulty during induction or maintenance of anaesthesia, such as an upper airway abnormality, which may make placement of an endotracheal tube difficult, or a spinal condition, which may hinder regional anaesthesia. Loose or prosthetic teeth will be identified and noted on the admission chart. The anaesthetist also evaluates possible sites for peripheral or central venous cannulation. After assessing the individual, the anaesthetist may prescribe any preoperative medications deemed necessary to be administered prior to surgery.

Informed consent

Before any operation is performed, the individual (or legal representative where appropriate) must provide their written **informed consent**, which must be freely given without coercion. Informed consent involves the surgeon providing the individual with enough information to understand the nature and consequences of the proposed procedure and informing the individual about the facts and possible risks relating to the surgery concerned, in terms that ensures understanding by the individual. The individual then consents, in writing, to have the operation. The surgeon and the individual must both sign a consent form, an important part of the documentation process that formalises the individual's agreement to undergo surgery (Seely et al 2022).

The nurse is not responsible for obtaining the individual's consent; however, part of the nursing role includes checking that informed consent has been obtained and making appropriate notifications if this is found not to be the case. In some agencies, nurses are asked to witness consent forms, but the act of witnessing only verifies that this is the person who signed the consent, and that it was given voluntarily. It does not relate to the individual's actual knowledge or understanding of the procedure. (More information on informed consent is provided in Chapter 2.)

Following discussion with the treating medical team, further interaction between the individual and the nurse should occur since knowledge and understanding promote feelings of being in control, and a sense of control may assist to relieve anxiety for the individual (Brown et al 2024). Through discussion with the individual, the nurse is able to identify any area of knowledge deficit about preoperative or postoperative nursing care requirements. It is important to note that any knowledge deficits identified that pertain to informed consent of the actual surgical procedure must be redirected back to the treating medical team (in particular the surgeon) for further conversation with the individual.

Laboratory and diagnostic testing

Laboratory and diagnostic tests help detect any risk factors or possible issues. Specific tests and studies performed depend on the individual's condition and on the nature and complexity of the surgery. Ideally, diagnostic tests are carried out with sufficient time before the scheduled procedure to allow for correction of any detected problems.

Tests can include, but are not limited to:

- blood type and cross-match, for procedures in which significant blood loss is anticipated or possible

TABLE 42.7 | Medical conditions that increase the risks of surgery

Type of condition	Reason for risk
Bleeding disorders (thrombocytopenia, haemophilia)	Increase risk of haemorrhaging during and after surgery.
Diabetes mellitus	Increases susceptibility to infection and impairs wound healing from altered glucose metabolism and associated circulatory impairment. Stress of surgery often causes increase in blood glucose levels.
Heart disease (recent myocardial infarction, arrhythmias, congestive heart failure) and peripheral vascular disease	Stress of surgery causes increased demands on myocardium to maintain cardiac output. General anaesthetic agents depress cardiac function.
Obstructive sleep apnoea	Administration of opioids increases risk of airway obstruction postoperatively. Individuals will desaturate as revealed by drop in O_2 saturation by pulse oximetry.
Upper respiratory infection	Increases risk of respiratory complications during anaesthesia (e.g. pneumonia and spasm of laryngeal muscles).
Liver disease	Alters metabolism and elimination of drugs administered during surgery and impairs wound healing and clotting time because of alterations in protein metabolism.
Fever	Predisposes individual to fluid and electrolyte imbalances and may indicate underlying infection.
Chronic respiratory disease (emphysema, bronchitis, asthma)	Reduces individual's means to compensate for acid–base alterations. Anaesthetic agents reduce respiratory function, increasing risk for severe hypoventilation.
Immunological disorders (leukaemia, acquired immune deficiency syndrome [AIDS], bone marrow depression and use of chemotherapeutic drugs or immunosuppressive agents)	Increase risk of infection and delayed wound healing after surgery.
Abuse of street drugs	Persons abusing drugs sometimes have underlying disease (HIV, hepatitis) that affects healing.
Chronic pain	Regular use of pain medications often results in higher tolerance. Increased doses of analgesics are sometimes necessary to achieve postoperative pain control.

(Potter et al 2023; Brown et al 2024)

- arterial blood gas and pH, to check respiratory function and oxygenation
- electrolytes urea creatinine (EUC), to check renal function
- full blood examination (FBE)
- prothrombin and/or plasma thromboplastin time, clotting factors, especially if the individual has been on anticoagulant therapy
- serum electrolytes, including sodium and potassium levels
- liver function studies
- chest X-ray
- electrocardiogram (ECG)
- pulmonary function studies
- urinalysis.

(Brown et al 2024; Queensland Health 2021)

Psychological preparation

To minimise anxiety and prepare the individual psychologically for the proposed procedure, the nurse must ensure that all relevant information is provided. People generally experience anxiety when they are facing the unknown, and anxiety may be minimised when accurate and relevant information is supplied. The nurse must ensure that the individual and the significant others are given opportunities to ask questions and to express any concerns they may have. It is important for the nurse to recognise that procedures that seem relatively minor or routine may not appear that way to individuals or to their significant others. The prospect of any surgical intervention may raise fears about body image alteration, loss of control, pain or even the possibility of death. The most common psychological factors are anxiety, fear and hope (Brown et al 2024). Some factors that the individual may be worried about include:

- What will happen while they are unconscious?
- Will they be anaesthetised before the surgery begins?
- Fear of experiencing severe pain.
- Length of hospital stay.
- Who will care for their family or pets?
- How long it will be before it is possible to return to work?

The family and/or significant others may also be worried, especially if the diagnosis is questionable or the outcome of the surgery is difficult to determine. If they choose to remain in the hospital while the operation is being performed, the nurse should ensure that the location of the waiting area and amenities are provided, and also where refreshments can be obtained. If the preference is to remain at home, family and/or significant others should be advised about the notification process (e.g. if the surgeon will contact them after the procedure, and whom and when they can call to obtain information).

Providing cultural safety

It is an expectation for nurses to provide healthcare to all individuals regardless of their cultural beliefs and background. Cultural safety is about providing care in a culturally sensitive and respectful manner (Nursing and Midwifery Board of Australia 2018). The traditional values and religious beliefs of members of Indigenous groups in Australia and New Zealand are emphasised in the literature on this concept, also referred to as cultural competence.

An example of this is outlined in an article on a Māori individual's wish to have an amputated limb returned to him and his family for burial, rather than sent for destruction as is the usual practice (Hoyle 2017). This requirement is not unique to Māori people, so nurses and other healthcare members in the perioperative environment need to be mindful of the policy and procedure for similar cases and be aware that there is usually a system in place for meeting most of the traditional beliefs of many cultures. Different individuals, with varying cultures, backgrounds and experience, may want different types of information (Brown et al 2024).

With knowledge of the likely traditional or religious beliefs affecting some individuals, with some forethought, many of these beliefs can be accommodated for in the perioperative environment. The responsibility for arranging any accommodations lies with all the stakeholders, from the individual to the ward staff and those working in the operating room. Case Study 42.4 provides an example of how traditional or religious beliefs should be accommodated. (See also Chapter 13 and Chapter 14.)

Teaching activities

Preoperative teaching (see Clinical Interest Box 42.4 for details) can help to reduce anxiety and stress, and teaching specific activities that the individual can undertake to promote their own recovery gives them a positive role to play. Preoperative teaching requires the nurse to consider a balance between the information that is required versus the risk of overwhelming the individual (Brown et al 2024).

CASE STUDY 42.4

Cultural case study

A Muslim woman was admitted to the holding bay of a public hospital prior to undergoing an elective cystoscopy for diagnostic purposes. She arrived wearing a head covering over her hospital-issued gown and a long-sleeved gown over that.

The ward staff indicated that she was unwilling to expose her hair or her limbs in public.

The perioperative nurse was happy for the individual to wear her scarf as long as she wore a paper cap over the top to which the individual was agreeable.

The (female) anaesthetist was able to reassure the individual that she would insert an IV access for the sedation into the back of her hand and therefore not expose her arms. The individual agreed that, should an emergency occur, she consented to exposure of other areas, like her chest, to allow resuscitation.

Problems occurred when the individual realised that she would have to expose her genital area to both the male scout nurse and the male urologist for the purposes of the cystoscopy. She stated that she expected that female staff only would be present in the theatre.

A female scout nurse was available from another theatre; however, the male urologist was the only one present on the day. The individual refused the procedure and was discharged to return another time when staffing could be arranged to suit.

1. Could this situation have been avoided? If so, how?
2. Was the situation handled appropriately? If not, explain why not.
3. Identify some interventions that could be made to improve cultural understanding in the perioperative environment and better prepare patients and staff for the perioperative experience.

CRITICAL THINKING EXERCISE 42.3

Identify the preoperative teaching you would provide for an individual who is having endoscopic surgery to remove part of the bowel (laparoscopic hemicolectomy).

Physical preparation

Ideal surgical conditions include an individual who is haemodynamically stable, with no current clinical infection, and with well-controlled pre-existing medical conditions. Depending on the individual's condition and the type of operation to be performed, specific measures may be implemented to minimise or eliminate any identified risks.

> **CLINICAL INTEREST BOX 42.4**
> **Teaching activities**
>
> - Deep breathing and coughing techniques to facilitate gas exchange and expectoration of accumulated mucus. The individual assumes a sitting position and takes several deep breaths followed by a short breath and cough. Alternatively, the individual may be taught to take a deep breath, hold it for 2–3 seconds then cough several times while exhaling. The individual will be taught to support any wounds with hands, or by splinting with a pillow, to reduce pain and facilitate deep breathing.
> - Leg exercises performed to stimulate blood circulation and enhance venous return to reduce the risk of a DVT. The individual is instructed how to bend the knees and contract the hamstring and quadriceps muscles, then to dorsiflex and plantar flex the feet (see Chapter 28 for further information).
> - Moving and changing position helps to prevent complications such as skin breakdown and DVT. The individual will be informed of any special equipment, or techniques that will be required for movement, and of any restrictions to movement.
>
> *(Berman et al 2020)*

For example, an individual with breathing difficulties may be required to undergo active therapy such as incentive spirometry (an exercise used to achieve maximum inspiratory capacity and reduce the risk of pulmonary consolidation).

An individual with pre-existing dehydration or poor nutritional status may be admitted for some time before surgery so that fluid and nutritional deficiencies may be corrected. A specific diet may be prescribed, such as low fibre before bowel surgery. A person with potential for infection may be administered prophylactic antibiotics prior to the operation. Physical preparation may also include cessation or modification of certain medication administration (2024 aspirin and other anticoagulant drugs) (Rothrock 2023). Cessation of smoking should also be encouraged. Other preoperative measures may include comprehensive preparation of the gastrointestinal tract and preparation of the skin. (For more information on physical preparation for surgery see Table 42.8.)

Preparation of the individual—Immediately prior to surgery

Although preparation during the 1–2 hours preceding an operation may vary slightly depending on the individual and type of operation, preparation generally involves standard procedures including the following:

- Measuring and documenting height and weight, including body mass index (BMI).
  - > Rationale: Knowledge of the individual's weight enables drug dosages to be calculated accurately. It is also useful for comparison as progress is monitored postoperatively, especially in relation to assessment of fluid balance status.
- Measuring and documenting vital signs.
  - > Rationale: These measurements are used as a baseline for postoperative comparison. Any deviation from previous results must be reported immediately and documented since abnormalities may result in postponement of the operation.
- Performing urinalysis. Any abnormalities must be reported immediately.
  - > Rationale: Since the kidneys excrete most drugs from the body, any sign of kidney dysfunction is significant.
- Ensuring that the individual is not wearing any nail polish, lipstick, talcum powder or other cosmetics.
  - > Rationale: The above could interfere with assessment of skin colour (pallor and cyanosis) or circulatory and oxygen saturation status.
- Ensuring that jewellery, hairpins, prosthetic devices, spectacles, contact lenses or hearing aids are removed (as appropriate) and stored safely. Spectacles and hearing aids are usually worn to the operating room then removed and kept for the individual in recovery. Each healthcare agency has its own policy regarding the wearing of wedding rings and earrings (e.g. these may be left on and secured in position with adhesive tape).
  - > Rationale: To prevent loss of, damage to or dislodgement as well as decreasing the risk of interference with surgical equipment.
- Dentures are usually left in situ, and based on the anaesthetist's instructions, but partial plates or bridges are removed before surgery. It is important to check the presence of any loose teeth for the same reason.
  - > Rationale: Consideration of the above to prevent dislodgement during endotracheal intubation.
- Attending to general hygiene and comfort needs by ensuring that appropriate clothing is worn and assisting the individual to dress if necessary. Generally, a plain cotton or paper open-back gown with tie-tapes is worn. A disposable paper cap is also worn to cover the individual's hair, and some facilities also provide disposable paper undergarments worn under the gown.
  - > Rationale: Provides modesty for individual and protects against potential transfer of microorganisms.
- Checking that the individual's identification bands (usually two) are correct and in situ. In some agencies, a red identification band is worn if the individual has any known allergies. It is also important to check all documents that will accompany the individual to the operating room.
  - > Rationale: Ensures the individual (and any identified allergies) are correctly identified.

Documentation

Each healthcare facility has its own preoperative forms and checklists. These checklists will require completion by the

TABLE 42.8 | Physical preparation for surgery

Preparation type	Method and rationale
Gastrointestinal	*Fasting:* To empty the stomach and prevent aspiration of stomach contents during anaesthesia. Individuals undergoing procedures under local anaesthetic may still be requested to fast in case a general anaesthetic needs to be used. Long-term fasting (more than 6 hours) will ensure a clear operative view of the internal bowel for open and endoscopic procedures. Fasting status of individual ensured by nurse. *Bowel cleansing:* Orally taken preparations (Picolax®, Fleet) will ensure the bowel is clear for gastrointestinal and some gynaecological procedures. Reduces contamination in open bowel procedures and allows clear view for colonoscopy and sigmoidoscopy. Bowel preparation undertaken by individuals at home prior to admission unless an inpatient where the nurse will ensure application of preparation. *Enema:* May be required for individuals suffering from depressed gastrointestinal activity to prevent postoperative constipation.
Skin	*Shower:* Individuals will be requested to shower before surgery; the nurse will ensure this for inpatient as part of the surgical preparation. Some surgeons require that the shower be performed using antibacterial preparations. *Removal of hair:* Clipping or shaving of hair near the operative site is done as near as possible to the time of surgery, usually in the operating room, to prevent bacterial colonisation due to possible skin scratches. Some authorities state that, unless hair is thick enough to interfere with the surgery, it is preferable to leave it intact. Hair removal is performed by the surgeon, the technician or the nurse. *Antiseptic preparation:* When individual is anaesthetised, and prior to draping, the operative site and beyond is painted with an antiseptic skin preparation of the surgeon's choice. Skin preps may have an aqueous or alcoholic base and are applied by the scrub nurse or the surgeon using sterile gauze pads.
Medication	*Individual's own:* The surgeon or anaesthetist may have temporarily discontinued some or all medications, or adjusted dosages. Otherwise, medications should be given as normal with a minimal amount of water. *Preoperative:* Some medications may be ordered for some individuals. These may be to reduce anxiety (rarely prescribed), reduce secretions (salivary, gastric and bronchial), open airways or provide local constriction of vessels for haemostasis. The nurse needs to be alert to any medications, such as sedation, that should not be given prior to giving instruction to individual, or gaining consent.

(Rothrock 2023; Potter et al 2023; Brown et al 2024)

ward nurse, the operating room nurses, and the PACU nurse. Included for checking on these lists are the other documents that are necessary to remain with the individual such as consent form, X-rays, medication charts, postoperative orders and others. See Figure 42.2 for an example of a preoperative checklist and Clinical Interest Box 42.5 for an example of information about paediatric individuals in the preoperative environment. The nurse must ensure that preoperative checklists are completed in accordance with the healthcare facility's policies and procedures.

INTRAOPERATIVE PHASE

Perioperative nurses undertake a variety of roles within the operating suite. These include circulating (scout) nurse, instrument (scrub) nurse, anaesthetic nurse and post anaesthetic (PACU) nurse (see Table 42.4). The circulating nurse is responsible for the documentation and management of all accountable items opened onto the sterile field. The scout supports the instrument nurse by being aware of the requirements of the surgical team and makes certain all supplies are deposited onto the surgical field aseptically. The circulating nurse performs the surgical count with the instrument nurse, and undertakes other responsibilities including individual positioning, individual safety issues, specimen collection, provision of equipment and being the communication link between theatre staff and those outside. The role of circulating or instrument nurse may be undertaken by an EN or RN. The instrument nurse is the one who assumes primary responsibility and accountability for all items used during the surgical procedure. The instrument nurse sets up all sterile instruments and supplies, and hands instruments to the operating team, anticipating their needs. The individual roles are dependent upon each other to work as part of a multidisciplinary team that aims to provide evidence-based best practice and optimal individual outcomes (ACORN 2023; Brown et al 2024).

Nursing interventions in the **intraoperative** phase also include establishing personal contact and supporting the

DO NOT WRITE IN THIS BINDING MARGIN

Queensland Government

Perioperative Patient Record
Pre-operative Checklist

Facility: ....

(Affix identification label here)

URN:

Family name:

Given name(s):

Address:

Date of birth: Sex: ☐ M ☐ F ☐ I

Date	Time	Weight	Height	BMI	Ward from	Ward to
/ /	:	kg	cm			

Check 1	Check 2 Confirmed	Check 2 Variance	Check 3 Confirmed	Check 3 Variance
Information provided by: ☐ Patient ☐ Substitute decision-maker ☐ Other Name: .... Relationship:				
1 Patient or substitute decision-maker to state full name and DOB and confirm full name, DOB and URN match ID band and medical record ☐ Yes ☐ No (document as variance) Patient's preferred name:				
2 Legal documentation (EPOA, ARP, AHD, other) ☐ Yes (document as variance) ☐ No				
3 Valid procedural consent form completed ☐ Yes ☐ No (document as variance)				
4 Patient or substitute decision-maker to state procedure in own words and confirm procedure stated corresponds with signed consent form ☐ Yes ☐ No (document as variance) Response:				
5 Intended surgical site marked by surgeon ☐ Yes ☐ No (document as variance)				
6 X-rays, medical imaging, PACS ☐ Yes (document as variance) ☐ No				
ALERTS				
7 Allergy or Adverse Drug Reaction ☐ Yes (document as variance) ☐ Nil known				
8 Infection precautions ☐ Yes (document as variance) ☐ No				
9 Cytotoxic medication administered in the last 7 days ☐ Yes (document as variance) ☐ No				
10 Anticoagulant, antiplatelet agent, thrombolytics or any complementary medicines (e.g. fish oil, turmeric) administered in the last 7 days ☐ Yes (document as variance) ☐ No				
11 Patient refuses blood products ☐ Yes (document as variance) ☐ No				
12 Pregnant ☐ Yes ☐ No ☐ Suspected or unknown (document as variance)				
13 Diabetic ☐ Yes (document as variance) ☐ No				
14 Skin assessment ☐ Intact ☐ Not intact (document as variance) ☐ Not assessed (document as variance) **Pressure risk assessment tool completed** ☐ Yes ☐ No (document as variance)				
15 Other alerts (e.g. falls, interpreter, aggression) ☐ Yes (document as variance) ☐ No				
16 Fasted ☐ Yes ☐ No (document as variance) Last food/non-clear fluid intake – Date: ___/___/___ Time: ___:___ Last clear fluid intake – Date: ___/___/___ Time: ___:___				
17 Pre-medication administered ☐ Yes (document as variance) ☐ No **Other usual medication withheld** ☐ Yes (document as variance) ☐ No				
18 Existing implants, prostheses ☐ Yes (document as variance) ☐ No				
19 Caps, crowns, loose teeth, braces or dentures ☐ Yes (document as variance) ☐ No				
20 Personal aids, items ☐ Yes (document as variance) ☐ No				
21 Preparation Surgical attire: ☐ Yes ☐ No (document as variance) Removed or taped jewellery, body jewellery, hair pins, make-up, nail polish, eye lashes: ☐ Yes ☐ No (document as variance) Procedure specific preparation complete: ☐ Yes ☐ No (document as variance) Bowel prep satisfactory: ☐ Not required ☐ Yes ☐ No (document as variance) Anti-embolic devices applied: ☐ Yes ☐ No (document as variance)				
22 Patient continent of urine ☐ Yes ☐ No (document as variance) ☐ IDC in-situ Last void – Time: ___:___				
23 Relevant documentation (e.g. medical record, medical chart, fluid order sheet, fluid balance chart, diabetic chart, 3 sheets of patient labels, observation sheet) ☐ Yes ☐ No (document as variance)				
24 Patient or substitute decision-maker agrees to clinicians discussing the procedure with the nominated support person ☐ Yes ☐ No (document as variance) Support person Name: .... Phone:				

Check 1	Print name:	Designation:	Signature:	Time: ___:___
Check 2	Print name:	Designation:	Signature:	Time: ___:___
Check 3	Print name:	Designation:	Signature:	Time: ___:___

Page 1 of 4

v8.00 - 06/2022
WINC Code: 1NY31477
SW068

PERIOPERATIVE PATIENT RECORD

Figure 42.2 Sample preoperative checklist

(Queensland Health Perioperative Patient Record Version 8.00. © State of Queensland (Queensland Health) 2022)

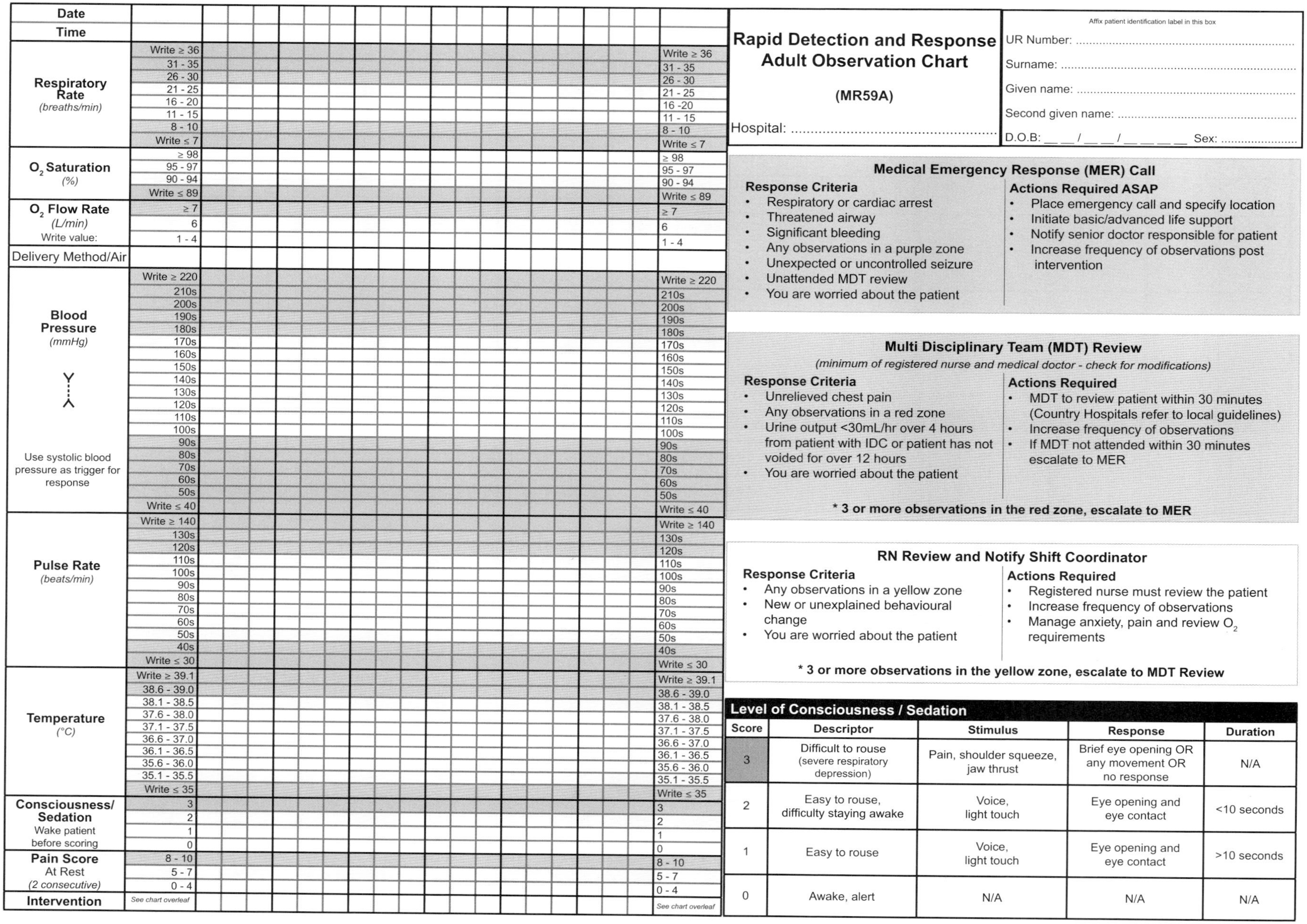

Rapid Detection and Response Adult Observation Chart

(MR59A)

Hospital: ....

Affix patient identification label in this box

UR Number: ....
Surname: ....
Given name: ....
Second given name: ....
D.O.B: __ __/__ __/__ __ __ __ Sex: ....

Date	
Time	
Respiratory Rate (breaths/min)	Write ≥ 36; 31 - 35; 26 - 30; 21 - 25; 16 - 20; 11 - 15; 8 - 10; Write ≤ 7
O_2 Saturation (%)	≥ 98; 95 - 97; 90 - 94; Write ≤ 89
O_2 Flow Rate (L/min) Write value:	≥ 7; 6; 1 - 4
Delivery Method/Air	
Blood Pressure (mmHg) Use systolic blood pressure as trigger for response	Write ≥ 220; 210s; 200s; 190s; 180s; 170s; 160s; 150s; 140s; 130s; 120s; 110s; 100s; 90s; 80s; 70s; 60s; 50s; Write ≤ 40
Pulse Rate (beats/min)	Write ≥ 140; 130s; 120s; 110s; 100s; 90s; 80s; 70s; 60s; 50s; 40s; Write ≤ 30
Temperature (°C)	Write ≥ 39.1; 38.6 - 39.0; 38.1 - 38.5; 37.6 - 38.0; 37.1 - 37.5; 36.6 - 37.0; 36.1 - 36.5; 35.6 - 36.0; 35.1 - 35.5; Write ≤ 35
Consciousness/ Sedation Wake patient before scoring	3; 2; 1; 0
Pain Score At Rest (2 consecutive)	8 - 10; 5 - 7; 0 - 4
Intervention	See chart overleaf

Medical Emergency Response (MER) Call

Response Criteria

- Respiratory or cardiac arrest
- Threatened airway
- Significant bleeding
- Any observations in a purple zone
- Unexpected or uncontrolled seizure
- Unattended MDT review
- You are worried about the patient

Actions Required ASAP

- Place emergency call and specify location
- Initiate basic/advanced life support
- Notify senior doctor responsible for patient
- Increase frequency of observations post intervention

Multi Disciplinary Team (MDT) Review

(minimum of registered nurse and medical doctor - check for modifications)

Response Criteria

- Unrelieved chest pain
- Any observations in a red zone
- Urine output <30mL/hr over 4 hours from patient with IDC or patient has not voided for over 12 hours
- You are worried about the patient

Actions Required

- MDT to review patient within 30 minutes (Country Hospitals refer to local guidelines)
- Increase frequency of observations
- If MDT not attended within 30 minutes escalate to MER

*** 3 or more observations in the red zone, escalate to MER**

RN Review and Notify Shift Coordinator

Response Criteria

- Any observations in a yellow zone
- New or unexplained behavioural change
- You are worried about the patient

Actions Required

- Registered nurse must review the patient
- Increase frequency of observations
- Manage anxiety, pain and review O_2 requirements

*** 3 or more observations in the yellow zone, escalate to MDT Review**

Level of Consciousness / Sedation

Score	Descriptor	Stimulus	Response	Duration
3	Difficult to rouse (severe respiratory depression)	Pain, shoulder squeeze, jaw thrust	Brief eye opening OR any movement OR no response	N/A
2	Easy to rouse, difficulty staying awake	Voice, light touch	Eye opening and eye contact	<10 seconds
1	Easy to rouse	Voice, light touch	Eye opening and eye contact	>10 seconds
0	Awake, alert	N/A	N/A	N/A

Figure 43.2 Rapid detection and response adult observation chart
(SA Health 2020)

Continued

Rapid Detection and Response Adult Observation Chart

(MR59A)

Hospital: ....

Affix patient identification label in this box

UR Number: ....
Surname: ....
Given name: ....
Second given name: ....
D.O.B: __ __ / __ __ / __ __ __ __ Sex: ....

Chart Number:

General Instructions

You must record appropriate observations:

- On admission
- At a frequency appropriate for the patient's clinical state but not less than once/shift for acute inpatients
- As per local procedures with a minimum of once daily for patients awaiting discharge placement.

You must record a set of observations including a minimum of respiratory rate, blood pressure, pulse rate, temperature, oxygen saturation and level of consciousness/sedation:

- If the patient is deteriorating or an observation is in a shaded area
- Whenever you are worried about the patient.

Review is required for unrelieved and unexpected pain that continues to trigger escalation for 2 consecutive values despite medication administration.

When graphing observations, place a dot (•) in the centre of the box which includes the current observation in its range of values and connect it to the previous dot with a straight line. If observations fall above or below graphic parameters, write the value in relevant box. For systolic blood pressure, use the symbol indicated on the graphic chart.

Whenever an observation falls within a shaded area, you must initiate the actions required for that colour, unless a modification has been made.

Modifications

If abnormal observations are to be tolerated for the patient's clinical condition, write the acceptable ranges and rationale (where a response will not be triggered) below. Duration of modification must be specified.

	Modification 1	Modification 2	Modification 3	Modification 4
Date	/ /	/ /	/ /	/ /
Time	:	:	:	:
Duration				
Observation(s) and acceptable range				
Brief Rationale *(Full description in medical record)*				
Doctor's Signature				
Doctor's Name *(print)*				
Doctor's Designation				
Nurse Signature				
Nurse Name *(print)*				
Nurse Designation				

Resuscitation Orders as Per Medical Records:

Full Resus: ☐ Modified Resus*: ☐ NFR*: ☐

Transcribed from Medical Records by: Signature .... Name..........

**If modified or NFR, look in patient's medical records.*

RDR Adult Observation Chart

MR59A

Rapid Detection and Response Adult Observation Chart

(MR59A)

Hospital: ....

Affix patient identification label in this box

UR Number: ....
Surname: ....
Given name: ....
Second given name: ....
D.O.B: __ __ / __ __ / __ __ __ __ Sex: ....

Additional Observations

Date																		
Time																		
Initials																		
Designation																		

Interventions or Review

If you administer an intervention or review, record here and note letter in intervention row over page in appropriate time column.		Initial *Please print*	Designation
a			
b			
c			
d			
e			
f			
g			
h			

Figure 43.2, cont'd

CLINICAL INTEREST BOX 43.2 Rapid detection and response escalation of care

Yellow zone

If an individual's observations enter the yellow zone, an RN must review the individual within 30 minutes and frequency of observations must be increased. Three or more observations in the yellow zone require escalation to the next level.

Red zone

If an individual's observations enter the red zone, an MDT review is required within 30 minutes, comprising at least a medical officer and an RN, and the frequency of observations must be increased. Three or more observations in the red zone require escalation to the next level.

Purple zone

If an individual's observations enter the purple zone, a medical emergency response is required, where clinical staff with advanced life support skills will be called to resuscitate the individual. In this instance, the senior doctor responsible for the individual must be notified of the event. Increase frequency of observations post intervention. Take advice from the medical emergency response team.

(SA Health 2020)

BASIC LIFE SUPPORT

Basic life support (BLS) is a temporary measure providing myocardial and cerebral oxygenation until **advanced life support (ALS)** personnel and equipment are available (Department of Health & Human Services 2021; Australian and New Zealand Committee on Resuscitation [ANZCOR] 2021e). Early detection of an individual's physiological deterioration and prevention of cardiac arrest are now key strategies recognised for individual survival rates in hospitals. Identification of an unresponsive individual using the acronym DRS ABCD (**d**angers, **r**esponsive, **s**end for help, open **a**irway, normal **b**reathing, start **C**PR, attach **d**efibrillator) should be followed (ANZCOR 2021e). (See Figure 43.3 and Clinical Interest Box 43.4.)

BLS includes airway management skills, rescue breathing techniques, external cardiac compressions and use of the automatic external defibrillator (AED) (ANZCOR 2021d; 2021e). The ARC states that for every minute that defibrillation is delayed there is an approximated 10% reduction in survival rate. It is recommended an AED is attached to the person as soon as possible. The application of an AED is a link in the chain of survival (ANZCOR 2021d). The Australian and New Zealand Committee on Resuscitation (ANZCOR) guideline 10.1 states that 'all those trained in CPR should refresh their skills annually' (ANZCOR 2023c). Clinical Interest Box 43.5 outlines the contents of a resuscitation trolley.

CLINICAL INTEREST BOX 43.3 Rapid response team flowchart

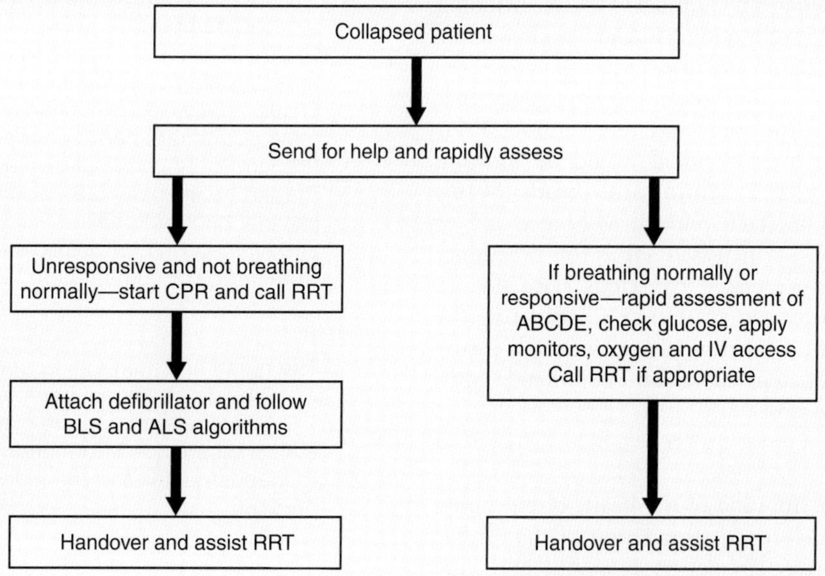

ALS = advanced life support; BLS = basic life support; CPR = cardiopulmonary resuscitation; RRT = rapid response team

(ARC 2024)

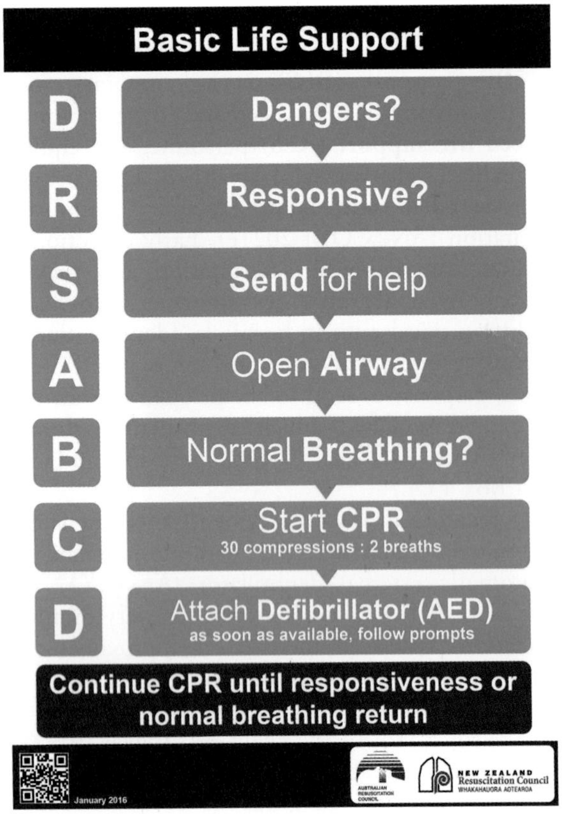

Figure 43.3 Basic life support
(ANZCOR 2023b)

Indications

Basic life support is indicated in cardiac or respiratory arrest.

Respiratory arrest

Respiratory arrest can result from a number of causes, including stroke, drug overdose, suffocation, foreign body airway obstruction, injuries, infection and myocardial infarction.

Respiratory arrest is a life-threatening emergency that requires immediate identification and intervention. Prior to a respiratory arrest, the individual would be showing signs of deterioration such as shortness of breath (SOB), increased respiratory rate (tachypnoea), associated use of accessory muscles due to increased effort of breathing, cyanosis, confusion or decreased conscious state due to hypoxia and decreased oxygen saturation. Considering the DRS ABCD algorithm, if breathing is not normal, ensure the establishment of a patent airway and commence compressions. (See Figure 43.3.)

Cardiac arrest

A **cardiac arrest** is the stopping of the heart, often caused by a disruption to the electrical stimulation of the cardiac muscle. In cardiac arrest, circulation is absent and vital organs are deprived of oxygen, resulting in death if not treated promptly. Effective CPR and application of an AED

CLINICAL INTEREST
BOX 43.4 Summary of guidelines for responding to the initial phase of resuscitation

First person present

1. Assess the area for danger.
2. Check the individual for response and conscious state.
3. If the individual is unresponsive, call for assistance and press the emergency bell to summon help.
4. Assess the airway, clear obstructions and perform airway-opening manoeuvre.
5. Check for normal breathing. If unresponsive and not breathing normally, commence CPR with 30 chest compressions followed by two ventilations.
6. Continue CPR until the MET team arrives or signs of life (responsiveness, starts moving and normal breathing) return.

Second person present

1. Collect the emergency trolley/AED.
2. Attach AED as soon as possible and follow its prompts. Ensure that the compressions are not interrupted while attaching the AED.
3. Connect bag-valve-mask and attach high-flow oxygen.
4. Assist with CPR.

Additional actions that may be taken by other staff during the initial phase of resuscitation

- Dial switchboard/emergency number and state as per institution protocol:
  - Type of emergency (e.g. MET, code blue medical).
  - Location of the emergency: ward, room and bed number.
- Get the individual's healthcare record and the nurse looking after the individual if this is not you.
- Ensure that working suction is available. Have at hand equipment needed for possible intubation.
- Prepare for IV cannulation if no IV cannula in situ. Prepare IV line with 0.9% sodium chloride.
- Have at hand adrenaline, atropine, lignocaine and amiodarone for possible administration.
- Commence documentation.

Other

- The nurse unit manager or senior nurse will:
  - Provide additional personnel if required.
  - Coordinate telephone communications.
- Staff shall provide information and support to friends/relatives of the individual who are present.

CLINICAL INTEREST BOX 43.5 Emergency trolley contents—adult

Note: Content and drawer location may differ slightly according to trolley used in hospital.

All components (gloves, masks, bagging circuits) on the arrest trolley should be latex free.

Top of trolley

- Defibrillator/monitor note: To be checked daily for 'OK' symbol
- Defibrillator pads (minimum three, check expiry)
- Packet ECG electrodes (in a plastic bag)
- ECG leads
- Self-inflating resuscitation bag-valve-mask system with PEEP valve, O_2 reservoir and tubing, size 5 clear face mask attached
- Sharps container (< ¾ full)/clinical waste bag
- Gloves/goggles/aprons/face shield

Side of trolley

- Emergency trolley contents list/checking folder/cardiac arrest record sheets
- C-size oxygen cylinder with Twin-O-Vac suction unit (**note:** Cylinder to be at least ¾ full pressure of 350 mmHg)
- Suction tubing with Yankauer sucker attached
- Nurse initiated ALS chart

Back of trolley

- IV pole
- 2 × tourniquets (latex free)
- Cardiac arrest backboard
- Bougie (a thin, flexible surgical instrument for exploring or dilating a passage of the body) (this must not be stored bent)

Airway and breathing drawer

- Yankauer sucker
- Y-suction catheters sizes 12F × 2 and 14F
- Endotracheal tubes: sizes 6, 7, 8, 9 introducing stylet
- Laryngoscope with size 4 blade attached (with spare batteries and globes)
- Laryngoscope with size 3 blade attached
- Magill intubating forceps
- Tracheostomy tubes sizes 6–10 mm
- Tracheal dilating forceps
- Cotton tape
- End-tidal CO_2 monitor
- Guarded artery forceps
- 10 mL syringe
- Oropharyngeal airways sizes 2, 3, 4, 5
- Nasopharyngeal airways sizes 6, 7
- Laryngeal mask sizes 4, 5
- Water-based lubricant sachets
- Scissors
- Cuff pressure manometer
- Lignocaine spray 10%

Note: Check that both laryngoscope blade globes are functioning.

Circulation drawer

- Heparinised blood gas syringes
- 21G, 23G, 25G and 18G drawing-up needles
- 10 mL syringes
- 10 mL 0.9% sodium chloride ampoules
- Interlink vial access cannula
- UEC/electrolyte vacutainer
- FBC vacutainer
- Blood cross-match vacutainer
- Vacutainer holder
- Vacutainer needle adaptor
- Alcohol wipes
- IV cannulas: 14G, 16G, 18G, 20G
- Intraosseous access
- Transpore tape
- Small transparent dressings
- Needleless access Luer lock
- 20 drops/mL solution infusion set
- Blood/solution administration pump
- Hartmann's 1000 mL
- Gelofusine 500 mL
- Dextrose 5% 1000 mL
- 0.9% sodium chloride 1000 mL

Medications drawer

First-line drugs

- Epinephrine/adrenaline 1 mg (1:10,000)
- Atropine 1 mg
- Amiodarone 150 mg ampoules and 5% glucose 100 mL
- Lignocaine 100 mg.

Intravenous medications

- Adenosine 6 mg
- Epinephrine/adrenaline 1 mg (1:10,000)
- Epinephrine/adrenaline 1 mg (1:1000)
- Amiodarone 150 mg ampoules
- Calcium chloride 10% 1 g/10 mL (6.8 mmol/10 mL)
- Diazepam 10 mg/2 mL
- Glucose 50%
- Magnesium sulphate 2.5 g/5 mL
- Midazolam 10 mg
- Naloxone hydrochloride 400 microg
- Potassium chloride
- Propofol 200 mg/20 mL
- Sodium bicarbonate 8.4% 100 mL
- Vasopressin 20 units/mL

Other medications/equipment

- Salbutamol 5 mg nebules
- Ipratropium 500 microg nebules

Continued

CLINICAL INTEREST BOX 43.5 Emergency trolley contents—adult—cont'd

- Nebuliser device and mask
- Sublingual GTN
- Aspirin 300 mg
- Furosemide/frusemide 20 mg
- Medication labels

Note: Check expiry date of all drugs.

Extras drawer

- Clear face masks: sizes 3, 4, 5
- Slide sheet for safe transfer
- Australian resuscitation guidelines

(Adapted from ARC 2014 and Queensland Health 2022)

are of the highest priority (ANZCOR 2021d). Cardiac arrest may occur both in and out of the hospital environment. Over 25,000 out-of-hospital cardiac arrests occur annually in Australia (Bray et al 2022). Implementation of the chain of survival is vital.

The causes of cardiac arrest are numerous. A 'heart attack' can lead to the development of a cardiac arrest but the two are different; this will be discussed later in the chapter.

The main precipitating conditions associated with cardiac arrest can be simplified by the 4Hs and 4Ts (ANZCOR 2021h):

- hypoxaemia
- hypovolaemia
- hyper/hypokalaemia (metabolic disorders)
- hypo/hyperthermia
- tension pneumothorax
- tamponade
- toxins/poisons/drugs
- thrombosis (pulmonary embolism or coronary thrombus leading to myocardial infarction).

Cardiac arrest can be associated with different cardiac rhythms:

- ventricular fibrillation (VF)
- pulseless ventricular tachycardia (VT)
- asystole
- other rhythms but without cardiac output—referred to as pulseless electrical activity (PEA).

Cardiopulmonary resuscitation

Cardiopulmonary resuscitation (CPR) is the technique of chest compressions and the delivery of rescue breaths to maintain sufficient circulation for perfusion of the brain until ALS is available.

CPR is initiated when the individual is unconscious and breathing is not normal. (See Clinical Skill 43.1.)

Defibrillation

Defibrillation is incorporated into BLS. The use of a defibrillator can revert some selected abnormal rhythms associated with cardiac arrest. Defibrillation is indicated for:

- ventricular fibrillation (VF)
- ventricular tachycardia (VT).

Defibrillation is the therapeutic delivery of electrical current to the myocardium. A defibrillator delivers a targeted burst of electrical energy that 'shocks' and produces near-simultaneous depolarisation of a mass of myocardial cells, momentarily ceasing all cardiac activity. The hope is that a functioning site in the heart's conduction system will then start a normal pattern of electrical activity (Goyal et al 2024).

Ventricular fibrillation (VF) (Figure 43.4) is a life-threatening cardiac arrhythmia. Rapid erratic electrical impulses that originate in the ventricles cause the ventricles to fibrillate, or quiver. There are no organised P waves or QRS complexes (ventricular contractions) and so there can be no **cardiac output**, which means there is no circulating blood to the brain and muscles, resulting in the individual becoming unconscious within seconds. The causes may include structural causes (resulting in myocardial ischaemia) or conditions such as electrolyte imbalances, acidosis, hypothermia, hypoxia, cardiomyopathies, alcohol use and electrical conduction abnormalities (Ludhwani et al 2024).

Ventricular tachycardia (VT) (Figure 43.5) is rapid arrhythmia (greater than 100 beats per minute) originating from the ventricles, resulting in wide QRS complexes (Foth et al 2024). Such a rapid heart rate means the ventricles are unable to adequately fill and therefore pump, leading to poor cardiac output, circulation and unconsciousness. VT is often a consequence of ischaemia and myocardial infarction, though it can also be triggered by electrolyte imbalance, sepsis and metabolic acidosis and can quickly deteriorate into VF (Foth et al 2024).

Asystole is characterised by the absence of any electrical activity. On the ECG monitor, this is sometimes referred to as 'flat line'. A flat line on a monitor can be due to operator error or equipment failure—always rapidly check the individual for signs of life before troubleshooting the monitor. Asystole cannot be treated with the defibrillator, so CPR should recommence and the team should focus on treating the reversible causes (4Hs and 4Ts) (ANZCOR 2021h).

Pulseless electrical activity (PEA) (previously known as electromechanical dissociation) occurs when an ECG rhythm that might normally be associated with having a cardiac output is observed on the electrocardiogram (ECG) but does not produce a pulse. PEA can come in many different forms. Sinus rhythm, tachycardia and bradycardia can all be seen with PEA. Again, check the individual first. Performing a pulse check after a rhythm/monitor check will ensure that you identify PEA in every situation. PEA usually has an underlying treatable cause. Hypoxia (due to respiratory failure) and hypovolaemia are high priority causes to address (Oliver et al 2024).

CLINICAL SKILL 43.1 Cardiopulmonary resuscitation/basic life support (BLS)

Please adhere to the policy and procedures of the facility/organisation prior to undertaking the skill. Ensure this skill is in your scope of practice.

NMBA Decision-making Framework considerations (refer to NMBA Decision-making framework for nursing and midwifery 2020):	**Equipment:**
1. Am I educated? 2. Am I authorised? 3. Am I competent? If you answer 'no' to any of these, do not perform that activity. Seek guidance and support from your teacher/a nurse team leader/clinical facilitator/educator.	Airway equipment (bag-valve-mask, pocket mask) PPE (goggles, disposable gloves, gown and face shield) Resuscitation trolley (if available) Automated external defibrillator

PREPARE FOR THE SKILL

(Please refer to the Standard Steps on pp. xviii–xx for related rationales.)
Mentally review the steps of the skill.
Discuss the skill with your instructor/supervisor/team leader, if required.
Confirm correct facility/organisation policy/safe operating procedures.
Validate the order in the individual's record.
Identify indication and rationale for performing the activity.
Assess for any contraindications.
Locate and gather equipment.
Perform hand hygiene.
Ensure therapeutic interaction.
Identify the individual using three individual identifiers.
Gain the individual's consent.
Assess for pain relief.
Prepare the environment.
Provide and maintain privacy.
Assist the individual to assume an appropriate position of comfort.

PERFORM THE SKILL

(Please refer to the Standard Steps on pp. xviii–xx for related rationales.)
Perform hand hygiene.
Apply PPE: gloves, eyewear, mask and gown as appropriate.
Ensure the individual's safety and comfort throughout skill.
Promote independence and involvement of the individual if possible and/or appropriate.
Assess the individual's tolerance to the skill throughout.
Dispose of used supplies, equipment, waste and sharps appropriately.
Remove PPE and discard or store appropriately.
Perform hand hygiene.

Skill activity	**Rationale**
Danger	
Recognise an emergency situation. Identify potential/real dangers. Ensure area is safe.	Ensures the environment is safe to attend BLS for self and others involved, including the individual.
Response	
Assess individual's conscious status by appropriate tactile and verbal stimulus (using a simple command [i.e. gently shaking and speaking loudly, giving simple commands such as 'Open your eyes, squeeze my hand']. Then grasp and squeeze the individual's shoulders firmly). Identify whether the individual is rousable or unconscious.	Assesses whether the individual is conscious or unconscious, and CPR is commenced appropriately. Using simple commands, and not shaking the individual, helps to maintain spinal precautions and prevent any further injuries.

Continued

CLINICAL SKILL 43.1 Cardiopulmonary resuscitation/basic life support (BLS)—cont'd

Send	
Identify how to send for help/trigger the alarm within the workplace. Describe the local clinical emergency response system protocols. Note the time. Identify the explicit relevant numbers used within the workplace for emergencies. If in a community setting, call emergency services.	Allows support to be activated and provides assistance and help with the individual. Allows for expert support to arrive quickly.
Airway	
Assess airway for obstruction. Clear airway (describing different methods [i.e. suction/ head turn, or roll individual on to their side]. Maintain C-spine precautions. Perform chin lift, jaw thrust or head tilt manoeuvre to open airway.	Assessing airway and removing debris allows for a patent airway and ensures oxygen/rescue breaths can effectively be administered to the individual. Only roll the individual if airway obstruction is seen; reduces time to start compressions, if required.
Breathing	
Maintain open airway. Assess breathing for maximum 10 seconds. Look, listen and feel technique performed. Look for chest rise and fall. Listen for outflow of air from mouth and/or nose. Feel outflow of air and chest movement.	Minimises the amount of time to assess individual's breathing, decreases the amount of downtime and oxygen-poor system. Reduces risk of hypoxia. Look, listen and feel technique is easy to perform and assesses breathing simultaneously.
Circulation	
In the absence of normal breathing commence CPR. For effective chest compressions the individual should be placed in a flat position, with a hard surface underneath. Commence compression using both hands on the centre of the chest. Correct hand position, one hand in centre of chest (heel of the hand) and the other hand on top. Maintain correct posture/alignment (arms straight and shoulder over chest, using hips as pivot point). Perform cardiac compression to one-third of the chest depth with a rate of 100–120/min. At 30 compressions, give two rescue breaths (1 second per breath) using appropriate workplace equipment. If unwilling/unable for perform rescue breaths, continue chest compressions only. Demonstrate appropriate mask positioning, showing good seal (two-person technique if required). Maintain cardiac compressions/rescue breaths at a ratio of 30:2. Demonstrate or state when the person performing compressions should be rotated (every 2-minute cycle, when two or more rescuers or signs of fatigue).	To provide effective cardiac compressions, hand placement is essential. One hand over the other, arms straight and shoulders over chest decreases the risk of fatigue and creates a greater chance of completing CPR for a 2-minute cycle. One hand wrapped around the dominant wrist is preferable. Compressions to one-third of the chest allow for effective pressure on the heart to pump blood around the body and deliver oxygen to vital organs. A hard surface increases compression depth; only place on hard surface if adequate staff present to do so efficiently, reducing lost compression time. A ratio of 30 compressions to two breaths maintains sufficient oxygen in the bloodstream to be pumped around the body. Proper mask positioning will ensure full delivery of oxygen or rescue breaths.

CLINICAL SKILL 43.1 Cardiopulmonary resuscitation/basic life support (BLS)—cont'd

Defibrillation	
Attach an automated external defibrillator (AED) as soon as able, turn on and follow voice prompts. Communicate safety considerations—pad placement (not over pacemaker), individual unconscious, not in contact with fluid, chest clear and dry (shave and dry chest before applying pads firmly if good contact is required between pads and individual), pads rolled onto chest, remove metal/medication patches. Demonstrate correct pad placement, sternum right parasternal 2nd intercostal space, apex: mid-axillary 6th intercostal space. Or anterior–posterior positioning. If shock advised: Scan the environment and individual for danger, ensure all persons are clear of individual and environment; verbalise before administering the shock to the individual. State safety considerations (oxygen removed, nil contact with metal, and individual is unresponsive at time of shock delivery). Safely administer shock as per AED prompts. When safe, immediately recommence CPR, post-delivery of shock. Continue to follow voice prompts until help arrives.	Immediately attach the AED when able (*while CPR is in progress*) to determine if individual needs to be shocked. The sooner the shocks can be administered, the better the outcome. Attaching the AED allows the machine to quickly identify a shockable rhythm and provide prompts. Rapid defibrillation is associated with long-term survival. Understanding the safety consideration for persons involved and the individual will ensure minimal risk of potential injuries/dangers. Correct pad placement ensures that the shock(s) are delivered more effectively. Consider safety precautions—environment is clear, persons involved are clear, oxygen is removed—to minimise the risk of potential risks/dangers. Oxygen removal also reduces risk of fire/explosion during defibrillation. Recommence CPR when safe, post shock delivery, to minimise the amount of time between effective CPR applications.
Communication	
Communicate to rapid response/ALS/ambulance team in ISBAR format. State when it is appropriate to cease BLS/CPR (response of life, medical officer pronounces time of death, physically impossible to continue, danger stopping any further rescue attempts). Communicate progress with relatives/significant others where appropriate.	Effective communication to further support services will help continue effective treatment of the individual. Understanding when it is appropriate to cease CPR/BLS avoids unnecessary length of CPR and decreases chance of injury to persons involved.

AFTER THE SKILL

(Please refer to the Standard Steps on pp. xviii–xx for related rationales.)
Communicate outcome to the individual any ongoing care and to report any complications.
Restore the environment.
Report, record and document assessment findings, details of the skill performed and the individual's response.
Report, record and document any abnormalities and/or inability to perform the skill.
Reassess the individual to ensure there are no adverse effects/events from the skill.

If the event occurs in a healthcare facility, document in healthcare record onset of arrest, medication and other treatments given, procedure performed and individual's response, plan of care (i.e. transferred to ICU). Include names and roles of staff present.	Informs all healthcare professionals of what occurred and allows for appropriate care to be planned and implemented. Accurate documentation is informative and supports the implementation of ongoing planning and care.

(ANZCOR 2021e; ARC 2024; Rebeiro et al 2021)

Initial steps of resuscitation in BLS

The initial steps of resuscitation can be remembered with DRS ABCD (ANZCOR 2021e).

Danger

Prior to commencing BLS personnel should consider safety:

- Check for hazards, electrical and fluid spills.
- Safely dispose of sharps.
- Appropriate personal protective equipment (PPE).
- Safe manual handling principles.

Response

Check for response of an individual who has collapsed by giving a loud, simple command, 'open your eyes', or squeeze their shoulder. If they are conscious and respond

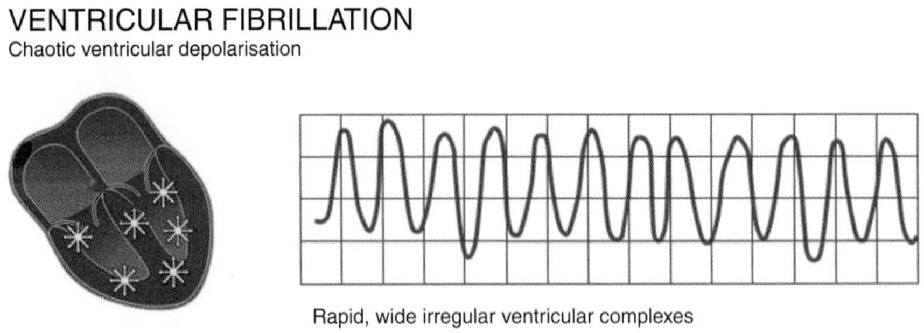

VENTRICULAR FIBRILLATION
Chaotic ventricular depolarisation
Rapid, wide irregular ventricular complexes

Figure 43.4 Ventricular fibrillation
(Malmivuo & Plonsey 1995, Fig 19.3C)

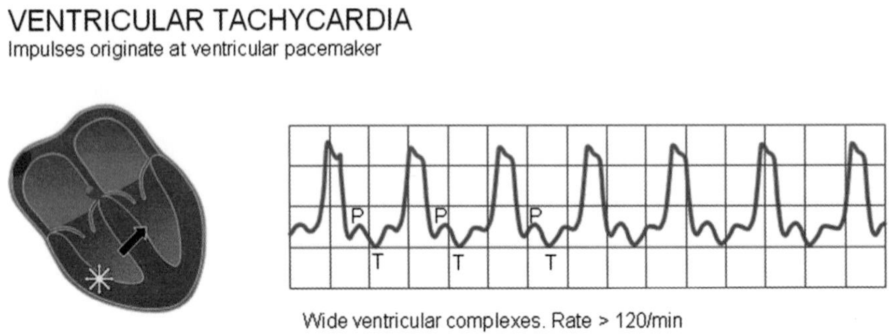

Impulses originate at ventricular pacemaker

Figure 43.5 Ventricular tachycardia
(Malmivuo & Plonsey 1995, Fig 19.3B)

to commands, keep the person in a comfortable and safe environment. Continue to observe closely—think of the ABCDE assessment described earlier.

If unresponsive—does not respond to verbal commands, does not move—continue DRS ABCD algorithm. (See Case Study 43.1.)

Send

Make sure help is coming—send someone to get help, or use a telephone. If in hospital, activate the emergency response system.

Airway

Ensure the individual is on their back and open their airway by using the head tilt-chin lift manoeuvre (ANZCOR 2021a). The mouth should be opened and turned slightly downwards to allow foreign material to drain. A finger sweep to remove observable foreign body obstruction may be done; however, there is risk of injury to the rescuer, so utilise suction if available (ANZCOR 2021a). The person may be turned on their side if the airway needs to be cleared. Consider: 'Airway management takes precedence over any suspected spinal injury' (ANZCOR 2021f).

Breathing

Once the airway has been opened, look, listen and feel for *normal* breathing:

- Look for chest movement of the upper abdomen/lower chest.
- Listen for air movement from nose and mouth.
- Feel for air movement at mouth and nose.

Be aware, individuals often emit *agonal gasps* during cardiac arrest (ANZCOR 2021b). This is not actually breathing—which is why the guidance is to assess for *normal* breathing.

Circulation

If a person is not breathing normally and is unresponsive, commence CPR. CPR should be commenced with 30 chest compressions followed by two breaths and continued with a ratio of 30:2.

- A resuscitation mask can be used with a one-way, non-return valve.
- If using a pocket mask, attach oxygen with a flow rate of 10 L/min.

The person performing chest compressions should:

- Place the heel of their hand in the *centre of the chest* with the other hand on top.
- Aim to depress approximately *one third the depth of the chest* each compression.
- Push at a rate of *100 to 120 compressions per minute.*

(ANZCOR 2021c)

Depth of compression

For compressions to be effective, they need to be deep enough to compress the heart. In an adult, this is ⅓ of the chest depth, which is about 5 cm. Inadequate chest compression depth is associated with poor outcomes. Complete recoil of the chest after each compression allows for filling of the heart. The time

CASE STUDY 43.1

As you walk into Mr Wilson's room and say good morning, you notice he doesn't give you the cheery greeting you are used to hearing from him, and he looks quite unwell. You decide to start an ABCDE assessment:

A—Mr Wilson's airway looks normal, with no foreign bodies or liquids and no swelling. His voice sounds normal.

B—You conduct a RATES assessment:
Respiratory rate—33 breaths/min
Air entry—bilateral normal breath sounds
Trachea—midline
Effort—no accessory muscle use

C—Mr Wilson's pulse feels week. The heart rate is 111 beats/min. You find his blood pressure is 88/47 mmHg.

D—Mr Wilson is responding to voice (aVpu).

E—You don't see any rashes, trauma or signs of bleeding. Temperature is 38.7°C.

1. Which important vital sign has not yet been assessed?
2. What could be causing this clinical picture? Think of three important causes.
3. What interventions would you consider for B and C?
4. While you are working with the team to assist Mr Wilson, you notice his eyes roll back, and he slumps back in the bed. What will you do?

allowed for recoil should be the same amount of time it takes to perform a chest compression (ANZCOR 2021c).

Rate of compressions

Chest compressions for all ages are at a rate of approximately 100–120/min. When performing compressions, if feasible, change rescuers at least every 2 minutes to prevent rescuer fatigue and deterioration in chest compression quality and depth, with consideration given to minimising interruptions to compressions (ANZCOR 2021c).

Rescue breathing during compressions

After 30 chest compressions have been performed, pause to deliver two rescue breaths, and then continue compressions (a ratio of 30:2). These may be mouth to mouth, mouth to mask or, if trained, preferably with a bag-valve-mask (ANZCOR 2021b).

Continue this management until circulation returns or the decision to stop resuscitation is made by the resuscitation team leader (ANZCOR 2021e). See Figure 43.3 for the ARC guideline on CPR.

Defibrillation

Attaching an automated external defibrillator (AED) is important for the individual receiving CPR. A defibrillator is more likely to be successful the earlier it is attempted and training is not required for its use.

The AED:

- automatically prompts the user regarding intervention.
- automatically analyses the heart rhythm.
- advises and prompts the user to deliver a shock only if needed.

(See Clinical Interest Box 43.6.)

Some AEDs have a manual override feature allowing responders with greater skill (e.g. critical care-trained staff) to have more control over defibrillation. The AED should be connected to the person once they are determined to be unconscious and not breathing normally (ANZCOR 2021d).

Preparation of skin prior to pad placement

- Ensure the surface of the individual's skin is dry.
- Remove chest hair if required.
- Do not delay defibrillation if shaving equipment is not available.
- Remove any medication patches.
- Remove jewellery.
- Check for implanted devices (pacemakers).

Placement of the pads

When applying AED pads (see Figure 43.6):

- Place one pad slightly below the collar bone on the right side of the chest and one below the armpit (the pads will have a picture to assist).
- Avoid placing pads over implantable devices (e.g. cardiac pacemaker), dressings or patches. If there is an implantable device, the defibrillator pad should be placed at least 8 cm from the device.
- In large-breasted women, the left electrode or paddle may be placed lateral to the left breast.

(ANZCOR 2021d)

Defibrillator safety

Follow the prompts of the device. Ensure no-one is touching the individual during delivery of a shock. After a shock, the AED will provide a prompt to continue CPR. If signs of life become evident, including the return of a palpable pulse,

CLINICAL INTEREST BOX 43.6 Use of AEDs

The use of AEDs by trained lay and professional responders is recommended to increase survival rates in victims with cardiac arrest. Check local organisation policy regarding AED training since usually annual training with demonstration of knowledge and skills assessment is a requirement. Please note the ANZCOR (2021d) states that 'AED use should not be restricted to trained personnel. Allowing the use of AEDs by individuals without prior formal training can be beneficial and may be lifesaving.'

(ANZCOR 2021d)

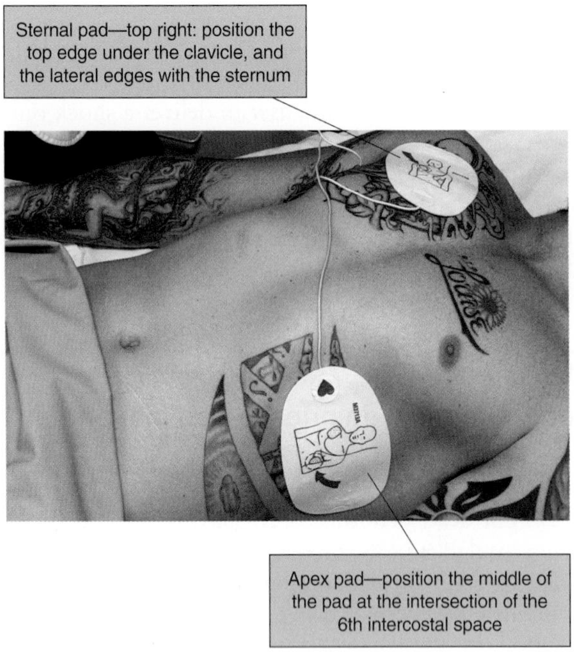
Sternal pad—top right: position the top edge under the clavicle, and the lateral edges with the sternum
Apex pad—position the middle of the pad at the intersection of the 6th intercostal space

Figure 43.6 AED pad placement

On large-breasted women, the left electrode may be placed lateral to or underneath the left breast.

(© Elsevier Australia)

successful resuscitation has occurred (at least temporarily) and post-resuscitation care can begin.

> **CRITICAL THINKING EXERCISE 43.2**
>
> Safety is important during a resuscitation. Imagine you discover an individual who has suffered a cardiac arrest while sitting out of bed in a chair. How will you resuscitate this individual and keep them, yourself and the team safe?

POST-RESUSCITATION CARE

Resuscitation does not stop after the return of a spontaneous circulation (ROSC)—these individuals are very unstable and may arrest again. It is important to assess them using the ABCDE algorithm. In addition:

- Continue supporting airway and breathing. Aim for SpO_2 94–98%.
- Aim for blood pressure greater than 100 mm/Hg—this may require medication or intravenous fluids.
- Continue to treat underlying cause/s, with consideration given to the 4Ts and 4Hs.
- Individuals who are unresponsive may require cooling to a targeted temperature to improve neurological outcomes post cardiac arrest.

(ANZCOR 2021i)

Detailed assessment of the individual and ongoing monitoring of:

- serum bloods to assess electrolyte, metabolic imbalances and blood glucose levels
- arterial blood gases to assess for hypoxia, hypocapnia (cerebral ischaemia) and acidosis.
- 12-lead electrocardiograph, to assess myocardial damage
- chest X-ray
- escalation of the person's care to a specific care unit such as intensive care (ICU), coronary care (CCU) or high dependency (HDU).

Emotional care

The EN may be involved in the care of an individual who suffers a cardiac arrest or clinical deterioration at any point. The EN may be present when medical staff explain to the family/carer or next of kin about the event and treatment plan. Nurses are skilled at helping family/significant others to understand and come to terms with a resuscitation event. Individuals who survive resuscitation can experience anxiety and depression as well as post-traumatic stress disorder (PTSD) related to the event and may need help in understanding what has happened to them, the immediate consequences and their future (Sawyer et al 2020). Nurses can provide care and support to individuals and family carers as it arises. Discussion of pastoral care services or a social worker are also within the scope of practice for the EN.

In-hospital medical emergency team documentation

The legal requirement for nurses to document individual care accurately and concisely is clear in the professional standards produced by governing and regulatory bodies. Treatment sequences including the 'who', 'what', 'where' and 'when' of interventions, and subsequent individual responses must be documented accurately; these standards specifically mention clinical handover and communication with members of the MDT (NMBA 2016). (See Figure 43.7.)

> **CRITICAL THINKING EXERCISE 43.3**
>
> If you saw the ECG tracing below, what would you do?

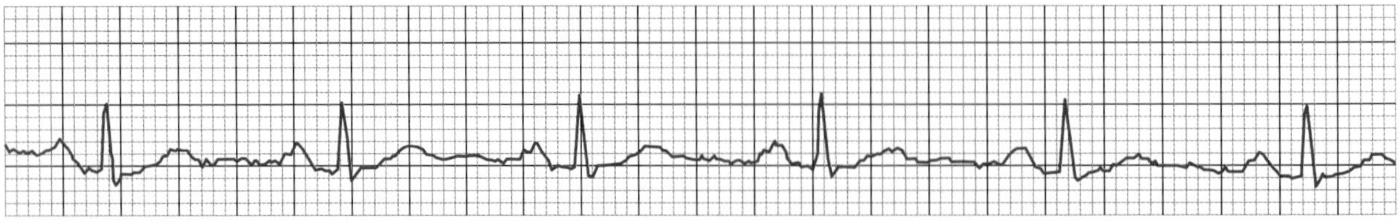

Respond MET Record

UR Number ______________________

Surname ______________________

Given Name(s) ______________________

Date of Birth ______________________

AFFIX PATIENT LABEL HERE

(Identify) Primary Nurse's name ______________ Date: ___ /___ /___ Time: _____ Ward: __________

(Situation) Why was the MET called?

- ☐ Obstructed airway
- ☐ Any difficulty breathing
- ☐ Breathing < 6 breaths / min
- ☐ Heart rate < 40 beats / min
- ☐ Patient cannot be roused
- ☐ Severe bleeding > 100 mls/hr
- ☐ Noisy breathing / Stridor
- ☐ SaO_2 < 90% despite 10L oxygen
- ☐ Breathing > 25 breaths / min
- ☐ Heart rate > 120 beats / min
- ☐ Prolonged seizures
- ☐ Worried / other ______________
- ☐ Problems with tracheostomy tube
- ☐ Urine output < 50mL in 4 hrs
- ☐ Systolic blood pressure < 90mmHg
- ☐ Sudden change in conscious state
- ☐ Severe / uncontrolled pain

(Background) Past History ______________________

____

Reasons for hospital admission ______________________

(Assessment)

____

ABBREVIATIONS FOR MANAGEMENT (below):

AIRWAY	Patient Maintained (PM), Guedel (G), Assisted Jaw Thrust/Chin Lift(AL), Intubated (ETT), Other (O)
BREATHING	Spontaneous breathing (SB), Bag Mask Ventilation (BMV), Mechanically Ventilated (MV), Non-Invasive Ventilation (NIV)
CIRCULATION	Rhythm: Sinus Rhythm (SR), Sinus Bradycardia (SB), Sinus Tachycardia (ST), Atrial Fibrillation/Flutter (AF), Supraventricular Tachycardia (SVT), Other (O)
NEUROLOGICAL	GCS Score or Alert (A), Responds to verbal stimuli (V), Responds to pain (P), Unconscious (U)

MANAGEMENT SEQUENCE:

Time	Airway	Breathing		Circulation			Neuro	Drug & Dose Additional Observations eg. O_2 Therapy, Temperature, BSL and Comments
		Mode & Rate	SpO_2	Rhythm	MR	BP		
								Initial values
								Continued on reverse

OUTCOME:

Transferred to ☐ ICU ☐ 5 EAST ☐ Emergency Department

OR ☐ Upgrade to Respond Blue OR ☐ Remained on ward / not transferred out

NEXT OF KIN NOTIFIED Name: ______________ Time: _____ BY WHOM ______________

PATIENT UNIT NOTIFIED: Doctor: ______________ Time: _____ BY WHOM ______________

Respond MET Record

M 16.13

Figure 43.7 In-hospital MET documentation

Documentation

The role of documenter/scribe is challenging and requires the staff member performing the role to have the following skills:

- confidence and assertiveness in communicating what they need to know, as well as what has occurred to ensure continuity of care
- knowledge of the roles of each staff member present
- knowledge of medications being given and correct documentation
- experience of resuscitation and the process and procedures involved.

The documenter should have no other role during the resuscitation so that full attention can be given to accurately completing all the documentation (Molan 2013).

Rationale for documentation

- Provides information that can guide continuing care for the individual.
- Helps to answer questions the family/carer may have about the event.
- Quality improvement, policy and procedure review opportunities.
- Statistical information for funding, staffing and resource allocation.
- Provides aggregate data that can be used to identify variances of concern and as the base for continuous quality improvement efforts.
- Identification of learning opportunities for staff.
- Provides the data to answer research questions.
- A successful outcome is the goal in any resuscitation. An unsuccessful outcome will be reviewed internally by the institution. The episode may even then be referred on to the coroner's court or civil court. It is vital that all documentation is completed, accurate and specific, avoids unacceptable abbreviations and documents the outcomes.

Overcoming barriers to accuracy of in-hospital cardiac arrest documentation

Knowledge of what needs to be documented and how to accurately document these events in a stressful situation is an important role of not only the 'scribe' nurse but also other members of the MDT. Healthcare facilities have specific policies in regards to what needs to be documented and by whom in situations involving a deteriorating individual.

Suggestions for documentation

Documentation differs from hospital to hospital. ISBAR is a clear format that ensures all aspects of an individual's care are discussed. Resuscitation documentation often follows this format as well as the ABCDE acronym.

ISBAR format

Most hospitals will have a template with guidelines for documentation. The record should include the following:

1. the individual's demographics (gender, DOB)
2. times of arrest, initiation of CPR, defibrillation and initiation of ALS (witnessed/unwitnessed)
3. doses and routes of administration of drugs
4. sequential cardiac monitoring/responses (rhythm, rate and event times)
5. counter-shocks delivered
6. special procedures such as airway support, chest drains or external cardiac pacing
7. vital signs and the individual's response to any interventions
8. the outcome at the end of resuscitation (ROSC, transfer to ICU).

Suggested critical time elements should be documented:

- time from collapse to the beginning of CPR
- time from collapse to first defibrillation when the initial rhythm is VF or pulseless VT
- time to advanced airway management
- time from collapse to first dose of resuscitation medications.

STAFF DEBRIEFING

Debriefing is a process that provides staff with the opportunity to discuss and reflect on the events. A debriefing should involve all staff that were involved. Ideally, some form of debrief should occur soon after the incident; this is referred to as a 'warm' debrief. A 'warm' debrief allows for reflection and having a clear view of events. A 'cold' debrief occurs up to a month after the incident/event and allows time for staff to reflect on how they feel and voice any concerns that they have, either personal or professional, related to the incident/event (Kessler et al 2015; Twigg 2020). Debriefing has been shown to have a positive psychological effect in association with the development of post-event stress and PTSD (Sawyer et al 2020). The use of a facilitator and formal format aid in ensuring all aspects of the event are covered: clinical management, teamwork and communication. The debrief should also highlight positive aspects of the event.

MANAGING SPECIFIC EMERGENCY SITUATIONS

Anaphylaxis

Anaphylaxis is the most severe form of allergic reaction—and is potentially life-threatening (ANZCOR 2019b). The Australasian Society of Clinical Immunology and Allergy (ASCIA) defines anaphylaxis as:

> *Any acute onset illness with typical skin features (urticarial rash or erythema/flushing, and/or angioedema), plus involvement of respiratory and/or cardiovascular and/or persistent severe gastrointestinal symptoms; or*
>
> *Any acute onset of hypotension or bronchospasm or upper airway obstruction where anaphylaxis is considered possible, even if typical skin features are not present.*
>
> (ASCIA 2023)

TABLE 43.2 Signs and symptoms of allergic reactions

Mild or moderate reactions	Anaphylaxis
Swelling of lips, face, eyes Hives or welts Tingling mouth Abdominal pain, vomiting (these are signs of anaphylaxis for insect sting or injected drug [medication] allergy)	Difficult/noisy breathing Swelling of tongue Swelling/tightness in throat Difficulty talking or hoarse voice Wheeze or persistent cough (unlike the cough in asthma, the onset of coughing during anaphylaxis is usually sudden) Persistent dizziness or collapse Pale and floppy (young children) Abdominal pain, vomiting—for insect stings or injected drug (medication) allergy

(ASCIA 2023)

See Table 43.2 for signs and symptoms of allergic reactions—and remember that not all cases will have a rash.

Treatment of anaphylaxis using the ABCDE approach includes:

- Removing the allergen (if still present).
- Laying the individual flat. Do not allow them to stand or walk. If breathing is difficult, allow them to sit.
- Administering an adrenaline injector. This is an intramuscular injection (IMI) of adrenaline (epinephrine) into outer mid-thigh without delay using an adrenaline auto-injector if available *or* adrenaline ampoule and syringe. Repeat in 5 minutes if necessary.
- Giving oxygen (if available).

(ASCIA 2023; ANZCOR 2019b)

Always give adrenaline auto-injector first, then asthma reliever if someone with known asthma and allergy to food, insects or medication has sudden breathing difficulty (including wheeze, persistent cough or hoarse voice), even if there are no skin symptoms.

If the person becomes unresponsive and stops breathing, commence CPR.

After giving adrenaline, monitor for relapse—this may be for up to 4 hours (or even longer) (ASCIA 2023).

Shock

Shock is the inadequate delivery of oxygen (and nutrients) to the tissues due to a loss of effective circulation (ANZCOR 2019a). If left untreated, it can cause life-threatening organ failure, and death.

Causes of shock

- *Hypovolaemic:* Insufficient volume for adequate circulation. This may be due to bleeding, burns, gastrointestinal loss (e.g. diarrhoea) or dehydration.
- *Cardiogenic:* Myocardial infarction or arrhythmia that causes the heart to fail as a pump.
- *Obstructive:* Pulmonary embolism, tension pneumothorax or tamponade disrupting blood flow. Can also occur in pregnancy if the uterus compresses the large abdominal veins.
- *Distributive:* Vasoregulation failure caused by sepsis, anaphylaxis, vasovagal episodes or neurogenic shock.

(ANZCOR 2019a; Haseer Koya & Paul 2024)

Stages of shock

Pre-shock or compensatory stage

Receptors detect the decrease in tissue perfusion, activating compensatory mechanisms. These include signs that can alert the nurse to the fact that the person may be in shock—including tachycardia, peripheral vasoconstriction and drops in blood pressure (Haseer Koya & Paul 2024).

Shock/progressive stage

Classic signs of shock appear. The compensatory mechanisms start to become insufficient.

End-organ dysfunction

Insult to organs due to hypoperfusion extend to irreversible organ dysfunction, and eventually multi-organ failure and death (Haseer Koya & Paul 2024).

Recognising the individual in shock

The early recognition and response to shock is vital for early escalation of care, identification of cause and effective treatment. Blood pressure alone cannot be used as an indicator of shock. Each person needs to be assessed individually (Tidy & Vakharia 2022). (See Table 43.3.)

Managing the individual in shock

- **A** Check patent airway.
- **B** Consider giving oxygen—in shock state insufficient oxygenated blood is being pumped to tissues.
- **C** Ensure intravenous access. Check Hb level. Consider giving blood products and/or intravenous fluid. *Severely shocked individuals may require large volumes.*
- **D** Monitor cerebral perfusion via neurological assessment.
- **E** Maintain body temperature. Ensure no further blood loss due to wounds, trauma, burns.

Consideration needs to be given to the following:

- continued assessment of the individual, including diagnostic scans
- ECG to assess cardiac function
- support of the individual and their family/carer
- communication of treatment and plan

TABLE 43.3 Stages of haemorrhagic shock

American College of Surgeons Advanced Trauma Life Support (ATLS) haemorrhagic shock classification	
Class 1	Up to 15% blood volume loss (750 mL). Heart rate is minimally elevated or normal. Typically, there is no change in blood pressure, pulse pressure or respiratory rate. Blood pressure maintained.
Class 2	15–30% blood volume loss (750–1500 mL). Heart rate and respiratory rate become elevated (100 beats/min to 120 beats/min, 20 breaths/min to 24 breaths/min). Pulse pressure begins to narrow, but systolic blood pressure may be unchanged to slightly decreased.
Class 3	30–40% blood volume loss (1500–2000 mL). Significant drop in blood pressure and changes in mental status occurs. Heart rate and respiratory rate are significantly elevated (more than 120 beats/min). Urine output declines. Capillary refill is delayed.
Class 4	Blood volume loss greater than 40% (> 2000 mL) Hypotension with narrow pulse pressure (less than 25 mmHg). Tachycardia becomes more pronounced (more than 120 beats/min), and mental status becomes increasingly altered. Urine output is minimal or absent. Capillary refill is delayed.

(Tidy & Vakharia 2022; Hooper & Armstrong 2024)

- accurate documentation of all observations, medications, fluids, blood and diagnostic procedures performed and person's response to treatment.

CARDIAC EMERGENCIES

Cardiovascular disease (CVD) was responsible for 600,800 hospital admissions in 2021 and for 42,700 deaths (25% of all deaths) (Australian Institute of Health and Welfare [AIHW] 2023). The WHO (2021) reports that CVD is the leading cause of death worldwide with 32% of all global deaths. CVD is defined by the WHO (2021) as 'the name for the group of disorders of the heart and blood vessels'.

CVD includes hypertension, stroke, coronary artery disease, peripheral vascular disease, heart failure, congenital heart disease and cardiomyopathies (WHO 2021).

Abnormalities in rate, rhythm, conduction, pumping and perfusion can disrupt normal cardiac function and cause the rapid deterioration of an individual. The EN needs to have a sound knowledge of the different clinical presentations and the care needs of those presenting with cardiac emergencies. This knowledge empowers the EN to recognise and respond to changes in the individual's condition and escalate care.

Myocardial infarction (MI) is the correct terminology for a 'heart attack'. MI and cardiac arrest are not the same. Myocardial infarction refers to injury to the myocardium usually due a blockage in an artery due to coronary artery disease, that is restricting blood flow to the myocardium, causing ischaemia, which results in cellular death and infarction (Ojha & Dhamoon 2024; Thygesen et al 2018). A *cardiac arrest* occurs when the heart stops pumping due to arrhythmia (American Heart Association 2022)—cessation of heart action occurs (ANZCOR 2021g). A MI can lead to a cardiac arrest (ANZCOR 2021g): as the disruption to the blood supply leads to development of cardiac arrhythmias, which may evolve into cardiac arrest. In clinical practice, the term acute coronary syndromes (ACS) is used. (See also Chapter 25.)

Acute coronary syndrome

Acute coronary syndrome (ACS) covers several potentially life-threatening conditions associated with ischaemia or infarction of the myocardium, generally caused by parts of an atherosclerotic plaque in coronary vessels producing thrombosis, thromboembolism and ischaemia (Alderman 2023; ANZCOR 2019c).

Clinically, there are three syndromes that are characterised by the presence or absence of ST elevation on the ECG. These syndromes are referred to as:

- ST elevation myocardial infarction (STEMI): Diagnosed by changes in the ST segment of the ECG accompanied by clinical signs and symptoms.
- Non-ST elevation myocardial infarction (NSTEMI): There may be non-specific changes on the ECG. Diagnosed by elevated biomarkers.
- Unstable angina—new symptoms (or a change in symptoms) of myocardial infarction, but without ECG changes or elevated biomarkers.

(Alderman 2023; ANZCOR 2019c)

The underlying cause is most often atherosclerosis—the formation of fatty plaques. Arteriosclerosis is the thickening and hardening of the artery walls. Atherosclerosis and arteriosclerosis are terms used interchangeably and can occur in any of the blood vessels; however, when it occurs in the arteries of the heart, it can cause a reduction in blood flow to the cardiac muscles, causing poor perfusion and ischaemia, and potentially damage the cardiac muscle, which can then impact on cardiac function and output.

Signs and symptoms include:

- chest pain or discomfort or heaviness which may radiate to the back
- pain in arms, jaw or epigastric area (especially on exertion)
- dyspnoea
- sweating
- nausea
- other symptoms.

(Ojha & Dhamoon 2024)

While these are 'classic' symptoms of myocardial infarction, they may not be present. The only way to diagnose myocardial infarction safely is through the use of ECG and blood tests.

As outlined previously, MI can precipitate a cardiac arrest; therefore, the ABCDE approach to assessment needs to be used in individuals with possible ACS.

Management of acute coronary syndrome

The ACSQHC (2019) has developed the acute coronary syndrome clinical care standards, which outline best practice in regard to treatment of individuals who present to health services with chest pain.

The specific recommendations of the clinical care standard for chest pain are:

- Performance and review of an ECG within 10 minutes of presentation.
- Insertion of intravenous access.
- Administration of 300 mg aspirin unless contraindicated.
- Collection of blood to assess cardiac markers such as troponin.
- For STEMI—to have percutaneous coronary intervention (to ease the blockage) within 90 minutes of presentation if a reperfusion service is available. If not, administer fibrinolysis.
- For NSTEMI—assess risk factors to determine whether to have coronary angiography to assess and treat blockages and treatment options.

(See also Chapter 25.)

The administration of oxygen is no longer recommended for all individuals with chest pain (Gibbs et al 2020). Oxygen administration should be guided by clinical assessment to maintain oxygen saturations > 93% (ANZCOR 2020).

In the clinical ward area, the EN would assess the individual with chest pain with consideration to the following:

- Summoning assistance and escalate care.
- Perform or assist with ABCDE assessment, including all vital signs and:
  - B—position for comfort and to reduce work of breathing.
  - C—12-lead ECG, cannula and taking bloods.
  - D—assess pain.
- Assessing history of chest pain, asking about:
  - Onset—what was the individual doing when the pain began?
  - Nature—how they describe the pain (e.g. crushing, heaviness, stabbing or bad heartburn) and location—where is the pain?
  - Radiation—does the pain go: to the jaw, arm or shoulder blades?
  - Intensity—pain on a scale of 1–10.
  - Duration—when did the pain start?
- Accurate documentation. (See Progress Note 43.1.)

Hypertensive emergencies

Hypertension is common, and it is known that controlling hypertension long term reduces the risk of cardiovascular disease. Decisions about treating acute hypertension can be more complicated since sudden lowering of blood pressure with medication may result in decreased cerebral or myocardial perfusion (Mangon et al 2022). A hypertensive emergency (or *crisis*) occurs when acutely elevated blood pressure is associated with signs of organ dysfunction (Alley & Schick 2024). Hypertensive crisis is not defined by specific deviations in blood pressure; however, the general consideration is:

- Systolic >180 mmHg and/or a diastolic >120 mmHg is hypertensive urgency.
- Systolic >220 mmHg and/or diastolic >140 mmHg is a hypertensive emergency with acute organ dysfunction.

(National Heart Foundation of Australia 2016)

In hypertensive emergencies, the elevated blood pressure is associated with signs of end-organ damage such as pulmonary oedema, cardiac ischemia, neurologic deficits, acute renal failure, eclampsia and aortic dissection (Alley & Schick 2024). During the assessment the EN may note symptoms such as headache, chest pain, dyspnoea, focal neurological signs, headache and visual impairment (Vallelonga et al 2020).

Nursing interventions

- Assess using ABCDE.
- Ensure BP cuff is a suitable correct size for the individual.
- An ECG may be helpful.
- Accurate documentation and escalation of care.
- Intravenous access and administration of medications to reduce blood pressure.
- Provide reassurance to the individual.

Asthma

While asthma is estimated to cause more than 1000 deaths per day globally, many of these deaths would be avoidable with better management and treatment (Global Asthma Network 2022). Asthma is a chronic condition associated with hypersensitivity and narrowing of the lower airways. Exposure to a trigger may cause bronchoconstriction, inflammation and mucus production (ANZCOR 2023a), resulting in increased work of breathing and impaired gas exchange.

Signs and symptoms

It is vital to recognise a severe asthma attack quickly by detecting:

- gasping for breath (with or without wheeze)
- inability to speak more than one or two words per breath
- severe chest tightness
- 'sucking in' of the throat and rib muscles, use of shoulder muscles or bracing with arms to help breathing

- blue discolouration around the lips
- pale and sweaty skin
- distress and anxiety
- decreased level of consciousness
- little or no improvement after using reliever medication/s
- symptoms rapidly getting worse or using reliever more than every 2 hours.

(ANZCOR 2023a)

Nursing interventions

- Undertake the ABCDE assessment and consider causes of similar symptoms (e.g. anaphylaxis).
- Position for comfortable breathing—this is usually sitting upright.
- Oxygen should be administered if saturations are low.
- Administer a bronchodilator, usually salbutamol. This is best given using an inhaler and spacer; however, may be given via a nebuliser especially for individuals with profound shortness of breath.
- Reassess respiratory rate, work of breathing and saturations regularly.
- Accurate documentation and escalation of care.

Oxygen is lifesaving for individuals who are hypoxic; however, many staff worry about administering it in case the individual has COPD and is a CO_2 retainer. Lower levels of 'normal' saturations may be tolerated in these individuals, but oxygen is still given if oxygen saturations are very low. It is important to monitor their saturations continuously and check respiratory rate and level of consciousness more frequently. (See also Chapter 25.)

Seizures

A seizure is defined as 'a transient occurrence of signs and/or symptoms due to abnormal excessive or synchronous neuronal activity in the brain' (BMJ Best Practice 2018c). Seizures are abnormal jerky or trembling body movements due to abnormal neuron activity in the brain (Anwar et al 2020) and may result in damage to organs including the brain. Seizures are not a disease; they are a symptom of many different disorders that can affect the brain.

The International League Against Epilepsy (ILAE) revised its classification of seizures in 2017 (Scheffer et al 2017). The terms 'partial' and 'grand mal' are no longer used. Seizures are classified into three main groups: focal onset, generalised onset and unknown onset. See Chapter 35 for further discussion on seizure disorders and classification of seizures.

Seizures may be 'unprovoked', such as in epilepsy. However, they can also be 'provoked' due to a variety of causes such as:

- electrolyte disturbances
- toxins (including some medications)
- alcohol or drug withdrawal
- infections or sepsis
- head trauma
- stroke
- neoplasm
- fever.

(Huff & Murr 2024)

Nursing interventions

Using the ABCDE assessment for initial nursing management during a seizure:

- Consider your own safety and the safety of the person, ensuring they do not harm themselves during the seizure; remove hazards.
- Take note of the time.
- Maintain airway, turn the individual on their side if possible and apply oxygen.
- Note type of seizure.
- Assist with intravenous administration of medications as ordered.
- Obtain blood glucose level.
- Assist with collection of bloods to assess electrolytes/infection/toxicity.
- Assist with ongoing assessment of individual including vital signs. Document accurately.

Post-seizure care of the individual:

- Repeat ABCDE, with particular attention to maintaining airway, assessing level of consciousness and blood glucose.
- Consider obtaining an ECG to check for cardiac causes of seizure.
- Assist with a head-to-toe examination—look for signs of secondary injury.
- Assist with gathering the individual's medical history.
- Maintain the individual's safety by reassuring them and reorient them.

(See also Chapter 35.)

Epilepsy

Epilepsy is a neurological disorder that is associated with recurrent seizures. Not everyone who has a seizure has epilepsy. The WHO states that epilepsy is one of the most common neurological diseases, with more than 50 million people worldwide having epilepsy (WHO 2019).

Terminology

'Status epilepticus' was historically defined as a generalised seizure lasting 30 minutes or longer. However, this definition has changed, and status epilepticus is considered a neurological and medical emergency defined as 5 or more minutes of either seizure activity or repeated convulsions without recovery of consciousness between each convulsion (Huff & Murr 2024). Untreated, this condition is fatal. The post-ictal phase is the period from the end of a seizure to the individual returning to baseline mental state, a period associated with transient altered consciousness (Huff & Murr 2024).

NURSING CARE PLAN 43.1

Assessment: Mr Jaymie Zeld, 27 yo, has been diagnosed with L leg deep vein thrombosis (DVT) and bilateral pulmonary embolism (PE) 24 hours ago.
Jaymie's past medical history includes:
Surgery 3 days ago for fractured L tibia after a fall from a ladder at work.

- smoker, obesity with a body mass index (BMI) of 37
- allergy to codeine, causing hallucinations
- recently, Jaymie has noted a productive cough in the mornings on waking.

Issue/s to be addressed: Decreased oxygenation due to PE.
Treatment with anticoagulant to reduce the risk of development of additional PE.
Goal/s: Reduction in clot to aid breathing and oxygenation, stabilisation of observations to within acceptable parameters.

Care/actions	Rationale
Monitor conscious state	Alterations in conscious state can be an indicator of cerebral hypoxia.
Measurement of vital signs 2-hourly	To monitor for hypoxia, assess RR and effort of breathing for dyspnoea. Goal of oxygen saturation 95% on air and RR $<$ 22 breaths/min.
Pain assessment	Reduction in pain to enhance breathing, reduce dyspnoea and increase individual comfort. Pain assessment 2-hourly with observations, as well as post administration of any required analgesia.
Skin assessment	Increased bed rest, monitor for alterations in skin integrity due to additional time in bed and from plaster back slab on L leg. Monitor skin 4-hourly.
Mobility	Encourage to mobilise as able, if not contraindicated. Encourage individual to sit out of bed to facilitate easier breathing. To enhance independence for discharge.
Education on use of anticoagulants	Educate individual about anticoagulant therapy. Advise about dosing and treatment goals. Advise about avoiding contact sports and razors for shaving while on anticoagulant. Advise what to do if blood noticed in stool or urine or has a bleeding nose.
Education on condition	Advise individual about future risks, signs and symptoms of VTE and prevention.

Evaluation:

CNS: Alert and oriented, individual educated on the signs and symptoms hypoxia.
Individual or family to report to staff any concerns they have.
CVS: Haemodynamically stable, vital signs maintained within parameters set by medical officer, warm and well perfused. TED stockings in situ.
RESP: Bilateral equal air entry all lung fields on auscultation. SpO_2 on room air 96%, exercise tolerance increasing gradually.
GIT: Bowels opened, and reports decreased appetite.
URO: Voiding good clear amounts of urine, advised to report if change in colour to urine (presence of blood).
INTEG: L leg elevated on pillows lengthways to assist with swelling. Advised individual to change position and sit out of bed (SOOB) to facilitate easier breathing.
Individual reports a reduction in chest pain and dyspnoea.

Nursing interventions:

Administer medications as per medication chart, observing for response and indication of side effects. Ask medical officer about contraindications of anticoagulant with anti-inflammatories that has been previously ordered. Explain medications including why they have been prescribed, the dose and any side effects.
Maintain an optimal fluid balance: A decreased volume can increase venous stasis.
Maintain adequate ventilation and circulation by positioning individual in semi-high Fowler's as tolerated to enhance chest expansion and oxygenation.
Provide education for the individual and significant other/s including the signs and symptoms of DVT and PE.
Explain the importance of risk reduction for the future, smoking cessation and weight loss.

Progress Note 43.1

20/04/24 1450 hrs	Nursing: At bed-to-bed handover, Jaymie's partner stated, 'Jaymie has been having some pain in his chest.' On assessment of pain, Jaymie stated it was 5/10 and had left-sided sharp pain, which was worse on inspiration. Pain was non-radiating, and there was no diaphoresis. Has had pain since 1300 hrs. Jaymie stated, 'I feel a bit out of breath, feel like I have run up the stairs.' Observations performed: RR 22 breaths/min, oxygen saturation 92% on air, T 36.6°C, HR 112 beats/min, BP 105/52 mmHg, alert and oriented. Team leader aware and care escalated to MDT review. *Tammy Aiya* (AIYA), *EN student*

DECISION-MAKING FRAMEWORK EXERCISE 43.1

Tammy is a student EN currently on placement in an acute surgical ward of the local hospital. She is working with an RN, Sarah, and they have been allocated four individuals to care for. Sarah is assisting the medical officer with another individual. Tammy has been asked to perform some vital signs on Jaymie, who has returned from radiology post CT pulmonary angiogram. While performing the observations, Jaymie asks when he is going to have the 'blood thinning' needle since they said they would do it on his return from the scan. Jaymie is very insistent that Tammy gives him the injection because he is worried about the clot in his leg getting worse. Tammy is aware that Jaymie has a left leg deep vein thrombosis (DVT). She checks his medication chart and confirms that Jaymie has not had his anticoagulant injection this morning. Tammy goes to speak to Sarah, who tells her that she is happy for her to administer the medication independently and unsupervised. Tammy says, 'You did one okay yesterday. I'm still busy and if he really wants it you will have to do it.'

Tammy is aware of the policy that students must be supervised for all administration of medications, but really likes Sarah.

Using the decision-making framework:

1. What should Tammy consider when deciding whether she should administer the medication?
2. Should Tammy give this medication? Please explain your answer.

Summary

Key elements of the role of the EN have been outlined in the many emergency situations in this chapter. The role of the EN includes the ability to use critical thinking in the thorough assessment of the individual receiving emergency care. Assessment requires underpinning knowledge and proficient clinical skills. It is this assessment that recognises a deteriorating individual. It then requires the nurse with the knowledge to detect deterioration to effectively communicate the need for an escalation of care for the deteriorating person, utilising communication tools such as ISBAR. Policy and procedures guide nurses in clinical practice. However, if a nurse is ever unsure of their scope of practice, they just need to ask themselves: Am I educated? Am I authorised? Am I competent? This is the basis of the decision-making framework and assists the nurse to consider, determine and self-assess their individual practice (NMBA 2020).

Review Questions

1. List the observations that should be included when performing a set of vital signs.
2. Provide a brief summary of your role in recognising and responding to deterioration in an individual.
3. You are working in the medical–surgical ward and are about to finish your morning shift. You decide to conduct a final check and discover Mrs Chenn slumped in her chair. When you enter the room, you notice the following:
   - Mrs Chenn is not moving.
   - The water jug has spilled on the floor.
     a. As the first responder, list your immediate priorities.
     b. Explain the assessment process when responding to an individual who is unresponsive.
4. Mrs Chenn's medical history includes type 1 diabetes mellitus and anaemia; she had reported before lunch that she 'felt weak'. There is no evidence in her progress notes that her concerns have been addressed or investigated. Her admission notes state that she was admitted the previous day for stabilisation of her blood sugars. Mrs Chenn has not had her vital signs measured since 1030 hours that morning. Reflect on this situation. What would your priorities have been in this situation?

Evolve® Answer guide for the Review Questions, Critical Thinking Exercises, Decision-making Framework Exercises and Critical Thinking Questions in Case Studies is hosted on Evolve: http//evolve.elsevier.com/AU/Koutoukidis/Tabbner.

References

Alderman, E., 2023. Acute coronary syndromes – ClinicalKey for nursing. Elsevier Point of Care. Available at: <https://www-clinicalkey-com-au.www.ezpdhcs.nt.gov.au/nursing/#!/content/clinical_overview/67-s2.0-d4363295-27ea-4b31-a1ff-70b751b3ece0>.

Alley, W., Schick, M., 2024. Hypertensive emergency. In *StatPearls*. Treasure Island (FL): StatPearls Publishing. Available at: <http://www.ncbi.nlm.nih.gov/books/NBK470371>.

American Heart Association, 2022. Heart attack and sudden cardiac arrest differences. Available at: <https://www.heart.org/en/health-topics/heart-attack/about-heart-attacks/heart-attack-or-sudden-cardiac-arrest-how-are-they-different>.

Anwar, H., Khan, Q., Nadeem, N., et al., 2020. Epileptic seizures. *Discoveries* 8(2), e110. Available at: <https://doi.org/10.15190/d.2020.7>.

Australian and New Zealand Committee on Resuscitation (ANZCOR), 2019a. Guideline 9.2.3 – Shock: First aid management of the seriously ill or injured person. Available at: <https://www.anzcor.org/home/new-guideline-page-2/guideline-9-2-3-shock-first-aid-management-of-the-seriously-ill-or-injured-person>.

Australian and New Zealand Committee on Resuscitation (ANZCOR), 2019b. Guideline 9.2.7 – First aid management of anaphylaxis. Available at: <https://www.anzcor.org/home/new-guideline-page-2/guideline-9-2-7-first-aid-management-of-anaphylaxis>.

Australian and New Zealand Committee on Resuscitation (ANZCOR), 2019c. Guideline 14 – Acute coronary syndromes. Available at: <https://www.anzcor.org/home/acute-coronary-syndromes/guideline-14-acute-coronary-syndromes>.

Australian and New Zealand Committee on Resuscitation (ANZCOR), 2020. Guideline 9.2.10 – The use of oxygen in emergencies. Available at: <https://www.anzcor.org/home/new-guideline-page-2/guideline-9-2-10-the-use-of-oxygen-in-emergencies/>.

Australian and New Zealand Committee on Resuscitation (ANZCOR), 2021a. Guideline 4 – Airway. Available at: <https://www.anzcor.org/home/basic-life-support/guideline-4-airway>.

Australian and New Zealand Committee on Resuscitation (ANZCOR), 2021b. Guideline 5 – Breathing. Available at: <https://www.anzcor.org/home/basic-life-support/guideline-5-breathing>.

Australian and New Zealand Committee on Resuscitation (ANZCOR), 2021c. Guideline 6 – Compressions. Available at: <https://www.anzcor.org/home/basic-life-support/guideline-6-compressions>.

Australian and New Zealand Committee on Resuscitation (ANZCOR), 2021d. Guideline 7 – Automated external defibrillation in basic life support. Available at: <https://www.anzcor.org/home/basic-life-support/guideline-7-automated-external-defibrillation-in-basic-life-support>.

Australian and New Zealand Committee on Resuscitation (ANZCOR), 2021e. Guideline 8 – Cardiopulmonary resuscitation (CPR). Available at: <https://www.anzcor.org/home/basic-life-support/guideline-8-cardiopulmonary-resuscitation-cpr>.

Australian and New Zealand Committee on Resuscitation (ANZCOR), 2021f. Guideline 9.1.6 – Management of suspected spinal injury. Available at: <https://www.anzcor.org/home/first-aid-management-of-injuries/guideline-9-1-6-management-of-suspected-spinal-injury>.

Australian and New Zealand Committee on Resuscitation (ANZCOR), 2021g. Guideline 9.2.1 – Recognition and first aid management of suspected heart attack. Available at: <https://www.anzcor.org/home/new-guideline-page-2/guideline-9-2-1-recognition-and-first-aid-management-of-suspected-heart-attack>.

Australian and New Zealand Committee on Resuscitation (ANZCOR), 2021h. Guideline 11.2 – Protocols for adult advanced life support. Available at: <https://www.anzcor.org/home/adult-advanced-life-support/guideline-11-2-protocols-for-adult-advanced-life-support>.

Australian and New Zealand Committee on Resuscitation (ANZCOR), 2021i. Guideline 11.8 – Targeted temperature management (TTM) after cardiac arrest. Available at: <https://www.anzcor.org/home/adult-advanced-life-support/guideline-11-8-targeted-temperature-management-ttm-after-cardiac-arrest>.

Australian and New Zealand Committee on Resuscitation (ANZCOR), 2023a. Guideline 9.2.5 – First aid for asthma. Available at: <https://www.anzcor.org/home/new-guideline-page-2/guideline-9-2-5-first-aid-for-asthma>.

Australian and New Zealand Committee on Resuscitation (ANZCOR), 2023b. Basic life support (flowchart). Available at: <https://www.anzcor.org/assets/Uploads/Basic-Life-Support-August-2023-1-v3.pdf>.

Australian and New Zealand Committee on Resuscitation (ANZCOR), 2023c. Guideline 10.1 – Basic life support (bls) training. Available at: <https://www.anzcor.org/home/education-and-implementation/guideline-10-1-basic-life-support-bls-training>.

Australian Resuscitation Council (ARC), 2024. Guideline 11.1 – Introduction to and principles of in-hospital resuscitation. Available at: <https://resus.org.au/download/guideline-11-1>.

Australasian Society of Clinical Immunology and Allergy (ASCIA), 2023. ASCIA Guidelines acute management of anaphylaxis. Available at: <https://allergy.org.au/hp/papers/acute-management-of-anaphylaxis-guidelines>.

Australian Commission on Safety and Quality in Health Care (ACSQHC), 2019. Acute Coronary Syndromes Clinical Care Standard. Available at: <https://www.safetyandquality.gov.au/sites/default/files/2019-12/acute_coronary_syndromes_ccs_-_december_2019.pdf#page=1.00&gsr=0>.

Australian Commission on Safety and Quality in Health Care (ACSQHC), 2021a. *National consensus statement: Essential elements for recognising and responding to acute physiological deterioration*, 3rd ed.

Australian Commission on Safety and Quality in Health Care (ACSQHC), 2021b. Recognising and Responding to Acute Deterioration Standard. In: *National safety and quality health service standards*, 2nd ed, 67–72.

Australian Commission on Safety and Quality in Health Care (ACSQHC), 2024. Clinical handover. Available at: <https://www.safetyandquality.gov.au/our-work/communicating-safety/clinical-handover>.

Australian Institute of Health and Welfare, 2023. Heart, stroke and vascular disease: Australian facts, all heart, stroke and vascular disease. Available at: <https://www.aihw.gov.au/reports/heart-stroke-vascular-diseases/hsvd-facts/contents/disease-types>.

Bray, J., Howell, S., Ball, S., et al., 2022. The epidemiology of out-of-hospital cardiac arrest in Australia and New Zealand: A binational report from the Australasian Resuscitation Outcomes Consortium (Aus-ROC). *Resuscitation* 172, 74–83. Available at: <https://doi.org/10.1016/j.resuscitation.2022.01.011>.

Brown, D., Edwards, H., Buckley, T., et al., 2024. *Lewis's medical-surgical nursing*, ANZ, 6th ed. Elsevier, Chatswood.

Buist, M., Bernard, S., Nguyen, T., et al., 2004. Association between clinically abnormal observations and subsequent in-hospital mortality: A prospective study. *Resuscitation* 62(2), 137–41. Available at: <https://doi.org/10.1016/j.resuscitation.2004.03.005>.

Burgess, A., van Diggele, C., Roberts, C., et al., 2020. Teaching clinical handover with ISBAR. *BMC Medical Education* 20(2), 459. Available at: <https://doi.org/10.1186/s12909-020-02285-0>.

Chua, W., Rahim, N., McKenna, L., et al., 2022. Intraprofessional collaboration between enrolled and registered nurses in the care of clinically deteriorating ward patients: A qualitative study. *Australian Critical Care* 35(1), 81–88. Available at: <https://doi.org/10.1016/j.aucc.2021.01.009>.

Considine, J., Casey, P., Omonaiye, O., et al., 2024. Importance of specific vital signs in nurses' recognition and response to deteriorating patients: A scoping review. *Journal of Clinical Nursing*. Available at: <https://doi.org/10.1111/jocn.17099>.

Department of Health & Human Services, 2021. Cardiopulmonary resuscitation (CPR). Available at: <http://www.betterhealth.vic.gov.au/health/conditionsandtreatments/cardiopulmonary-resuscitation-cpr>.

Dresser, S., Teel, C., Peltzer, J., 2023. Frontline nurses' clinical judgment in recognizing, understanding, and responding to patient deterioration: A qualitative study. *International Journal of Nursing Studies* 139, 104436. Available at: <https://doi.org/10.1016/j.ijnurstu.2023.104436>.

Drost-de Klerck, A., Olgers, T., Van De Meeberg, E., et al., 2020. Use of simulation training to teach the ABCDE primary assessment: An observational study in a Dutch university hospital with a 3–4 months follow-up. *BMJ Open* 10(7), e032023. Available at: <https://doi.org/10.1136/bmjopen-2019-032023>.

Foth, C., Gangwani, M., Ahmed, I., et al., 2024. Ventricular tachycardia. In: *StatPearls*. Treasure Island (FL): StatPearls Publishing. Available at: <http://www.ncbi.nlm.nih.gov/books/NBK532954>.

Gibbs, L., Pham, K., Langston, S., et al., 2020. Supplemental oxygen therapy for nonhypoxemic patients with acute coronary syndrome. *American Family Physician* 101(11), 687–88.

Global Asthma Network, 2022. The Global Asthma Report 2022. *The International Journal of Tuberculosis and Lung Disease* 26(1), 1–104. Available at: <https://doi.org/10.5588/ijtld.22.1010>.

Goyal, A., Chhabra, L., Sciammarella, J., et al., 2024. Defibrillation. In: *StatPearls*. Treasure Island (FL): StatPearls Publishing. Available at: <http://www.ncbi.nlm.nih.gov/books/NBK499899>.

Haseer Koya, H., Paul, M., 2024. Shock. In: *StatPearls*. Treasure Island (FL): StatPearls Publishing. Available at: <http://www.ncbi.nlm.nih.gov/books/NBK531492>.

Hooper, N., Armstrong, T., 2024. Hemorrhagic shock. In: *StatPearls*. Treasure Island (FL): StatPearls Publishing. Available at: <http://www.ncbi.nlm.nih.gov/books/NBK470382>.

Huff, S., Murr, N., 2024. Seizure. In: *StatPearls*. Treasure Island (FL): StatPearls Publishing. Available at: <http://www.ncbi.nlm.nih.gov/books/NBK430765>.

Kessler, D., Cheng, A., Mullan, P., 2015. Debriefing in the emergency department after clinical events: A practical guide. *Annals of Emergency Medicine* 65(6), 690–98. Available at: <https://doi.org/10.1016/j.annemergmed.2014.10.019>.

Ludhwani, D., Goyal, A., Jagtap, M., 2024. Ventricular fibrillation. In: *StatPearls*. Treasure Island (FL): StatPearls Publishing. Available at: <http://www.ncbi.nlm.nih.gov/books/NBK537120>.

Mangon, A., Jarmuzewska, E., Gabb, G., et al., 2022. Blood pressure elevations in hospital. *Australian Prescriber* 45(6). Available at: <https://doi.org/10.18773/austprescr.2022.068>.

Molan, E., 2013. Scribe during emergency department resuscitation: Registered nurse domain or up for grabs? *Australasian Emergency Nursing Journal: AENJ* 16(2), 45–51. Available at: <https://doi.org/10.1016/j.aenj.2013.03.001>.

National Heart Foundation of Australia, 2016. Guideline for the diagnosis and management of hypertension in adults. Available at: <https://www.heartfoundation.org.au/for-professionals/hypertension>.

Nursing and Midwifery Board of Australia (NMBA), 2020. Decision-making framework for nursing and midwifery. Available at: <https://www.nursingmidwiferyboard.gov.au/codes-guidelines-statements/frameworks.aspx>.

Nursing and Midwifery Board of Australia (NMBA), 2016. *Enrolled nurse standards for practice*. Available at: <https://

www.nursingmidwiferyboard.gov.au/Codes-Guidelines-Statements/Professional-standards/enrolled-nurse-standards-for-practice.aspx>.

Ojha, N., Dhamoon, S., 2024. Myocardial infarction. In: *StatPearls*. Treasure Island (FL): StatPearls Publishing. Available at: <http://www.ncbi.nlm.nih.gov/books/NBK537076>.

Oliver, T., Sadiq, U., Grossman, S., 2024. Pulseless electrical activity. In: *StatPearls*. Treasure Island (FL): StatPearls Publishing. Available at: <http://www.ncbi.nlm.nih.gov/books/NBK513349>.

Peran, D., Kodet, J., Pekara, J., et al., 2020. ABCDE cognitive aid tool in patient assessment – development and validation in a multicenter pilot simulation study. *BMC Emergency Medicine* 20(1), 95. Available at: <https://doi.org/10.1186/s12873-020-00390-3>.

Queensland Health, 2022. Resuscitation trolley checklist. Available at: <https://www.health.qld.gov.au/__data/assets/pdf_file/0026/1066625/RRESS_resus_trolley_checklist.pdf>.

Rebeiro, G., Wilson, D., Fuller, S., 2021. *Fundamentals of nursing: Clinical skills workbook*, 4th ed. Elsevier, Chatswood.

Resuscitation Council UK, 2024. The ABCDE approach. Available at: <https://www.resus.org.uk/library/abcde-approach>.

Romero-Brufau, S., Gaines, K., Nicolas, C., et al., 2019. The fifth vital sign? Nurse worry predicts inpatient deterioration within 24 hours. *JAMIA Open* 2(4), 465–70. Available at: <https://doi.org/10.1093/jamiaopen/ooz033>.

SA Health, 2020. Rapid detection and response observation charts. Department for Health and Ageing, Government of South Australia. Available at: <https://www.sahealth.sa.gov.au/wps/wcm/connect/ff3a769a-e8f0-45db-970e-12281b2891b2/MR59A%2B-%2BAdult%2BObservation%2BChart%2B-%2BEXAMPLE+%281%29.pdf?MOD=AJPERES&CACHEID=ROOTWORKSPACE-ff3a769a-e8f0-45db-970e-12281b2891b2-oun4qXB>.

Sawyer, K., Camp-Rogers, T., Kotini-Shah, P., et al., 2020. Sudden cardiac arrest survivorship: A scientific statement from the American Heart Association. *Circulation* 141(12), e654–85. Available at: <https://doi.org/10.1161/CIR.0000000000000747>.

Scheffer, I., Berkovic, S., Capovilla, G., et al., 2017. Position paper of the ILAE Commission for Classification and Terminology. *Epilepsia* 58(4), 512–21. Available at: <https://doi.org/10.1111/epi.13709>.

Smith, D., Bowden, T., 2017. Using the ABCDE approach to assess the deteriorating patient. *Nursing Standard* 32, 51–63. Available at: <https://doi.org/10.7748/ns.2017.e11030>.

Soltan, M., Kim, M., 2016. The ABCDE approach explained. *BMJ* 355, i4512. Available at: <https://doi.org/10.1136/sbmj.i4512>.

Sydney Local Health District, 2014. ISBAR. Available at: <https://www.slhd.nsw.gov.au/BTF/ISBAR.html>.

Thygesen, K., Alpert, J., Jaffe, A., et al., 2018. Fourth universal definition of myocardial infarction. *Journal of the American College of Cardiology* 72(18), 2231–2264. Available at: <https://doi.org/10.1016/j.jacc.2018.08.1038>.

Tidy, C., Vakharia, K., 2022. Resuscitation in hypovolaemic shock. Patient info. Available at: <https://patient.info/doctor/resuscitation-in-hypovolaemic-shock>.

Trauma Victoria, 2023. Early trauma care – secondary survey. Available at: <https://trauma.reach.vic.gov.au/guidelines/early-trauma-care/secondary-survey>.

Twigg, S., 2020. Clinical event debriefing: A review of approaches and objectives. *Current Opinion in Pediatrics* 32(3), 337–42. Available at: <https://doi.org/10.1097/MOP.0000000000000890>.

Vallelonga, F., Carbone, F., Benedetto, F., et al., 2020. Accuracy of a symptom-based approach to identify hypertensive emergencies in the emergency department. *Journal of Clinical Medicine* 9(7), 2201. Available at: <https://doi.org/10.3390/jcm9072201>.

World Health Organization (WHO), 2021. Cardiovascular diseases (CVDs). Available at: <https://www.who.int/news-room/fact-sheets/detail/cardiovascular-diseases-(cvds)>.

World Health Organization (WHO) and International Committee of the Red Cross (ICRC), 2018. *Basic emergency care (BEC): Approach to the acutely ill and injured*. Available at: <https://iris.who.int/bitstream/handle/10665/275635/9789241513081-eng.pdf?sequence=1>.

Recommended Reading

Bogossian, F., Cooper, S., Cant, R., et al., 2014. Undergraduate nursing students' performance in recognising and responding to sudden patient deterioration in high psychological fidelity simulated environments: An Australian multi-centre study. *Nurse Education Today* 34(5), 691–696.

Christ, M., Dierschke, W., Von Auenmueller, K., et al., 2014. Cardiac arrest teams and time of day: Effects on surviving in-hospital resuscitation. *International Journal of General Medicine* 2014(7), 319–323. Available at: <https://doi.org/10.2147/IJGM.S66609>.

Cooper, A., Gorman, J., Wilson, M., et al., 2015. Improving observation with new technology. *Nursing Times* 111(15), 12–14.

Cardona-Morrell, M., Nicholson, M., Hillman, K., 2015. Vital signs: From monitoring to prevention of deterioration in general wards. In: Vincent, J.-L., (ed.), *Annual update in intensive care and emergency medicine 2015*, pp. 533–45. Springer International Publishing, Cham. Available at: <https://doi.org/10.1007/978-3-319-13761-2_39>.

Heart Foundation, 2019. Heart disease in Australia. Available at: <https://www.heartfoundation.org.au/about-us/what-we-do/heart-disease-in-australia>.

Kantamineni, P., Emani, V., Saini, A., et al., Cardiopulmonary resuscitation in the hospitalized patient: Impact of system-based variables on outcomes in cardiac arrest. *The American Journal of the Medical Sciences* 348(5), 377–81. Available at: <https://doi.org/10.1097/MAJ.0000000000000290>.

Martin, P., 2017. 7 pulmonary embolism nursing care plans. Available at: <https://nurseslabs.com/pulmonary-embolism-nursing-care-plans>.

McMeekin, D.E., Hickman, R.L., Douglas, S.L., et al., 2017. Stress and coping of critical care nurses after unsuccessful cardiopulmonary resuscitation. *American Journal of Critical Care* 26(2), 128–135. Available at: <https://doi.org/10.4037/ajcc2017916>.

Wheatley, I., 2018. Respiratory rate 5: Using this vital sign to detect deterioration. *Nursing Times* 114(10), 45–46.

Online Resources

Australian and New Zealand Committee on Resuscitation (ANZCOR): <https://www.anzcor.org>.

Australian Commission on Safety and Quality in Health Care (ACSQHC): <www.safetyandquality.gov.au>.

Australian Resuscitation Council (ARC): <www.resus.org.au>.

CHAPTER 44

Maternal and newborn care

Vanessa Cashen-McNally and Kate Stainton

Key Terms

amenorrhoea
antenatal
Apgar score
birth
Braxton Hicks contractions
breast milk
caesarean
colostrum
foetal heart rate
foetus
gestation
haemolytic disease
hyperbilirubinaemia
jaundice
labour
lactation
lanugo
lochia
meconium
morning sickness
postnatal
quickening
Rhesus (D) blood type
stages of labour
thermoregulation
trimester
uterine enlargement
vernix caseosa

Learning Outcomes

At the completion of this chapter and with further reading, learners should be able to:

- Define the key terms.
- Describe the physiology of pregnancy.
- Describe the physiological changes that occur during pregnancy.
- Describe the importance of the first antenatal visit and screening that is included.
- Explain the postnatal care of a woman following the birth of her newborn.
- Describe the newborn assessment at birth.
- Describe medications recommended to newborns at birth and why they are recommended.
- Identify activities that should be included in a daily care plan for a normal newborn.
- Explain positioning and attachment in breastfeeding a newborn to assist a mother to successfully breastfeed.
- Explain normal newborn behaviours in the initial period post birth and in the postnatal period.

CHAPTER FOCUS

Maternity nursing involves the care of a woman during her pregnancy and labour, and the care of both the woman and her baby during and after birth. Maternity care is based on an awareness and/or assessment of the physical, emotional, social, cultural and spiritual wellbeing of both the woman and her infant/s (Australian College of Midwives [ACM] 2021). Although midwifery is a specialised profession, requiring the learner midwife to undertake a separate educational program, the Enrolled Nurse (EN) may be required to assist in the provision of maternity care. It is therefore important that the EN has a basic knowledge of human growth and development and the processes of normal pregnancy and labour, and an understanding of the immediate and subsequent care of the mother and the newborn infant. The actual work and scope of practice of the individual EN is influenced by the employment setting, their level of competency and employer policy requirements.

The birth of a baby follows a woman's pregnancy and the process of labour. The first part of this chapter focuses on the physiology of pregnancy and the indicators and methods of confirming pregnancy and pregnancy care, which includes preparing for the birth. Later, the four stages of labour, and nursing measures for mother and baby during the postnatal period, are explained.

LIVED EXPERIENCE

Lola, 34 years old, delivered her daughter Imogen 3 days ago. On entering her room, Kat found Lola is in tears, sitting looking at her sleeping baby. Lola tells Kat that she misses her mother who passed away from breast cancer 6 months ago. Lola goes on to tell Kat that after her mother was diagnosed with breast cancer, she was tested for the BRCA gene, and as a result had a bilateral mastectomy. Her baby was the result of an embryo donor as she did not want to pass the gene on to her baby. Lola is worried she might not bond with her baby since she is unable to breastfeed.

Lola, mother of 3-day-old Imogen, talking to Kat, an Enrolled Nurse

PREGNANCY

Pregnancy (**gestation**) lasts for approximately 40 weeks or 280 days, measured from the date of the woman's last normal menstrual period (LNMP).

A term pregnancy is from 37 to 42 weeks' gestation; prior to this, the newborn is considered premature. Pregnancy can occur naturally by sexual intercourse or via assisted reproductive technology.

A pregnancy is divided into three **trimesters**:

- First trimester—conception (week 1) until week 12. This is the embryonic phase.
- Second trimester—weeks 13–27. This is the foetal phase of development.
- Third trimester—week 28 until term.

In the first trimester, the **foetus'** body and organs develop, and the placenta also develops. Generally, placenta development is complete by week 10.

In the second trimester, the foetus' organs mature; in the third trimester, the foetus grows and lays down fat stores (Blackburn 2018; Davidson et al 2020). The gender and inherited characteristics of the newborn baby are decided at conception. The estimated due date/date of delivery/date of birth (EDD/EDB) is determined based on the date of the woman's last normal menstrual period (LNMP) and the first accurate ultrasound examination. The estimated date of delivery/birth (EDD/EDB) or estimated agreed due date (ADD) of the birth is an estimate and newborns will be born across the gestational weeks due to a variety of circumstances; some circumstances are still not understood (Department of Health & Aged Care 2020; Safer Care Victoria 2021).

Physiological changes

Pregnancy involves major physiological changes so the woman's body can support the growth and development of her baby, both in utero and in the postnatal period.

Most of these changes are temporary and most are the result of hormone action. These changes prepare the mother's body to protect the developing embryo and foetus, provide for the demands of the foetus, and prepare to feed the baby when it is born. Profound endocrine changes occur that are essential for maintaining pregnancy, normal foetal growth, and post-partum recovery.

The hormones predominantly associated with pregnancy include but are not limited to:

- hCG—human chorionic gonadotrophin
- hPL—human placental lactogen
- oestrogen
- progesterone.

A detailed list of these hormones of pregnancy is available in Table 44.1.

The uterus is a pelvic organ until 10–12 weeks' gestation. As a result, a Doppler cannot hear the foetal heartbeat prior to this time. With the use of ultrasound, the foetal heart can be visualised and heard as early as 4–6 weeks'

TABLE 44.1 | Hormonal factors in pregnancy

Source	Hormone	Actions
Ovary	Oestrogens and progesterone during the first few weeks of pregnancy	Oestrogens influence: • uterine growth • breast growth • water and sodium retention • pituitary hormone release • maternal blood flow with the uterus and placenta to ensure oxygen and nutrients to the foetus and removal of foetal waste. Progesterone influences: • relaxation of smooth muscle (e.g. uterus, blood vessels) • softening of connective tissue (e.g. cervix, ligaments and nipples) • development of mammary ducts and alveolar tissue in the breast • immune system—enables the woman's body to tolerate foreign DNA (e.g. foetus).
Placenta	Oestrogens and progesterone	When the placenta is fully developed.
	Human placental lactogenic (hPL) hormone	• Commences 5–10 days after implantation; levels continue to increase and peak just prior to term. • Facilitates growth and development of the foetus. • Stimulates development of the breasts. • Plays a role in foetal metabolism. • Changes maternal metabolism to maximise the availability of nutrients to the foetus. • Anti-insulin properties.
	Relaxin	Has a relaxant effect, especially on connective tissue (e.g. ligaments in the pelvis), softens the cervix.
Pituitary	Thyroid-stimulating hormone (TSH)	Small amount of TSH crosses the placenta to maintain normal foetal thyroid function for up to 12 weeks' gestation when the foetus' thyroid begins to function. Critical role in foetal development of the brain and nervous system. Stimulates release of thyroxine to maintain increased metabolism.
	Oxytocin	Contraction of the uterus (at the end of pregnancy). Excretion of milk (after birth).
	Prolactin	Initiates lactation (after baby is born). Prepares the breast tissue for lactation.
Parathyroids	Parathormone	Maintains normal calcium ion concentration.
Adrenals	Adrenal hormones (e.g. glucocorticoids and aldosterone)	Increased secretion maintains increased metabolism. Steroids released are used by the placenta to produce oestrogen.

(Blackburn 2018; Pairman et al 2023)

gestation. An ultrasound is not routinely performed at this gestation unless there are associated concerns (e.g. vaginal bleeding that is not menstrual period). An ultrasound is not attended with the view to listen to and visualise the heart at an early gestation.

In the last trimester of pregnancy, **vernix caseosa** naturally occurs over the foetal skin. Vernix caseosa (or vernix as it is commonly called in clinical practice) is produced by the foetal sebaceous glands. It is a waxy, cheese-like substance found on the skin of newborns, protecting the foetal skin from amniotic fluid in utero. The amniotic fluid has many roles, one being to protect the foetus from infection.

As foetal gestation advances, the amount of vernix on the foetus reduces. Once born, if there is any vernix on the newborn's skin, this does not need to be washed off/removed. It assists to moisturise and protect the newborn's skin and assist with **thermoregulation**.

Thermoregulation is the ability to balance heat loss with heat production through normal thermoregulatory mechanisms in order to maintain body temperature within a normothermic range (The Royal Children's Hospital Melbourne 2019).

Some newborns may be born with fine hair on their body, particularly their shoulders and upper arms. This is called **lanugo**. The earlier the gestation, the more lanugo is present. Lanugo initially develops at approximately 18–20 weeks' gestation and often disappears by weeks 36–40. Lanugo assists to protect the foetal skin and provides the ability for the vernix caseosa to adhere to the foetal skin.

Adaptation to pregnancy involves all of a woman's body systems. The mother's physical response is assessed in relation to normal expected alterations. Women can experience varying signs that can signify pregnancy. The maternal physiological changes during pregnancy are listed in Table 44.2.

Psychological changes

During pregnancy a woman's psychological status may alter (e.g. she may experience anxiety and emotional lability). The pregnant woman's psychological status depends on many factors, including her basic personality, whether the pregnancy was planned and is desired, the strength of her social and family support systems and her self-concept. A number of emotional problems can arise during pregnancy or after the birth. Anxiety or depression can occur antenatally or postnatally (see also Chapter 39).

Confirmation of pregnancy

The signs of pregnancy are divided into three general groups: possible, probable and positive.

Possible indicators of pregnancy

Signs of possible pregnancy are those from which a definite diagnosis of pregnancy cannot be confirmed. Signs and

TABLE 44.2 | Physiological changes in pregnancy

Area of change	Description
Uterus	Increase in size to about 30 × 22 × 20 cm (at term). The uterus is five times its normal size by term. Increase in mass to about 1 kg (at term). Cervix becomes softer (in preparation for labour). A plug of mucus (the operculum) is formed by, and remains in, the cervix from the eighth week until labour begins. The uterus forms into two segments; the lower segment is thinner and becomes soft and dilated towards the end of pregnancy. Painless, irregular contractions (Braxton Hicks contractions) occur throughout pregnancy.
Vagina	In early pregnancy, the vagina (and cervix) change in colour from pink to dark red/blue. The amount of acidic vaginal secretions increases. Thickness increases, due to venous dilation.
Breasts	Increase in size and mass. Nipples enlarge and become more prominent and darker in colour. Areolae become darker. Prominent sebaceous glands (Montgomery's tubercles) appear on the areolae at about 12 weeks. Surface blood vessels more visible due to increased circulation. Increased sensation and tingling. Colostrum (the fluid secreted during pregnancy) can be expressed at 16 weeks.
Skin	Darker pigmentation in the nipples and areolae, on the face (chloasma) and on the abdominal midline (linea nigra). Stretch marks may appear on the abdomen, breasts and buttocks. Spider naevi (bright red lesions with minute radiating branches) may appear on the face and upper chest.
Musculoskeletal system	Spinal curvature changes to compensate for the abdominal enlargement, resulting in arching of the back. The symphysis pubis and sacroiliac joints become mobile, and the pelvis becomes wider, due to softening of the connective tissue in preparation for labour due to the effects of relaxin.

TABLE 44.2 | Physiological changes in pregnancy—cont'd

Area of change	Description
Urinary tract	Relaxation of smooth muscle causes the ureters to become dilated, elongated. These changes may lead to stasis of urine and infection. Frequency of micturition may occur in the early months, as the uterus occupies more of the pelvis. Reduced muscle tone in the pelvic floor, and increased pressure from the growing foetus, may result in stress incontinence towards the end of pregnancy.
Gastrointestinal tract	Hormonal and mechanical changes (e.g. increased hormonal levels and reduced intestinal motility) may result in morning sickness, gastric acid reflux and constipation due to the hormonal effects on relaxing the smooth muscles.
Cardiovascular system	Blood volume increases by 30–50%. A pregnant woman has up to 1.5 L extra blood at full term. Cardiac output is increased because of increased heart rate by about 15 beats/minute and an increase in stroke volume (amount of blood pumped out of the heart in a single beat). Haemodilution (due to increased plasma volume) results in lowered haemoglobin level as, although there is a constant red blood cell increase, the increase in blood plasma volume is larger, resulting in dilution. Total volume of red blood cells increases by 18% due to the increased oxygen requirements of the mother, foetus and placenta. Coagulability of blood is slightly increased. Reduced tone in blood vessels may result in varicose veins.
Respiratory tract	Ventilation rate is increased to obtain the higher amounts of oxygen required.
Basal metabolic rate (BMR)	In the second half of pregnancy, BMR increases by 15–25% to cope with the increased demands.
Body mass	Weight gain is due partially to the growth of the uterus and breasts, the uterine contents, increase in maternal blood volume and interstitial fluid and maternal storage of fats and proteins.
Weight gain	Average gain in the first 3 months is 0.5–2 kg for everyone. Recommended weight gain over the whole pregnancy: BMI $<$18.5: 12.5–18 kg; BMI 18.5–24: 11.5–16 kg; BMI 25–29: 7–11.5 kg; BMI $>$30: 5–9 kg.

(Blackburn 2018; Department of Health & Aged Care 2020; Pairman et al 2023)

symptoms during this stage can often be caused by other conditions. The indications of possible pregnancy are:

- amenorrhoea—missed period
- nausea and vomiting
- breast enlargement and tenderness
- frequency of micturition, especially at night
- quickening
- cravings for some foods, distaste for other foods usually liked
- a sour or metallic taste persisting even when not eating
- fatigue.

(Perry et al 2022)

Amenorrhoea (the cessation of menses) in a sexually active healthy woman is often the first indication of pregnancy (Lowdermilk et al 2020). However, other factors may cause amenorrhoea, such as eating disorders (anorexia nervosa, bulimia), excessive exercise or changes in metabolism and endocrine function. Some women may experience a 'light' period around the time of their expected period, not realising this is not a period but is evidence of uterine implantation by the embryo.

The symptoms of nausea and vomiting, which can occur at any time of the day, are often referred to as **morning sickness**. Nausea often occurs between 6 and 14 weeks' gestation but may continue until 32 weeks, or longer for some women. It is believed to be a result of high quantities of placental hormones (progesterone, oestrogen, hCG and hPL) (Lowdermilk et al 2020).

Breast enlargement and tenderness are a result of the placental hormones stimulating the breast ductal system in preparation for breastfeeding. Some women experience similar symptoms premenstrually and pregnancy is often overlooked for this reason.

Increased pigmentation of the skin occurs over the face (chloasma), breasts (darkening of the areolae) and abdomen (linea nigra—a dark line extending from the umbilicus to the symphysis pubis).

Frequency of micturition occurs at the start of pregnancy and then again in the third trimester. In the first trimester, the enlarging uterus competes for space in the pelvic cavity and exerts pressure on the urinary bladder. In the later stage of pregnancy, the descending foetal part of the uterus moves into the pelvic cavity in preparation for birth.

Quickening is the result of foetal movement and is first perceived at 16–20 weeks' gestation. The sensation is felt by the mother and is described as gentle fluttering in the lower abdomen (Pairman et al 2023; Perry et al 2022).

Fatigue is common in early pregnancy due to the increased production of progesterone, which slows down metabolism and is necessary to maintain the pregnancy and for early foetal growth.

The woman's energy level often increases at approximately 16–20 weeks' gestation, when the placenta has established its function. However, iron deficiency anaemia may be another reason for this symptom.

Probable indicators of pregnancy

Abdominal **uterine enlargement**, the presence of Braxton Hicks contractions and a positive pregnancy test are indicators that a woman is probably pregnant. However, on very rare occasions there may be other conditions or factors (uterine tumours, medications, or premature menopause) that cause these events.

Abdominal and uterine enlargement occurs around the 12th week of pregnancy. At this stage, the fundus of the uterus can be located just above the symphysis pubis and extends to the umbilicus between weeks 20 and 22.

Braxton Hicks contractions are irregular, painless uterine contractions that first occur in the second trimester (Lowdermilk et al 2020). They are more pronounced in multiparas (women who have had more than one child) and can be mistaken for labour contractions.

A pregnancy test may be performed after the first missed menstrual cycle. Pregnancy tests use maternal blood or urine to determine the presence of the placental hormone hCG. hCG is the earliest biologic marker for pregnancy (Lowdermilk et al 2020). Levels of hCG rise steeply in the first trimester of pregnancy and then fall to low levels for the remainder of the pregnancy. A positive result from a pregnancy test is considered an indicator of probable pregnancy. Sandwich-type immunoassay testing is the most popular method of testing for pregnancy and is the basis for most home pregnancy tests. The accuracy of the results of home pregnancy testing is related to following the instructions correctly. The main reason for incorrect results is the test being performed too soon following a suspected 'missed' period before a significant rise in hCG level; this can cause a false-negative result (Lowdermilk et al 2020).

Professional pregnancy tests based on urine or blood serum are even more reliably accurate. The most highly reliable test is the radioimmunoassay (RIA), a technique in radiology that can accurately identify pregnancy as early as 1 week after ovulation. Blood tests are 99% accurate. A quantitative blood test measures the exact amount of hCG in the blood, providing an estimate of gestation. The qualitative blood test checks for the presence of hCG in the blood. While attributed with high levels of accuracy, pregnancy tests cannot be classed as absolutely certain indicators because there are factors that may interfere with the reliability of test results. These factors include premature menopause, the effects of taking some particular medications (anticonvulsants or anti-anxiety drugs) and the presence of a malignant ovarian tumour.

Haematuria or a urinary tract infection (UTI), a recent birth or miscarriage, a faulty test kit or a dirty, contaminated collection cup may also interfere with the reliability of the test results (Murray et al 2023).

Positive indicators of pregnancy

The most positive sign of pregnancy is a growing and developing baby (Perry et al 2022). The foetal heartbeat can be detected as early as 4–6 weeks of gestation using equipment such as a pelvic ultrasound. This scan enables (allows) the examiner to detect and record the foetal heart rate and therefore confirm pregnancy. The Doppler can be used to listen to the baby's heart rate from 12–14 weeks' gestation onwards.

Foetal body parts can be felt by an educated examiner (obstetrician or midwife) from the later part of the second trimester onwards. This gives the examiner an indication of the position of the foetus, which is vital during the third trimester when discussing birthing options.

Estimated due date/estimated agreed due date

The date when the baby is due—EDD/ADD—may be calculated by LNMP dates or by use of an ultrasound. Ultrasound scanning is most accurate in determining gestational age between 8 and 14 weeks of pregnancy; after 24 weeks of pregnancy, the date of the last menstrual period is used (Department of Health & Aged Care 2020).

An estimated ADD should be made as soon as possible in pregnancy.

The evidence suggests that:

- If the LNMP was certain and menstruation regular, then the following need to be considered:
  - If the woman has had an ultrasound between 6 and 13 weeks of gestation and the two EDD differ by 5 days or less, use the LNMP EDD. If the two dates differ by more than 5 days, use the ultrasound EDD.
  - If the woman has had an ultrasound between 13 and 24 weeks of gestation and the two EDD dates differ by 10 days or less, use the LNMP EDD. If the two dates differ by more than 10 days, use the ultrasound EDD.
- If the woman has not had an ultrasound between 6 and 24 weeks of gestation, use the LNMP EDD.
- If the LNMP was not certain or she had irregular menstrual periods (e.g. because of lactational amenorrhoea), use the EDD estimate from an ultrasound performed between 6 and 24 weeks of gestation.

(Department of Health & Aged Care 2020; Lowdermilk et al 2020; Safer Care Victoria 2021)

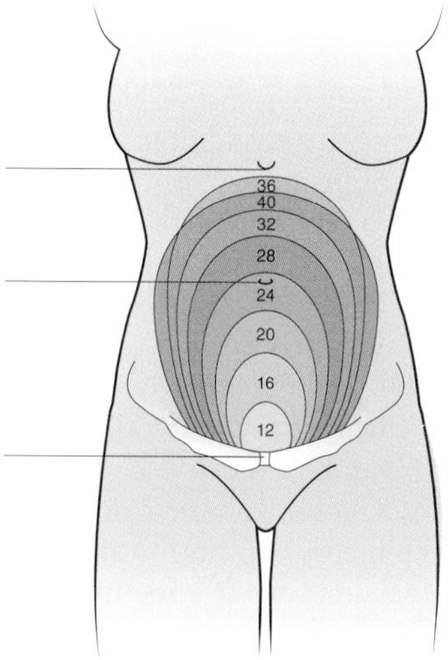

Figure 44.1 Fundal height of the uterus

Calculation by dates to determine the estimated due date is made by ascertaining the first day of the last known menstrual period and adding 9 months and 7 days.

Fundal height is used to indirectly measure foetal growth in relation to gestational age. Calculation by assessing the fundal height (Figure 44.1) is made by measuring the height of the upper border of the fundus from the upper border of the symphysis pubis. If the woman's bladder is empty at the time of measurement, from gestational weeks 18 to 30, the height of the fundus in centimetres is approximately the same as the number of weeks of gestation (± 2 gestational weeks) (Lowdermilk et al 2020).

Minor discomforts associated with pregnancy

The pregnant woman may experience one or more minor disorders or discomforts, many of which are the result of increased secretion of hormones or pressure from the uterus and its contents on other body structures. Table 44.3 lists the potential discomforts and outlines guidelines that can be used to increase comfort levels.

TABLE 44.3 | Health education: Management of minor discomforts during pregnancy

Discomfort	Management guidelines
Morning sickness	Small, frequent dry meals. Fluids in-between meals. Something to eat (e.g. a dry biscuit) before getting out of bed in the morning. Avoid fried and heavily spiced foods. Before bed, eat food that contains protein.
Indigestion	Small frequent meals. Avoid spicy foods or greasy foods. Avoid drinking coffee. Avoid smoking cigarettes. Elevate the head of the bed.
Constipation	High-fibre foods. Adequate fluids. Exercise every day.
Fainting	Avoid sudden postural changes. Avoid constrictive clothing. Avoid lying on the back during late pregnancy. Avoid fatigue.
Backache	Maintain correct posture. Daily rest periods. Wear low-heeled shoes. Sleep on a firm surface (e.g. place a board under the mattress). Warm pack on back. Back massage.
Varicose veins	Avoid long periods of standing. Avoid constrictive clothing. Elevate the legs whenever possible. Wear supportive stockings. Avoid sitting or standing with the legs crossed.
Urinary tract infection	Adequate fluids. Perineal hygiene measures (e.g. wiping from front to back after elimination).
Leg muscle cramps	Avoid standing for long periods. Elevate the legs whenever possible. Relieve symptoms by pulling upwards on toes. Diet with adequate calcium, iron and potassium.
Haemorrhoids	Avoid constipation—eat plenty of fruit and vegetables and drink plenty of fluids. Relieve discomfort by applying cold compresses or ice packs. Lying down for periods of time.

(Lowdermilk et al 2020; Pairman et al 2023; Perry et al 2022)

Gravidity and parity

An understanding of the following terms used to describe pregnancy and the woman who is pregnant assists in the provision of maternity care:

- gravida: a woman who is pregnant
- gravidity: pregnancy
- nulligravida: a woman who has never been pregnant and is not currently pregnant
- primigravida: a woman who is pregnant for the first time
- multigravida: a woman who has had two or more pregnancies
- parity: the number of pregnancies in which the foetus or foetuses have reached 20 weeks of gestation, not

the number of foetuses (e.g. twins) born; parity is not affected by whether the foetus is born alive or is stillborn (i.e. showing no signs of life at birth)
- nullipara: a woman who has not completed a pregnancy with a foetus or foetuses who have reached at least 20 weeks of gestation
- primipara: a woman who has completed one pregnancy with a foetus or foetuses who have reached 20 weeks of gestation or more
- multipara: a woman who has completed two or more pregnancies to 20 weeks of gestation or more.

(Lowdermilk et al 2020)

PRENATAL CARE AND PREPARATION

Prenatal (or **antenatal**) means before birth. The aims of prenatal care are to:
- promote a healthy pregnancy and normal labour
- promote the birth of a healthy, living baby
- prepare the woman and her partner/support person for labour and birth
- detect and manage any complications.

The initial consultation

The woman's initial consultation concerning her pregnancy may be with her general practitioner, obstetrician or a midwife, and involves obtaining a comprehensive health and social history, performing a thorough physical examination, and discussing where the woman wishes to give birth (Perry et al 2022).

The physical examination includes checking the blood pressure, heart and lungs, palpating the abdomen, and assessing weight, height, body build and skin colour. Samples of urine and blood are obtained and tested. Urine is tested to diagnose pregnancy and to detect the presence of abnormalities (e.g. glucose or protein or signs of asymptomatic bacteraemia). Blood is tested to determine blood group and Rhesus (Rh) factor status, haemoglobin level and the presence of rubella antibodies. Maternal serum screening testing will also be discussed and offered to the woman, screening for some foetal abnormalities (e.g. trisomy 18 and 21).

Testing will be done to exclude certain disorders, such as blood-borne viruses (e.g. human immunodeficiency virus [HIV] and hepatitis B and C) and sexually transmitted infections (e.g. syphilis), and to gauge vitamin D levels. Glucose tolerance testing to screen for gestational diabetes and a vaginal swab to test for group B streptococcal (GBS) infection will also be discussed and attended (or a risk factor-based approach to prevention taken), depending on organisational policy.

Approximately 1:7 (17%) of women are **Rhesus (D)** negative blood type. While this is generally not an issue, during pregnancy, the woman with Rhesus (D) negative blood requires/is recommended to have additional monitoring, and prophylactic treatment during the antenatal period (with the woman's consent) is required. In addition, in the postnatal period, if the newborn baby's blood is tested and found to be Rhesus (D) positive, additional treatment for the mother is required/recommended.

During pregnancy, if the foetus' blood is Rhesus (D) positive, there is a small risk of maternal sensitisation to the Rhesus (D) positive blood. Maternal sensitisation occurs when there has been in utero mixing of the maternal Rhesus (D) negative blood with the Rhesus (D) positive blood of the foetus, either during pregnancy or at the birth. The woman's body develops antibodies to the Rhesus (D) positive blood. In a first pregnancy if no sensitisation occurs, the foetus will not be affected. However, in subsequent pregnancy/s with a foetus with Rhesus (D) positive blood, if this sensitising event has occurred, antibodies to Rhesus (D) positive blood will attack the red blood cells of the foetus, causing **haemolytic disease** of the foetus and/or newborn (HDFN). This can result in serious complications and even death of the foetus or newborn due to severe anaemia.

To minimise this sensitisation event, research recommends that all women who have Rhesus (D) negative blood receive prophylactic administration of Rh (D) (anti-D) immunoglobulins via injection at 28 and 34 weeks' gestation pregnancy. In addition, within 72 hours of birth, if the newborn is Rhesus (D) positive, the woman receives a further injection of Rh (D) (anti-D) immunoglobulin.

Rh (D) (anti-D) immunoglobulin administration may also be required to be administered to Rhesus (D) negative women if during pregnancy they have a potentially sensitising event (e.g. miscarriage, termination of pregnancy, amniocentesis or abdominal trauma) (Australian Red Cross Lifeblood 2017; RANZCOG 2019a).

A cervical smear and/or cervical swabs may be obtained if the woman has not had regular cervical screening tests or if infection is suspected. This may be delayed until the woman has her 6-week post-birth check-up.

If pregnancy is confirmed, the obstetrician or midwife will discuss with the woman possible options regarding the birth. The woman may choose to give birth in a hospital or in a birthing centre or have a home birth; she may also choose not to continue with the pregnancy (Pairman et al 2023).

Prenatal education may be provided by the obstetrician, midwives or childbirth educators. The educational aspects of prenatal care are listed in Table 44.4.

Subsequent consultations

The frequency with which subsequent visits occur depends on the model of care chosen, which may include obstetrician, team midwives or GP/shared care, and the needs of the woman. The usual practice is to schedule visits 4-weekly until 28 weeks, then 2-weekly until 36 weeks, then weekly until birth. Women with low-risk pregnancies may have fewer routine prenatal visits, whereas those at risk for complications may be seen more frequently.

TABLE 44.4 | Prenatal education

Aspect	Description
Diet	A balanced diet designed to meet the nutritional requirements of pregnancy: • Vegetables/legumes/beans: 5 daily serves. • Fruit: 2 daily serves. • Grains: 8 daily serves if < 19 yrs; 8.5 daily serves if > 19 yrs. • Lean meat, chicken, fish: 2.5 daily serves. • Eggs, nuts and seeds. • Milk, yoghurt, cheese: 2.5 daily serves if < 19 yrs; 3.5 daily serves if > 19 yrs. • Folic acid: Supplement 400 microg per day when planning a pregnancy and in the first trimester. • Iodine: Increased requirement during pregnancy, daily supplement of 150 microg of iodine recommended as most food in Australia is low in iodine (most pregnancy multivitamins contain this. Kelp tablets contain too much iodine). • Iron: Supplement if blood tests suggest low iron levels. • Calcium: 100 mg/100 mL. • Vitamin D: A supplement is suggested if blood test is low or if the woman is at risk of vitamin D deficiency (e.g. darker skin, covers most of body in clothing or spends most of time indoors). • Vitamin B12: People who do not eat meat, eat little dairy or eggs or none at all are at risk. A supplement may be suggested depending on blood test levels. • Listeria: Avoid foods that may contain this bacterium (e.g. sandwich meat, soft cheese, soft-serve ice cream, prepared salads, pate, smoked salmon, uncooked seafood). Freshly cooked seafood is safe. Cooking food to boiling point destroys listeria, so if reheating, make sure the food is steaming hot. • Alcohol: Nil is safest. • Fish: 3 serves a week; however, limit shark/marlin/broadbill or swordfish—no more than 2 serves/fortnight. Deep sea perch or catfish—one serve/week and eat no other fish that week due to the high mercury levels. • Caffeine: Safe in moderation, 1–3 cups a day depending on strength and up to 5 cups of tea a day. Limit energy drinks. • Liver/vitamin A: Liver up to 50 g/week. • Toxoplasmosis: Cook meat thoroughly. Use of gloves when handling kitty litter. Wash hands after handling pets or after gardening. • *Salmonella:* Avoid uncooked meats and eggs to minimise the risk of *Salmonella* infection.
Exercise	• Pregnancy is not a time to begin more intense exercise programs; continue and/or modify established programs. • Avoid overheating—pregnancy increases body temperature; avoid hot humid weather and poorly ventilated rooms. • Exercise should not be commenced or stopped suddenly. • Avoid long periods of motionlessness. • Avoid high-intensity exercise and increasing heart rate above 140 beats/min. • If stretching is part of exercise routine, in second and third trimester, gently stretch due to effects of relaxin.
Rest	• Fatigue should be avoided by obtaining sufficient sleep and by having numerous short rest periods during the day.
Hygiene	• Normal hygiene practices should be continued. Vaginal douching is to be avoided.
Clothing	• Wear comfortable non-constrictive garments and shoes with low heels. • Maternity girdles are available, which provide support for just above the symphysis pubis and the lower back.
Preparation for labour and birth	• Midwives or physiotherapists conduct education on childbirth and relaxation techniques on an individual or group basis. The woman's partner/support person is encouraged to attend the childbirth education program, which prepares the couple for labour and birth. The classes include instruction in relaxation techniques. • The couple is also informed of the physiology of labour and encouraged to discuss all aspects of pregnancy, birth, and care of the baby.

Continued

TABLE 44.4 | Prenatal education—cont'd

Aspect	Description
Manifestations of complications	The woman is advised to contact her obstetrician or the hospital immediately if there is: • vaginal bleeding • abdominal or 'menstrual-type' pain • severe headaches • drainage of fluid from the vagina • excessive vomiting • blurred vision • difficulty in passing urine • swelling of the hands, feet or face • reduced or altered foetal movements.
Manifestations of labour	The couple are informed of the manifestations of the onset of labour: • regular, painful, rhythmical contractions • vaginal 'show' (bloodstained mucus).
Breasts	• Maternity bras are designed to support the breasts as they increase in size and mass.
Sexual activity	• Sexual activity may be continued throughout the pregnancy, unless there are known pregnancy complications as advised by the obstetrician/midwife (e.g. placenta praevia). • If the woman has a history of spontaneous abortion, she may be advised to avoid sexual intercourse during the first 3 months of pregnancy.
Environmental hazards	Factors potentially harmful to the pregnancy should be avoided: • Smoking is linked to abortion, intrauterine growth retardation and perinatal death. • Alcohol is linked to physical and mental foetal abnormalities and foetal growth retardation. • Many drugs, prescribed and unprescribed, may be linked to foetal harm. • Exposure to microorganisms (e.g. rubella) in the first 3 months may result in foetal abnormalities. • Immunisations—influenza and the whooping cough (pertussis) vaccine are both encouraged during pregnancy. • Exposure to radiation during the early weeks of pregnancy may inhibit normal cell division. • Exposure to pesticides and other chemicals may result in foetal abnormalities.

(Department of Health & Aged Care 2020; Lowdermilk et al 2020; Murray et al 2023)

Prenatal care involves:

- gestation and estimated due date (EDD)
- blood pressure check
- maternal weight
- fundal height measurement
- foetal movements
- auscultation of the foetal heart with Doppler from 20 weeks
- abdominal palpation.

The standard antenatal check provides the basis for routine biophysical screening, assessment, referral and education (Pairman et al 2023). Blood tests or other investigations (e.g. ultrasonic examination) may be performed as part of routine care or when other tests or physical symptoms indicate there is a need. Ultrasound examination between 18 and 20 weeks' gestation allows assessment of foetal development and anatomy. It is also used to estimate gestational age when this has not been assessed in the first trimester (Department of Health & Aged Care 2020).

LABOUR

Labour is the process in which the woman has uterine contractions to assist with her baby's birth. The process also includes the vaginal birth of the placenta and membranes. Normal labour occurs spontaneously at 37–42 weeks of pregnancy. Towards the end of pregnancy, women may experience an increase in the intensity of Braxton Hicks contractions and an increase in vaginal discharge/mucus. There will be further descent of the foetal head into the pelvis and episodes of increasing uterine activity. Labour and birth are a normal process; the woman should be encouraged to listen to and trust her body, to rest and eat/drink as required with the support of professional midwifery/obstetric care. Avoidance of unnecessary intervention is beneficial to most women during their labour and birth. Because the management of, and attitudes towards, labour and birth differ widely among different cultures, expectant women, obstetricians and midwives, practices are adjusted according to individual needs, knowledge and experience.

The length of labour will vary from one woman to another.

Factors that may result in spontaneous onset of normal labour include changes in hormonal levels, uterine distension, foetal pressure and a sudden reduction of intrauterine pressure when the membranes rupture (Davidson et al 2020; Murray et al 2023; Pairman et al 2023).

Traditionally, there are four **stages of labour**. Table 44.5 lists the characteristics of each stage. However, labour is a continuous process with changes in the emotional and physical wellbeing of the woman.

During labour, the uterus contracts rhythmically to dilate and efface (take up) the cervix and push the foetus through the birth canal. After the baby is born, the uterus continues contracting to aid in the birth of the placenta and membranes.

The following section addresses the general aspects of care and support throughout labour and birth.

The first stage

Latent stage

Latent stage is difficult to define and understand, and there is no consensus regarding the length of time that the latent phase may take; however, this is often the longest stage of labour, particularly for a woman having her first baby. During this stage, the woman's body is preparing for birth. The cervix may begin to soften and become quite thin (efface) and may start to open (dilate). This can go on for hours or days. Some women feel nothing during this time; eventually, many women start to feel some pain and discomfort but there is no regularity or pattern to the contractions.

During this phase, the contractions are short and irregular, and the woman is easily distracted, able to sleep for short periods of time, often still feels hungry and is still connected to and has awareness of her surroundings (Pairman et al 2023).

Active or established first stage

During this stage of labour, the contractions are increasing in intensity, frequency and duration and becoming regular. The woman needs to move around more and may be unable to rest in one position for any length of time. The woman is often less connected to her surroundings and less able to talk through contractions and will 'go into herself'. The woman may not wish to eat.

On abdominal palpation, the baby has moved further into the pelvis and, on vaginal examination, the cervical effacement has continued to increase, the cervix continues to soften and dilate, and the baby's head is lower in the pelvis. At this time, women often want continuous support (Pairman et al 2023).

Care during the first stage involves monitoring the progress of labour, monitoring the condition of the woman and unborn baby (foetus) and promoting physical and psychological comfort. Progress of labour is monitored by assessing the strength, frequency and duration of contractions, by palpating the abdomen to assess the position and descent of the foetus and by performing vaginal examinations only when deemed necessary to assess the degree of cervical dilation and the position of the presenting part of the foetus. The condition of the woman and her response to labour are monitored by checking her vital signs, by observing urinary output and by observing her for the manifestations of fatigue, discomfort or pain.

The health of the unborn baby is monitored by assessing the foetal heart. Because the **foetal heart rate** and rhythm is the main indicator of the baby's health, the heartbeat is regularly assessed during labour. The heart rate should remain between 110 and 160 beats per minute

TABLE 44.5 | Stages of labour

Stage	Characteristics
First	Contractions occur at fairly regular intervals, from about every 10 minutes at the onset of labour to about every 2 minutes at the end of the first stage. The cervix is effaced (raised up). The foetal head begins to descend in the pelvis. The cervix is gradually dilated. The membranes may rupture and release amniotic fluid.
Second	Strong contractions occur, lasting about 60 seconds and becoming expulsive, and the woman experiences a desire to bear down. The woman uses abdominal muscles and the diaphragm to assist in pushing the foetus down the birth canal. The muscles of the pelvic floor are displaced by the advancing foetal head. The vagina is dilated, and the perineum is thinned and flattened by the advancing head. The vulva and vaginal orifice bulge and the anus dilates as the head advances. The baby is born.
Third	After a brief period, the placenta separates from the uterine wall. Uterine contractions restart to expel the placenta and membranes. Signs of separation and descent of the placenta are: • A small gush of blood from the vagina • The cord lengthens at the vulva • The uterus is firmly contracted, and the height of the fundus drops to umbilical level.
Fourth	In the 2 hours after birth of the baby and expulsion of the placenta and membranes, the uterus begins the process of involution. Involution is the return of the uterus to its normal size. The fourth stage of labour completes when the mother's body has returned to physiological stability.

(Davidson et al 2020)

and the beat should remain strong and regular. Assessment may be performed by listening to the heart through a foetal Doppler placed on the woman's abdomen or by using a foetal monitoring device, such as electronic foetal monitoring, known as a cardiotocograph. Foetal monitoring devices provide an audible and/or visual record of the foetal heartbeat (Pairman et al 2023; Perry et al 2022; RANZCOG 2019b).

Another way to assess the condition of the foetus is by observing the drainage of 'liquor' from the woman's vagina, if the membranes have ruptured either spontaneously or artificially. Normally, the liquor remains clear or pink-coloured, though at times it may be green or yellow in colour. This is called **meconium**-stained liquor and means that at some stage the foetus has passed meconium in the amniotic fluid, giving it a green/yellow colour. This may be a normal physiological response but may also be an indicator of an episode of hypoxia for the foetus; however, if this is the case, it cannot be directly determined when such an event may have occurred (Victorian Newborn Resuscitation Project 2014).

Promoting comfort

Unless there are factors that may compromise the condition of the woman or her baby, the woman is encouraged to do whatever will contribute to her comfort. She may choose to walk around or may prefer to sit or lie down. The woman may like to engage in some form of activity, such as reading, watching television or listening to music. Some women find that frequent warm showers/baths enhance their comfort, while others may prefer to have their partner or the midwife massage their abdomen and back.

During the first stage, the woman may need to be encouraged and supported to use the relaxation techniques learned in prenatal classes. She is encouraged to empty her bladder at least every 2 hours since a full bladder can inhibit uterine action. The woman is also encouraged to consume fluids and a light diet as tolerated. Because the absorption of food is slowed down during labour, women often do not feel like eating and often feel nauseated and/or may vomit.

Fatigue is minimised by encouraging rest and relaxation and by relieving discomfort or pain.

Strong contractions may be painful, and the measures used to minimise and relieve discomfort will vary according to the needs and choices of each woman. Measures to relieve pain aim to reduce pain and tension without any harmful effects to the woman or baby. Measures include practising relaxation techniques, assuming the most comfortable position, back and abdominal massage, using music as a distraction and medications. Medications such as analgesics may be prescribed. Analgesic medications may be administered by inhalation (e.g. nitrous oxide and oxygen), intramuscular injection (e.g. morphine/pethidine) or injection of local anaesthetic solution into the epidural/spinal space surrounding the spinal cord, from which the nerves supplying the uterus or cervix arise (epidural/spinal analgesia).

Throughout the first stage, the midwife should provide emotional support and encouragement (Murray et al 2023; Pairman et al 2023; Perry et al 2022).

Transitioning to second stage

This is the final stage of the first stage of labour. At this point, the cervix is progressing from 7 cm to 10 cm (fully dilated); it is the shortest but hardest part of birth and is when women may doubt their ability to birth their baby and will often request pain relief. At this point, the woman is almost at the pushing stage. She may worry about how long her labour will last and how much more intense it will become. Women can be very vulnerable at this stage and will often accept interventions they previously had stated they did not want. During this stage, the woman needs lots of emotional support and guidance and should be encouraged to rest between contractions. The woman may have a heavy, bloodstained mucus 'show' and a sensation of pressure in her bowel, with an urge to push. For some women at this stage, their contractions slow down and they can rest and/or sleep in-between contractions.

Second stage of labour

Traditionally, and currently, the definition of second stage labour commencement is described as when the cervix is fully dilated. The duration of second stage is therefore based on when the woman is diagnosed as being fully dilated by the midwifery or medical staff.

Although it may be accompanied by some anxiety, the second stage of labour signals the imminent birth of the baby and concludes with the actual birth of the baby (Murray et al 2023). Progress of labour and the condition of the unborn baby are monitored as in the first stage, but at more frequent intervals. During contractions the midwife and/or partner should offer encouragement. As the foetal head reaches the pelvic floor, most women experience the urge to push (Murray et al 2023). The woman will automatically begin to exert pressure downwards by contracting her abdominal muscles while relaxing her pelvic floor. This bearing-down reflex is an involuntary reflex response to the pressure of the presenting part on stretch receptors of pelvic muscles. The midwife then encourages the woman to push when the urge to push is felt, rather than giving a long-prolonged push on command.

Between contractions the woman may wish to have her lower back massaged and should be encouraged to rest. Small sips of fluid or ice chips should be offered to moisten her mouth, and the woman may wish to have her face wiped at frequent intervals. The woman is encouraged to adopt the position in which she feels the most comfortable for the birth. Physical support may be needed to maintain the woman in a suitable position.

The birth

The **birth** of the baby may take place with the mother lying down, standing, squatting or kneeling. Some maternity units and birth centres are equipped to accommodate the woman and her partner in a home-like environment, with some women choosing to have a water birth. During birth of the baby, the obstetrician or midwife assists by gently controlling the emergence of the head to prevent perineal damage. In some instances, an episiotomy (incision into the perineum to enlarge the vaginal opening) may be necessary. Sometimes the application of obstetric forceps to the foetal head may be necessary to assist in its passage through the birth canal.

During an uncomplicated birth, after the baby's head has cleared the vagina, the shoulders and the rest of the baby's body are gently pushed out. Immediately after birth, the baby is generally placed on the mother's abdomen. The umbilical cord is clamped in two places and cut between the clamps (Davidson et al 2020). Although 96–97% of babies present headfirst, a small number are born buttocks first (breech presentation) (Lowdermilk et al 2020).

The second stage is completed when the baby is born, which is an emotional time for everyone involved in the birth process. The baby is placed on the mother's abdomen, and both she and her partner can look at and caress their infant. The obstetrician or midwife remains nearby so that the condition of both mother and baby can be monitored. The midwife encourages the mother to initiate skin-to-skin contact with her baby: the baby is placed at her breast and encouraged to suckle. This is thought to help establish the attachment process between mother and baby, and suckling promotes uterine contractions, necessary for expulsion of the placenta.

Caesarean birth

A **caesarean** birth is the birth of the baby through a surgical abdominal incision. The incision is usually made just above the pubic bone in the lower part of the abdomen. When the uterus is cut through the lower part, this approach is referred to as a lower uterine segment caesarean section (LUSCS). Some caesarean births are planned (elective caesarean) because of existing problems with the pregnancy. These may include presentation of the foetus, maternal diseases, prolapsed umbilical cord or placenta praevia. In other cases, the decision to perform a caesarean is made during labour. This is called an emergency caesarean. An emergency caesarean section may be indicated for a variety of reasons, including maternal complications, such as severe bleeding or preeclampsia, foetal distress or failure to progress in labour. Most women who have had a LUSCS are eligible for a vaginal birth after caesarean (VBAC) in the future (Murray et al 2023; Perry et al 2022).

The third stage

During this stage, the placenta and membranes are expelled. In most settings, oxytocic medications such as Syntocinon or Syntometrine are given (if the woman does not have hypertension) to promote uterine contraction and reduce the risk of post-partum haemorrhage. After expulsion of the placenta, the woman's vulva and vagina are inspected for any lacerations or tears. Lacerations or an episiotomy may be repaired. Some lacerations may not need repairing if they are limited in size, the wound edges approximate and the laceration is not bleeding. A perineal pad is applied (often with an ice pack to assist with swelling and pain) to collect the vaginal discharge. The woman is assessed for signs of haemorrhage and for any adverse effects of the birth. To assist with involution (decrease in size of the uterus), the midwife will massage the uterine fundus through the abdominal wall to promote contraction and retraction. The placenta and membranes are assessed to see if they are normal and complete. If they are incomplete, there may be fragments retained in the uterus, preventing uterine contraction, and increasing the potential for post-partum haemorrhage or infection (Davidson et al 2020). (See Case Study 44.1.)

The fourth stage

The fourth stage of labour is the first 2 hours after birth of the placenta, or until the woman has regained physiological stability (Lowdermilk et al 2020). During this time, the midwife's role includes monitoring the woman for her emotional health and wellbeing, levels of pain, bladder function, blood loss and recovery from anaesthesia. The midwife will support skin-to-skin contact between mother and baby and support the initiation of breastfeeding. Observations of the newborn's adaptation to extrauterine life will be observed by monitoring the newborn's colour, respirations, heart rate and temperature.

The midwife's role also includes providing emotional support that may be necessary for the woman, family, or significant others. It should be acknowledged that not all women will have partners and not all will have the family support they may desire, and this may be a time when sensitivity is required.

CASE STUDY 44.1

Ben and Emily

Emily had been in labour for 12 hours and delivered a 3.9 kg male infant vaginally after a normal pregnancy, labour and delivery. Emily and her husband Ben have another son at home aged 18 months. Emily had just transferred into the ward an hour before and the report you received was that all her assessments were normal. She uses her call bell and when you go to answer, you find her sitting on the toilet. She shows you her pad, which is saturated and full. When she stands up you notice a trickle running down her leg. She tells you it has been like that since she left the bed to go to the toilet. As you help her back to bed, you notice a large blood-soaked area on the sheets.

What nursing actions should you take?

Cultural influences on birthing practices

The woman's cultural background may influence her needs and wishes during pregnancy, labour and the postnatal period. This may be very different from that of the midwife but must be understood and respected. Australia is a multicultural society and providing for the many different cultural preferences of women requires flexibility on the part of midwives and nurses. Over one-quarter (27%) of mothers who gave birth in 2018 were born in a mainly non-English-speaking country compared with 26% of women of reproductive age in the population (AIHW 2020). There are differing cultural beliefs of significant importance to women concerning:

- who should be present during the labour and birth
- showering or bathing after birth
- what is considered an appropriate diet for a new mother
- how long and how much a woman should rest after the birth
- what should happen to the baby (e.g. when breastfeeding should begin, what clothing and adornments should be used)
- specific rituals and practices that promote healing of the body
- what should happen to the placenta.

Cultural attitudes vary enormously. For example, in over 50 known cultures, including Filipino, Vietnamese, Korean and Mexican, it is not the cultural norm for women to give infants colostrum, and breastfeeding is delayed until the milk has come in (Ladewig et al 2017). In most Southeast Asian cultures, it is seen as essential that the woman is not exposed to anything cold after the birth since this is believed to risk the onset of arthritis and bladder problems. Many people of Vietnamese culture believe that showering and washing the hair too soon after giving birth leads to recurring headaches and hair dropping out quickly in old age. Many people in Hmong culture believe that when a person dies, they must collect the person's placenta (termed 'black jacket') and put it on the deceased so they can be allowed entry into heaven. For this reason, a Hmong woman may be very anxious about what is happening to her placenta and may request that it be given to the family for burial at the woman's home. Clinical Interest Box 44.1 provides examples of cultural influences on infant feeding.

When midwives/nurses understand the beliefs behind cultural practices, the risk of confusion and conflict concerning what the woman chooses to do during and after the birth of her baby is reduced (Pairman et al 2023). However, care should be taken not to generalise about what happens in particular cultures because attitudes, values, beliefs and practices can vary significantly even within each cultural group (see Chapter 13). In addition, the process of assimilation into a new culture may alter traditional beliefs and practices. Clinical Interest Box 44.2

CLINICAL INTEREST BOX 44.1 Cultural influences on infant feeding

Infant feeding may be influenced by cultural beliefs and practices. Many cultures only begin breastfeeding after the milk has 'come in' and do not give colostrum to newborns. These include Asian, Latin American and sub-Saharan African cultures. Some rationales for this practice include a concern that because colostrum volume is small, the baby may be at risk for dehydration, or that non-milk feeds are needed to 'cleanse' the gastrointestinal tract for digestion.

A recent study of Chinese immigrant women in Australia reported that Chinese women were more likely to combine breastfeeding with formula and introduce solids earlier than the general Australian population (Kuswara et al 2016). Chinese mothers shared that although they supported exclusive breastfeeding, grandparents frequently pressured them to use formula, believing that 'a fat baby is a healthy baby'. Similar findings were found in Somali women where early formula supplementation and the introduction of early water feedings is common. Somali culture apparently favours 'chubby' babies, and formula is seen as the best way to ensure this.

(Kuswara et al 2016; Speedie & Middleton 2022; Wandel et al 2016)

CLINICAL INTEREST BOX 44.2 Pregnancy care guidelines for Aboriginal and Torres Strait Islander women

While many Aboriginal and Torres Strait Islander women experience healthy pregnancies, poor health and social complexity contribute to worse overall perinatal outcomes than those experienced by non-Aboriginal and Torres Strait Islander women. The Department of Health & Aged Care (2019) provides evidence-based recommendations to support health professionals to provide high-quality, safe pregnancy care for Aboriginal and Torres Strait Islander women and cover the following topics:

- providing woman-centred care
- understanding the woman's context
- cultural safety
- improving women's experience of antenatal care:
  - taking an individualised approach
  - providing information and support so that women can make decisions
  - Aboriginal community worker involvement
- successful models of antenatal care
- birthing on country
- adolescent mothers
- improving outcomes.

(Department of Health & Aged Care 2019)

provides pregnancy care guidelines for Aboriginal and Torres Strait Islander women.

However, not only are there cultural and religious beliefs to consider, the family unit may not consist of the 'traditional family' of a mother, father and sibling/s depending on the gender identity and sexual orientation a person may identify as.

Pregnancy is becoming increasingly more common among couples who are lesbian, gay, bisexual, transgender, or queer/questioning, intersex and asexual (LGBTQIA+) (Lowdermilk et al 2020). Evidence suggests that the LGBTQIA+ community experience poorer health outcomes and reduced social engagement in services due to either actual or perceived prejudice from others, including health professionals. For many couples, challenges around conception, sharing the news and facing intrusive questioning from friends, family, colleagues and even health professionals, is followed by difficulties accessing appropriate supports and services during pregnancy (Centre of Perinatal Excellence [COPE] 2023a). Engagement and appropriate use of language and communication involves utilising language that is free from words/tones that reflect prejudice, discrimination or stereotypes (Victorian Government 2021).

People who identify with the LGBTQIA+ community may not identify as female but may have been born with a uterus and may or may not be undergoing gender reassignment but are able to give birth.

As surrogacy and alternative parenting options are growing, there is the need to acknowledge that women planning to breastfeed may not be the birthing parent of the newborn.

For this group of women, support and education associated with establishing breastfeeding with the 'adoptive' female parent is an area that as a nurse you will be required to assist with in a non-judgmental and non-biased manner. Clearly, developing skills in communication is paramount to providing successful healthcare irrespective of people's choices and identities.

CRITICAL THINKING EXERCISE 44.1

You are caring for Winnie, a young woman who came to Australia from China a year ago. She gave birth to her first baby earlier today. The midwife has instructed her to get up to have a shower. Winnie is crying and distressed and tells you that 'the midwife doesn't understand'.

1. What do you think might be the reason for Winnie's distress?
2. How could this misunderstanding have been avoided?
3. What will you do now to relieve Winnie's distress?
4. What other cultural issues need to be explored to ensure that care is culturally appropriate?

POSTNATAL CARE

The postpartum period is the time between the birth and return of the reproductive organs to their pre-pregnancy state (Lowdermilk et al 2020). Depending on the model of care they have chosen, women generally return home within hours or days of the birth. It is important to provide as much help and education as possible before discharge. While this section focuses mostly on care in the birthing centre or hospital, the ongoing needs of the woman, baby and family should be considered so that support required after discharge home can be planned as required.

Care of the woman

The degree of care required will depend on a variety of factors, such as where the birth occurred, how long the woman remains in the maternity unit or birth centre, whether the birth was full or preterm, if it was uncomplicated, whether there were multiple births and whether there are any postnatal discomforts or complications. In addition, care must be adapted to meet any specific cultural needs. The woman who has had a caesarean birth must also be assessed like any other postoperative person. **Postnatal** care is directed at promoting the health of both mother and baby, providing education, and preparing for care of the infant and services available in the community. Aspects of care include promoting:

- the establishment of infant feeding (breastfeeding or artificial)
- comfort
- reduced risk of infection
- bonding and attachment with the infant
- adequate rest and nutrition of the mother
- knowledge and confidence in caring for the baby.

(Murray et al 2023; Perry et al 2022)

Assessment is made of the **lochia**, the vaginal discharge that occurs after birth. Lochia consists of blood and broken-down endometrium and is discharged for up to 6 weeks after birth. At first it is bright red in colour (rubra), then becomes pink (serosa) and, ultimately, presents as a colourless or white discharge (alba). Flow of lochia usually increases with ambulation and breastfeeding. Lochia tends to pool in the vagina when the woman is lying in bed; the woman then can experience a gush of blood when she stands. This gush should not be confused with haemorrhage (Lowdermilk et al 2020). Lochia should not have an offensive odour or contain any blood clots; the presence of either indicates the possibility that products of conception have been retained in the uterus. Observe for character, colour, odour and presence of clots. Clinical Interest Box 44.3 outlines the assessment of lochia. Nursing Care Plan 44.1 outlines the care of a postnatal woman and Progress Note 44.1 shows an example of an entry into progress notes.

Perineal lacerations and episiotomies can increase the risk for infection as a result of interruption in skin integrity (Lowdermilk et al 2020). Perineal care involves twice daily showering or perineal wash to cleanse the area, wiping from front to back after toileting and frequent changing of perineal pads to reduce the risk of infection and promote healing. Educate the woman to identify and report any

CLINICAL INTEREST BOX 44.3 Changes in lochia that cause concern

Change

- Presence of clots
- Persistent lochia rubra or return of lochia rubra when this had ceased
- Offensive discharge

Possible problem

- Inadequate uterine contractions that allow bleeding from vessels at the placental site
- Inadequate uterine contractions; retained placental fragments; infection

Nursing action

- Assess location and firmness of fundus (performed by a registered midwife)
- Assess lochia (pad) for colour, texture, volume, frequency, odour
- Assess voiding pattern
- Assess activity pattern
- Assess for signs of infection
- Record and report findings of nursing actions

(Ladewig et al 2017; Lowdermilk et al 2020)

changes. If a perineal tear occurred or if an episiotomy was performed, nursing staff must check and document the appearance at least once every 24 hours or if the woman voices concerns. Care is needed to reduce discomfort and prevent infection around the area. Local care may involve the application of cold/ice packs to the area, education regarding position of comfort and analgesic medications such as paracetamol and non-steroidal anti-inflammatories may be prescribed. Observe for haematoma and oedema.

Vital signs are assessed with abnormalities reported. The extremities are evaluated for signs of thrombophlebitis. The bladder is observed for fullness, output, burning and pain. The bowels are assessed to determine passage of flatus and bowel sounds, and for normal bowel function for that woman.

If the woman has had a caesarean birth, vital signs, incision, fundus and lochia are assessed according to hospital policies, procedures or protocols. Fundal height is not routinely checked following a caesarean section due to discomfort.

For women who have not delivered by caesarean section, fundal height will be assessed and documented once a day, or as required, by the midwife to monitor involution of the uterus. It may be necessary to massage the fundus to promote uterine contraction. The height of the fundus decreases by about 1 cm each day until, by the 11th or 12th day, it can no longer be palpated abdominally. The firmness, height and location are evaluated. (See Figure 44.2.)

If the woman is breastfeeding and/or expressing, the breasts and nipples are assessed each day for any red areas, oedema, cracking or bleeding. The mother is taught to palpate each breast and identify any areas of change (e.g. hardness, warmth, redness) that may indicate blocked milk ducts.

Postnatal exercises are started gently within the first day or two. They are designed to strengthen the pelvic floor and abdominal muscles. An instruction sheet illustrating the

NURSING CARE PLAN 44.1

Assessment: Maddy and Mark Jones delivered a 3.5 kg female infant earlier this morning. Maddy had an epidural anaesthetic during a 12-hour labour. She had a greater than normal blood loss at delivery. The midwife has asked you to get her up and walk her to the toilet. She says she has full return of sensation to her legs but feels a little light-headed. As she stands up, Maddy says she feels weak and dizzy. Her gait is unsteady, so you lower her back to bed to prevent her from fainting.
Issue/s to be addressed: Risk of injury related to postural hypotension.
Goal/s: To remain free of complications related to mobilisation post-delivery.

Care/actions	Rationale
Allow Maddy to rest before attempting mobilisation. Assist with ambulation.	Rest will allow dizziness to pass and circulation to stabilise. Orthostatic hypotension may occur, and having someone present helps prevent injury.
Check Maddy's blood pressure before getting her out of bed again. Instruct Maddy to bend her knees and move her feet when she first stands. Initiate measures to prevent injury if Maddy were to faint.	A decrease of 15–20 mmHg in systolic pressure on rising indicates postural hypotension. Will increase venous return from the lower extremities.

Evaluation: Maddy requested assistance when ambulating initially and sustained no injury during her postnatal stay.

(Murray et al 2023)

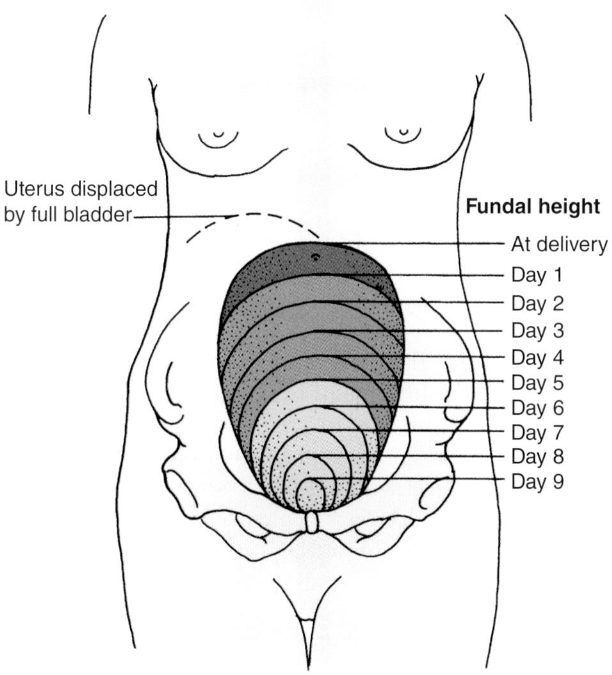

Figure 44.2 The height of the uterine fundus changes each day as involution progresses
(Leifer 2023)

exercises to be performed is generally given to the mother and explained by the midwife or physiotherapist.

Evaluation of the woman's emotional status involves observing family interaction and support and any signs of a depressive state. The woman should also be observed for interest in and interaction with the newborn, eye contact, touch contact and the ability to respond to the infant's cries (Davidson et al 2020). In the early days following birth, up to 80 per cent of women may experience a temporary condition commonly known as 'the baby blues'. The baby blues usually occur between the third to the fifth day after birth and are due to the sudden change in hormone levels following the birth (COPE 2023b). Signs of the baby blues include being teary, irritable, overly sensitive in interactions with others and moody. The baby blues usually clear up after a few days with no other treatment except support and understanding. If the woman's mood does not lighten, it may be a sign of another type of mental health condition like postnatal depression or postnatal anxiety (see Chapter 39).

Postnatal teaching covers topics such as nutrition, rest, breast care, exercise, activity, urinary and bowel function, blood loss, perineal care, contraception, sexual activity, postnatal signs and symptoms that should be reported, infant care and feeding, postnatal depression, available resources and follow-up care (Murray et al 2023).

A balanced diet, which provides adequate nutrients and fibre for the woman's health and energy—particularly taking note of levels of iodine, vitamin B12, iron and calcium—is advised (National Health and Medical Research Council [NHMRC] 2013). If the woman is fully breastfeeding in the first 6 months, she should consume an extra 2000 kJ/day above the requirements of pregnancy. The lactating mother is advised to continue to eat the foods she ate while pregnant. The extra demands on nutrients required during breastfeeding are often compensated for by the woman's body being more efficient at utilising available nutrients in foods. In addition, an increase in appetite during the breastfeeding period increases the amount of food consumed, and the woman's body accesses the additional fat stores laid down during pregnancy from the reduced energy used in the later stages of pregnancy (Australian Breastfeeding Association 2021).

The woman who wishes to breastfeed should also be advised of the substances that may be excreted in **breast milk**. Substances that should be avoided include:

- nicotine
- alcohol
- caffeine
- some anti-infective agents (most antibiotics are safe during breastfeeding)
- sedatives.

Minor postnatal discomforts

Some discomforts are associated with the postnatal period (Murray et al 2023). These include after-pains, constipation, difficulty with passing urine and engorged breasts. After-pains are cramps that may occur for a few days after birth, as the uterine muscles contract during the process of involution. They are increased during breastfeeding due to the release of oxytocin, required for the 'let-down' mechanism for breast milk releasing from the breast, which also activates the muscles of the uterus to contract (Australian Breastfeeding Association 2021). Mild pain relief medication may be prescribed.

Constipation may result from inadequate fibre or fluid intake. The woman may also be afraid to go to the toilet post birth since it may increase her levels of pain and discomfort. Increasing fibre in the diet and maintaining a high fluid intake is important and, if necessary, a stool-softening medication may be prescribed. Analgesia may also be given prior to the woman going to the toilet.

Difficulty in voiding may be experienced initially because of loss of bladder tone, bruising of the urethra or perineal soreness. Some women may find that initially voiding in the shower post birth assists with passing urine. If there is significant perineal trauma or after a caesarean birth, an indwelling catheter (IDC) may be inserted until the swelling to the perineal area is reduced and mobility increased. One must be mindful that an IDC creates a potential for infection so should be removed as soon as practical and the area kept clean with water in the shower and regular perineal pad changes.

Engorged breasts may occur a few days after the birth because of increased blood supply to the breasts when beginning lactation. The breasts may become full, distended, hard and uncomfortable. The midwife should advise mothers that this is not unusual and that wearing a supportive nursing bra, even during the night, will help, provided that it is not too tight. Breastfeeding the baby at frequent intervals, as demanded by the newborn, assists with minimising the possibilities of engorgement, together with correct positioning and attachment of the newborn to the breast. Frequent breastfeeding (2-hourly or more often) is normal newborn behaviour in the early postnatal period. The woman needs to be reassured of this and that frequent feeding is a normal process of breastfeeding.

The midwife or a lactation consultant may be included for further management and advice as required (The Royal Women's Hospital 2020; WHO 2018).

Breastfeeding

Breastfeeding is the optimal method of feeding the baby. The World Health Organization (WHO) (2018) recommends breastfeeding exclusively for the first 6 months of the newborn's life. A woman should be advised of the benefits of breastfeeding and provided with support and assistance to correctly position and attach her newborn at the breast using the 'hands off technique' (HOT) and encouraging lots of skin-to-skin contact (The Royal Women's Hospital 2020; UNICEF UK nd; WHO 2018).

Lactation

During pregnancy, placental hormones, oestrogen, progesterone, hCG and hPL stimulate the development of glandular tissue and ducts in the breasts. **Colostrum** is the fluid secreted by the breasts during pregnancy and the first few days after birth. It is a thin, yellow serous fluid consisting of water, protein, fat, carbohydrates and immunologically active substances. When the placenta is expelled after birth of the baby, the anterior pituitary gland releases prolactin, which activates the mammary cells to produce milk, and oxytocin, which enables the 'let-down reflex' (Davidson et al 2020).

Lactation depends on the maintenance of milk production and on the let-down reflex, whereby milk is ejected from the breasts. A neurogenic reflex stimulates the let-down reflex, with oxytocin released from the pituitary gland in response to suckling, forcing milk out of the alveoli in the breasts. The let-down reflex, which generally occurs a short time after the baby begins to suck on the nipple, can also be stimulated when the mother sees, hears or thinks about her baby. Conversely, the reflex can be inhibited by anxiety, fear or tension.

Breastfeeding has advantages for both the mother and the baby. Breast milk is free from microorganisms, is easily digested, contains all the essential nutrients necessary for the baby's development and contains immunoglobulins and other substances that protect the infant from many infections while the immune system is underdeveloped. Breastfeeding aids involution of the uterus and is generally emotionally satisfying for the mother. Breastfeeding is also convenient and economical.

There are many breastfeeding benefits for both the mother and the newborn. Benefits for the mother include:

- Breast milk is always fresh, clean and at the right temperature; it is healthy and economical.
- No preparation or sterilisation is required.
- Frequent and exclusive breastfeeding can delay the return of fertility (lactational amenorrhoea).
- The uterus returns to normal size and blood loss reduces more quickly.
- Women who breastfeed are more likely to return to their pre-pregnant weight.
- Risks of reproductive cancers, particularly uterine cancer, are reduced if a woman breastfeeds for 6 months or longer, and this protection increases with breastfeeding duration.
- Women who breastfeed for a total of 2 years or more reduce their risk of breast cancer by 24%; with an increased lifetime of breastfeeding, the overall risk of breast cancer in premenopausal and post-menopausal women is decreased, particularly for premenopausal women.
- Breastfeeding decreases ovulatory age and therefore decreases the risk of ovarian cancer.
- The risk of osteoporosis is decreased fourfold compared with a woman who has not breastfed, and the risk of hip fractures is lower.
- Breastfeeding reduces the risk for, and incidence of, thyroid cancer.
- Women who breastfeed for at least 24 months over their reproductive years have a 25% lower risk of developing heart disease and a 23% reduction in coronary artery disease.
- New studies provide evidence that breastfeeding protects against type 2 diabetes and a woman who has gestational diabetes and breastfeeds after that pregnancy also has a reduced likelihood of developing type 2 diabetes mellitus.

(BFHI 2020; WHO 2018)

Management

Breastfeeding basics:

1. A breastfeed should always be started with a calm newborn. This may mean leaving nappy changes until midway during a breastfeed rather than at the start of a breastfeed.
2. Look for early feeding cues:
   - stirring
   - mouth opening
   - turning head, seeking and rooting
   - turning head side to side.
3. Medium to late feeding cues include:
   - stretching
   - increased physical movement
   - hand to mouth
   - crying
   - agitated body movements
   - colour turning red.
4. If the newborn is crying, the following tips are suggested to relax the newborn before breastfeeding commences:
   - cuddling
   - skin to skin on chest

- talking
- letting the newborn suck on a clean finger until they settle
- gentle rocking movements
- stroking the newborn's back in one direction and awaiting early cues to feed.

5. The newborn will start to lift and bob head around looking for the nipple.
6. The newborn will dig the chin into the breast, reach up with an open mouth, attach to the breast and commence sucking. (See Figure 44.3.)

Attachment to the breast

1. The woman needs to sit comfortably with their back and feet well supported.
2. Unwrap the baby and hold close; the mother/newborn combination are chest to chest.
3. Do not hold the occiput of the newborn's head as this creates a reflex response, and the newborn will 'pull away' from the breast.
4. Turn newborn on their side with the chest towards the woman and the head tilted slightly back at the same level as the breast. The newborn's nose should be at nipple level.
5. Gently brush the newborn's mouth with the underside of the areola.
6. Wait for the newborn to open their mouth wide; the tongue is forward and over the lower gums.
7. Quickly bring the newborn to the breast with the areola and nipple angled to the roof of the newborn's mouth.
8. As the mouth closes, a large mouthful of the mother's breast should enter the newborn's mouth, stimulating a sucking response.
9. Ways to assess for correct attachment include:
   - The newborn's chin is pressed into the breast, nose clear of the breast, though it may still be touching the breast.
   - The lower lip of the newborn is turned out over the breast.
   - The newborn's tongue is forward and over the lower gum.
   - Much of the areola is in the mouth, particularly on the chin side of the newborn.
   - The woman has no pain with attachment and sucking by newborn.
   - The whole jaw of the newborn moves as they suck, including wiggling of the ears.

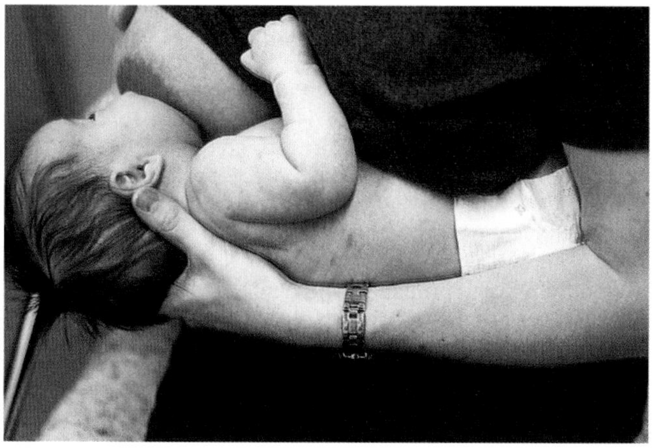

Figure 44.3 Cross-cradle position
(Courtesy of Dr Jack Newman, International Breastfeeding Centre, Toronto Canada)

Any damage or pain during any part of the breastfeed is suggestive that the newborn is inadequately attached/ positioned to the breast.

Take the newborn off the breast by inserting a clean little finger in the corner of the mouth to break the suction. Reattach newborn to the breast following the process above and seek assistance from the midwife and/or lactation consultant.

If the woman's nipples are creased, ridged or squashed, blistered, cracked or bleeding, the newborn is inadequately attached to the breast and the latch is not deep enough, resulting in the nipple 'rubbing' on the hard palate of the newborn's mouth and resulting in pain and/or damage (Australian Breastfeeding Association 2021; La Leche League nd).

The woman should ensure that her nipples are clean and dried. Expressed breast milk is rubbed into the nipple after the feed then allowed to dry to assist with nipple soreness; however, the only remedy for sore and/or damaged nipples is correct attachment and positioning of the newborn to the breast.

Demand feeding or 'baby-led' feeding is the recommendation for feeding a newborn, reducing engorgement, and encouraging and maintaining lactation. The frequency and length of breastfeeds will be unpredictable and different in both length and frequency from one feed to the next. This is very normal breastfeeding behaviour.

The baby and mother establish their own feeding routine, and the mother's milk supply adjusts according to demand.

Breast milk may be expressed, either manually or with a breast pump, if necessary. Expression may be necessary to relieve discomfort if the breasts are overfull, to help stimulate milk production or if the newborn is premature and/or unwell and in a special care nursery.

At times, women may experience some challenges associated with breastfeeding (e.g. oversupply, damaged nipples); however, with adequate support, time, correct information and assistance these issues can be overcome. Organisations such as the Australian Breastfeeding Association provide support and advice on a range of topics associated with breastfeeding and provide peer support and breastfeeding groups for women and their newborn babies.

Artificial bottle feeding is the method of infant feeding women choose if not breastfeeding their babies. Artificial feeds are generally based on cow's milk, although other preparations are available, such as soy-based formulas. Formula selection is generally based upon parental request but, on occasion, specific formula products are required due to a medical condition, such as phenylketonuria.

The mother must have formula preparation and sterilisation of bottles together with milk storage demonstrated and discussed with the midwife if she chooses to bottle feed her newborn. The woman should be provided with information regarding management of her breasts as she may lactate despite choosing not to breastfeed.

As a response to the falling breastfeeding initiation and retention rates worldwide, UNICEF/WHO first published the *Ten Steps to Successful Breastfeeding* in the early 1990s. (See also Clinical Interest Box 44.4 and Case Study 44.2.)

CRITICAL THINKING EXERCISE 44.2

You are caring for Katerina, a 28-year-old woman, who 3 days ago gave birth to her first baby. She tells you her breasts feel really heavy, hot and tight and the baby is finding it difficult to effectively attach to the breast. Katerina states she has tried to help the baby latch by expressing some milk before putting the baby to the breast but 'Nothing is coming out and my baby keeps crying. Maybe the baby is not getting enough milk, and needs some formula.'

1. What might be the likely reason for this sudden fullness?
2. What could you suggest to Katerina to help her adjust to her breast changes?
3. What advice would be appropriate in relation to encouraging Katerina to continue to breastfeed?
4. What are your responsibilities as an Enrolled Nurse in this situation?

Immediate care of the baby

Immediately after birth, the newborn is placed on the mother's chest, skin to skin, enabling the baby to seek the breast and initiate breastfeeding.

During the first few minutes of life, the midwife or obstetrician will observe the newborn for evidence that the newborn is adapting to extrauterine life (i.e. that the newborn is adjusting to life outside of the uterus).

If the newborn is breathing normally and its colour is improving, the newborn remains skin to skin with its mother, where it will continue to adjust to life outside of the uterus. The midwife assists in supporting the mother to initiate breastfeeding. Both mother and newborn should be left for at least 1 hour or until after the first breastfeed. Because the newborn baby has a limited ability to regulate its body temperature in relation to the environment, care is taken to ensure that it does not become cold by maintaining skin-to-skin contact under a warm blanket with the newborn's mother or, if this is not appropriate at the time, with the mother's partner/support person.

CLINICAL INTEREST BOX 44.4 Baby Friendly Health Initiative (BFHI)

The BFHI is a global initiative introduced by the WHO and the United Nations International Children's Emergency Fund (UNICEF) to implement practices that protect, promote and support breastfeeding. These practices include the following:

1. Have a written infant feeding policy that is routinely communicated to all healthcare staff and parents.
2. Ensure that staff have sufficient knowledge, competence and skills to support breastfeeding.
3. Discuss the importance and management of breastfeeding with women who are pregnant and their families.
4. Facilitate immediate and uninterrupted skin-to-skin contact and support mothers to initiate breastfeeding as soon as possible after birth.
5. Support women to initiate and maintain breastfeeding and manage common difficulties.
6. Do not provide breastfed newborns any food or fluids other than breast milk, unless medically indicated.
7. Enable mothers and their infants to remain together and to practise rooming-in 24 hours a day.
8. Support mothers to recognise and respond to their infants' cues for feeding.
9. Counsel mothers on the use and risks of feeding bottles, teats and dummies.
10. Coordinate discharge so that parents and their infants have timely access to ongoing support and care.

(BFHI Australia 2020; WHO 2018)

CASE STUDY 44.2

Molly, Alex and Thomas

Alex and I had Thomas 2 days ago. I had to have a caesarean delivery since he was breech. I was worried that I wouldn't get to bond with him, but as soon as he was delivered, they quickly dried him and gave him to me for a cuddle for a few minutes. I didn't realise that this would be possible and was really happy when the midwife was able to stay with me in the recovery area and gave Thomas to me for skin-to-skin contact before helping me with the first breastfeed. I was worried I wouldn't be able to do any of this so soon after delivery because of the caesarean. With the midwives' help, he went on first go. I couldn't believe it! We are doing really well, and with help from the midwives, I've been able to get the hang of breastfeeding him. Now that I'm up and about, we are managing ourselves most of the time, but the midwives are available to help if I need them.

Molly, first-time mum,
talking about breastfeeding her infant

How can the midwife help Molly establish breastfeeding during the initial breastfeeding session?

There are many benefits to encouraging skin-to-skin contact with mother and newborn at birth and following birth. These benefits include the following:

- assists the newborn to adjust to life outside of the uterus
- calms and relaxes both the mother and her newborn
- regulates the newborn's heart rate and breathing
- regulates the newborn's temperature
- stimulates hormones in the mother to be released to support breastfeeding and mothering
- colonisation of the newborn's skin with the mother's friendly bacteria, providing protection against infection for the newborn.

(Australian College of Midwives 2016; WHO 2018b)

Breathing in the newborn is initiated in response to high blood CO_2 level, stimulating the respiratory centre in the medulla. In the first few breaths, air is drawn in to expand the alveoli in the lungs, thus oxygenating the blood. Eighty-five per cent of babies who are term or near term initiate spontaneous respirations and commence breathing within 30 seconds of birth and 95% commence within 44 seconds of birth. Immediate and ongoing assessment of the baby starts at birth and continues, depending on the adaptation of the newborn to extrauterine life (Queensland Health 2022).

At 1, 3 and 5 minutes after birth, and then every 5 minutes until the heart rate is normal and respiration has been established (or full ventilator assistance is being given), the **Apgar score** is assessed and recorded. The Apgar scoring system is a valuable method to determine the condition of the newborn immediately after birth (see Table 44.6).

Should a newborn not respond to life outside of the uterus (i.e. it does not establish respirations, has poor muscle tone and colour), do not wait for the Apgar score result before initiating neonatal resuscitation.

TABLE 44.6 | Apgar scoring

Factor	Score		
	2	1	0
Heart rate	>100 beats/min	Slow (<100 beats/min)	Absent
Respiratory effort	Good, strong cry	Irregular, slow weak cry	Absent
Colour	Pink all over	Body pink, blue extremities	Blue, pale
Muscle tone	Well flexed	Fair (some flexion of extremities)	Limp
Reflex Irritability	Cry, sneeze	Grimace	No response

(Lowdermilk et al 2020; Murray et al 2023; Speedie & Middleton 2022; Queensland Government 2022)

Apgar scoring is determined by allocating a score of 0, 1 or 2 to five simple criteria:

1. colour (appearance)
2. heart rate (pulse)
3. reflex irritability (grimace)
4. muscle tone (activity)
5. respiratory effort (breathing).

(Speedie & Middleton 2022)

A total score of 10 indicates that the infant is in optimal condition; if the newborn is flat, floppy, blue, not initiating respirations and/or no heart rate, immediate attention and active resuscitation is commenced.

A score of 7–10 indicates the absence of difficulty in adapting to extrauterine life, a score of 4–6 indicates moderate difficulty, while a score of 0–3 indicates severe distress in the newborn and its adaptation to extrauterine life. Many healthy newborns do not achieve a score of 10 because the body is not completely pink.

Any score lower than 7 indicates the newborn needs assistance. Scores below 5 indicate that the newborn needs immediate assistance in adjusting to their new environment. However, a newborn who has a low score at 1 minute and a normal score at 5 minutes should not have any long-term problems (Queensland Government 2022; Speedie & Middleton 2022).

In a healthcare setting such as a hospital or birth centre, an identification band is placed on the baby's wrist and ankle. This identification procedure must be performed before the baby is removed from the mother and is a legal requirement and part of the Australian Commission on Safety and Quality in Health Care's (ACSQHC) National Safety and Quality Health Service Standards 'Comprehensive Care' Standard (ACSQHC 2021).

The baby may be weighed and measured, preferably not before the first breastfeed, and the information documented (Perry et al 2022). It is recommended that every baby is given an intramuscular injection of vitamin K as a preventative measure against haemorrhagic disease of the newborn (see Clinical Interest Box 44.5).

An initial examination of the baby is performed after the birth so that any concerns can be escalated to the appropriate medical officer (e.g. a paediatrician for review and follow-up as required). Table 44.7 outlines the findings expected in a normal newborn and the presence of any obvious abnormalities. Later, a more thorough examination is performed. (See also Figure 44.4.)

Subsequent care of the baby

Care of the baby in the period immediately after birth is directed towards keeping the baby adequately nourished, clean, warm and free from infection. Careful observation is necessary to detect any problems should they occur. Rooming-in, where the baby remains in the same room as the mother, is encouraged and is part of the Baby Friendly Health Initiative (BFHI) recommendations. The mother

CLINICAL INTEREST BOX 44.5 The role of vitamin K

Vitamin K is needed by humans to cause blood to clot. Without vitamin K, small cuts can go on bleeding for a long time, small injuries can cause a lot of bruising, and bleeding can occur in many parts of the body, including in the brain, causing a stroke.

Vitamin K is mostly made by bacteria in our gut because humans are unable to make vitamin K themselves.

Vitamin K at birth

All newborn babies have low levels of vitamin K. Only a little vitamin K goes through the placenta to the baby, and at birth a baby's gut is sterile (there are no bacteria in the gut).

After birth, there is little vitamin K in breast milk and breastfed babies can be low in vitamin K for several weeks until the gut bacteria start to make it.

Infant formula has added vitamin K, but formula-fed babies have very low levels of vitamin K for several days.

Why is vitamin K given?

Shortly after birth, vitamin K is administered to prevent haemorrhagic disease of the newborn. The intestinal flora synthesises vitamin K; however, because the newborn's intestine is sterile at birth, vitamin K levels are insufficient. A dose of vitamin K provides protection until the newborn's intestinal flora is established, which usually occurs by 3 to 4 days of age. It is recommended that all babies are given vitamin K at birth to prevent haemorrhagic disease of the newborn. This bleeding is rare even when babies are not given extra vitamin K, but if it happens it can cause severe harm to a baby, including death or severe brain damage.

(NHMRC 2010; Pairman et al 2023; Speedie & Middleton 2022)

gets to know, and gains confidence in caring for, her baby (Figure 44.5). The midwife is available to offer guidance and encouragement in all aspects of infant care.

Supporting thermoregulation

Maintenance of body temperature is vital. The core temperature of the term newborn is 36.5–37.5°C (Blackburn 2018). Hypothermia can cause problems such as hypoglycaemia, as the newborn uses glucose to generate heat, and respiratory distress, because the metabolic rate is higher and consumes more oxygen. The first bath is not undertaken until the newborn is at least 24 hours of age.

Obtaining vital signs

- Respiratory rate: It is best to obtain respiratory rate before disturbing the baby. Count the respirations for a minute. The rate can be auscultated with a stethoscope, or a hand can be placed lightly over the abdomen—watch for the rise and fall.
- Heart rate: Assess using a stethoscope at the apex of the heart. Count for 1 minute.
- Temperature: Axillary temperatures are most commonly used for the well newborn infant. A thermometer is placed in the axilla, parallel to the chest wall.

Table 44.8 gives the vital sign parameters for a healthy newborn.

TABLE 44.7 | The usual characteristics of a newborn

Anatomy	Usual characteristics
Head	Head circumference 33–35 cm. Anterior fontanelle—diamond shaped, no tension or depression. Posterior fontanelle—triangular, palpable. May be elongated from moulding as the skull bones glide over each other during passage through the birth canal.
Face	Nose and cheeks may have tiny white spots (milia).
Skin	Normal colour for race. May be covered with lanugo (fine downy hair). May be vernix (white, greasy protective substance) in the skin folds. Mongolian blue spot may be present.
Eyes	Lids usually oedematous. Dark blue; white sclera. Blink reflex present.
Thorax	Average circumference 34 cm. Expands symmetrically with ventilations. Breast tissue palpable in males and females.
Abdomen	Cylindrical in shape. Prominent but not distended. Moves up and down with ventilations. Umbilical cord blue/white at birth with two arteries and one vein.
Limbs	Symmetrical, warm, rounded. Move freely. Hands and feet may be slightly cyanosed.
Back	Spine straight, intact, easily flexed.
Genitalia	Male: Large in relation to body, scrotum contains both testes, foreskin adheres to glans, urethral meatus central on tip of penis. Female: Prominent labia and clitoris, vaginal opening visible.
Anus	Patent.

(Davidson et al 2020; Hockenberry et al 2019)

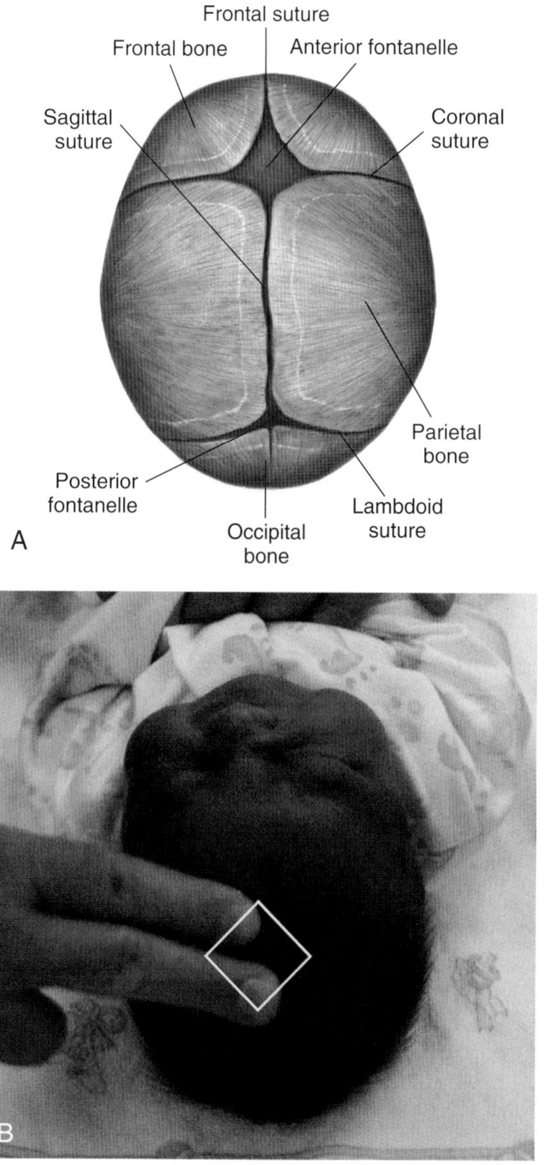

Figure 44.4 Fontanelles and suture lines
(Crisp et al 2021)

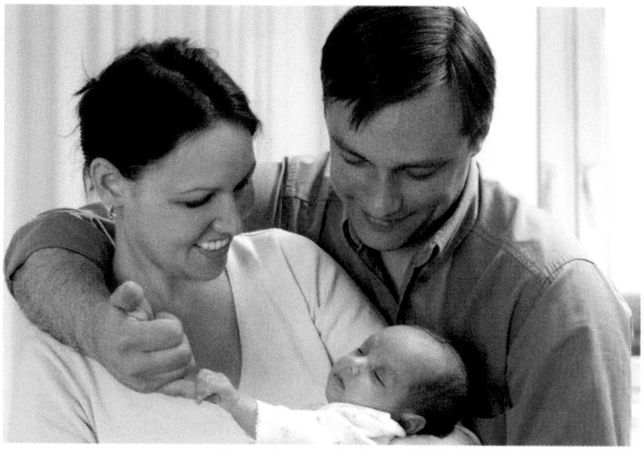

Figure 44.5 Parent–child nurturing
(© privilege/Shutterstock)

TABLE 44.8 | Newborn vital signs

Vital sign	Normal range
Pulse	110–160 beats/min. During sleep as low as 100 beats/min; if crying, up to 180 beats/min. Apical pulse counted for 1 full minute.
Respirations	30–60 respirations/minute. Predominantly diaphragmatic but synchronous with abdominal movements. Respirations are counted for 1 full minute.
Temperature	Normal range: 36.5–37.5°C performed per axilla.

(Ladewig et al 2017; Murray et al 2023; Speedie & Middleton 2022)

Hygiene and skin care

The baby is usually bathed daily or second-daily. The initial newborn bath is best delayed for at least 24 hours until thermal and cardiorespiratory stabilisation has been achieved and the opportunity for initial skin-to-skin holding and breastfeeding is complete (Speedie & Middleton 2022). It is important that the infant's skin is kept clean and dry, with special attention being paid to the scalp, skin folds and genitals. The buttocks and groin area are washed with plain water. Disposable or cloth nappies may be used; however, generally, in the hospital environment, disposable nappies are used.

The bath is a good time to observe the newborn for general wellbeing, activity and behaviour.

If the baby's fingernails are long, the infant may scratch their face so mittens may be worn to prevent the infant from scratching.

Umbilical cord care

Care is aimed at preventing infection. The remnant of the cord is observed every time a nappy is changed, until it has separated, and the umbilicus has healed. It is kept clean by washing the cord stump in the bath each day and patting dry the cord stump after the bath. The cord stump is observed for any bleeding or signs of infection. It becomes dry and brownish black as it dries. The cord remnant separates from the umbilicus by a process of dry necrosis, with an average separation time of 5 to 15 days (Speedie & Middleton 2022).

The parents are taught to keep the base clean and dry, to observe for any signs of infection and report redness of the area or a moist or a foul-smelling cord. (See Figure 44.6.)

Elimination

Most newborns void within 24 hours of birth. A normal breastfed baby will have one wet nappy per day of life in the first 4 days after birth. This means one on the first day,

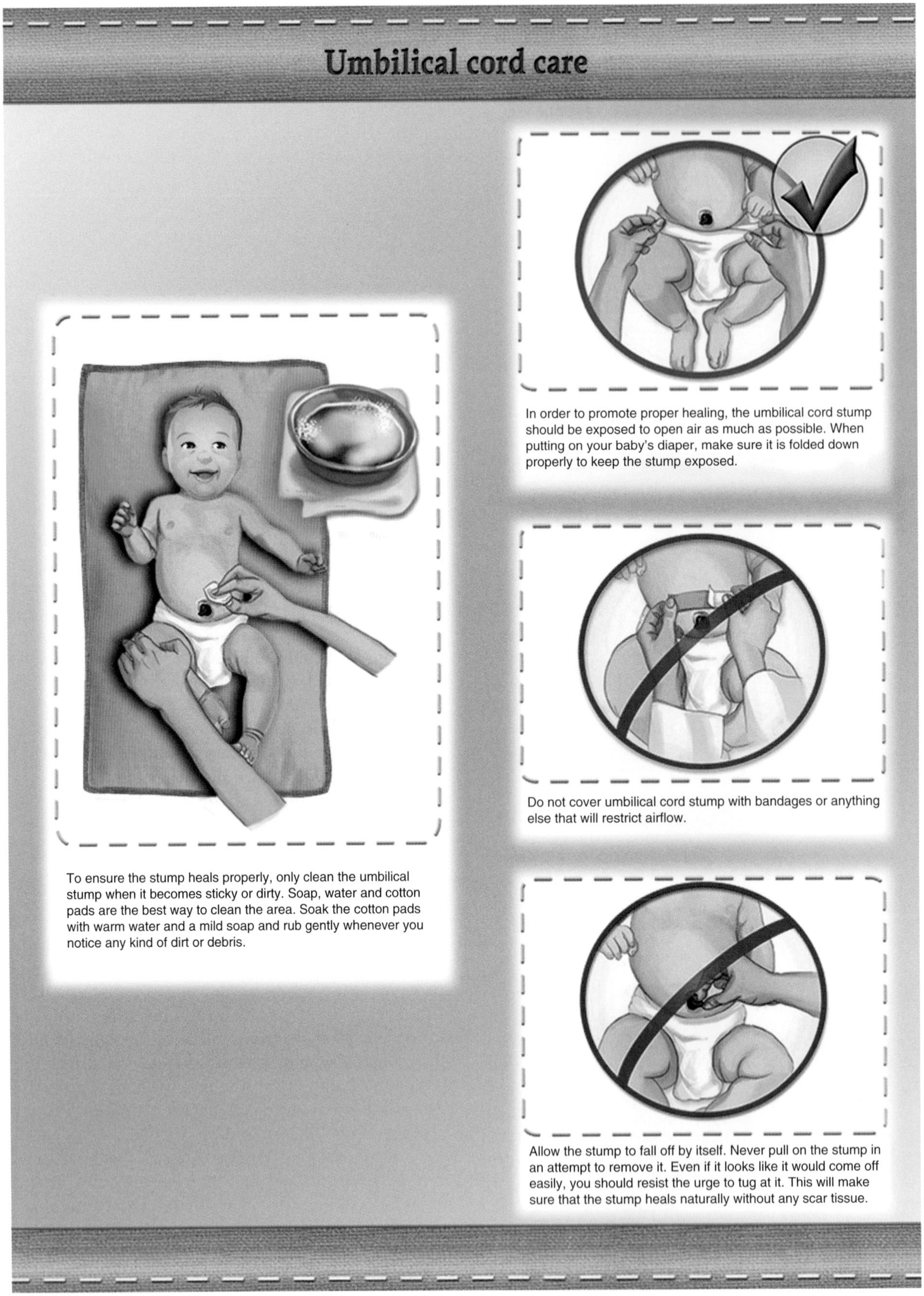
Umbilical cord care
In order to promote proper healing, the umbilical cord stump should be exposed to open air as much as possible. When putting on your baby's diaper, make sure it is folded down properly to keep the stump exposed.
To ensure the stump heals properly, only clean the umbilical stump when it becomes sticky or dirty. Soap, water and cotton pads are the best way to clean the area. Soak the cotton pads with warm water and a mild soap and rub gently whenever you notice any kind of dirt or debris.
Do not cover umbilical cord stump with bandages or anything else that will restrict airflow.
Allow the stump to fall off by itself. Never pull on the stump in an attempt to remove it. Even if it looks like it would come off easily, you should resist the urge to tug at it. This will make sure that the stump heals naturally without any scar tissue.

Figure 44.6 Umbilical cord care

two on the second and so on. From day 5 onwards, a baby will have at least 5 heavy wet single-use nappies in each 24-hour period. The urine should be clear or very pale (Australian Breastfeeding Association 2021). In the first few days, the newborn's nappy may have a rusty, orange-red stain present. These are salts of uric acid (urates) and are normal up to day 4. If urates are found after day 4, referral to a midwife and/or medical officer for review of the newborn is recommended.

Meconium is a black/dark green tarry substance that fills the lower intestine at birth. Most healthy term infants pass meconium within the first 12 to 24 hours after birth, with almost all passing meconium by 48 hours. The stool changes in colour, consistency and frequency during the first week, being most numerous between the third and sixth days. Newborns fed early pass stools sooner (Lowdermilk et al 2020). From day 5 onwards, the newborn will usually pass 3 or more bowel motions every 24 hours, until at least 6 weeks (Australian Breastfeeding Association 2021). See Clinical Interest Box 44.6. The stools of an infant who is formula-fed are yellow to light brown, firmer consistency and have a stronger odour than breast milk stools. They are generally fewer in number.

Sometimes, if the mother has damaged nipples and she is breastfeeding, there may be some blood in the stools. Improvement in breastfeeding positioning and attachment is required to resolve this issue if the newborn is otherwise well. If the baby is not breastfed, or the mother's nipples are not damaged when breastfeeding, a medical officer should review this.

CLINICAL INTEREST BOX 44.6 Stool patterns of newborns

Meconium

- Passage of meconium should occur within the first 24–48 hours after birth, although it can be delayed up to 7 days in very low birth weight infants. Passage of meconium can occur in utero and can be a sign of foetal distress.

Transitional stools

- Usually appear by third day after initiation of feeding.
- Greenish brown to yellowish brown; thin and less sticky than meconium; can contain some milk curds.

Milk stools

- Usually appear by the fourth day.
- Breast milk: Yellow to golden, pasty in consistency; resemble a mixture of mustard and cottage cheese, with an odour similar to sour milk.
- Commercial infant formula: Stools pale yellow to light brown, firmer consistency, stronger odour than breast milk stools.

(Lowdermilk et al 2020)

CRITICAL THINKING EXERCISE 44.3

You are working in the postnatal unit when a parent asks you if their baby should have had a wet or dirty nappy yet. It is 48 hours since the baby was born. What would you do in this situation?

Nutrition

The baby is fed on demand—baby-led feeding. Frequent feeding is encouraged with limitless access to the breast by the newborn.

Regimented frequent feedings may be indicated if the newborn is demonstrating signs of hypoglycaemia. Signs of hypoglycaemia in the newborn include jitteriness, poor muscle tone, sweating, respiratory difficulty, low temperature, poor suck, high-pitched cry, lethargy and seizures. A heel stick is performed when obtaining capillary blood for glucose screening.

Weighing and measuring

The newborn is generally weighed at birth and then on the day of discharge. Most newborns weigh 2700 to 4000 grams, with the average weight being about 3400 grams. Accurate birth weights and lengths are important because they provide a baseline for assessment of risk status and future growth (Speedie & Middleton 2022). Most newborns have lost weight by their weigh at 48 hours old. A loss of up to 10% of the birth weight is normal in the first 3–4 days; after this, the baby should begin to gain weight. It is expected that the baby will be back to its birth weight within 10–14 days (Pairman et al 2023).

The length and head circumference are routinely measured at birth. The average length of the newborn is 48 to 53 cm and for the full-term infant, average head circumference is between 33 and 35 cm (Speedie & Middleton 2022).

Infection control

Infections that are harmless to adults may be fatal to the newborn because of the immaturity of their immune system. The baby is protected from infection by normal hygiene practices, the most important aspect of which is washing the hands thoroughly before attending to the baby. Anyone with an infection is advised not to have contact with the newborn. Parent/s and close family members are advised regarding influenza vaccination during pregnancy as influenza can cause serious complications in a woman who is pregnant. It has been found that vaccination against influenza during pregnancy can provide protection to the newborn for the first 6 months after birth. Influenza vaccination is recommended in each pregnancy, at any stage of the pregnancy.

Pertussis (whooping cough) vaccination (Boostrix vaccine) during each pregnancy is ideally recommended at 20–32 weeks' gestation or postpartum before discharge from hospital to minimise infection of the newborn. Adult household contacts and carers of infants <6 months of age are recommended to receive pertussis-containing vaccine at least 2 weeks before they have close contact with the infant if their last dose was more than 10 years ago (Department of Health & Aged Care 2023).

Breastfeeding is one of the best protective factors for infection prevention in newborns.

Temperature control

As the neonate's temperature-regulating centre is not fully functional, the baby must be protected from extremes of environmental temperature. Conduction, convection and radiation can be used to add heat to the body. Maintaining the room at an even, comfortable temperature, dressing the baby in suitable clothes and wrapping the infant in warm lightweight wraps can achieve this.

Overheating is also avoided as a measure to prevent sudden infant death syndrome (SIDS). Parents are taught how to wrap and position their infant as part of health education prior to discharge (Red Nose 2023). (See Clinical Interest Box 44.7.)

Screening tests

Newborn bloodspot screening (NBS) is a publicly funded system for testing newborn babies' blood for a number of medical conditions. All newborn babies are offered screening in Australia. The blood test is taken by heel prick, usually between 48–72 hours after birth regardless of gestational age, weight, feeding or health status. Collection of several bloodspots is made onto an absorbent card and sent for analysis. After the dried blood has been tested, it will be stored in the laboratory for varying periods, depending on which state of Australia the test has occurred. The more common well-known conditions tested for include phenylketonuria (PKU), congenital hypothyroidism, cystic fibrosis (CF) and a number of other extremely rare conditions. Some of these conditions can result in physical and/or intellectual problems if not treated promptly, and are often referred to as inborn errors of metabolism (Hall et al 2022; Pairman et al 2023).

Newborn hearing testing is a free universal hearing screening that has been in use in Australia since 2000. Where possible, screening of hearing is best attended any time after the newborn is 24 hours old and before discharge from the hospital.

CLINICAL INTEREST BOX 44.7 Safe sleeping

- Sleep baby on the back from birth, not on the tummy or side.
- Sleep baby with head and face uncovered.
- Keep baby smoke free before birth and after.
- Provide a safe sleeping environment night and day.
- Sleep baby in their own safe sleeping place in the same room as an adult caregiver for the first 6 months.
- Breastfeed baby.

(Red Nose 2023)

Neonatal disorders

Only brief mentions of some of the disorders that can affect neonates are included here. For detailed information, the nurse should refer to a current paediatric text. Disorders may be minor and temporary, major and permanent or life-threatening. They include:

- prematurity
- low birth weight
- jaundice
- hypoxia
- hyaline membrane disease
- hypoglycaemia
- persistent vomiting
- birth injuries
- congenital abnormalities
- macrosomia
- infant of a woman with diabetes.

The term **hyperbilirubinaemia** refers to an excessive level of accumulated bilirubin in the blood and is characterised by **jaundice**, a yellowish discoloration of the skin and other organs (Hockenberry et al 2019). There are two main types of neonatal jaundice: physiological and pathological. Physiological jaundice is due to the inability to break down bilirubin due to immaturity of the liver. It appears 2–5 days after birth and lasts for 1–2 weeks. It is commonly treated with phototherapy. Pathological jaundice can occur if there is an incompatibility of the mother's and neonate's blood group (Hall et al 2022; Pairman et al 2023).

Clinical Interest Box 44.8 outlines the procedure for assessing the newborn for jaundice.

Many hospital settings will perform an assessment of neonatal jaundice using a transcutaneous bilirubinometer and, pending the result of this, request a blood test to accurately determine the serum bilirubin rate (SBR).

Offer parents or carers information about treatment for hyperbilirubinaemia, including the anticipated duration of treatment and that breastfeeding, nappy-changing and cuddles can usually continue. Encourage mothers of breastfed babies with jaundice to breastfeed frequently, and to wake the baby for feeds if necessary.

Treatment for phototherapy is dependent on the SBR levels and the age of the newborn, and often further blood test investigations will be carried out as part of the management of jaundice (National Institute for Clinical Evidence [NICE] 2016). (See Figure 44.7.)

CLINICAL INTEREST BOX 44.8 Assessing for jaundice

- Check the naked infant in bright and preferably natural light.
- Press skin with thumb until the skin lightens.
- Observe colour of the sclera and gums.
- Consider other factors including infant alertness, intake (feeding) and output (elimination).

(NICE 2016; Speedie & Middleton 2022)

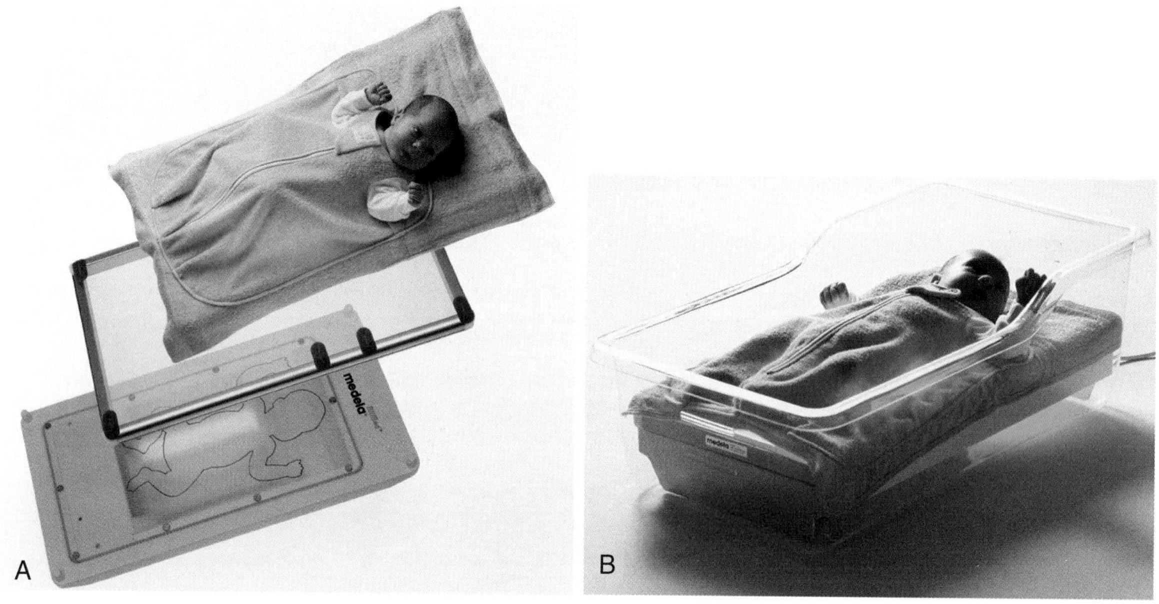

Figure 44.7 Bilibed
(Leifer 2023)

Progress Note 44.1

12/04/2024 1030 hrs	Nursing: Maddy supervised with mobilisation to toilet as feeling light-headed getting out of bed for first time after delivery. BP checked and no postural drop noted. Instructed to call for assistance when next wanting to mobilise. Call bell left within reach. Maddy stated she will do this. *L Adams* (ADAMS), *EN*

DECISION-MAKING FRAMEWORK EXERCISE 44.1

Kat, a newly graduated EN, is working in the postnatal unit with Kym, a midwife. They are sharing the care of six mothers/babies and collectively reviewing the events for the shift.

Since Baby A is 48 hours old at midday, Kym asks Kat if she could discuss with the mother the need to weigh the baby, obtain consent for the newborn bloodspot screening and attend the test.

Kat is not familiar with the consent process for the newborn bloodspot screening and does not know where the information is for the mother to read prior to the test.

In addition, Kat has not been educated regarding performing blood tests on newborns and is uncertain if this is within her scope of practice.

Using the decision-making framework, how will Kat determine what her scope of practice is in relation to this scenario and how will she then manage this scenario?

Summary

A nurse may be required to assist registered midwives in the care of women and their newborn babies. This chapter has briefly outlined the basic knowledge that is essential for the nurse who undertakes this role: the processes of normal pregnancy, labour and birth and the postnatal care of the mother and her baby. It is recommended that nurses gain an understanding of cultural differences in birthing beliefs and practices of the women they care for during and after the birth of their babies. It is also recommended that nurses access current paediatric textbooks to gain or enhance knowledge of neonatal care and disorders that may be encountered in the areas of maternal and child health nursing.

Review Questions

1. Describe the physiological changes of pregnancy.
2. How and why is fundal height measured during antenatal visits?
3. Provide an overview of the stages of labour.
4. Immediately after the birth of a baby an assessment is performed on the neonate. What is this called and what does it entail?
5. What assessments are performed on the newborn baby after birth?
6. What assessments of the mother are made in the post-partum period?
7. Why is skin-to-skin contact so important after birth and what measures might you take to achieve this?
8. What measures would you put in place to assist a woman to establish her breastfeeding relationship with her newborn?
9. What is newborn bloodspot screening and when is the ideal time for this to be attended?
10. Which of the following factors are considered protective factors for sudden infant death syndrome (SIDS)?
    A. Side sleeping position, breastfeeding, updated childhood immunisation status
    B. Supine sleeping position, breastfeeding, smoke free before and after birth
    C. Prone sleeping position, exposure to maternal tobacco use, smoke free before and after birth
    D. Supine sleeping position, breastfeeding, updated childhood immunisation status

Evolve® Answer guide for the Review Questions, Critical Thinking Exercises, Decision-making Framework Exercises and Critical Thinking Questions in Case Studies is hosted on Evolve: http://evolve.elsevier.com/AU/Koutoukidis/Tabbner.

References

Australian College of Midwives (ACM), 2021. National Midwifery Guidelines for Consultation and Referral. Available at: <https://midwives.org.au/common/Uploaded%20files/_ADMIN-ACM/National-Midwifery-Guidelines-for-Consultation-and-Referral-4th-Edition-(2021).pdf>.

Australian Breastfeeding Association, 2021. Breastfeeding: An introduction booklet. Available at: <www.breastfeeding.asn.au>.

Australian Commission on Safety and Quality in Health Care (ACSQHC), 2021. National safety and quality health service standards, 2nd ed. ACSQHC, Sydney.

Australian Institute of Health and Welfare (AIHW), 2020. Australia's mothers and babies 2018—in brief. Available at: <https://www.aihw.gov.au/reports/mothers-babies/australias-mothers-and-babies-2018-in-brief/summary>.

Australian Red Cross Lifeblood, 2017. You and your baby: Important information for Rh(D) negative women. Available at: <https://www.lifeblood.com.au/sites/default/files/resource-library/2021-12/99.-000135-RhD-Brochures-Update-You-and-your-baby-A5-8p-NoREF_V1.pdf>.

Baby Friendly Health Initiative (BFHI) Australia, 2020. Maternity facilities: 10 steps to successful breastfeeding. Available at: <https://bfhi.org.au/maternity-facilities/>.

Blackburn, S., 2018. *Maternal, fetal and neonatal physiology: A clinical perspective*, 5th ed. WB Saunders, Sydney.

Centre of Perinatal Excellence (COPE), 2023a. LGBTIQ+ parents. Available at: <https://www.cope.org.au/new-parents/lgbtiq-parents>.

Centre of Perinatal Excellence (COPE), 2023b. Recovery from birth. Available at: <https://www.cope.org.au/preparing-for-birth/the-days-following-birth>.

Crisp, J., Douglas, C., Rebeiro, G., et al. (eds), 2021. *Potter and Perry's fundamentals of nursing*, 6th ed. Elsevier, Sydney.

Davidson, M., London, M., Ladewig, P., 2020. *Old's maternal-newborn nursing and women's health across the lifespan*, 11th ed. Prentice Hall, Upper Saddle River.

Department of Health and Aged Care, 2019. Pregnancy care guidelines: Pregnancy care for Aboriginal and Torres Strait Islander women. Available at: <https://www.health.gov.au/resources/pregnancy-care-guidelines/part-a-optimising-pregnancy-care/pregnancy-care-for-aboriginal-and-torres-strait-islander-women>.

Department of Health and Aged Care, 2020. Clinical practice guidelines: Pregnancy care. Available at: <https://www.health.gov.au/resources/pregnancy-care-guidelines>.

Department of Health and Aged Care, 2023. National immunisation program schedule. Available at: <https://beta.health.gov.au/health-topics/immunisation/immunisation-throughout-life/national-immunisation-program-schedule>.

Hall, H., Glew, P., Rhodes, J., 2022. *Fundamentals of nursing and midwifery: A person-centred approach to care*, 4th ed. Lippincott Williams & Wilkins, Sydney.

Hockenberry, M., Wilson, D., Rodgers, C. (eds.), 2019. *Wong's nursing care of infants and children*, 11th ed. Mosby, St Louis.

Kuswara, L., Kremer, et al., 2016. The infant feeding practices of Chinese immigrant mothers in Australia: A qualitative exploration. *Appetite* 105, 375–384.

La Leche League (Canada), nd. Positioning and latching. Available at: <https://www.lllc.ca/sites/default/files/Positioning%20and%20latching-1.pdf>.

Ladewig, P.W., London, M.L., Davidson, M.R., 2017. *Contemporary maternal-newborn nursing care*, 9th ed. Pearson Prentice Hall, Upper Saddle River.

Leifer, G., 2023. *Introduction to maternity and pediatric nursing*, 9th ed. WB Saunders, Philadelphia.

Lowdermilk, D.L., Perry, S.E., Cashion, K., et al., 2020. *Maternity & women's health care*, 12th ed. Mosby Elsevier, St Louis.

Murray, S.S., McKinney, E.S., Holub, K., et al., 2023. *Foundations of maternal-newborn and women's health nursing*, 8th ed. Saunders Elsevier, St Louis.

National Health and Medical Research Council (NHMRC), 2010. Joint statement and recommendations on vitamin K administration to newborn infants to prevent vitamin K deficiency bleeding in infancy. Available at: <https://nhmrc.gov.au/about-us/publications/vitamin-k-administration-newborns-joint-statement>.

National Health and Medical Research Council (NHMRC), 2013. Australian dietary guidelines. National Health and Medical Research Council, Canberra. Available at: <https://www.health.gov.au/sites/default/files/australian-dietary-guidelines.pdf>.

National Institute for Clinical Excellence (NICE), 2016. Neonatal jaundice. RCOG Press, London.

Pairman, S., Tracy, S., Dahlen, H., et al., 2023. *Midwifery: Preparation for practice*, 5th ed. Elsevier, Sydney.

Perry, S.E., Hockenberry, M.J., Lowdermilk, D., et al., 2022. *Maternal child nursing care*, 7th ed. Mosby, St Louis.

Queensland Government, 2022. Clinical practice procedure—assessment/Apgar score. Available at: <https://www.ambulance.qld.gov.au/docs/clinical/cpp/CPP_APGAR%20score.pdf>.

Queensland Health, 2022. Queensland clinical guideline: Neonatal resuscitation. Available at: <https://www.health.qld.gov.au/__data/assets/pdf_file/0011/140600/g-resus.pdf>.

Red Nose, 2023. Safe sleeping: Red nose six safe sleep recommendations. Available at: <https://rednose.org.au/article/red-nose-six-safe-sleep-recommendations>.

Royal Australian and New Zealand College of Obstetricians and Gynaecologists (RANZCOG), 2019a. Guidelines for the use of Rh (D) immunoglobulin (anti-D) in obstetrics. Available at: <https://ranzcog.edu.au/wp-content/uploads/2022/05/Anti-D-guidelines_July-2021.pdf>.

Royal Australian and New Zealand College of Obstetricians and Gynaecologists (RANZCOG), 2019b. Intrapartum Fetal Surveillance (IFS) Clinical Guideline. Available at: <https://fsep.ranzcog.edu.au/what-we-offer/2-clinical-guideline>.

Safer Care Victoria, 2021. Accurate pregnancy dating (estimated due date). Available at: <https://www.safercare.vic.gov.au/clinical-guidance/maternity/accurate-pregnancy-dating-estimated-due-date>.

Speedie, L., Middleton, A. 2022. *Wong's nursing care of infants and children – for students*, Elsevier Australia.

The Royal Children's Hospital Melbourne, 2019. Clinical guidelines: Temperature management. Available at: <https://www.rch.org.au/rchcpg/hospital_clinical_guideline_index/Temperature_Management>.

The Royal Women's Hospital, 2020. Clinical guidelines: Breastfeeding the healthy term baby. Available at: <https://thewomens.r.worldssl.net/images/uploads/downloadable-records/clinical-guidelines/infant-feeding-breastfeeding-the-healthy-term-baby_280720.pdf>.

UNICEF UK, nd. Skin-to-skin contact. Available at: <https://www.unicef.org.uk/babyfriendly/baby-friendly-resources/implementing-standards-resources/skin-to-skin-contact>.

Victorian Government, 2021. LGBTIQ+ Inclusive language guide. Available at: <https://www.vic.gov.au/inclusive-language-guide>.

Wandel, T., Nguyen, C., et al., 2016. Breastfeeding among Somali mothers living in Norway: Attitudes, practices and challenges. *Women and Birth* 29, 487–493.

World Health Organization (WHO), 2018. Implementation guidance: Protecting, promoting and supporting breastfeeding in facilities providing maternity and newborn services – the revised Baby-friendly Hospital Initiative. Geneva. Available at: <https://www.who.int/publications/i/item/9789241513807>.

Recommended Reading

Kramer, L.I., 1969. Advancement of dermal icterus in the jaundiced newborn. *American Journal of Diseases of Children* 118, 454–458.

Queensland Health, 2015. Cultural dimensions of pregnancy, birth and postnatal care. Available at: <www.health.qld.gov.au/multicultural/health_workers/Chinese-preg-prof.pdf> and <https://www.health.qld.gov.au/__data/assets/pdf_file/0027/159561/sudanese-preg-prof.pdf>.

Royal Australian and New Zealand College of Obstetricians and Gynaecologists (RANZCOG), 2017. Maternity care in Australia: A framework for a healthy new generation of Australians, 1st ed. Available at: <https://ranzcog.edu.au/wp-content/uploads/2022/01/Maternity-Care-in-Australia-Web.pdf#:,:text=This%20document%20aims%20to%20set%20out%20a%20framework,the%20centre%20of%20planning%2C%20as%20it%20should%20be.>.

The Royal Women's Hospital, nd. Clinical guidelines: Good nutrition for pregnancy. Available at: <https://www.thewomens.org.au/health-information/pregnancy-and-birth/a-healthy-pregnancy/food-nutrition-in-pregnancy>.

The Royal Women's Hospital, 2021. Weight gain during pregnancy. Available at: <https://thewomens.r.worldssl.net/images/uploads/fact-sheets/Weight-gain-during-pregnancy_2021.pdf>.

Online Resources

Australian College of Midwives: <https://www.midwives.org.au>.

Baby Friendly Health Initiative Australia: <https://bfhi.org.au>.

Beyond Blue: <www.beyondblue.org.au>.

Centre of Perinatal Excellence: <https://www.cope.org.au>.

KidsHealth: <www.kidshealth.org>.

LGBTIQ+ Health Australia: <https://www.lgbtiqhealth.org.au>.

National Institute of Diabetes, Digestive and Kidney Diseases. Pregnancy and thyroid disease: <https://www.niddk.nih.gov>.

Post and Antenatal Depression Association (PANDA): <https://panda.org.au>.

Pregnancy, Birth and Baby: <https://www.pregnancybirthbaby.org.au>.

Red Nose: <https://rednose.org.au>.

Victorian Children's Tool for Observation and Response (ViCTOR): <victor.org.au>.

CHAPTER 45

Community, rural and remote

Ellie Kirov

Key Terms

community-based healthcare
community health nursing
geographical isolation
Indigenous health
models of care
person-centred care
primary care
primary healthcare
primary healthcare nursing
public health
remote area health services
remote area nurses (RANs)
rural health services
rural nurses
telehealth

Note: The term 'Indigenous' is used interchangeably with the term 'Aboriginal and Torres Strait Islander Peoples' throughout this chapter to assist readability.

Learning Outcomes

At the completion of this chapter and with further reading, learners should be able to:

- Define the key terms.
- Explain the role of public health in community-based care.
- Discuss primary healthcare and primary care.
- Describe the role of the primary health nurse and community health nurse.
- Identify the models of care used in community health practice.
- Explain the issues that affect nurses who are involved in home care.
- Describe the common competencies and skills of the primary health and community health nurse.
- Define person-centred care.
- Compare and contrast health status and needs between urban, rural and remote communities.
- Identify how regions are classified as rural or remote in Australia.
- Identify the key infrastructures for effective healthcare service delivery in remote settings.
- Identify and discuss potential sources of stress related to working in a remote health context.
- Describe the characteristics of rural and remote area nursing.
- Describe the challenges a nurse may face when providing nursing care to people living in rural and remote areas.

CHAPTER FOCUS

There is increased focus on primary healthcare in the community. A continuing shift of healthcare delivery from hospital to the community has increased the acuity and complexity of care provided in the community, including the home. These changes have occurred as a result of public health policies aimed at maintaining health and preventing illness, a consumer push for more healthcare options, earlier discharge from acute hospitals and containment of costs. In addition, rural and remote nursing is any type of nursing practice that involves the provision of nursing care in a centre or area that is geographically removed from a major city. This can present a unique set of challenges to nursing staff and the provision of quality care.

This chapter discusses the diverse role of the nurse who works in the community in Australia, including the role of, and challenges faced by, the rural and remote nurse. It explains the principles of primary healthcare and how they are practised in the context of the public health paradigm, and community health and healing are also explored. The factors that impact the health of individuals, families and communities are discussed, and the role, skills and competencies of the primary health and community health nurse are broadly examined. In addition, an overview of rural and remote nursing in healthcare environments, focusing on related workforce development and health service delivery in Australia is discussed, and key factors such as geographical isolation and sociological and cultural challenges are explored.

LIVED EXPERIENCE

I wouldn't work anywhere else. Where else could I care for a person with a snakebite at the beginning of my shift, assist with the plaster cast on a gentleman with a broken arm, attend a community immunisation clinic before lunch and provide a talk to school children on looking out for a mate with epilepsy in the afternoon? No other nursing job would allow me to be in all these places, it would be multiple positions, not as I love it ... it is my every day.

Joan, Enrolled Nurse

INTRODUCTION

Community healthcare is changing. Previously, community healthcare involved disease-recovery nursing care for transitioning individuals as they moved out of the hospital environment and into the community context. More attention is now directed to the provision of early intervention, prevention, maintenance and education about self-management. Early intervention measures for people living with chronic conditions are focused on preventing hospitalisation and readmission into the acute healthcare system by minimising adverse effects and promoting continued health and wellbeing (Australian Institute of Health and Welfare [AIHW] 2022). Community nurses increasingly assist individuals and their carers/families to self-manage their health situation within their community and home environment, which require a person-centred approach to care (McCormack et al 2021; Giusti et al 2020). **Person-centred care** is a model of care where individuals are seen as active participants and partners in healthcare (Byrne et al 2020).

A social view of health considers determinants of health that include economic and social factors (AIHW 2022). The social determinants of health have been recognised and asserted by the World Health Organization (WHO 1978). 'Health for all', a philosophy developed by the WHO, has been promoted in many countries (WHO 1978). An example of this within Australian society can be seen in Aboriginal and Torres Strait Islander populations where chronic conditions are the leading cause of the health gap compared with non-Indigenous Australians; 34% of this gap was explained by socioeconomic factors, such as household income and employment status (AIHW 2022). A social view of health impacts on the provision of care for people in the community.

CRITICAL THINKING EXERCISE 45.1

Mr McHugh, 32 years old, is homeless and spends most nights sleeping in the park. He has asthma and chronic bronchitis. Sometimes he drops in at the local charity food kitchen. He likes to pay his way and usually offers to help with the clean-up. Recently he has been short of breath. What interventions would you consider to improve Mr McHugh's health and quality of life?

Illness is influenced by how an individual experiences medically diagnosed pathophysiology, which may have characteristic signs and symptoms (Clendon et al 2022). The interactions between factors affecting health are illustrated in Figure 45.1.

According to Moore (2016), the 'extension of health services beyond the medical treatment model to a social model, and beyond the institutional to the community context, has seen "patients" now described also by terms used in social settings as "clients"'. Service users include the individual and their primary carers who access a service

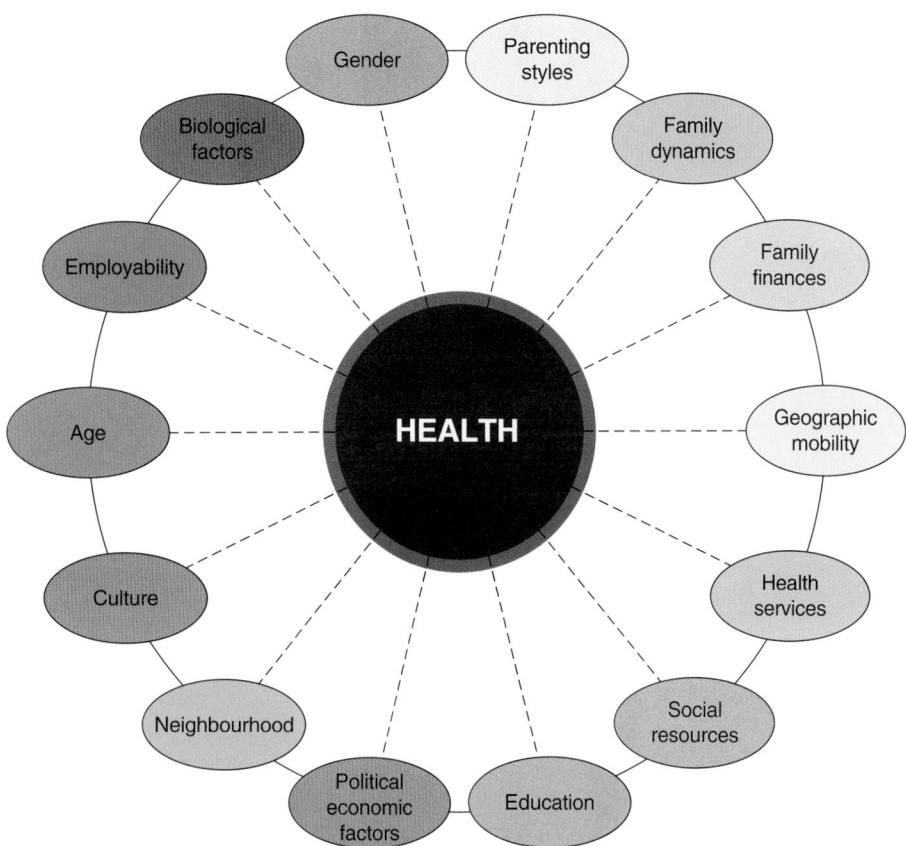

Figure 45.1 Interactions between factors affecting health
(Clendon et al 2022)

with the individual's consent. With the introduction of the National Safety and Quality Health Service Standards (Australian Commission on Safety and Quality in Health Care [ACSQHC] 2021; 2022), and in particular the 'Partnering with Consumers' Standard, this has evolved to also include the term 'consumer'. Such a change illustrates an increased focus on active partnerships between health service organisations and consumers and focuses on responding to consumer needs (ACSQHC 2021; 2022).

In Australia, community-based services are focusing more on specific at-risk sub-groups, such as 'socioeconomic groups; rural and remote populations; culturally and linguistically diverse populations; people with disability; lesbian, gay, bisexual, transgender and intersex people; veterans; and prisoners' (AIHW 2022).

The health of a community

Clendon et al (2022) state that 'the field of community health concentrates on the self-identified needs of individuals and families within communities'. It embodies:

An ideal where all community members strive towards a common state of health. The role of nurses and other health practitioners in promoting community health includes advocating, teaching, and enabling health based on local knowledge and understanding of the community's health goals.

These concepts are illustrated in the model for community healing in Figure 45.2.

A number of factors have been identified that impact on the context of community care:

- the changing and diverse complexity of illness and disease comorbidities that people experience as they live longer
- the increasing number of people who want to be cared for in their homes
- healthcare delivery that is becoming more complex with multiple services that require multidisciplinary team approaches to care provision and complex policy and strategic guidance to ensure quality and safe outcomes.

(Frost et al 2020)

People with chronic illness face many challenges. Helping a person to be more empowered is the role of any nurse. Empowerment is beneficial as it enhances a person's capacity to develop personal resources to manage their particular situation.

Public health

The drivers of **public health** are both economic and philosophical. Philosophically, the values for public health are based on notions of health for all, social justice, and

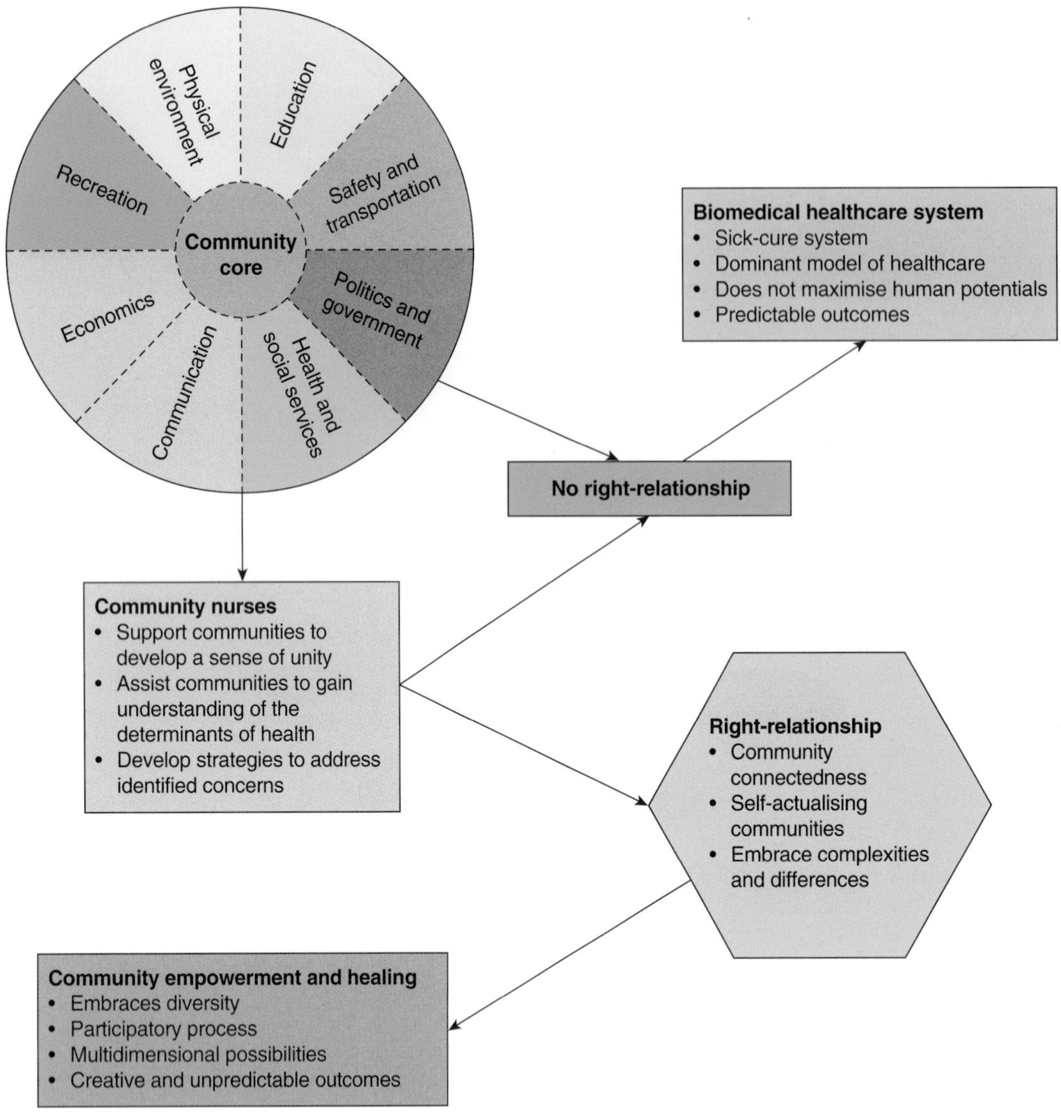

Figure 45.2 Model for community healing
(Francis et al 2013)

equity. Economic drivers work to reduce the cost of illness and treatment by preventing ill-health, promoting and protecting the public's health and maintaining a healthy workforce (Keleher 2023).

Public health seeks to protect and improve population health through education and the promotion of healthy lifestyles. Public health services aim to look at the health of a community and work to prevent people falling ill in the first place (Fleming & Baldwin 2023). Public health action has had a significant impact on improvements in the health of the Australian population. Key issues such as control of infectious diseases, environmental health, improved maternal and child health, better food and nutrition, mental health promotion, sexual and reproductive health, physical activity, injury prevention, cancer screening and chronic disease prevention are all contributing factors to improved population health (AIHW 2022; Keleher 2023).

Fleming and Parker (2023) suggest that 'Public health is about preventing disease, illness and injury, together with promoting the quality of life of human populations. This is a very complex process and requires the committed skills and expertise of many different professional disciplines.'

These authors have summarised the roles and functions of the public health workforce as:

- understanding the context for public health activity and its role and functions
- providing clarity around political impacts on public health
- applying a range of methodological approaches to understand data

- having a theoretical understanding of the disciplines that underpin public health and their contribution to strategy selection
- understanding a range of skills around surveillance, prevention, promotion and restoration of the population's health
- developing and analysing policy
- planning, implementation and evaluation
- using evidence-based practice
- using advocacy, communication and negotiation skills
- working intersectorally and with multidisciplinary groups
- demonstrating ethical practice.

(Fleming & Parker 2023)

Community health nursing and primary care nursing

Primary care is the first level of contact that individuals, families and communities have with the healthcare system (Hales 2020a). **Primary healthcare** is a model of community-based health service delivery that is part of the publicly funded health system in Australia. It focuses on decreasing the burden of chronic disease, decreasing the burden on hospitals and health services, and increasing equity in access to healthcare (Dawda & True 2023). Primary healthcare reflects care that transitions health system boundaries and focuses attention on community needs (Dawda & True 2023). Primary healthcare takes a person-centred approach, which minimises the potential for harm because the individual's values and preferred approaches to health are respected (ACSQHC 2021; 2022). The outcomes of primary healthcare, apart from better health, should be empowerment and self-reliance. Primary healthcare should be holistic in its approach and works on the premise that health is created and maintained in the context of settings of people's lives. Members of the community are empowered by the knowledge and the expectation that they will be full participants in health decision-making (Clendon et al 2022).

Primary healthcare nursing refers to nursing that takes place within a range of primary healthcare settings, each sharing the characteristic that they are part of the first level of contact with the health system (Australian Primary Health Care Nurses Association [APNA] 2024). In Australia, Nurse Practitioners, Registered Nurses (RNs) and Enrolled Nurses (ENs) practise in primary healthcare in a range of clinical and non-clinical roles, in urban, rural and remote settings, including maternal and child health, general practice, community health, school health and mental health (Clendon et al 2022). (See Clinical Interest Box 45.1.)

Primary healthcare nursing encompasses population health, health promotion, disease prevention, wellness care, first point of contact care and disease management across the lifespan. The setting and the ethnic and cultural grouping of the people determine models of practice.

CLINICAL INTEREST BOX 45.1 Primary healthcare nursing settings and roles

- Community settings—including community-controlled health services, correctional facilities (including juvenile and adult), refugee health, the community health sector and roles within social service settings
- General practice
- Domiciliary settings in the home, including residential aged care, custodial/detention settings, boarding houses and outreach to homeless people
- Educational settings, including preschool, primary and secondary school, vocational and tertiary education settings
- Occupational settings, occupational health and safety and workplace nursing
- Informal and unstructured settings, including ad hoc roles in daily life, such as sports settings and community groups

Roles of nurses may include:

- health promotion
- illness prevention
- healthy ageing
- antenatal and postnatal care
- child and family health nursing
- treatment and care of sick people
- rehabilitation and palliation
- community development
- population and public health
- education and research
- policy development and advocacy.

(APNA 2024)

Partnerships with people, individuals, families, communities and populations to achieve the shared goal of health for all is central to primary healthcare nursing. However, with significant policy changes in the primary healthcare arena, the focus remains firmly on general practice and increasing the scope of the practice nurse in community-based healthcare (Dawda & True 2023).

Community-based healthcare is a primary healthcare system that provides health-related services within the context of people's everyday lives and is directed towards a specific group within the geographical neighbourhood. To be effective it needs to:

- Provide easy access to care.
- Be flexible in responding to the care needs that individuals and families identify.
- Promote care between and among healthcare agencies through improved communication mechanisms.
- Provide appropriate support for family caregivers.
- Be affordable.

(Hales 2020a)

A range of services delivered in community-based settings in Australia are designed to provide early intervention to maximise health and wellbeing outcomes and prevent or slow the progression of ill-health. These services are funded by the state and federal governments, private services and volunteer-led and community-based organisations and play an important role in meeting the needs of people with, or at risk of, poorer health (AIHW 2022). The scope and organisation of services vary between states and territories. In Victoria, community health services provide priority access for people with specific health needs, with a schedule of fees that depends on the individual's circumstances. Services are provided through a mixture of independent community health centres and services that are part of rural or metropolitan public health services (Ridgeway et al 2021). In Western Australia, community health services focus on community nursing. They provide child and school health, Indigenous health, refugee health and immunisation. They are organised through state-run metropolitan and rural health services (Swerissen & Duckett 2018). In New South Wales (NSW), community nurses perform diverse roles such as generalist community nurses (GCN), early childhood nurses (ECN) and nurses involved in palliative care, mental health, home care, paediatrics, aged care, Indigenous health and women's health, as well as domiciliary midwives (Koff & Lyons 2020).

Australia also has many not-for-profit home nursing organisations, Bolton Clarke being one of many that delivers general and specialised nursing and healthcare in individuals' homes, and which is 'committed to improving and maintaining our clients' quality of life and independence by providing tailored care to meet their individual needs' (Bolton Clarke 2024). **Community health nursing** focuses on promoting and preserving the health of population groups (Hales 2020a).

THE COMMUNITY HEALTH NURSE'S ROLE

Community nurses provide comprehensive nursing care that allows recipients of care to remain in their communities. Services are diverse and wide ranging and include palliative care; mental health assessment and support; wound care; hospital in the home; prenatal and postnatal care; child and family care; complex, aged and chronic care; women's and men's health services; immunisation services; and Indigenous health (Blay et al 2021). The APNA (2017) statement in Clinical Interest Box 45.2 encapsulates the role of the community health nurse in Australia.

According to Clendon et al (2022), the community health nurse's role is different from that of a nurse working in a healthcare institution. Institutional care focuses on an episode of illness, whereas community health nursing involves preventing illness, protecting people from harm or worsening health, and recovery and rehabilitation following illness. Caring for the community itself is also a central premise, which may involve fostering health literacy and empowering the community to make decisions to 'maintain the community's viability and capability to cope with future challenges' (Clendon et al 2022, p. 3). Community health nurses need to be creative, adaptable and responsive to a variety of norms, cultures and value systems whether they are working with individuals, families or community groups.

CLINICAL INTEREST BOX 45.2 The role of the community health nurse

The community health nurse works to prevent illness and to promote health by identifying barriers to healthy lifestyles and general wellness. Working with families and communities, they deliver evidence-based nursing care to individuals, families, significant others and defined communities; empower individuals to change unhealthy lifestyles; provide post-acute care to people in their homes; and support self-reliance in recovery from illness and in managing chronic and terminal conditions. Nurses in community health work as part of an interdisciplinary team to provide an interpretative bridge between the acute sector and community services. They embrace a social model of health to advocate, and give a voice to, the community accessing care. In a system that is often complex and hard to navigate, nurses in community health can simplify the health systems, referral pathways and access to care.

(APNA 2017)

Teamwork in community care

Being healthy in any community means having equitable access to resources, empowerment, cultural inclusiveness, healthy environments and participation in decision-making (Clendon et al 2022). Partnerships between community members and healthcare professionals are critical for collaborative decisions that promote awareness and understanding of a community's health needs (Khan et al 2022; Larsson et al 2022).

To achieve better health and care outcomes, current models of practice require community health nurses and other health practitioners to be integral members of multidisciplinary teams to provide community-based healthcare, both in centres and in people's homes. Interdisciplinary team members can include nurses, doctors and allied health practitioners, such as social workers, occupational therapists and physiotherapists (Clendon et al 2022). Collaborative working relationships between healthcare workers, institutions and agencies are essential for providing coordinated care for individuals in the community. Competencies identified as being vital for collaboration include effective communication skills, mutual respect and trust, and a team decision-making process with shared responsibility for the outcome (Hales 2020a).

Home care and support

The terms used to describe the provision of nursing care in people's homes vary but can include domiciliary nursing, ambulatory care, community health nursing, district nursing, hospital in the home and home care. Regardless of the title, home care requires specialised skill sets of advanced nursing care since nurses may work in an environment which necessitates that they work independently, and includes coordination of services, provision of direct care, assessment, consulting, education, administration and research activities (Hales 2020b).

The RN working in home care may also be responsible for the direction and supervision of unregulated care workers as well as the EN. The role of the home health nurse includes being advocate, carer, educator, case manager or coordinator. The home care nurse also needs to consider other perspectives related to working in a person's home environment: the person's safety, legal and ethical issues, infection prevention and control, and nurse safety (Hales 2020b).

MODELS OF CARE IN COMMUNITY HEALTH

As the community changes, there are also changes in the way that healthcare is aligned, organised and delivered. Key areas of reform include Commonwealth reforms such as the National Disability Insurance Scheme (NDIS), aged care and the establishment of Primary Health Networks (PHNs). Various approaches are emerging to address community health, such as integrated health, community initiatives, coalitions, managed care, case management and outreach programs (Hales 2020a). Community and primary healthcare nursing applies a social model of healthcare that addresses the health needs of individuals and communities while considering the social, economic and environmental factors affecting their health (Fisher et al 2022). See Clinical Interest Box 45.3 for a summary of these **models of care**.

CLINICAL INTEREST BOX 45.3 Models of care

- Integrated healthcare system—makes all levels of care (primary, secondary and tertiary) available in an integrated form.
- Community initiatives—members of the community establishing health priorities, goals and actions to achieve goals.
- Community coalitions—individuals and groups having a shared purpose of improving community health.
- Managed care—multidisciplinary teams working together to provide cost-effective and quality healthcare across the care continuum with the managed care organisation liaising between individuals, provider and payer.
- Case management—tracks individuals' needs and helps them access services through a variety of care settings to ensure continuity. Case management is defined as a collaborative process of assessment, planning, facilitation and advocacy for options and services to meet an individual's health needs through communication and available resources to promote quality cost-effective outcomes. It is a dominant model used in community mental healthcare.
- Outreach programs—link people who have difficulty accessing services with the formal healthcare system.
- Solution-focused nursing—considers the sociocultural as well as the individual world of a person with nurses being proactive in promoting health and wellbeing rather than reacting to palliate symptoms.

(Hales 2020a; Orr 2023; McAllister 2010; McAllister et al 2006; Moore 2016)

ISSUES FOR COMMUNITY HEALTH NURSES IN HOME CARE

Isolation is an issue for some community nurses. Rural and remote community nurses work in diverse settings, often in isolated practice in resource-poor environments, with their practice influenced by the geography of the community, communication, issues of transportation and personal safety (Baldwin et al 2013; Cox et al 2023).

In addition to incident management and reporting, the community nurse has mandatory reporting requirements as part of their duty of care to the individual. These requirements include reporting for suspected incidences of child abuse and neglect to government authorities. Each state and territory in Australia has enacted legislation commonly known as 'mandatory reporting laws'. The types of child abuse or neglect that must be reported by nurses within each state and territory vary between each jurisdiction, and can include physical abuse, sexual abuse, psychological/emotional abuse, neglect and exposure to domestic violence (Staunton & Chiarella 2024).

Giving culturally safe care is an integral requirement in community healthcare. Cultural safety means providing an environment in which individuals feel spiritually, socially and emotionally safe, as well as being physically safe. Cultural safety is about the person who is providing care reflecting on their own assumptions. In 2018, the Nursing and Midwifery Board of Australia (NMBA) and the Congress of Aboriginal and Torres Strait Islander Nurses and Midwives (CATSINaM) issued a joint statement on culturally safe and respectful care to remind nurses and midwives of their responsibility to provide care that is free of bias and racism, challenges belief based upon assumption and is culturally safe and respectful for Aboriginal and Torres Strait Islander Peoples (NMBA 2018b). Culturally safe nursing accommodates and respects a diverse range of views on health and healing (Stein-Parbury 2021). Refer to Chapter 13 for further reading on cultural diversity in healthcare.

Aboriginal and Torres Strait Islander health workers are vital in Indigenous health services as they are better equipped to provide services to Indigenous populations, and to bridge the gap with non-Indigenous health professionals in their community (Mackean et al 2020b; Pearson et al 2020). In addition, 'disconnection from country, culture, language and family are cited as major contributors to endemic proportions of chronic disease' in Aboriginal and Torres Strait Islander Peoples due to intergenerational trauma accrued from systemic removal of children from their cultural land and the subsequent erasure of cultural identity (Gatwiri et al 2021). See Chapter 14 for further reading on Indigenous health.

Personal safety is an important consideration for the nurse who makes home visits. Strategies to eliminate or manage risks must be implemented. Risks include working as a sole practitioner; being 'on call' in remote communities; gender bias (where most community health nurses are female); dealing with hazards in the home such as obstructions and debris; aggressive dogs; having to use mobile telephones, especially in rural Australia; dealing with angry and aggressive individuals and domestic violence; driving; needlestick incidents; and working alone (APNA 2015; Orr 2023). See Clinical Interest Box 45.4 for home care personal safety considerations.

CLINICAL INTEREST BOX 45.4 Personal safety considerations for home visits

Consideration must be given to:

- the time of day of the service
- communication with practice staff around time of departure and expected time of return
- individual patient issues (infectious disease/immune status/mental health)
- adequate/safe parking at the residence
- access to and location of residence
- other household residents
- pets
- nurse's natural instinct for unsafe environments and danger/risk
- injury to nurse while in the patient's home (tripping, slipping)
- what to do in case of an accident or road rage
- safe driving
- unsecured equipment in vehicle
- adverse weather (flood, fire, fog, storms)
- equipping the nurse with a personal duress alarm
- attending a nurse home visit in a pair, particularly where volatile behaviour is likely or unpredictable.

(APNA 2015)

CRITICAL THINKING EXERCISE 45.2

The community health nurse role involves case management and can be challenging. As an Enrolled Nurse working in this environment, what are the key components of your role?

STANDARDS AND SCOPE OF PRACTICE OF THE COMMUNITY AND PRIMARY HEALTHCARE NURSE

Internationally, there is growing emphasis on building strong primary healthcare nursing workforces to meet the challenges of rising chronic and complex disease (Lukewich et al 2020). Indeed, further work is required to develop and test robust standards that can communicate the skills and knowledge required of nurses working in primary healthcare settings to policy-makers, employers, other health professionals and consumers (Scammel et al 2020). Competency standards are important tools for communicating the role of nurses to consumers and other health professionals, as well as defining this role for employers, policy-makers and educators. Various professional practice/competency standards have been developed to support nurses working in primary healthcare (Beasleigh et al 2024).

Community nurses must be compliant with the legal and regulatory requirements of the jurisdictions in which they practise. ENs who work in community and primary healthcare settings must work within their scope of practice under the supervision of the RN. Over time, and in collaboration with education providers, community nurses, and the Australian Nursing and Midwifery Federation (ANMF), a number of practice standards for community health nurses have been developed (see Clinical Interest Box 45.5). There is a consistent distinction between the competencies of the beginning practitioner and the practitioner with advanced skills, and the need for integration of advanced competencies into Nurse Practitioner programs (Chan et al 2020; Torrens et al 2020; Whitehead et al 2022).

In 2014, the Australian Nursing and Midwifery Federation (ANMF) released the *National Practice Standards for Nurses in General Practice*, which were developed to accompany the NMBA standards for practice. Specifically focusing on the RN and EN workforce in Australian general practice and reflecting the aspects of the nursing role unique to the general practice context, these standards are different from those expected of the nurse in other clinical settings. At the time of releasing these standards, it was acknowledged that further work is required and that some other groups of primary healthcare nurses who are working outside general practice are yet to have professional practice

CLINICAL INTEREST BOX 45.5 Practice standards for community health nurses, Victoria

Domain one: Professional practice

Standard 1: Demonstrates a comprehensive knowledge of community health nursing incorporating population health, primary healthcare, and health promotion.
Standard 2: Advocates for individuals/groups/communities and their rights for community health nursing service, primary healthcare, health equity and healthy environments, policies and legislation.
Standard 3: Practises within an ethical and professional nursing framework.
Standard 4: Practises in accordance with legislation affecting community health nursing practice and primary healthcare.
Standard 5: Demonstrates leadership in the development, coordination and management of systems and processes to anticipate and facilitate safe quality health and wellbeing services.

Domain two: Critical thinking and analysis

Standard 6: Participates in continuing professional development (CPD) of self and others.
Standard 7: Practises within an evidence-based framework.

Domain three: Provision and coordination of care

Standard 8: The community health nurse (CHN) conducts comprehensive and systematic assessment, planning, implementation and evaluation in an ongoing way in collaboration with the individual, family, group, team and community.
Standard 9: Coordinates, organises and provides integrated health promotion (IHP) considering a whole of community approach.
Standard 10: Facilitates a physical, emotional, social and cultural environment that promotes individual/group/community safety, security, respect and health and wellbeing.

Domain four: Communication and collaboration

Standard 11: Establishes, maintains and concludes therapeutic relationships with individuals, groups and communities.
Standard 12: Collaborates with the multidisciplinary team to provide community health nursing.

(Ward et al 2013; Chan et al 2020; Torrens et al 2020; Whitehead et al 2022)

standards developed specifically for their clinical setting (ANMF 2014). Nurses should check with the relevant organisations to ensure that they are using the most recent and complete version of these practice standards.

Nurses working to their full scope of practice as part of an interdisciplinary team can enable more integrated, efficient and accessible healthcare (APNA 2017). To facilitate integration between team members and optimise the distribution of care provision across the team, it is important that all team members have an awareness of the scope of practice and competence of each of the professions that comprise the team. Barriers to optimal scope of practice for primary healthcare nurses are listed in Clinical Interest Box 45.6.

The APNA's Career and Education Frameworks for Nurses in Primary Health Care (Clinical Interest Box 45.7) aim to improve the recruitment and retention of the nursing workforce within primary healthcare. The RN and EN Frameworks and associated tools have been developed to improve and promote the employment opportunities, build capacity and support the transferability of nursing skills across primary healthcare settings (APNA 2018).

THE NURSING PROCESS AND COMMUNITY NURSING

The nursing process is used in community health and community-based nursing, as in many other areas of nursing care. See Chapter 7 for further reading on the nursing process. As a logical framework for nursing care, the steps of assessment, nursing identification of issues, planning, implementation and evaluation are particularly useful for individuals receiving care in the community. The nursing process is instructive in providing a formalised and documented problem-solving strategy (Ingham-Broomfield 2020). Using tools designed to help in decision-making, such as the NMBA decision-making framework, is recommended (NMBA 2020). (See Case Study 45.1.) Nurses in community care also use critical-thinking skills to resolve issues, manage risks and make appropriate referrals (Ingham-Broomfield 2020). Community nurses need to reflect at the analytical and personal levels about the individuals in their care and the larger community, and also about themselves and their own role and function in the community they serve. See Chapter 6 for further reading on critical thinking, problem-based learning and reflective practice.

CLINICAL INTEREST BOX 45.6 Barriers to optimal scope of practice for primary healthcare nurses

- Primary healthcare nurse financing
- Intradisciplinary and interdisciplinary support and awareness of full scope of practice
- Formal education, training and career frameworks

(APNA 2017)

CLINICAL INTEREST BOX 45.7
APNA Career and Education Frameworks for Nurses in Primary Health Care—Enrolled Nurses

APNA has developed Career and Education Frameworks for Nurses in Primary Health Care, funded by the Commonwealth Department of Health. The Enrolled Nurse Frameworks and associated tools have been developed to improve and promote the employment opportunities, build capacity and support the transferability of nursing skills across primary healthcare settings.

(APNA 2018)

CLINICAL INTEREST BOX 45.8
Program snapshot: Refugee health program, Victoria

The Refugee Health Program (formerly Refugee Health Nurse Program) provides a coordinated approach using community nurses who have expertise in working with culturally and linguistically diverse and marginalised communities. These nurses work in community health services with high refugee populations. The program has three aims: increase refugee access to primary health services; improve the response of health services to refugees' needs; and enable individuals, families and refugee communities to improve their health and wellbeing.

(Victorian Refugee Health Network, http://refugeehealthnetwork.org.au)

CASE STUDY 45.1

Rebecca is an Enrolled Nurse who works in a community-based nursing service. In a typical day, Rebecca sees 10–15 individuals in their homes. The activities she is involved in include hygiene assistance, wound care, monitoring blood glucose levels and assisting individuals with the application of compression stockings.

Rebecca is responsible for organising her own day, which starts at the office base with a handover and ends there with time allowed to debrief with the coordinator and other staff. Rebecca's days are not often the same and she finds herself regularly involved in providing health education and emotional support to individuals and carers, as well as information on other services that are available in the community.

1. What are some of the community services in existence that could benefit the individuals Rebecca cares for?
2. What are some relevant health promotion/education programs that could benefit the individuals Rebecca cares for?
3. One of the individuals Rebecca cares for in the community has a BGL of 27.9 mmol. What action would she take?
4. When assisting an individual in the shower, Rebecca notices significant bruising on her arms. When questioned, the individual tells Rebecca that her son did this but that he didn't mean to hurt her. What is Rebecca's responsibility in this scenario?
5. What are some of the key personal safety strategies Rebecca would implement when working in community nursing?

Nurses working in the community or home setting have the opportunity to observe individuals in their own environment, enabling a more holistic assessment (Clinical Interest Box 45.8). The focus on a person's choice and autonomy means that individuals and families are encouraged to participate actively in the nursing process. As a result, the individual and their family may be more proactive in the implementation phase, significantly contributing to the success of the care plan as they work towards their own goals. An example of a care plan has been provided in Nursing Care Plan 45.1.

DECISION-MAKING FRAMEWORK EXERCISE 45.1

You have just been employed at a large, busy general practice surgery. You have been asked to undertake a day shift under the supervision of a senior Enrolled Nurse who has worked at the practice for the past 4 years. The general practitioner on shift has said they are happy to provide support if needed. You have been asked to perform all wound care appointments, triage of walk-ins and follow-up phone calls of the clinic's individuals with diabetes.

Using the decision-making process address the following:

1. Do you accept this allocation of duties?
2. Considering the staff on this shift, is the model of nursing care appropriate?
3. What (if any) are the issues that could potentially result in you working outside of your scope of practice?
4. Identify the potential and/or actual flaws within this scenario.

NURSING CARE IN RURAL AND REMOTE AREAS

Nurses represent the largest component of the health workforce in rural and remote Australia. Health inequities

NURSING CARE PLAN 45.1

Assessment: Community medication review.
Issue/s to be addressed: Medication compliance in elderly person recently discharged from hospital after an acute myocardial infarction.
Goal/s: Ensure individual understands all medications, what they are for, when and how they should be taken.

Care/actions:	Rationale:
Explain discharge medications. Discuss blister packs for ease of medication management. Discuss possible MedsCheck with local pharmacist. Help write a daily/weekly medication plan for the individual.	To increase individual's understanding and compliance with medications to help prevent readmission to hospital or a negative health outcome related to medication mismanagement.

Evaluation:
Medications taken as directed.
MedsCheck undertaken.
Blister packs in situ.
Nil further readmission related to medication management.
Referrals to pharmacist and general practitioner regarding medication review.

exist, with rural and remote communities experiencing poorer health outcomes than their city counterparts (AIHW 2023b). The concept of remoteness, and of understanding the role of the nurse in a rural or remote setting, is interesting and complex. Central to rural and remote health practice is learning how nursing care and community interaction is important while working in the setting.

A common distinction between **rural health services** and **remote area health services** usually involves the presence (rural) or absence (remote) of a medical officer. In addition, rural communities usually always have a 24-hour healthcare facility with medical service capabilities, whereas most remote areas rely on health centres that are open during office hours and an on-call service after hours (Whitehead & Quinn 2019).

Significant factors for the role of the **rural nurse** are the context of the environment; its location and distance from a tertiary referral centre; the size of the facility; the healthcare team in which nurses work; the working conditions; and the profile of the rural community in which the nurses care, work and reside (Whitehead & Quinn 2019). For example, for a resident of Yuendumu in the Western Desert, Northern Territory, access to health services and education and the degree of perceived 'remoteness' will differ from that of someone in a regional centre such as Alice Springs or a rural town like Goondiwindi. There will also be variations over time—for example, when the Yuendumu road is washed out or when drought occurs. For health professionals at Yuendumu, perceived remoteness would also differ. An Aboriginal health worker is likely to be in their home community and therefore close to family, albeit far from most formal educational opportunities. However, the **remote area nurses (RANs)** are likely to be distant from family and professional support, as well as being physically remote from the closest regional centre. For many nurses, the opportunity to provide nursing care within or near their hometown locality is appealing and provides a rewarding and challenging career pathway.

Within Aboriginal and Torres Strait Islander communities in Australia, the opportunity for Aboriginal health workers and health practitioners to engage within their community and work with and for the community is available. This is achieved through the role of the Aboriginal health worker and health practitioner. They are trained specifically in the needs of the Aboriginal and Torres Strait Islander populations to work within the healthcare team for Aboriginal and Torres Strait Islander Peoples.

Several classifications are used in Australia to define 'rural' and 'remote' and these are often used to allocate both services and resources. The most commonly used systems are:

- Accessibility/Remoteness Index for Australia (ARIA or ARIA+) classification.
- Australian Standard Geographical Classification (ASGC) Remoteness Areas classification. This is based on the road distance to the service centres
- Modified Monash Model (MMM). Differentiates rural locations with inner and outer regional Australia, based on town size.

These classification systems do not take into account the socioeconomic status, population size or cultural factors (Roberts & Guenther 2021; Brown et al 2023).

The proportion of rural and remote Indigenous populations in Australia is high, at 32%, comparative to non-Indigenous population at 1.7%, who have indicated they are not of Aboriginal and Torres Strait Islander origin (AIHW 2024). Between 2013 and 2021, the number of Indigenous medical practitioners registered in Australia increased from 247 to 604 (from 31 to 69 per 100,000), while the number of Indigenous nurses and midwives registered in Australia increased from 2833 to 6160 (324 to 701 per 100,000) (AIHW 2023a). Among Indigenous-specific primary healthcare organisations and maternal/child health services, 46% of full-time equivalent (FTE) health staff in 2021–2022 were Indigenous (2305 FTE), the majority being Aboriginal health practitioners/Aboriginal health workers (960 FTE, 99.5%) and other health workers (1114 FTE, 52%), with lower proportions for general practitioners (GPs) (42 FTE, 6.1%) and nurses and midwives (189 FTE, 15%) (AIWH 2023).

The promotion of cultural safety is a key area of consideration in efforts to support individuals utilising the healthcare setting in a manner that is consistent with local traditions, culture and needs. There are often cultural and cross-cultural issues distinguishing service provision in rural and remote areas. The principles of respect, relationships and responsibility underpin many frameworks that describe cultural safety in nursing and health more generally (Mackean et al 2020a). The need to enact and uphold these values is important and reliant on the professional nature of those working in the setting.

Collaboration with Aboriginal health workers and health practitioners is an important aspect of the role. The role of the Aboriginal health worker forms the base of a cultural broker between health professionals and the individual (Drummond 2022). They act to guide and protect non-Indigenous workers in rural and remote settings, (Drummond 2022). In many remote settings it is the remote area nurse who works collaboratively with the Aboriginal health worker.

In any culture, there exists a set of values, beliefs, rituals and practices; understanding and adapting to these is often a complex and difficult pathway. Working as a non-Indigenous nurse within an Indigenous community can highlight many differences in ideals, expectations and understanding of the healthcare setting (Ramsamey 2022). These can vary according to the location and remoteness of the setting; however, they are reliant on the nurse being able to understand and adapt. Often the support structures are limited and require the nurse to become familiar with tradition and culture and adapt work practices to achieve this. Sometimes this results in an inability to work within the area and a high mobility or transient characteristic in the workforce. Positive work relations can be developed and grown with local Elders within the community and in the inclusion and support that can be provided by an Aboriginal health worker. Getting to know and understand the community that you work within is important to gaining a better understanding of and socialisation within a rural or remote area.

Resourcing within remote centres differs greatly from that provided within a tertiary referral setting. The availability of public (and often private) transport decreases with increasing remoteness. Coupled with poorer socioeconomic status, unsealed and sometimes unmaintained roads, and seasonal variations in road access, access to health and other services is often poorer (Whitehead & Quinn 2019).

Health services in remote areas have distinctive features. One of these is that they tend to be supply driven. That is, access is constrained by the availability of suitably experienced staff and appropriately resourced clinics. In urban and many rural areas, services are more demand driven. The population exists for a variety of services and access to these is within driving or public transport distances. In other words, with a better supply (and diversity) of health staff and facilities, persons can access doctors, health clinics and allied health professionals as often as they need and can afford. Additionally, remote health services are predominantly state/territory government funded, whereas in urban and most rural areas there is a greater private component, and a greater use of Medicare funding.

REMOTE AND RURAL AUSTRALIA

The remote areas of Australia generally pose particular challenges for consumers and providers of health services. The Australian rural and remote setting (or 'the outback') is characterised by large distances, extremes of climate, formidable geography, poor health status, diverse cultures, sparse population and tenuous infrastructure. This concept of living in a rural locality creates a sense of life on a farm, fresh food, water and the great outdoors; however, according to the Australian health-related statistics, individuals in rural areas are at greater risk than those in urban areas of health-related problems (AIHW 2023b).

Significant issues

Government

In Australia, the majority of remote health services are provided or funded by state and territory governments. In cross-border regions, there are differences and difficulties over policies, laws and historic traditions. Superimposed are the Commonwealth, state and local government divisions of responsibility, which also vary from area to area. The Commonwealth has responsibility for some aspects of health, such as general practice services, immunisation and some **Indigenous health** services; however, the state government has authority over most areas of health service. The Commonwealth and the states and territories may also have jurisdiction over land, particularly Crown land, mining and conservation (Best & Fredericks 2022). It is these government boundaries that require additional communication and planning for people from within health services to achieve an outcome for an individual.

In many ways, the bush is the battleground on which the issues of state and federal politics are fought. It is also the place where the lack of defined responsibilities for the different tiers of government in areas such as health is more apparent. Medicare services versus state-government-funded health services, native title, mining, fishing rights, forestry, environmental control and conservation are a few of the major issues in remote and rural Australia (Best & Fredericks 2022). See Chapter 4 for further reading on Australia's healthcare system.

Health resources

The health status of people living in remote areas is significantly worse than those living in urban areas. The poorer health outcomes are attributable to high proportions of Indigenous populations with high disease burdens and inequitable access to health services (AIHW 2023a). People living in remote areas have less access to health resources and have traditionally had services delivered mainly by remote area nurses; hence, they have had little or no access to the Medicare Benefits Schedule (MBS) and the Pharmaceutical Benefits Scheme (PBS) funding. Findings of the AIHW (2023) include:

- The supply of GPs and retail pharmacists falls sharply in remote zones.

- Nurses provide a higher proportion of healthcare in rural and remote Australia than in metropolitan Australia.
- The number of medical specialists in remote areas per capita is substantially lower.
- Nursing home availability decreases with increasing remoteness.
- Medicare data indicates that people living in rural and remote zones are using fewer services than those living in metropolitan zones.
- Overall hospitalisation rates are highest for those living in the remote zone.

Comparison of health needs of urban, rural and remote communities

Internationally, there is a disparity in health status in favour of urban populations and Australia reflects this trend, with current morbidity and mortality data showing a significant rural/remote-urban differential. Examples of this include:

- Australia's farming population has a distinctive illness/injury profile, characterised by high rates of unintentional injury and fatality.
- Geographically, the healthcare workforce is unevenly distributed, and problems of access extend beyond 'mere distances to services'.
- Rural and remote health services are more dependent on primary healthcare services with medical support provided by general practitioners (GPs).
- People living in rural and remote areas generally receive a smaller share of overall health spending; there are fewer GPs, specialist nurses and health professionals; and more limited access to specialist services.
- People living in rural and remote areas are often required to travel large distances to attend medical appointments, with even greater distances to seek specialised treatments.

(AIHW 2023b)

HEALTH AND ILLNESS PATTERNS IN RURAL AND REMOTE AUSTRALIA

Australian statistics identify disadvantaged comparisons in rural and remote Australia that include income and poverty levels, unemployment rates, education and living costs. The rural/remote population also experiences poorer health than their urban counterparts, with health status and life expectancy decreasing the further the individual resides from an urban centre. Needless to say, there is less access to health services and specialist services are rare. Rural and remote Australians also display higher rates of disability, premature mortality, morbidity, hypertension and mental health illnesses. Health risk factors such as smoking, alcohol consumption and environmental dangers are greater in rural areas, as are rates of injury including particularly high rates of child accidents, and chronic conditions, especially asthma and diabetes (AIHW 2023b; Best & Fredericks 2022).

These higher morbidity and mortality rates are exacerbated by poor infrastructure supports (inferior roads, long distances to services and lack of transport options) and are often a deterrent to help-seeking behaviours, thus further impacting on health outcomes.

Indigenous Australians experience not only significantly lower life expectancy rates than their non-Indigenous counterparts but also higher rates of most ill-health and trauma, particularly higher rates of chronic conditions and accidents.

Rural/remote Australia, population health and provision of services

Healthcare provision and access is one of the most significant issues for rural and remote Australia. Despite the evident health needs (as briefly outlined above), health services in rural and remote Australia remain stretched and underfunded and there is a widespread lack of specialist services. Inaccessible areas, particularly small, remote communities, are likely to have a poorer health status and poorer standard of care (AIHW 2023b). This corresponds with less availability of services or ability to access services. There are many reasons for this, with the biggest being the size of the area that needs to be serviced and the distance between the services that are currently offered.

Rural/remote populations have greater difficulty accessing basic services, including GPs. There is considerable evidence of service paucity and overstretched resources, with patterns indicating declining service provision at the same time that demand is increasing. Health disadvantage and poorer standards of service delivery are well-established factors of rural/remote life in small communities throughout Australia, yet government policy responses generally do not seem to be able to ameliorate this issue, thereby limiting appropriate and effective responses (AIHW 2023b; Whitehead & Quinn 2019). It is a complex issue and one that is not easily resolved. Given the enormity of distance that health services are required to cover, it is an ongoing debate and dilemma for any government in power.

Positively, living in a rural or remote setting provides health workers and the local community with a sense of community. There is a noted reliance on each other, the community and the service providers that do have services in town. In the event of trauma, natural disaster or illness, it is not uncommon for communities to focus on 'getting ready' to help out in many and varied ways, although decreased disaster resilience is linked to geographic remoteness (Parsons et al 2021; Ryan et al 2020).

This sense of community provides psychological support and reassurance for community members and also for healthcare workers, who can sometimes be caught between the professional requirements of the registration standards of an Enrolled or Registered Nurse and that of community member. As a nurse there is a privacy privilege that allows for the disclosure of personal medical and personal information relevant to the provision of care; however, there remain distinct confidentiality requirements of professionals (Taylor 2017). In 'tight-knit' communities this requires health professionals to be discreet and have the ability to maintain confidentiality and trust in all conversations.

There is an increasingly well-documented, uneven geographical distribution of the healthcare workforce. There are fewer doctors per capita in rural and remote areas compared with urban areas; the contribution and importance of other health professionals must not be underestimated. However, the need for individuals to travel is high due to the lack of specialists in the setting.

Nursing and health schools now focus attention on clinical placements within rural and remote settings in an aim to showcase the positives of working within these. For many students, this is their first experience of a rural locality and for some it offers the chance of future work opportunities. For many, it is the opportunity to become part of the community, learning from Enrolled Nurses and Registered Nurses within the area. Learning in the rural setting is a unique opportunity for students since it enables a closer connection with community unlike the experience in an urban setting.

The recruitment and retention of staff in rural and remote settings is often difficult due to locality and long distances from an urban setting (Liu et al 2023). Retention is impacted by a number of factors: isolation, since often the nurse is the sole provider; there may be periods of blurred professional and personal boundaries; and the requirement for a broad range of skills and limited opportunities for professional development (Whiteing et al 2021). In 2019, Services for Australian Rural and Remote Allied Health (SARRAH) was commissioned by the NSW Ministry of Health to develop a paper outlining strategies that have been proven effective or ineffective for increasing the efficacy of allied health rural recruitment and retention in Australia. The report identified 'limited quality evidence to demonstrate the impact of recruitment and retention interventions on workforce outcomes across individual professions or the allied health workforce as a whole' (Battye et al 2019, p. 4). The most common positive extrinsic incentives to recruiting healthcare professionals into the rural context were rural lifestyle and diversity of caseload (Battye et al 2019). Access to professional development, professional isolation and insufficient supervision were the most commonly identified negative extrinsic factors that might inhibit recruitment.

The diversity of situations that rural nurses work in requires them to make decisions independent of other health professionals. This requires that nurses are prepared, skilled and educated in contemporary practice to manage and coordinate situations from outpatient clinics to multi-trauma life-threatening situations (Calleja et al 2022). Coupled with this demand is the geographical barrier to accessing education; however, the improvement in **telehealth** and internet accessibility has slightly diminished this barrier.

Rural and remote health is a complex problem that does not have one neat fix, nor does it belong to one government department. There is a need for a whole-of-government response: a national, coordinated approach that takes into consideration the needs and diversity of the population.

Geography, space, place and health

Health status comparisons are typically assessed through rates of life expectancy, morbidity and mortality. As referred to previously, life expectancy rates have been found to be significantly higher in urban areas compared with rural and remote areas. The rates range from 80 years (males) and 85 years (females) in major cities to 67 years (males) and 69 years (females) in very remote areas (AIHW 2023b). Therefore, it is not surprising that all-cause mortality rates of Australian people increased with the level of remoteness. Most rural males are hard workers in the agricultural sector—and the appropriate services may not be available to them nor affordable to access in another locality. Likewise, property landholders may struggle with workload requirements resulting in the inability to take time 'off the land' to attend to health ailments. Within rural industry, time off leaves properties unattended or with less than the required staff to enable functioning of the property, with resultant loss of income. This, as well as the ongoing struggle that nature presents with drought, flood and fire, and the political landscape with mining and changes in export market requirements, adds greater pressure to those working and managing rural properties.

The common leading causes of death in rural areas include cardiovascular and respiratory diseases, as well as injury (e.g. poisonings, motor vehicle accidents and suicide) (AIHW 2023b). A recurring theme in rural and remote demography is that population density is low and dispersed. These characteristics impact on healthcare services, particularly the ability to sustain healthcare services at accessible locations.

While an increase in local hospital closures in rural and remote locations has resulted in a reduction of primary care and an increase in travel, this has not been the sole rural healthcare issue. Additional healthcare concerns include quality of care, specialisation of services, ambulatory care and emergency treatment: all factors that can negatively impact the health of rural people. In large part, distance, isolation and dispersed populations have been the leading causes of these problems. These common characteristics have led to difficulties in recruiting, as well as retaining qualified and skilled professionals. The urban and more prosperous areas are disproportionately home to the skilled healthcare workforce in most, if not all, countries around the world.

Many promising health service initiatives in rural and remote areas have not been sustained, with the result that many communities still lack adequate health services and residents often forgo care at times of need. It is appropriate to consider the critical factors driving the need for changes in healthcare models and what impediments exist to achieving equitable access to healthcare regardless of geographical or socioeconomic circumstances (AIHW 2023a; Whitehead & Quinn 2019).

For many reasons, there is a growing diversity of rural and remote populations and a high level of unemployment and welfare dependency. The factors that have shaped and continue to shape the culture of rural and remote areas include the movement of people in and out of such areas, changes in agricultural prosperity, workforce changes, globalisation (growth of the international marketplace) and 'detraditionalisation' and diversity of rural and remote areas. More than two decades ago, Welch (2000) wrote about the determinants of rural health and much of what she discussed is still the case today. Her argument is that while Australia is one of the most highly urbanised countries in the world, the economy is still dependent, to some degree, on the rural sector. The general perception of rural Australia as a homogenous mass of people, experiencing health and healthcare in a similar way is not the case in reality.

CRITICAL THINKING EXERCISE 45.3

There are many challenges facing nurses working in the area of rural and remote health (geographical isolation and environmental, sociological or cultural factors). These challenges often create barriers to care provision.

1. Discuss why the following factors are a challenge to individuals living in a rural or remote area.
   - Geographical isolation
   - Environment (population size)
   - Sociological issues (e.g. employment)
   - Cultural diversity
2. What individual nurse practice changes do you need to consider in care delivery and decision-making to be an effective nurse providing quality care in the rural or remote setting?
3. What communication strategies can be utilised with the inclusion of telehealth in assessing and planning for care in a rural setting?

REMOTE AREA AND RURAL NURSING

In any healthcare service in Australia, nurses make up the greatest number of health professionals in the workforce, and this is even more so in rural and remote areas. Nurses working in these areas must possess high-level clinical skills across a range of specialty areas (Berman et al 2020).

The healthcare team within a rural community is made up of different members including medical officers, nurses, allied health professionals (e.g. physiotherapists, dietitians and speech pathologists), a general practitioner or Royal Flying Doctor Service clinic doctor/nurse, community health and, within some communities, Aboriginal health workers and the increasing possibility of a Nurse Practitioner. Interestingly, not all members of the team will be located within a given local area. Some members of the team will be accessed via telehealth systems and sometimes via a visiting practitioner who periodically comes to town. This approach provides the benefits of holistic and culturally sensitive health services without the need for individuals to travel large distances.

The inclusion of Aboriginal health workers aims to achieve better health outcomes and better access to health services for Indigenous people. These quite distinctive healthcare providers communicate and plan care, often by telehealth or phone consultation, to achieve the optimal outcome for residents residing in rural and remote localities. The role of the Registered Nurse and Enrolled Nurse often comes with advanced practice opportunities to ensure that the people being cared for have access to services that are usually offered by other members of the healthcare team. For example, RNs within rural and remote areas may have prescribing rights for some medications and are able to perform cervical screening tests and, in some areas, X-rays. Advanced practice standing differs between the Registered Nurse and Enrolled Nurse; however, opportunities are offered that are not available within regional or metropolitan areas.

Remote area nursing

Nurses in remote areas are required to manage medical emergencies and trauma, usually with assistance via telephone or, in some instances, telehealth, from medical colleagues hundreds, or even thousands, of kilometres away. Nurses also need to be sensitive to the needs and cultural norms of the individuals they care for. Having knowledge and understanding of the customs and practices of the local culture requires a level of respect, understanding and preparation to ensure care is completed in a culturally respectful manner (Mackean et al 2020a). See Chapter 13 and Chapter 14 for further reading on cultural competence, safety and diversity, as well as Aboriginal and Torres Strait Islander health and principles of cultural safety respectively.

Remote area nurses provide the following care:

- age-appropriate wellness check-ups and healthcare
- detection and monitoring of chronic disease
- end-of-life care
- examination and diagnosis, and prescribing (in Australia only) and dispensing medications as part of routine practice
- follow-up nursing and medical care after transfer back to the local area from a regional or tertiary health facility
- community development and health promotion activities
- public health programs (e.g. screening and surveillance).

This care often occurs in a cross-cultural environment that operates with languages, knowledge and cultural systems different from those of the healthcare providers (Power et al 2018). An understanding of culture, context and space is needed in preparing non-Indigenous health professionals for work in a culturally respectful way to ensure that there is a positive contribution that addresses health disparities and prejudices (Power et al 2018).

Rural nursing

The lack of other healthcare professionals will determine the scope of practice of the rural nurse. In Australia, and internationally, rural nurses have a more generalist role as the population declines and nurses have to work with remotely located allied healthcare and medical practitioners. Rural nurses also require a broad range of skills and knowledge (Brown et al 2023). The team comprises RNs, ENs and Aboriginal health workers and Aboriginal health practitioners. Each member of the nursing team provides care within their level and scope of practice. For many years, nursing within rural and remote areas has been identified with a 'bush' nursing model of care. That is, a generalist yet expert role that has extended beyond nursing care realms of those working in larger centres, with inclusions of prescribing rights and extended assessment and treatment plans, to name a couple of areas.

Extensions now exist to these roles of nurses in rural and remote settings and the role of the Nurse Practitioner has evolved (Gum et al 2020; McCullough et al 2020). Often it is these services led by a nurse that now provide a greater ability within a health service to provide frontline care and referral within rural and remote communities. This positive inclusion within the workforce is not in all areas but, where evident, it is key to prompt and efficient care delivery, coordination, and referral without delays in service delivery (Gum et al 2020; McCullough et al 2020).

Characteristics of remote and rural nursing

The characteristics of remote area and rural nursing in Australia are usually not experienced in other nursing contexts (see Clinical Interest Box 45.9 for examples of rural and remote nursing characteristics).

The need for remote area and rural nurses to work at an advanced practice level increases as the size of the healthcare service decreases. Clinical Interest Box 45.10 outlines some of the activities that remote area and rural nurses undertake.

The professional support available to remote area and rural nurses is outlined in Clinical Interest Box 45.11.

EFFECTIVE HEALTHCARE SERVICE DELIVERY IN REMOTE SETTINGS

Effective healthcare service delivery in remote settings can involve working in teams and in partnership. Health professionals need to share problems and be prepared to resolve differences. The key to achieving successful partnerships is a willingness to consider and respect the perspectives and needs of others (Brown et al 2023).

CLINICAL INTEREST BOX 45.9 Characteristics of remote area and rural nursing

- Providing care to small, dispersed and highly mobile populations
- Delivering care when climatic extremes exist
- Providing care to populations with high morbidity and mortality
- Working in the context of a lack of social and human services infrastructure
- Working in isolation (whether geographical, social, professional and cultural)
- A strongly multidisciplinary approach with flexible professional boundaries, often with a horizontal style of management
- Advanced and collaborative practice utilising telehealth and digital health spaces
- Lack of boundaries between home and work
- On-call arrangements with small diverse working cultures
- High level of traumatic events
- Autonomy and flexibility
- Cross-cultural environment
- Frequently lacking formal preparation for the advanced and extended practice role
- Primary healthcare approach

(Battye et al 2019; Brown et al 2023; Badu et al 2020)

CLINICAL INTEREST BOX 45.10 Nursing activities for remote area and rural nurses

- Assessment, diagnosis and treatment of acute conditions
- Early detection and co-management of chronic disease
- Midwifery, postnatal, child health and growth and development monitoring of 0–5-year-olds
- Health promotion and community engagement activities (immunisation programs, outbreak control, depression, anxiety, and sexually transmitted infection control), environmental health and nutrition programs
- Collaborative medication management practices
- Management of acute trauma and medical emergencies
- Evacuating an individual via road, sea or air, telehealth practices and referrals

(Brown et al 2023; Calleja et al 2022; Whitehead & Quinn 2019)

CLINICAL INTEREST BOX 45.11 Professional support for remote area and rural nurses

In Australia, the following organisations support remote area and rural nurses:

- CRANAplus is the professional organisation representing health professionals of all disciplines who work in rural and remote areas: <https://crana.org.au>.
- The Rural Nursing and Midwifery Faculty of the Royal College of Nursing Australia provides professional support for rural nurses: <https://www.acn.edu.au/membership/faculty/rural-remote-nursing>.
- The National Rural Health Alliance represents 51 national organisations working to improve the health and wellbeing of people in rural and remote Australia: <https://www.ruralhealth.org.au>.

(Brown et al 2023)

Working in health teams and partnerships in rural and remote contexts

Successful teamwork is an essential ingredient for providing an effective health service in rural and remote contexts. Proficient teamwork can also enhance satisfaction, productivity and survival, whereas dysfunctional teams compound the considerable challenges that already exist for rural and remote health professionals and the consumers of the service. (See Case Study 45.2.)

There are many leadership styles, and a number are seen in healthcare. Historically, nursing has seen autocratic leadership or a 'top-down' style of leadership, with tasks and skills delegated as deemed relevant. Stanley and Stanley (2019) explored the notion that leadership is a critical role for all health professionals in the rural and remote context. It is the effect of leadership that will determine an organisation's ability to change and learn, and it is the organisation's willingness that will promote or inhibit change. This creates challenges for nurses since they have to balance their leadership role between resolving immediate and conflicting clinical pressures, as well as continuing to make progress in staff development and the identification and implementation of the latest evidence within their nursing practice. Through development and promotion of clinical nursing leaders for the future, rural facilities can aim to achieve the goal of providing quality nursing care within supportive work environments that use evidence to guide their nursing practice.

Successful leadership in healthcare is greater than defining and engaging a specific leadership style. Through research conducted by Stanley (2009), a model of congruent leadership was developed. Stanley (2009, p. 19) affirmed that it is congruent leadership that 'responds to challenges and critical problems with actions and activities in accordance with staff values and belief'. The elements of clinical leadership identified by Stanley (2009) remain today. Giles et al (2018) explored the notion of clinical leadership and the ability of the nurse to work across organisations and disciplines, with the nurse seen as the central authority in care collaboration. The nurse leader in the rural or remote setting has a powerful impact on change in clinical practice with greater autonomy in practice and the capacity for decision-making. According to Stanley and Stanley (2019), nurse leaders are seen as the catalyst for change: the professional with the inherent link with community, caring and with the ability to be the decision-maker, communicator and negotiator in care and care decision-making.

Features of remote health teams

Rural and remote health teams have a number of features, some of which they share with teams in urban areas and some that are unique to the rural and remote context. Generally, they operate in areas of high morbidity and mortality (and hence have a greater health need); in extreme isolation; in harsh environments; and often in cross-cultural contexts including the city/bush cultural divide, with a highly transitory, cross-discipline membership. These factors provide not only the greatest challenges but also the greatest potential accomplishments of teams in rural and remote areas. The experience of operating effectively as a team member enhances interpersonal skills, problem-solving capacity, conflict management skills and mutual support. It is common for rural and remote team members to become long-term friends. The intense teamwork experience creates friendship and support that can extend into the future.

Working within a rural and remote health setting can be rewarding and provide opportunities that cannot be experienced in any other setting. However, it is the reward that encourages staff to continue to work in these settings, the satisfaction that all that could be done has been done. It is the sense of belonging and the sense of community that holds nurses in high regard in these settings. As an example of how one nurse describes it, see the Lived Experience box here.

LIVED EXPERIENCE

I completed a clinical placement at this hospital. Towards the end of my diploma, I applied for a graduate program in the rural health setting. I started work here about 9 months ago. I've never lived in a rural area but now I love it. I was scared when I first started since the whole nursing team was so much smaller with a lot more responsibility. This has been a rewarding experience. Each day I learn new things and each day I am able to help people in my new local community. There is such a strong spirit in the town, even though the drought has meant many people and their businesses are struggling. I can see myself working here for a long time.

Jessie, Enrolled Nurse

CASE STUDY 45.2

Working in teams is complex and multifaceted, irrespective of the clinical setting. Teamwork requires all members of the team to listen, participate and respond to each other in amicable ways. In nursing, teamwork also requires a 'hands on' assistance approach to achieving individualised care in timely and efficient ways.

Below, a remote area nurse describes how the health centre staff were having some communication problems and needed to look at new ways of building their team in a more positive way. A new assistant director of nursing position was being advertised and it was hoped that this role would assist the team to improve the following team concerns. This is how the team did not work:

- We had an old-fashioned, vertical structure. The doctor was above the nurse, the nurse was above the Aboriginal health worker (AHW) and we were all above the community and anybody from outside the community. There was division along professional, gender, cultural and experience lines. So each of us needed to 'divide to rule' or to at least have a say. This was a very unhappy team ...
- The team did not build a sense of community. The health centre was not then a community health place; it was a 'sickness' place—the place of last resort. Things looked efficient; everyone knew their place (like it or not). The trains ran on time; the problem was there was no-one on the train, only the drivers, and the community got nowhere.
- This situation manifested in late presentations. Families and individuals delayed at home ill, so the children came very late, often when they were too sick to treat locally. The traditional healer would not come near the health centre since they clearly felt uncomfortable and culturally unsafe.

A successful appointment was made to the team and a new nurse took charge of the team and negotiated a change of focus and leadership style. This led to the following experiences:

- The nurses and AHWs together with the visiting doctor worked collaboratively and developed a plan to manage children who did not appear to be growing well. Mothers with sick children would come to the health centre a lot. The children presented as very weak and undernourished, usually with an associated infection. The nurse and the AHW would examine the child, undertake the relevant investigations for the presentation and, if necessary, refer to the doctor for further review, examination and tests. This is where the senior clinician would take the lead.
- Sometimes the child would be referred back since the main issue seemed that there were problems with access to food. Questions would be asked as to why: was it an issue of money, understanding or home situation? This was where the AHWs would take the lead. Together, the health staff would visit the home and talk to the family but the AHWs took the lead on this. 'First to speak, first to walk into the home.'
- Sometimes the numbers of children would get too big for the team to manage effectively. Too many children were malnourished or were not adequately recuperating after an acute illness. So the health staff took the information to the community. The community leaders started looking at funding programs for child feeding and maternal education. Then they looked at the community and family issues that were directly impacting on the health and wellbeing of the kids and used the state of the children as a springboard for a range of actions. This is where the community took the lead.

1. How would you describe this leadership change in focus for the healthcare team?
2. What benefits does the shift in leadership have for a nurse working in the setting?
3. What benefits do the shift in leadership and resultant outcomes have for the individual using the health service?

Multidisciplinary team

Rural and remote health teams are multidisciplinary, involving Aboriginal health workers and practitioners, doctors, nurses, community welfare and allied and other professional groups, as well as administrative and management staff. They require each member to have specific areas of expertise as well as advanced generalist skills and the capacity to support and complement each other. The inclusion of the Aboriginal health worker seeks to provide the key link between culture, the people and their health.

It is through a combined team approach that care is coordinated and provided to those in need or to those who require primary health strategies within the community setting. Nurses provide the dominant service within rural and remote communities from both a preventative and an illness or injury management perspective. This often overlaps with roles and responsibilities of other members of the healthcare team; however, it is unavoidable due to the nature of the work. This is commonly a source of conflict in those teams whose members originate from traditional practice backgrounds of urban hospitals and private practice and are more familiar and comfortable with the models of clear boundaries between professional roles, responsibilities and authority.

From a positive perspective, multidisciplinary teams with overlapping roles reduce professional barriers and barriers between individuals and increase the team's capacity to deal effectively with the greater demands of the service, while utilising individual expertise appropriately.

Teamwork is highly valued within the rural and remote health context (Khan et al 2023; Stanley & Stanley 2019). As in so many other areas of rural and remote practice, there is a huge learning curve (and unlearning in terms of past hierarchical team processes) to come to grips with. In summary, teamwork is about constant adaptation and change: adaptation to new members and rapidly changing circumstances as well as health systems. In the vortex of external change, the team needs to be a haven of support for the individual health professional, a motivator through shared visions of the future, a creator of learning opportunities and be a way to realistically test expectations.

LIVED EXPERIENCE

I've worked in the rural setting for the last 5 years. Prior to this job I worked for 3 years in a metropolitan hospital in a medical unit. I started here as a novice EN as my previous experience only partially prepared me for the challenges of rural nursing. The team I work with have embraced me and I have learnt so much on the job. I've learnt that each day is something different, my practice is more autonomous than previous positions and, mostly, the community I now live and work in embrace me. I have the best of both worlds—my personal community involvement and my professional work and the love of learning new things.

Andrea, Registered Nurse, rural practice

STRESS RELATED TO WORKING IN A REMOTE HEALTH CONTEXT

Stress reactions can be described as a process of adaptation, a concept that can apply to stress associated with rural and remote practice. When health professionals begin work in a situation they have not worked in before, a period of adjustment is expected. The adjustment process will give rise to varying levels of stress (i.e. psychological 'strain'). This will persist until the health practitioner gains a level of mastery (i.e. become comfortable and effective) in their new environment.

High turnover of staff in rural and remote areas prevents the development of an experienced workforce whose members have completed their adaptation process and become effective health professionals (Bailey et al 2020). This means that the bulk of the rural and remote workforce is at the beginning of their learning curve. Collective memory of what has gone on before, what works and what does not work tends to be short, resulting in the same mistakes being made repeatedly. It is difficult to establish or maintain efficient and effective remote health services when health professionals are constantly being replaced (Naden et al 2023).

What is stressful about remote practice?

Stress is an issue that impacts on all health professionals, regardless of where they work, whether in towns, cities or the bush.

Commonly accepted sources of stress in rural and remote work environments can be:

- the job (e.g. workload [too much or too little], role ambiguity, lack of control and conflict)
- the organisation, for example, working conditions, lack of recognition and support and unsuitable staffing levels
- organisational change, changes to procedures, new technologies and expectations of transfer or retrenchment
- violence and other traumatic events in the workplace.

While stressors in the rural and remote work environment, such as fire, flood, pestilence and commodity price falls are easy to recognise, many of the causes of stress may not be so obvious. The interactions between these concepts are illustrated in Figure 45.3. Health professionals may be stressed by uncertainty about their roles, by the responsibilities they carry, by their workload, by the way their working lives are organised, by the content of their jobs or by the network of interpersonal relationships that characterise their day-to-day existence.

Lack of anonymity and personal privacy

Life in small remote communities is sometimes described as 'living in a fishbowl'; that is, all areas of the remote health professional's life may come under scrutiny and provoke comment from local residents, not just about their professional abilities.

Many people value the interconnectedness of small communities, particularly if there is a community culture of helping each other out in hard times. Many would suggest that urban dwellers miss out on this sense of community (e.g. many urban dwellers might not even know their neighbours).

However, like most things in remote areas, knowing everybody and everyone knowing the nurse is a two-edged sword. In some situations, it is considered beneficial (a 'blessing'). In others, it may be considered detrimental (a 'curse'). A familiarity with a healthcare professional can be seen as a conflict of interest in the rural healthcare setting but it can also provide a sense of comfort and relief.

Lack of anonymity of health professionals and individuals (and their families) in small communities may raise issues about confidentiality. For example, a common rule of thumb in terms of maintaining confidentiality has been that workers may talk about work-related issues with others (e.g. colleagues or partner), but only if they can do so in a way that does not identify those involved. This is hard to achieve in small communities when most people know most of what goes on and may know the people involved.

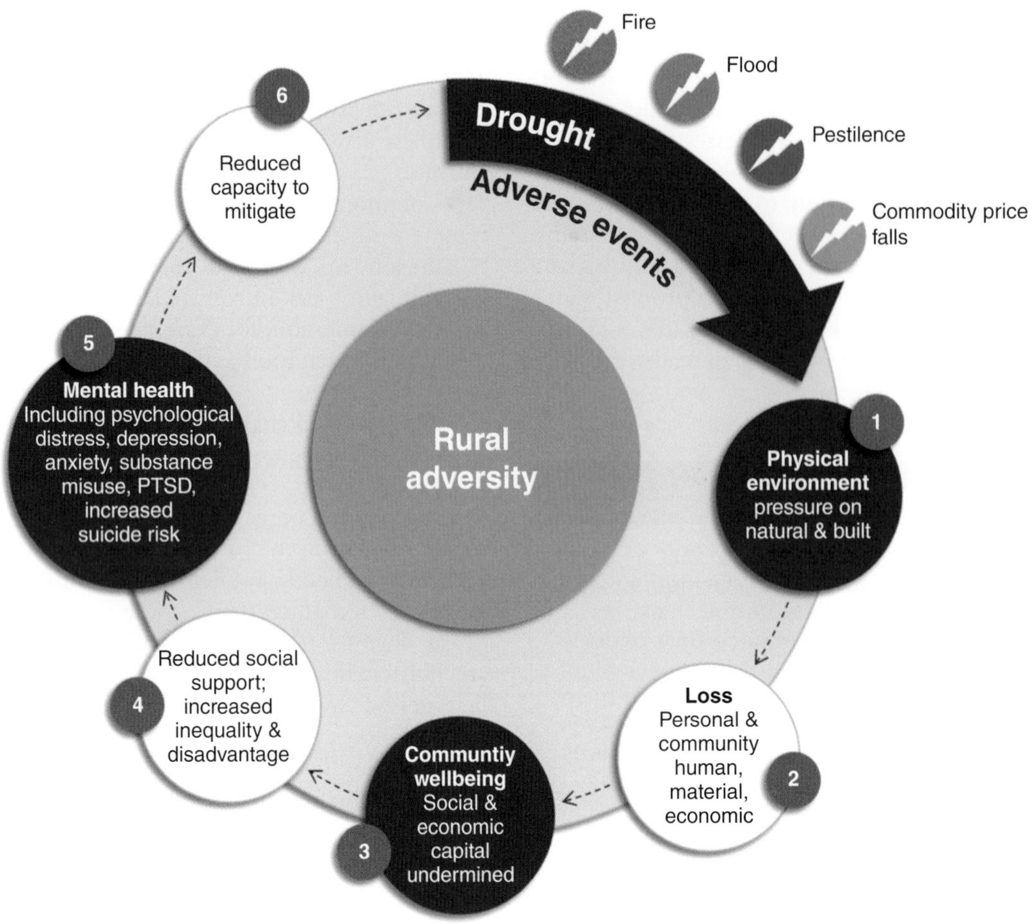

Figure 45.3 A dynamic conceptual model of rural adversity showing the impact of adverse events on the environment, community wellbeing and individual mental health
(Adapted from Hart et al 2011)

Opportunities for health professionals to talk about their work with others or to safely express any anger or frustration may be restricted as a result. Yet, the need to talk over work-related issues is recognised as an important part of debriefing following a stressful day.

Lack of anonymity of health professionals and individuals may also pose ethical challenges. For example, health professionals are generally discouraged from providing health services to friends and family. Ethical guidelines for professional practice have been developed to suit urban health professionals, who usually deal with individuals who are strangers to them. While practising in small community settings, nurses may find themselves in breach of the ethical guidelines set down by their professional body.

Lack of anonymity also impacts on the health professional's ability to maintain privacy and personal space (Swan & Hobbs 2021). In some instances, on-site health professionals may be seen as a community resource, with the expectation that they will be there to meet the health needs of the community at any time of the day or night. On-site health professionals may be accessed by health service consumers wherever they are in the community, regardless of what they are doing, such as shopping or socialising.

This might be a negative or positive experience, depending on whether the health professional finds this level of trust and responsibility to be enriching or whether they see it as an intrusion.

LIVED EXPERIENCE

As a local locum to the area, it is difficult as a doctor. I don't know the community or the range of health conditions that they present with. Each of the staff I work with already has a rapport and knows the conditions that many of the people come to see me with. It's been good to get to know people, although a little tough learning about each person. Each day there is a new challenge, with new patients and many who seem to know a lot about me, [more] than I know about them. My position is for 3 months, and it's only been 1 month so far.

John, General Practitioner

If you have grown up in a small community, this may not seem a big issue to you. If you are not accustomed to these levels of connectedness and visibility, then a period of adjustment will be necessary before a level of comfort is achieved. It is about being comfortable with being uncomfortable in new surroundings and with new challenges.

Lack of boundaries between work and home

The division between the nurse as a person and the nurse as the health professional tends to be less clear-cut in small rural and remote communities. This is partly due to the lack of natural circuit breakers between work and home, and between the personal and professional boundaries.

City workers and health professionals who provide visiting health services can do their job and then leave their professional role behind and return home to personal lives relatively unconnected to their work. They may have a choice of recreational activities to participate in, and access to a range of other people, friends and acquaintances that are not connected to their workplace. This allows some downtime to relax following work demands.

In small and remote communities, work and home life are less easily differentiated. Home may be just a stroll away from work or may be in living quarters in the hospital grounds. If the health professional is on call, their movements may be restricted. Rural and remote communities tend not to offer the same range of recreational activities available in town. In addition, friends and acquaintances tend to be drawn from contacts made in the workplace. Areas of common interest may be work-related.

For health professionals who live on-site in the remote community, the lack of boundaries between work and home may become particularly apparent when they are required to be on call. Their home becomes part of the workplace; people knock on their door to request assistance.

In such contexts, it may be difficult for remote health professionals to find time and personal space to just be themselves and to escape from their professional roles. This can impact on their ability to achieve rest time and to express parts of themselves not related to their work.

Housing issues

The difficulties in establishing personal boundaries sometimes extend to the health professional's living space. Housing issues in rural and remote areas traditionally have been longstanding sources of conflict and stress for many health professionals. While health professionals recruited from outside the community may be provided with accommodation, local people (e.g. health workers) may not have accommodation provided (yet they may share the same issues of inadequate and overcrowded housing as others in Indigenous communities).

In some instances, the lack of guest accommodation in remote communities (e.g. motels or guesthouses) means that there may be an expectation that health professionals will provide accommodation for other health professionals and others that visit the community.

Some health professionals are required to leave the remote community to access annual or other leave so that the relieving/locum health professional can use their accommodation.

Unrelenting demands

Health professionals who have grown up in the community may find the demands on them from friends, families and health service individuals to be unrelenting.

LIVED EXPERIENCE

I work in a multidisciplinary health service within an Indigenous community. I'm a single parent and live with my four children just out of town and work 4 days a week within the service. Many of the individuals in the community are family to me and this makes it difficult when I see the decisions they make that then leads to complications to their renal function and diabetes management. Sometimes it is hard to differentiate between nurse and family member; it tears me apart.

Deb, Enrolled Nurse, Indigenous health

The unrelenting nature of remote work is a particular issue for on-site health professionals who may be required to be on call frequently. Sole health professionals may be on call 24 hours a day, 7 days a week.

LIVED EXPERIENCE

Sue received a call alerting her to a vehicle rollover out of town. The ambulance was sent and staff began preparing the clinic's rooms awaiting the arrival of the injured. A man arrived and said, 'No, it's nothing, it was just me', and he had a broken hand. Sue relaxed a bit. About half an hour later noise was heard outside, and 17 further people presented—they were all in the vehicle rollover. The event required the whole nursing team, a 24-hour shift, and six people evacuated.

Keast 2014, p. 19

Sleep deprivation may become an issue at times for the remote worker health practitioner. Even losing a single night's sleep can impair performance. Both short-term and long-term memory are affected after a night without sleep, and performance is slower (Fietze et al 2022). Without enough sleep, individuals can have problems paying attention, and they can miss information due to lapses in attention (Fietze et al 2022). People deprived of sleep also tend to be more irritable than usual.

Cultural adaptation

All rural and remote communities have their own culture, whether agricultural, fishing, Indigenous, mining, railway or tourist. Being familiar with the culture and the demand that this makes on being able to successfully work and reside in an area requires attention, discretion and understanding. Working within, and with, cultures and building community trust are inherent features within the *Code of Conduct for Nurses* (Nursing and Midwifery Board of Australia [NMBA] 2018a).

Culture shock can be a significant issue confronting healthcare workers in any healthcare setting, but more so in the rural and remote space. Non-Indigenous healthcare professionals working within Indigenous communities are of particular interest since culture shock is not just about the healthcare worker and adjustments to the culture, but also the adjustment of the people in the area to a new worker from perhaps a differing background, culture or ethnicity (Battye et al 2019). In transitioning into a setting, priority needs to be given to gaining an understanding of the community expectations, the practices and ideologies of the community; introducing yourself and attending appropriate social events to engage in local heritage; listening to the local conversations; working with staff with experience in the area; and sharing your experience and knowledge where it is deemed appropriate.

Indigenous communities

The greater the difference between the health professional's cultural background and the community's culture(s), the greater the adaptation required before they master the new environment sufficiently to become effective and competent. This is particularly apparent for non-Indigenous health professionals recruited to work in remote Indigenous communities (Battye et al 2019; Best & Fredericks 2022). Adjustment (and readjustment) is likely to occur when a health professional begins work in a remote area for the first time. For example, when a local from the remote community begins work within the bureaucratic environment of the health department, when a health professional moves from one remote community to another or during periods of organisational change.

LIVED EXPERIENCE

I have chosen to work in a rural setting ... I came here after graduation and am now part of the community 5 years on. At first the adjustment was hard; often you are on your own, you need to be able to adapt, think on your feet and when you finish work engage in the community while maintaining high levels of confidentiality. This is a special privilege and an isolating one at the same time.

Joanne, Registered Nurse, isolated practice, 2019

Some health professionals feel they must exchange their own cultural values for the cultural values of the remote community they are living or working in. This is not so, nor is it necessarily desirable. Living one's own life according to one's own cultural values helps to maintain a sense of security, meaning and identity. However, this concept applies to individuals accessing health services as well as health professionals.

The emphasis on the remote health professional to develop sufficient understanding of the culture(s) of the remote community and the impact of their own behaviours is vital to ensure effective and culturally safe work practice within the cultural context(s) of a particular community. Living and/or working in a culture other than your own can be a disorienting experience. Some speak of experiencing 'culture shock' while adjusting to living and working in a culture other than their own.

As health professionals learn new knowledge, skills and attitudes and adapt to the remote community over time, it is almost inevitable that they will be changed in some ways. It can be disconcerting for some health professionals working in rural or remote environments to find that a period of re-adaptation is required upon returning to the city or 'mainstream' nursing environments. Many report feeling uncomfortable and out of place for a while until they re-adapt to their own culture and the non-remote setting.

Issues of isolation

Isolation in remote communities can occur at several levels: geographical, professional and cultural. **Geographical isolation** is something that cannot usually be changed and is by definition part of remote health work (Swan & Hobbs 2021). For those who grew up in the remote community, it may not necessarily be seen as unusual or a hardship.

A sense of isolation may be relative. A person's sense of geographical isolation may be reduced by roads being upgraded, frequency of air services, owning their own vehicle, networking with outside organisations, or maintaining contact with others, both inside and outside the community.

For community members, the need for accurate and timely healthcare is important. The need for preventative health information is also important. How to balance and manage the needs of individuals within communities can be assisted with the inclusion of information sourced and accessed via the internet or telephone. It is these services that can be updated and managed remotely that can assist communities to gather information to prevent health concerns or to assist in their management. It is also a key link to understanding a diagnosis or treatment plan. Healthdirect Australia is one of the services available via the internet, or via a phone app. Healthdirect Australia offers the community within Australia resources in relation to symptoms, conditions, medications and treatments with an 1800 telephone number for health-related questions or advice. The service also offers information and guidance to healthcare professionals working in areas of isolation or rurality. Through the use of the internet or smartphone applications, access to this service has become easier; however, there are still barriers within levels of literacy or the lack of suitable phone or internet coverage.

Healthdirect Australia is also a source of information for nurses working in the remote setting and is an ideal way of sharing reliable and evidence-based information with the community. Often, working alone, without colleagues to consult or discuss clinical and other issues with, can increase the stress associated with many situations. Some remote health professionals may feel isolated within their own professions. Remote workers are not only minorities within the population, but also within their own professions. Urban health professionals may have different agendas and issues of concern.

A sense of professional isolation can be reduced by, for example, joining and participating in professional bodies that contain remote health professionals, networking with other remote health professionals, subscribing to professional journals or undertaking further study. If the health professional has not grown up in the cultural context of a particular community—be it mining, tourism, railway or Indigenous—then a sense of isolation may arise, particularly until they learn enough to feel comfortable or become competent within that particular cultural context. This is commonly cited as a barrier to recruitment and retention of remote health professionals (Liu et al 2023). Certainly, for new graduates or those new to remote area work practice, it may be difficult to access ongoing supervision and mentoring, which is necessary as the healthcare professional adjusts to their new role.

A sense of cultural isolation can arise as a consequence of being a member of a minority culture within a larger cultural group. This can be felt not only when recruited from outside the community, but also when working in an organisational setting that has different values to the health professional, cultural or otherwise. A sense of cultural isolation may be reduced, and a sense of security and identity maintained, by keeping links with the health professional's own culture, particularly during the early stages of cultural adaptation.

CRITICAL THINKING EXERCISE 45.4

Take a piece of paper. List the positive aspects of working in a remote context on one side of the page and list the negative aspects of working in a remote context on the other side. How many factors appear on both lists? That is, do the 'blessings' (benefits) of remote practice also contain the potential to become 'curses' (detriments)? Do the positives outweigh the negatives?

Trauma and violence

Traumatic events are those in which the individual experiences some form of threat to their own or others' lives or are exposed to the threat of, or actual death of, others, particularly under violent, shocking or horrific circumstances, and may also involve exposure to gruesome images. During or after the event the individual may feel an overwhelming sense of horror, terror or helplessness.

Individuals who are exposed to such events may experience a characteristic set of psychological and behavioural reactions that have their roots in the human stress response. Considering the great diversity of human nature and cultures, the uniformity of the experience of traumatic stress reactions is remarkable and suggests a biological basis to the reaction pattern, and also that the reaction pattern is a form of adaptation which has survival value.

As in day-to-day stress, a traumatic event is a combination of the actual event, which contains the potential to traumatise, whether the health professional perceives the event to be personally traumatic and the health professional's reactions during and after the event. The experience of traumatic stress is an essentially human and normal response to extremely stressful situations.

Violence against health professionals is not uncommon in remote areas (Topp et al 2022). The effects of social tensions and violence in the remote community can also impact on the workplace. The emotional aftermath, although a normal reaction following such events, can be a difficult and challenging experience. While early intervention strategies, such as psychological support and debriefing, aim to prevent long-term psychological harm from occurring, some health professionals may become overwhelmed by their experience and go on to develop post-traumatic stress disorder.

While employers have a duty of care to prevent traumatic events where possible, and to support workers in their recovery, it is also important that health professionals accept responsibility for their own role in maximising their recovery following such events.

Living and working within a rural or remote setting can be difficult, particularly when traumatic events occur. The role of healthcare worker can involve being a provider, community support and personal involvement. The importance of identifying personal boundaries and the maintenance of an individual's scope of practice and ethical conduct is complex (Badu et al 2020). The support that a nurse requires during these times is also complex (e.g. deciding who to talk with when the involvement is widespread in the community). Such is often the case when a major road trauma or suicide occurs within the community resulting in the 'loss of a local'. Support for nurses and the awareness of ethical and legislative boundaries are vital; however, these are often limited in the rural and remote space (NMBA 2018b).

The key importance in dealing with traumatic events is the post-event debrief that should be conducted within the healthcare team at a time and place suitable to participants. Boundaries should be established and the ability to grieve, converse and gain a sense of closure should be established for individuals participating. Often this is a complex process given the professional and personal boundary blur. The *Code of Conduct for Nurses* in Australia sets out the legal requirements, professional behaviour and conduct expectations for all nurses, in all practice settings, in Australia (NMBA 2018a).

CRITICAL THINKING EXERCISE 45.5

What are your views on being accessible after hours—for example, while shopping or at a community social event? What are your personal guidelines regarding what you see as acceptable and not acceptable in relation to this issue?

ACCESS TO HEALTH SERVICES IN RURAL AND REMOTE AREAS

Telehealth

One of many strategies currently being used to deliver healthcare services to rural and remote communities is telehealth. Telehealth is defined by the World Health Organization (WHO) as 'the use of information communication technology applications to provide health and long-term care services over a distance' (Berman et al 2020). There have been many reported examples of ongoing use of telehealth in Australia and clinical reports of positive results for people suffering from ongoing effects of acute illness and chronic illness and for their carers and rural and remote health service providers. It is anticipated that improved communications through teleconference and videoconference facilities will be the basis of strategies to ensure equitable access to healthcare and form the framework for future healthcare provision in rural and remote Australia (Berman et al 2020).

Telehealth is being extended into rural Australia as the use of digital infrastructure improves. There are many advantages for the nurse working in a rural or remote facility; for example, nurses can communicate with experts in trauma centres in relation to individual care situations as they present rather than managing a person based on the team's knowledge or limited prior exposure. This provides a sense of security for healthcare teams in rural and remote areas and also provides the best possible approach to timely, lifesaving or immediate advice from a specialist consultant from a tertiary setting.

Telemedicine refers to the practice of a medical consultant having communication, consultation and the provision of advice or care planning and medical intervention in a setting outside the area usually within rural or remote facilities (Hand 2022).

The challenges that present within a rural setting are often complex and require a nurse to manage the situation until medical assistance arrives. As a nurse working in a rural setting, it is important that the provision of care for a person and their carer is completed in partnership. Decision-making processes, the model of care used in the setting and the delegation and responsibility of all staff within their scope of practice are vital to positive outcomes (Stanley & Stanley 2019). Individuals using health services should participate in making decisions about their own healthcare.

In the provision of care, consideration needs to be given to the individual roles of the healthcare team and the required resources of each health service organisation. The National Safety and Quality Health Service Standards identify key processes to ensure that there is early recognition of the deteriorating person and prompt and effective management of individuals in these circumstances (Australian Commission on Safety and Quality in Health Care 2021). Time is a critical factor in managing a deteriorating individual and, for nurses in rural and remote health areas, the access to more specialised services can sometimes be complex. This is where telehealth can prove very advantageous to the healthcare team.

Telehealth and telemedicine have been used in Australia as a means of reducing inequity in access to healthcare, addressing health professional shortages, and augmenting other service delivery models in rural and remote areas (Perimal-Lewis et al 2021). Telehealth, however, does not encompass the same holistic experience that face-to-face consultations provide; therefore, in order to enhance the virtual care approach, the need for supportive adjunct services, connections to local community services, and service provision expansion is essential (Mathew et al 2023). Consideration of these factors has been linked to the long-term improvement of clinical care models, patient experience, medical costs, and patient safety. In addition, the effective use of existing technologies with integration and blending of innovative technologies, may serve to enhance the virtual care environment and improve the patient experience. Future developments need to consider technology integration, care models, workflow, workforce skills, funding models, policy, standards, guidance, safety and quality, standards of care, patient engagement, continuity of care, privacy and security (Calleja et al 2022; Perimal-Lewis et al 2021). The interactions between these concepts in virtual care are illustrated in Figure 45.4.

Transferring to regional or metropolitan health services

At times, people in rural and remote areas are required to travel to a regional or metropolitan specialist health centre. This process can often be a source of great anxiety and stress for the person, their family and community. As a nurse working in urban, regional, rural or remote communities, it is important to have an understanding of the issues relating to transfer for treatment (Berman et al 2020).

The Royal Flying Doctor Service (RFDS) supports residents in rural and remote communities requiring access to high-level care. In one day in Australia, the RFDS flies more than 65,000 km and performs more than 100 medical evacuations, and over 85,000 consultations are conducted each year. The RFDS provides more than emergency retrieval and transfer services; it plays a key role in the provision of telehealth, health prevention and screening programs and general practice clinics run in isolated areas on a regular basis (Berman et al 2020).

Angel Flight is a charity service that provides flights for non-urgent travel to and from medical appointments. The staff and pilots are volunteers, and the service relies on

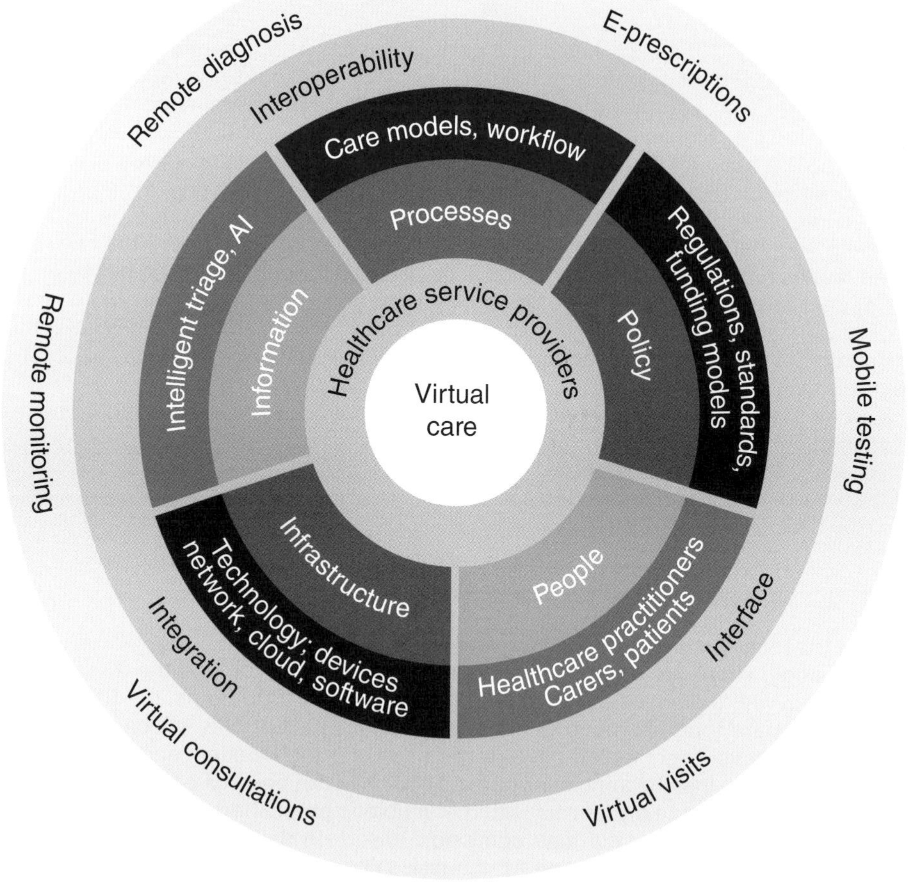

Figure 45.4 The construction of virtual care and its components *(Perimal-Lewis et al 2021)*

fundraising to exist. A referral must be completed and submitted to Angel Flight up to 2 weeks before the required travel, depending on the location. This can be completed by a nurse, doctor, or allied health professional. This service is not for individuals with acute care needs as no medical assistance is provided onboard the plane but is for people needing to attend medical appointments.

For community members in a rural or remote location within Australia there exists in each state a transport system of support. The level of support is both physically and financially driven for those needing medical care outside their local community. The patient-assisted travel schemes (PATS) provide a subsidy to help with travel, escort and accommodation expenses incurred by those living within a rural or remote area. The scheme is available to individuals who need to travel to medical appointments or hospitals more than 100 km from where they live. As a nurse, it is important to communicate with individuals about the scheme and how to apply for assistance during times when medical referral away from home is needed.

Links to these schemes are available within the list of Online Resources at the end of this chapter.

When someone in your care is being transferred to another healthcare service and requires retrieval services take the following into consideration: Does the person have anyone to travel with them, or meet them at the destination? How will they get to their destination? What is the anticipated length of stay? Whether they require accommodation for support person and/or themselves? Do arrangements need to be made for their home, work or family? Do they have necessary items such as a small amount of money, toiletries and a change of clothes, contact details or identification documents? And whether there are any weight requirements or size restrictions of the transfer vehicle (Berman 2020). Case Study 45.3 asks you to consider support mechanisms that could be provided in the rural and remote setting.

CRITICAL THINKING EXERCISE 45.6

Consider the community health nurse competencies described in this chapter. Which of the competencies would be within the scope of practice of the Enrolled Nurse?

CASE STUDY 45.3

You have applied and successfully been appointed to a position within a rural hospital located 1100 km west of where you currently live. You have visited the town only once before and do not know anyone except the director of nursing (DON) and one staff member who you met at the interview. Your first shift commences, and you start to introduce yourself to the other staff and the people that you will be caring for. A woman arrives at the front counter and asks how her husband is today. You ask her who he is and she responds with, 'Why don't you know and who are you anyway?'

1. What is your response?

Later in the evening you notice the same woman crying as she makes herself a cup of tea. You go to see if she is okay. She responds by telling you that their farm is not doing so well; the drought has meant they have had to sell a large number of cattle and feed is running low for those animals that remain. She tells you she has been hiding the severity of the feed issue from her husband since he is so unwell. By now, you know that her husband is 60 years old with a recent diagnosis of bowel cancer, who has been transferred back to the local hospital from a long stay for surgery, radiotherapy and chemotherapy in a tertiary facility. He remains in hospital because he is still receiving treatment for an infection within his bowel.

2. How do you respond to this woman and what support mechanisms can you see that could be provided in the rural and remote setting?

DECISION-MAKING FRAMEWORK EXERCISE 45.2

It is an evening shift at the local hospital, and you are working with a Registered Nurse (RN) who is busy in the office area with an upcoming audit. There are a total of 11 inpatients allocated to you and the RN. One of these inpatients was admitted 24 hours ago with a diagnosis of urinary tract infection. At 1800 hours, the RN asks you to complete a set of observations and prepare the next round of antibiotics for this patient (this will be the fifth dose) and she will be with you in a minute. You have just completed the observations for the inpatient and notice that this person has a temperature of 38.6°C. You notice that the antibiotics due at 1400 have not been given. You have only just finished your medication endorsement and are not really familiar with the antibiotic prescribed.

Complete the following care plan for the new admission based on the following information: According to the admission notes, the care plan requires completing for the late shift. You notice that Mrs Jones is wearing her nightie inside-out and she appears pale and quiet. When you enquire how her day has been, she says she is waiting to go home.

1. What key assessments must be considered in Mrs Jones's care for the evening? Complete the table below.

<table>
<tr><td colspan="2">Assessment:
Issue/s to be addressed:
Goal/s:</td></tr>
<tr><td>Care/actions:</td><td>Rationale:</td></tr>
<tr><td colspan="2">Evaluation:</td></tr>
</table>

A number of questions arise for you to consider:

2. What handover do you provide the RN to alert them of the clinical situation evolving?
3. What is your responsibility in relation to the clinical error that has been identified with the omission of a medication at 1400 hours?
4. Within the scope of the EN, what are the supervision requirements relating to the administration of IV antibiotics?

DECISION-MAKING FRAMEWORK EXERCISE 45.3

You are working with a Registered Nurse (RN) in the emergency area of a rural health facility. The staffing in the area is yourself as Enrolled Nurse (EN) and the RN; the ward area attached to the emergency area has an RN and EN working alongside a ward assistant. The morning has been extremely busy, and you are aware that the RN is with an acutely unwell person in the resuscitation bay. A local resident arrives at the triage desk and informs you they have cut themselves with a machete knife while harvesting broccoli. Their arm is currently wrapped in a towel; however, there

DECISION-MAKING FRAMEWORK EXERCISE 45.3—cont'd

are traces of blood evident on the towel. You take the person's details and move them to a cubicle where they can be seen and let the RN know what has occurred. The RN tells you to deal with the situation, assess the wound and let her know what needs to happen.

1. Do you assess the person's arm?
2. What strategies can you use within the EN scope of practice in caring for this person?
3. Considering the staff in the whole facility at the time of this presentation, what other strategies could you utilise?
4. How would you effectively discuss these strategies with the RN and maintain harmony within the team?
5. What assessments could you undertake to communicate to the RN the need for an assessment by them?

Summary

There has been an increased focus on preventative care and wellbeing promotion in recent years. Primary healthcare and community care is increasingly helping individuals transition from acute services to care and enabling services in the community. The philosophy of public healthcare and the practice of primary healthcare underpin the delivery of community health services in Australia. Integral to this service are the roles of remote area and rural nurses, including the recognition that these nurses require a high level of knowledge and clinical skills. Additionally, the acknowledgment that advances in technology may have a substantial future impact on the ability of Australians living in remote and rural areas to receive healthcare in their home communities with a reduced need to travel for specialist or follow-up support services is essential. These factors have the ability to empower communities to become healthy, while addressing the non-traditional determinants of health such as social and economic factors. Primary health and community nurses have particular competencies and skills that are now being formally recognised. Nurses providing care in community settings, and in particular home care, have specific issues, which impact on their practice. The nursing process informs care delivery along with applying critical thinking strategies and decision-making tools to assist to manage risks and resolve problems.

In this chapter, a broad comparison of the health status and needs of urban, rural and remote communities was provided, and some of the features of remote environments were outlined. The key infrastructures for effective healthcare service delivery in rural and remote settings in general were examined, and potential sources of stress related to working in a remote health context were discussed. Several case studies illustrating particular aspects of community-based, rural and remote healthcare were provided.

Review Questions

1. What is meant by a social view of health?
2. What are the philosophical values of public health?
3. What influence does public health aim to have on the Australian healthcare system?
4. What are some of the key benefits of primary healthcare?
5. List some models of care used in community health.
6. Define community health nurse as an occupation.
7. What are some of the issues community nurses face in home care?
8. Describe 'cultural safety'.
9. What are the steps in the nursing process?
10. What indicators would you use to define remoteness? Think about these in order of priority for you as a health professional working in a remote location.
11. List four to six key features of rural or remote healthcare environments in Australia.
12. What are the key factors and processes that have led to poorer health service delivery in rural and remote areas than in urban areas?
13. List the common characteristics of rural and remote nursing.
14. What are the key determinants of health affecting the rural or remote geographical areas in Australia and how do these impact on the care provided in rural facilities?
15. Identify key ways of engaging with the rural or remote community to minimise culture shock and to become part of the rural or remote setting.

16. Outline the cultural safety practices that a nurse must consider when working in a rural or remote community.
17. What nursing codes of practice relate to the nurse working in Australia? Discuss the impact of the *Code of Conduct for Nurses* (NMBA 2018a) on nurses in rural and remote settings.
18. Telehealth and telemedicine are more widely available in rural and remote settings in Australia with greater digital infrastructure.
    a. What advantages and disadvantages does this have on care in the rural or remote setting?
    b. What advantages does this have on nursing practice in the rural or remote setting?

Evolve® Answer guide for the Review Questions, Critical Thinking Exercises, Decision-making Framework Exercises and Critical Thinking Questions in Case Studies is hosted on Evolve: http://evolve.elsevier.com/AU/Koutoukidis/Tabbner.

References

Australian Commission on Safety and Quality in Health Care (ACSQHC), 2021. National safety and quality primary and community healthcare standards. Available at: <https://www.safetyandquality.gov.au/sites/default/files/2021-10/national_safety_and_quality_primary_and_community_healthcare_standards.pdf>.

Australian Commission on Safety and Quality in Health Care (ACSQHC), 2022. National safety and quality primary and community healthcare standards guide for healthcare services. Available at: <https://www.safetyandquality.gov.au/sites/default/files/2022-12/draft_national_safety_and_quality_primary_and_community_healthcare_standards_guide_for_healthcare_services.pdf>.

Australian Institute of Health and Welfare (AIHW), 2022. Australia's health 2022: Data insights. Australia's health series no. 18. AUS 240. AIHW, Canberra. Available at: <https://www.aihw.gov.au/getmedia/c91a05ef-307f-4c18-8ed3-dfe33d0c603d/aihw-aus-240.pdf?v=20230919120233&inline=true>.

Australian Institute of Health and Welfare (AIHW), 2023a. Cultural safety in health care for Indigenous Australians: Monitoring framework. Available at: <https://www.aihw.gov.au/reports/indigenous-australians/cultural-safety-health-care-framework/contents/summary>.

Australian Institute of Health and Welfare (AIHW), 2023b. Rural and remote health. Available at: <https://www.aihw.gov.au/reports/rural-remote-australians/rural-and-remote-health>.

Australian Institute of Health and Welfare (AIHW), 2024. Aboriginal and Torres Strait Islander health performance framework summary report. Available at: <https://www.indigenoushpf.gov.au/getattachment/90249f39-4473-4479-9c45-33a41f6ddfeb/2024-march-hpf-summary-report.pdf>.

Australian Nursing and Midwifery Federation (ANMF), 2014. National practice standards for nurses in general practice. Available at: <https://www.anmf.org.au/media/idvfkhng/anmf_national_practice_standards_for_nurses_in_general_practice.pdf>.

Australian Primary Health Care Nurses Association (APNA), 2015. APNA nurse home visit guidelines. Available at: <https://www.apna.asn.au/files/DAM/3%20Knowledge%20Hub/NurseHomeVisitGuidelines.pdf>.

Australian Primary Health Care Nurses Association (APNA), 2017. APNA position statement: Scope of practice. Available at: <https://www.apna.asn.au/docs/bb75968b-dee1-ea11-80d9-005056be66b1/APNAPositionStatement-ScopeofPracticeSep2017.pdf>.

Australian Primary Health Care Nurses Association (APNA), 2018. APNA career and education framework for nurses in primary health care—enrolled nurses. Available at: <https://www.apna.asn.au/files/DAM/8.%20Nursing%20Tools/Career%20and%20Education%20Framework/APNA%20Career%20and%20Education%20Framework%20for%20Nurses%20in%20Primary%20Health%20Care%20-%20Enrolled%20Nurses.pdf>.

Australian Primary Health Care Nurses Association (APNA), 2024. What is primary health care nursing? Available at: <https://www.apna.asn.au/profession/what-is-primary-health-care-nursing>.

Badu, E., O'Brien, A., Mitchell, R., 2020. Workplace stress and resilience in the Australian nursing workforce: A comprehensive integrative review. *International Journal of Mental Health Nursing* 29(1), 5–34. doi: 10.1111/inm.12662.

Bailey, J., Blignault, I., Carriage, C., et al., 2020. We are working for our people. Growing and strengthening the Aboriginal and Torres Strait Islander health workforce: Career pathways project report. Available at: <https://www.lowitja.org.au/content/Image/Career_Pathways_Report_Working_for_Our_People_2020.pdf>.

Baldwin, R., Stephens, M., Sharp, D., et al., 2013. Issues facing aged care services in rural and remote Australia. Aged and Community Services Australia, Canberra.

Battye, K., Roufeil, L., Edwards, M., et al., 2019. Strategies for increasing allied health recruitment and retention in Australia: A rapid review. Services for Australian Rural and Remote Allied Health (SARRAH). Available at: <https://pub-b0561b18fd0b407ba7c21f42b2d2de7e.r2.dev/rapid_review_-_recruitment_and_retention_strategies_-_final_web_ready.pdf>.

Beasleigh, S., Bish, M., Mahoney, A.M., 2024. The learning needs and clinical requirements of post graduate critical care nursing students in rural and regional contexts: A scoping review. *Australian Critical Care* 37(2), 326–337. doi: 10.1016/j.aucc.2023.06.001.

Berman, A., Frandsen, G., Snyder, S., et al., 2020. *Kozier and Erb's fundamentals of nursing*, 5th ed. Pearson, Frenchs Forest.

Best, O., Fredericks, B., 2022. *Yatdjuligin: Aboriginal and Torres Strait Islander nursing and midwifery care*, 3rd ed. Cambridge University Press, Melbourne.

Blay, N., Sousa, M.S., Rowles, M., Murray-Parahi, P., 2021. The community nurse in Australia. Who are they? A rapid systematic review. *Journal of Nursing Management* 31(1), 154–168. doi: 10.1111/jonm.13493.

Bolton Clarke, 2024. Home and community support. Available at: <https://www.boltonclarke.com.au/support-at-home>.

Brown, D., Edwards, H., Seaton, L., 2023. *Lewis's medical–surgical nursing*, 6th ed. Elsevier, Sydney.

Byrne, A.L., Baldwin, A., Harvey, C., 2020. Whose centre is it anyway? Defining person-centred care in nursing: An integrative review. *PLoS ONE* 15(3), e0229923. doi: 10.1371/journal.pone.0229923.

Calleja, P., Wilkes, S., Spencer, M., et al., 2022. Telehealth use in rural and remote health practitioner education: An integrative review. *Rural and Remote Health* 22, 6467. doi: 10.22605/RRH6467.

Chan, T.E., Lockhart, J.S., Thomas, A., et al., 2020. An integrative review of nurse practitioner practice and its relationship to the core competencies. *Journal of Professional Nursing* 36(4), 189–199. doi: 10.1016/j.profnurs.2019.11.003.

Clendon, J., Munns, A., McMurray, A., 2022. *Community health and wellness: Primary health care in practice*, 7th ed. Elsevier, Sydney.

Cox, R., Robinson, T., Rossiter, R., et al., 2023. Nurses transitioning to primary health care in Australia: A practice improvement initiative. *SAGE Open Nursing* 10(9), 23779608231165695. doi: 10.1177/23779608231165695.

Dawda, P., True, A., 2023. Primary health care in Australia. In: Reynolds, L., Debono, D., Travaglia, J. (eds.), *Understanding the Australian health care system*, 5th ed. Elsevier, Australia.

Drummond, A., 2022.Working with Aboriginal and Torres Strait Islander health workers and health practitioners. In: Best, O., Fredericks, B. (eds.), *Yatdjuligin: Aboriginal and Torres Strait Islander nursing and midwifery care*, 3rd ed. Cambridge University Press, Melbourne, pp. 155–176.

Fietze, I., Rosenblum., L., Salanitro, M., et al., 2022. The interplay between poor sleep and work-related health. *Frontiers in Public Health* 10 (20220701), 866750. doi: 10.3389/fpubh.2022.866750.

Fisher, M., Freeman, T., MacKean, T., et al., 2022. Universal health coverage for non-communicable diseases and health equity: Lessons from Australian primary healthcare. *International Journal of Health Policy Management* 11(5), 690–700. doi: 10.34172/ijhpm.2020.232.

Fleming, M., Baldwin, L., 2023. *Introduction to public health*, 5th ed. Elsevier, Sydney.

Francis, K., Chapman, Y., Hoare, K., et al. (eds.), 2013. *Australia and New Zealand community as partner: Theory and practice in nursing*, 2nd ed. Wolters Kluwer Health/ Lippincott Williams & Wilkins, Sydney.

Frost, R., Rait, G., Wheatley, A., et al., 2020. What works in managing complex conditions in older people in primary and community care? A state-of-the-art review. *Health & Social Care in the Community* 28(6), 1915–1927. doi: 10.1111/hsc.13085.

Gatwiri, K., Rotumah, D., Rix, E., 2021. BlackLivesMatter in healthcare: Racism and implications for health inequity among Aboriginal and Torres Strait Islander peoples in Australia. *International Journal of Environmental Research and Public Health* 18, 4399. doi: 10.3390/ijerph18094399.

Giles, M., Parker, V., Conway J., et al., 2018. Knowing how to get things done: Nurse consultants as clinical leaders. *Journal of Clinical Nursing* 27, 1981–1993. doi: 10.1111/ jocn.14327.

Giusti, A., Nkhoma, K., Petrus, R., et al., 2020. The empirical evidence underpinning the concept and practice of person-centred care for serious illness: A systematic review. *BMJ Global Health* 5, e003330. doi:10.1136/bmjgh-2020-003330.

Gum, L.F., Sweet, L., Greenhill, J., Prideaux, D., 2020. Exploring interprofessional education and collaborative practice in Australian rural health services. *Journal of Interprofessional Care* 34(2), 173–183, doi: 10.1080/ 13561820.2019.1645648.

Hales, M., 2020a. Community health. In: Berman, A., Frandsen, G., Snyder, S., et al. (eds.), *Kozier and Erb's fundamentals of nursing: Concepts, process and practice*, 5th ed, vol. 1. Pearson Education, Frenchs Forest.

Hales, M., 2020b. Home care. In: Berman, A., Frandsen, G., Snyder, S., et al. (eds.), *Kozier and Erb's fundamentals of nursing: Concepts, process and practice*, 5th ed, vol. 1. Pearson Education, Frenchs Forest.

Hand, L.J., 2022. The role of telemedicine in rural mental health care around the globe. *Telemedicine and e-Health* 28(3), 285–294. doi: 10.1089/tmj.2020.0536.

Hart, C.R., Berry, H.L., Tonna, A.M., 2011. Improving the mental health of rural New South Wales communities facing drought and other adversities. *Australian Journal of Rural Health* 19, 231–238.

Ingham-Broomfield, B., 2020. Critical thinking and the nursing process. In: Berman, A., Frandsen, G., Snyder, S., et al. (eds.), *Kozier and Erb's fundamentals of nursing: Concepts, process and practice*, 5th ed, vol. 1. Pearson Education, Frenchs Forest.

Keast, K., 2014. Nursing beyond the bush. *Australian Nursing and Midwifery Journal* 22(3), 18–22.

Keleher, H., 2023. Public health in Australia. In: Reynolds, L., Debono, D., Travaglia, J. (eds.), *Understanding the Australian health care system*, 5th ed. Elsevier, Australia.

Khan, A.I., Barnsley, J., Harris, J.K., et al., 2022. Examining the extent and factors associated with interprofessional teamwork in primary care settings. *Journal of Interprofessional Care* 36(1), 52–63. doi: 10.1080/13561820.2021.1874896.

Koff, E., Lyons, N., 2020. Implementing value-based health care at scale: The NSW experience. *Medical Journal of Australia* 212(3), 104–106. doi:10.5694/mja2.50470.

Larsson, R., Erlingsdóttir, G., Persson, J., et al., 2022. Teamwork in home care nursing: A scoping literature review. *Health and Social Care in the Community* 30(6), e3309–e3327. doi: 10.1111/hsc.13910.

Liu, X.L., Wang, T., Bressington, D., et al., 2023. Factors influencing retention among regional, rural and remote undergraduate nursing students in Australia: A systematic review of current research evidence. *International Journal of Environmental Research and Public Health* 20(5), 3983. doi: 10.3390/ijerph20053983.

Lukewich, J., Allard, M., Ashley, L., et al., 2020. National competencies for registered nurses in primary care: A Delphi study. *Western Journal of Nursing Research* 42(12), 1078–1087. doi:10.1177/0193945920935590.

Mackean, T., Fisher, M., Friel, S., et al., 2020a. A framework to assess cultural safety in Australian public policy. *Health Promotion International* 35(2), 340–351. doi: 10.1093/heapro/daz011.

Mackean, T., Withall, E., Dwyer, J., et al., 2020b. Role of Aboriginal health workers and liaison officers in quality care in the Australian acute care setting: A systematic review. *Australian Health Review* 44(3), 427–433. doi: 10.1071/AH19101.

McAllister, M., 2010. Solution focused nursing: A fitting model for mental health nurses working in a public health paradigm. *Contemporary Nurse* 34(2), 149–157.

McAllister, M., Moyle, W., Iselin, G., 2006. Solution focused nursing: An evaluation of current practice. *Nurse Education Today* 26(5), 439–447.

McCormack, B., McCance, T.V., Bulley, C., et al., 2021. *Fundamentals of person-centred healthcare practice*, John Wiley, New York.

McCullough, K., Whitehead, L., Bayes, S., et al., 2020. The delivery of primary health care in remote communities: A grounded theory study of the perspective of nurses. *International Journal of Nursing Studies* 102, 103474. doi: 10.1016/j.ijnurstu.2019.103474.

Moore, E., 2016. Systems diversity in case management: Characteristics, models and dimensions. In: Moore, E. (ed.), *Case management inclusive community practice*, 2nd ed. Oxford University Press Australia and New Zealand, Melbourne.

Naden, K., Hampton, D., Walke, E., et al., 2023. Growing our own rural, remote and Aboriginal health workforce: Contributions made, approaches taken and lessons learnt by three rural Australian academic health departments. *Australian Journal of Rural Health* 31(3), 589–595. doi: 10.1111/ajr.12972.

Nursing and Midwifery Board of Australia (NMBA), 2018a. Code of conduct for nurses. NMBA, Canberra.

Nursing and Midwifery Board of Australia (NMBA), 2018b. NMBA and CATSINaM joint statement on culturally safe care. Available at: <https://www.nursingmidwiferyboard.gov.au/Codes-Guidelines-Statements/Position-Statements/joint-statement-on-culturally-safe-care.aspx>.

Nursing and Midwifery Board of Australia (NMBA), 2020. Decision-making framework for nursing and midwifery. Available at: <https://www.nursingmidwiferyboard.gov.au/Codes-Guidelines-Statements/Frameworks.aspx>.

Orr, F., 2023. Mental health and recovery-oriented mental health services. In: Reynolds, L., Debono, D., Travaglia, J. (eds.), *Understanding the Australian health care system*, 5th ed. Elsevier, Sydney.

Parsons, M., Reeve, I., McGregor, J., et al. 2021. Disaster resilience in Australia: A geographic assessment using an index of coping and adaptive capacity. *International Journal of Disaster Risk Reduction* 62, 102422. doi: 10.1016/j.ijdrr.2021.102422.

Pearson, O., Schwartzkopff, K., Dawson, A., 2020. Aboriginal community controlled health organisations address health equity through action on the social determinants of health of Aboriginal and Torres Strait Islander peoples in Australia. *BMC Public Health* 20(1859). doi: 10.1186/s12889-020-09943-4.

Power, T., Virdum, C., Gorman, E., et al., 2018. Ensuring Indigenous cultural respect in Australian undergraduate students. *Higher Education Research and Development* 37(4), 837–851. doi: 10.1080/07294360.2018.1440537.

Ramsamey, N., 2022. Remote area nursing practice. In: Best, O., Fredericks, B. (eds.), *Yatdjuligin: Aboriginal and Torres Strait Islander nursing and midwifery care*, 3rd ed. Cambridge University Press, Melbourne, pp. 139–154.

Ridgeway, L., Hackworth, N., McKenna, L., 2021. Working with families: A systematic scoping review of family-centred care in universal, community-based maternal, child, and family health services. *Journal of Child Health Care* 25(2), 268–289. doi: 10.1177/1367493520930172.

Ryan, B., Johnston, K.A., Taylor, M., et al., 2020. Community engagement for disaster preparedness: A systematic literature review. *International Journal of Disaster Risk Reduction* 49, 101655. doi: 10.1016/j.ijdrr.2020.101655.

Scammel, J.M.E., Apostolo, J.L.A., Bianchi, M., 2020. Learning to lead: A scoping review of undergraduate nurse education. *Journal of Nursing Management* 28(3), 756–765. doi: 10.1111/jonm.12951.

Stanley, D., 2009. Leadership: Behind the mask. *ACORN: The Journal of Perioperative Nursing in Australia* 22(1), 14.

Stanley, D., Stanley, K., 2019. Clinical leadership and rural and remote practice: A qualitative study. *Journal of Nursing Management* 27(6), 1314–1324. doi: 10.1111/jonm.12813.

Staunton, P., Chiarella, M., 2024. *Law for nurses and midwives*, 10th ed. Elsevier, Sydney.

Stein-Parbury, J., 2021. *Patient and person: Interpersonal skills in nursing*, 7th ed. Elsevier, Sydney.

Swan, M.A., Hobbs, B.B., 2021. Lack of anonymity and secondary traumatic stress in rural nurses. *Online Journal of Rural Nursing and Health Care* 21(1). doi: 10.14574/ojrnhc.v21i1.651.

Swerissen, H., Duckett, S., 2018. Mapping primary care in Australia. Available at: <https://grattan.edu.au/wp-content/uploads/2018/07/906-Mapping-primary-care.pdf>.

Taylor, P., 2017. The privilege of nursing: An interview with Whitney Harris. *AACN Bold Voices* 9(8), 12–13.

Topp, S., Tully, J., Cummins, R., et al., 2022. Rhetoric, reality and racism: The governance of Aboriginal and Torres Strait Islander health workers in a state government health service in Australia. *International Journal of Health Policy Management* 11(12), 2951–2963.

Torrens, C., Campbell, P., Hoskins, G., et al., 2020. Barriers and facilitators to the implementation of the advanced nurse practitioner role in primary care settings: A scoping review. *International Journal of Nursing Studies* 104, 103443. doi: 10.1016/j.ijnurstu.2019.103443.

Ward, M., Aumann, O., Di Stefano, G., et al., 2013. Community Health Nurses Special Interest Group ANF (Vic Branch) (issuing body.) Practice standards for Victorian community health nurses. [Carlton, Victoria] Community Health Nurses Special Interest Group ANF (Vic Branch). Available at: <https://www.apna.asn.au/files/DAM/3%20Knowledge%20Hub/PracticeStandardsForVictorianCommunityHealthNurses.pdf>.

Welch, N., 2000. Understanding of the determinants of rural health. National Rural Health Alliance Online. Available at: <https://www.ruralhealth.org.au/sites/default/files/documents/nrha-policy-document/policy-development/dev-determinants-rural-health-01-feb-2000.pdf>.

Whitehead, L., Quinn, R., 2019. Improving health outcomes in rural and remote Australia: Optimising the contribution of nurses. *The Collegian* 26, 407–414. doi: 10.1016/j.colegn.2019.03.002.

Whitehead, L., Twigg, D.E., Carman, R., et al., 2022. Factors influencing the development and implementation of nurse practitioner candidacy programs: A scoping review. *International Journal of Nursing Studies* 125, 104133. doi: 10.1016/j.ijnurstu.2021.104133.

Whiteing, N., Barr, J., Rossi, D.M., 2021. The practice of rural and remote nurses in Australia: A case study. *Journal of Clinical Nursing* 31(11–12), 1502–1518. doi: 10.1111/jocn.16002.

World Health Organization (WHO), 1978. Declaration of Alma-Ata. Online. Available at: <https://cdn.who.int/media/docs/default-source/documents/almaata-declaration-en.pdf?sfvrsn=7b3c2167_2>.

Recommended Reading

Aljassim, N., Ostini, R., 2020. Health literacy in rural and urban populations: A systematic review. *Patient Education and Counseling* 103(10), 2142–2154. doi: 10.1016/j.pec.2020.06.007.

Australian Government, 2021. National Aboriginal and Torres Strait Islander Health Plan 2021–2031. Commonwealth of Australia, Canberra. Available at: <https://www.health.gov.au/sites/default/files/documents/2022/06/national-aboriginal-and-torres-strait-islander-health-plan-2021-2031.pdf>.

Berman, A., Frandsen, G., Snyder, S., et al., 2020. *Kozier and Erb's fundamentals of nursing: Concepts, process and practice*, 5th ed, vol. 1. Pearson Education, Frenchs Forest.

Brayley, A., 2013. Bush nurses—inspiring true stories of nursing bravery and ingenuity in rural and remote Australia. *The Lamp* 70(6), 43.

Collett, M.J., Fraser, C., Thompson, S.C., 2020. Developing the future rural nursing workforce: Report on a nursing roundtable. *Collegian* 27(4), 370–374. doi: 10.1016/j.colegn.2019.10.007.

Cosgrave, C., 2020. The whole-of-person retention improvement framework: A guide for addressing health workforce challenges in the rural context. *International Journal of Environmental Research and Public Health* 17(8), 2698. doi: 10.3390/ijerph17082698.

Crisp, J.C., Douglas, C., Rebeiro, G., et al. (eds.), 2020. *Potter & Perry's fundamentals of nursing*, Australian version, 6th ed. Elsevier, Sydney.

David, S., Karen, S., Bindu, S., 2020. Bullying and threats to belonging: Cultural challenges in rural and remote nursing practice. *Nursing & Primary Care* 4(1), 1–7.

Guzys, D., Brown, R., Halcomb, E., et al., 2020. *An introduction to community and primary health care*, 3rd ed. Cambridge University Press, Port Melbourne.

Hines, S., Wakerman. J., Carey, T.A., et al., 2020. Retention strategies and interventions for health workers in rural and remote areas: A systematic review protocol. *JBI Evidence Synthesis* 18(1), 87–96. doi: 10.11124/JBIS-RIR-2017-004009.

Kenny, A., Dickson-Swift, V., DeVecchi, N., et al., 2021. Evaluation of a rural undergraduate nursing student employment model. *Collegian* 28(2), 197–205. doi: 10.1016/j.colegn.2020.07.003.

Kralik, D., Trowbridge, K., Smith, J. (eds.), 2008. *A practice manual for community nursing in Australia*. Wiley Australia, Milton.

Kralik, D., van Loon, A. (eds.), 2021. *Community nursing in Australia*, 2nd ed. Wiley Australia, Milton.

Mathew, S., Fitts, M.S., Liddle, Z., et al., 2023. Telehealth in remote Australia: A supplementary tool or an alternative model of care replacing face-to-face consultations? *BMC Health Services Research* 23(341). doi: 10.1186/s12913-023-09265-2.

Oldland, E., Botti, M., Hutchinson, A.M., et al., 2020. A framework of nurses' responsibilities for quality healthcare – exploration of content validity. *Collegian* 27(2), 150–163. doi: 10.1016/j.colegn.2019.07.007.

Osborne, S.R., Alston, L.V., Bolton, K.A., et al., 2020. Beyond the black stump: Rapid reviews of health research issues affecting regional, rural and remote Australia. *Medical Journal of Australia* 213 (s11), s3–s32. doi: 10.5694/mja2.50881.

Perimal-Lewis, L., Williams, P.A.H., Mudd, G., et al., 2021. Virtual care: The future of telehealth. In: Maeder A.J., Higa, C., Van Den Berg, M.E.L., et al., (eds.), *Telehealth innovations in remote healthcare services delivery: Global telehealth 2020*. IOS Press Ebooks, Amsterdam.

Quilliam, C., Wong, S.A., Corboy, D., et al., 2023. Design and implementation characteristics of research training for rural health professionals: A qualitative descriptive study. *BMC Medical Education* 23(1), 200. doi: 10.1186/s12909-023-04169-5.

Roberts, P., Guenther, J., 2021. Framing rural and remote: Key issues, debates, definitions, and positions in constructing rural and remote disadvantage. In: Roberts, P., Fuqua, M. (eds.), *Ruraling education research*. Springer, Singapore.

Russell, D., Mathew, S., Fitts, M., et al., 2021. Interventions for health workforce retention in rural and remote areas: A systematic review. *Human Resources for Health* 19(1), 103. doi: 10.1186/s12960-021-00643-7.

Ryan, A.A., McKenna, H., 2015. 'It's the little things that count.' Families' experience of roles, relationships and quality of care in rural nursing homes. *International Journal of Older People Nursing* 10(1), 38–47. doi: 10.1111/opn.12052.

Smith, S., Lapkin, S., Sim, J., et al., 2020. Nursing care left undone, practice environment and perceived quality of care in small rural hospitals. *Journal of Nursing Management* 28(8), 2166–2173. doi: 10.1111/jonm.12975.

van de Mortel, T.F., Nilsson, J., Lepp, M., 2021. Validating the nurse professional competence scale with Australian baccalaureate nursing students. *Collegian* 28(2), 244–251. doi: 10.1016/j.colegn.2020.06.010.

Wong, S.A., Quilliam, C., Corboy, D., et al., 2022. What shapes research and research capacity building in rural health services? Context matters. *Australian Journal of Rural Health* 30(3), 410–421. doi: 10.1111/ajr.12852.

Online Resources

Angel Flight: <https://www.angelflight.org.au>.

Australian Health Practitioner Regulation Authority (Ahpra): <https://www.ahpra.gov.au>.

Australian Indigenous HealthInfoNet: <https://healthinfonet.ecu.edu.au>.

Australian Primary Health Care Nurses Association (APNA): <www.apna.asn.au>.

Bolton Clarke: <https://www.boltonclarke.com.au>.

CRANAplus: <www.crana.org.au>.

Department of Health Western Australia: <https://www.health.wa.gov.au/Articles/F_I/Health-Networks>.

Healthdirect: <http://www.healthdirect.gov.au>.

Health Victoria: <https://www2.health.vic.gov.au/primary-and-community-health>.

National Rural Health Alliance: <www.ruralhealth.org.au>.

New South Wales (NSW) Health: <https://www.health.nsw.gov.au/regional/Pages/default.aspx>.

Northern Territory Government: <https://nt.gov.au/wellbeing/remote-health>.

Public Health Association of Australia: <www.phaa.net.au>.

Queensland Health: <https://www.health.qld.gov.au/public-health/groups/rural-and-remote-health>.

Royal Flying Doctor Service: <https://www.flyingdoctor.org.au>.

Services for Australian Rural and Remote Allied Health (SARRAH): <https://sarrah.org.au>.

Tasmanian Department of Health: <https://www.health.tas.gov.au/health-topics/ageing-and-aged-care>.

Victorian Refugee Health Network: <http://refugeehealthnetwork.org.au>.

Credits

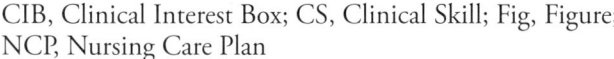

CIB, Clinical Interest Box; CS, Clinical Skill; Fig, Figure; NCP, Nursing Care Plan

CASE STUDY

Case Study 1.1, Australian Health Practitioner Regulation Agency (Ahpra), 2021. Former enrolled nurse fined after Ahpra prosecution. Available at: <https://www.ahpra.gov.au/News/2021-02-21-Former-enrolled-nurse-fined.aspx>. **Case Study 10.2,** NSW Health, 2019. Clinical handover. Policy directive. Available at: <https://www1.health.nsw.gov.au/pds/ActivePDSDocuments/PD2019_020.pdf>. **Case Study 13.1,** Agency for Clinical Innovation (ACI), 2023a. Consumer enablement guide: Culturally and linguistically diverse communities. Available at: <https://aci.health.nsw.gov.au/projects/consumer-enablement/how-to-support-enablement/culturally-responsive-practice/culturally-and-linguisticallydiverse-communities>; General Practice Training Queensland (GPTQ), 2020. Indigenous health in-practice guide, vol 1–3. Available at: <https://www.gptq.qld.edu.au/indigenous-health-in-practice-guides>; State of Queensland, Queensland Health, 2015. Sad news, sorry business: Guidelines for caring for Aboriginal and Torres Strait Islander people through death and dying, v. 2. Available at: <https://www.health.qld.gov.au/__data/assets/pdf_file/0023/151736/sorry_business.pdf>.

CLINICAL INTEREST BOXES

CIB 1.1, The Nightingale Pledge. Available at: <https://www.truthaboutnursing.org/press/pioneers/lystra_gretter.html#pledge&gsc.tab=0>. **CIB 1.2,** Scrubs, nd. A list of rules for nurses from 1887. Available at: < http://scrubsmag.com/a-list-of-rules-for-nurses-from-1887>. **CIB 1.3,** Australian Army Nursing Service (AANS) Pledge of Service, 1935. © Commonwealth of Australia. **CIB 1.4,** Benner, P., 1984. *From novice to expert: Excellence and power in clinical nursing practice.* Addison-Wesley, Nursing Division, Menlo Park. **CIB 1.5,** Nursing and Midwifery Board of Australia (NMBA), 2020. Decision-making framework summary: Nursing. Available at: <https://www.nursingmidwiferyboard.gov.au/codesguidelines-statements/frameworks.aspx>. **CIB 1.6,** Wiggins, D., Downie, A., Engel, R.M. Brown, B.T., 2022. Factors that influence scope of practice of the five largest health care professions in Australia: A scoping review. *Human Resources for Health* 20(87). Available at: <https://human-resources-health.biomedcentral.com/articles/10.1186/s12960-022-00783-4>. **CIB 1.7,** Nursing and Midwifery Board of Australia (NMBA), 2016. Continuing professional development guidelines, 2016. Available at: <https://www.nursingmidwiferyboard.gov.au/Codes-Guidelines-Statements/Codes-Guidelines.aspx>. **CIB 1.8,** NSW Health, 2020. Between the flags. Available at: < http://www.cec.health.nsw.gov.au/patient-safety-programs/adultpatient-safety/between-the-flags>; Nursing and Midwifery Board of Australia (NMBA), 2016. Continuing professional development guidelines, June 2016. Available at: <https://www.nursingmidwiferyboard.gov.au/Codes-Guidelines-Statements/Codes-Guidelines.aspx>. **CIB 1.9,** Nursing and Midwifery Board of Australia (NMBA), 2018. Code of conduct for nurses, March 2018. Available at: <https://www.nursingmidwiferyboard.gov.au/Codes-Guidelines-Statements/Professional-standards.aspx>; International Council of Nurses (ICN), 2012. The ICN code of ethics for nurses. Available at: <https://ipe.umn.edu/sites/health1.umn.edu/files/2021-08/2012_icn_codeofethicsfornurses_eng.pdf>.**CIB 1.10,** Friberg, E., 2024. Theories and frameworks for professional nursing practice. *Conceptual foundations: The bridge to professional nursing practice*, 8th ed, edited by Friberg, E., Saewert, K., pages 44–59, ISBN 978-0-323-84713-1. Available at: < http://dx.doi.org/10.1016/B978-0-323-84713-1.00014-9>. **CIB 2.1,** Berman, A., Frandsen, G., Snyder, S., et al., 2021. *Kozier and Erb's fundamentals of nursing*, 5th ed. Pearson, Melbourne. **CIB 2.3,** Nursing and Midwifery Board of Australia (NMBA), 2018. Code of professional conduct for nurses. Available at: < http://www.nursingmidwiferyboard.gov.au/Codes-Guidelines-Statements/Codes-Guidelines.aspx>. **CIB 2.4**, Allan, S., 2020. *Law & ethics for health practitioners.* Elsevier Australia, Chatswood; Atkins, K., De Lacey, S., Ripperger, B., Ripperger, R., 2020. *Ethics and law for Australian Nurses*, 4th ed. Cambridge University Press, Cambridge. **CIBs 2.5, 2.8, 2.9, 2.15,** Atkins, K., De Lacey, S., Ripperger, B., Ripperger, R., 2020. *Ethics and law for Australian nurses*, 4th ed. Cambridge University Press, Cambridge. **CIBs 2.6, 2.7, 2.11, 2.13,** Staunton, P.J., Chiarella, M., 2020. *Law for nurses and midwives*, 9th ed. Elsevier, Chatswood. **CIB 2.10,** Nursing and Midwifery Board of Australia (NMBA), 2014. Guidelines for

mandatory notification. Available at: < http://www.nursingmidwiferyboard.gov.au/Codes-Guidelines-Statements/Codes-Guidelines/Guidelines-for-mandatory-notifications.aspx>. **CIB 2.12,** Department of Health, Government of Western Australia, 2019. Clinical incident management policy. Patient Safety Surveillance Unit, Perth. **CIB 2.14,** Queensland Courts, Coroners Court, 2021. Reportable deaths. The State of Queensland. Available at: <https://www.courts.qld.gov.au/courts/coroners-court/coroners-process/reportable-deaths>. **CIB 2.16,** Allan, S., 2020. *Law & ethics for health practitioners*. Elsevier Australia, Chatswood. **CIB 2.17,** Beauchamp, T.L., Childress, J.F., 2013. *Principles of biomedical ethics*, 7th ed. Oxford University Press, USA. **CIB 2.18,** Daly, J., Jackson, D., 2020. *Contexts of nursing*, 6th ed. Elsevier Australia, Chatswood. **CIB 2.19,** Baillie, L., 2017. An exploration of the 6Cs as a set of values for nursing practice. *British Journal of Nursing* 26(10), 558–563. **CIB 2.20,** Atkins, K., De Lacey, S., Ripperger, B., Ripperger, R., 2020. Ethics and law for Australian nurses, 4th ed. Cambridge University Press, Cambridge; Johnstone, M.J., 2019. *Bioethics: A nursing perspective*, 7th ed. Elsevier, Chatswood. Crisp, J., Douglas, C., Rebeiro, G., et al. (eds.), 2021. *Potter & Perry's fundamentals of nursing*, 6th ed. Elsevier, Chatswood. **CIB 2.21**, Johnstone, M.J., 2019. *Bioethics: A nursing perspective*, 7th ed. Elsevier, Chatswood. Crisp, J., Douglas, C., Rebeiro, G., et al. (eds.), 2021. *Potter & Perry's fundamentals of nursing*, 6th ed. Elsevier, Chatswood. **CIB 2.22,** Staunton, P.J., Chiarella, M., 2020. *Law for nurses and midwives*, 9th ed. Elsevier, Chatswood; Crisp, J., Douglas, C., Rebeiro, G., et al. (eds.), 2021. *Potter & Perry's fundamentals of nursing*, 6th ed. Elsevier, Chatswood. **CIB 2.24,** Berman, A., Frandsen, G., Snyder, S., et al., 2021. *Kozier and Erb's fundamentals of nursing*, 5th ed. Pearson, Melbourne. **CIB 3.4,** Richardson-Tench, M., Nicholson, P., 2022. *Research in nursing, midwifery and allied health: Evidence for best practice*, 7th ed. Cengage Learning, Melbourne; Whitehead, D., Ferguson, C., et al., 2020. *Nursing and midwifery research: Methods & appraisal for evidence-based practice*, 6th ed. Elsevier, Sydney. **CIB 3.5,** Gray, J., Grove, S., 2021. *Burns and Grove's The practice of nursing research: Appraisal, synthesis, and generation of evidence*, 9th ed. Elsevier, St Louis; Richardson-Tench, M., Nicholson, P., 2022. *Research in nursing, midwifery and allied health: Evidence for best practice*, 7th ed. Cengage Learning, Melbourne; Whitehead, D., Ferguson, C., et al., 2020. *Nursing and midwifery research: Methods & appraisal for evidence-based practice*, 6th ed. Elsevier, Sydney. **CIBs 3.6, 3.7, 3.8,** Jackson, D., Halcomb, E., Walthall, H., 2023. *Navigating the maze of research,* 6th ed. Elsevier. **CIB 4.1,** Swerissen, H., Duckett, S., 2018. *Mapping primary care in Australia*. Grattan Institute, Carlton. **CIB 4.3,** Australian Institute of Health and Welfare (AIHW), 2023. Health expenditure Australia 2021–22. Available at: <https://www.aihw.gov.au/reports/health-welfare-expenditure/health-expenditure-australia-2021-22/contents/about>.
CIB 5.1, Australian Institute of Health and Welfare (AIHW), 2016. Australia's health 2016. Australia's health series no. 15. Cat. no. AUS 199. Canberra: AIHW. **CIB 5.2,** Australian Bureau of Statistics (ABS), 2019. National health survey: Health literacy. Available at: <https://www.abs.gov.au/statistics/health/health-conditions-and-risks/national-health-survey-health-literacy/latest-release>. **CIB 5.4,** World Health Organization (WHO), 1986. The Ottawa Charter for Health Promotion. WHO, Geneva. Available at: < http://www.who.int/healthpromotion/conferences/previous/ottawa/en>. **CIBs 5.5, 5.6,** Taylor, J., O'Hara, L., Talbot, L., et al., Verrinder, G., 2021. *Promoting health: The primary health care approach*, 7th ed. Elsevier, Sydney. **CIB 5.7,** Harding, M., Kwong, J., Hagler, D., 2023. *Lewis's medical-surgical nursing*, 12th ed. Elsevier, Missouri. **CIB 6.1,** Kaya, H., Senyuva, E., Bodur, G., 2017. Developing critical thinking disposition and emotional intelligence of nursing students: A longitudinal research. *Nurse Education Today* 48(1), 72–77; Noone, T., Seery, A., 2018. Critical thinking dispositions in undergraduate nursing students: A case study approach. *Nurse Education Today* 68, 203–207; Seibert, S.A., 2021. Problem-based learning: A strategy to foster generation Z's critical thinking and perseverance. *Teaching and Learning in Nursing* 16(1), 85–88. **CIB 6.2,** Crisp, J., Douglas, C., Rebeiro, G., et al. (eds.), 2021. *Potter & Perry's fundamentals of nursing*, 6th ed. Elsevier, Chatswood. **CIB 6.3,** Seibert, S.A., 2021. Problem-based learning: A strategy to foster generation Z's critical thinking and perseverance. *Teaching and Learning in Nursing* 16(1), 85–88; Toney-Butler, T.J., Thayer, J.M., 2022. Nursing process. International Library of Medicine. StatPearls Publishing, 2022. **CIBs 6.4, 6.5,** Levett-Jones, T., Reid-Searl, K. 2022. *The clinical placement: An essential guide for nursing students*, 5th ed. Elsevier Australia, Chatswood, Australia. **CIBs 7.1, 7.2** Stromberg, H., 2023. *Medical-surgical nursing*, 5th ed. Elsevier Health Science, USA. **CIB 7.3,** Crisp, J., Douglas, C., Rebeiro, G., et al. (eds.), 2021. *Potter & Perry's fundamentals of nursing*, 6th ed. Elsevier, Chatswood. **CIB 7.4**, Wilson, S.F., Giddens J.F., 2022. *Health assessment for nursing practice*, 7th ed. Elsevier Health Sciences, USA. **CIB 7.5,** Australian Human Rights Commission, 2019. Terminology. Available at: <https://humanrights.gov.au/our-work/lgbti/terminology>. **CIB 7.8,** Brown, D., Edwards, H., Buckley, T., et al., 2020. *Lewis's medical-surgical nursing*, 5th ed. Elsevier, Chatswood. **CIB 8.1,** Australian Commission on Safety and Quality in Health Care (ACSQHC), nd. Documenting information: Communicating for safety resource portal. ACSQHC, Sydney. Available at: <https://c4sportal.safetyandquality.gov.au/documenting-information>; Manias, E., Bucknall, T., Hutchinson, A., et al., 2017. *Improving documentation at transitions of care for complex patients*. Australian Commission on Safety and Quality in Health Care, Sydney. **CIB 8.2,** Australian Government, 2022. *Privacy Act 1988*. No. 119, 1988. Compilation No. 93. Amendment Registered December

2022. Office of Parliamentary Counsel, Canberra. Available at: Federal Register of Legislation. Available at: <https://www.legislation.gov.au/Details/C2022C00361>. **CIB 8.3,** Crisp, J., Douglas, C., Rebeiro, G., et al. (eds.), 2021. *Potter & Perry's fundamentals of nursing*, 6th ed. Elsevier, Chatswood; New South Wales (NSW) Government, 2021. Documentation in the Health Care Record. South Eastern Sydney Local Health District (SESLHD). Procedure Document Number SESLHDPR/336; Staunton, P.J., Chiarella, M., 2020. *Law for nurses and midwives*, 9th ed. Elsevier, Chatswood. **CIB 8.6,** McBride, S., Tietze, M., 2019. *Nursing informatics for the advanced practice nurse: Patient safety, quality, outcomes, and interprofessionalism*, 2nd ed. New York: Springer Publishing Company USA; Nelson, R., Staggers, N., 2018. *Health informatics: An interprofessional approach*, 2nd ed. Elsevier, St Louis. **CIB 8.7,** Australian Commission on Safety and Quality in Health Care (ACSQHC), nd. Documenting information: Communicating for safety resource portal. ACSQHC, Sydney. Online. Available at: <https://c4sportal.safetyandquality.gov.au/documenting-information>; Manias, E., Bucknall, T., Hutchinson, A., et al., 2017. *Improving documentation at transitions of care for complex patients*. Australian Commission on Safety and Quality in Health Care, Sydney. **CIB 8.9,** Data from Australasian Institute of Digital Health (AIDH), 2022. Australian Informatics Competency Framework. 2nd ed. South Melbourne, Australia. Available at: <https://digitalhealth.org.au/wp-content/uploads/2022/06/AHICFCompetencyFramework.pdf>. **CIBs 8.10, 8.11,** Australian Nursing and Midwifery Federation (ANMF), 2015. National informatics standards for nurses and midwives. Australian Government Department of Health and Ageing. Available at: <https://anmf.org.au/documents/National_Informatics_Standards_For_Nurses_And_Midwives.pdf>. **CIB 8.13,** Australian Commission on Safety and Quality in Health Care (ACSQHC), 2019b. Emergency Department Clinicians' Guide to My Health Record. ACSQHC, Sydney; Australian Digital Health Agency (ADHA). 2018. Australia's National Digital Health Strategy. Australian Government. <https://www.digitalhealth.gov.au/sites/default/files/2020-11/Australia%27s%20National%20Digital%20Health%20Strategy%20-%20Safe%2C%20seamless%20and%20secure.pdf>. **CIB 8.14,** Crisp, J., Douglas, C., Rebeiro, G., et al. (eds.), 2021. *Potter & Perry's fundamentals of nursing*, 6th ed. Elsevier, Chatswood; McBride, S., Tietze, M., 2019. *Nursing informatics for the advanced practice nurse: patient safety, quality, outcomes, and interprofessionalism*, 2nd ed. Springer Publishing Company, New York; Nelson, R., Staggers, N., 2018. *Health informatics: An interprofessional approach*, 2nd ed. Elsevier, St Louis. **CIB 8.15,** Department of Human Services, 2022. Your right to privacy. Available at: < http://www.humanservices.gov.au/customer/information/privacy>. **CIB 8.16,** Australian Cyber Security Centre (ACSC), 2023. Passwords and passphrases. Available at: <https://www.cyber.gov.au/protect-yourself>. **CIB 8.17,** McBride, S., Tietze, M., 2019. *Nursing informatics for the advanced practice nurse: Patient safety, quality, outcomes, and interprofessionalism*, 2nd ed. New York: Springer Publishing Company USA. **CIB 8.18,** Crisp, J., Douglas, C., Rebeiro, G., et al. (eds.), 2021. *Potter & Perry's fundamentals of nursing*, 6th ed. Elsevier, Chatswood. **CIB 8.19,** Crisp, J., Douglas, C., Rebeiro, G., et al. (eds.), 2021. *Potter & Perry's fundamentals of nursing*, 6th ed. Elsevier, Chatswood; Nelson, R., Staggers, N., 2018. *Health informatics: An interprofessional approach*, 2nd ed. Elsevier, St Louis. **CIB 9.1,** Department of Health, 2021. Victoria State Government. Collecting patient reported outcome measures. Available at: <https://www.health.vic.gov.au/quality-safety-service/collecting-patient-reported-outcome-measures>. **CIBs 9.2, 9.3,** Australian Commission on Safety and Quality in Health Care (ACSQHC), 2021. National safety and quality health service standards, 2nd ed. Available at: <https://www.safetyandquality.gov.au/sites/default/files/2021-05/national_safety_and_quality_health_service_nsqhs_standards_second_edition_-_updated_may_2021.pdf>. **CIB 10.2,** Stein-Parbury, J., 2021. *Patient and person: Interpersonal skills in nursing*, 7th ed. Elsevier, Sydney. **CIB 10.4,** Dwyer, J., 2020. *Communication for business and the professions: Strategies and skills*, 7th ed. Pearson, Australia. **CIB 10.5,** Moss, B., 2020. *Communication skills in nursing, health & social care*. Sage Publications, Melbourne. **CIB 10.7,** National Institute on Deafness and Other Communication Disorders, 2019. Assisted devices for people with hearing, voice, speech or language disorders. Available at: <https://www.nidcd.nih.gov/health/assistive-devices-people-hearing-voice-speech-or-language-disorders>. **CIB 10.8,** Moss, B., 2020. *Communication skills in nursing, health & social care*. Sage Publications, Melbourne, Australia; O'Toole, G., 2020. *Communication: Core interpersonal skills for health professionals*, 4th ed. Elsevier; Neimeyer, R.A., 2023. Grief therapy as a quest for meaning. Steffen, E.M., Milman, E., Neimeyer, R. (eds), *The handbook of grief therapies*. Sage Publishing, London; Torrens-Burton, A., Goss, S., Sutton, E., et al., 2022. 'Empty and lost': The challenges of being bereaved during the COVID-19 pandemic. *Palliative Medicine* 36(1), 62. Available at: <https://pesquisa.bvsalud.org/global-literatureon-novel-coronavirus-2019-ncov/resource/fr/covidwho-1916791?lang=en>. **CIB 10.9,** O'Toole, G., 2020. *Communication: Core interpersonal skills for health professionals*, 4th ed. Elsevier, Sydney; Stein-Parbury, J., 2021. *Patient and person: Interpersonal skills in nursing*, 7th ed. Elsevier, Sydney. **CIB 10.10,** Australian Commission on Safety and Quality in Health Care (ACSQHC), 2021. National Safety and Quality Primary and Community Healthcare Standards, 2nd ed. Available at: <https://www.safetyandquality.gov.au/publications-and-resources/resource-library/national-safety-and-quality-health-service-standards-second-edition>; Australian Commission on Safety and Quality in Health Care (ACSQHC), 2023.

Communicating for safety standard. Communication at clinical handover. Available at: <https://www.safetyandquality.gov.au/standards/nsqhs-standards/communicating-safety-standard/communication-clinical-handover>. **CIB 10.11,** Australian Commission on Safety and Quality in Health Care (ACSQHC), 2023. Communicating for safety standard. Communication at clinical handover. Available at: <https://www.safetyandquality.gov.au/standards/nsqhs-standards/communicating-safety-standard/communication-clinical-handover>. **CIBs 11.1, 11.10,** Berman, A., Synder, S., Levett-Jones, T., et al., 2021. *Kozier and Erb's fundamentals of nursing*, 5th ed, vol. 2. Pearson, Melbourne. **CIB 11.2,** Cummings, G.G., Lee, S., Tate, K., et al., 2021. The essentials of nursing leadership: A systematic review of factors and educational interventions influencing nursing leadership. *International Journal of Nursing Studies* 115. doi: 10.1016/j.ijnurstu.2020.103842; Weintraub, P. McKee, M. 2019. Leadership for innovation in healthcare: An exploration. *International Journal of Health Policy and Management* 8(3), 138–144. doi: 10.1517/ijhpm.2018.122. **CIB 11.5,** McLeod, C., Jokwiro, Y., Gong, Y., et al., 2021. Undergraduate nursing student and preceptors' experiences of clinical placement through an innovative clinical school supervision model. *Nurse Education in Practice* 51. doi: 10.1016/j.nepr.2021.102986. **CIBs 11.6, 11.7** Crisp, J., Douglas, C., Rebeiro, G., et al., 2020. *Potter and Perry's fundamentals of nursing*, 6th ed. Elsevier, Chatswood. **CIB 11.8,** Berman, A., Synder, S., Levett-Jones, T., et al., 2021. *Kozier and Erb's fundamentals of nursing*, 5th ed, vol. 2. Pearson, Melbourne; Dimock, M. 2019. *Defining generations: Where Millennials end and Generation Z begins.* Pew Research Centre. **CIB 11.9,** Australian Bureau of Statistics (ABS), 2022. Estimates of Aboriginal and Torres Strait Islander Australians. Available at: <https://www.abs.gov.au/statistics/people/aboriginal-andtorres-strait-islander-peoples/estimates-aboriginal-andtorres-strait-islander-australians/latest-release>; Berman, A., Synder, S., Levett-Jones, T., et al., 2021. *Kozier and Erb's fundamentals of nursing*, 5th ed, vol. 2. Pearson, Melbourne. **CIB 12.1,** Australian Nursing and Midwifery Federation, 2023. Clinical placement tips. Available at: <https://otr.anmfvic.asn.au/articles/clinical-placement-tips>. **CIB 12.4,** Carson, K.D., Carson, P.P., Fontenot, G., Burdin Jr, J.J., 2005. Structured interview questions for selecting productive, emotionally mature, and helpful employees. *The Health Care Manager* 24(3), 209–215. **CIB 12.6,** Crane, P.J., Ward, S.F., 2016. Self-healing and self-care for nurses. *AORN Journal* 104(5), 386–400. **CIB 12.7,** Australian College of Nursing, 2021. 4 tips to bounce back from a tough day of placement. Available at: <https://www.acn.edu.au/nurseclick/4-tips-to-bounce-back-from-a-tough-day-of-placement>. **CIB 13.1,** Daly, J., 2021. *Contexts of nursing*, 6th ed. Elsevier, Australia; Jacobsen, K.H. 2023, *Introduction to global health,* 4th ed. Jones & Bartlett Learning, Burlington, MA. Available at: <https://search.ebscohost.com/login.aspx?direct=true&scope=site&db=nlebk&db=nlabk&AN=3387884>. **CIB 13.2,** Medical Journal of Australia (MJA), 2019. Getting it right: Validating a culturally specific screening tool for depression (a PHQ-9) in Aboriginal and Torres Strait Australians. Medical Journal of Australia 211 (1), 24–30. Available at: <https://www.mja.com.au/journal/2019/211/1/getting-it-right-validating-culturally-specific-screening-tool-depression-aphq-9>. **CIB 13.3,** Australian Institute of Family Studies (AIFS), 2022, LGBTIQA+ glossary of common terms CFCA Resource Sheet-February 2022, Australian Government, Australia. Available at <https://aifs.gov.au/resources/resource-sheets/lgbtiqa-glossary-common-terms>; State of Victoria, Australia, Department of Families, Fairness and Housing, 2022. Inclusive Victoria – State disability plan 2022–2026. Available at: <https://healthinfonet.ecu.edu.au/healthinfonet/getContent.php?linkid=677191&title=Inclusive+Victoria%3A+state+disability+plan+2022%E2%80%932026+&contentid=44880_1>; O'Shea, A., Latham, J., Beaver, S., et al., 2020. More than Ticking a Box: LGBTIQA+ People with disability talking about their lives. Geelong: Deakin University. Available at: <https://rainbowinclusion.org.au/wp-content/uploads/2022/12/More-than-ticking-a-Box.pdf>. **CIB 13.4,** Australian Institute of Family Studies (AIFS), 2022. LGBTIQA+ glossary of common terms CFCA Resource Sheet-February 2022, Australian Government, Australia. Available at <https://aifs.gov.au/resources/resource-sheets/lgbtiqa-glossary-common-terms>; Clendon, J., Munns, A., 2023. *Community health and wellness: Principles of primary health care*, 7th ed. Elsevier, Australia; O'Shea, A., Latham, J., Beaver, S., et al., 2020. More than ticking a box: LGBTIQA1 people with disability talking about their lives. Deakin University, Geelong. Available at: <https://rainbowinclusion.org.au/wp-content/uploads/2022/12/More-than-ticking-a-Box.pdf>; State of Victoria, Australia, Department of Families, Fairness and Housing, 2022. Inclusive Victoria – state disability plan 2022–2026. Available at: <https://healthinfonet.ecu.edu.au/healthinfonet/getContent.php?linkid5677191&title5Inclusive1Victoria%3A1state1disability1plan12022%E2%80%9320261&contentid544880_1>. **CIB 13.5,** Dune, T., McLeod, K., Williams, R. (eds.), 2021. *Culture, diversity and health in Australia: Towards culturally safe health care.* Taylor & Francis Group, Milton; Williams, D.R., Lawrence, J.A., Davis, B.A., 2019. Racism and public health: Evidence and needed research. *Annual Review of Public Health* 40, 105–15. Available at: <https://www.annualreviews.org/doi/pdf/10.1146/annurev-publhealth-040218-043750>. **CIB 13.6,** Dowling, A., Enticott, J., Kunin, M., et al., 2019. The association of migration experiences on the self-rated health status among adult humanitarian refugees to Australia: An analysis of a longitudinal cohort study. Available at: <https://equityhealthj.biomedcentral.com/articles/10.1186/s12939-019-1033-z>; NSW Health, 2019. Multicultural health week 2019: a focus on new and emerging communities. Available at: <https://www.health.nsw.gov.au/news/Pages/20190902_00.aspx>; Australian Bureau of Statistics (ABS), 2022. Cultural diversity: Census. Available at: <https://www.abs.gov.au/statistics/people/people-and-communities/cultural-diversity-census/2021>. **CIB 13.7,** NSW Health, 2019. Working with people from new and emerging communities. Available at: <https://www.mhcs.health.nsw.gov.au/events/multicultural-health-week/working-with-people-from-new-and-emerging-communities>. **CIB 13.8,** Dowling, A., Enticott, J., Kunin, M., et al., 2019. The association of migration experiences on the self-rated health status among adult humanitarian refugees to Australia: An analysis of a longitudinal cohort study. Available at: <https://equityhealthj.biomedcentral.com/articles/10.1186/s12939-019-1033-z>; UNHCR- The UN Refugee Agency, 2023. Refugee data Finder. Available at: <https://www.unhcr.org/refugee-statistics>. All Clinical Interest Boxes have had NSQHS Standards attached to each box – these are drawn from the main page given below some individual pages have been listed separately under the References list. Australian Commission on Safety and Quality in Health Care (ACSQHC) 2022c. The NSQHS Standards Available at: <https://www.safetyandquality.gov.au/standards/nsqhs-standards>. **CIB 14.1,** NAHSWP 1989, p. ix. **CIB 14.2,** Kidd, R., 2002. *Black lives, government lies.* UNSW Press, Sydney. **CIB 14.3,** Australian Government, Department of the Prime Minister and Cabinet, 2019. **CIB 15.1,** Crisp, J.C., Douglas, C., Rebeiro, G., et al. (eds), 2020. *Potter & Perry's fundamentals of nursing*, Australian ed, 6th ed. Elsevier, Sydney; Australian Commission on Safety and Quality in Health Care (ACSQHC), 2021. National safety and quality health service standards, 2nd ed. Available at: <https://www.safetyandquality.gov.au/sites/default/files/migrated/National-Safety-and-Quality-Health-Service-Standards-second-edition.pdf>. **CIB 15.2,** Lewis, P., Foley, D., 2020. *Health assessment in nursing*, Australian and New Zealand ed, 3rd ed. Wolters Kluwer, Macquarie Park, NSW. **CIB 15.3,** Berman, A., Kozier, B., Erb, G.L., 2021. *Kozier and Erb's fundamentals of nursing*, 5th ed. Pearson, Melbourne; Potter, P.A., Perry, A.G., Stockert, P.A., Hall, A., 2021. *Potter & Perry's essentials of nursing practice*, Sae, ebook. Elsevier Health Sciences. **CIB 15.4,** Perry, A. G., Potter, P. A., Ostendorf, W. R., Laplante, N., 2021. *Clinical nursing skills and techniques.* Elsevier Health Sciences. **CIB 15.5,** Department of Health, Government of Western Australia, nd. Advance health directives (AHD). Available at: <https://ww2.health.wa.gov.au/Articles/A_E/Advance-Health-Directives>; Department of Justice, Government of Western Australia, 2022. Advance health directives. Available at: <https://www.publicadvocate.wa.gov.au/A/advance_health_directives.aspx>. **CIBs 16.1, 16.2, 16.6, 16.7, 16.8,** Vafeas, C., Slatyer, S., 2021. *Gerontological nursing.* Elsevier Australia. **CIBs 16.3, 16.5,** Crisp, J., Douglas, C., Rebeiro, G., et al., 2021. *Potter & Perry's fundamentals of nursing*, 6th ed. Elsevier, Sydney. **CIB 16.9,** The Royal Children's Hospital, Melbourne, 2019. Clinical guidelines (nursing) temperature management. Available at: <https://www.rch.org.au/rchcpg/hospital_clinical_guideline_index/Temperature_management>. **CIB 16.10,** Australian Commission on Safety and Quality in Health Care (ACSQHC), 2022. Sepsis Clinical Care Standard. Available at: <https://www.safetyandquality.gov.au/standards/clinicalcare-standards/sepsis-clinical-care-standard>. **CIB 17.1,** Stern, T.A., Fava, M., Wilens, T.E. et al., 2016. *Massachusetts general hospital comprehensive clinical psychiatry*, 2nd ed. Elsevier, London. **CIBs 17.2, 17.3,** Brown, D., Buckley, T., Aitken, R., Edwards, H. 2023. *Lewis's medical-surgical nursing: Assessment and management of clinical problems.* Elsevier, Chatswood; Crisp, J., Douglas, C., Rebeiro, G., Waters, D., 2021. *Potter and Perry's fundamentals of nursing*, 6th ed. Elsevier, Chatswood. **CIB 17.4,** Barkemeyer, B., 2015. Discharge planning. *Pediatric Clinics of North America* 62(2), 545–556; Crisp, J., Douglas, C., Rebeiro, G., Waters, D., 2021. *Potter and Perry's fundamentals of nursing*, 6th ed. Elsevier, Chatswood; White, J., Plompen, R., Osadnik, C., et al., 2018. The experience of interpreter access and language discordant clinical encounters in Australian health care: A mixed methods exploration. *International Journal for Equity in Health* 17(1), 151. Available at: <https://equityhealthj.biomedcentral.com/articles/10.1186/s12939-018-0865-2>. **CIB 17.5,** Mental Health Commission, 2015. *Consumer handbook to the Mental Health Act 2014.* Available at: <https://www.mhc.wa.gov.au/media/1437/consumer-handbook-to-the-mental-health-act-2014-version-2-1.pdf>; Stern, T.A., Fava, M., Wilens, T.E. et al., 2016. *Massachusetts general hospital comprehensive clinical psychiatry*, 2nd ed. Elsevier, London. **CIB 17.6,** Brown, D., Buckley, T., Aitken, R., Edwards, H. 2023. *Lewis's medical-surgical nursing: Assessment and management of clinical problems.* Elsevier, Chatswood; Crisp, J., Douglas, C., Rebeiro, G., Waters, D., 2021. *Potter and Perry's fundamentals of nursing*, 6th ed. Elsevier, Chatswood; Australian Institute of Health and Welfare (AIHW), 2023. Elective surgery waiting times 2022–23: Australian hospital statistics. Available at: <https://www.aihw.gov.au/reportsdata/myhospitals/intersection/access/eswt>. **CIB 18.1,** Food Standards Australia New Zealand, 2023. Safe Food Australia, 4th ed. Available at: <https://www.foodstandards.gov.au/publications/pages/safefoodaustralia3rd16.aspx>; NSW Government, 2013. Guidelines for bringing occasional food for patients. Available at: <https://www.cclhd.health.nsw.gov.au/wp-content/uploads/Guidelines_for_Bringing_Occasional_Food_to_Patients.pdf>; Australian Capital Territory (ACT) Government, 2021. Guidelines for bringing food into hospital. 2021. Available at: <https://www.canberrahealthservices.act.gov.au/__data/assets/pdf_file/0009/1949670/Guidelines-for-bringing-food-to-hospital_Accessible_FA.pdf>. **CIB 18.2,** Modified from Crisp, J., Douglas, C., Rebeiro, G., et al. 2021. *Potter and*

Perry's fundamentals of nursing, 6th ed. Elsevier, Chatswood. **CIB 18.3,** Modified Harding, M., Kwong, J., Hagler, D., 2023. *Lewis's medical-surgical nursing: assessment and management of clinical problems*, 12th ed. Elsevier Health Sciences, St Louis. **CIB 18.4,** Modified from Health Vic 2015. Comprehensive health assessment of the older person. Available at: <https://www.health.vic.gov.au/residential-aged-care/comprehensive-health-assessment-of-the-older-person>; The Royal Children's Hospital Melbourne, 2022. Clinical guidelines: Nursing assessment. Available at: < http://www.rch.org.au/rchcpg/hospital_clinical_guideline_index/Nursing_Assessment>. **CIB 18.5,** National Health and Medical Research Council (NHMRC), 2019. Australian guidelines for the prevention and control of infection in healthcare. Available at: <https://www.nhmrc.gov.au/about-us/publications/australian-guidelines-prevention-and-control-infection-healthcare-2019>; Victorian Government. 2020. Coronavirus (COVID-19) Infection prevention and control guidelines. Available at: <https://www.health.vic.gov.au/covid-19/infection-prevention-control-resources-covid-19#infection-control-guidelines>. **CIB 18.6,** Adapted from Australian Commission on Safety and Quality in Health Care (ACSQHC), 2022. Guidance for Health Services Organisation: Covid-19 Infection Prevention and Control Risk Management. Available at: <https://www.safetyandquality.gov.au/covid-19>. **CIB 18.8,** Modified from Crisp, J., Douglas, C., Rebeiro, G., et al. 2021. *Potter and Perry's fundamentals of nursing*, 6th ed. Elsevier, Chatswood. **CIB 18.9,** Modified from National Health and Medical Research Council (NHMRC), 2019. Australian guidelines for the prevention and control of infection in healthcare. **CIB 19.2,** Hill, R., Hall, H., Glew, P., 2022. *Fundamentals of nursing and midwifery*, 4th ed. Lippincott Williams and Wilkins, North Ryde. **CIB 20.1,** Adapted from Touhy, T.A., Jett, K.F., 2020. *Ebersole & Hess' toward healthy ageing: Human needs & nursing response*, 10th ed. Elsevier, St Louis. **CIB 20.2,** Broyles, B., Reiss, B., Evans, M., et al., 2019. *Pharmacology in nursing* – Australian and New Zealand ed, 3rd ed. Cengage Learning Australia, Melbourne; Knights, K., Darroch, S., Rowland, A., et al., 2023. *Pharmacology for health professionals*, 6th ed. Elsevier, Sydney; Ritter, J.M., Flower, R.J., Henderson, G., et al., 2023. *Rang and Dale's pharmacology*, 10th ed. Elsevier, Spain. **CIB 20.3,** Frotjold, A., Bloomfield, J. 2021. Medication therapy. In: Crisp, J., Douglas, C., Rebeiro, G., et al. (eds.), *Potter and Perry's fundamentals of nursing*, ANZ ed. 6th ed. Elsevier, Chatswood; Broyles, B., Reiss, B., Evans, M., et al., 2019. *Pharmacology in nursing*, Australian and New Zealand edition, 3rd ed. Cengage Learning Australia, Melbourne. **CIB 20.4,** Frotjold, A., Bloomfield, J. 2021. Medication therapy. In: Crisp, J., Douglas, C., Rebeiro, G., et al. (eds.), *Potter and Perry's fundamentals of nursing*, ANZ ed. 6th ed. Elsevier, Chatswood; Department of Health and Wellbeing, Government of South Australia, 2023. South Australian Paediatric Clinical Practice Guidelines. Available at: <https://www.sahealth.sa.gov.au/wps/wcm/connect/fbce826b-e137-4716-a2c0-72c7e70a0e3c/Intravenous+%28IV%29+Fluid+Management+in+Children_Paed_v1_0.pdf?MOD=AJPERES&CACHEID=ROOTWORKSPACE-fbce826b-e137-4716-a2c0-72c7e70a0e3c-ocQI.X2>; Kliegman, R.E., St Geme, J.W., et al. (eds.), 2019. *Nelson textbook of pediatrics*, 21st ed. Elsevier, US. **CIBs 20.5, 20.6, Adapted** from Frotjold, A., Bloomfield, J., 2021. Medication therapy. In: Crisp, J., Douglas, C., Rebeiro, G., et al. (eds.), *Potter and Perry's fundamentals of nursing*, ANZ ed. 6th ed. Elsevier, Chatswood; Broyles, B., Reiss, B., Evans, M., et al., 2019. *Pharmacology in nursing*, Australian and New Zealand ed, 3rd ed. Cengage Learning Australia, Melbourne. **CIB 21.2,** Australian Institute of Health and Welfare (AIHW), 2020. Overweight and obesity among Australian children and adolescents. Available at: <https://www.aihw.gov.au/reports/overweight-obesity/overweight-obesity-australian-children-adolescents/summary>; Australian Institute of Health and Welfare (AIHW), 2023. Overweight and obesity. Available at: <https://www.aihw.gov.au/reports/overweight-obesity/overweight-and-obesity/contents/about>. **CIB 21.3,** Department of Health and Aged Care, 2022. The national obesity strategy 2022–2032. Available at: <https://www.health.gov.au/sites/default/files/documents/2022/03/national-obesity-strategy-2022-2032_0.pdf>. **CIB 21.4,** Hockenberry, M.J., Wilson, D., Rodgers, C.C., 2022. *Wong's essentials of paediatric nursing*, 11th ed. Mosby, St Louis. **CIB 22.1,** L Leifer, G., 2023. *Introduction to maternity and pediatric nursing*, 9th ed. WB Saunders, Philadelphia. **CIB 22.2,** Australian Institute of Health and Welfare (AIHW), 2020. Overweight and obesity among Australian children and adolescents. Available at: <https://www.aihw.gov.au/reports/overweight-obesity/overweight-obesity-australian-children-adolescents/summary>. **CIBs 24.1, 24.2, 24.4, 24.5, 24.12, 24.17,** Crisp, J., Douglas, C., Rabeiro, G., et al., 2021. *Potter and Perry's fundamentals of nursing*, 6th ed. Elsevier, Australia; Eliopoulos, C., 2021. *Gerontological nursing*, 10th ed. Lippincott Williams & Wilkins, Philadelphia. **CIBs 24.3, 24.9,** 24.13, Crisp, J., Douglas, C., Rabeiro, G., et al., 2021. *Potter and Perry's fundamentals of nursing*, 6th ed. Elsevier, Australia. **CIB 24.6,** Bub, L., 2019. Loss and end-of-life issues. In: Meiner, S.E., Yeager, J.J. (eds.). *Gerontologic nursing*, 6th ed. Elsevier, St Louis. **CIB 24.7,** Dementia Australia, 2023. Available at: <https://www.dementia.org.au>. **CIB 24.10,** Aged Care Quality and Safety Commission. Available at: <https://wwwagedcarequality.gov.au/older-australians/safety-care/minimising-restrictive-practices. **CIB 24.14,** Roberts, H., Lim, S., Cox, N., Ibrahim, K., 2019. The challenge of managing undernutrition in older people with frailty. *Nutrients* 11, 808. doi:10.3390/nu11040808; Murphy, J., 2022. Prevention, identification and management of malnutrition in older people in the community. *Nursing Standard* 37(8), 75–81. doi: 10.7748/ns.2022.e11891.

PMID: 35786674. **CIB 24.15,** Williams, P., 2021. *Fundamental concepts and skills for nursing*, 6th ed. WB Saunders, Philadelphia. **CIB 24.16,** Adapted from Molloy, W., 2014. Standardised mini-mental state examination (SMMSE)—Guidelines for administration and scoring instructions. Independent Hospital Pricing Authority, Commonwealth of Australia. Available at: <https://www.ihpa.gov.au/sites/g/files/net636/f/publications/smmse-guidelines-v2.pdf>; © Commonwealth of Australia 2014. **CIB 25.2,** Boltz, M. (ed.) 2021. *Evidence-based geriatric nursing protocols for best practice*, 6th ed. Springer Publishing Company, New York, New York. **CIB 25.3,** World Health Organization (WHO), 2020. A guide to EHO's Guidance on COVID-19. WHO, Geneva. Available at: <https://www.who.int/emergencies/diseases/novel-coronavirus-2019/technical-guidance>. **CIB 25.4,** Perry, A.G., Potter, P.A., Ostendorf, W., Laplante, N., 2022. *Nursing interventions and clinical skills*, 10th ed. Elsevier Inc, St Louis. **CIB 25.5,** Crisp, J., Douglas, C., Rebeiro, G., et al. (eds.), 2021. *Potter and Perry's fundamentals of nursing*, 6th ed. Elsevier, Australia and New Zealand, New South Wales. **CIB 25.6,** Perry, A.G., Potter, P.A., Ostendorf, W., Laplante, N., 2022. *Nursing interventions and clinical skills*, 10th ed. Elsevier Inc, St Louis. **CIB 26.1,** Hall, H., Glew, P., Rhodes, J., 2022. *Fundamentals of nursing and midwifery: A person-centred approach to care*, 4th ANZ ed. Lippincott Williams & Wilkins, Sydney. **CIB 26.2,** LeMone, P., Bauldoff, G., Gubrud-Howe, P., et al., 2020. *Medical–surgical nursing: Critical thinking in person-centred care*, 4th ed. Pearson, Australia; Schub, T., Oji, O., 2018. Hydration: Maintaining oral hydration in older adults. CINAHL Nursing Guide. Evidence-Based Care Sheet, T700987. **CIB 26.5,** Ashraf, M., Rea, R., 2017. Effect of dehydration on blood tests. *Practical Diabetes* 34(5), 169–171. Available at: <https://doi.org/10.1002/pdi.2111>; Brown, D., Edwards, H., Buckley, T., et al., 2020. *Lewis's medical–surgical nursing. Assessment and management of clinical problems*, 5th ed. Elsevier, Sydney; Crisp, J., Douglas, C., Rebeiro, G., et al. (eds.), 2021. *Potter and Perry's fundamentals of nursing*, 6th ed. Elsevier. **CIB 26.6,** Banasik, J., 2022. *Pathophysiology*, 7th ed. Elsevier, St Louis; Brown, D., Edwards, H., Buckley, T., et al., 2020. *Lewis's medical–surgical nursing. Assessment and management of clinical problems*, 5th ed. Elsevier, Sydney; Crisp, J., Douglas, C., Rebeiro, G., et al. (eds.), 2021. *Potter and Perry's fundamentals of nursing*, 6th ed. Elsevier. **CIB 26.7,** Brown, D., Edwards, H., Buckley, T., et al., 2020. *Lewis's medical–surgical nursing. Assessment and management of clinical problems*, 5th ed. Elsevier, Sydney; Kear, T.M., 2017. Fluid and electrolyte management across the age continuum. *Nephrology Nursing Journal* 44(6) 491–497. **CIB 26.8,** Kear, T.M., 2017. Fluid and electrolyte management across the age continuum. *Nephrology Nursing Journal* 44(6), 491–497. **CIB 26.9,** Brown, D., Edwards, H., Buckley, T., et al., 2020. *Lewis's medical–surgical nursing. Assessment and management of clinical problems*, 5th ed. Elsevier, Sydney; Kear, T.M., 2017. Fluid and electrolyte management across the age continuum. *Nephrology Nursing Journal* 44(6) 491–497. **CIB 26.13,** Knight, B.P., Waseem, M,. 2023. Pediatric Fluid Management. In: StatPearls [Internet]. Treasure Island (FL): StatPearls Publishing; 2023 Jan-. Available at: <https://www.ncbi.nlm.nih.gov/books/NBK560540>. **CIB 26.14,** Australian Commission for Safety and Quality in Health Care (ACSQHC), 2021. Management of peripheral intravenous catheters clinical care standard. Available at: <https://www.safetyandquality.gov.au/standards/clinical-care-standards/management-peripheral-intravenous-catheters-clinical-care-standard>; Williams, L.S., Hopper, P.D., 2019. *Understanding medical surgical nursing*, 6th ed. F.A. Davis Company, Philadelphia. **CIB 26.18,** Sommers, M.S., 2023. *Davis's diseases and disorders: A nursing therapeutics manual*, 7th ed. F.A. Davis Company, Philadelphia. **CIB 27.1,** Adapted from Berman, A., Snyder, S.J., Levett-Jones, T., et al., 2020. *Kozier and Erb's fundamentals of nursing*, 5th ed. Pearson, Melbourne; Cooper, K., Gosnell, K., 2022. *Foundations and adult nursing*, 18th ed. Elsevier, St Louis; Gordon, C., 2021. *Fostering sleep*. In: Crisp, J., Douglas, C., Rebeiro, G., et al. (eds.), *Potter and Perry's fundamentals of nursing*, 6th ed. Elsevier, Australia. **CIBs 27.2, 27.4, 27.10,** Adapted from Cooper, K., Gosnell, K., 2022. Foundations and adult nursing, 18th ed. Elsevier, St Louis; Gordon, C., 2021. Fostering sleep. In: Crisp, J., Douglas, C., Rebeiro, G., e t al. (eds.), *Potter and Perry's fundamentals of nursing*, 6th ed. Elsevier, Australia. **CIBs 27.3, 27.15,** Adapted from Berman, A., Snyder, S.J., Levett-Jones, T., et al., 2020. *Kozier and Erb's fundamentals of nursing*, 5th ed. Pearson, Melbourne. **CIBs 27.5, 27.6, 27.12, 27.13,** Gordon, C., 2021. Fostering sleep. In: Crisp, J., Douglas, C., Rebeiro, G., et al. (eds.), *Potter and Perry's fundamentals of nursing*, 6th ed. Elsevier, Australia. **CIB 27.8,** Cooper, K., Gosnell, K., 2022. *Foundations and adult nursing*, 8th ed. Elsevier, St Louis. Gordon, C., 2021 Fostering sleep. In: Crisp, J., Douglas, C., Rebeiro, G., et al. (eds.), *Potter and Perry's fundamentals of nursing*, 6th ed. Elsevier, Australia. **CIB 27.9** Sleep Health Foundation, 2023. Shiftwork. Available at: <https://www.sleephealthfoundation.org.au/shiftwork.html>. **CIB 27.11,** Cooper, K., Gosnell, K., 2022. *Foundations and adult nursing*, 8th ed. Elsevier, St Louis. Gordon, C., 2021. Fostering sleep. In: Crisp, J., Douglas, C., Rebeiro, G., et al. (eds.), *Potter and Perry's fundamentals of nursing*, 6th ed. Elsevier, Australia; Tiziani, A., 2022. Harvard's nursing guide to drugs, 11th ed. Elsevier, Sydney. **CIB 27.14,** Adapted from Gordon, C., 2021. Fostering sleep. In: Crisp, J., Douglas, C., Rebeiro, G., et al. (eds.), *Potter and Perry's fundamentals of nursing*, 6th ed. Elsevier, Australia. **CIB 28.1,** Adapted from Marieb, E. N., Keller, S.M., 2022. *Essentials of human anatomy & physiology*, 13th ed. Pearson, New York; Patton, K. T., Thibodeau, G. A., 2019. *Anatomy and physiology*, 10th ed. Mosby Elsevier, St Louis. CIB 28.2, Adapted from Marieb, E.N., Keller, S.M., 2022. *Essentials of human* *anatomy and physiology*, 13th ed. Pearson, New York. **CIB 28.3,** Adapted from Goldman, L., Schafer, A.I., 2019. *Goldman-Cecil medicine*, 26th ed. Elsevier Saunders, New York. **CIB 28.4,** Adapted from Crisp, J., Douglas, C., Rebeiro, G., et al., 2021. *Potter and Perry's fundamentals of nursing*, Australian ed, 6th ed. Elsevier, Sydney. **CIB 29.1,** Ahangar, P., Woodward, M., Cowin, A.J., 2018. Advanced wound therapies. *Wound Practice & Research* 26(2), 55–68; Wu, S., Carter, M., Cole, W., et al, 2023. Best practice for wound repair and regeneration: Use of cellular, acellular and matrix-like products (CAMPs). *Journal of Wound Care* 32(4 suppl B), S1–S32. **CIB 29.2,** Haesler, E., Carville, K., 2023. *Australian standards for wound prevention and management*, 4th ed. Australian Health Research Alliance, Wounds Australia and WA Health Translation Network. **CIB 29.3,** International Wound Infection Institute (IWII), 2022. *Wound infection in clinical practice: Principles of best practice.* Wounds International. Available at: <https://woundinfection-institute.com/wp-content/uploads/IWII-CD-2022-web-1.pdf>. **CIB 29.4,** Adapted from International Wound Infection Institute (IWII), 2022. *Wound infection in clinical practice: Principles of best practice.* Wounds International. Available at: <https://woundinfection-institute.com/wp-content/uploads/IWII-CD-2022-web-1.pdf>; Australian Commission on Safety and Quality in Health Care (ACSQHC), 2023. Antimicrobial stewardship. Available at: <https://www.safetyandquality.gov.au/our-work/antimicrobial-stewardship>. **CIB 29.5,** Carville, K., 2023. *Wound care manual*, 8th ed. Silver Chain Nursing Association, Perth, West Australia; International Wound Infection Institute (IWII), 2022. *Wound infection in clinical practice: Principles of best practice.* Wounds International. Available at: <https://woundinfection-institute.com/wp-content/uploads/IWII-CD-2022-web-1.pdf>. **CIB 29.6,** Holman, M., 2023. Using tap water compared with normal saline for cleansing wounds in adults: A literature review of the evidence. *Journal of Wound Care* 32(8), 507–512; Sibbald, R.G., Elliot, J.A., Persaud-Jaimangal, R., et al., 2021. Wound Bed Preparation 2021. *Advances in Skin & Wound Care* 34(4), 183–195; Weir, D., Swanson, T., 2019. Back to basics: Clean it like you man it! International Wound Infection Institute Newsletter, May 2019. **CIB 29.7,** Carville, K., 2023. *Wound care manual*, 8th ed. Silver Chain Nursing Association, Perth, West Australia. **CIB 29.8,** Adapted from European Pressure Ulcer Advisory Panel (EPUAP), National Pressure Injury Advisory Panel (NPIAP) and Pan Pacific Pressure Injury Alliance (PPIA), Haesler, E. (ed.), 2019. *Prevention and treatment of pressure ulcers/injuries: Clinical practice guidelines*, 3rd ed. EPUAP/NPIAP/PPPIA. **CIB 29.9,** Finch, K., Osseiran-Moisson, R., Carville, K., et al., 2018. Skin tear prevention in elderly patients using twice-daily moisturiser. *Wound Practice and Research* 26(2), 99–109. **CIB 29.10,** Australian Commission on Safety and Quality in Health Care (ACSQHC), 2017. Approaches to Surgical Site Infection Surveillance. Available at: <https://www.safetyandquality.gov.au/sites/default/files/2019-06/approaches-to-surgical-site-infection-surveillance.pdf>; The-Association for Safe Aseptic Practice (The-ASAP), 2019. Aseptic Non Touch Technique (ANTT), The ANTT clinical practice framework V4.0. Available at: <https://www.antt.org/antt-practice-framework.html>. **CIB 30.1,** Ferri, F. 2022. Clinical overview: Constipation in older adults. Available at: <https://clinicalkey.com.au>. **CIB 30.2,** Ayerbe, J., Hauser, B., Salvatore, S., Vandenplas, V., 2019. Diagnosis and management of gastroesophageal reflux disease in infants and children: From guidelines to clinical practice. *Pediatric Gastroenterology, Hepatology & Nutrition* 22(2), 107–121; Tang, M., Adolphe, S., Rogers, S., Frank, D., 2021. Failure to thrive or growth faltering: Medical, developmental/behavioural, nutritional, and social dimensions. *Pediatrics in Review* 42(11), 590–603. Available at: <https://doi.org/10.5223/pghn.2019.22.2.107>. **CIB 30.3,** Agarwal, E., Ferguson, M., Banks, M., et al., 2010. Nutritional status and dietary intake of acute care patients: results from the Australasian day survey. *Clinical Nutrition* 31, 41–47; Woodward, T., Josephson, C., Ross, L. et al., 2020. A retrospective study of the incidence and characteristics of long-stay adult inpatients with hospital-acquired malnutrition across five Australian public hospitals. *European Journal of Clinical Nutrition* 74, 1668–1676. Available at: <https://doi.org/10.1038/s41430-020-0648-x>. **CIB 30.4,** Garofolo, A., Qiao, L., dos Santos Maia-Lemos, P,. 2020. Approach to nutrition in cancer patients in the context of the coronavirus disease 2019 (COVID-19) pandemic: Perspectives. *Nutrition and Cancer* 73(8), 1293–1301. Available at: <https://doi.org/10.1080/01635581.2020.1797126>; Holdoway, A. 2020 Nutritional management of patients during and after COVID-19 illness. *British Journal of Community Nursing* 25(Sup8), S6–S10. doi: 10.12968/bjcn.2020.25.Sup8.S6; Tsagari, A., Kyriazis, I., 2021 Nutritional care of the COVID-19 patient. *International Journal of Caring Sciences* 14(1), 794–799; World Health Organization (WHO) 2023. Timeline: WHO's COVID-19 response. Available at <https://www.who.int/emergencies/diseases/novel-coronavirus-2019/interactive-timeline#!>. **CIB 31.1,** Adapted from Continence Foundation of Australia, 2023. Continence in Australia: a snapshot. Continence Foundation of Australia, Melbourne. Available at: <https://continence.org.au/data/files/Reports/Continence_in_Australia_Snapshot.pdf>. **CIB 31.2,** Department of Health and Aged Care, 2022. National aged care mandatory quality indicator program (QI) program manual 3.0 – Part A. Commonwealth of Australia. **CIB 31.3,** Adapted from Cooper, K., Gosnell, K., 2023. *Adult health nursing*. 9th ed. Elsevier. **CIB 32.1,** Crisp, J., Douglas, C., Rebeiro, G., et al., 2021. *Potter and Perry's fundamentals of nursing*, 6th ed. Elsevier, Sydney. **CIB 32.2,** Williams, P., 2021. *Fundamental concepts and skills for nursing*, 6th ed. Elsevier, St Louis. **CIBs 33.1, 33.2,** Crisp, J., Douglas, C., Rebeiro, G., et al., 2021. *Potter and Perry's fundamentals of nursing*, 6th ed. Elsevier,

Sydney. **CIB 33.3,** Schofield, P., 2018. The assessment of pain in older people: UK national guidelines. *Age and Ageing* 47(1), i1–i22. doi: 10.1093/ageing/afx192. **CIB 33.4, Craft**, J., Gordon, C., Heuther, S., et al., 2023. *Understanding pathophysiology*, 4th ed. Elsevier, Sydney. **CIB 33.5,** Knights, K., et al., 2023. *Pharmacology for health professionals*, 6th ed. Elsevier, Sydney. **CIBs 34.1, 34.2,** Crisp, J., Douglas, C., Rebeiro, G., et al., 2020. *Potter and Perry's fundamentals of nursing*, 6th ed. Elsevier, Sydney; Brown, D., Edwards, H., Buckley, T., et al., 2020. *Lewis's medical-surgical nursing*, 5th ed. Elsevier, Sydney. **CIB 34.3,** Berman, A., Franden, G., Snyder, S., et al. 2021. *Kozier and Erb's fundamentals of nursing*, 5th ed. Pearson Australia, Melbourne. **CIB 34.4,** Crisp, J., Douglas, C., Rebeiro, G., et al., 2020. *Potter and Perry's fundamentals of nursing*, 6th ed. Elsevier, Sydney; Brown, D., Edwards, H., Buckley, T., et al., 2020. *Lewis's medical-surgical nursing*, 5th ed. Elsevier, Sydney; *McCance & Huether's pathophysiology*, 9th ed. Copyright © 2023, 2019, 2014, 2010, 2006, 2002, 1998, 1994, 1990 Elsevier, Missouri. **CIB 34.5,** Glaucoma Australia, 2023. What Is Glaucoma?. Available at: <http://www.glaucoma.org.au>. **CIB 34.7,** Perry, A., Potter, P., Ostendorf, W., 2020. *Nursing interventions and nursing clinical skills: Care of the eye and ear*, 7th ed. Elsevier, St Louis, Ch. 12, pp. 283–298. **CIBs 35.1, 35.2,** 35.5, LeMone, P., Burke, K., Dwyer, T., et al., 2017. *Medical–surgical nursing. Critical thinking in person-centred care*, 4th ed. Pearson, Frenchs Forest. **CIB 35.3,** Crisp, J., Douglas, C., Rebeiro, G., et al. (eds.), *Potter and Perry's fundamentals of nursing*, 5th ed. Elsevier, Chatswood. **CIB 35.6,** Independent Living Centre NSW, 2017. Assistive technology. Available at: <https://at-aust.org/home/assistive_technology/assistive_technology>. **CIB 36.1,** Crawford, A. H., 2023. Endocrine problems. In: Harding, M. M., Kwong, J., Hagler, D., et al., *Lewis's medical-surgical nursing*, 12th ed. Elsevier, St Louis; Medical News Today 2023. What is the difference between hypothyroidism and hyperthyroidism? Available at: <https://www.medicalnewstoday.com/articles/hypothroidism-vs-hyperthyroidism>; National Institute of Diabetes and Digestive and Kidney Diseases (NIDDK), 2021b. Hyperthyroidism (Overactive thyroid). Available at: <https://www.niddk.nih.gov/health-information/endocrine-diseases/hyperthyroidism>. **CIB 36.2,** Crawford, A. H., 2023. Endocrine problems. In: Harding, M. M., Kwong, J., Hagler, D., et al., *Lewis's medical-surgical nursing*, 12th ed. Elsevier, St Louis; Johns Hopkins Medicine 2023. Cushing's Syndrome. Available at: <https://www.hopkinsmedicine.org/health/conditions-and-diseases/cushings-syndrome>; Waugh, A., Grant, A., 2022. *Ross & Wilson anatomy and physiology in health and illness*, 14th ed. Elsevier, Glasgow. **CIB 36.3,** Crawford, A. H., 2023. Endocrine problems. In: Harding, M. M., Kwong, J., Hagler, D., et al., *Lewis's medical-surgical nursing*, 12th ed. Elsevier, St Louis; Waugh, A., Grant, A., 2022. *Ross & Wilson Anatomy and physiology in health and illness*, 14th ed. Elsevier, Glasgow. **CIB 36.4,** Craft, J., Gordon, C., McCance, K.L., et al., 2023. *Understanding pathophysiology*, Australia and New Zealand ed, 4th ed. Elsevier, Chatswood; Crawford, A.H., 2023. Endocrine problems. In: Harding, M.M., Kwong, J., Hagler, D., et al., *Lewis's medical-surgical nursing*, 12th ed. Elsevier, St Louis; Endocrine Society of Australia, 2023. Polycystic ovarian syndrome (PCOS). Available at: <www.hormones-australia.org.au/endocrine-diseases/polycyctic-ovarian-syndrome-pcos>. **CIB 36.5,** Dickinson, J.K., 2023. Diabetes in Lewis's medical-surgical nursing, 12th ed. Elsevier: Australia. Miller, B., 2022. Diabetes Mellitus – Pathophysiology in Pathophysiology, 7th ed. Elsevier, United States. National Diabetes Services Scheme (NDSS), 2022. Continuous glucose monitoring, Available at: <https://www.ndss.com.au/wp-content/uploads/fact-sheets-continuous-glucose-monitoring.pdf>. **CIB 37.1,** Adapted from Healthy Male, 2021. Testicular cancer. Available at: <https://www.healthymale.org.au/mens-health/testicular-cancer>. **CIB 37.2,** Hechtman, L., 2019. *Clinical naturopathic medicine*, 2nd ed. Elsevier, Chatswood. **CIB 37.3,** Blackburn, S.T., 2018. *Maternal, fetal & neonatal* physiology, 5th ed. Elsevier, St Louis. **CIB 37.4,** Lab Tests Online, 2022. Human chorionic gonadotropin. Available at <https://www.labtestsonline.org.au/learning/test-index/hcg>. **CIB 37.6,** HPV Vaccine, 2023. The HPV vaccine program. Available at < http://www.hpvvaccine.org.au/the-hpv-vaccine/has-the-program-been-successful.aspx>. **CIB 37.8,** Cancer Council NSW, 2022. Breast cancer. Available at <https://www.cancercouncil.com.au/breast-cancer>.**CIB 37.9,** Cancer Council Australia, 2023. Cervical cancer. Available at <https://www.cancer.org.au/about-cancer/types-of-cancer/cervical-cancer.html#jump_3>. **CIB 38.1,** Palliative Care Australia 2022. National palliative care standards for all health professionals and aged care services. Available at: <https://palliativecare.org.au/publication/national-palliative-care-standards-for-all-health-professionals-and-aged-care-services>. **CIB 38.2,** Based on Palliative Care Australia, 2022. National palliative care standards for all health professionals and aged care services. Available at: <https://palliativecare.org.au/publication/national-palliative-care-standards-for-all-health-professionals-and-aged-care-services>. **CIB 38.3,** World Health Organization, 2019. WHO definition of palliative care. Available < http://www.who.int/cancer/palliative/definition/en>. **CIB 38.7,** Based on Sinha, A., Deshwal, H., Vashisht, R., 2023. End-of-life evaluation and management of pain. In: StatPearls [Internet]. Treasure Island (FL): StatPearls Publishing. PMID: 33760512. **CIB 39.1,** Hercelinskyj, G., Alexander, L., 2022. *Mental health nursing*, enhanced edition, 1st ed. Cengage; LGBTIQ1 Health Australia, 2023. Available at: <www.lgbtiqhealth.org.au>. **CIB 39.2,** American Psychiatric Association, 2022. *Diagnostic and statistical manual of mental disorders*, 5th ed. Text revision. American Psychiatric Association, Washington, USA; National Alliance on Mental Illness, 2023. Available at: <www.nami.org>;

Hercelinskyj, G., Alexander, L., 2022. *Mental health nursing*, enhanced edition, 1st ed. **CIB 39.3,** Australian Institute of Family Studies (AIFS), 2022. Understanding the mental health and help-seeking behaviours of refugees. Available at: <https://aifs.gov.au/resources/shortarticles/understanding-mental-health-and-help-seekingbehaviours-refugees#:~:text=For%20a%20range%20of%20reasons,is%20low%20and%2For%20problematic>; Foster, K., Marks, P., O'Brien, A., Raeburn, T., 2020. *Mental health in nursing – Theory and practice for clinical settings*. Elsevier; Hungerford, C., Hodgson, D., Clancy, R., et al., 2020. *Mental health care: An introduction for health professionals*, 4th ed. Wiley, China.; Steele, D. 2023. *Keltner's psychiatric nursing*, 9th ed. Elsevier. **CIBs 39.4, 39.6, 39.8, 39.9, 39.12,** Foster, K., Marks, P., O'Brien, A., Raeburn, T., 2020. *Mental health in nursing – Theory and practice for clinical settings*. Elsevier; Hungerford, C., Hodgson, D., Clancy, R., et al., 2020. *Mental health care: An introduction for health professionals*, 4th ed. Wiley, China.; Steele, D. 2023. *Keltner's psychiatric nursing*, 9th ed. Elsevier. **CIB 39.5,** Hercelinskyj, G., Alexander, L., 2022. *Mental health nursing*, enhanced edition, 1st ed. Cengage; Foster, K., Marks, P., O'Brien, A., Raeburn, T., 2020. *Mental health in nursing – Theory and practice for clinical settings*. Elsevier. **CIBs 39.7** Foster, K., Marks, P., O'Brien, A., Raeburn, T., 2020. *Mental health in nursing – Theory and practice for clinical settings*. Elsevier; Hungerford, C., Hodgson, D., Clancy, R., et al., 2020. *Mental health care: An introduction for health professionals*, 4th ed. Wiley, China.; Steele, D. 2023. *Keltner's psychiatric nursing*, 9th ed. Elsevier; Beyond Blue: <https://www.beyondblue.org.au>. **CIB 39.10,** Dementia Australia, 2018. Dementia statistics. Australian Government Department of Social Services. Available at: <https://www.dementia.org.au/statistics>. **CIB 39.11,** Hercelinskyj, G., Alexander, L., 2022. *Mental health nursing*, enhanced edition, 1st ed. Cengage. **CIB 39.13,** Halter, M.J., 2017. *Varcarolis' foundations of psychiatric mental health nursing*, 8th ed. Elsevier, USA. **CIB 40.3,** Brown, D., Edwards, H., Buckley, T. et al. 2020. *Lewis's medical-surgical nursing*, ANZ ed, 5th ed. Elsevier; Chang, E., Johnson, A., 2022. *Living with chronic illness & disability: Principles for nursing practice*, 4th ed. Elsevier, Chatswood; Cifu, D., 2020. Braddom's physical medicine and rehabilitation, 6th ed. Elsevier, Philadelphia. **CIB 40.5,** Brown, D., Edwards, H., Buckley, T. et al. 2020. *Lewis's medical-surgical nursing*, ANZ, 5th ed. Elsevier; Crisp, J., Douglas, C., Rebeiro, G., et al. (eds.), 2021. *Potter and Perry's fundamentals of nursing*, 6th ed. Elsevier, Sydney. **CIB 40.6,** Labeit, B., Ahring, S., Boehmer, M. et al. 2022. Comparison of simultaneous swallowing endoscopy and videofluoroscopy in neurogenic dysphagia. *Journal of the American Medical Directors Association* 23(8), 1360–1366. doi: 10.1016/j.jamda.2021.09.026. **CIB 41.1,** Pederson, C.L., Gorman-Ezell, K., Brookings, J.B., 2020. Psychological distress among postural tachycardia syndrome patients in the Fennell Crisis phase. *Fatigue: Biomedicine, Health & Behavior* 8(2), 108–118. **CIB 41.2,** Livneh, H., 2022. Psychosocial adaptation to chronic illness and disability: An updated and expanded conceptual framework. *Rehabilitation Counseling Bulletin* 65(3), 171–184; Van Wilder, L., Pype, P., Mertens, F., et al., 2021. Living with a chronic disease: insights from patients with a low socioeconomic status. *BMC Family Practice* 22, 1–11. **CIB 41.3,** Livneh, H., 2022. Psychosocial adaptation to chronic illness and disability: An updated and expanded conceptual framework. *Rehabilitation Counseling Bulletin* 65(3), 171–184. **CIB 41.4,** Agaronnik, N., Campbell, E.G., Ressalam, J., Iezzoni, L.I., 2019. Communicating with patients with disability: Perspectives of practicing physicians. *Journal of General Internal Medicine* 34, 1139–1145; Australian Federation of Disability Organisations, 2023. Communication with people with disabilities. Available at: <https://www.afdo.org.au/resource-communication-withpeople-with-disabilities>. **CIB 41.5**, Francisco, M.P.B., Hartman, M., Wang, Y., 2020. Inclusion and special education. *Education Sciences* 10(9), 238; Collins, A., Rentschler, R., Williams, K., Azmat, F., 2022. Exploring barriers to social inclusion for disabled people: Perspectives from the performing arts. *Journal of Management & Organization* 28(2), 308–3028; Maguire-Rosier, 2016; Dimov, S., Devine, A., Shields, M., et al., 2022. Improving disability employment study (IDES): Methods of data collection and characteristics of study sample; Macleod, K., Kamruzzaman, L., Musselwhite, C., 2022. Transport and health equity, social inclusion and exclusion. *Journal of Transport & Health* 27, 101543; Australian Building Codes Board, 2022. Access for people with a disability. Available at: <https://ncc.abcb.gov.au/editions/2019-a1/ncc-2019-volume-one-amendment-1/section-d-access-and-egress/part-d3-access-people>; Australian Communications and Media Authority, 2023. Available at: <https://www.acma.gov.au/compliance-priorities>. **CIB 41.6,** Chang, E., Johnson, A., 2021. *Living with chronic illness and disability: Principles for nursing practice*. Elsevier Health Sciences; Gutenbrunner, C., Stievano, A., Nugraha, B., et al., 2022. Nursing–a core element of rehabilitation. *International Nursing Review* 69(1), 13–19. **CIB 41.7,** McCormack, B., McCance, T., Bulley, C., et al., 2021. *Fundamentals of person-centred healthcare practice*. John Wiley & Sons. **CIB 41.8,** Germani, A. C.C.G., de Mello Cahú, F.G., Miranda, F.E.S., et al., 2022. Health promotion to people with disabilities: Case report from two university extension projects. *Research, Society and Development* 11(1), e56111124956–e56111124956; Rural Heath Information Hub, 2023. Health promotion and disease prevention in rural communities. Available at: <https://www.ruralhealthinfo.org/toolkits/health-promotion/1/introduction>. **CIBs 42.1, 42.2,** LeMone, P., Bauldoff, G., Gubrud-Howe, P., et al., 2020. Medical–surgical nursing: critical thinking in person-centred care, 4th ed. Pearson, Melbourne. **CIB 42.3,** Brown, D., Edwards, H., Buckley, T., Aitken, R., 2024. Lewis's medical-surgical nursing, 6th ed. Elsevier; The Royal Children's Hospital Melbourne, 2020. Central venous access device management. Available at: <https://www.rch.org.au/policy/public/Central_Venous_Access_Device_Management>. **CIBs 42.4,** Berman, A., Frandsen, G., Snyder, S., et al., 2020. *Kozier and Erb's fundamentals of nursing*, 5th ed. Pearson, Melbourne. **CIB 42.5,** Sutherland-Fraser, S., Davies, M., Gillespie, B. M., Lockwood, B., 2022. *Perioperative nursing: An introduction*, 3rd ed. Elsevier, Sydney. **CIB 42.6,** Images: Courtesy of Cardinal Health. © 2007 Cardinal Health. All rights reserved. © Bellovac. © Surimex; Berman, A., Frandsen, G., Snyder, S., et al., 2020. *Kozier and Erb's fundamentals of nursing*, 5th ed. Pearson, Melbourne. **CIB 43.1,** Peran, D., Kodet, J., Pekara, J., et al., 2020. ABCDE cognitive aid tool in patient assessment – development and validation in a multicenter pilot simulation study. *BMC Emergency Medicine* 20(1), 95. Available at: <https://doi.org/10.1186/s12873-020-00390-3>; Resuscitation Council UK, 2024. The ABCDE approach. Available at: <https://www.resus.org.uk/library/abcdeapproach>. **CIB 43.2,** SA Health, 2020. Rapid detection and response observation charts. Department for Health and Ageing, Government of South Australia. Available at: <https://www.sahealth.sa.gov.au/wps/wcm/connect/ff3a769a-e8f0-45db-970e-12281b2891b2/MR59A%2B-%2BAdult%2BObservation%2BChart%2B-%2BEXAMPLE1%281%29.pdf?MOD5AJPERES&CACHEID5ROOTWORKSPACEff3a769a-e8f0-45db-970e-12281b2891b2-oun4qXB>. **CIB 43.3,** Australian Resuscitation Council (ARC), 2024. Guideline 11.1 – Introduction to and principles of in-hospital resuscitation. Available at: <https://resus.org.au/download/guideline-11-1>. **CIB 43.5,** Australian Resuscitation Council (ARC), 2024. Guideline 11.1 – Introduction to and principles of in-hospital resuscitation. Available at: <https://resus.org.au/download/guideline-11-1>; Queensland Health, 2022. Resuscitation trolley checklist. Available at: <https://www.health.qld.gov.au/__data/assets/pdf_file/0026/1066625/RRESS_resus_trolley_checklist.pdf>. **CIB 43.6,** Australian and New Zealand Committee on Resuscitation (ANZCOR), 2021d. Guideline 7 – Automated external defibrillation in basic life support. Available at: <https://www.anzcor.org/home/basic-life-support/guideline-7-automated-external-defibrillation-in-basic-life-support>. **CIB 44.1,** Kuswara, L., Kremer, et al., 2016. The infant feeding practices of Chinese immigrant mothers in Australia: A qualitative exploration. *Appetite* 105, 375–384; Speedie, L., Middleton, A. 2022. *Wong's nursing care of infants and children* – for students, Elsevier Australia; Wandel, T., Nguyen, C., et al., 2016. Breastfeeding among Somali mothers living in Norway: Attitudes, practices and challenges. *Women and Birth* 29, 487–493. **CIB 44.2,** Department of Health & Aged Care, 2019. Pregnancy Care Guidelines: Pregnancy care for Aboriginal and Torres Strait Islander women. Available at: <https://www.health.gov.au/resources/pregnancy-care-guidelines/part-a-optimising-pregnancy-care/pregnancy-care-for-aboriginal-and-torres-strait-islander-women>. **CIB 44.3,** Ladewig, P.W., London, M.L., Davidson, M.R., 2017. *Contemporary maternal-newborn nursing care*, 9th ed. Pearson Prentice Hall, Upper Saddle River; Lowdermilk, D.L., Perry, S.E., Cashion, K., et al., 2020. *Maternity & women's health care*, 12th ed. Mosby Elsevier, St Louis. **CIB 44.4,** Baby Friendly Health Initiative (BFHI) Australia, 2020. Maternity facilities: 10 steps to successful breastfeeding. Available at: <https://bfhi.org.au/maternity-facilities>; World Health Organization (WHO), 2018. Implementation guidance: protecting, promoting and supporting breastfeeding in facilities providing maternity and newborn services – the revised Baby-friendly Hospital Initiative. Geneva. Available at: <https://www.who.int/publications/i/item/9789241513807>. **CIB 44.5,** National Health and Medical Research Council (NHMRC), 2010. Joint statement and recommendations on vitamin K Administration to newborn infants to prevent vitamin K deficiency bleeding in infancy. Available at: <https://nhmrc.gov.au/about-us/publications/vitamin-k-administration-newborns-joint-statement>; Pairman, S., Pincombe, J., Tracy, S., et al., 2023. *Midwifery: Preparation for practice*, 5th ed. Elsevier, Sydney; Speedie, L., Middleton, A. 2022. *Wong's nursing care of infants and children* – for students, Elsevier Australia. **CIB 44.6,** Lowdermilk, D.L., Perry, S.E., Cashion, K., et al., 2020. *Maternity & women's health care*, 12th ed. Mosby Elsevier, St Louis. **CIB 44.7,** Red Nose 2023. Safe sleeping. Available at: <https://rednose.org.au/article/red-nose-six-safe-sleep-recommendations>. **CIB 44.8,** National Institute for Clinical Excellence (NICE), 2016. Neonatal jaundice. RCOG Press, London; Speedie, L., Middleton, A., 2022. *Wong's nursing care of infants and children* – for students, Elsevier Australia. **CIBs 45.1,** Australian Primary Health Care Nurses Association (APNA), 2024. What is primary health care nursing? Available at: <https://www.apna.asn.au/profession/what-is-primary-health-care-nursing>. **CIBs 45.2, 45.6,** Australian Primary Health Care Nurses Association (APNA), 2017. APNA position statement: Scope of practice. Available at: <https://www.apna.asn.au/docs/bb75968b-dee1-ea11-80d9-005056be66b1/APNAPositionStatementScopeofPracticeSep2017.pdf>. @Refs:@Refs:**CIB 45.3,** Hales, M., 2020. Community health. In: Berman, A., Frandsen, G., Snyder, S., et al. (eds.), *Kozier and Erb's fundamentals of nursing: Concepts, process and practice*, 5th ed, Australian ed, vol 1. Pearson Education, Frenchs Forest; Orr, F., 2023. Mental health and recovery-oriented mental health services. In: Reynolds, L., Debono, D., Travaglia, J. (eds.), *Understanding the Australian health care system*, 5th ed. Elsevier, Sydney; McAllister, M., 2010. Solution focused nursing: A fitting model for mental health nurses working in a public health paradigm. *Contemporary Nurse* 34(2), 149–157; McAllister, M., Moyle, W., Iselin, G., 2006. Solution focused nursing: An evaluation of current practice. *Nurse Education Today* 26(5), 439–447; Moore, E., 2016.

Systems diversity in case management: characteristics, models and dimensions. In: Moore, E. (ed.), *Case management inclusive community practice*, 2nd ed. Oxford University Press Australia and New Zealand, Melbourne. **CIB 45.4,** Australian Primary Health Care Nurses Association (APNA), 2015. APNA nurse home visit guidelines. Available at: <https://www.apna.asn.au/files/DAM/3%20Knowledge%20Hub/NurseHomeVisitGuidelines.pdf>. **CIB 45.5,** Ward, M., Aumann, O., Di Stefano, G., et al., 2013. Community Health Nurses Special Interest Group ANF (Vic Branch) (issuing body.) Practice standards for Victorian community health nurses. [Carlton, Victoria] Community Health Nurses Special Interest Group ANF (Vic Branch). Available at: <https://www.apna.asn.au/files/DAM/3%20Knowledge%20Hub/PracticeStandardsForVictorianCommunityHealthNurses.pdf>; Chan, T. E., Lockhart, J. S., Thomas, A., et al., 2020. An integrative review of nurse practitioner practice and its relationship to the core competencies. *Journal of Professional Nursing* 36(4), 189–199. doi: 10.1016/j.profnurs.2019.11.003; Torrens, C., Campbell, P., Hoskins, G., et al., 2020. Barriers and facilitators to the implementation of the advanced nurse practitioner role in primary care settings: A scoping review. *International Journal of Nursing Studies* 104, 103443. doi: 10.1016/j.ijnurstu.2019.103443. **CIB 45.6,** Australian Primary Health Care Nurses Association (APNA), 2017. APNA position statement: Scope of practice. Available at: <https://www.apna.asn.au/docs/bb75968bdee1-ea11-80d9-005056be66b1/APNAPositionStatement-ScopeofPracticeSep2017.pdf>. **CIB 45.7,** Australian Primary Health Care Nurses Association (APNA), 2018. APNA career and education framework for nurses in primary health care—enrolled nurses. Available at: <https://www.apna.asn.au/files/DAM/8.%20Nursing%20Tools/Career%20and%20Education%20Framework/APNA%20Career%20and%20Education%20Framework%20for%20Nurses%20in%20Primary%20Health%20Care%20-%20Enrolled%20Nurses.pdf>. **CIB 45.8,** Victorian Refugee Health Network. Available at: <http://refugeehealthnetwork.org.au>. **CIBs 45.9,** Battye, K., Roufeil, L., Edwards, M., et al., 2019. Strategies for increasing allied health recruitment and retention in Australia: a rapid review. Services for Australian Rural and Remote Allied Health (SARRAH). Available at: <https://pub-b0561b18fd0b407ba7c21f42b2d2de7e.r2.dev/rapid_review_-_recruitment_and_retention_strategies_-_final_web_ready.pdf>; Brown, D., Edwards, H., Seaton, L., 2023. *Lewis's medical–surgical nursing*, 6th ed. Elsevier, Sydney; Badu, E., O'Brien, A. P., Mitchell, R., 2020. Workplace stress and resilience in the Australian nursing workforce: A comprehensive integrative review. *International Journal of Mental Health Nursing* 29(1), 5-34. doi: 10.1111/inm.12662. **CIB 45.10,** Brown, D., Edwards, H., Seaton, L., 2023. *Lewis's medical-surgical nursing*, 6th ed. Elsevier, Sydney; Calleja, P., Wilkes, S., Spencer, M., et al., 2022. Telehealth use in rural and remote health practitioner education: An integrative review. *Rural and Remote Health* 22, 6467. doi: 10.22605/RRH6467; Whitehead, L., Quinn, R., 2019. Improving health outcomes in rural and remote Australia: optimising the contribution of nurses. *The Collegian* 26, 407–414. doi:10.1016/j.colegn.2019.03.002. **CIB 45.11,** Brown, D., Edwards, H., Seaton., L., 2023. *Lewis's medical-surgical nursing*, 6th ed. Elsevier, Sydney.

CLINICAL SKILLS

CS 5.1, Burgess, A., van Diggele, C., Roberts, C. et al., 2020. Tips for teaching procedural skills. *BMC Medical Education* 20(2), 458. Available at: <https://doi.org/10.1186/s12909-020-02284-1>; Crisp, J., Douglas, C., Rebeiro, G., et al. (eds.), 2021. *Potter and Perry's fundamentals of nursing*, 6th ed. Elsevier, Sydney; Tollefson, J., Watson, G., Jelly, E., et al., 2022. *Essential clinical skills: Enrolled nurses*, 5th ed. Cengage Learning, Australia. **CS 8.1,** Crisp, J., Douglas, C., Rebeiro, G., et al. (eds.), 2021. *Potter & Perry's fundamentals of nursing*, 6th ed. Elsevier, Chatswood; Perry, A., Potter, P., Ostendorf, W., 2020. *Nursing interventions and clinical skills*, 7th ed. Elsevier, St Louis; Tollefson, J., Hillman, E., 2022. *Clinical psychomotor skills*, 8th ed. Cengage Learning, Melbourne. **CS 8.2,** Australian Nursing and Midwifery Federation (ANMF), 2015. National informatics standards for nurses and midwives. Australian Government Department of Health and Ageing. Available at: <https://anmf.org.au/documents/National_Informatics_Standards_For_Nurses_And_Midwives.pdf>; Honey, M., Collins, E., Britnell, S., 2018. *Guidelines: Informatics for nurses entering practice*. Auckland, New Zealand. Available at: < http://doi.org/10.17608/k6.auckland.7273037>; Hunter, K. M., McGonigle, D.M., Hebda, T.L., 2013. TIGER-based measurement of nursing informatics competencies: The development and implementation of an online tool for self-assessment. *Journal of Nursing Education and Practice* 3(12), 70–80. Available at: <https://doi.org/10.5430/jnep.v3n12p70>; Kleib, M., Nagle, L., 2018. Development of the Canadian nurse informatics competency assessment scale and evaluation of Alberta's registered nurses' self-perceived informatics competencies. *CIN: Computers Informatics Nursing* 36(7), 350–358. Available at: <https://doi.org/10.1097/CIN.0000000000000435>; Rahman, A., 2015. Development of a nursing informatics competency assessment tool (NICAT). ProQuest Dissertations Publishing. Walden University. Available at: <https://scholarworks.waldenu.edu/cgi/viewcontent.cgi?article=2849&context=dissertations>; Yoon, S., Shaffer, J. A., Bakken, S., 2015. Refining a self-assessment of informatics competency scale using Mokken scaling analysis. *Journal of Interprofessional Care* 29(6), 579–586. Available at: <https://doi.org/10.3109/13561820.2015.1049340>. **CS 10.1**, Crisp, J., Douglas, C., Rebeiro,

G., et al. (eds.), 2021. *Potter and Perry's fundamentals of nursing*, 6th ed. Elsevier, Sydney; NSW Health, 2019. Clinical Handover. Policy Directive. Available at: <https://www1.health.nsw.gov.au/pds/ActivePDSDocuments/PD2019_020.pdf>; Rebeiro, G., Wilson, D., Fuller, S., 2021. *Potter and Perry's fundamentals of nursing workbook*, 4th ed. Elsevier, Chatswood., Tollefson, J., Hillman, E., 2021. *Clinical psychomotor skills: Assessment tools for nurses*, 8th ed. Cengage Learning, Melbourne; Tollefson, J., Watson, G., Jelly, E., et al., 2021. *Essential clinical skills: Enrolled nurses*, 5th ed. Cengage Learning, Australia. **CS 15.1,** Adapted from Australian Commission on Safety and Quality in Health care (ACSQHC), 2021. National safety and quality health service standards, 2nd ed. Available at: <https://www.safetyandquality.gov.au/sites/default/files/2021-05/national_safety_and_quality_health_service_nsqhs_standards_second_edition_-_updated_may_2021.pdf>; European Pressure Ulcer Advisory Panel, National Pressure Injury Advisory Panel and Pan Pacific Pressure Injury Alliance (EPUAP/NPIAP/PPPIA), 2019. Prevention and treatment of pressure ulcers/injuries: quick reference guide. In: Haesler, E. (Ed.). EPUAP/NPIAP/PPPIA; Jensen, S., Smock, R., 2022. *Nursing health assessment: A clinical judgment approach*. Lippincott Williams & Wilkins. **CS 15.2,** Adapted from Australian Commission on Safety and Quality in Health Care (ACSQHC), 2021. National safety and quality health service standards, 2nd ed. Available at: <https://www.safetyandquality.gov.au/sites/default/files/2021-05/national_safety_and_quality_health_service_nsqhs_standards_second_edition_-_updated_may_2021.pdf>; Chambers, M., 2017. *Psychiatric and mental health nursing: The craft of caring*, 3rd ed. Routledge; Jensen, S., Smock, R., 2022. *Nursing health assessment: A clinical judgment approach*. Lippincott Williams & Wilkins. **CS 15.3,** Adapted from Australian Commission on Safety and Quality in Health Care (ACSQHC), 2021. National safety and quality health service standards, 2nd ed. Available at: <https://www.safetyandquality.gov.au/sites/default/files/2021-05/national_safety_and_quality_health_service_nsqhs_standards_second_edition_-_updated_may_2021.pdf>; Department of Health, Government of Western Australia, 2014. Falls risk assessment and management plan. Available at: <https://ww2.health.wa.gov.au/Articles/F_I/Falls-Risk-Assessment-and-Management-Plan>; Jensen, S., Smock, R., 2022. *Nursing health assessment: A clinical judgment approach*. Lippincott Williams & Wilkins. **CS 15.4,** Adapted from Australian Commission on Safety and Quality in Health care (ACSQHC), 2021. National safety and quality health service standards, 2nd ed. Available at: <https://www.safetyandquality.gov.au/sites/default/files/2021-05/national_safety_and_quality_health_service_nsqhs_standards_second_edition_-_updated_may_2021.pdf>; Jensen, S., Smock, R., 2022. *Nursing health assessment: A clinical judgment approach*. Lippincott Williams & Wilkins; NSW Government, Ministry of Health, 2017. Nutrition care. Available at: <https://www1.health.nsw.gov.au/pds/ActivePDSDocuments/PD2017_041.pdf>. **CS 15.5,** Adapted from Australian Commission on Safety and Quality in Health Care (ACSQHC), 2021. National safety and quality health service standards, 2nd ed. Available at: <https://www.safetyandquality.gov.au/sites/default/files/2021-05/national_safety_and_quality_health_service_nsqhs_standards_second_edition_-_updated_may_2021.pdf>; Jensen, S., Smock, R., 2022. *Nursing health assessment: A Clinical judgment approach*. Lippincott Williams & Wilkins; NSW Government, Ministry of Health, 2017. *Nutrition care*. Available at: <https://www1.health.nsw.gov.au/pds/ActivePDSDocuments/PD2017_041.pdf>. **CS 15.6,** Adapted from Australian Commission on Safety and Quality in Health Care (ACSQHC), 2021. National safety and quality health service standards, 2nd ed. Available at: <https://www.safetyandquality.gov.au/sites/default/files/2021-05/national_safety_and_quality_health_service_nsqhs_standards_second_edition_-_updated_may_2021.pdf>. Jensen, S., Smock, R., 2022. *Nursing health assessment: A clinical judgment approach*. Lippincott Williams & Wilkins. **CS 16.1, 16.2,** Crisp, J., Douglas, C., Rebeiro, G., et al., 2021. *Potter & Perry's fundamentals of nursing*, 6th ed. Elsevier, Sydney; Forbes, H., Watt, E., 2021. *Jarvis's physical examination and health assessment*, 3rd ed. Elsevier, Australia. **CS 16.3, 16.4, 16.5,** Crisp, J., Douglas, C., Rebeiro, G., et al., 2021. *Potter & Perry's fundamentals of nursing*, 6th ed. Elsevier, Sydney; Forbes, H., Watt, E., 2021. *Jarvis's physical examination and health assessment*, 3rd ed. Elsevier, Australia; Scott, K., Webb, M., Kostelnick, C., 2018. Chapter 11: Health assessment. In: *Long-term caring*, 4th ed. Elsevier, Australia, ch 11, pp. 236–252; Sorrentino, S., Remmert, L., 2017. Oxygen needs. In: *Mosby's textbook for nursing assistants*, 9th ed. Elsevier, ch 39, pp. 642–657. **CS 17.1,** Crisp, J., Douglas, C., Rebeiro, G., Waters, D., 2021. *Potter and Perry's fundamentals of nursing*, 6th ed. Elsevier, Chatswood; Williams & Walker 2022. *Lippincott's nursing procedures*, 8th ed. Wolters Kluwer, Philadelphia; Perry, A., Potter, P., Ostendorf, M., 2019. *Nursing interventions and clinical skills*, 7th ed. Elsevier, St Louis; Tollefson, J., Watson, G., Jelly, E., et al., 2021. *Essential clinical skills*, 5th ed. Cengage Learning, Melbourne. **CSs 18.1, 18.2, 18.3,** Berman, A., Frandsen, G., Snyder, S., Levett-Jones, T., et al., 2021. *Kozier & Erb's fundamentals of nursing concepts, process and practice*, 5th ed. Pearson, Frenchs Forest; Berman, A., Snyder, S., Levett-Jones, T., et al., 2021. *Skills in clinical nursing*, 2nd ed. Pearson, Frenchs Forest; National Health and Medical Research Council (NHMRC), 2019. Australian guidelines for the prevention and control of infection in healthcare. Available at: <https://www.nhmrc.gov.au/about-us/publications/australian-guidelines-prevention-and-control-infection-healthcare-2019>; Rebeiro, G., Wilson, D., Fuller, S., 2021. *Fundamentals of nursing: Clinical skills workbook*, 4th ed. Elsevier, Chatswood; Tollefson, J., Hillman, E., 2022.

Clinical psychomotor skills: Assessment skills tools for nurses, 8th ed. Cengage Learning Australia, South Melbourne, Victoria; World Health Organization (WHO), 2009. Guidelines on hand hygiene in healthcare. Available at: <https://www.who.int/gpsc/5may/tools/9789241597906/en>. **CS 19.1,** Australian Commission on Safety and Quality in Health Care (ACSQHC), 2021. National safety and quality health service standards, 2nd ed. Available at: <https://www.safetyandquality.gov.au/sites/default/files/2021-05/national_safety_and_quality_health_service_nsqhs_standards_second_edition_-_updated_may_2021.pdf>; Joanna Briggs Institute, 2022. Bathing and showering techniques. (JBI13750.) Available at: <https://joannabriggs.org.au>; Joanna Briggs Institute, 2022. Hygiene management. (JBI2021.) Available at: <https://joannabriggs.org.au>; Rebeiro, G., Wilson, D., Fuller, S., 2021. *Fundamentals of nursing: Clinical skills workbook*, 4th ed. Elsevier; Wilkinson, J., Treas, L., Barnett, K., Smith, M.H., 2019. *Fundamentals of nursing: Thinking, doing and caring*, 4th ed, vol. 2. F.A. Davis Company. **CS 19.2,** Australian Commission on Safety and Quality in Health Care (ACSQHC), 2021. National safety and quality health service standards, 2nd ed. Available at: <https://www.safetyandquality.gov.au/sites/default/files/2021-05/national_safety_and_quality_health_service_nsqhs_standards_second_edition_-_updated_may_2021.pdf>; Joanna Briggs Institute, 2022. Bathing and showering techniques. (JBI13750.) Available at: <https://joannabriggs.org.au>; Joanna Briggs Institute, 2022. Hygiene management. (JBI2021.) Available at: <https://joannabriggs.org.au>; Rebeiro, G., Wilson, D., Fuller, S., 2021. *Fundamentals of nursing: Clinical skills workbook*, 4th ed. Elsevier; Wilkinson, J., Treas, L., Barnett, K., Smith, M.H., 2019. *Fundamentals of nursing: Thinking, doing and caring*, 4th ed, vol. 2. F.A. Davis Company. **CS 19.3,** Australian Commission on Safety and Quality in Health Care (ACSQHC), 2021. National safety and quality health service standards, 2nd ed. Available at: <https://www.safetyandquality.gov.au/sites/default/files/2021-05/national_safety_and_quality_health_service_nsqhs_standards_second_edition_-_updated_may_2021.pdf>; Joanna Briggs Institute, 2019. Eye cleansing. (JBI1022.) Available at: https://joannabriggs.org>; Joanna Briggs Institute, 2022. Eye toilet: Older person. (JBI2133.) Available at: <https://joannabriggs.org.au>; Rebeiro, G., Wilson, D., Fuller, S., 2021. *Fundamentals of nursing: Clinical skills workbook* (4th ed.). Elsevier. **CS 19.4,** Australian Commission on Safety and Quality in Health Care (ACSQHC), 2021. National safety and quality health service standards, 2nd ed. Available at: <https://www.safetyandquality.gov.au/sites/default/files/2021-05/national_safety_and_quality_health_service_nsqhs_standards_second_edition_-_updated_may_2021.pdf>; JBI, 2022. Dementia: Oral hygiene care. (JBI681). Available at: < http://jbi.global/ebp>; JBI, 2022. Oral hygiene in adults: General principles. (JBI23021). Available at: < http://jbi.global/ebp>; JBI, 2022. Stroke: Oral hygiene. (JBI20454). Available at: < http://jbi.global/ebp>; Rebeiro, G., Wilson, D., Fuller, S., 2021. *Fundamentals of nursing: Clinical skills workbook*, 4th ed. Elsevier. **CS 19.5,** Australian Commission on Safety and Quality in Health Care (ACSQHC), 2021. National safety and quality health service standards, 2nd ed. Available at: <https://www.safetyandquality.gov.au/sites/default/files/2021-05/national_safety_and_quality_health_service_nsqhs_standards_second_edition_-_updated_may_2021.pdf>; Joanna Briggs Institute. 2022. Oral hygiene in adults: General principles. (JBI23021.) Available at: <https://joannabriggs.org.au>; Rebeiro, G., Wilson, D., Fuller, S., 2021. *Fundamentals of nursing: Clinical skills workbook*, 4th ed. Elsevier. **CS 19.6,** Australian Commission on Safety and Quality in Health Care (ACSQHC), 2021. National safety and quality health service standards, 2nd ed. Available at: <https://www.safetyandquality.gov.au/sites/default/files/2021-05/national_safety_and_quality_health_service_nsqhs_standards_second_edition_-_updated_may_2021.pdf>. Joanna Briggs Institute, 2022. Bed making. (JBI2299.) Available at: <https://joannabriggs.org.au>; Rebeiro, G., Wilson, D., Fuller, S., 2021. *Fundamentals of nursing: Clinical skills workbook*, 4th ed. Elsevier. **CS 19.7,** Australian Commission on Safety and Quality in Health Care (ACSQHC), 2021. National safety and quality health service standards, 2nd ed. Available at: <https://www.safetyandquality.gov.au/sites/default/files/2021-05/national_safety_and_quality_health_service_nsqhs_standards_second_edition_-_updated_may_2021.pdf>; Joanna Briggs Institute, 2022. Bed making. (JBI2299.) Available at: <https://joannabriggs.org.au>; Rebeiro, G., Wilson, D., Fuller, S., 2021. *Fundamentals of nursing: Clinical skills workbook*, 4th ed. Elsevier, Chatswood. **CS 19.8,** Australian Commission on Safety and Quality in Health Care (ACSQHC), 2021. National safety and quality health service standards, 2nd ed. Available at: <https://www.safetyandquality.gov.au/sites/default/files/2021-05/national_safety_and_quality_health_service_nsqhs_standards_second_edition_-_updated_may_2021.pdf>; Joanna Briggs Institute, 2022. Bed making. (JBI2299.) Available at: <https://joannabriggs.org.au>; Rebeiro, G., Wilson, D., Fuller, S., 2021. *Fundamentals of nursing: Clinical skills workbook*, 4th ed. Elsevier. **CS 20.1,** Australian Commission on Safety and Quality in Health Care (ACSQHC), 2012. Medication safety action guide. Available at: <https://www.safetyandquality.gov.au/sites/default/files/migrated/1.1-Medication-Safety.pdf>; Australian Commission on Safety and Quality in Health Care (ACSQHC), 2019. NIMC user guide. Available at: <https://www.safetyandquality.gov.au/publications-and-resources/resource-library/national-inpatient-medication-chart-nimc-user-guide>; Frotjold, A., Bloomfeild, J., 2021. Medication therapy. In: Crisp, J. Douglas, C., Rebeiro, G., et al. (eds.), *Potter and Perry's fundamentals of nursing*, ANZ ed, 6th ed. Elsevier, Chatswood; JBI, 2022. Medication administration: Oral. (JBI2144.) Available at:

<https://jbi.global/ebp>; Rebeiro, G., Wilson, D., Fuller, S., 2021. *Potter and Perry's fundamentals of nursing* workbook, 4th ed. Elsevier, Chatswood; The Society of Hospital Pharmacists of Australia (SHPA), 2022. *Don't rush to crush*, 4th ed. SHPA, South Melbourne; Tollefson, J., Watson, G., Jelly, E., et al., 2022. *Essential clinical skills: Enrolled nurses*, 5th ed. Cengage Learning, Australia. **CS 20.2,** Australian Commission on Safety and Quality in Health Care (ACSQHC), 2012. Medication safety action guide. Available at: <https://www.safetyandquality.gov.au/sites/default/files/migrated/1.1-Medication-Safety.pdf>; Australian Commission on Safety and Quality in Health Care (ACSQHC), 2019. NIMC user guide. Available at: <https://www.safetyandquality.gov.au/publications-and-resources/resource-library/national-inpatient-medication-chart-nimc-user-guide>; JBI, 2022b. Enteral tube: Administration of medication. (JBI23655.) Available at: <https://jbi.global/ebp>; Williams, P.A., 2022. *DeWit's fundamental concepts and skills for nursing*, 6th ed. Elsevier Saunders, Philadelphia; The Agency for Clinical Innovation and the Gastroenterological Nurses College of Australia, 2015. A clinician's guide: Caring for people with gastrostomy tubes and devices. Available at: <https://aci.health.nsw.gov.au/__data/assets/pdf_file/0017/251063/ACI-Clinicians-guide-caring-eoplegastrostomy-tubes-devices.pdf>; The Society of Hospital Pharmacists of Australia (SHPA), 2022. *Don't rush to crush*, 4th ed. SHPA, South Melbourne; Tollefson, J., Watson, G., Jelly, E., et al., 2022. *Essential clinical skills: Enrolled nurses*, 5th ed. Cengage Learning, Australia. **CS 20.3,** Australian Commission on Safety and Quality in Health Care (ACSQHC), 2012. Medication safety action guide. Available at: <https://www.safetyandquality.gov.au/sites/default/files/migrated/1.1-Medication-Safety.pdf>; Australian Commission on Safety and Quality in Health Care (ACSQHC), 2019. NIMC user guide. Available at: <https://www.safetyandquality.gov.au/publications-and-resources/resource-library/national-inpatient-medication-chart-nimc-user-guide>; JBI, 2022a. Enema: Disposable (older adult). (JBI2129.) Available at: <https://jbi.global/ebp> ; Rebeiro, G., Wilson, D., Fuller, S., 2021. *Potter and Perry's fundamentals of nursing workbook*, 4th ed. Elsevier, Chatswood; Tollefson, J., Watson, G., Jelly, E., et al., 2022. Essential clinical skills: Enrolled Nurses, 5th ed. Cengage Learning, Australia. **CS 20.4,** Australian Commission on Safety and Quality in Health Care (ACSQHC), 2012. Medication safety action guide. Available at: <https://www.safetyandquality.gov.au/sites/default/files/migrated/1.1-Medication-Safety.pdf>; Australian Commission on Safety and Quality in Health Care (ACSQHC), 2019. NIMC user guide. Available at: <https://www.safetyandquality.gov.au/publications-and-resources/resource-library/national-inpatient-medication-chart-nimc-user-guide>; Australian Commission on Safety and Quality in Health Care (ACSQHC), 2023. APINCHS classification of high risk medicines. Available at: <https://www.safetyandquality.gov.au/our-work/medication-safety/high-risk-medicines/apinchs-classification-of-high-risk-medicines>; JBI, 2021. Intramuscular injection. (JBI2138.) Available at: <https://jbi.global/ebp>; JBI, 2022. Subcutaneous injection. (JBI1964.) Available at: <https://jbi.global/ebp>. Rebeiro, G., Wilson, D., Fuller, S., 2021. *Potter and Perry's fundamentals of nursing workbook*, 4th ed. Elsevier, Chatswood; The Society of Hospital Pharmacists of Australia, (SHPA), 2023. *The Australian Injectable Drugs Handbook*, 8th ed. SHPA, South Melbourne; Tollefson, J., Watson, G., Jelly, E., et al., 2022. Essential clinical skills: Enrolled Nurses, 5th ed. Cengage Learning, Australia. **CS 20.5,** Australian Commission on Safety and Quality in Health Care (ACSQHC), 2012. Medication safety action guide. Available at: <https://www.safetyandquality.gov.au/sites/default/files/migrated/1.1-Medication-Safety.pdf>; Australian Commission on Safety and Quality in Health Care (ACSQHC), 2015. National standard for user-applied labelling of injectable medicines, fluids and lines. Available at: <https://www.safetyandquality.gov.au/wp-content/uploads/2015/09/National-Standard-for-User-Applied-Labelling-Aug-2015.pdf>; Gorski, L.A., 2023. Phillips's manual of IV therapeutics: evidence based practice for infusion therapy, 8th ed. F.A. Davis Company, Philadelphia; Queensland Health, 2018. Guideline: Peripheral Intravenous Catheter (PIVC). Available at: <https://www.health.qld.gov.au/__data/assets/pdf_file/0025/444490/icare-pivc-guideline.pdf>. Rebeiro, G., Wilson, D., Fuller, S., 2021. *Potter and Perry's fundamentals of nursing workbook*, 4th ed. Elsevier, Chatswood; Tollefson, J., Watson, G., Jelly, E., et al., 2022. Essential clinical skills enrolled nurses, 5th ed. Cengage Learning, Australia. **CS 20.6,** Australian Commission on Safety and Quality in Health Care (ACSQHC), 2012. Medication safety action guide. Available at: <https://www.safetyandquality.gov.au/sites/default/files/migrated/1.1-Medication-Safety.pdf>; Australian Commission on Safety and Quality in Health Care (ACSQHC), 2015. National standard for user-applied labelling of injectable medicines, fluids and lines. Available at: <https://www.safetyandquality.gov.au/wp-content/uploads/2015/09/National-Standard-for-User-Applied-Labelling-Aug-2015.pdf>; Gorski, L.A., 2023. *Phillips's manual of IV therapeutics: Evidence based practice for infusion therapy*, 8th ed. F.A. Davis Company, Philadelphia; Queensland Health, 2018. Guideline: Peripheral Intravenous Catheter (PIVC). Available at: <https://www.health.qld.gov.au/__data/assets/pdf_file/0025/444490/icare-pivc-guideline.pdf>; Rebeiro, G., Wilson, D., Fuller, S., 2021. *Potter and Perry's fundamentals of nursing workbook*, 4th ed. Elsevier, Chatswood; Tollefson, J., Watson, G., Jelly, E., et al., 2022. *Essential clinical skills: Enrolled nurses*, 5th ed. Cengage Learning, Australia; South Eastern Sydney Local Health District (SESLHD), 2019. Infective Complications- Mandatory reporting requirements of peripheral intravenous cannula (PIVC) or central venous access device (CVAD) infections in the incident

information management systems (IIMS). Available at: <https://www.seslhd.health.nsw.gov.au/sites/default/files/documents/SESLHDPD%20280.pdf>. **CS 20.7,** Australian Commission on Safety and Quality in Health Care (ACSQHC), 2012. Medication safety action guide. Available at: <https://www.safetyandquality.gov.au/sites/default/files/migrated/1.1-Medication-Safety.pdf>; Australian Commission on Safety and Quality in Health Care (ACSQHC), 2015. National standard for user-applied labelling of injectable medicines, fluids and lines. Available at: <https://www.safetyandquality.gov.au/wp-content/uploads/2015/09/National-Standard-for-User-Applied-Labelling-Aug-2015.pdf>; Australian Commission on Safety and Quality in Health Care (ACSQHC), 2024. APINCHS classification of high risk medicines. Available at: <https://www.safetyandquality.gov.au/our-work/medication-safety/high-risk-medicines/apinchs-classification-of-high-risk-medicines>; Gorski, L.A., 2023. *Phillips's manual of IV therapeutics: Evidence based practice for infusion therapy*, 8th ed. F.A. Davis Company, Philadelphia; Queensland Health, 2018. Guideline: Peripheral intravenous catheter (PIVC). Available at: <https://www.health.qld.gov.au/__data/assets/pdf_file/0025/444490/icare-pivc-guideline.pdf>; Rebeiro, G., Wilson, D., Fuller, S., 2021. *Potter and Perry's fundamentals of nursing workbook*, 4th ed. Elsevier, Chatswood; The Society of Hospital Pharmacists of Australia, (SHPA), 2023. *The Australian Injectable Drugs Handbook*, 8th ed. SHPA, South Melbourne; Tollefson, J., Watson, G., Jelly, E., et al., 2022. *Essential clinical skills: Enrolled nurses*, 5th ed. Cengage Learning, Australia; South Eastern Sydney Local Health District (SESLHD) 2019 Infective Complications- Mandatory reporting requirements of peripheral intravenous cannula (PIVC) or central venous access device (CVAD) infections in the incident information management systems (IIMS). Available at: <https://www.seslhd.health.nsw.gov.au/sites/default/files/documents/SESLHDPD%20280.pdf>. **CS 20.8,** Gorski, L.A., 2023. *Phillips's manual of IV therapeutics: Evidence based practice for infusion therapy*, 8th ed. F.A. Davis Company, Philadelphia; JBI, 2022. Peripheral intravenous cannula: Removal. (JBI14047.) Available at: <https://jbi.global/ebp>.
Queensland Health. 2018. Guideline: Peripheral Intravenous Catheter (PIVC). Available at: <https://www.health.qld.gov.au/__data/assets/pdf_file/0025/444490/icare-pivc-guideline.pdf>. **CS 20.9,** Australian Commission on Safety and Quality in Health Care (ACSQHC), 2012. Medication safety action guide. Available at: <https://www.safetyandquality.gov.au/sites/default/files/migrated/1.1-Medication-Safety.pdf>; Australian Commission on Safety and Quality in Health Care (ACSQHC), 2015. National standard for user-applied labelling of injectable medicines, fluids and lines. Available at: <https://www.safetyandquality.gov.au/wp-content/uploads/2015/09/National-Standard-for-User-Applied-Labelling-Aug-2015.pdf>; Australian & New Zealand Society of Blood Transfusions Ltd, 2019. *Guidelines for the administration of blood products*, 3rd ed. Australian & New Zealand Society of Blood Transfusion Ltd, Sydney; Department of Health, 2018. Royal Melbourne Hospital blood component prescription includes consent. Available at: <https://www.health.vic.gov.au/publications/royal-melbourne-hospital-blood-component-prescription-includes-consent-pdf>; Department of Health, 2021. Infection control - standard and transmission-based precautions. Available at: <https://www.health.vic.gov.au/infectious-diseases/infection-control-standard-and-transmission-based-precautions>; Gorski, L.A., 2023. *Phillips's manual of IV therapeutics: Evidence based practice for infusion therapy*, 8th ed. F.A. Davis Company, Philadelphia. Joanna Briggs Institute (JBI), 2021. Transfusion: blood or blood product. (JBI1846.) Available at: <joannabriggs.org>; Rebeiro, G., Wilson, D., Fuller, S., 2021. *Potter and Perry's fundamentals of nursing workbook*, 4th ed. Elsevier, Chatswood; South Eastern Sydney Local Health District (SESLHD) 2019 Infective Complications- Mandatory reporting requirements of peripheral intravenous cannula (PIVC) or central venous access device (CVAD) infections in the incident information management systems (IIMS). Available at: <https://www.seslhd.health.nsw.gov.au/sites/default/files/documents/SESLHDPD%20280.pdf>.
CS 20.10, Australian Commission on Safety and Quality in Health Care (ACSQHC), 2012. Medication safety action guide. Available at: <https://www.safetyandquality.gov.au/sites/default/files/migrated/1.1-Medication-Safety.pdf>; Australian Commission on Safety and Quality in Health Care (ACSQHC), 2015. National standard for user-applied labelling of injectable medicines, fluids and lines. Available at: <https://www.safetyandquality.gov.au/wp-content/uploads/2015/09/National-Standard-for-User-Applied-Labelling-Aug-2015.pdf>; Australian Commission on Safety and Quality in Health Care (ACSQHC), 2023. APINCHS classification of high risk medicines. Available at: <https://www.safetyandquality.gov.au/our-work/medication-safety/high-risk-medicines/apinchs-classification-of-high-risk-medicines>; Gorski, L.A., 2023. *Phillips's manual of IV therapeutics: Evidence based practice for infusion therapy*, 8th ed. F.A. Davis Company, Philadelphia; Queensland Health, 2018. Guideline: Peripheral intravenous catheter (PIVC). Available at: <https://www.health.qld.gov.au/__data/assets/pdf_file/0025/444490/icare-pivc-guideline.pdf>; Rebeiro, G., Wilson, D., Fuller, S., 2021. *Potter and Perry's fundamentals of nursing workbook*, 4th ed. Elsevier, Chatswood; The Society of Hospital Pharmacists of Australia, (SHPA), 2023. *The Australian Injectable Drugs Handbook*, 8th ed. SHPA, South Melbourne; Tollefson, J., Watson, G., Jelly, E., et al., 2022. *Essential clinical skills: Enrolled nurses*, 5th ed. Cengage Learning, Australia. **CS 20.11,** Australian Commission on Safety and Quality in Health Care (ACSQHC), 2012. Medication safety action guide. Available at: <https://www.safetyandquality.gov.au/sites/default/files/migrated/1.1-Medication-Safety.pdf>;

Australian Commission on Safety and Quality in Health Care (ACSQHC), 2019. NIMC user guide. Available at: <https://www.safetyandquality.gov.au/publications-and-resources/resource-library/national-inpatient-medication-chart-nimc-user-guide>; Joanna Briggs Institute (JBI), 2022. Topical medications. (JBI1962.) Available at: <joannabriggs.org>; Rebeiro, G., Wilson, D., Fuller, S., 2021. *Potter and Perry's fundamentals of nursing workbook*, 4th ed. Elsevier, Chatswood; Tollefson, J., Watson, G., Jelly, E., et al., 2022. *Essential clinical skills: Enrolled nurses*, 5th ed. Cengage Learning, Australia. **CS 20.12,** Australian Commission on Safety and Quality in Health Care (ACSQHC), 2012. Medication safety action guide. Available at: <https://www.safetyandquality.gov.au/sites/default/files/migrated/1.1-Medication-Safety.pdf>; Australian Commission on Safety and Quality in Health Care (ACSQHC), 2019. NIMC user guide. Available at: <https://www.safetyandquality.gov.au/publications-and-resources/resource-library/national-inpatient-medication-chart-nimc-user-guide>; Rebeiro, G., Wilson, D., Fuller, S., 2021. *Potter and Perry's fundamentals of nursing workbook*, 4th ed. Elsevier, Chatswood; Tollefson, J., Watson, G., Jelly, E., et al., 2022. *Essential clinical skills: Enrolled nurses*, 5th ed. Cengage Learning, Australia. **CS 20.13,** Australian Commission on Safety and Quality in Health Care (ACSQHC), 2012. Medication safety action guide. Available at: <https://www.safetyandquality.gov.au/sites/default/files/migrated/1.1-Medication-Safety.pdf>; Australian Commission on Safety and Quality in Health Care (ACSQHC), 2019a. NIMC user guide. Available at: <https://www.safetyandquality.gov.au/publications-and-resources/resource-library/national-inpatient-medication-chart-nimc-user-guide>; Joanna Briggs Institute (JBI), 2021. Eye medication: administration. (JBI2172.) Available at: <joannabriggs.org>; Rebeiro, G., Wilson, D., Fuller, S., 2021. *Potter and Perry's fundamentals of nursing workbook*, 4th ed. Elsevier, Chatswood; Tollefson, J., Watson, G., Jelly, E., et al., 2022. *Essential clinical skills: Enrolled nurses*, 5th ed. Cengage Learning, Australia. **CS 20.14,** Australian Commission on Safety and Quality in Health Care (ACSQHC), 2012. Medication safety action guide. Available at: <https://www.safetyandquality.gov.au/sites/default/files/migrated/1.1-Medication-Safety.pdf>; Australian Commission on Safety and Quality in Health Care (ACSQHC), 2019. NIMC user guide. Available at: <https://www.safetyandquality.gov.au/publications-and-resources/resource-library/national-inpatient-medication-chart-nimc-user-guide>; Joanna Briggs Institute (JBI), 2023. Ear drops instillation. (JBI2337.) Available at: <joannabriggs.org>; Rebeiro, G., Wilson, D., Fuller, S., 2021. *Potter and Perry's fundamentals of nursing workbook*, 4th ed. Elsevier, Chatswood; Tollefson, J., Watson, G., Jelly, E., et al., 2022. *Essential clinical skills: Enrolled nurses*, 5th ed. Cengage Learning, Australia. **CS 20.15,** Australian Commission on Safety and Quality in Health Care (ACSQHC), 2012. Medication safety action guide. Available at: <https://www.safetyandquality.gov.au/sites/default/files/migrated/1.1-Medication-Safety.pdf>; Australian Commission on Safety and Quality in Health Care (ACSQHC), 2019. NIMC user guide. Available at: <https://www.safetyandquality.gov.au/publications-and-resources/resource-library/national-inpatient-medication-chart-nimc-user-guide>; Joanna Briggs Institute (JBI), 2021. Vaginal medication. (JBI1999.) Available at: <joannabriggs.org>; Rebeiro, G., Wilson, D., Fuller, S., 2021. *Potter and Perry's fundamentals of nursing workbook*, 4th ed. Elsevier, Chatswood; Tollefson, J., Watson, G., Jelly, E., et al., 2022. *Essential clinical skills: Enrolled nurses*, 5th ed. Cengage Learning, Australia. **CS 20.16,** Australian Commission on Safety and Quality in Health Care (ACSQHC), 2012. Medication safety action guide. Available at: <https://www.safetyandquality.gov.au/sites/default/files/migrated/1.1-Medication-Safety.pdf>; Australian Commission on Safety and Quality in Health Care (ACSQHC), 2019. NIMC user guide. Available at: <https://www.safetyandquality.gov.au/publications-and-resources/resource-library/national-inpatient-medication-chart-nimc-user-guide>; Australian Commission on Safety and Quality in Health Care (ACSQHC), 2020. Managing intranasal administration of medicines for patients during COVID-19. Available at <https://www.safetyandquality.gov.au/sites/default/files/2020-05/covid-19_-_position_statement_-_intranasal_medicines.pdf>; Department of Health, 2021. Infection control - standard and transmission-based precautions. Available at: <https://www.health.vic.gov.au/infectious-diseases/infection-control-standard-and-transmission-based-precautions>; Joanna Briggs Institute (JBI), 2021. Inhalation therapy (nebulizer). (JBI2149.) Available at: <joannabriggs.org>; Tollefson, J., Watson, G., Jelly, E., et al., 2022. *Essential clinical skills: Enrolled nurses*, 5th ed. Cengage Learning, Australia. **CS 20.17,** Australian Commission on Safety and Quality in Health Care (ACSQHC), 2012. Medication safety action guide. Available at: <https://www.safetyandquality.gov.au/sites/default/files/migrated/1.1-Medication-Safety.pdf>; Australian Commission on Safety and Quality in Health Care (ACSQHC), 2019. NIMC user guide. Available at: <https://www.safetyandquality.gov.au/publications-and-resources/resource-library/national-inpatient-medication-chart-nimc-user-guide>; Australian Commission on Safety and Quality in Health Care (ACSQHC), 2020. Managing intranasal administration of medicines for patients during COVID-19. Available at <https://www.safetyandquality.gov.au/sites/default/files/2020-05/covid-19_-_position_statement_-_intranasal_medicines.pdf>; Department of Health, 2021. Infection control - standard and transmission-based precautions. Available at: <https://www.health.vic.gov.au/infectious-diseases/infection-control-standard-and-transmission-based-precautions>; Joanna Briggs Institute (JBI), 2021. Aerosol inhaler (puffer) techniques. (JBI2115.) Available at: <joannabriggs.org>; Rebeiro, G., Wilson, D., Fuller, S., 2021. *Potter and Perry's fundamentals of nursing workbook*, 4th ed. Elsevier, Chatswood; Tollefson, J.,

Watson, G., Jelly, E., et al., 2022. *Essential clinical skills: Enrolled nurses*, 5th ed. Cengage Learning, Australia. **CS 20.18,** Australian Commission on Safety and Quality in Health Care (ACSQHC), 2012. Medication safety action guide. Available at: <https://www.safetyandquality.gov.au/sites/default/files/migrated/1.1-Medication-Safety.pdf>; Australian Commission on Safety and Quality in Health Care (ACSQHC), 2019. NIMC user guide. Available at: <https://www.safetyandquality.gov.au/publications-and-resources/resource-library/national-inpatient-medication-chart-nimc-user-guide>; Department of Health, 2021. Infection control - standard and transmission-based precautions. Available at: <https://www.health.vic.gov.au/infectious-diseases/infection-control-standard-and-transmission-based-precautions>; Joanna Briggs Institute (JBI), 2022. Nasal medications. (JBI1968.) Available at: <joannabriggs.org>; Rebeiro, G., Wilson, D., Fuller, S., 2021. *Potter and Perry's fundamentals of nursing workbook*, 4th ed. Elsevier, Chatswood; Tollefson, J., Watson, G., Jelly, E., et al., 2022. *Essential clinical skills: Enrolled nurses*, 5th ed. Cengage Learning, Australia. **CS 25.1,** Aitken, L.M., Marshall, A., Chaboyer, W. (eds.), 2019. *Critical care nursing*, 4th edition, Elsevier Australia, Chatswood, NSW; Menzies-Gow, E., 2018. How to record a 12-lead electrocardiogram. *Nursing Standard* 33 (2) 38–42. doi: 10.7748/ns.2018.e11066; Perry, A.G., Potter, P.A., Ostendorf, W., Laplante, N., 2022. *Nursing interventions and clinical skills*, 10th ed. Elsevier Inc, St Louis; Rebeiro, G., Wilson, D., Fuller, S., 2021. *Potter and Perry's fundamentals of nursing workbook*, 4th ed. Elsevier, Chatswood. **CS 25.2,** Crisp, J., Douglas, C., Rebeiro, G., et al. (eds.), 2021. *Potter and Perry's fundamentals of nursing*, 6th ed. Elsevier, Australia and New Zealand, New South Wales Sydney; Perry, A.G., Potter, P.A., Ostendorf, W., Laplante, N., 2022. *Nursing interventions and clinical skills*, 10th ed. Elsevier Inc, St Louis. **CS 25.3,** Carter, C., Notter, J., 2024. *Handbook for registered nurses.* Elsevier Ltd; Perry, A.G., Potter, P.A., Ostendorf, W., Laplante, N., 2022. *Nursing interventions and clinical skills*, 10th ed. Elsevier Inc, St Louis. **CS 25.4,** Perry, A.G., Potter, P.A., Ostendorf, W., Laplante, N., 2022. *Nursing interventions and clinical skills*, 10th ed. Elsevier Inc, St Louis. **CS 25.5,** Perry, A.G., Potter, P.A., Ostendorf, W., Laplante, N., 2022. *Nursing interventions and clinical skills*, 10th ed. Elsevier Inc, St Louis; Rebeiro, G., Wilson, D., Fuller, S., 2021. *Potter and Perry's fundamentals of nursing workbook*, 4th ed. Elsevier, Chatswood. **CS 25.6,** Berman, A., Kozier, B., Erb, G.L., 2020. *Kozier and Erb's fundamentals of nursing: Concepts, process and practice*, Australian ed, 5th ed. Pearson Australia, Melbourne; Carter, C., Notter, J., 2024. *Handbook for registered nurses.* Elsevier Ltd; Perry, A.G., Potter, P.A., Ostendorf, W., Laplante, N., 2022. *Nursing interventions and clinical skills*, 10th ed. Elsevier Inc, St Louis; Rebeiro, G., Wilson, D., Fuller, S., 2021. *Potter and Perry's fundamentals of nursing workbook,* 4th ed. Elsevier, Chatswood. **CS 25.7,** Carter, C., Notter, J., 2024. *Handbook for registered nurses*, Elsevier Ltd; Knapp, R., (ed.), 2019. *Respiratory care made incredibly easy!*, 2nd ed. Wolters Kluwer, Philadelphia, Pennsylvania; Perry, A.G., Potter, P.A., Ostendorf, W., Laplante, N., 2022. *Nursing interventions and clinical skills*, 10th ed. Elsevier Inc, St Louis; Rebeiro, G., Wilson, D., Fuller, S., 2021. *Potter and Perry's fundamentals of nursing workbook*, 4th ed. Elsevier, Chatswood. **CS 25.8,** Carter, C., Notter, J., 2024. *Handbook for registered nurses.* Elsevier Ltd; Perry, A.G., Potter, P.A., Ostendorf, W., Laplante, N., 2022. *Nursing interventions and clinical skills*, 10th ed. Elsevier Inc, St Louis; Rebeiro, G., Wilson, D., Fuller, S., 2021. *Potter and Perry's fundamentals of nursing workbook*, 4th ed. Elsevier, Chatswood. **CS 26.1,** Berman, A., Frandsen, G., Snyder, S., et al., 2020. *Kozier and Erb's fundamentals of nursing*, 5th ed. Pearson, Melbourne; Crisp, J., Douglas, C., Rebeiro, G., et al. (eds.), 2021. *Potter and Perry's fundamentals of nursing*, 6th ed. Elsevier, Chatswood; Simpson, D., McIntosh, R., 2021. Measuring and monitoring fluid balance. *British Journal of Nursing* 20(12) 706 –710. **CS 28.1,** Crisp, J., Douglas, C., Rebeiro, G., et al., 2021. *Potter and Perry's fundamentals of nursing*, Australian ed, 6th ed. Elsevier, Sydney; Rebeiro, G., Wilson, D. Fuller, S., 2021. *Fundamentals of nursing: Clinical skills workbook*, 4th ed. Elsevier, Chatswood; Tollefson, J. Hillman, E. , 2022. *Clinical psychomotor skills: Assessment tools for nursing students*, 8th ed. Cengage Learning Australia, South Melbourne, Victoria. **CS 28.2,** Perry, A.G., Potter, P.A., Ostendorf, W.R., 2019. *Nursing interventions and clinical skills*, 7th ed. Elsevier, St Louis; Rebeiro, G., Wilson, D., Fuller, S., 2021. *Fundamentals of nursing: Clinical skills workbook*, 4th ed. Elsevier, Chatswood; Tollefson, J., Hillman, E., 2022. *Clinical psychomotor skills: Assessment tools for nursing students*, 8th ed. Cengage Learning Australia, South Melbourne, Victoria. **CS 28.3,** Crisp, J., Douglas, C., Rebeiro, G., et al., 2021. *Potter and Perry's fundamentals of nursing*, Australian ed, 5th ed. Elsevier, Sydney; Rebeiro, G., Wilson, D., Fuller, S., 2021. *Fundamentals of nursing: Clinical skills workbook*, 4th ed. Elsevier, Chatswood. **CSs 29.1, 29.2, 29.4, 29.5, 29.6,** Adapted from Australian College for Infection Prevention and Control (ACIPC), 2015. Aseptic technique policy and practice guidelines. Available at: <https://www.acipc.org.au/aseptic-technique-resources>; LeMone, P., Bauldoff, G., Gubrud-Howe, P., et al., 2020. *Medical-surgical nursing: Critical thinking in person-centred care*, 4th ed. Pearson, Melbourne; Berman, A., Snyder, S., Levett-Jones, T., et al., 2020. *Kozier and Erb's fundamentals of nursing*, 5th ed. Pearson, Melbourne; International Wound Infection Institute (IWII), 2022. Wound infection in clinical practice: principles of best practice. *Wounds International.* Available at: <https://woundinfection-institute.com/wp-content/uploads/IWII-CD-2022-web-1.pdf>; Lynn, P., 2022. *Taylor's clinical nursing skills. A nursing process approach*, 6th ed. Wolters Kluwer Lippinott Williams & Wilkins, Philadelphia; The Association for Safe Aseptic Practice (The-ASAP), 2015. Aseptic Non touch Technique: The

ANTT Clinical Practice Framework ... for all invasive Clinical Procedures from Surgery to Community Care version 4. Available at: <www.antt.org>. **CS 29.3,** Adapted from Australian College for Infection Prevention and Control (ACIPC), 2015. Aseptic technique policy and practice guidelines. Available at: <https://www.acipc.org.au/aseptic-technique-resources>; LeMone, P., Bauldoff, G., Gubrud-Howe, P., et al., 2020. *Medical–surgical nursing: Critical thinking in person-centred care*, 4th ed. Pearson, Melbourne; Berman, A., Snyder, S., Levett-Jones, T., et al., 2020. *Kozier and Erb's fundamentals of nursing*, 5th ed. Pearson, Melbourne; International Wound Infection Institute (IWII), 2022. Wound infection in clinical practice: principles of best practice. *Wounds International.* Available at: <https://woundinfection-institute.com/wp-content/uploads/IWII-CD-2022-web-1.pdf>; LeBlanc, K., Campbell, K., Beeckman, D., et al., 2018. Best practice recommendations for prevention and management of skin tears in aged skin: An overview. *Journal of Wound, Ostomy, and Continence Nursing* 45(6), 540–542; Lynn, P., 2022. *Taylor's clinical nursing skills. A nursing process approach*, 6th ed. Wolters Kluwer Lippinott Williams & Wilkins, Philadelphia; The Association for Safe Aseptic Practice (The-ASAP), 2015. Aseptic Non touch Technique: The ANTT Clinical Practice Framework ... for all invasive Clinical Procedures from Surgery to Community Care version 4. Available at: <www.antt.org>. **CS 29.7,** LeMone, P., Bauldoff, G., Gubrud-Howe, P., et al., 2020. *Medical-surgical nursing: Critical thinking in person-centred care*, 4th ed. Pearson, Melbourne; LeBlanc, K., Campbell, K., Beeckman, D., et al., 2018. Best practice recommendations for prevention and management of skin tears in aged skin: An overview. *Journal of Wound, Ostomy, and Continence Nursing* 45(6), 540–542; Lynn, P., 2022. *Taylor's clinical nursing skills. A nursing process approach*, 6th ed. Wolters Kluwer Lippinott Williams & Wilkins, Philadelphia; The Association for Safe Aseptic Practice (The-ASAP), 2015. Aseptic Non touch Technique: The ANTT Clinical Practice Framework ... for all invasive Clinical Procedures from Surgery to Community Care version 4. Available at: <www.antt.org>. **CS 30.1,** Berman, A., Snyder, S., Levett-Jones, T., et al., 2020. *Kozier and Erb's fundamentals of nursing*, 5th ed. Pearson, Frenchs Forest; Hall, H., Glew, P., Rhodes, J., 2022. *Fundamentals of nursing and midwifery: A person-centred approach to care*, 4th ed. Australian and New Zealand ed. Lippincott Williams & Wilkins Australia, Sydney; NSW Department of Health, 2017. Policy directive: Nutrition care. Pd2017_041. NSW Health, Sydney. Available at: <https://www1.health.nsw.gov.au/pds/ActivePDSDocuments/PD2017_041.pdf>. **CSs 30.2, 30.3,** Berman, A., Snyder, S., Levett-Jones, T., et al., 2020. *Kozier and Erb's fundamentals of nursing*, 5th ed. Pearson, Frenchs Forest; Crisp, J., Douglas, S., Rebeiro, G., et al. (eds.), 2021. *Potter and Perry's fundamentals of nursing*, 6th ed. Elsevier, Sydney; Hall, H., Glew, P., Rhodes, J., 2022. *Fundamentals of nursing and midwifery: A person-centred approach to care*, 4th ed. Australian and New Zealand ed. Lippincott Williams & Wilkins Australia, Sydney; LeMone, P., Burke, K., Bauldoff, G., et al., 2020. Medical–surgical nursing: Critical thinking for person-centred care, 4th ed. Pearson, Melbourne; NSW Health, 2023. Guideline: Insertion and management of nasogastric and orogastric tubes in adults. Available at: <https://www1.health.nsw.gov.au/pds/Pages/doc.aspx?dn=GL2023_001>; Rebeiro, G., Wilson, D., Fuller, S., 2021. *Fundamentals of nursing: Clinical skills workbook*, 4th ed. Elsevier, Chatswood. **CSs 31.1, 31.8,** Patton, K.T., Bell, F., Thompson, T., Williamson, P., 2024. *The human body in health and disease.* 8th ed. Elsevier, Missouri, pp. 571–598; Watt, E., 2021. Maintaining continence. In: Crisp, J., Douglas, C., Rebeiro, G., et al. (eds.), 2021. *Potter and Perry's fundamentals of nursing,* 6th ed. Elsevier, Sydney, pp. 1043–1089. **CSs 31.2, 31.4,** Patton, K.T., Bell, F., Thompson, T., Williamson, P., 2024. *The human body in health and disease*, 8th ed. Elsevier, Missouri, pp. 571–598; Rebeiro, G., Wilson, D., Fuller, S., 2021. *Potter & Perry's fundamentals of nursing workbook*, 4th ed. Elsevier, Chatswood; Watt, E., 2021. Maintaining continence. In: Crisp, J., Douglas, C., Rebeiro, G., et al. (eds.), 2021. *Potter and Perry's fundamentals of nursing,* 6th ed. Elsevier, Sydney, pp. 1043–1089. **CS 31.3,** Patton, K.T., Bell, F., Thompson, T., Williamson, P., 2024. *The human body in health and disease.* 8th ed. Elsevier, Missouri, pp. 571–598; Potter, P., Perry, A.G., Stockert, P.A., et al., 2023. *Fundamentals of nursing,* 11th ed. Elsevier, Missouri; Watt, E., 2021. Maintaining continence. In: Crisp, J., Douglas, C., Rebeiro, G., et al. (eds.), 2021. *Potter and Perry's fundamentals of nursing,* 6th ed. Elsevier, Sydney, pp. 1043–1089. **CS 31.5,** Australian Commission on Safety and Quality in Health Care (ACSQHC), 2021. National safety and quality health service standards, 2nd ed. ACSQHC, Sydney; , K.T., Bell, F., Thompson, T., Williamson, P., 2024. T*he human body in health and disease*, 8th ed. Elsevier, Missouri, pp. 571–598; Watt, E., 2021. Maintaining continence. In: Crisp, J., Douglas, C., Rebeiro, G., et al. (eds.), 2021. *Potter and Perry's fundamentals of nursing,* 6th ed. Elsevier, Sydney, pp. 1043–1089; Patton. **CSs 31.6, 31.7,** Australian Commission on Safety and Quality in Health Care (ACSQHC), 2021. National safety and quality health service standards, 2nd ed. ACSQHC, Sydney; Cooper, K., Gosnell, K., 2023. *Adult health nursing*, 9th ed. Elsevier, Missouri; Rebeiro, G., Wilson, D., Fuller, S., 2021. *Potter & Perry's fundamentals of nursing workbook*, 4th ed. Elsevier, Chatswood; Watt, E., 2021. Maintaining continence. In Crisp, J., Douglas, C., Rebeiro, G., et al. (eds.), 2021. *Potter and Perry's fundamentals of nursing,* 6th ed. Elsevier, Sydney, pp. 1043–1089. **CS 32.1,** Australian Council of Stoma Associations Inc, 2021. Colostomy hints and tips. Available at: <https://australianstoma.com.au/wp-content/uploads/HInts-and-Tips-for-Colostomy.pdf>; Rebeiro, G., Wilson, D., Fuller, S., 2021. *Potter and Perry's fundamentals of nursing workbook*, 4th ed. Elsevier,

Chatswood; Tollefson, J., Watson, G., Jelly, E., Tambree, K., 2022. *Essential clinical skills: Enrolled nurses*, 5th ed. Cengage Learning, Australia. **CS 32.2,** Linton, A.D., Matteson, M.A., 2023. *Introduction to medical-surgical nursing*, 8th ed. Elsevier Saunders, St Louis. **CS 33.1,** Brown, D., Edwards, H., Buckley, T., et al., 2020. *Lewis's medical-surgical nursing*, 5th ed. Elsevier, Sydney; Crisp, J., Douglas, C., Rebeiro, G., et al., 2021. *Potter and Perry's fundamentals of nursing*, 6th ed. Elsevier, Sydney; Rebeiro, G., Wilson, D., Fuller, S., 2021. *Fundamentals of nursing: Clinical skills workbook*, 4th ed. Elsevier, Chatswood. **CS 34.1,** Australian Commission on Safety and Quality in Health Care (ACSQHC), 2021. National safety and quality health service standards, 2nd ed updated. ACSQHC, Sydney; Berman, A., Frandsen, G., Snyder, S., et al., 2021 *Kozier and Erb's fundamentals of nursing*, 5th ed. Pearson Education Australia, Melbourne; Tollefson, J., Watson, G., Jelly, E., et al., 2022. *Essential clinical skills of enrolled nurses*, 5th ed. Cengage, Melbourne. **CS 34.2,** Australian Commission on Safety and Quality in Health Care (ACSQHC), 2021. National safety and quality health service standards, 2nd ed updated. ACSQHC, Sydney; Berman, A., Frandsen, G., Snyder, S., et al., 2021 *Kozier and Erb's fundamentals of nursing*, 5th ed. Pearson Education Australia, Melbourne; Stromberg, H., 2023. *Medical-surgical nursing: Concepts and practice*, 5th ed. Elsevier Inc, St Louis; Tollefson, J., Watson, G., Jelly, E., et al., 2022. *Essential clinical skills of enrolled nurses*, 5th ed. South Melbourne, Melbourne. **CS 35.1,** Australian Commission on Safety and Quality in Health Care, (ACSQHC), 2021a. National safety and quality health service standards, 2nd ed. ACSQHC, Sydney. Available at: <https://www.safetyandquality.gov.au/publications-andresources/resource-library/national-safety-and-quality-healthservice-standards-second-edition>; Berman, A., Fandsen, G., Snyder, S., Levett-Jones, T., et al., 2021. *Kozier and Erb's fundamentals of nursing: Concepts, process and practice*, 5th ed. Pearson, Melbourne; Crisp, J., Douglas, C., Rebeiro, D., et al., 2021. *Potter & Perry's fundamentals of nursing*, Australian and New Zealand edition, 6th ed. Elsevier, Chatswood; Hall, H., Glew. P., Rhodes, J., 2022. *Fundamentals of nursing and midwifery: A person-centred approach to care*, 4th ed. Lippincott Williams & Wilkins, North Ryde; LeMone, P., Bauldoff, G., Gubrud-Howe, P., et al., 2020. *Medical–surgical nursing: Critical thinking for person-centred care*, 4th ed. Pearson, Melbourne; Rebeiro, G., Wilson, D., Fuller, S., 2021. *Fundamentals of nursing: Clinical skills workbook*, 4th ed. Elsevier, Chatswood. **CS 35.2,** Berman, A., Fandsen, G., Snyder, S., Levett-Jones, T., et al., 2021. *Kozier and Erb's fundamentals of nursing: Concepts, process and practice*, 5th ed. Pearson, Melbourne; Crisp, J., Douglas, C., Rebeiro, D., et al., 2021. *Potter & Perry's fundamentals of nursing*, Australian and New Zealand edition, 6th ed. Elsevier, Chatswood; Hall, H., Glew. P., Rhodes, J., 2022. *Fundamentals of nursing and midwifery: A person-centred approach to care*, 4th ed. Lippincott Williams & Wilkins, North Ryde; LeMone, P., Bauldoff, G., Gubrud-Howe, P., et al., 2020. *Medical–surgical nursing: Critical thinking for person-centred care*, 4th ed. Pearson, Melbourne. **CS 36.1,** Australian Commission on Safety and Quality in Health Care (ACSQHC), 2021. National safety and quality health service standards, 2nd ed. ACSQHC, Sydney. Available at: <https://www.safetyandquality.gov.au/publications-andresources/resource-library/national-safety-and-qualityhealth-service-standards-second-edition>; Crawford, A.H., 2023. Endocrine problems. In: Harding, M. M., Kwong, J., Hagler, D., et al., *Lewis's medical-surgical nursing*, 12th ed. Elsevier, St Louis; Dickinson, J.K., 2023. Diabetes. In: Harding, M.M., Kwong, J., Hagler, D., et al., Lewis's medical-surgical nursing, 12th ed. Elsevier, St Louis; Miller, B., 2022. Diabetes mellitus – pathophysiology. In: Banasik, J., *Pathophysiology*, 7th ed. Elsevier, St Louis. **CS 38.1,** Crisp, J., Douglas, C., Rebeiro, G., et al. (eds.), 2021. *Potter & Perry's fundamentals of nursing*, 6th ed. Elsevier, Chatswood; Hospice UK, 2022. Care after death, 4th ed. Available at: <https://www.hospiceuk.org/publications-and-resources/care-after-death>; Marie Curie, 2022. Providing care after death. Available at: <https://www.mariecurie.org.uk/professionals/palliativecare-knowledge-zone/final-days/care-after-death>; Perry, A., Potter, P., Ostendorf, W., Laplante, N., 2022. *Clinical nursing skills and techniques*, 10th ed. Elsevier Inc; Queensland Health, 2019. Care plan for the dying person: Health professional guidelines. Available at: <https://www.health.qld.gov.au/__data/assets/pdf_file/0023/833315/cpdp-care-plan-hp-guidelines.pdf#:,:text5%E2%80%A2%20Recognition%20that%20the%20person%20is%20in%20the,advocate%20immediately%20after%20death%20is%20dignified%20%26%20respectful>. **CS 42.1,** Carter, C., Notter, J., 2024. Handbook for Registered Nurses, Elsevier, London; Crisp, J., Douglas, C., Rebeiro, G., et al., 2021. *Potter and Perry's fundamentals of nursing* – ANZ edition, 6th ed. Elsevier, Sydney; Tollefson, J., Hillman, E., 2021. *Clinical psychomotor skills: Assessment tools for nurses*, 8th ed. Cengage Learning, Australia. **CS 42.2,** Crisp, J., Douglas, C., Rebeiro, G., et al., 2021. *Potter and Perry's fundamentals of nursing* – ANZ edition, 6th ed. Elsevier, Sydney; The Royal Children's Hospital Melbourne, 2020. Central venous access device management. Available at: <https://www.rch.org.au/policy/public/Central_Venous_Access_Device_Management>; Tollefson, J., Hillman, E., 2021. Clinical psychomotor skills: Assessment tools for nurses, 8th ed. Cengage Learning, Australia. **CS 42.3,** Berman, A., Frandsen, G., Snyder, S., et al., 2020. *Kozier and Erb's fundamentals of nursing*, 5th ed. Pearson, Melbourne; Crisp, J., Douglas, C., Rebeiro, G., et al., 2021. *Potter and Perry's fundamentals of nursing* – ANZ edition, 6th ed. Elsevier, Sydney; Rebeiro, G., Wilson, D., Fuller, S., 2021. *Fundamentals of nursing: Clinical skills workbook*, 4th ed. Mosby Elsevier, Sydney. **CS 43.1,** Australian and New Zealand Committee on Resuscitation (ANZCOR), 2021e. Guideline 8 – Cardiopulmonary resuscitation (CPR). Available at: <https://www.anzcor.org/home/basic-life-support/guideline-8-cardiopulmonaryresuscitation-cpr>; Australian Resuscitation Council (ARC), 2024. Guideline 11.1 – Introduction to and principles of in-hospital resuscitation. Available at: <https://resus.org.au/download/guideline-11-1>.; Rebeiro, G., Wilson, D., Fuller, S., 2021. *Fundamentals of nursing: Clinical skills workbook*, 4th ed. Mosby Elsevier, Sydney.

FIGURES

Fig 1.1, Australian War Memorial. **Figs 1.2,** Nursing and Midwifery Board of Australia (NMBA), 2020. Decision-making framework for nursing and midwifery. Available at: <https://www.nursingmidwiferyboard.gov.au/Codes-Guidelines-Statements/Frameworks.aspx>. **Fig 2.1,** Adapted from Staunton, P.J., Chiarella, M., 2020. *Law for nurses and midwives*, 9th ed. Elsevier, Chatswood. **Fig 2.2,** Adapted from Varkey, B., 2021. Principles of clinical ethics and their application to practice. *Medical Principles and Practice* 30, 17–28. doi: 10.1159/000509119. **Fig 3.1,** Hopkins, J., 2015. CRAAP evaluation checklist. Available at: <https://researchguides.ben.edu/source-evaluation>. With kind permission from Benedictine University Library. **Fig 3.2,** Hoffmann, T., Bennett, S., Del Mar, C., 2024. *Evidence-based practice across the health professions*, 4th ed. Elsevier Australia. **Figs 4.1, 4.2,** Health Workforce Australia, 2014. Australia's future health workforce: Nurses detailed report. Department of Health, Canberra, ACT. **Figs 4.3,** Australian Institute of Health and Welfare (AIHW), 2023. Health care quality & performance. Available at: <https://www.aihw.gov.au/reports-data/health-welfare-overview/healthcare-quality-performance/coordination-of-health-care>; Australian Institute of Health and Welfare (AIHW), 2023. Health expenditure Australia 2021–22. Available at: <https://www.aihw.gov.au/reports/health-welfare-expenditure/health-expenditure-australia-2021-22/contents/about>. **Fig 4.4,** Australian Institute of Health and Welfare (AIHW), 2023. Health expenditure Australia 2020–2021. Available at: <https://www.aihw.gov.au/reports/health-welfare-expenditure/health-expenditure-australia/contents/about>. **Fig 5.1,** Australian Institute of Health and Welfare (AIHW), 2020. Australia's health 2020: in brief. Cat. No. AUS 231. AIHW, Canberra. Available at: <https://www.aihw.gov.au/getmedia/be95235d-fd4d-4824-9ade-34b7491dd66f/aihw-aus-231.pdf?inline=true>. **Fig 5.2,** Adapted from Labonté, R., 1992. Heart health inequities in Canada: Models, theory and planning. *Health Promotion International* 7(2), 119–121. **Figs 5.3, 5.4,** Taylor, J., O'Hara, L., Talbot, L., et al., 2021. *Promoting health: The primary health care approach*, 7th ed. Elsevier, Sydney. **Fig 5.5,** Illness-Wellness Continuum © 1972, 1981, 1988, 2004 by John W. Travis, MD. Reproduced with permission from *Wellness workbook: How to achieve enduring health and vitality*, 3rd ed, by John Travis and Regina Sara Ryan, Celestial Arts, 2004. <http://www.wellnessworkbook.com>. **Fig. 7.1,** Levett-Jones, T., Reid-Searl, K., 2022. *The clinical placement: An essential guide for nursing students*, 5th ed. Elsevier Australia, Chatswood, Australia. **Fig. 7.2,** Modified from Potter, P.A., Perry, A.G., Stockert, P.A., et al., 2021. Fundamentals of nursing, 10th ed. Elsevier Health Sciences, USA. **Fig. 7.3,** Crisp, J., Douglas, C., Rebeiro, G., et al. (eds.), 2021. *Potter & Perry's fundamentals of nursing*, 6th ed. Elsevier, Chatswood. **Fig 8.2,** © *Emerging Systems, a Telstra Health Business.* **Fig 8.3,** *Sample Chart: Adult Observation and Response Chart, MR 140A Form. WA Country Health Service.* **Figs 8.4, 8.5,** © *Emerging Systems, a Telstra Health Business.* **Fig 8.6,** *Sample chart. Telephone Communication Record: Medical Emergency Response Call. WA Country Health Service.* **Figs 8.7, 8.8,** *Raghunathan, K., 2024.* **Fig 8.9,** © *InterMetro Industries Corporation.* **Fig 8.10,** *Reprinted with permission from Xplore Technologies Corporation of America. Photographer: Scott Van Osdol. © 2010.* **Fig 8.11,** Raghunathan, K., 2024. Figs 8.12, 8.13, © 2016 Orion Health. **Figs 8.14, 8.15,** © *My Health Record System Operator, Australian Digital Health Agency.* **Fig 9.1,** Adapted from Reason, J., 2000. Human error models and management. *British Medical Journal* 320(7237), 768–770. Available at: < http://www.ncbi.nlm.nih.gov/pmc/articles/PMC1117770>. **Fig 10.1,** Phlsph7; Wikipedia Commons, 2022. SMCR Model. Available at: <https://commons.wikimedia.org/wiki/File:SMCR_model_-_full.svg>. **Fig 10.2,** Boggs, K.U., 2023. *Interpersonal relationships: Professional communication skills for* nurses, 9th ed. Elsevier, Sydney. **Fig 10.3,** Harding, M., Kwong, J., Hagler, D., 2023. *Lewis's medical-surgical nursing: Assessment and management of clinical problems*, 12th ed. Elsevier Health Sciences, St Louis. **Fig 10.4,** Adapted from Implementation toolkit: Standard key principles for clinical handover, NSW Department of Health 2009. **Fig 12.1,** Peden, C.J., Fleisher, L.A., Englesbe, M., 2023. *Perioperative quality improvement.* Elsevier Inc, New York. **Fig 12.2,** Based on Wilding, P.M., 2008. Reflective practice: A learning tool for student nurses. *British Journal of Nursing* 17(11), 720–724. **Fig 14.1,** © Ningura Naspurrla. Available at: <www.sydneycatholic.org/news/latest_news/2014/201455_750.shtml>. **Fig 14.2,** © Morris Gibson Tjapaltjarri licensed by Aboriginal Artists Agency Ltd. Image courtesy Papunya Tula Artists Pty Ltd. **Fig 14.3,** Photographer Sharmila Wood, courtesy FORM, Ngarluma Ngurra: Aboriginal culture on the map. **Fig 14.4,** Australian Bureau of Statistics, 2016. Census of population and housing: reflecting Australia—stories from the Census, 2016. Aboriginal and Torres Strait Islander population. 2016 Census data summary. Available at: <https://www.abs.gov.au/ausstats/abs@.nsf/Lookup/by%20Subject/2071.0,2016,Main%20Features,Cultural%20Diversity%20Data%20Summary,30>. **Fig 14.5,** © Fairfax Media/Contributor. **Fig 14.6,** Photo by Justin Brierty. **Figs 14.7, 14.8,** © Western Desert Nganampa Walytja Palyantjaku

Tjutaku Aboriginal Corporation. **Fig 15.1,** Courtesy of Melbourne Health. **Figs 16.1, 16.2,** Reproduced with permission from Adult Deterioration Detection System (ADDS) chart with blood pressure table, developed by the Australian Commission on Safety and Quality in Health Care (ACSQHC), 2012. ACSQHC, Sydney). **Fig 16.3,** Gilder, R., 2015. **Fig 16.4,** Kostelnick, C., 2020. *Mosby's textbook for long-term care nursing assistants*, 8th ed. Elsevier Inc, St Louis. **Fig 16.5,** Bonewit-West, K., 2024. *Clinical procedures for medical assistants*, 11th ed. Elsevier Inc, Philadelphia. **Fig 16.6,** Bowen, D.M., Pieren, J.A., 2020. *Darby and Walsh dental hygiene: Theory and practice*, 5th ed. Elsevier Inc, St Louis. **Fig 16.7,** McKinney, E.S., James, S.R., Murray, S.S, et al., 2022. *Maternal-child nursing*, 6th ed. Elsevier Inc, St Louis. **Fig 16.9,** Zenith, 2016. *Medical assisting module D eBook*, 4th ed. Elsevier Inc, St Louis. **Fig 16.10,** Fairchild, S.L., O'Shea, R., 2023. *Pierson and Fairchild's principles and techniques of patient care*, 7th ed. Elsevier Inc, St Louis. **Fig 16.12,** Williams, P.A., 2023. *Fundamental concepts and skills for nursing*, 6th ed. Elsevier Inc, St Louis. **Fig 16.13,** Gilder, R., 2015. **Fig 16.15,** ©Image Source/GettyImages. **Fig 17.1,** Medical illustration, RMH. **Fig 17.2,** iStockphoto/Mutlu Kurtbas. **Fig 17.3,** Broadmeadows Health Service. Modified from the original, with permission. **Fig 17.4,** Reproduced with permission of the Alfred Hospital, Melbourne. **Fig 17.5,** Courtesy of the Royal Brisbane and Women's Hospital. **Fig 18.1,** Reproduced from Centers for Disease Control and Prevention, Updated May 2012. *Principles of epidemiology in public health practice*, 3rd ed. Department of Health and Human Services, Atlanta. **Fig 18.2,** Australian Commission on Safety and Quality in Health Care (ACSQHC), 2015. Standardised infection control and prevention signs. Available at: < http://www.safetyandquality.gov.au/our-work/healthcare-associated-infection/infection-control-signage>. **Figs 18.3, 18.4, 18.5, 18.6,** Reproduced with permission of the World Health Organization. **Fig 18.8,** Stewart, K., Adler, A., Carlton, R., 2023. *Introduction to radio-logic & imaging sciences & patient care*, 8th ed. Elsevier. **Fig 18.9, 18.13, 18.14, 18.15,** Courtesy of Teresa Lewis. **Fig 18.10,** Printed with kind permission of www.antt.org. ANTT clinical practice framework 2024. The Association for Safe Aseptic Practice. **Fig 18.11, 18.12** The Association for Safe Aseptic Practice (The-ASAP), 2015. Aseptic Non-Touch Technique (ANTT), The ANTT clinical practice framework V4.0. Available at: < http://www2.nphs.wales.nhs.uk:8080/WHAIPDocs.nsf/61c1e930f9121fd080256f2a004937ed/e4528983f2eddd3a80257f10003dd2f3/$FILE/ANTT%20Framework%20v4.0pdf>. **Fig 18.16,** Victorian Aged Care Response Centre, 2020. Putting on (donning) PPE: Entering confirmed COVID-19 resident red zone. Available at <https://www.health.gov.au/sites/default/files/documents/2020/10/coronavirus-covid-19-putting-on-and-taking-off-personal-protective-equipment-posters.pdf>. **Fig 18.17,** Victorian Aged Care Response Centre, 2020. Taking off (doffing) PPE: Leaving confirmed COVID-19 resident red zone. Available at <https://www.health.gov.au/sites/default/files/documents/2020/10/coronavirus-covid-19-putting-on-and-taking-off-personal-protective-equipment-posters.pdf>. **Fig 19.1A**: www.argo.com; **B**: www.alertmedical.com; **C**: © iStockphoto/ Kameleon007; **D**: © B. Brown/ Shutterstock; **E**: Image used with permission of Arjo Inc.; **F**: Walker, S.H., 2013. Elimination of faeces. In: Brooker, C., Waugh, A. (eds.), *Foundations of nursing practice: Fundamentals of holistic care*, 2nd ed. Elsevier Ltd, Oxrod; **G**: www.breezemobility.com.au. **Fig 19.4A:** https://www.aidacare.com.au/globalassets/knowledge/resources-page/aspire/aspire_lifecomfort_active_air_mattresses_brochure.pdf; **B**: © iStock/Hippo1971; **C**: © ST Design Studio/ Shutterstock. **Figure 19.5A:** deWit, S.C., Williams, P.A., 2014. *Fundamental concepts and skills for nursing*, 4th ed. Elsevier Inc, St Louise.; Remmert, L., Sorrentino, S.A., 2023. *Mosby's essential for nursing assistants*, 7th ed. Elsevier Inc, St Louis; Stein, L.N.M, Hollden, C.J., 2024. *Concept-based clinical nursing skills*, 2nd ed. Elsevier Inc, St Louis. **Fig 19.6,** Kostelnick, C., 2015. *Mosby's textbook for long-term care nursing assistants*, 7th ed, Mosby, St Louis, Mosby. **Fig 19.7,** Potter, P.A., Perry, A.G., Stockert, P., et al., 2023. *Fundamentals of nursing*, 11th ed. Mosby, St Louis. **Fig 19.8,** Swartz, M.H., Phrampus, P.E., 2021. The acutely ill or injured patient. In: Swartz, M.H. (ed.), *Textbook of physical diagnosis: History and examination.* 8th ed. Elsevier, pp. 612–623. **Fig 20.1,** Department of Health and Aged Care, 2023. National medicines policy. Available at: <https://www.health.gov.au/resources/publications/national-medicines-policy>. **Fig 20.2,** Frotjold, A., Bloomfield, J., 2021. Ensuring medication safety. In: Crisp, J., Douglas, C., Rebeiro, G., et al. (eds.), *Potter and Perry's fundamentals of nursing*, ANZ ed. 6th ed. Elsevier, Sydney, pp. 547–637. **Fig 20.3, 20.9, 20.10, 20.11, 20.12, 20.13, 20.14, 20.15, 20.16, 20.17,** Potter, P.A., Perry, A.G., Stockert, P., et al., 2023. *Fundamentals of nursing*, 11th ed. Elsevier, St Louis. **Fig 20.4, 20.6, 20.19, 20.20,** McCuistion, L.E., DiMaggio, K.V., Winton, M.B., Yeager, J.J., 2023. *Pharmacology: A patient-centered nursing process approach*, 11th ed. Elsevier, Missouri. **Fig 20.5A:** Australian Commission on Safety and Quality in Health Care (ACSQHC), 2019c. National inpatient medication chart: NIMC (acute). Available at: <https://www.safetyandquality.gov.au/sites/default/files/2019-08/saq8404_nimc_shortstay_v3_film_nofileinfo.pdf>; **B:** Australian Commission on Safety and Quality in Health Care (ACSQHC), 2022. National subcutaneous insulin chart. Available at: <https://www.safetyandquality.gov.au/publications-and-resources/resource-library/national-subcutaneousinsulin-chart>. **Fig 20.7,** Australian Commission on Safety and Quality in Health Care (ACSQHC), 2019c. National inpatient medication chart: NIMC (acute). Available at: <https://www.safetyandquality.gov.au/sites/default/files/2019-08/saq8404_nimc_shortstay_v3_film_nofileinfo.pdf>. **Fig 20.18,** © BD. **Fig 20.21,** Knights, K., Darroch, S.,

Rowland, A., et al., 2023. *Pharmacology for health professionals*, 6th ed. Elsevier, Sydney. **Fig 20.22,** Courtesy Manrex Pty Ltd, WebsterCare 2023. Available at: <https://www.webstercare.com.au/shop/item/community-webster-pak>. **Fig 21.1, 21.3, 21.6,** Moore, K.L, Persaud, T.V.N., Torchia, M.G., 2015. *The developing human: Clinically oriented embryology*, 10th ed. Saunders, Philadelphia. **Fig 21.2,** Keenan-Lindsay, L., Sams, C., O'Connor, C., 2022. *Perry's maternal child nursing care in Canada*, 3rd ed, Elsevier Canada. **Fig 21.5,** ID 71617401 © Pablo Fernandez Rivera, Dreamstime.com. **Fig 21.7,** Centers for Disease Control and Prevention—reproduced with permission from the National Center for Health Statistics. **Fig 21.8,** Modified from Leifer, G., 2019. *Introduction to maternity and pediatric nursing*, 8th ed. Elsevier, St Louis. **Fig 22.1,** Dinulos, J., 2021. *Habif's clinical dermatology: A color guide to diagnosis and therapy*, 7th ed. **Fig 22.2,** Leifer, G., 2023. *Introduction to maternity and pediatric nursing*, 9th ed. WB Saunders, Philadelphia; Redrawn from photographs of JM Tanner, MD, Institute of Child Health, Department of Growth and Development, University of London, England, 2020. **Fig 22.3**, Court, P., 2022. *Psychologist's guide to adolescents and social media*. Elsevier. **Fig 25.1,** Patton, K., Thibodeau, G., 2019. *Anatomy and physiology*, Adapted international edition. Elsevier Ltd. **Fig 25.8,** Craft, J., Gordon, C., McCance, K. L., et al., 2023. *Understanding pathophysiology*, Australia and New Zealand ed, 4th ed. Elsevier, Chatswood. **Figs 25.18,** Magee, D., 2014. *Orthopedic physical assessment*, 6th ed. Elsevier Inc. **Fig 25.19,** *Haematology: An illustrated colour text*, 4th ed. © 2013 Elsevier Ltd. **Fig 25.20,** Lewis, S.M., Dirksen, S.R., Heitkemper, M.M., 2014. *Medical–surgical nursing. Assessment and management of clinical problems*, 9th ed. Mosby, St Louis. **Figs 25.21, 25.22, 25.28, 25.29,** Potter, P.A., Perry, A.G., Stockert, P., et al., 2023. *Fundamentals of nursing*, 11th ed. Mosby, St Louis. **Fig 25.24,** Stein, L., Hollen, C., 2024. *Concept-based clinical nursing skills: Fundamental to advanced competencies*, 2nd ed. Elsevier Inc. **Fig 25.25, 25.26,** Ignatavicius, D., Workman, M., Rebar, C., et al., 2021. *Medical-surgical nursing: Concepts for interprofessional collaborative care*, 10th ed. Elsevier Inc. **Fig 25.30,** Images of Carnét® Oxygen Pressure Regulators (AS and BS) courtesy of BOC Limited, a member of the Linde group. **Fig 26.2,** Waugh, A., Grant, A., 2023. *Ross & Wilson anatomy and physiology in health and illness*, 14th ed. Elsevier. **Fig 26.3, 26.8,** Craft, A.J., Gordon, C.J., Huether, S.E., et al., 2023. *Understanding pathophysiology*, 4th ed. Elsevier, Sydney. **Fig 26.4,** LadyofHats, Wikimedia Commons. Available at: < http://commons.wikimedia.org/wiki/File:Osmotic_pressure_on_blood_cells_diagram.svg>. **Figs 26.5, 26.11,** Crisp, J., Douglas, C., Rebeiro, G., et al. (eds.), 2021. *Potter & Perry's fundamentals of nursing*, 6th ed. Elsevier, Chatswood. **Fig 26.6,** Adapted from Crisp, J., Douglas, C., Rebeiro, G., et al., 2021. *Potter and Perry's fundamentals of nursing*, Australian ed, 6th ed. Elsevier, Sydney. **Figs 26.7,** Herlihy, B., Maebius, N., 2011. *The human body in health and disease*, 4th ed. Saunders, Philadelphia. **Fig 26.9,** Potter, P.A., Perry, A.G., 2021. *Fundamentals of nursing*, 10th ed. St. Louis, Mosby. **Fig 26.10**, Patton, K.T., Williamson, P., Thompson, T., et al 2024. *The human body in health & disease*, 8th ed. Elsevier. **Fig 27.1,** Webb, M., Scott, K., 2023. Promoting and maintaining health and wellness. In: Scott, K. *Long-term caring*, 5th ed. Elsevier Australia. **Fig 28.1,** Crisp, J., Douglas, C., Rebeiro, G., et al., 2021. *Potter and Perry's fundamentals of nursing*, Australian ed, 5th ed. Elsevier, Sydney. **Fig 28.2,** McHugh Pendleton, H., Schultz-Krohn, W., 2018. *Pedretti's occupational therapy*, 8th ed. Elsevier, St Louis. **Fig 28.3,** © Christine Ingram. **Fig 28.5**, © The State of Queensland (Queensland Health) 1996–2016. **Figs 28.7, 28.9,** © Dorothy Lanyon. **Fig 28.8,** Fig. 28.4 from Yoost, B.L., Crawford, L.R. (eds.) *Fundamentals of nursing: Active learning for collaborative practice*. Elsevier Inc. 2022. ISBN 978-0-323-29557-4. **Fig 28.10A**: Williamson, P., Thompson, T., Bell, F., Patton. K., 2024. *The human body in health & disease*, 8th ed. Elsevier, St Louis; **B: Cooper, T.**, Bischoff, L.L., Schoene, D., et al., 2019. A multi-component exercise intervention to improve physical functioning, cognition and psychological well-being in elderly nursing home residents: A study protocol of a randomized controlled trial in the PROCARE (prevention and occupational health in long-term care) project. *BMC Geriatrics* 19(1), 369–369. **Fig 28.11,** Courtesy of Lanny L. Johnson, MD, East Lansing, MI. Used with permission. **Fig 28.12** Silvestri, A., Silverstri, L., 2023. *Saunders comprehensive review for the NCLEX-RN Examination*, 9th ed, Elsevier, St Louis. **Fig 28.13,** Fig 17.8 from Perry, A.G., Potter, P.A., Ostendorf, W.R., 2019. *Nursing interventions and clinical skills*, 7th ed. Elsevier, St Louis. **Figs 28.14, 28.16, 28.20,** Potter, P.A., Perry, A.G., Stockert, P.A., et al., 2023. *Fundamentals of nursing*, 11th ed. Elsevier/Mosby, St Louis. **Fig 28.15**, Richards, J., Whittle, M., Levine, D., 2023. Whittle's Gait Analysis, 6th ed, Elsevier, St Louis. **Fig 28.17, 28.19,** Sehgal, M., Silvestri, L., 2023. *Saunders comprehensive review for the NCLEX-RN Examination*, 9th ed. Elsevier, St Louis. **Fig 28.18,** © Norman Lanyon. **Fig 29.1,** Zenith, 2018. *Medical assisting module A textbook*. Elsevier Inc, St Louis. **Fig 29.2,** Singh, R., Kumar, A., Solanki, P., et al., 2024. *Nanotechnological aspects for next-generation wound management*. Elsevier Inc, St Louis. **Fig 29.3,** Hockenberry, M., Duffy, E., Gibbs, K., 2024. *Wong's nursing care of infants and children*, 12th ed. Elsevier Inc, St Louis. **Fig 29.4,** Potter, P.A., Perry A.G., Stockert, P.A. et al., 2013. *Fundamentals of nursing*, 8th ed. Mosby, St Louis. **Fig 29.5,** Zerwekh J., Garneau A., Miller C.J., 2017. *Digital collection of the memory notebooks of nursing*, 4th ed. Nursing Education Consultants Inc, Chandler. **Fig. 29.6,** International Wound Infection Institute, 2022. **Fig 29.7,** Fillit, H.M. 2017. *Brocklehurst's textbook of geriatric medicine and gerontology*, 8th ed. Elsevier Ltd, London. **Fig 29.9,** European Pressure Ulcer Advisory Panel (EPUAP), National Pressure Injury Advisory Panel and

Pan Pacific Pressure Injury Alliance, Haesler, E. (ed.), 2019. Prevention and treatment of pressure ulcers/injuries: clinical practice guidelines, 3rd ed. EPUAP/NPIAP/PPPIA. **Fig 29.10,** Deans, C., Paterson, H., 2024. *Core topics in general and emergency surgery: A companion to specialist surgical practice*, 7th ed. Elsevier Ltd. **Fig 29.11,** LeBlanc, K., Baranoski, S., Holloway, S., et al., 2013. Validation of a new classification system for skin tears. *Advances in Skin and Wound Care* 26(6), 263–265. **Fig 29.12,** Curtis, P., Duane L., 1965. Treatment of burns. *Current Problems in Surgery* 2(3), 1–40. ISSN 0011-3840. Available at: <https://doi.org/10.1016/S0011-3840(65)80012-0>. **Fig 30.1,** NSW Department of Health, 2017. Policy directive: Nutrition care. Pd2017_041. NSW Health, Sydney. Available at: <https://www1.health.nsw.gov.au/pds/ActivePDSDocuments/PD2017_041.pdf>. **Fig 30.2,** National Health and Medical Research Council (NHMRC), 2013. The Australian guide to health eating. Guidelines for healthy foods and drinks supplied in school canteens. Available at: <https://www1.health.gov.au/internet/publications/publishing.nsf/Content/nhsc-guidelines,aus-guide-healthy-eatinghttps://www1.health.gov.au/internet/publications/publishing.nsf/Content/nhsc-guidelines,aus-guide-healthy-eating>. **Fig 30.3,** National Health and Medical Research Council (NHMRC), 2019. How to understand food labels. Available at: <https://www.eatforhealth.gov.au/eating-well/how-understand-food-labels>. **Fig 30.4,** National Health and Medical Research Council (NHMRC), 2015. Serve sizes. Available at: <https://www.eatforhealth.gov.au/food-essentials/how-much-do-we-need-each-day/serve-sizes>. **Fig 30.5,** National Health and Medical Research Council (NHMRC), 2013. Clinical practice guidelines for the management of overweight and obesity in adults, adolescents and children in Australia. NHMRC, Canberra. **Fig 30.6,** Djachenko, A. **Fig 30.7,** Crisp, J., Douglas, S., Rebeiro, G., et al. (eds.), 2021. *Potter and Perry's Fundamentals of nursing*, 6th ed. Elsevier, Sydney. **Figs 31.4, 31.8,** Crisp, J., Douglas, C., Rebeiro, G., et al. (eds.), 2021. *Potter and Perry's fundamentals of nursing*, 6th ed. Elsevier, Sydney. **Fig 31.5,** Continence Foundation of Australia, 2021. Bladder Diary with instructions | Continence Foundation of Australia. Available at: <https://www.continence.org.au/resource/bladder-diary-instructions?v=8452>. **Fig 31.9,** Fairchild, S.L., O'Shea, R.K., Washington, R.D., 2022. *Pierson and Fairchild's principles and techniques of patient care*, 7th ed. Elsevier, St Louis. **Fig 32.1,** Monahan, F.D., Neighbours, M., 1998. *Medical-surgical nursing*, 2nd ed. Saunders, Philadelphia. **Fig 32.2,** Solomon, E.P., 2016. *Introduction to human anatomy and physiology*, 4th ed. Saunders Elsevier, St Louis. **Fig 32.3,** Odom-Forren, J., 2024. *Drain's perianaesthesia nursing*, 8th ed. Elsevier, St Louis. **Fig 32.4,** Shiland, B.J., 2022. *Mastering healthcare terminology*, 7th ed. Elsevier, St Louis. **Fig 32.5,** Rogers, J.L. 2023. *McCance & Huether's pathophysiology*, 9th ed, Elsevier, St Louis. **Fig 32.6,** Waugh, A., Grant, A., 2023. *Ross and Wilson anatomy and physiology in health and illness*, 14th ed. Elsevier, Edinburgh. **Fig 32.7,** Meiner, S.E., Yeager, J.J., 2019. Gerontologic nursing, 6th ed. St Louis, Elsevier. **Fig 32.8,** I Davis, K., Guerra, A., 2022. *Mosby's® pharmacy technician: Principles and practice*, 6th ed. Elsevier, St Louis. **Figs 32.9,** Harding, M., Kwong, J., Hagler, D., Reinisch, C., 2023. *Lewis's medical-surgical nursing*, 12th ed. Elsevier, St Louis. **Fig 32.10,** Linton, A.D., Matteson, M.A., 2023. *Introduction to medical-surgical nursing*, 8th ed. Elsevier Saunders, St Louis. **Fig 32.12**, Harding, M., Kwong, J., Hagler, D., Reinisch, C., 2023. *Lewis's medical-surgical nursing*, 12th ed. Elsevier, St Louis. **Fig 32.13**, Leonard, P., 2022. *Building a medical vocabulary: With Spanish translations*, 11th ed. Elsevier, St Louis. **Fig 32.14,** Hagler, D., Harding, M., Kwong, J., et al., 2022. *Clinical companion to medical-surgical* nursing, 12th ed. Elsevier, St Louis. **Figs 33.1, 33.2, 33.3, 33.4, 33.9,** Craft, J., Gordon, C., Heuther, S., 2023. *Understanding pathophysiology*. Elsevier, Sydney. **Fig 33.5**, Acute Pain Management Guideline Panel, 1992. Acute pain management in adults: Operative procedures. Quick reference guide for clinicians, AHCPR Pub No. 92-0019. Agency for Health Care Policy and Research, Rockville, MD. **Fig 33.6,** Abbey, J., Piller, N., DeBellis, A., et al., 2004. The Abbey Pain Scale. A 1-minute numerical indicator for people with late-stage dementia. *International Journal of Palliative Nursing* 10(1), 6–13. **Fig 33.7,** Workman, M., LaCharity, L., 2024. *Understanding pharmacology: Essentials for medication safety*, 3rd ed. Elsevier Inc. **Fig 33.8,** McKenry, L, Tessier, E, Hogan, M., 2006. *Mosby's pharmacology in nursing*, 22nd ed. Mosby, St Louis. **Figs 34.1, 34.5, 34.6, 34.8,** Patton, K., Thibodeau, G.A., 2024. *The human body in health and disease*, 8th ed. Elsevier, St Louis. **Fig 34.3,** Ball, J., Dains, J., Flynn, J., et al., 2023. *Seidel's guide to physical examination*, 10th ed. Elsevier, St Louis. **Fig 34.4,** Applegate, E., 2011. *The anatomy and physiology learning system*, 4th ed. St Louis, Saunders. **Fig 34.7,** Silvestri, L.A., Silvestri, A., 2023. *Saunders comprehensive review for the NCLEX-RN® examination*, 9th ed. St. Louis, Saunders. **Fig 35.1A:** Patton, K.T., Bell, F.B., Thompson, T., Williamson, P.L., 2024. *The human body in health & disease*, 8th ed. Elsevier Inc, St. Louis; **B: Applegate, E., 2011.** *The anatomy and physiology learning system*, 4th ed. Saunders, St Louis. **Fig 35.2,** Patton, K.T., Bell, F.B., Thompson, T., Williamson, P.L., 2024. *The human body in health & disease*, 8th ed. Elsevier Inc, St. Louis. **Figs 35.3,** Patton, K.T., Thibodeau G.A., 2018. The human body in health & disease, 7th ed. Elsevier Inc., St. Louis. **Fig 35.4A:** Patton et al 2022; B: Banasik, J.L., Copstead, L.E.C., 2019. Pathophysiology, 6th ed. Elsevier Inc, St. Louis. **Figure 35.5,** Patton et al 2022. **Figure 35.6,** Hall, J.E., Hall, M.E., 2021. *Guyton and Hall textbook of medical physiology*, 14th ed. Elsevier Inc, St Louis. **Fig 35.7,** Rollins, J.H., Long, B.W., Curtis, T., 2023. *Merrill's atlas of radiographic positioning and procedures*, 15th ed. Elsevier Inc, Mosby. **Fig 35.8,** Stein, L.N.M., Hollen, C.J., 2024. *Concept-based clinical nursing skills*, 2nd ed. Elsevier Inc,

St Louis. **Fig 35.9,** deWit, S.C., Kumagai, C.K., 2013. *Medical-surgical nursing*, 2nd ed. Saunders, St Louis. **Figs 36.1,** Harding, M. M., Kwong, J., Hagler, D., Reinisch, C., 2023. *Lewis's medical-surgical nursing*, 12th ed. Elsevier, St Louis. **Fig 36.2,** Lough, M. E., 2024. Endocrine clinical assessment and diagnostic procedures. In: Urden, L., Stacy, K., Sanchez, K., et al., *Priorities in critical care nursing*, 9th ed. Elsevier, St Louis. **Fig 36.3,** Modified from Herlihy, B., Maebius, N.K., 2007. *The human body in health and illness*, 3rd ed. Saunders, St Louis. **Fig 36.4,** Williamson, P., Thompson, T., Bell, F., Patton, K.T., 2022. *Anatomy & physiology*, 11th ed. Elsevier, St Louis. **Fig 36.5,** Dover, J., Fairhurst, K., Innes, J., 2024. *Macleod's clinical examination*, 15th ed. Elsevier, St Louis. **Fig 36.6A,** Belchetz, P., Hammond, P., 2003. *Mosby's color atlas and text of diabetes and endocrinology*. Mosby, Edinburgh. **Fig 36.6B,** Crawford, A.H., 2023. Endocrine problems. In: Harding, M.M., Kwong, J., Hagler, D., et al., *Lewis's medical-surgical nursing*, 12th ed. Elsevier, St Louis. **Fig 36.7,** Khurana, I., Khurana, A., 2020. *Medical physiology for undergraduate students*, 2nd ed. Elsevier, St Louis. **Fig 36.8,** Damjanov, I., 2006. *Pathology for the health-related profession*, 3rd ed. WB Saunders, Philadelphia. **Fig 36.9,** Tchang, B. G., 2021. Diabetes mellitus. In: Leppert, B., Kelly, C., *Netter's integrated review of medicine*. Elsevier, St Louis. **Fig 36.10,** Iaquinto, J.M., Leslie, M.E., 2023. Neurological foot pathology. In: Ledoux, E., Telfer, S., *Foot and ankle biomechanics*. Elsevier, St Louis. **Fig 36.11,** Copyright Eli Lilly and Company. All rights reserved. Used with permission. **Fig 36.12,** Atway, S.A., DiMassa, N.V., 2020. Debridement and negative pressure wound therapy. In: Roy, S., Das, A., Bagchi, D., *Wound healing, tissue repair, and regeneration in diabetes*. Elsevier, St Louis. **Fig 37.1,** Anderson, A. 2023. *Mosby's® textbook for medication* assistants, 2nd ed, Elsevier Inc. **Fig 37.2,** Moore K., Persaud, T., Torchia, M., 2016. *The developing human: clinically oriented embryology*, 10th ed. Saunders, Philadelphia. **Fig 37.3A:** Anderson, A. 2023. *Mosby's® textbook for medication assistants*, 2nd ed, Elsevier Inc; **B**: Drake, R., Vogl, A.W., Mitchell, A., et al., 2020. *Gray's atlas of anatomy*, 3rd ed. Churchill Livingstone, Philadelphia, **Fig 37.4**, Standring, S., 2021. *Gray's anatomy*, 42nd ed. Elsevier, London. **Fig 37.5,** McKenry, L., Tessier, E., Hogan, M.A., 2006. *Mosby's pharmacology in nursing*. 22nd ed. Mosby, St Louis. **Fig 37.6,** Stewart, R., Dains, J., Ball, J., Solomon, B., Flynn, J., 2023. *Seidel's guide to physical examination: An interprofessional approach*, 10th ed. Elsevier Inc. **Fig 37.7,** Perry, A., Stockert, P., Hall, A., Ostendorf, W., Potter, P., 2023. *Fundamentals of nursing*, 11th ed. Elsevier, St Louis. **Fig 37.8,** Grimm, J., 2025. Oncologic and hematologic problems. In: Silvestri, A.E., Bowser, A.E., Silvestri, L.A., et al., *Saunders comprehensive review for the NCLEX-PN® examination*, 9th ed. Elsevier Inc, Philadelphia. **Fig 38.1,** Crisp, J., Douglas, C., Rebeiro, G., et al. (eds.), 2021. *Potter & Perry's fundamentals of nursing*, 6th ed. Elsevier, Chatswood.

Fig. 40.1, Pendleton, H.M., Schultz-Krohn, W., 2018. *Pedretti's occupational therapy: Practice skills for physical dysfunction*, 8th ed. Elsevier Inc, St Louis. **Fig. 40.2,** Wellcome Photo Library. **Fig. 40.3,** Patterson Medical USA. **Fig. 40.4,** Patterson Medical USA. **Fig. 40.5,** Patterson Medical USA. **Fig 41.1,** das Neves Júnior, T.T., de Queiroz, A.A.R., de Carvalho, E.A., et al., 2023. Clinical and sociodemographic profile of users with chronic diseases in primary health care. *Enfermería Global* 22(1), 271–282. **Fig 41.2,** Epping-Jordan, J., Pruitt, S., Bengoa, R., et al., 2004. Improving the quality of health care for chronic conditions. *BMJ Quality & Safety* 13(4), 299–305. **Figure 42.1,** Black, J.M., Hokanson Hawks, J., Malarvizhi, S., et al., 2019. *Black's medical-surgical nursing: Clinical management for positive outcomes*, First South Asia ed. RELX India Pvt. Ltd, India. **Fig 42.2,** Queensland Health Perioperative Patient Record Version 8.00. © State of Queensland (Queensland Health), 2022. **Fig 42.3,** This checklist has been adapted from the World Health Organization Surgical Safety Checklist by the Royal Australasian College of Surgeons in consultation with the Australian and New Zealand College of Anaesthetists, the Royal Australian and New Zealand College of Ophthalmologists, the Royal Australian and New Zealand College of Obstetricians and Gynaecologists, the Australian College of Operating Room Nurses and the Perioperative Nurses College of the New Zealand Nurses Organisation; it is not intended to be comprehensive, additions and modifications to fit local practice are encouraged [Oct 09]. Based on the WHO Surgical Safety Checklist, © World Health Organization 2009. All rights reserved. **Fig 43.1,** Sydney Local Health District, 2014. ISBAR. Available at: <https://www.slhd.nsw.gov.au/BTF/ISBAR.html>. **Fig 43.2,** SA Health, 2020. Rapid detection and response observation charts. Department for Health and Ageing, Government of South Australia. Available at: <https://www.sahealth.sa.gov.au/wps/wcm/connect/ff3a769a-e8f0-45db-970e-12281b2891b2/MR59A%2B-%2BAdult%2BObservation%2BChart%2B-%2BEXAMPLE1%281%29.pdf?MOD5AJPERES&CACHEID5ROOTWORKSPACEff3a769a-e8f0-45db-970e-12281b2891b2-oun4qXB>. **Fig 43.3,** Australian and New Zealand Committee on Resuscitation (ANZCOR), 2023. Basic life support (flowchart). Available at: <https://www.anzcor.org/assets/Uploads/Basic-Life-Support-August-2023-1-v3.pdf>. **Figs 43.4,** Malmivuo & Plonsey 1995, Fig 19.3C. **Fig 43.5,** Malmivuo & Plonsey 1995, Fig 19.3B. **Fig 43.6,** © Elsevier Australia. **Fig 44.2,** Leifer, G., 2023. *Introduction to maternity and pediatric nursing*, 9th ed. WB Saunders, Philadelphia. **Fig 44.3** Courtesy of Dr Jack Newman, International Breastfeeding Centre, Toronto Canada. **Fig 44.4,** Crisp, J., Douglas, C., Rebeiro, G., et al. (eds.), 2021. *Potter and Perry's fundamentals of nursing*, 6th ed. Elsevier, Sydney. **Fig 44.5,** © privilege/Shutterstock.

Fig 44.7, Leifer, G., 2023. *Introduction to maternity and pediatric nursing*, 9th ed. WB Saunders, Philadelphia. **Fig 45.1,** Clendon, J., Munns, A., McMurray, A. 2022. *Community health and wellness: Primary health care in practice*, 7th ed. Elsevier, Sydney. **Fig 45.2,** Francis, K., Chapman, Y., Hoare, K., et al., 2013. *Community as partner: Theory and practice in nursing*. Lippincott Williams & Wilkins, Sydney. **Fig 45.3,** Adapted from Hart, C.R., Berry, H.L., Tonna, A.M., 2011. Improving the mental health of rural New South Wales communities facing drought and other adversities. *Australian Journal of Rural Health* 19, 231–238. **Fig 45.4,** Perimal-Lewis, L., Williams, P. A. H., Mudd, G., et al., 2021. Virtual care: The future of telehealth. In Maeder A. J., Higa, C., Van Den Berg, M. E. L., et al., (eds.), *Telehealth innovations in remote healthcare services delivery: Global telehealth 2020.* IOS Press Ebooks, Amsterdam.

NURSING CARE PLANS

NCP 13.1, Barkway P., O'Kane, D., 2020. *Psychology: An introduction for health professionals*. Elsevier, Australia; Gonzalez, L., Curry, K., 2020. Understanding each other: Communication and culture, ch 5, 52–65. In: Balzer, R.J., *Communication in nursing*, 9th ed. Elsevier, Australia; Encyclopaedia Britannica, 2022. Uyghur: People. Available at: <https://www.britannica.com/topic/Uyghur>; Minnican, C., O'Toole, G., 2020. Exploring the incidence of culturally responsive communication in Australian Healthcare: The first rapid review on this concept. *BMC Health Services Research* 20(1). doi: 10.1186/s12913-019-4859-6. Available at: <https://web.p.ebscohost.com/ehost/pdfviewer/pdfviewer?vid51&sid5a753764c-5a18-498f-bef6-b9b54609eea1%40redis>. **NCP 20.1,** Broyles, B., Reiss, B., Evans, M., et al., 2019. *Pharmacology in nursing*, Australian and New Zealand ed, 3rd ed. Cengage Learning Australia, Melbourne. **NCP 27.1,** Flynn Makic, M.B., Martiknez-Kratz, M.R., 2022. *Ackley and Ladwig's nursing diagnosis handbook*, 13th ed. Elsevier Ltd; Carpineto, L.J., 2022. *Handbook of nursing diagnosis: Application to clinical practice*, 16th ed. Lippincott Williams & Wilkins, Philadelphia; Gordon, C., 2021. Fostering sleep. In: Crips, J., Douglas, C., Rebeiro, G., et al. (eds.), *Potter and Perry's fundamentals of nursing*, 6th ed. Elsevier, Chatswood. **NCP 28.1,** Adapted from Australian Commission on Safety and Quality in Health Care (ACSQHC), 2021. National safety and quality health service standards, 2nd ed. ACSQHC, Sydney; Crisp, J.C., Douglas, C., Rebeiro, G., et al., (eds.), 2021. *Potter and Perry's fundamentals of nursing*, Australian ed, 6th ed. Elsevier, Australia; Gulanick, M., Myers, J.L., 2022. *Nursing care plans: Diagnoses, interventions, and outcomes*, 10th ed. Elsevier Mosby, St Louis. **NCP 28.2,** Crisp, J.C., Douglas, C., Rebeiro, G., et al., (eds.), 2021. *Potter and Perry's fundamentals of nursing*, Australian ed, 6th ed. Elsevier, Australia; Gulanick, M., Myers, J.L., 2022. *Nursing care plans: Diagnoses, interventions, and outcomes*, 10th ed. Elsevier Mosby, St Louis; Touhy, T.A., Jett, K., 2019. *Ebersole & Hess's toward healthy aging*, 10th ed. Elsevier, St Louis. **NCP 29.1,** Australian Commission on Safety and Quality in Health Care (ACSQHC), 2020. Preventing pressure injuries and wound management. Available at: <https://www.safetyandquality.gov.au/sites/default/files/2020-10/fact_sheet_-_preventing_pressure_injuries_and_wound_management_oct_2020.pdf>; European Pressure Ulcer Advisory Panel (EPUAP), National Pressure Injury Advisory Panel (NPIAP), Pan Pacific Pressure Injury Alliance (PPPIA), Haesler, E. (ed.), 2019. *Prevention and treatment of pressure ulcers/injuries: Clinical practice guidelines*, 3rd ed. EPUAP/NPIAP/PPPIA. **NCP 35.1,** Berman, A., Fandsen, G., Snyder, S., Levett-Jones, T., et al., 2021. *Kozier and Erb's fundamentals of nursing: Concepts, process and practice*, 5th ed. Pearson, Melbourne; LeMone, P., Bauldoff, G., Gubrud-Howe, P., et al., 2020. *Medical–surgical nursing: Critical thinking for person-centred care*, 4th ed. Pearson, Melbourne. **NCP 39.1,** Hercelinskyj, G., Alexander, L., 2022. *Mental health nursing*, enhanced edition, 1st ed. Cengage. **NCP 40.1,** Chang, E., Johnson, A., 2022. *Living with chronic illness & disability: Principles for nursing practice*, 4th ed. Elsevier, Chatswood; Crisp, J., Douglas, C., Rebeiro, G., et al. (eds.), 2021. *Potter and Perry's fundamentals of nursing*, 6th ed. Elsevier, Sydney. **NCP 44.1,** Murray, S.S., McKinney, E.S., Holub, K., 2023. *Foundations of maternal-newborn and women's health nursing*, 8th ed. Saunders Elsevier, St Louis.

TABLES

Table 1.1, Crisp, J., Douglas, C., Rebeiro, G., et al. (eds.), 2013, *Potter and Perry's fundamentals of nursing*, 5th ed. Elsevier, Chatswood; Royal College of Nursing, Australia (RCNA), 2011. Media release, 30 November. Available at: <www.acn.org.au>; Hansard Source, 2008; CATSINaM, 2023; CDNM, 2016. **Table 2.1,** Australian Human Rights Commission (AHRC), 2014. Good practice, good business: A quick guide to Australian discrimination laws. Fact sheets. Available at: <https://humanrights.gov.au/our-work/employers/good-practice-good-business-factsheets>. **Table 2.2,** Australian Commission on Safety and Quality in Health Care (ACSQHC), 2017. National Safety and Quality Health Service Standards, 2nd ed. ACSQHC, Sydney; NSW Government, 2020. Health Records and Information Manual for Community Health Facilities, Ministry of Health, Sydney. **Table 2.3,** Australian Commission on Safety and Quality in Health Care (ACSQHC), 2013. Australian Open Disclosure Framework. ACSQHC, Sydney. **Table 2.4,** Crisp, J., Douglas, C., Rebeiro, G., et al. (eds.), 2021. *Potter & Perry's fundamentals of nursing*, 6th ed. Elsevier, Chatswood; Daly, J., Jackson, D., 2020. *Contexts of Nursing*, 6th ed. Elsevier Australia, Chatswood; Mathews, B., Kenny, M.C., 2008. Mandatory reporting legislation in the United States, Canada, and Australia: A cross-jurisdictional review of key features, differences, and issues. *Child Maltreatment* 13 (1), 50–63.

Smith, J.D., 2016. *Australia's rural, remote and Indigenous health*, 3rd ed. Elsevier, Chatswood; Staunton, P.J., Chiarella, M., 2020. *Law for nurses and midwives*, 9th ed. Elsevier, Chatswood; Willis, J.M., Black, K., 2016. Ethical and legal issues in critical care nursing. In: Sole, M.L., Klien, D.G., Moseley, M.J. (eds.), *Introduction to critical care nursing*, 7th ed. Elsevier Saunders. **Table 2.5,** Adapted from Allan, S., 2020. *Law & ethics for health practitioners*, Elsevier Australia: Chatswood. **Table 3.1,** Australian Research Data Commons (ARDC), 2019. What is research data? Available at: <ardc.edu.au/guides/what-is-research-data>; Australian Bureau of Statistics, nd. Variables. Available at: <https://www.abs.gov.au/statistics/understanding-statistics/statistical-terms-and-concepts/variables>; Creswell, J.W., Creswell, J.D., 2023. *Research design: Qualitative, quantitative, and mixed methods approaches*, 6th ed. SAGE Publications; Ellis, P., 2022. *Understanding research for nursing students*, 5th ed. Transforming nursing practice. Learning Matters. SAGE Publications; Galvan, J.L., Galvan, M., 2017. *Writing literature reviews: A guide for students of the social and behavioural sciences*, 7th ed. Routledge, Taylor & Francis Group; Merriam-Webster, nd. 'Research'. In Merriam-Webster.com dictionary. Available at: <https://www.merriam-webster.com/dictionary/research>; Moule, P., 2020. *Making sense of research in nursing, health and social care*, 7th ed. SAGE Publications. **Table 3.2,** Creswell, J.W., Creswell, J.D., 2023. *Research design: Qualitative, quantitative, and mixed methods approaches*, 6th ed. SAGE Publications; Jolley, J., 2020. *Introducing research and evidence-based practice for nursing and healthcare professionals*, 3rd ed. Routledge. Available at: <https://doi.org/10.4324/9780429329456>; Moule, P., 2020. *Making sense of research in nursing, health and social care*, 7th ed. SAGE Publications. **Table 3.3,** Creswell, J.W., Creswell, J.D., 2023. *Research design: Qualitative, quantitative, and mixed methods approaches*, 6th ed. SAGE Publications; Moule, P., 2020. *Making sense of research in nursing, health and social care*, 7th ed. SAGE Publications; Ellis, P., 2022. *Understanding research for nursing students*, 5th ed. Transforming nursing practice. Learning Matters. SAGE Publications. *Table 3.5,* Moule, P., 2020. *Making sense of research in nursing, health and social care*, 7th ed. SAGE Publications; Creswell, J.W., Creswell, J.D., 2023. *Research design: Qualitative, quantitative, and mixed methods approaches*, 6th ed. SAGE Publications. **Table 3.6,** Creswell, J.W., Creswell, J.D., 2023. *Research design: Qualitative, quantitative, and mixed methods approaches*, 6th ed. SAGE Publications; Jolley, J., 2020. *Introducing research and evidence-based practice for nursing and healthcare professionals*, 3rd ed. Routledge. Available at: <https://doi.org/10.4324/9780429329456>; Moule, P., 2020. Making sense of research in nursing, health and social care, 7th ed. SAGE Publications; Ellis, P., 2022. *Understanding research for nursing students*, 5th ed. Transforming nursing practice. Learning Matters. SAGE Publications. **Table 3.7,** Creswell, J.W., Creswell, J.D., 2023. *Research design: Qualitative, quantitative, and mixed methods approaches*, 6th ed. SAGE Publications. **Table 4.1,** World Health Organization (WHO), 2023. Global health observatory. WHO, Geneva. **Table 4.2,** World Health Organization (WHO), 2023b. Global Health Workforce statistics database. WHO, Geneva. **Table 4.3A, 4.3B,** Australian Bureau of Statistics, 2018. Self-assessed health status. Available at: <https://www.abs.gov.au/statistics/health/health-conditions-and-risks/self-assessed-health-status/2017-18>. **Table 6.1,** Levett-Jones, T., Reid-Searl, K., 2022. *The clinical placement: An essential guide for nursing students*, 5th ed. Elsevier Australia, Chatswood, Australia. **Table 7.1,** Wilson, S.F, Giddens J.F., 2022. *Health assessment for nursing practice*, 7th ed. Elsevier Health Sciences, USA. **Tables 7.2, 7.3,** Crisp, J., Douglas, C., Rebeiro, G., et al. (eds.), 2021. *Potter & Perry's fundamentals of nursing*, 6th ed. Elsevier, Chatswood. **Table 8.1,** Australian Government Department of Health, 2021. Australian National Aged Care Classification (AN-ACC): AN-ACC Reference Manual including AN-ACC Assessment Tool (Appendix 1). Australian Government. Available at: <https://www.health.gov.au/resources/publications/an-acc-reference-manual-and-an-acc-assessment-tool?language=en>; Australian Government Department of Health and Aged Care, 2023. Care Minutes and 24/7 Registered Nurse Responsibility Guide. Australian Government. Available at: <https://www.health.gov.au/sites/default/files/2023-03/care-minutes-and-24-7-registered-nurse-responsibility-guide.pdf>. **Table 8.3,** Adapted from Australian Commission on Safety and Quality in Health Care (ACSQHC), nd. Documenting information: Communicating for safety resource portal. ACSQHC, Sydney. Available at: <https://c4sportal.safetyandquality.gov.au/documenting-information>. **Table 8. 4,** Crisp, J., Douglas, C., Rebeiro, G., et al. (eds.), 2021. *Potter & Perry's fundamentals of nursing*, 6th ed. Elsevier, Chatswood. **Table 8.5,** JBI, 2018. Evidence summaries: Documentation at transition of care. (JBI159.) Available at: <https://jbi.global/ebp>; Manias, E., Bucknall, T., Hutchinson, A., et al., 2017. Improving documentation at transitions of care for complex patients. Australian Commission on Safety and Quality in Health Care, Sydney. **Table 8.6,** McBride, S., Tietze, M., 2019. *Nursing informatics for the advanced practice nurse: Patient safety, quality, outcomes, and interprofessionalism*, 2nd ed. New York: Springer Publishing Company USA; Sewell, J.P., 2019. *Informatics and nursing: Opportunities and challenges*, 6th ed. Wolters Kluwer, Philadelphia. **Table 8.7,** McBride, S., Tietze, M., 2019. *Nursing informatics for the advanced practice nurse: Patient safety, quality, outcomes, and interprofessionalism*, 2nd ed. New York: Springer Publishing Company USA. **Table 8.8,** McBride, S., Tietze, M., 2019. *Nursing informatics for the advanced practice nurse: Patient safety, quality, outcomes, and interprofessionalism*, 2nd ed. Springer Publishing Company, New York; Nelson, R., Staggers, N., 2018. *Health informatics: An interprofessional approach*, 2nd ed. Elsevier, St Louis. **Table 8.9,** McBride,

S., Tietze, M., 2019. *Nursing informatics for the advanced practice nurse: Patient safety, quality, outcomes, and interprofessionalism*, 2nd ed. Springer Publishing Company, New York; Nelson, R., Staggers, N., 2018. *Health informatics: An interprofessional approach*, 2nd ed. Elsevier, St Louis; Office of the National Coordinator for Health Information Technology (ONC), 2017. Standard nursing terminologies: A landscape analysis. Available at: <https://www.healthit.gov/sites/default/files/snt_final_05302017.pdf>. **Table 8.10,** Adapted from Nelson, R., Staggers, N., 2018. *Health informatics: An interprofessional approach*, 2nd ed. Elsevier, St Louis. **Table 8.11,** Reproduced with permission from Emergency department clinicians' guide to My Health Record, developed by the Australian Commission on Safety and Quality in Health Care (ACSQHC), 2019. ACSQHC, Sydney. **Table 9.1,** Kellerman, T. **Table 9.2,** Victorian Department of Health, 2023. Major trauma guidelines and education: Trauma Victoria. Teamwork and communication. Available at: <https://trauma.reach.vic.gov.au/guidelines/teamwork-and-communication/dealing-with-issues>. **Table 10.1,** Boggs, K.U., 2023. *Interpersonal relationships: Professional communication skills for nurses*, 9th ed. Elsevier, Sydney; O'Toole, G., 2020. *Communication: Core interpersonal skills for health professionals.* 4th ed. Elsevier, Sydney. **Table 10.2,** Based on Speech Pathology Australia, 2023. Communication disability and communication access. Available at: <https://www.speechpathologyaustralia.org.au/SPAweb/whats_on/Speech_Pathology_Week/Communication_Disability/SPAweb/What_s_On/Speech_Pathology_Week/Communication_disability.aspx?hkey=19fa3a7d-521d-4cf6-a728-e10c560e1e5e>. **Table 10.3,** Dryden, P., Greenshields, S., 2020. Communicating with children and young people. *British Journal of Nursing* 29(20). Available at: <https://www.britishjournalofnursing.com/content/clinical/communicating-with-children-and-young-people>; The Royal Children's Hospital Melbourne, 2021. *Communicating procedures to children*. Available at: <https://www.rch.org.au/clinicalguide/guideline_index/Communicating_procedures_to_families>; Boggs, K.U., 2023. *Interpersonal relationships: Professional communication skills for nurses*, 9th ed. Elsevier, Sydney; Speedie, L., Middleton, A. 2023. *Wong's nursing care of infants and children* – for students. Elsevier Australia. **Table 10.4,** Based on Caresearch, 2022. Communication with patients, carers and families. Available at:<https://www.caresearch.com.au/tabid/7440/Default.aspx>. **Table 10.5,** Adapted from Vision Australia, 2023. Tips on communicating to patients with vision loss. Available at: <https://www.visionaustralia.org/news/tips-communicating-patients-vision-loss>. **Table 10.6,** Victory, J., 2020. Communication tips for talking to people with hearing loss. Available at: <https://www.healthyhearing.com/report/51744-Communication-strategies-when-talking-to-individuals-with-hearing-loss>. **Table 10.7,** Based on Dementia Australia, 2022. Communication. Available at: <https://www.dementia.org.au/national/support-and-services/carers/managing-changes-in-communication>. **Table 10.8,** Alruwaily, A.K.K., 2021. The effectiveness of the situation, background, assessment and recommendations (SBAR): Framework in improving patient safety outcomes in the nursing context. *Diversity and Equality in Health and Care* 18(9). Available at: <https://www.proquest.com/openview/b5f9237c381e930a480c411090643775/1.pdf?pq-origsite5gscholar&cbl52033334>; Institute for Healthcare Improvement, 2017. SBAR: Situation-background-assessment-recommendation. Available at: https://www.mhanet.com/mhaimages/SQI/3_IHI%20SBAR%20tool.pdf#:,:text=The%20SBAR%20%28Situation-Background-Assessment-Recommendation%29%20technique%20provides%20a%20framework%20for,ones%2C%20requiring%20a%20clinician%E2%80%99s%20immediate%20attention%20and%20action.>. **Table 11.1,** Adapted from Berman, A., Synder, S., Levett-Jones, T., et al., 2021. *Kozier and Erb's fundamentals of nursing*, 5th ed, vol. 2. Pearson, Melbourne. **Table 11.2,** Adapted from Crisp, J., Douglas, C., Rebeiro, G., et al., 2021. *Potter and Perry's fundamentals of nursing*, 6th ed. Elsevier, Chatswood. **Table 12.1,** Australian College of Nursing, 2021. Managing conflict on clinical placement. Available at: <https://www.acn.edu.au/nurseclick/managing-conflict-on-clinical-placement>. **Table 13.1,** Brown, D., Edwards, H., Buckley, T., Aitken, R.L., 2020. *Lewis's medical-surgical nursing*, ANZ 5th ed. Elsevier, Au; Harding, M.M., 2023. *Lewis's medical-surgical nursing*, 12th ed. Elsevier, Canada. **Tables 14.1, 14.2,** Australian Bureau of Statistics (ABS), 2022. Population: Census. Available at: <https://www.abs.gov.au/statistics/people/population>. **Table 15.1,** Adapted from Crisp, J.C., Douglas, C., Rebeiro, G., et al., (eds.), 2021. *Potter and Perry's fundamentals of nursing* – Australian ed, 5th ed. Elsevier, Australia; Gordon, M., 2016. *Manual of nursing diagnosis*, 13th ed. Jones and Bartlett Learning, an Ascend learning company, Burlington. **Table 15.2,** Centre for Culture, Ethnicity & Health, 2011. *Cultural considerations in health assessment.* Available at: <https://www.ceh.org.au/resource-hub/cultural-considerations-in-health-assessment-tip-sheet>. **Table 15.3,** Jarvis, C., 2021. *Jarvis's physical examination & health assessment*, 3rd ed. Elsevier, Sydney. **Table 16.1,** Crisp, J., Douglas, C., Rebeiro, G., et al., 2021. *Potter & Perry's fundamentals of nursing*, 6th ed. Elsevier, Sydney; Douglas, C., Booker, C., Fox, R., et al., 2016. Nursing physical assessment for patient safety in general wards: Reaching consensus on core skills. *Journal of Clinical Nursing* 25(13–14), 1890–1900. **Table 16.2,** Forbes, H., Watt, E., 2021. *Jarvis's physical examination and health assessment*, 3rd ed. Elsevier, Australia. **Table 16.3,** Celler, B.G., Butlin, M., Argha, A., et al., 2021. Are Korotkoff sounds reliable markers for accurate estimation of systolic and diastolic pressure using brachial cuff sphygmomanometry?, IEEE *Transactions on Biomedical Engineering* 68(12), 3593–3601. **Table 16.4,** Craft, J.A.,

Gordon, C.J., Huether, S.E., et al., 2023. *Understanding pathophysiology*, 4th ed. Elsevier, Australia. **Tables 16.5, 16.6** Craft, J.A., Gordon, C.J., Huether, S.E., et al., 2023. *Understanding pathophysiology*, 4th ed. Elsevier, Australia; Crisp, J., Douglas, C., Rebeiro, G., et al., 2021. *Potter & Perry's fundamentals of nursing*, 6th ed. Elsevier, Sydney. **Table 17.1,** Crisp, J., Douglas, C., Rebeiro, G., Waters, D., 2021. *Potter and Perry's fundamentals of nursing*, 6th ed. Elsevier, Chatswood; Rullander, A.C., Lundstrom, M., Lindkvist, M., et al., 2016. Stress symptoms among adolescents before and after scoliosis surgery: Correlations with postoperative pain. *Journal of Clinical Nursing* 25(7–8), 1086–1094. **Table 18.1,** Adapted from Berman, A., Frandsen, G., Snyder, S., Levett-Jones, T., et al., 2021a. *Kozier & Erb's fundamentals of nursing*, 5th ed. Pearson, Frenchs Forest; Lee, G., Bishop, P., 2016. *Microbiology and infection control for health professionals*, 6th ed. Pearson, Frenchs Forest. **Table 18.2,** Modified from Williams, P., 2020. *Fundamental concepts and skills for nursing*, 6th ed. Elsevier Saunders, Philadelphia. **Tables 18.3, 18.4,** Modified from Berman, A., Frandsen, G., Snyder, S., Levett-Jones, T., et al., 2021. *Kozier & Erb's fundamentals of nursing*, 5th ed. Pearson, Frenchs Forest. Lee, G., Bishop, P., 2016. *Microbiology and infection control for health professionals*, 6th ed. Pearson, Frenchs Forest. **Table 18.5,** Modified from Berman, A., Frandsen, G., Snyder, S., Levett-Jones, T., et al., 2021a. *Kozier & Erb's fundamentals of nursing*, 5th ed. Pearson, Frenchs Forest; Health Vic 2015. Comprehensive health assessment of the older person. Available at: https://www.health.vic.gov.au/residential-aged-care/comprehensive-health-assessment-of-the-older-person; The Royal Children's Hospital Melbourne, 2022. *Clinical guidelines: Nursing assessment*. Available at: <http://www.rch.org.au/rchcpg/hospital_clinical_guideline_index/Nursing_Assessment>. **Table 18.6,** Australian Technical Advisory Group on Immunisation (ATAGI). *Australian immunisation handbook*, 2022. Australian Government Department of Health, Canberra. Available at: <https://immunisationhandbook.health.gov.au>. **Table 18.7,** Reproduced with permission from Use of standard and transmission-based precautions, developed by the Australian Commission on Safety and Quality in Health Care (ACSQHC), 2022. ACSQHC, Sydney. **Table 20.1,** Adapted from Frotjold, A., Bloomfield, J. 2021. Medication therapy. In: Crisp, J., Douglas, C., Rebeiro, G., et al., (eds.), *Potter and Perry's fundamentals of nursing*, 6th ed. Elsevier, Sydney; Broyles, B., Reiss, B., Evans, M., et al., 2019. *Pharmacology in nursing*, Australian and New Zealand ed, 3rd ed. Cengage Learning Australia, Melbourne; Knights, K., Darroch, S., Rowland, A., et al., 2023. *Pharmacology for health professionals*, 6th ed. Elsevier, Sydney. **Table 20.2,** Reproduced with permission from APINCHS classification of high risk medicines, 'APINCHS safety improvement list', developed by the Australian Commission on Safety and Quality in Health Care (ACSQHC), 2024. ACSQHC, Sydney. **Table 20.3,** Based on content from Department of Health and Aged Care, Therapeutic Goods Administration (TGA), 2023. The Poisons Standard (the SUSMP). Available at: <https://www.tga.gov.au/how-we-regulate/ingredients-and-scheduling-medicines-and-chemicals/poisons-standard-and-scheduling-medicines-and-chemicals/poisons-standard-susmp>. **Table 20.4,** Adapted from Frotjold, A., Bloomfield, J. 2021. Medication therapy. In: Crisp, J., Douglas, C., Rebeiro, G., et al., (eds.), *Potter and Perry's fundamentals of nursing*, 6th ed. Elsevier, Sydney. **Table 20.5,** Adapted from Broyles, B., Reiss, B., Evans, M., et al., 2019. *Pharmacology in nursing* – Australian and New Zealand ed, 3rd ed. Cengage Learning Australia, Melbourne; Gorski, L., Hadaway, L., Hagle, M. et al. 2021. *Infusion nursing: Infusion therapy standards of practice*, 8th ed. Infusion Nurse Society, USA. **Table 20.6,** Adapted from Frotjold, A., Bloomfield, J., 2021. Medication therapy. In: Crisp, J., Douglas, C., Rebeiro, G., et al., (eds.), *Potter and Perry's fundamentals of nursing*, 6th ed. Elsevier, Sydney; Broyles, B., Reiss, B., Evans, M., et al., 2019. *Pharmacology in nursing* – Australian and New Zealand ed, 3rd ed. Cengage Learning Australia, Melbourne. Gorski, L., Hadaway, L., Hagle, M. et al. 2021. *Infusion nursing: Infusion therapy standards of practice*, 8th ed. Infusion Nurse Society, USA. **Table 20.7,** Adapted from South Eastern Sydney Local Health District (SESLHD), 2019 Infective Complications – Mandatory reporting requirements of peripheral intravenous cannula (PIVC) or central venous access device (CVAD) infections in the incident information management systems (IIMS). Available at: <https://www.seslhd.health.nsw.gov.au/sites/default/files/documents/SESLHDPD%20280.pdf>. **Table 28.8,** Adapted from Knights, K., Darroch, S., Rowland, A., et al., 2023. *Pharmacology for health professionals*, 6th ed. Elsevier, Sydney;. Tiziani, A., 2022. *Harvard's nursing guide to medications*, 11th ed. Mosby, Australia. **Table 21.1,** Lowdermilk, D.L., Cashion, K., Alden, K.R., et al., 2024. *Maternity & women's health care*, 13th ed. Mosby Elsevier, St Louis. **Table 21.2,** Figures reproduced from Moore, K.L., Persaud, T.V.N., Torchia, M.G., 2015. *The developing human: Clinically oriented embryology*, 10th ed. Saunders, Philadelphia; Table reproduced from Leifer, G., Fleck, E., 2022. *Growth and development across the lifespan*, 3rd ed. Elsevier, St Louis. **Tables 21.3, 21.4, 21.5, 21.8, 21.9, 21.10, 22.11,** Hockenberry, M.J., Wilson, D., Rodgers, C.C., 2022. *Wong's essentials of paediatric nursing*, 11th ed. Mosby, St Louis. **Tables 21.6, 21.7,** Speedie, L., Middleton, A. 2022. *Wong's nursing care of infants and children* – for students, Elsevier Australia. **Tables 22.1,** Hockenberry, M.J., Wilson, D., 2019. *Wong's nursing care of infants and children*, 11th ed. Mosby, St Louis. **Table 22.2,** Speedie, L., Middleton, A. 2022. *Wong's nursing care of infants and children* – for students, Elsevier, Sydney. **Table 22.3,** Leifer, G., 2023. *Introduction to maternity and pediatric nursing*, 9th ed. WB Saunders, Philadelphia. **Table 22.4,** Maaks, D., Starr, N., Brady, M., et al., 2019. (eds.), *Pediatric primary care*, 7th ed. Elsevier, Sydney.

Table 22.5, Modified from Crisp, J., Douglas, C., Rebeiro, G., et al. (eds.), 2021. *Potter and Perry's fundamentals of nursing*, 6th ed. Elsevier, Sydney. **Table 23.1** Adapted from Jarvis, C., Forbes, H., Watt, E., 2021. *Jarvis's health assessment and physical examination*, 3rd ed. Elsevier, Chatswood; Levinson D., 1978. *The seasons of a man's life*. Norton, New York. **Table 23.2** Australian Institute of Health and Welfare (AIHW), 2022. Australian burden of disease study 2022. AIHW, Canberra. **Table 23.3** Australian Institute of Health and Welfare (AIHW), 202b. Deaths in Australia. AIHW, Canberra. **Table 23.4,** Adapted from Crisp, J., Douglas, C., Rebeiro, G., et al., 2021. *Potter and Perry's fundamentals of nursing*, 6th ed. Elsevier, Chatswood; Erikson, E. H.,1982. *The life cycle completed: A review*. Norton, New York; Levinson D., 1978. *The seasons of a man's life*. Norton, New York; Tyler, S., 2020. *Human behaviour and the social environment*. University of Arkansas. **Table 23.5** Australian Institute of Health and Welfare (AIHW), 2022i. *Chronic conditions and multimorbidity*. **Table 23.6** Australian Bureau of Statistics. (ABS), 2022. Deaths, Australia. Available at: <https://www.abs.gov.au/statistics/people/population/deaths-australia/latest-release>; Australian Institute of Health and Welfare (AIHW), 2022. Deaths in Australia. Available at: <https://www.aihw.gov.au/reports/life-expectancy-death/deaths-in-australia>. **Table 23.7** Australian Bureau of Statistics. (ABS), 2022. Deaths, Australia. Available at: <https://www.abs.gov.au/statistics/people/population/deaths-australia/latest-release>; Australian Institute of Health and Welfare (AIHW), 2022. Deaths in Australia. Available at: <https://www.aihw.gov.au/reports/life-expectancy-death/deaths-in-australia>. **Table 23.8,** Australian Institute of Health and Welfare (AIHW), 2018. Australia's health 2018. Available at: < http://www.aihw.gov.au/reports/austraias-health/australias-health-2018/contents/table-of-contents>; Australian Bureau of Statistics (ABS). 2022, Long-term health conditions. **Table 23.9** Australian Institute of Health and Welfare (AIHW), 2018. Australia's health 2018; Australian Bureau of Statistics. (ABS), 2022. Health conditions prevalence. Available at: <https://www.abs.gov.au/statistics/health/health-conditions-and-risks/health-conditions-prevalence/latest-release>. **Table 23.10,** Berman, A., Snyder, S., Levett-Jones, T., et al., 2020. *Kozier and Erb's fundamentals of nursing*, 5th ed. Pearson, Melbourne; Crisp, J., Douglas, C., Rebeiro, G., et al., (eds.) 2021. *Potter and Perry's fundamentals of nursing*, 6th ed. Elsevier, Chatswood; World Health Organization (WHO), 2022. *Adolescent and young adult health*. **Table 24.1** Adapted from Department of Health: Differential diagnosis – depression, delirium and dementia. Available at: <https://www.health.vic.gov.au/patient-care/differential-diagnosis-depression-delirium-and-dementia>. **Table 24.2,** Grada, A., Phillips, T., 2022. Pressure Injuries. *The Merck manual professional edition*. Merck Sharp and Dohme Corp, New Jersey. Available at: <https://www.msdmanuals.com/professional/dermatologic-disorders/pressure-injury/pressure-injuries>; Adapted from Norton, D., 1989. Calculating the risk: Reflections on the Norton Scale. *Decubitus* 2, 24. **Table 25.2,** Hartley, J., 2018. Respiratory rate 2: Anatomy and physiology of breathing. *Nursing Times* 104 (6), 43–44. **Table 25.4,** Ignatavicius, D., Workman, M., Rebar, C., et al., 2021. *Medical-surgical nursing: concepts for interprofessional* collaborative care, 10th ed. Elsevier Inc; Pinsky, M., Teboul, J., Vincent J., (eds.), 2019. *Hemodynamic monitoring*. Springer International Publishing, Cham; Potter, P.A., Perry, A.G., Stockert, P., et al., 2023. *Fundamentals of nursing*, 11th ed. Mosby, St Louis. **Table 26.2,** Adapted from Craft, A.J., Gordon, C.J., Huether, S.E., et al., 2023. *Understanding pathophysiology*, 4th ed. Elsevier, Sydney; Active transport image © Balint Radu/Fotolia.com. **Table 26.3,** Adapted from Brown, D., Edwards, H., Buckley, T., et al., 2020. *Lewis's medical–surgical nursing: Assessment and management of clinical problems*, 5th ed. Elsevier, Sydney. **Table 26.4,** Brown, D., Edwards, H., Buckley, T., et al., 2020. *Lewis's medical–surgical nursing: Assessment and management of clinical problems*, 5th ed. Elsevier, Sydney; Craft, A.J., Gordon, C.J., Huether, S.E., et al., 2023. *Understanding pathophysiology*, 4th ed. Elsevier, Sydney. **Table 26.5,** Craft, A.J., Gordon, C.J., Huether, S.E., et al., 2023. *Understanding pathophysiology*, 4th ed. Elsevier, Sydney; Shrimanker, I., Bhattarai, S., 2023. Electrolytes. In: StatPearls [Internet]. Treasure Island (FL): StatPearls Publishing; 2023 Jan-. Available at: <https://www.ncbi.nlm.nih.gov/books/NBK541123>. **Table 26.6,** The Royal College of Pathologists of Australia, nd. RCPA Manual – Online. *ISSN 1449-8219*. <https://www.rcpa.edu.au/Manuals/RCPA-Manual>. **Table 26.7,** Schub, T., Oji, O., 2018. Hydration: maintaining oral hydration in older adults. CINAHL Nursing Guide. Evidence-Based Care Sheet, T700987. **Table 26.8,** Data from Shrimanker, I., Bhattarai, S., 2023. Electrolytes. In: StatPearls [Internet]. Treasure Island (FL): StatPearls Publishing. Available at: <https://www.ncbi.nlm.nih.gov/books/NBK541123>. **Table 26.12,** Children's Health Queensland Hospital and Health Service. 2023. Queensland paediatric emergency care: Skill sheets. CHQ-NSS-51004 Hydration Assessment v2.0 Developed by the State-wide Emergency Care of Children Working Group. Queensland Government. Available at: <https://www.childrens.health.qld.gov.au/wp-content/uploads/PDF/qpec/nursing-skill-sheets/hydration-assessment.pdf>; Knight, B.P, Waseem, M,. 2023. Pediatric fluid management. In: StatPearls [Internet]. Treasure Island (FL): StatPearls Publishing. Available at: <https://www.ncbi.nlm.nih.gov/books/NBK560540>. **Table 26.16,** Williams, L.S., Hopper, P.D., 2019. *Understanding medical surgical nursing*, 6th ed. F.A. Davis Company, Philadelphia. **Table 26.17,** Adapted from Sydney Children's Hospital Network (SCHN), 2017. Intravenous fluid and electrolyte therapy—SCH, practice guideline. Available at: <https://www.schn.health.nsw.gov.au/_policies/pdf/2013-7033.pdf>. **Table 26.18,** The Royal College of Pathologists of Australia. nd. RCPA Manual

– Online. ISSN 1449-8219. <https://www.rcpa.edu.au/Manuals/RCPA-Manual>. **Table 26.19,** Craft, A.J., Gordon, C.J., Huether, S.E., et al., 2023. *Understanding pathophysiology*, 4th ed. Elsevier, Sydney. **Table 28.1,** Adapted from Hockenberry, M.J., Wilson, D., Rodgers, C.C., 2022. *Wong's essentials of pediatric nursing*, 11th ed. Elsevier, St Louis. **Tables 28.2, 28.3,** Adapted from Crisp, J., Douglas, C., Rebeiro, G., et al., 2021. *Potter and Perry's fundamentals of nursing*, Australian ed, 6th ed. Elsevier, Sydney; Marieb, E.N., Keller, S.M., 2022. *Essentials of human anatomy and physiology*, 13th ed. Pearson, New York; Patton, K.T., Thibodeau, G.A., 2019. *Anatomy & physiology*, 10th ed. Mosby Elsevier, St Louis. **Table 29.1,** Paul, W., Sharma, C.P., 2021. *Tissue and organ regeneration: An introduction*. In: Sharma CP Regenerated Organs. Academic Press. Available at: <https://www.sciencedirect.com/science/article/pii/B9780128210857000014?via%3Dihub>; Wu, S., Carter, M., Cole, W., et al, 2023. Best practice for wound repair and regeneration: Use of cellular, acellular and matrix-like products (CAMPs). *Journal of Wound Care* 32(4 suppl B), S1–S32. **Table 29.2,** Bishop, A., Witts, S., Martin, T., 2018. The role of nutrition in successful wound healing. *Journal of Community Nursing* 32(4), 44–50; Ahuja, K., Lio, P., 2023. The role of trace elements in dermatology: A systematic review. *Journal of Integrative Dermatology*. Available at: <https://www.jintegrativederm.org/article/73228-the-role-of-trace-elements-in-dermatology-a-systematic-review>. **Table 29.3,** International Wound Infection Institute (IWII), 2022. Wound infection in clinical practice: Principles of best practice. *Wounds International*. Available at: <https://woundinfection-institute.com/wp-content/uploads/IWII-CD-2022-web-1.pdf>. **Table 29.4,** Adapted from Carville, K., 2023. *Wound care manual*, 8th ed. Silver Chain Nursing Association, Perth, West Australia; International Wound Infection Institute (IWII), 2022. Wound infection in clinical practice: Principles of best practice. *Wounds International*. Available at: <https://woundinfection-institute.com/wp-content/uploads/IWII-CD-2022-web-1.pdf>. **Table 29.5,** Adapted from Carville, K., 2023. *Wound care manual*, 8th ed. Silver Chain Nursing Association, Perth, West Australia; Gibb, M., 2023. *A to almost A of wound dressings*, 1st ed. Wound Specialist Services Pty Ltd, Samford QLD; International Wound Infection Institute (IWII), 2022. Wound infection in clinical practice: principles of best practice. *Wounds International*. Available at: <https://woundinfection-institute.com/wp-content/uploads/IWII-CD-2022-web-1.pdf>. **Table 29.6,** Addapted from Carville, K., 2023. *Wound care manual*, 8th ed. Silver Chain Nursing Association, Perth, West Australia; Edwards, H., Finlayson, K., Parker, C., et al., 2019. Champions for skin integrity wound dressing guide. Queensland University of Technology, Brisbane. Available at: <https://research.qut.edu.au/ccm>. **Table 29.7,** Adapted from Gawkrodger, D.J., Arden-Jones, M.R., 2021. *Dermatology: An illustrated colour text*, 7th ed. Elsevier, Edinburgh; Patton, K.T., Thibodeau, G.A., 2019. Skin – Anatomy and Physiology, in Patton, K.T., (eds.), *Anatomy and physiology*, Adapted International ed, Elsevier, St Louis. **Table 29.8,** © Barbara Braden and Nancy Bergstrom, 1988. Reprinted with permission. All Rights Reserved. **Table 29.9,** Carville, K., 2023. *Wound care manual*, 8th ed. Silver Chain Nursing Association, Perth, Western Australia. **Table 29.10,** Trauma Victoria, 2023. Burns. Available at: <https://trauma.reach.vic.gov.au>; Victorian Adult Burns Service, 2019. Burns Management Guidelines. Available at: <www.vicburns.org.au>. **Table 30.1,** Pirlich, M., Norman, K., 2018. Bestimmung des Ernährungszustands (inkl. Bestimmung der Körperzusammensetzung und ernährungsmedizinisches Screening) in Biesalski, rnährungsmedizin. Georg Thieme Verlag KG; Stuttgart, Germany; Esper, D.H., 2015. Utilization of nutrition-focused physical assessment in identifying micronutrient deficiencies. *Nutrition in Clinical Practice* 30, 194–202. Doi: 10.1177/0884533615573054. **Table 30.2,** Mann, J., Truswell, A.S., 2017. *Essentials of human nutrition*, 5th ed. Oxford University Press, New York. **Table 30.3,** Crisp, J., Douglas, S., Rebeiro, G., et al. (eds.), 2021. *Potter and Perry's fundamentals of nursing*, 6th ed. Elsevier, Sudney; Patton, K.T., Thibodeau, G.A., 2019. *Anatomy and physiology*, 10th ed. Mosby Elsevier, St Louis. **Table 30.4,** Raymond, J., Morrow, K., 2023. *Krause and Mahan's food and the nutrition care process*, 16th ed. Elsevier, St Louis. **Table 31.1,** Adapted from Jarvis, C., Eckhardt, A., 2021. *Jarvis's health assessment and physical examination*, 8th ed. Elsevier, Chatswood, pp. 692–710; Brandt, C.L., 2022. Disorders of the lower urinary tract – pathophysiology. In: Banasik, J., 2022. *Pathophysiology*, 7th ed. Elsevier, Missouri, pp. 620–635. **Table 31.2,** Adapted from Cardozo, L., Rovner, E., Wein, A., Abrams, P. (eds.), 2023. *Incontinence*, 7th ed. ICI-ICS, International Continence Society, Bristol. **Table 31.3,** Kirov. E., Needham, A., 2023. *Foundations of anatomy and physiology*. Elsevier Chatswood. **Table 31.4,** Adapted from The Royal College of Pathologists of Australasia, 2019. Manual. Available at: <https://www.rcpa.edu.au/Manuals/RCPA-Manual/Pathology-Tests/U/Urinalysis>; Watt, E., 2021. Maintaining continence. In: Crisp, J., Douglas, C., Rebeiro, G., et al. (eds.), 2021. *Potter and Perry's fundamentals of nursing*, 6th ed. Elsevier, Sydney, pp. 1043–1089. **Table 32.1,** Berman, A., Frandsen, G., Snyder, S.J., Levett-Jones, T., Burston, A., Dwyer, T., et al., 2020. *Kozier and Erb's fundamentals of nursing*, 5th ed. Pearson Australia, Melbourne. **Table 32.2,** Tiziani, A., 2021. *Havard's nursing guide to drugs*, 11th ed. Elsevier, Chatswood. **Table 33.1,** Berman, A., Snyder, S., Levett-Jones, T., et al., 2020. *Kozier and Erb's fundamentals of nursing*, 5th ed. Pearson Australia, Melbourne; Crisp, J., Douglas, C., Rebeiro, G., et al. (eds.), 2021. *Potter and Perry's fundamentals of nursing*, 6th ed. Elsevier, Sydney; International Association for the Study of Pain (IASP), 2021. IASP terminology—pain terms. Available at: <https://www.iasp-pain.org/Education/Content.

aspx?ItemNumber=1698>. **Table 33.2,** Adapted from Crisp, J., Douglas, C., Rebeiro, G., et al. (eds.), 2021. *Potter and Perry's fundamentals of nursing*, 6th ed. Elsevier, Sydney. **Tables 33.3, 33.4,** Adapted from Brown, D., Edwards, H., Buckley, T., et al., 2020. *Lewis's medical-surgical nursing*, 5th ed. Elsevier, Sydney; Adapted from Crisp, J., Douglas, C., Rebeiro, G., et al. (eds.), 2021. *Potter and Perry's fundamentals of nursing*, 6th ed. Elsevier, Sydney. **Tables 33.5, 33.6,** Adapted from Knights, K. et al., 2023. *Pharmacology for health professionals*, 6th ed. Elsevier, Sydney; Tziani, A., 2022. *Havard's nursing guide to drugs*, 11th ed. Elsevier, Sydney. **Table 34.1,** Patton, K., Thibodeau, G.A., 2018. *The human body in health and disease*, 7th ed. Elsevier, St Louis. **Table 34.2,** Vision Australia Foundation, 2023. <www.visionaustralia.org.au>. **Table 34.3,** Brown, D., Edwards, H., Buckley, T., et al., 2020. *Lewis's medical-surgical nursing*, 5th ed. Elsevier, Sydney. Crisp, J., Douglas, C., Rebeiro, G., et al. (eds.), 2021. *Potter and Perry's fundamentals of nursing*, 6th ed. Elsevier, Sydney. **Table 34.4,** Soundfair, 2023. Available at: <www.soundfair.org.au>. **Table 35.1,** Marieb, E., Keller, S., 2021. *Essentials of human anatomy & physiology*, 13th ed. Pearson, London; Patton, K., Thibodeau, G., Douglas, M., 2012. *Essentials of anatomy & physiology*. Elsevier Mosby, St Louis. **Table 35.2,** Jain, S., Iverson, L., 2023. Glasgow coma scale. National Library of Medicine. **Table 35.3,** Berman, A., Fandsen, G., Snyder, S., Levett-Jones, T., et al., 2021. *Kozier and Erb's fundamentals of nursing: Concepts, process and practice*, 5th ed. Pearson, Melbourne; Epilepsy Action Australia, 2023. What do you wish people knew about epilepsy? Available at: <https://www.epilepsy.org.au/about-epilepsy/what-do-you-wish-people-knewabout-epilepsy>; LeMone, P., Bauldoff, G., Gubrud-Howe, P., et al., 2020. *Medical–surgical nursing: Critical thinking for person-centred care*, 4th ed. Pearson, Melbourne. **Table 35.4,** LeMone, P., Bauldoff, G., Gubrud-Howe, P., et al., 2020. *Medical–surgical nursing: Critical thinking for person-centred care*, 4th ed. Pearson, Melbourne. **Tables 35.5, 35.6, 35.7, 35.8,** Brown, D., Edwards, H., Buckley, T., et al., 2020. *Lewis's medical-surgical nursing*, 5th ed. Elsevier, Sydney. **Table 36.1,** Crawford, A. H., 2023. Endocrine problems. In: Harding, M. M., Kwong, J., Hagler, D., et al., *Lewis's medical-surgical nursing*, 12th ed. Elsevier, St Louis; Waugh, A., Grant, A., 2022. *Ross & Wilson Anatomy and physiology in health and illness*, 14th ed. Elsevier, Glasgow. **Table 36.2,** Banasik, J., 2022. *Pathophysiology*, 7th ed. Elsevier, St Louis; Medical News Today 2023. What is the difference between hypothyroidism and hyperthyroidism? Available at: <https://www.mmedicalnewstoday.com/articles/hypothroidism-vs-hyperthyroidism>. **Table 37.1,** Adapted from Andrology Australia, 2018. Erectile dysfunction. Fact sheet online. Available at: <https://www.healthymale.org.au/files/resources/erectile_dysfunction_fact_sheet_healthy_male_2019.pdf>. **Table 37.2,** Adapted from Andrology Australia, 2018. Testicular cancer. Fact sheet online. Available at: <https://www.healthymale.org.au/files/resources/testicular_cancer_fact_sheet_healthy_male_2019.pdf>. **Table 37.3,** Adapted from Andrology Australia, 2018. BPH prostate enlargement. Fact sheet online. Available at: <https://www.healthymale.org.au/files/resources/bph_prostate_enlargement_fact_sheet_healthy_male_2019.pdf>. **Table 37.4,** Adapted from Ferri, F.F., 2020. *Ferri's clinical advisor 2020*, Elsevier, Philadelphia. © Copyright 2020 by Elsevier Inc. **Table 37.5,** IVF Australia, 2023. Menstrual cycle. Available at: <https://www.ivf.com.au/planning-for-pregnancy/female-fertility/female-fertility-factors/menstrual-cycle#phase-1-the-follicular-phase>. **Table 37.6,** Adapted from Better Health Channel, 2021. Prolapsed uterus. Available at: <https://www.betterhealth.vic.gov.au/health/ConditionsAndTreatments/prolapsed-uterus>. **Table 37.7,** Adapted from Jean Hailes, 2023. Polycystic ovarian syndrome. Available at: <http://jeanhailes.org.au/health-a-z/pcos>. **Table 37.8,** Ovarian Cancer Australia, 2023. Know ovarian cancer. Available at: <https://ovariancancer.net.au/about-ovarian-cancer>; **Table 37.9,** Cancer Council Australia, 2023. Cervical cancer. Available at: <https://www.cancer.org.au/about-cancer/types-of-cancer/cervical-cancer.html#jump_3>. **Table 37.10,** The American College of Obstetricians and Gynaecologists, 2021. Hysterectomy. Available at: <https://www.acog.org/Patients/FAQs/Hysterectomy?IsMobileSet=false#different>. **Table 37.11,** Family Planning NSW, 2020. Reproductive and sexual health: an Australian clinical practice handbook, 4th ed. Family Planning NSW, Ashfield; Family Planning NSW, nd. Contraception fact sheets. Available at: <https://www.fpnsw.org.au/health-information/individuals/contraception>; Family Planning NSW, Family Planning Victoria and True Relationships and Reproductive Health, 2016. Contraception: an Australian clinical practice handbook, 4th ed. Family Planning NSW, Ashfield. **Table 37.12,** Adapted from Andrology Australia, 2018. Male infertility. Fact sheet online. Available at: <https://www.healthymale.org.au/files/resources/male_infertility_fact_sheet_healthy_male_2019.pdf>. **Table 37.13,** Family Planning NSW, 2020. *Reproductive and sexual health: an Australian clinical practice handbook*, 4th ed. Family Planning NSW, Ashfield. **Table 38.1,** Lind, S., Bengtsson, A., Alvariza, A., Klarare, A., 2022. Registered nurses' experiences of caring for patients in hospitals transitioning from curative to palliative care: A qualitative study. *Nursing & Health Sciences*, 24(4), 820– 827. Available at: <https://doi.org/10.1111/nhs.12982>; National Institute on Aging, 2022. Providing care and comfort at the end of life. Available at: <https://www.nia.nih.gov/health/providing-comfort-end-life>; Department of Health, Victoria, nd. Managing physical symptoms during palliative care. Available at: <https://www2.health.vic.gov.au/hospitals-and-health-services/patient-care/older-people/palliative/palliative-physical>. **Table 39.1,** American Psychiatric Association, 2022. Diagnostic and statistical manual of mental disorders, 5th ed. Text revision. American

Psychiatric Association, Washington, USA; Halter, M.J., 2021. *Varcarolis' foundations of psychiatric-mental health nursing*, 9th ed. A clinical approach. Elsevier, USA; Hercelinskyj, G., Alexander, L., 2022. *Mental health nursing*, enhanced edition, 1st ed. Cengage. **Table 39.2,** World Health Organization (WHO), 2022. Mental disorders. Available at: <https://www.who.int/news-room/fact-sheets/detail/mental-disorders>; Hercelinskyj, G., Alexander, L., 2022. *Mental health nursing*, enhanced edition, 1st ed. Cengage. **Tables 39.3, 39.4, 39.5, 39.7, 39.10, 39.11,** Foster, K., Marks, P., O'Brien, A., Raeburn, T., 2020. *Mental health in nursing – Theory and practice for clinical settings*. Elsevier; Halter, M.J., 2021. *Varcarolis' foundations of psychiatric-mental health nursing*, 9th ed. A clinical approach. Elsevier, US; Hungerford, C., Hodgson, D., Clancy, R., et al., 2020. *Mental health care: An introduction for health professionals*, 4th ed. Wiley, China; Steele, D., 2023. *Keltner's psychiatric nursing*, 9th ed. Elsevier; Hercelinskyj, G., Alexander, L., 2022. *Mental health nursing*, enhanced edition, 1st ed. Cengage. **Table 39.6,** Steele, D. 2023. *Keltner's psychiatric nursing*, 9th ed. Elsevier. **Table 39.8,** Hercelinskyj, G., Alexander, L., 2022. *Mental health nursing*, enhanced edition, 1st ed. Cengage. Table 39.9, Foster, K., Marks, P., O'Brien, A., Raeburn, T., 2020. *Mental health in nursing – Theory and practice for clinical settings*. Elsevier; Hungerford, C., Hodgson, D., Clancy, R., et al., 2020. *Mental health care: An introduction for health professionals*, 4th ed. Wiley, China. Table 39.12, Dementia Australia, 2022. Dementia statistics. Australian Government Department of Social Services. Available at: <https://www.dementia.org.au/statistics>; Fortinash, K.M., Holoday Worret, P.A., 2011. *Psychiatric nursing care plans*, 5th ed. Mosby, St Louis. **Table 41.1,** Adapted from National Disability Service, 2022. Disability types and description. Available at: <https://www.nds.org.au/disability-types-and-descriptions>. **Table 41.2,** Australian Bureau of Statistics, 2019. Disability, ageing and carers, Australia: Summary of findings. Available at: <https://www.abs.gov.au/statistics/health/disability/disability-ageing-and-carers-australia-summary-findings/latest-release#disability>. **Table 41.3,** National Disability Service, 2022. Disability types and description. Available at: <https://www.nds.org.au/disability-types-and-descriptions>. **Table 41.4,** Alonso-Sardón, M., Iglesias-de-Sena, H., Fernández-Martín, L.C., Mirón-Canelo, J.A., 2019. Do health and social support and personal autonomy have an influence on the health-related quality of life of individuals with intellectual disability? *BMC Health Services Research* 19(1), 1–10; Proescher, E., Aase, D.M., Passi, H.M., et al., 2022. Impact of perceived social support on mental health, quality of life, and disability in post–9/11 US military veterans. *Armed Forces & Society* 48(1), 115–135; Ogawa, M., Fujikawa, M., Jin, K., et al., 2021. Acceptance of disability predicts quality of life in patients with epilepsy. *Epilepsy & Behavior* 120, 107979; Zhang, Q., Shan, X., Ling, Y., et al., 2019. Psychosocial predictors of adjustment to disability among patients with breast cancer: A cross-sectional descriptive study. *Journal of Nursing Research* 27(2), e15; Dunn, D. S., Wehmeyer, M. L., 2022. *The positive psychology of personal factors: Implications for understanding disability*, 15; Bollier, A., Sutherland, G., Krnjacki, L., et al., 2021. Attitudes Matter: national survey of community attitudes toward people with disability in Australia. Victoria: Centre of Research Excellence in Disability and Health; Kim, G.M., Lim, J.Y., Kim, E.J., Park, S.M., 2019. Resilience of patients with chronic diseases: A systematic review. *Health & Social Care in the Community* 27(4), 797–807; Lim, K.K., Matchar, D.B., Tan, C.S., et al., 2020. The association between psychological resilience and physical function among older adults with hip fracture surgery. *Journal of the American Medical Directors Association* 21(2), 260–266; World Health Organization, nd. Quality of care. Available at: <https://www.who.int/health-topics/quality-of-care#tab5tab_1>. **Table 41.6,** Drury, V., 2021. Models of care. In: Chang, E., Johnson, A., (eds.), *Living with chronic illness and disability: Principles for nursing practice*. Elsevier Health Sciences. **Table 41.7,** Drury, V., Aw, A.T., 2020. Nursing care: Chronic illness and disability. In: Koutoukidis, G., Stainton, K., (eds.), *Tabbner's nursing care: Theory and practice*, 8th ed. Elsevier Health Sciences, Australia; Drury, V.B., Aw, A.T., Shiow, L.H.P., 2017. *Self-Management of vision impairments. promoting self-management of chronic health conditions: Theories and practice*. **Table 41.8,** Del Rio Szupszynski, K.P., de Ávila, A.C., 2021. The transtheoretical model of behavior change: Prochaska and DiClemente's model. Psychology of Substance Abuse: Psychotherapy, clinical management and social intervention, 205–216; DiClemente, C.C., Graydon, M.M., 2020. 10 Changing Behavior Using the Transtheoretical Model. The Handbook of Behavior Change, 136; Prochaska, J.O., Norcross, J.C., 2001. Stages of change. *Psychotherapy: Theory, Research, Practice, Training* 38(4), 443. **Table 41.9,** Miller, W.R., Rollnick, S., 2012. *Motivational interviewing: Helping people change*. Guilford Press, New York; Williams, L., 2023. Motivational interviewing. In: Cooper, D., *Alcohol use: Assessment, withdrawal management, treatment and therapy: Ethical practice*, pp. 363–380. Springer. **Table 41.10,** Legano, L.A., Desch, L.W., Messner, S.A., et al., 2021. Maltreatment of children with disabilities. *Pediatrics* 147(5); Nagaratnam, K., Nagaratnam, N., 2019. *Elderly abuse and neglect. Advanced age geriatric care: A comprehensive guide*, 19–24. **Tables 42.1, 42.2,** LeMone, P., Bauldoff, G., Gubrud-Howe, P., et al., 2020. *Medical–surgical nursing: Critical thinking in person-centred care*, 4th ed. Pearson, Melbourne. **Table 42.3,** Al-Khafaji, A.H., 2020. Multiple organ dysfunction syndrome in sepsis. Medscape. Available at: <https://emedicine.medscape.com/article/169640-overview#a4>. **Table 42.4** Sutherland-Fraser, S., Davies, M., Gillespie, B. M., Lockwood, B., 2022. *Perioperative nursing: An introduction*, 3rd ed. Elsevier, Sydney. **Table 42.5,** Rothrock, J., 2023. *Alexander's care of the patient in surgery*, 16th ed. Elsevier, St Louis; Potter, P.A., Perry,

A.G., Stockert, P., et al., 2023. *Fundamentals of nursing*, 11th ed. Elsevier, St Louis; Brown, D., Edwards, H., Buckley, T., Aitken, R., 2024. *Lewis's medical-surgical nursing*, 6th ed. Elsevier. **Tables 42.6, 42.7,** Potter, P.A., Perry, A.G., Stockert, P., et al., 2023. *Fundamentals of nursing*, 11th ed. Elsevier, St Louis; Brown, D., Edwards, H., Buckley, T., Aitken, R., 2024. *Lewis's medical-surgical nursing*, 6th ed. Elsevier. **Table 42.8,** Rothrock, J., 2023. *Alexander's care of the patient in surgery*, 17th ed. Elsevier, St Louis; Potter, P.A., Perry, A.G., Stockert, P., et al., 2023. *Fundamentals of nursing*, 11th ed. Elsevier, St Louis; Brown, D., Edwards, H., Buckley, T., Aitken, R., 2024. *Lewis's medical-surgical nursing*, 6th ed. Elsevier. **Table 42.9,** Bouyer-Ferullo, S., 2013. Preventing perioperative nerve injuries. *AORN Journal* 97(1), 110–124; Rothrock, J., 2023. *Alexander's care of the patient in surgery*, 17th ed. Elsevier, St Louis; Potter, P.A., Perry, A.G., Stockert, P., et al., 2023. *Fundamentals of nursing*, 11th ed. Elsevier, St Louis; Brown, D., Edwards, H., Buckley, T., Aitken, R., 2024. *Lewis's medical-surgical nursing*, 6th ed. Elsevier. **Table 42.10,** Sutherland-Fraser, S., Davies, M., Gillespie, B. M., Lockwood, B., 2022. *Perioperative nursing: An introduction*, 3rd ed. Elsevier, Sydney. **Table 42.11,** Crisp, J., Douglas, C., Rebeiro, G., et al., 2021. *Potter & Perry's fundamentals of nursing* – ANZ ed, 6th ed. Elsevier; Marieb, E.N., Hoehn, K.N., 2018. *Human anatomy and physiology*, 11th ed. Pearson, Boston; Brown, D., Edwards, H., Buckley, T., Aitken, R., 2024. *Lewis's medical-surgical nursing*, 6th ed. Elsevier. **Table 42.12,** Rothrock, J., 2023. *Alexander's care of the patient in surgery*, 17th ed. Elsevier, St Louis; Brown, D., Edwards, H., Buckley, T., Aitken, R., 2024. *Lewis's medical-surgical nursing*, 6th ed. Elsevier. **Table 43.2,** Australasian Society of Clinical Immunology and Allergy (ASCIA), 2023. ASCIA Guidelines acute management of anaphylaxis. Available at: <https://allergy.org.au/hp/papers/acute-management-of-anaphylaxis-guidelines>. **Table 43.3,** Tidy, C., Vakharia, K., 2022. Resuscitation in hypovolaemic shock. Patient info. Available at: <https://patient.info/doctor/resuscitation-in-hypovolaemic-shock>. **Table 44.1,** Blackburn, S., 2018. *Maternal, foetal and neonatal physiology: A clinical perspective*, 44th ed. WB Saunders, Sydney; Pairman, S., Pincombe, J., Tracy, S., et al., 2023. *Midwifery: Preparation for practice*, 5th ed. Elsevier, Sydney. **Table 44.2,** Blackburn, S., 2018. *Maternal, foetal and neonatal physiology: A clinical perspective*, 44th ed. WB Saunders, Sydney; Department of Health and Aged Care, 2020. Clinical Practice Guidelines: Pregnancy Care. Available at: <https://www.health.gov.au/resources/pregnancy-care-guidelines>; Pairman, S., Pincombe, J., Tracy, S., et al., 2023. *Midwifery: Preparation for practice*, 5th ed. Elsevier, Sydney. **Table 44.3,** Lowdermilk, D.L., Perry, S.E., Cashion, K., et al., 2020. *Maternity & women's health care*, 12th ed. Mosby Elsevier, St Louis; Pairman, S., Pincombe, J., Tracy, S., et al., 2023. *Midwifery: Preparation for practice*, 5th ed. Elsevier, Sydney; Perry, S.E., Hockenberry, M.J., Lowdermilk, D., et al., 2022. *Maternal child nursing care*, 7th ed. Mosby, St Louis. **Table 44.4,** Department of Health and Aged Care, 2020. Clinical Practice Guidelines: Pregnancy Care. Available at: <https://www.health.gov.au/resources/pregnancy-care-guidelines>; Lowdermilk, D.L., Perry, S.E., Cashion, K., et al., 2020. *Maternity & women's health care*, 12th ed. Mosby Elsevier, St Louis; Murray, S.S., McKinney, E.S., Holub, K., 2023. *Foundations of maternal-newborn and women's health nursing*, 8th ed. Saunders Elsevier, St Louis. **Table 44.5,** Davidson, M., London, M., Ladewig, P., 2020. *Old's maternal-newborn nursing and women's health across the lifespan*, 11th ed. Prentice Hall, Upper Saddle River. **Table 44.6,** Lowdermilk, D.L., Perry, S.E., Cashion, K., et al., 2020. *Maternity & women's health care*, 12th ed. Mosby Elsevier, St Louis; Murray, S.S., McKinney, E.S., Holub, K., 2023. *Foundations of maternal-newborn and women's health nursing*, 8th ed. Saunders Elsevier, St Louis; Speedie, L., Middleton, A. 2022. *Wong's nursing care of infants and children – for students.* Elsevier Australia; Queensland Government, 2022. Clinical practice procedure—assessment/Apgar score. Available at: <https://www.ambulance.qld.gov.au/docs/clinical/cpp/CPP_APGAR%20score.pdf>. **Table 44.7,** Davidson, M., London, M., Ladewig, P., 2020. *Old's maternal-newborn nursing and women's health across the lifespan*, 11th ed. Prentice Hall, Upper Saddle River; Hockenberry, M., Wilson, D., Rodgers, C. (eds.), 2019. *Wong's nursing care of infants and children*, 11th ed. Mosby, St Louis. **Table 44.8,** Ladewig, P.W., London, M.L., Davidson, M.R., 2017. *Contemporary maternal-newborn nursing care*, 9th ed. Pearson Prentice Hall, Upper Saddle River; Murray, S.S., McKinney, E.S., Holub, K., 2023. *Foundations of maternal-newborn and women's health nursing*, 8th ed. Saunders Elsevier, St Louis; Speedie, L., Middleton, A. 2022. *Wong's nursing care of infants and children – for students*, Elsevier Australia.

Index

A

B

D

E

F

G

H

M

N

P

Q

S

T

U

V

W

X

Y

Z